MEDICAL-SURGICAL NURSING

Common health problems of adults
and children across the life span

MEDICAL-SURGICAL NURSING

Common health problems of adults and children across the life span

DIANE McGOVERN BILLINGS, RN, MSEd

Associate Professor, Indiana University
School of Nursing,
Indianapolis, Indiana

LILLIAN GATLIN STOKES, RN, MSN

Associate Professor, Indiana University
School of Nursing,
Indianapolis, Indiana

*with **713** illustrations*

The C. V. Mosby Company

ST. LOUIS • TORONTO • LONDON   1982

MOSBY

A TRADITION OF PUBLISHING EXCELLENCE

Editor: Pamela L. Swearingen
Assistant editor: Bess Arends
Manuscript editor: Teri Merchant
Book design: Kay Kramer
Cover design: Diane Beasley
Production: Jeanne Bush

with contributed work by

Janet Miller Barber, RN, MS

Captain, USAF, Wilford Hall USAF Medical Center (AFSC),
Lackland Air Force Base, Texas

Marchusa Huff, RN, MSN

Associate Professor, Indiana University
School of Nursing,
Indianapolis, Indiana

The C.V. Mosby Company
11830 Westline Industrial Drive, St. Louis, Missouri 63141

Library of Congress Cataloging in Publication Data

Billings, Diane McGovern.
    Medical-surgical nursing.

    Bibliography: p.
    Includes index.
        1. Nursing.   I.   Stokes, Lillian Gatlin.
II.   Title.   III.   Title: Common health problems of
adults and children across the life span.   [DNLM:
1. Nursing process.   WY 100 B599m]
RT41.B54   610.73   81-16856
ISBN   0-8016-0736-1   AACR2

GW/VH/VH   9   8   7   6   5   4   3   2   1   03/D/349

Consultant board

Preface

Medical-Surgical Nursing: Common Health Problems of Adults and Children across the Life Span is written for students and nurses engaged in nursing in varied health care settings. Client situations differ as a result of the nature of the situation, individual differences, or the manner in which a client or family member may perceive or react to a given situation. The nurse must therefore use an approach that will facilitate responses to situations on an individualized basis for clients of all ages. This care requires the ability to make comprehensive *assessments,* to *analyze the data,* and to use the data as the basis for *planning* and *implementing* care. Once these steps have been taken, the client outcomes are *evaluated,* so that changes can be made in the plan of care. Each stage is dynamic, because data uncovered in one stage may alter the significance of data uncovered in previous stages.

Nursing practice also requires a body of knowledge about common health problems that will supply the basic information for using the nursing process in nursing activities. No attempt has been made to exhaust all medical and surgical problems of children and adults; as implied by the title, *Common Health Problems,* we have carefully selected problems that, according to morbidity and mortality reports, are common and recurrent across the life span. Significant information related to growth and development, pathophysiology, sociology, nutrition, pharmacology, and psychodynamics has been incorporated, but the reader may wish to refer to comprehensive texts to review or supplement content in these areas.

This book is divided into 21 chapters. The first 8 chapters provide the framework of theoretical foundations about man, environment, health, and nursing. The remaining portion is organized by body systems to facilitate arrangement of content and health assessment. In each of these clinical nursing chapters, components of the nursing process are clearly identified with this symbol ☞ to focus the reader's attention on the process of nursing as well as on the knowledge used to provide nursing care. It is indicative of how we apply the nursing process. Throughout all chapters, emphasis is directed toward nursing activities for promotion, maintenance, and restoration of the client's optimum level of health.

The reader may recognize philosophical and conceptual elements from *Adult and Child Care: A Client Approach to Nursing.* We continue to be com-

Preface

mitted to the client approach to nursing and acknowledge the contributions of Janet Barber and colleagues.

We wish to extend our appreciation to:

Colleagues Cheryl Ashbaucher, RN, Mary Jane Lundburg, RN, and Mary Van Allen, RN, who critiqued sections of the manuscript and Janet Barber, RN, and Marchusa Huff, RN, who contributed content.

Consultants Connie Bobick, RN, Judy Masiak, RN, Susan Pierce, RN, and Terry Valiga, RN.

Secretaries Cindy Allen, Brenda Eseray, Winnie Green, Carol Hash, Lorna Medley, Dorothy Pock, and Paula Stant.

Artist Jeanne Robertson.

Editors Pamela Swearingen, Bess Arends, and Teri Merchant.

Our families for the understanding, support, and time to accomplish this task.

Diane McGovern Billings
Lillian Gatlin Stokes

Contents

Contents

MEDICAL-SURGICAL NURSING

Common health problems of adults
and children across the life span

PART ONE

FOUNDATIONS OF CLINICAL PRACTICE: Man, environment, health, and nursing

1 Perspectives for nursing across the life span

Nursing is a dynamic interaction with clients in various stages of individual and family development. Nurses therefore necessarily use theoretical frameworks from physical and social sciences that provide perspectives of human growth and development. The purpose of this chapter is to characterize several theoretical frameworks useful to nurses' understanding of man's behavior across the life span.

Universal theories, such as general systems, basic needs, and stress adaptation, provide insights into man's relationships with internal and external environments. On the other hand, developmental theories, such as psychosocial levels, developmental tasks, and family systems, focus on critical stages at which growth and development are facilitated. Since no one theory totally characterizes the nature of man, the chapter concludes with a discussion of holistic man and philosophical orientations requisite for nurses to respond to man's uniqueness and his universality.

Universal theories

GENERAL SYSTEM THEORY

The general system theory describes relationships between component parts and the whole.[9] A system can be defined as something that is made up of a number of separate parts or elements; the parts or elements of the system rely on each other, are interrelated, have a common purpose, and together form a collective entity or wholeness. Effective systems are characterized by being efficient, reliable, repeatable, and purposeful.[1]

A cybernetic system, or one that uses feedback to control behavior, has four components: (1) the inputs, (2) the throughputs or transformation processes, (3) the outputs, and (4) feedback or knowledge of results. Feedback provides data about the consequences of action and the state of achievement in relation to a goal. It is also a source of motivation to sustain performance.[1]

3

Foundations of clinical practice

Living systems are classified as open systems because they exchange matter, energy, and information with the environment. This exchange fosters heterogeneity and organization and assures order.

Open systems are contained by boundaries describing the system and differentiating suprasystems (contained outside the system) and subsystems (component parts of the system). The boundaries of open systems are semipermeable to allow exchange between the system and internal and external environments.

Open systems maintain a steady state, or equilibrium, by adapting to the environment. Adaptation assures evolution from undifferentiated states to increasing differentiation and integration.

Systems theory provides a mechanism for understanding the nature of man and his relationship with the environment. In this schema relationships of biophysical man and social man can be perceived. Levels of system activity of biophysical man may be cells, tissues, organs, organ systems, and the human organism. Levels of activity for social man may include groups (families), communities, cultures, nations, worlds, and universes. Systems theory then, views man's internal environment as subsystems and the external environments as the suprasystem (Fig. 1-1).

Systems theory is also useful in understanding development across the life span. As systems mature, they tend to evolve from general and diffuse movements to purposeful and specific responses. Subsystems become increasingly articulated between subsystems; input stimuli are perceived more

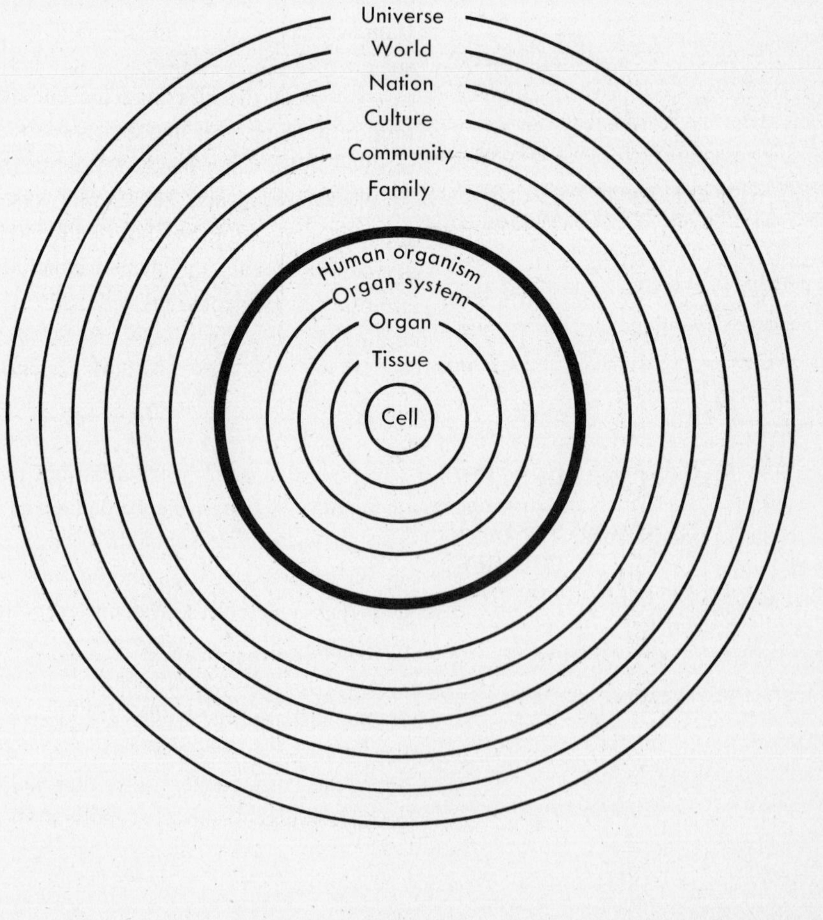

FIG. 1-1
Man's physical and social systems.

4

discretely, and output behaviors are focused toward goal achievement; flexible problem-solving behaviors emerge; and the system becomes more independent of the suprasystem. These behaviors are discussed in Chapter 2 as they relate to human growth and development.

The purpose of human systems is to obtain optimal use of energy exchange between the system and the environment. Disequilibrium occurs as energy differentials shift from the environment or system. According to general system theory, the goal of nursing is to identify disequilibrium and facilitate the return of the human system to the steady state.

BASIC NEED THEORY Basic need theory was first described by Abraham Maslow, who views man as a system of basic needs.[6] Basic needs include physiological needs of oxygen, water, nutrition, elimination, rest and sleep, and sex. Higher-level needs include those of safety and security, love and belonging, self-esteem, and self-actualization.

Needs can be placed in a hierarchical order (Fig. 1-2). Lower-order needs must be met before higher-order needs can emerge. Human needs are also interrelated, and disturbances in one area of functioning will cause reciprocal disequilibrium in other areas.

Needs are motivators, and man constantly strives to maintain equilibrium in his environment by meeting basic needs. Priorities have been established for meeting these needs, and physiological needs require continuous refilling before the individual can engage himself in satisfying experiences with higher-level needs, such as love and belonging or self-esteem. The ultimate goal is developing the human potential for self-actualization, which according to Maslow few attain.

Throughout the life span certain needs become dominant concerns during various developmental periods. In infancy when the tasks relate to achievement of trust, the need for safety and security is dominant. As childhood growth becomes rapid and autonomy increasingly important, the need for activity and rest deserves special consideration. In adolescence and young adulthood sexual role functioning is primary. Maintenance needs—oxygen, nutrition, and elimination—are symbolic of adulthood stability.

According to basic need theory, the goal of nursing is to help the client meet his basic needs. Disturbances in lower-level needs preclude achieving higher-level needs and ultimately self-actualization. Meeting needs in a consistent, dependable way is therefore necessary for fostering growth and development

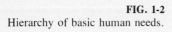

FIG. 1-2
Hierarchy of basic human needs.

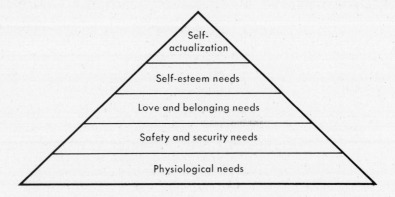

throughout the life span. The resources and energies of nursing can be used to help the client achieve this goal.

STRESS ADAPTATION THEORY

Another view of the human system is offered by Hans Selye, who describes the goal of man as adaptation to stress. Stress is a response to a demand and may be positive (eustress) or negative (distress). Stress is necessary for growth and development throughout the life span, and man's ability to adapt to stress evolves with maturity.

Stress is always present but increases when there is a change or threat to the human system. The factor or agent precipitating the change or threat is known as a *stressor* and may be biological, environmental, or social. Thus stress is a syndrome of change in a biological system as a result of a stressor.[4,7]

Stress occurs when the stressor exceeds the limits of the organism's coping abilities. Therefore, stress is a function of both the stressor and the coping abilities of the organism. Stress occurs in three stages: alarm, resistance, and exhaustion.[8] Reduction of stress can occur at any stage.

Adaptation is the organism's response to stress and serves to return the organism to the steady state. Adaptation occurs at physiological, psychological, and sociocultural levels and is referred to as the general adaptation syndrome in which the organism's energies are mobilized to cope with the stressor by modifying internal or external environments. The viability of the organism depends on the mediation of environmental demands and adaptive energies.[2]

According to the stress adaptation view of man, health is a state of adaptation to stress. In this framework the goal of nursing is to help the client identify stressors and coping mechanisms and achieve positive adaptation. These are discussed when appropriate throughout the text.

Developmental theories

PSYCHOSOCIAL DEVELOPMENTAL LEVELS

Erik Erikson believes that the personality of the human organism develops throughout the life span. He has identified eight stages of man at which basic tasks of personality development occur.[4] Erikson believes that individuals attain levels of development at their own rate. Failure to achieve levels of psychological and social development, however, leads to negative counterparts. The opposing forces cause a crisis to which the individual must respond and resolve before proceeding to the next level (Table 1-1).

As a helping profession, nursing can help clients accomplish basic tasks of psychosocial development and resolve conflict of negative counter-

TABLE 1-1
Psychosocial developmental levels

Developmental level	Task	Negative counterpart
1. Infant	Trust	Mistrust
2. Toddler	Autonomy	Shame and doubt
3. Preschooler	Initiative	Guilt
4. School-ager	Industry	Inferiority
5. Adolescent	Identity	Role confusion
6. Young adult	Intimacy	Isolation
7. Middlescent	Generativity	Stagnation
8. Older adult	Ego integrity	Despair

From Erikson, Erik: Childhood and society, ed. 2, New York, 1963, W.W. Norton & Co., Inc.

parts. Specific nursing actions and developmental levels are discussed in Chapter 2.

DEVELOPMENTAL TASKS Robert Havighurst, like Erikson, views man's emergence across the life span. Havighurst describes man's development as a series of tasks necessary for healthy physical, psychological, and social development.[5] Tasks arise at certain critical periods in the individual's life and are described for six age periods (see outline that follows). Achievement of the tasks leads to happiness and success with future tasks, while failure leads to unhappiness, disapproval by society, and difficulty with later tasks. Tasks may arise because of physical maturation, cultural pressure, or personal goals. Some tasks are age specific; others recur across the life span.

Nurses can help clients and families identify critical periods of task achievement. According to Havighurst, there is at these times a "teachable

---

DEVELOPMENTAL TASKS

1. Infancy and early childhood
   a. Learn to walk
   b. Learn to take solid food
   c. Learn to talk
   d. Control elimination of body wastes
   e. Learn sex differences and sexual modesty
   f. Form concepts and learning language to describe social and physical reality
   g. Get ready to read
   h. Learn to distinguish right and wrong and begin to develop a conscience
2. Middle childhood
   a. Learn physical skills necessary for ordinary games
   b. Build wholesome attitudes toward oneself as a growing organism
   c. Learn to get along with age-mates
   d. Learn an appropriate masculine or feminine social role
   e. Develop fundamental skills in reading, writing, and calculating
   f. Develop concepts necessary for everyday living
   g. Develop conscience, morality, and a scale of values
   h. Achieve personal independence
   i. Develop attitudes toward social groups and institutions
3. Adolescence
   a. Achieve new and more mature relations with age-mates of both sexes
   b. Achieve a masculine or feminine social role
   c. Accept one's physique and use body effectively
   d. Achieve emotional independence of parents and other adults

e. Prepare for marriage and family life
f. Prepare for economic career
g. Develop an ideology—a set of values and an ethical system as a guide to behavior
h. Achieve socially responsible behavior
4. Early adulthood
   a. Select a mate
   b. Learn to live with a marriage partner
   c. Start a family
   d. Rear children
   e. Manage a home
   f. Start an occupation
   g. Assume civic responsibility
   h. Find a congenial social group
5. Middle age
   a. Assist children to become responsible and happy adults
   b. Achieve adult social and civic responsibility
   c. Attain and maintain satisfactory performance in occupation
   d. Develop adult leisure-time activities
   e. Relate to spouse as a person
   f. Accept and adjust to physiological changes
   g. Adjust to aging parents
6. Later maturity
   a. Adjust to decreasing physical strength and health
   b. Adjust to retirement and reduced income
   c. Adjust to death of spouse
   d. Establish affiliation with one's age group
   e. Adopt and adapt to social roles in a flexible way
   f. Establish satisfactory physical living arrangements

From Havighurst, Robert: Developmental tasks and education, ed. 3. Copyright © 1972 by Longman, Inc. Reprinted by permission of Longman, Inc., New York.

Foundations of clinical practice

moment'' or unique readiness to learn the task. The role of the nurse in fostering human development and task achievement is discussed specifically in Chapter 2 and when appropriate throughout the text.

THE FAMILY SYSTEM

While previous theorists have described relationships of man's internal and external environments or stages of development, Evelyn Duvall focuses on the individual within the family system.[3] The stages of family life are illustrated by eight tasks that must be accomplished at each stage for the growth of the individual and the family's own system (see outline that follows).

THE FAMILY SYSTEM

A. Stages
   1. Married couple
   2. Childbearing family
   3. Family with preschool children
   4. Family with school-age children
   5. Family with teenagers
   6. Family as a launching center
   7. The ''empty nest'' family
   8. The aging family

B. Tasks of each stage
   1. Physical maintenance
   2. Allocation of resources
   3. Division of labor
   4. Socialization of family members
   5. Reproduction, recruitment, and release
   6. Maintenance of order
   7. Placement of members into the larger society
   8. Maintenance of motivation and morale

From Duvall, Evelyn M.: Family development, ed. 4, Philadelphia, 1971, J.B. Lippincott Co. Reprinted by permission of Harper & Row, Inc.

The nurse must recognize that clients are members of family systems and that a change in one member creates reciprocal changes in the family group. Nursing care is planned to support family growth and facilitate task accomplishment at each stage. Nursing actions for supporting family growth are discussed in detail in Chapter 3 and when appropriate throughout the text.

HOLISTIC MAN

Systems, needs, stages, and tasks often are inadequate descriptors of man, for man is indeed more than the sum of his parts. Man is a biopsychosocial being, a harmony of internal and external environments. Holism is a concept that describes man as integrating all factors to maintain system integrity. Man's responses to the environment, to health and health problems, and to the health care system occur in holistic modes. The young child with tonsillitis, for example, is not only a physical organism with a health problem, adapting to stress, but also an individual with basic human needs, dealing with psychosocial tasks of industry versus inferiority, accomplishing developmental tasks of middle childhood, as well as a member of a family, social group, culture, and nation.

Nurses respond to holistic man when planning nursing care that considers the entirety of the client's concerns as opposed to a focus on subsystems or stages. Holistic nursing care is derived from a broad theory base and applied with concern for the uniqueness of the individual. Holistic nursing care facilitates growth and development throughout the life span and supports each individual as he seeks his own maximum potential for health.

Summary   Theoretical frameworks help nurses explain, predict, or validate the behaviors of man as he evolves during the life span. The general system theory views man's relationships with internal and external environments, whereas the basic need theory views man's need to satisfy lower-level needs in order to facilitate the ultimate goal, self-actualization. Stress adaptation theory provides insights into man's reaction to biological and environmental or social stressors and describes man's facilities for coping and adapting. Developmental theories focus on levels and stages of physical and psychosocial growth of individuals and families. Though all theoretical frameworks are useful, none encompasses the entire concept of man's being. Therefore, nurses may find a holistic view of man necessary for facilitating the individual's optimal potential during each stage of human development.

References
1. Bailey, June, and Claus, Karen: Decision making in nursing: tools for change, St. Louis, 1975, The C.V. Mosby Co.
2. Byrne, Marjorie, and Thompson, Lida: Key concepts for the study and practice of nursing, ed. 2, St. Louis, 1978, The C.V. Mosby Co.
3. Duvall, Evelyn M.: Family development, ed. 4, Philadelphia, 1971, J.B. Lippincott Co.
4. Erikson, Erik: Childhood and society, ed. 2, New York, 1963, W.W. Norton & Co., Inc.
5. Havighurst, Robert: Developmental tasks and education, ed. 3, New York, 1972, David McKay Co., Inc.
6. Maslow, Abraham H.: Motivation and personality, New York, 1954, Harper & Row, Publishers, Inc.
7. Schuster, Clara, and Ashburn, Shirley: The process of human development: a holistic approach, Boston, 1980, Little, Brown and Co.
8. Selye, Hans: The stress of life, New York, 1956, McGraw-Hill Book Co.
9. Von Bertalanffy, Ludwig: General system theory, New York, 1968, George Braziller, Inc.

Additional readings
Fuller, Sarah: Holistic man and the science and practice of nursing, Nurs. Outlook **26:**706-704, 1978.
Laszlo, Ervin: The systems view of the world, New York, 1972, George Braziller, Inc.
Laszlo, Ervin, editor: The world system, models, norms, variations, New York, 1973, George Braziller, Inc.
Saxton, Dolores, and Hyland, Patricia: Planning and implementing nursing intervention: stress and adaptation applied to patient care, ed. 2, St. Louis, 1979, The C.V. Mosby Co.
Sutherland, John: A general systems philosophy for the social and behavioral sciences, New York, 1973, George Braziller, Inc.

2 Client development across the life span

Human life unfolds in predictable patterns across the life span. These patterns have been described as stages[5] or seasons[11] and are commonly denoted as neonate, infant, toddler, preschool child, school-age child (middle childhood), preadolescent, adolescent, young adult, middle-aged adult (adulthood), and older adult (later maturity). The purpose of this chapter is to provide a foundation of principles of growth and development from which the nurse can plan health care. The chapter begins with an eclectic theory base and includes approaches to assessing growth and development and a description of each developmental stage, including norms and unique hazards of development. Death is considered by some as the final stage of life,[10] and the chapter concludes with a discussion of coping with death.

Theories of human development

Theories of growth and development can be used to explain or predict human behavior throughout the life span. Several have particular relevance as they provide insight into specific aspects of development such as intellectual or moral development; others are useful for their global viewpoints. Theories by nature are generalizations about human growth and development, and nurses must be cognizant of individual differences and those owing to ethnic background (culture) or socioeconomic status. It is however, valuable for nurses to understand the classical theoretical orientations to human development that have influenced the direction of parenting, child-rearing practices, and aging. No single theory addresses itself to all aspects of human behavior; therefore, contemporary thinking regarding developmental concepts is largely a synthesis of ideas that have been adapted from the following theorists.

2   Client development across the life span

SIGMUND FREUD: PSYCHOANALYTIC THEORY

Sigmund Freud was the classical founder of the psychoanalytic theory of human development. He maintained that man as an organism had two unconscious drives—sexual energy and self-destruction (that is, death wish). According to Freud, at birth the infant is operating at the *id* level, or exclusively according to the *pleasure principle*. Immediate gratification is the infant's quest. Later on, through day-to-day experiences, he finds that there is another operant phenomenon, the *reality principle,* which is fundamental to the origin of the *ego*. Subsequently, the child acquires a social consciousness and a moral framework; this stage marks advent of the *superego*. This cognitive developmental process does not occur in a vacuum but is established during a series of motivational changes called "psychosexual stages" of development.

Freud reminds us that motivations remain constant throughout life. Only their mode of expression changes. Gratification of the id is accomplished in different ways during development. As an infant it is obtained orally; thus infancy constitutes the *oral stage,* with the components of sucking, eating, and biting. Eating is both sexually pleasurable and destructive, according to Freud. The breast and the mother provide pleasure; and since ingestion is destructive (because elements are consumed), it also satisfies the death wish.

The toddler obtains gratification through controlling the anus as he learns to retain or expel feces at will. This time period Freud calls the *anal stage*. This developmental phase characteristically encompasses considerable preoccupation with the anal region, and Freud relates behavioral facets accordingly. They include toilet training, frequent spankings because of defiant behavior (pleasurable stimulation of the area), and stool smearing (destruction).

Preschool years Freud calls the *phallic stage,* when gratification sources move to the genitalia, and the classic Oedipus and Electra complexes occur when boys and girls, respectively, want to destroy the parent of the same sex and marry the parent of the opposite sex. The goal of gratification is mixed with the fear of retaliation, which includes "castration" anxiety, from the parent to be destroyed. This kind of conflict is ultimately resolved; and by the age of about 5, the child enters the sexual *latency period,* which persists until adolescence, when mature sexual expression dominates the developmental tasks.

ERIK ERIKSON: STAGES OF MAN

Freudian notions, according to some psychologists, are more useful in explaining pathological behavior than they are in explaining regular events of normal development. However, at least one of Freud's followers is worthy to note. He is Erik Erikson, who devised the Eight Stages of Man, which are described in later portions of this chapter. These stages are descriptive of the success or failure to resolve the developmental conflicts at various points of life. Below is a comparison of Freud's and Erikson's stages of development.

Freud	Erikson
Oral stage or infancy	Trust versus mistrust
Anal stage or toddlerhood	Autonomy versus shame and doubt
Phallic stage or preschool	Initiative versus guilt
Latency or school age	Industry versus inferiority
Adolescence	Identity versus diffusion or role confusion
Young adulthood	Intimacy versus isolation
Adulthood	Productivity versus self-absorption or stagnation
Later maturity	Integrity versus despair

JEAN PIAGET: COGNITIVE DEVELOPMENT

Piaget, a Swiss psychologist, is recognized primarily for his psychology of cognition according to a developmental point of view.[12] This theorist advocates that there are functional and structural aspects of intellectual behavior. Organization of experience and adaptive processes of accommodation and assimilation are important tenets. Perception of information or stimuli that enter the system influences how it is incorporated into the individual or how it is used. These input and processing phenomena change all subsequent related perceptual experiences, with the individual making fine differentiations, but always in terms of the original experience. Piaget believes that human adaptation comprises a balance between assimilation and accommodation.

Structural developmental units are associated with Piaget's theory. Essentially, they serve as frameworks for sensory input. These units are (1) sensorimotor, (2) preconceptual, (3) intuitive thought, (4) concrete operations, and (5) formal operations. Play, language development, personality formation, acquisition of morals, and life-space considerations are important elements in the latter phases. Piaget professes that the sequence of development is always the same with different children, who proceed through them at varying rates. Each subsequent state is characterized by the most recently acquired capability, and the dynamic process of structural building continues as environmental experiences emerge. In Piaget's theory, the ultimate cognitive development is achieved when the child can deal with his environment on a symbolic level and when he conceptualizes his social world in terms of responsible interaction with it. Table 2-1 is an abbreviated outline of Piaget's schemata of early development.

TABLE 2-1
Piaget's schemata of development

Sensorimotor development	Cognitive development
Birth to 1 month Reflexive behavior: Behavior dependent on reflexes and innate performance capacities.	**2 to 4 years** Preconceptual stage: Uses symbolism to represent absent objects and to form basis for memory. "Let's pretend" games are popular. Feelings may be worked out through play. May try to change reality. Thoughts lack generality and individuality. Classification behavior is inconsistent. Tends to be illogical. Uses transductive reasoning.
1 to 4 months Primary circular reactions: Behavior revolves around "self." No time-space reality. Perceptual recognition begins by association in repetitive acts.	
4 to 8 months Secondary circular reactions: The external world is recognized. Repetition and self-reinforcement remain important. Child discovers that he can cause things to happen. Develops awareness that objects come and go, and can perceive those not in sight.	**4 to 7 years** Intuitive stage: Perceptions, not logic, rule thought processes. Centers attention on one part of a complex whole. May ignore important elements and relationships between them. Does not comprehend process reversal.
8 to 12 months Coordination of secondary schemata: Cause-effect notion is expanded. Exhibits ability to employ others as a means to an end. Attempts to overcome barriers to attain object.	**7 to 11 years** Concrete operational stage: Grasps concepts of reversing, and expands beyond centering and egocentricity. Develops understanding of conservation; that is, objects are not altered in number, volume, or size simply because they are reshaped or rearranged. Skilled at classification schemes.
12 to 18 months Tertiary circular reactions: Uses trial and error tactics to explore objects. Employs variable modes of manipulation to evoke new responses. Discovers that there may be more than a singular means to an end.	**11 to 15 years** Formal operational stage: Capable of solving complex and abstract problems. Can formulate and test hypotheses within the laws of the scientific method.
18 to 24 months Invention of new means through mental combination: Can manipulate and invent new means to an end with extensive trial and error. Imitates objects and animals, even when not visible. Works out play before initiation.	

2 Client development across the life span

Recent research on adult development has resulted in various frameworks for the study of this life period. Although there are variations in theme and labeling, in each theory certain patterns emerge that divide adult life into phases and stages based on chronological age.

Levinson and his associates recognize that there are no sharp divisions between the various stages of life; rather, there are phases of "entering," "transition," and "culmination" that should be noted.[11] Each division is permitted plus or minus 2 years within this description.

17-22, early adult transition: The individual abandons the preadult world and initiates the tasks of early adulthood.

22-28, entering the adult world: There is an exploration of adulthood, and efforts are focused on the creation of a stable structure.

28-33, transition: A reappraisal process takes place. Life's dream is formed, and mentor relationships are created. Career, love relationships, marriage, and family are crucial elements during this phase.

33-40, settling down: A niche in society is established, and the individual endeavors toward advancement of goals. Later in this phase there is increasing independence in becoming one's own man. Mentor relationships may be vulnerable during this time. Affirmation is sought, and many "culminating" events are occurring. Several hazards exist during this time. The failure to resolve career goals, personal strife in business or intimate relationships, and anxiety about life's direction can create developmental vulnerability.

40-45, midlife transition: During this phase the individual reviews his life and makes modifications in occupation, dreams, and personal-social relationships. Some theorists refer to this time as the "midlife crisis." The failure to resolve key problems can initiate a long process of frustration and a feeling of failure.

45-50, entering middle adulthood: Middle adulthood is ideally marked by a satisfactory life structure, since earlier crises have been resolved. Mastery and personal satisfaction are paramount.

50-55, transition

55-60, culmination of middle adulthood

60-65, late adult transition

65 and over, late adulthood

Robert Peck is noted for his contribution of refining the crucial issues of middle age and old age more precisely than earlier theorists, whose stages encompassed essentially all of the years of maturity.[7] Peck divides these years into two periods and deals with seven central developmental issues.

The middle years are characterized by four challenges: (1) valuing wisdom versus valuing physical powers, (2) socializing versus sexualizing in human relationships, (3) cathectic (emotional) flexibility versus cathectic impoverishment, and (4) mental flexibility versus mental rigidity.

In older adulthood there are three challenges: (1) ego differentiation versus work-role preoccupation, (2) body transcendence versus body preoccupation, and (3) ego transcendence versus ego preoccupation. Peck believes that older adults can transcend retirement, body frailty, and even their own deaths by finding new satisfactions in activity, creativity, human interaction, and the joy of anticipation of leaving behind their lives' significance with others.

THEORIES OF AGING

Three theories of aging deserve some consideration as they relate to the study of older clients: the theories of (1) disengagement, (2) activity, and (3) continuity.[3]

Disengagement

The basis for this theory arises from the fact that man is mortal and must eventually leave his place and role in society. Preparation for this exit requires that there be planning to ensure an orderly transition of power and responsibilities from older to younger members before disability, inefficiency, or death of the older person affects operations. This process has essentially become institutionalized, and a set of norms has been established for sorting out which older individuals should be replaced and when the disengagement should commence. Thus ages have been identified for compulsory retirement, for collecting pensions, and for obtaining Social Security benefits, for example. Society expects that persons, especially those in key positions, can carry out their roles until their successor is selected. Elaborate rituals and mechanisms exist in industry, business, and academia for this transitionary process. Care is taken in filling important positions to ensure that the individual selected has a high probability of uninterrupted functioning before leaving the post because of aging or health problems. It is easy to appreciate that the accepted group norms do not always coincide with the needs or desires of the individual.

Individuals disengage by gradually withdrawing from certain roles and activities and become, in turn, more self-centered. This process of disengagement may be because of declining energy, as the older person becomes aware that his life span and life space have certain limitations. It may also be a result of awareness of the inevitable imposed disengagement, and the desire of the individual to be in control of what is happening, as opposed to being controlled. Disengagement, like other changes, is more easily accepted if it is self-initiated and self-controlled rather than imposed from external sources. A satisfactory compromise is reached when there is a sharing of decision making that relates to disengagements, with both the individual and the society assuming certain responsibilities based on mutual needs. Obviously, the time period for the disengagement may vary from days to years, depending on the circumstances.

Activity

The activity theory of aging assumes that the same norms exist for all mature individuals. Therefore, the standards of functional activity that are characteristic for the middle aged are also used as a measuring device or standard for persons much older. The degree to which the individual "acts like" or "looks like" a middle-aged model is the determinant of the aging process. Successful aging occurs when one seems most middle aged and exhibits the fewest signs and symptoms of earlier or later stages of life. One must constantly struggle to remain functional (that is, middle aged) and take on new activities to replace lost ones. There is no provision for legitimate disengagement.

Continuity

The continuity theory of aging accounts for the continuous flow of phases in the life cycle and does not limit itself to change. It assumes that persons will remain the same unless there are factors that stimulate change or necessitate adaptation. Habits, preferences, and associations would be static without externally or internally imposed biological and psychological influences. Obviously these influential factors cannot be avoided during life processes, and thus dynam-

14

TABLE 2-2
Biological theories of aging

Theory	Explanation
Wear and tear	The body is like a machine. Parts wear out and the machine breaks down.
Rate of living	The body has a fixed rate of potential for living. The faster one lives, the sooner one ages and dies.
Waste theory	Chemical wastes collect in the body and produce deterioration by interfering with cellular functioning.
Collagen theory	Collagen stiffens with age, producing loss of elasticity in organs, skin, tendons, blood vessels, and so forth. The resultant stiffness adversely affects function.
Autoimmune theory	Cellular mutations that occur with aging cause protein production, which acts as a foreign substance, thus stimulating the production of antibodies.
Mutation theory	With lifelong cellular division, successive mutations occur that adversely affect organ functioning. Mutations increase steadily with aging, and biological errors occur.

Data from Atchley, R.C.: The social forces in later life: an introduction to social gerontology, Belmont, Calif., 1972, Wadsworth Publishing Co., Inc., pp. 44-47.

ic changes are subtly but constantly occurring. Since all individuals have unique experiences, aging is likewise a unique phenomenon for everyone.

Biological theories of aging are summarized in Table 2-2.

Other theories

There are some other theoretical ideas that relate to aging.[3] One of these proposes that older persons are essentially a *subculture* and must relate and interact primarily with each other, at least within their own social class. Another advocates that the aged are a *minority group;* and because of a biological trait that identifies them on sight (that is, being old), they are discriminated against through isolation and prejudice. This theory is further substantiated by the fact that many of our older citizens are poor and have few opportunities for a high quality of life. A final idea relates to aging as an *identity crisis.* The crisis occurs because an individual is unable to adjust to a revised identity (self-concept and self-image) that is congruent with aging and with the changes in position that accompany the process.

Like theories about most subjects, none is entirely acceptable and all require considerably more investigation. However, they supply a useful framework for the discussion of growth and developmental considerations pertinent to the older adult in our society.

LAWRENCE KOHLBERG: A THEORY OF MORAL DEVELOPMENT

The moral development of individuals is based on a series of life experiences that stimulate and shape problem solving regarding value systems. Since human behavior is largely influenced by moral reasoning, it is valuable to understand the development of morality. Lawrence Kohlberg has formulated a theory that divides the process into three major levels and six substages (Table 2-3).[6,9]

The *preconventional level* is based on the premise that moral behavior is primarily determined by a system of rewards and punishments. Individuals at stage 1 weigh the consequences of action according to the goal of avoiding punishment from those in power. Later, during stage 2, a modified perspective emerges characterized by an exchange of favors. Actions are justified if they satisfy one's personal needs and sometimes the needs of others. Moral behavior is tempered by "what's in it for me" rather than by the blind obedience of stage 1. Children and delinquent adults operate resentfully at this preconventional

TABLE 2-3

Stages of moral development according to Kohlberg

I. Preconventional level	Behavior abides by cultural rules because of punishment or reward consequences.
Stage 1: The punishment and obedience orientation	Good and bad and right and wrong are thought of in terms of consequences of action. Avoidance of punishment.
Stage 2: The instrumental realistic orientation	Right action is whatever satisfies one's own needs and occasionally the needs of others. Exchange of favors. "Do for me and I do for you."
II. Conventional level	Behavior is self-controlled due to expectations of others and desire to conform and accept social expectations.
Stage 3: Interpersonal acceptance of "good boy, nice girl" social concept	Good behavior is what pleases and is approved by others. Response to stereotype; social units are loose and flexible.
Stage 4: The "law and order" orientation	Right behavior accepts and shows respect for authority. Doing one's duty for the good of the social order; laws are permanent and not likely to change.
III. Postconventional, autonomous, or principled level	Effort to define moral values and principles that are valid beyond the authority of the group and even beyond the self.
Stage 5: The social contract, utilitarian orientation	Adherence to legal rights commonly agreed upon by society but with laws subject to interpretation and change in terms of rational consideration for the rights of the individual while maintaining respect of self and others.
Stage 6: The universal ethical principle orientation	Right behavior is defined in terms of ethical principles based on logical comprehensiveness, universality, and consistency, and respects the inherent dignity of human beings as individuals.

From Kaluger, George, and Kaluger, Meriem Fair: Human development: the span of life, ed. 2, St. Louis, 1979, The C.V. Mosby Co. Based on data from Kohlberg, L.: Stage and sequence: the cognitive-development approach to socialization. In D. Goslin (Ed.), Handbook of socialization: theory and research, Chicago, 1969, Rand McNally & Co.

level with self-interests and material considerations taking precedence within their value system and related behaviors.

The *conventional level* is dominated by social expectations. Maintenance of a social system and loyalty to established institutions or social relationships shapes moral behavior. Stage 3 is marked by approval of others or stereotyped majority behavior. Individual ties and primary groups are paramount. Stage 4, although still dominated by social approval, reaches into secondary groups (such as community or nation). There is a pronounced respect for "law and order," the stabilizing schemes of the larger society. Most adults operate within these conventional moral constructs. Few adults devote primary time to the weighty task of developing "principled" moral reasoning that stems from prolonged self-study of integrated values.

The *postconventional*, or *principled, level* defined moral behavior in terms of what is right according to "social contract." Equality and mutual obligation of the fraternity of mankind receive emphasis. Stage 5 recognizes that rules may be changed by democratic reform, provided that there is attention to liberty, equal rights, and brotherhood. Stage 6 is an extension of Stage 5 and can be defined as consisting of self-selected, abstract ethical principles that have inherent logic and are comprehensive, universal, and consistent. The dignity of the life of man is paramount. The principled level of moral behavior is not situation bound but reflects an inherent belief that society and social relationships can be arranged in many ways to accommodate particular values. Nonconformity is acceptable and authority may be questioned, but behaviors must abide by social norms insofar as human values are served. The latter represents the essence of moral obligation, according to Kohlberg.

A careful study of the levels and stages reveals that they are not defined by opinions or judgments; rather, they represent ways of thinking about moral matters and bases of choice. Throughout adult development, individuals are subject to repeated opportunities to modify and upgrade their moral behavior based on cognitive acquisition. The quality of life experiences, human interaction, and education determine the operating morals of adults in our society.

Principles of growth and development

Before exploration of specific concepts and principles, it is imperative to distinguish the three frequently used terms growth, maturation, and development.

Growth is merely an increase in body mass, the person becoming taller or heavier.

Maturation is biological development that permits new behaviors. It can occur with growth, but growth in size or weight is not a corequisite. Maturation precedes new behavior and determines the amount of growth or modification possible for the organism. For example, maturation of certain neurological structures must take place before sphincter control of the bowel and bladder can be learned and achieved by the young child.

Development is new behavioral patterns made possible through physical growth and maturation. Since growth and development occur together in most instances, the terms are often used synonymously.

Growth is a continuous and orderly process. All individuals proceed through the same sequential growth pattern, but there is considerable variation in the rate, or tempo, of their progression. Most growth charts permit a wide range of individual differences to fall within the scope of "normal."

Growth is essential to the initiation of many functional behaviors that are termed development. Although growth may not be evident in a given situation, development is a dynamic process. For example, the peak of physical growth is reached during adolescence, but coordination and body control continue to be improved and refined.

Development proceeds from simple to complex, from homogeneous to heterogeneous, and from general to specific. Gross movements of limbs precede controlled movements. An infant can move his arms (a simple, homogeneous, and general act) before he can wave bye-bye with his hand or grasp and throw an object (complex, heterogeneous, and specific acts).

The sequence of developmental activity occurs in cephalocaudal and proximal-distal directions. Early developmental activities center around the head and upper portion of the body, for example, eating, smiling, and hand-grasping an object. Later developmental aspects include the lower portion of the body, for example, standing, walking, and bowel and bladder control. Proximal-distal direction refers to the fact that controlled movements close to the trunk (head, arms, and legs) are possible before movements of the distal portions (hands, fingers, feet, and toes) can be voluntarily controlled.

There are many guidelines that define normal growth and developmental capabilities at various age intervals, but it is important to recall that considerable latitude is possible within the acceptable ranges for normalcy. Developmental guidelines are cited only to demonstrate the usual for the most children and are not meant to exclude the fact that healthy variations are bound to occur when we deal with a heterogeneous population of unique human beings.

FIG. 2-1
Head circumference for boys from birth to 18 years of age. There is a similar graph for females. (From Hughes, James G.: Synopsis of pediatrics, ed. 5, St. Louis, 1980, The C.V. Mosby Co.)

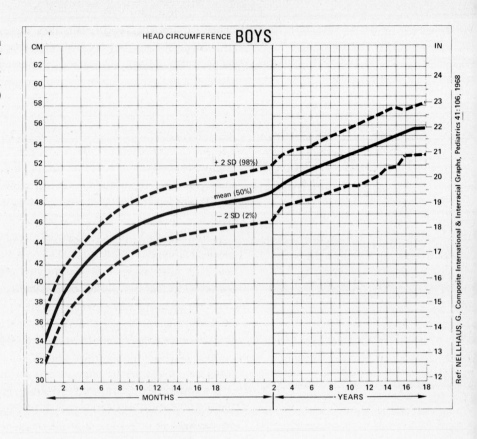

HEAD CIRCUMFERENCE **BOYS**

+ 2 SD (98%)

mean (50%)

− 2 SD (2%)

MONTHS — YEARS

Ref: NELLHAUS, G., Composite International & Interracial Graphs, Pediatrics 41:106, 1968

FIG. 2-2
Head circumference is an objective indication of a growth pattern. (Courtesy March of Dimes Birth Defects Foundation.)

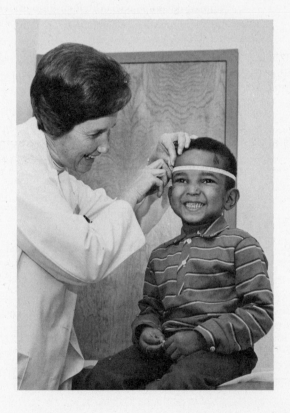

2 Client development across the life span

A descriptive summary of growth and development for children and adults is presented in Table 2-6 and the accompanying illustrations at the end of this chapter.

Assessing growth and development
GROWTH

A significant part of the nurse's role in health management is a thorough understanding of human growth and development. Such knowledge is important in determining whether a given client's biological equipment is functioning properly and whether or not his behavioral characteristics are congruent with the normal patterns for his age group. If discrepancies are noted, they may be indicative of physical or emotional health problems.

Normal growth patterns are well established, and a number of ways exist to appraise this growth. They include objective measurements of (1) weight and height, (2) head, chest, and abdominal circumference, (3) osseous development, and (4) dentition. Growth charts that allow comparison of progress against the range of normal instead of merely an average are extremely valuable tools. Some charts illustrate growth patterns by percentile graphs in which the progress of a given client can be considered as he relates to ninety-nine others of his age group.

The rate of growth is a better indicator of development than merely size measurements at a given time.

Osseous development and dentition are valuable indicators of growth because they follow a definite pattern, which can be closely related to physiological growth. If abnormalities in rate or sequence are noted, they may be indicative of disease.

A thorough evaluation of special organs and senses also contributes to assessment of growth and development. Detailed data on such assessments are provided in subsequent chapters. For examples of growth charts, see Appendix A.

TABLE 2-4

Assessment factors, gestational age

Characteristic	Premature (below 37 weeks)	Term (37 to 38 weeks)	Postmature (above 38 weeks)
Vernix caseosa	Absent	Present	Absent
Skin	Fragile, translucent	Pale, smooth	Parchment like
Breast nodule	2 mm	4 mm	7 mm
Hair (body)	Predominant on forehead, back, shoulders	Some body hair	Absent
Hair (scalp)	Fine	Fine	Coarser and silky
Nails	Soft, extend to fingertips	Cyanotic, do not extend beyond fingertips	Yellowish brown, may extend beyond fingertips
Sole creases*	Anterior transverse crease only	Creases in anterior two thirds	Many creases
External ear	No cartilage	Some cartilage	Thick cartilage
Genitalia (female)	Clitoris and labia minora prominent; labia majora widely separated	Labia majora cover labia minora	
Genitalia (male)	Testes in inguinal canal; few scrotal rugae	Intermediate	Pendulous testes; scrotum full with many rugae
Reflexes (see Chapter 10)			

*This factor is invalid in black neonates

TABLE 2-5
Apgar scoring chart

Sign	Score 0	Score 1	Score 2
Heart rate	Absent	Slow (below 100)	Over 100
Respiratory effort	Absent	Slow, irregular; hypoventilation	Good; crying lustily
Muscle tone	Flaccid	Some flexion of extremities	Active motion, well flexed
Reflex irritability	No response	Cry; some motion	Vigorous cry
Color	Blue, pale	Body pink, hands and feet blue	Completely pink

From Hughes, James G.: Synopsis of pediatrics, ed. 5, St. Louis, 1980, The C.V. Mosby Co., p. 238.

Assessing gestational age

The maturity of an infant does not always reflect the gestational history of the pregnancy. It is important to assess the neonate for objective evidence of development and not to rely on weeks of reported gestation or weight to determine whether prematurity or postmaturity actually exists. Criteria useful in judging gestational age include: (1) appearance and characteristics of the skin, hair, and nails, (2) cartilage development of the ear, (3) appearance of external genitalia, and (4) reflexes (Table 2-4).

Assessing the neonate

The neonate should be assessed in the delivery room at 1 and 5 minutes after birth. A popular tool to use in this evaluation is the Apgar score card, which facilitates categorizing the infant quickly into a normal, depressed, or high-risk group on the basis of five factors: heart rate, respiratory effort, muscle tone, reflex irritability, and color (Table 2-5). This scoring method helps physicians and nurses in determining the immediate management priorities of the neonate.

DEVELOPMENT

Consistent observations of various age groups have provided a series of characteristic behavioral patterns that seem to be operant during a particular time in growth. Both the sequence in which patterns of development occur and the age at which given patterns appear are highly predictable. For example, 1-year-olds usually display a pincer grasp while manipulating small objects; whereas a 28-week-old infant will ordinarily rake an object toward him, a cruder method of retrieval. We know, therefore, that most "normal" infants develop this one element of fine motor coordination in the second 6 months of life.

Developmental landmarks are not to be used in an absolute sense. A person does not "fail" a test if he does not display a certain characteristic simultaneously with the norming peers of his age group. It merely means that the examiner should note this, and during a subsequent test, progress in fine motor skills should be observed closely.

Children may at times be ahead of their chronological age in developmental manifestations of any of the subgroups of behaviors. For example, language behavior may be quite advanced, but perhaps gross motor behavior is typical or even retarded. Since the tempo of development is uneven, developmental diagnosis is never based on an isolated factor. It is important to compare the child's developmental pattern with himself as well as with the thousands of others used to establish behavioral guidelines. The major reason that developmental assessments are performed is to ensure that orderly progress is being made toward achieving maturity. If singular or multiple identifications of re-

20

tarded development are demonstrated through several testings, tempo and trend causative factors should be searched for and a remedial program planned to enhance environmental, physical, and social stimulation related to developmental advances.

There are five major areas of behavior that represent different aspects of growth: (1) adaptive behavior, (2) gross motor behavior, (3) fine motor behavior, (4) language behavior, and (5) personal-social behavior.[8]

Adaptive behavior is concerned with the organization of stimuli, the perception of relationships, the dissection of wholes into their component parts, and the reintegration of these parts in a meaningful fashion. Problem-solving activities relating to objects and situations (that is, hand-eye coordination in reaching and manipulating) are considered adaptive.

Gross motor behavior includes postural reactions, head balance, sitting, standing, creeping and walking.

Fine motor behavior consists of the use of the hands and fingers in the prehensory approach to grasping and manipulation of an object.

Language behavior includes all visible and audible forms of communication, whether by facial expression, gesture, postural movements, vocalizations, words, phrases, or sentences. It also encompasses mimicry and comprehension of the communications of others.

Personal-social behavior comprises the child's personal reactions to the social culture in which he lives. Training and social conventions, along with the child's neuromotor maturity, strongly influence eventual attainment of these behaviors.

Behavioral observation must include qualitative and quantiative evaluation and be accompanied by adequate social and medical data gathering.

A popular tool used to assess development is the Denver Developmental Screening Test (see Appendix B).

Developmental hazards

A study of human growth and development would not be complete without a discussion of phenomena that can interfere with the normal progression of life experiences. *The potential for physical and mental growth is determined before birth, but it is the dynamics of heredity and environment that determine development.* Developmental achievement is dependent on the nature and functioning of the biological equipment that a person possesses, the quality of his environment, and the significance of his experiences with the physical and social world. In this section we discuss some of the hazards of human development and consider ways in which nurses and other members of the health team can help clients avoid the hazards or at least minimize their effects on subsequent developmental patterns.

CONCEPT OF THE CRITICAL PERIOD

In the previous discussion of developmental tasks we emphasized that if certain behaviors or achievements are not accomplished at specific points in the life experience, they are difficult or even impossible to attain at a later time. Conversely, having selected learnings or experiences at a given age period may make some behaviors more certain in future years. However, identical experiences, depending on when they occur and what has preceded them, may have very different effects. For example, long-term hospitalization will have varying impacts on the lives of neonates, infants, preschoolers, adolescents, or mature adults. Even within these various age groups, hospitalization will produce highly individual responses, since no two persons have had exactly the same genetic endowment, environment, or human experiences.

Early childhood and the beginning of adolescence are critical periods because change is most dynamic at these times. Therefore, any serious interferences with the physical organism or its environment should receive special attention from the health team. *Since all tasks are intricately related to each other on a highly complex continuum, what occurs at any given point affects eventual development.*

PRENATAL HAZARDS

At the moment of conception a significant number of genetic and environmental factors become operational to determine the existence and quality of new human life. Although intrauterine development is not easily controlled, it can be assessed and understood in terms of certain physiological realms. Fetal life and growth processes can be studied with techniques such as amniotic fluid and blood chemistry studies, ultrasonics, radiography, and electromonitoring. The analysis of cause-effect relationships concerning intrauterine environmental factors and the subsequent appearance of developmental anomalies, or pathophysiology, has led to the identification of certain hazards of fetal life and in some cases to successful medical or surgical intervention by highly skilled specialists called fetologists.

Factors that adversely affect the development of the fetus can be genetic, maternally influenced, or idiopathic. Some of the more significant elements that can be responsible for adverse fetal effects are discussed below.

Age and health habits of the mother

Statistics demonstrate that babies born out of wedlock and to teenage mothers have twice the average risk of being abnormal in some respect. Mothers under 18 or over 35 years of age are considerably more likely to deliver a child with a physical or mental handicap. The presence of a hereditary or chronic maternal illness and poor nutrition seem to also adversely affect the developing fetus. Cardiovascular, metabolic, or renal disorders, venereal diseases, excessive smoking or alcohol consumption, prolonged stress, or the ingestion of addicting drugs cannot be overlooked in prenatal management, since they produce demonstrable changes in the intrauterine environment.

Mechanical disturbances and trauma

The developing fetus must depend on the maternal pelvis to permit its growth, support its life processes, and facilitate its delivery at the appropriate time. Fetal-pelvic disproportion, abdominal trauma, or similar mechanical disturbances are likely to cause physiological distress for the growing fetus or impair its delivery at the moment of "readiness."

Specific diseases and drugs

A number of specific illnesses and medications are important to note for their implications in fetal pathophysiology. Some affect the uterine environment to the degree that they result in an abortion or premature delivery. Unfortunately, some of the adverse effects of drugs and maternal illness are not so profound and may not be identified for several months or years after birth.

Viruses such as the cytomegalovirus, coxsackievirus, herpesvirus, and influenza, hepatitis, and mumps viruses have been shown to contribute to intrauterine infections resulting in developmental anomalies or in newborn illness and death. *Rubella* is a serious infection that affects the fetus, especially during the first trimester of pregnancy. Up to one third of the fetuses who are in the early developmental stage are adversely influenced by this viral infection. Among the resultant anomalies are central nervous system damage, hypoplasia of the myocardium and other cardiac anomalies, hearing loss, cataracts, and dermatological manifestations. Skeletal defects are seldom attributed to a congenital rubella infection. *Rubeola* may also be responsible for an increase in the perinatal death rate. Although malformations are uncommon, abortions and premature deliveries (especially when the disease is contracted in the third trimester of pregnancy) often occur.

Syphilis if untreated causes abortion, fetal death, premature deliveries, and congenital anomalies. A serological test for this infection is essential at the first obstetrical visit, and if it is positive, rigorous therapy must be instituted at once.

Drugs or vaccines administered to the mother during pregnancy have potential effects on the fetus, including a variety of pathological conditions, anomalies, and death. Some are clearly linked to their neonatal effects, such as thalidomide, chloramphenicol, streptomycin, Sabin polio vaccine, and smallpox vaccine. Several others are suspected of having adverse effects on the developing fetus. Radiation and other high-energy sources also are capable of producing negative fetal effects, especially in the early weeks of pregnancy. Congenital addicts whose mothers are regular users of ''hard'' drugs such as heroin have a perinatal mortality of up to 20%. Most physicians are especially cautious in the administration of medications to pregnant women. Nurses should take every opportunity for teaching potential mothers the hazards of self-medication during pregnancy and urging them to consult their physician if they feel they need drug management for any problem.

Other human developmental phenomena

THE ADOPTED CHILD

There are more than 2 million adopted children under age 18 in the United States. Most were placed before they were 1 year old. Motives for adoption are unique for every couple (or person) and encompass biological, social, and psychological phenomena.

Adoption is a process by which a child is placed in a desirable permanent home and family setting in preference to institutionalization, thus providing more satisfaction and security for the child. In many communities the demands exceed the supply of adoptable babies because an increasing number of unwed mothers are keeping their children and contraception and abortion are practiced with increasing regularity. If more than one child is desired, parents must be willing, in some cases, to adopt a baby of another race or one who is biracial or handicapped.

When the child reaches the age to raise questions about his adoption, he should be answered with honesty; for example, ''We wanted a baby, so a few weeks after you were born, you were brought to live with us.'' There is little or no advantage in giving the child a long, complicated answer mentioning that ''he is very special,'' or ''was selected from all the rest.'' These explanations, although useful for parents in their confession and ventilation of tensions, only provoke anxiety in the child. How can he possibly live up to his parents' expectations of being ''special''? How can he ever repay them for their noble gesture of ''taking him in''? Furthermore, attempting to explain details of his biological parents' circumstances may raise an additional concern: "if abandoned and unwanted once, could I be abandoned again?"

Despite many widely held opinions, adopted children are governed by the same forces as their nonadopted counterparts—heredity and environment. Since adoptive parents cannot alter heredity, their emphasis must be on making their home an ideal place for a child to grow and develop.

MULTIPLE BIRTHS

In the United States about 1 out of 75 or 80 pregnancies results in a multiple birth, primarily twins.

Because of the unusual distension of the uterus, the onset of labor is usually premature, yielding small, high-risk infants. Although the incidence of severe congenital anomalies is higher in multiple births, the overall survival rate is comparable to that of single births of the same weight.

Families find it fascinating to rear twins and observe similarities and differences in their developmental patterns. Although twins are often alike in appearance and behavior, they should be regarded as separate entities rather than a pair of children. Individualization in dress and activities is especially important in later childhood when the self-concept becomes more clearly defined. It is usually a traumatic experience for everyone when twins are separated, since they tend to be highly interdependent.

The infant

Infancy, or the first year of life, is marked by rapid physical growth and near total dependence on parents or other adults for meeting the basic needs of life. The role of *mother* becomes the most important factor in the world around him. It is mother who feeds him, keeps him warm, makes him feel secure, and is always near to determine his needs. The mother role may be assumed by either

FIG. 2-3
The infant responds with pleasure to mother's face. (From The first and second years of life, Columbus, Ohio, Ross Laboratories.)

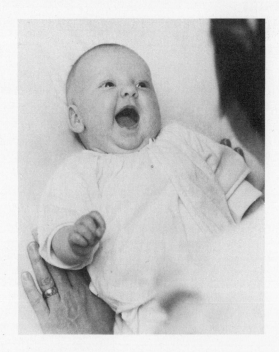

parent, grandparents, other relatives, or even a friend, depending on the life-style of the family into which the child is born.

Maternal figures play a highly significant role in the life of an infant. In addition to bearing the responsibility for meeting the infant's physical needs, the mother must interact with the child on a consistent basis to provide stimulation necessary for physical as well as mental and emotional growth (Fig. 2-3). Any incident that causes prolonged separation from the mother may disturb the child's developmental progression.

During the first year of life, learning is essentially accomplished by trial and error based on the "pain-pleasure" principle and the process of conditioning. The infant discovers that he is a separate entity and not linked absolutely to this mother on whom he depends so much. He realizes that he can be miserable without her if he is wet, hungry, or cold but that when she reappears and does things for him he becomes comfortable and happy. It is these experiences of tension and relief of tension (pain and pleasure) that contribute to the formation of associations that ultimately comprise the *trust* relationship, the major goal of infancy. Without mother, tension and pain are possible. With mother near to meet his needs, tension is relieved and a pleasurable sensation returns.

There is no self-concept and therefore no identity during infancy, but the experiences of these first months of life are presumed to be recorded on an unconscious level and can contribute to the development of feelings of well-being, security, confidence, and wholeness.

Infancy is a self-centered, or egocentric, stage of life. The singular psychic structure element present at this time is the *id* (inherited reservoir of drives). It is mostly unconscious and is aimed at immediate satisfaction of libidinal urges. A helpless child demands much for meeting his needs but is able to return little except a smile or a coo. Self-gratification is paramount. Nourishment, warmth, and the security of a mother figure are the essential elements required to make the baby thrive physically and mentally.

Infancy is a stage of development characterized by the instability that accompanies rapid growth. The biological equipment at birth is not fully ready to cope with the stresses of the extrauterine environment. Mechanisms that protect, integrate, and regulate body systems are still in the process of maturation. Emotional as well as physical responses are often generalized and unpredictable and, at times, lack unity of purpose. An infant shows that he is pleased not only by smiling or laughing but also by waving his arms and moving his entire body in delight. A moment later he may cry or appear uninterested in the person or object that so recently provoked an obvious response of pleasure. The fact that the various experiences with emotional overtones seem to evoke but a transient response does not mean they are not significant. *An infant is capable of lasting impressions* and is likely to establish habits based on even a single experience. This phenomenon is operant in all phases of development in which rapid changes are occurring, and this helps explain why they are known as the "critical periods."[4] Feelings are more easily perceived than attitudes. Words have meaning largely in terms of the ways they are used rather than in terms of their specific meaning. The infant derives information from his "feeling" perception as opposed to his intellectual perception of verbal communication. Tenderness in caring for the infant and soft-spoken words promote reassurance and the sense of basic trust.

Foundations of clinical practice

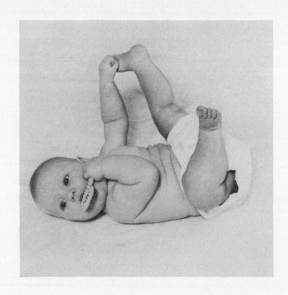

The basic human needs of the infant are essentially the same ones characteristic in older children and adults. However, the needs for sucking, mouthing, and biting are predominant, and the most important sensory input is derived from the mouth. As previously mentioned, infancy is the *oral stage* of development (Fig. 2-4).

Infant learning is primarily the result of conditioning. When a baby is hungry and unsatisfied, he cries out in frustration. Mother, eager to return the infant to a state of satisfaction, feeds him or provides a toy or pacifier to mouth and suck. Very early in life the association between his cry of distress and the appearance of mother who comforts him is established, and learning has taken place. The conditioning type of learning is most effective when the pattern of stimuli and response is a consistent time relationship that the infant can detect and, perhaps most important, when he can derive a high degree of satisfaction during the response period. The infant and mother both become conditioned to certain aspects of feeding, sleeping, and elimination. This points out the need for routines related to bathing, elimination, eating, and even discipline at an early age so that association necessary for learning can be fostered.

An infant's emotional development is largely dependent on the quality of relationships present during his early learnings. Mother and the routines that she has made meaningful to the infant are the two most important components of this developmental stage whose major goal is the establishment of a trusting relationship. The greatest hazard during infancy is that discontinuities in care may exaggerate a natural sense of loss as the child discovers his separateness from his mother and may lead to a basic *mistrust* persisting throughout life.

The infant is more interested in the process rather than the results of his "doing." For example, he derives considerable pleasure from games like peekaboo and pat-a-cake. Much activity occurs simply out of the joy of movement. Infants demonstrate curiosity about their environment and respond readily to new or more complex stimuli.

The infant is egocentric and demanding, requiring close attention of a mother or maternal substitute to meet his needs during his early months of life.

He is unstable physically and emotionally because of his rapid growth pattern, and fluctuations in behavioral patterns should be anticipated.

The developmental tasks of the infant are combined with those of the toddler.

The toddler

The child from 1 to 3 years of age is termed a toddler. Many believe this time to be one of the most delightful periods of childhood because of the "cute" things toddlers do as they strive to be autonomous in a social and physical environment seemingly dominated by adults and other big and tall things—often just out of their reach. The toddler starts out seeing many things from below but soon learns that he can see things from above merely by climbing to a new vantage point. This is but one example of toddler behavior that demonstrates his striving for independence, or *autonomy*—that happy "I can do it" feeling.[13]

The toddler delights in his new-found freedom that comes from his ability to walk and manipulate objects. He is extremely active in exploration of his environment. Naturally he ventures farther from his mother than ever before and discovers that he can do certain things without her but yet must not alienate the individual with whom he has established a trusting relationship. Since he is unsure of his power and control, it seems advisable to maintain and enhance his association with mother. The toddler will exhibit specific behavior designed to please mother, who seems to be protecting and guiding him in his activities as he grows, experiments, and learns. Parents usually find it necessary to set limits that curtail some of the toddler's behavioral urges. He soon incorporates into his learning the concept of a "no-no." Realizing that disapproval of an act may be accompanied by physical discomfort such as having his hands spanked is a step forward in forming his tiny conscience. Finding that autonomy brings with it responsibility in behavior places him in a conflict situation. He wants to be independent, but is it worth the discomfort of being bossed, disciplined, or possibly rejected by those he needs the most? Temper tantrums, obstinate behavior, and negativism are common manifestations of the conflict that accompanies early autonomy.

During the second year of life the neurological maturation of the bowels and bladder makes toilet training possible. At about 18 months of age the toddler becomes aware of sensations related to elimination and finds these somewhat pleasurable. He is likely to discover that soiled and wet diapers are uncomfortable and annoying, especially when he wants to run and play. It also becomes apparent to him that mother finds his soiled diapers equally distasteful and replaces them with clean, dry ones. Since he wants to please her, this discovery is an important motivation toward toilet training. (For a discussion of toilet training see Chapter 18).

The toddler begins to learn the value of language as he deals with his family and his environment. He learns basic words to communicate his needs, such as "milk," "potty," and "drink," and nouns for important people like "Mamma," "Dada," and "me." Evidence of conceptual thinking appears in words like "hot," "cold," "up," "down," "big," "fast," "boy," and "girl." Father as an individual takes on a new importance with the toddler.

The toddler can be quite a charming individual as he acts flirtatious, coy, or cute. Although he enjoys the attention he gets from showing off for others, his interests are basically egocentric. It is extremely important that he master certain tasks during this developmental stage to avoid feelings of *shame and doubt,* which can accompany new encounters. For example, if he does not master autonomy associated with toilet training, or the *anal stage,* he realizes that he is not ready for new experiences and skills. His response may be *withdrawal* from new stimuli, resulting in interferences with socialization and further developmental achievements.

Toddlerhood is a period of exciting changes in behavior, which bridge infancy and the preschool years. Learning how to achieve a judicious balance of autonomy and self-control is the developmental order. This stage is a trying time for parents as well as the child because motor skills outweigh language development and judgment.

DEVELOPMENTAL TASKS OF THE INFANT AND TODDLER

1. Learning to eat solid foods.
2. Learning to walk and use fine muscles.
3. Learning approved habits of elimination.
4. Learning to communicate.[4]

The preschool child

The preschool years, 3 to 6, are truly the carefree years of childhood. There are few limitations physically or socially, and spontaneity is possible and acceptable. Behavior acquires purpose and direction, with increased motor capabilities and coordination. Performance is equally as vivid in the world of fantasy as it is in the world of reality. The preschool child is in the *initiative* stage of development where he tests his ego in a widening social climate (Fig. 2-5).

FIG. 2-5
The preschooler joins his older brothers in a game to test his ego strength in group activity.

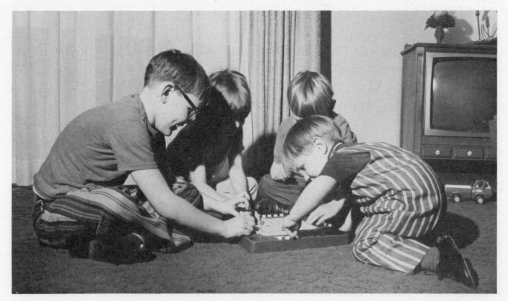

2 Client development across the life span

The psychoanalytical school of thought terms the preschool stage *phallic* because basic sexual conflicts appear during this time. As the child becomes increasingly aware of his body's anatomy, a sexual identity forms of "maleness" or "femaleness." As Freud explained, romantic interest in parents of the opposite sex also occurs. This romantic interest is considered normal, since seemingly all children of this age group form a special attachment to the parent of the opposite sex and feel a concurrent rejection of the parent of the same sex.

Sexual identity is important to the preschooler in his play. Although boys may play with dolls and girls may be cowboys, the child feels an increasing need to be role oriented according to sex at this age.

The preschool child is developing a value system and a working conscience in harmony with the expectations of society. Concepts of right and wrong and good and bad become meaningful determinants of behavior.

DEVELOPMENTAL TASKS

1. Attaining independence in self-care.
2. Learning sexual role identity and modesty.
3. Forming reality concepts.
4. Learning and internalizing concepts of right and wrong.
5. Learning to identify with family members and others.[4]

The environment for success with these tasks must be stable and stimulating and characterized by an atmosphere of acceptance and love. Failure to reinforce the preschooler's initiative with parental attention and affection may seriously interfere with learning and socialization. If exploration and curiosity are curtailed, the child may feel that he is bad and unacceptable, feelings that lead to a sense of *guilt* within the growing personality structure. Furthermore, deprivation of sensual experiences such as hugging, rocking, and swinging may lead to difficulty in expressing affection in later years.

DEVELOPMENTAL HAZARDS

Numerous behavioral manifestations of childhood may indicate that the child is experiencing a developmental problem with which he cannot cope easily. These behaviors are often associated with the type and amount of need gratification throughout the formative years. Some of these disturbances can be attributed to environmental situations such as maternal deprivation or overindulgence or to other factors that interfere with a legitimate quantity of need gratification at any period of development.

Fixations in certain periods can occur, causing the child not to be willing or able to progress beyond a certain point. He may be so satisfied with his own world of self-indulgence that he fails to become socially involved with those around him or so pleased with the attention of being fed and diapered that he shows little interest in learning to feed himself or accomplish bowel and bladder control.

Another basic problem is developmental regression. The child advances to the next stage of development or independence only to fall back into old established patterns again. Children become toilet trained but are incontinent in situations of stress or insecurity. Those who can eat independently refuse to do so, demanding to be fed or even given a bottle. Other examples are the return to baby talk after speech formation has been progressing, resuming body play after becoming pleased with toys, or establishing destructive behavioral patterns after constructive ones have been apparent for some time. Such regressions can be attributed to fatigue, illness, anxiety, or pain. Temporary regressions are normal throughout development, but prolonged regressions may indicate the presence of a serious developmental hazard.

Sibling rivalry

For many reasons, sibling relations can become a source of anxiety in the home. Jealousy among children is not uncommon and, if dealt with wisely, probably does not cause a serious threat to any siblings. One of the more frequent causes of sibling rivalry is the introduction of a new member into the nuclear family. An infant poses a threat to other children, especially the firstborn or only child (Fig. 2-6), and is often the reason for developmental regression. One who has received the primary amount of attention suddenly feels that he is competing for position within the family. Parents should avoid making comparative statements about children in their presence. Such comparisons usually place one of the siblings in a situation in which he feels jealous, and his behavior is met with verbal admonishments, criticisms, or shame from parents. This only reinforces his feelings of unworthiness, rejection, and loss of esteem in the eyes of his parents.

Parents should endeavor to prepare their children for the arrival of a baby through frequent and progressive discussions. The other children should be permitted to share in plans for the new arrival, such as shopping for the furniture and clothes or decorating the room. When the infant is a reality in the home, parents should involve the older child or children in his care when feasible. It is helpful to set aside a specific time each day for the older sibling when he alone is the focus of attention. This tends to reinforce the idea that he is an important member of the family and has not been replaced by the new arrival.

FIG. 2-6
Sibling rivalry often occurs when an infant poses a threat to the firstborn who has previously enjoyed the exclusive attention of his parents.

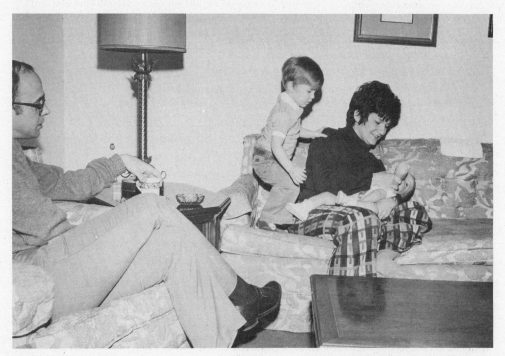

2 Client development across the life span

It is normal for infants to suck thumbs, fingers, pacifiers, blankets, or toys; this is the first act in which he can coordinate his efforts to achieve an act of self-gratification. However, if sucking persists into the preschool years, it requires attention.

Thumb-sucking is usually abandoned spontaneously during toddlerhood when the child finds new sources of pleasure. Attempts by parents to interrupt thumb-sucking earlier are of little avail and usually reinforce the habit rather than halt it. Putting "hot" solutions on the thumb that taste offensive to the child, teasing, shaming, or scolding only appear to frustrate the child further.

Some authorities have contended that thumb-sucking is a response to deprivation of the sucking drive during the oral stage of development. Nipples that allow feeding to be accomplished too quickly and early weaning have been cited as causative factors. On the other hand, many believe that overgratification of the sucking urge, with long hours of practice, leads to yet a stronger need to continue sucking thumbs.

It seems important not to frustrate the drive in infancy when it is especially strong, but weaning should not be delayed. Prolonged thumb-sucking can result in problems of dentition that require special attention.

Parents and nurses should know when thumb-sucking occurs, how long it persists, and in what special circumstances it seems to be especially prevalent. This may provide clues to whether or not it is a symptom of an internalized conflict related to need satisfaction.

Enuresis

Enuresis, or bed-wetting, is usually considered in relation to the child who is 4 or older. It is a symptom, not a disorder. Before this time, most children achieve both daytime and nighttime continence, with only occasional accidents. Enuresis is usually confined to sleep in the older child but may occur during waking hours in a few cases. However, if the child continues in his incontinence beyond this time, consideration must be given to the reason.

Assuming that the child is organically healthy, with a normal urinary tract free of infection, injury, or disease, let us consider some aspects of the problem. Faulty toilet training begun before the child is physiologically capable of continence (15 to 18 months of age), desires to regress to the dependence of infancy, sexual fantasies, and childhood neuroses are among the suspected causes of enuresis.

The first measure to be undertaken in dealing with the incontinent child is a thorough physical examination. If there is no evidence of abnormality of the urinary tract structure, causes of emotional origin should be considered. Tension in the home, sibling rivalry, problems with school or friends, or parents who expect too much of the child are commonly related problems.

Since enuresis is a serious concern for the child and his development, he must be assured that others want to help him with his problems. It is important to assure him that he is physically normal and that he is not an ill child with "weak kidneys" or a "bad bladder." Shaming, bribing, or scolding should be avoided. This only tends to increase his feelings of anxiety, guilt, and fear. Limiting fluids after the evening meal is helpful in some cases. He should be toileted immediately before retiring. If incontinence occurs at about the same time during the night, it may be helpful to awake him just before this time for voiding. Electronic conditioning devices in which an alarm sounds when the bed linens become damp are of questionable value. Keeping dry for the night is a valuable reinforcement for the bed-wetting child, especially if coupled with praise from his parents.

If enuresis is not controlled as the child approaches adolescence, serious emotional conflicts tend to ensue. The child becomes a social isolate laden with fear that an enuretic episode will embarrass him. He may avoid staying with relatives and friends, fear falling asleep away from home, and even become preoccupied with his genitalia. Prolonged bed-wetting should be vigorously pursued in terms of physical or psychogenic causes.

The school-age child

The changes in the life of the child from 6 to 9 or 10 years of age are characterized by three phenomena: (1) movement of the child from the home and into the peer group, (2) introduction to the world of games and work requiring specific skills, and (3) entry into the realm of concepts, logic, and symbolism.

Although the child may have had previous experiences with nursery school or kindergarten, the elementary school program makes new and greater demands for achievement and self-control. The teacher takes a place alongside mother as an authority figure whom he feels obligated to respect, obey, and even love.

The school-age child is characterized by a sense of *industry* necessary to be accepted into group work and to achieve academic success. Rewards and recognition for significant accomplishments are most important in helping the child feel adequate and worthy. If a sense of *inferiority* pervades these years, it will significantly alter his chances for a fulfilled adolescence and adulthood.

As mentioned, Freud called middle childhood a time of *latency,* because of the relative quiescence of sexual impulses at this time. Although this child is curious about certain aspects of sex—especially regarding where babies come from—interests are directed toward peer group activities and relationships.

Parents usually enjoy the school-age child, since he is basically self-reliant and self-controlled. Because acceptance and approval are extremely important to a child of this age, discipline is a lesser problem than it will be during adolescence. A well-developed conscience assists in regulating behavior.

Middle childhood includes the needs for (1) direction, (2) clear understanding of appropriate conduct, (3) help in accepting one's sex role, (4) play space and materials, and (5) education that does not arouse hostility.[4] The parents and the school join forces to meet these needs and to help the child build ego strength.

Physical growth slows during the school-age period, or middle childhood. The body is quiescent, awaiting the onset of adolescence. However, maturation, learning, and practice result in refined motor skills and improved manipulation, timing, and hand-eye coordination. The trunk, head, and extremities more closely approximate adult proportions, although the body may appear weak and clumsy. Hair becomes coarse and less manageable. The nose enlarges, and as dentition becomes complete, the lower portion of the face enlarges. These changes, coupled with the child's disinterest in his appearance, often contribute to a certain unattractiveness.

General health during middle childhood is excellent. Although the child of this age is prone to childhood illnesses such as measles, chickenpox, and mumps, he encounters them with ease and seldom has any adverse or lasting sequelae. Accidents are the major cause of death in this age group.

2 Client development across the life span

SOCIAL CONSIDERATIONS

Middle childhood is a time of increasing one's social horizons at school and in club or neighborhood activities. "The attitudes of co-operation, competition, aggressiveness or agreeableness the child develops are also, in part, a function of learning what one's particular social group values are and copying the kind of behavior revealed by one's models."[4]

Competition in group activities is important in the development of a cooperative spirit with others in reaching a common goal. Self-development occurs within the group as one's power and influence as well as abilities are tested in intragroup relations. Popularity in the school-age period seems to be a result of good looks, health, game skills, academic success, and friendliness.

INTELLECTUAL DEVELOPMENT

Middle childhood is marked by rapid intellectual achievement. Language skills play a significant role in this facet of development, and these seem to be greatly influenced by family cultural experiences as well as innate ability. In general girls and children from high socioeconomic strata exceed boys and those from lower strata in vocabulary and sentence structure abilities.[4] This difference occurs partly because girls spend more time in the home associating with adults and because children from the higher strata are exposed to more stimulating resources in the home and community—books, newspapers, cultural events, and the arts. Intellectual growth seems to be linked closely with social and emotional growth. For example, children who are unusually dependent on their parents make fewer gains in intelligence testing than those who are more independent from their parents.

A series of psychological, intelligence, and achievement tests are used during the school years to identify assets or limitations in learning abilities.

DEVELOPMENTAL TASKS

1. Acquiring game skills.
2. Learning to relate positively with peers.
3. Building a wholesome self-concept.
4. Developing a sense of conscience.
5. Refining skills of communication.[4]

This last task of childhood is extremely important. Reading, writing, and speaking meaningfully and grammatically correctly are essential to academic achievement. Children develop interests in communicating only when they are assured that they have something worthy to say and that others care about them and their experiences. Schools often have highly individualized programs to enhance language skills of pupils. Listening exercises, reading groups, and audiovisual aids are used to arouse interest in communication improvement.

The school-age child acquires knowledge and social attitudes that are useful tools in his everyday life. Refined family life experiences and peer group relationships become important socialization experiences and a testing ground for his developing conscience.

DEVELOPMENTAL HAZARDS

Autism

Autism is a severe behavioral disorder of children characterized primarily by withdrawal from people and an unusual, even affectionate attachment to objects. Although autistic tendencies may be noted as early as the fourth or fifth month of life, they become most pronounced at a later age when language skills and motor abilities revolve around the desire for socialization.

Foundations of clinical practice

The autistic pattern of the preschool child includes a characteristic syndrome of introversion and self-indulgence. He is distinctly uninterested in relating with others, and previously learned language skills are no longer needed because words are used to satisfy internal needs rather than to communicate. The vocabulary may cease to grow, although learning and memory are not impaired. In fact, memory is often amazing. Some autistic children derive considerable pleasure from mechanical recitation of poems, rhymes, and prayers. However, environmental noises (not self-produced) seem to disturb these youngsters, and they often cover their ears to shut out monotonous conversation, music, or other sound stimuli.

Obsessive-compulsive behavior is often noted. There is a desire for sameness about such things as the arrangement of toys in the room and a dining or bedtime ritual. A slight deviation may evoke considerable agitation.

Although the autistic child seldom finds pleasure in activities enjoyed by most children, there are a few things from which he seems to receive real ecstasy. Body rocking, head banging, and spinning himself around and around elicit glee for long periods of time.

The cause of autism in children is unknown, but most authorities do not attribute it to organic brain disease. It is thought to be the result of faulty nurturing. Mothers and fathers of these youngsters are usually highly intelligent and aloof but seem to lack the warmth essential for fostering satisfying human relationships.

When the autistic child is identified, a psychiatric evaluation should be planned. Long-term professional help may avert the high risk of later development of schizophrenia.

Other behavioral problems

Other behavioral disturbances of childhood, if left unchecked, can create serious developmental hazards. Among these are nail-biting, destructiveness, breath holding, teeth grinding, and sleep disorders. The causes and manifestations are highly variable, but they should be coped with in the same manner as thumb-sucking and enuresis. Warm, helpful responses are considerably more fruitful in evoking positive change than punitive measures, which tend to increase anxiety and impulsiveness. Parents and health care workers must understand the cause of the problem before they can effectively participate in correcting it.

Learning disorders

Many biological, sociocultural, and psychological factors affect one's ability to learn. These may include brain damage, sensory and motor disturbances, anxiety, deprivation, poor nutrition, faulty child-rearing practices, substandard economic and housing levels, and low self-concept. It is impossible to discuss all the interrelated variables that affect learning, but some selected ones of childhood are explored here, since they pose a hazard to normal growth and development.

Modern society is achievement oriented, and achievement is virtually impossible without learning. As a child begins the learning process in the home, his motivation is derived chiefly from the monitoring and feedback of parents. If adults do not respond to their role in his learning or if they are unable to cope with it because of their preoccupation with stresses in their own tumultuous world, they will not be much help. Although the child has adequately functioning biological equipment for learning, he depends on human contact for using his innate resources. Poverty and minority status are often associated with slow learning, primarily because of deprivation that affects the attainment of language skills and adaptive behaviors. Since evidence strongly indicates that maternal deprivation and faulty nurturing are occurring more often in *all* socioeconomic classes, these fundamental problems appear to deserve added attention. It is estimated that over one half of all children with learning disorders have as their core problem the lack of adequate monitoring, feedback, and motivation, which must be chiefly derived from the home.

Because physical defects can contribute to learning disorders, it is imperative that all children have thorough health examinations throughout their early years. Defective vision, impaired hearing, malnutrition, neurological problems, and their attendant emotional disturbances account for many barriers to learning. No health maintenance program for school-age children is complete unless it includes assessment of classroom adjustment and learning progress. For example, some left-handed children with right hemispheric language dominance of the brain have a natural tendency to read from right to left, and thus they often reverse word order or read backwards. Early recognition and intervention can be highly advantageous in alleviating some learning handicaps.

Boys and girls reach school age at the same chronological age but not at the same developmental age. A girl's autonomic nervous system reactivity is more stable than a boy's, and her reading skills are usually superior. In addition to these factors, most elementary school teachers are female, and much of the subject matter is feminine. Mathematics is often the only course in the curriculum that boys like, and so other subjects tend to bore boys and create physical restlessness. Their activity needs are also higher than those of girls, and yet the typical educational structure places them in passive learning situations. They may tend to become hyperactive and eventually unorganized in their behavior.

If school achievement does not meet expectations of teachers and parents, the child often becomes an unfortunate victim of misdirected pressures. Children do not like to ask for help, because they fear this may indicate a sign of weakness and dependence. Parents also are reluctant to place their child in specialized learning groups because they view themselves as part of the problem of a slow learner. They see their own status in jeopardy in an achievement-oriented society, and this takes precedence over the special needs of the child. They prefer to add more pressure to their youngster to increase his performance to meet their expectations. When unrealistic goals for achievement are maintained, they are likely to increase the factors of failure for the child. He fears asking for help, taking risks to learn, disappointing parents and teachers, and exposing himself to his peers as ''dumb'' or ''stupid.''

Psychological testing is valuable for preschoolers as well as school-age children. Functional problems such as ambivalence or hostility toward parents and other authority figures, low self-esteem, confusion in sexual role identity, and excessive dependency may be revealed. Most larger educational institutions have incorporated psychological testing programs in their routine evaluation of pupil readiness and progress and as an aid in diagnosis of learning disorders. Intelligence and achievement testing may be done in conjunction with batteries of other tests for sensory-motor skills, language development, visual perception, higher cognitive functions, and auditory perception. A wide range of tests has been designed to evaluate these factors and has been adapted for use with children of many age groups.

Foundations of clinical practice

Nursing implications. Most learning disorders that are not of an organic origin can be well controlled if they are discovered early in the developmental process and are managed by the appropriate specialists. The goal is to match the learning environment with the child's needs and potential.

Nurses often are in contact with total families and thus are able to assess more completely all variables that might relate to learning. As the child is seen periodically for evaluation of physical growth, health supervision, or intervention, specific steps should be taken to assess emotional responses and evidence of learning. If problems are perceived, they should be discussed with the physician who in turn must deal openly and frankly with parents in this regard. If special evaluation is deemed necessary, referrals may be made for the child and his parents. It is not uncommon for nurses to act as a liaison among teachers, family, and various helping agents.

Since emotional problems almost always exist concurrently with learning disabilities, environmental and social manipulation should assure the child a secure, relaxed, and happy experience in which learning is not the sole reason for his being and his acceptance. Parents and teachers should understand what things are important to the child, and time should be set aside for them at regular intervals. Childhood should not be marred by making achievement the core of all life experiences.

The majority of learning disorders among children can be, at least in part, alleviated or compensated for with early recognition, high-quality intervention,

FIG. 2-7
Nurses as well as teachers should be cognizant of behavior that indicates lack of involvement in learning experiences.

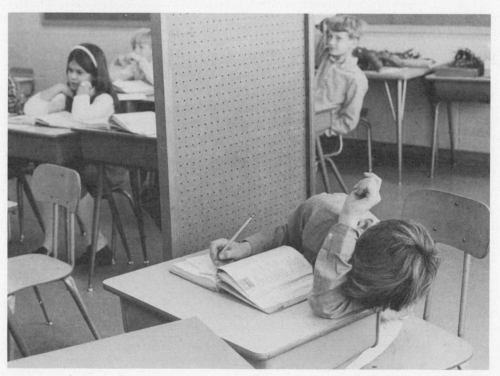

and instruction. Nurses assume a key role in these events if they are truly client and family centered in their profession (Fig. 2-7).

PSYCHOSEXUAL DISTURBANCES

The school-age child has a natural curiosity about sex. Fears and fantasies are common. A lack of sexual information will reinforce fears and may lead to negative or rigid sexual values. Since information gained from peers may be misleading, parents should assume the initiative to provide answers to the child's questions or concerns. The school-age child who relates openly with parents about sexual matters will be more likely to gain a healthy sexual identity.

The preadolescent

The period of preadolescence, which encompasses the ages of 9 or 10 through 13, is one that has seemingly been forgotten in many considerations of growth and development. Few people have shown special interest in this age range, but more preadolescents than any other age group are referred to child guidance clinics. Although many who work with children find babies a joy to care for or adolescents a significant challenge, the preadolescent does not seem to possess similar appeal. Let us examine why children of this age are a truly unique group with characteristics and special needs that require consideration.

Preadolescence is not a stage when growth and development are static, but a time when linear growth is somewhat dormant, awaiting the adolescent "growth spurt," and refinement of behavior is limited. It is evident that change, rather than improvement, is taking place.

Theorists believe that the well-structured pattern of childhood behavior must be disintegrated before adolescence and an entirely new adult structure formed. During this upheaval in casting off childhood ways, some long-repressed behaviors of earlier years surface again before their final disappearance. This accounts for the irritating habits of the preadolescent, such as physical restlessness, nail-biting, baby talk, and obstinate behavior toward siblings and parents. They seem to lose their sense of shame or guilt and delight in telling gory stories or dirty jokes, belching loudly merely for a laugh from peer group members, or openly criticizing their parents in front of the rest of the family and others. At the point when parents and teachers think their children have learned some proper social conduct and know how to use it, they act ostentatiously at every opportunity and enjoy it. Manners, courtesy, and self-control are reserved for special occasions.

"Perhaps the outstanding development of the preadolescent is his interaction with the peer group, where he learns much about himself, other people, and ideas of conduct and human relationship."[4] Child society forms with some of the same fundamental codes as adult society. Friends are carefully selected for their help in presenting a united front against the adult world, as an extension and reinforcement of the child's own nebulous identity, or because of common skills and interests. Gang behavior is a collective force to strike back at the adult society and what it represents to the child. Thus the negative behavior toward their own parents is probably only a manifestation of negativism toward adult society as a whole rather than a particular loss of respect for the parents or their role. Temporarily, the loyalty to the peer group supercedes even loyalty to parents. Leadership in the peer group is more important than any other guidance, even if it is poorly directed toward experimentation with alcohol, drugs, tobacco, or delinquency. Gang codes evolve in varying degrees, and these take precedence over everything. They may range from a group pact to not make good grades on a certain test at school to agreeing to lie to protect a member who has stolen someone else's wallet. In nearly every case the gang code is characterized by collective action against adults and their system.

When children have been thoroughly indoctrinated in their early years to conform to adult codes and expectations, the shift to peer codes is not without considerable anxiety. Preadolescents still love and respect their parents but cannot take the chance of being cast out by peers as a coward, "chicken" or "sissy." The conflict is so great for some members of this age group that it creates emotional problems of a serious nature. Whether they choose to cling to parental expectations or shift to the gang's patterns, they will be, in effect, rejecting an important aspect of their developmental life.

Girls usually are ahead in their physical development at these ages, but soon the boys catch up and exceed them in both height and weight. Being ahead or behind the peer group in development seems to be a source of embarrassment and uneasiness in either sex group. Modesty is mixed with curiosity. They want to know if their bodies are changing like those of the others in their age group but tend to not want anyone, even their parents, to watch them dress or bathe.

Personality development of the preadolescent is aimed toward ego strength and integration. Concern is primarily centered on his role in the peer group, but some recognition of his place in the larger society is apparent. Boy-girl interests develop, with girls usually assuming the aggressor role. They love attention, and to gain it, they are boisterous, noisy, rowdy, and show-offs. In the presence of parents and teachers the preadolescent may display good humor, self-control, and tolerance. The superego seems well established, and he can be a good companion to adults as well as peers if he chooses. It is through interaction of the peer group, however, that he learns most about himself, others, and the mechanisms of human relationships.

Nurses as well as parents must be aware of the typical behavior of preadolescents and understand ways to cope with the attendant problems. Adults must be prepared for their hyperactive nature, pranks, and smart-aleck remarks. Adults should not fight what they see or hear, but strive to interpret what these preadolescents are really feeling. Perhaps they are expressing disgust with adults and their attitudes or displeasure at leaving the carefree days of childhood behind in change for responsibility. They, like toddlers, look for discipline as an aid in checking out their superego, and their actions may be a cry for outside intervention when they feel loss of their own inner control. Their experiments in living in a new code system should not be squelched; adults should plan for their children's freedom to test new ideas and get feedback. When discipline must be used, adults need to be creative. Nurses and parents should not revert to childish methods of rewards, punishment, or threats but should be constantly on the lookout for pathological behavior that seems inappropriate or out of line with expected preadolescent phenomena. A major personality reorganization is going on, and severe problems requiring special attention may present themselves at this time.

DEVELOPMENTAL TASKS

1. Breaking free from primary identification with adults.
2. Forming relationships with peers.

3. Clarifying the world of adulthood.
4. Developing morality.
5. Identifying with one's psychosocial-biological sex role.
6. Attaining new motor patterns.
7. Learning ways of studying and mastering the physical world.
8. Refining symbol systems and conceptual abilities.
9. Relating to the cosmos.[4]

Achievement of the developmental tasks is in a large part dependent on peer group relationships, especially with those of the same sex. Discipline and household rules must be relaxed so that the child has an opportunity to make decisions without fear of repression, but parental guidance should be evident if he expresses a need for support. Freedom to explore, experiment, and make mistakes is necessary for learning, and opportunities within the family and community should be provided so that the preadolescent can ask his own questions and seek his own answers.

PSYCHOSEXUAL DISTURBANCES

The preadolescent is faced with new concerns about sexual identity, physiological sexual responses, and body image. Parents who provide little or no information about such matters or who set rigid limits about sexual behavior may thwart the child's development of self-confidence. On the other hand, setting no limits may contribute to a delay in the child's development of an internal sexual value system. Parents who overreact to a preadolescent's sexual experiences may find that their child is not gaining a feeling of wholesomeness about sexual matters, including body image and physiological functioning. An ongoing, open dialogue between the adult and the child is vital for psychosexual development at this phase of rapid physical and social changes.

The adolescent

SOCIOCULTURAL IMPLICATIONS

Adolescence is a conceptual age period extending from puberty to early adulthood and considered to envelop the teenage years. It is primarily a phenomenon of the Western world in the twentieth century. Although physical changes are significant factors in this period, the cultural milieu seems to play a larger part in the role of adolescence. In some societies at puberty the child automatically becomes an adult, with the attendant privileges and responsibilities. However, in the United States we have forced our teenagers into a long period of economic, social, and intellectual dependence. Modern conveniences have limited the role of the adolescent as a helper in the home, and our educational system requires their spending many years in formal education programs.

Our general standard of living, especially our nutrition, has accelerated physical maturity. Bodies become ready for adult roles before minds and emotions are ready. Sexual maturity is occurring earlier, but marriage must be put off until education is complete. The many years of waiting for sexual fulfillment are responsible for a lot of conflict in the adolescent. Despite our seeming relaxation in socialization processes and value systems, it is still looked on with favor—particularly where girls are concerned—to reserve intimate sexual experiences, especially intercourse, for adult marriage. Consequences of such intimacies outside a conjugal relationship include social repercussions related to morality, venereal disease, and unwanted pregnancies. Even if couples choose to marry in their teens, they are seldom prepared to be financially solvent, and considerable strain is placed on the personal relationship. Meaningful social experiences must be provided to indirectly satiate sexual desires.

The typical adolescent enjoys the acquiring and spending of money, but there is a minimum amount of suitable employment for the teenager. Business and industry prefer hiring persons with their high school educations complete. If a teenager drops out of school, his chances of finding suitable employment are quite limited, with the result that many adolescents drift aimlessly while waiting for a job. Much delinquency can be attributed to the frustrated teenager who is unemployed and seeking some form of stimulation or a way to obtain money to purchase the necessities of the age—cars, gasoline, clothes, and entertainment.

The culture of adolescence is unique and has been created in order that teenagers may achieve an identity apart from that of the child and adult worlds. Their clothes, habits, behavior, and language are best understood in terms of their obstinacy. Adults claim that they do not understand the adolescent and his world and have difficulty in communicating with him. This gap is sometimes referred to as the *generation gap*. Parents of today faced different experiences in their teens than their children do in today's complex world. A thorough study of the forces that have created the American adolescent is useful in gaining an appreciation of the teenager.

Women have traditionally been more influential in shaping lives of young people because of their roles as teachers and mothers. They have primarily controlled the home during the time when father is away for employment and recreational purposes. Schoolteachers are predominantly women, especially in elementary school. It has become apparent that male adult role models in the home and school are lacking.

Teenagers are confronted with two worlds—idealism and realism. Their intellectual sophistication makes them painfully aware of the incongruence in our society. Many become activists for selected causes related especially to social justice. Much of their dismay stems from the awareness that the adults who control them are responsible, at least in part, for the ills of the society. Their reactions include an admixture of frustration, hostility, resentment, and despair. They realize that all too quickly they will be part of this adulthood, which has made their life rich with material experiences but is at the same time very anxiety provoking.

PHYSICAL GROWTH   Adolescence is characterized by marked physical growth. For several years certain organs have been rather dormant and undergoing slow maturation, which enables the dramatic physiological phenomena of adolescence to occur.

There are great increases in height and weight of both sexes. Girls, on the average, are about 2 years ahead of boys in their physical development, experiencing the greatest spurt just before menarche. The most dramatic growth occurs early in the accelerated period, and some teenagers may gain as much as 25 pounds in weight and grow several inches taller within a 3- or 4-month period.

"The activity of the pituitary gland, which is primarily responsible for growth is inhibited by the hormones from the gonads and growth rates of bodily mass are sharply decelerated."[4] This phenomenon is Nature's way of controlling the growth rate but ensuring that satisfactory secondary sexual characteristics are present before the growth spurt is interrupted.

Ovarian and testicular hormones are active in the promotion of secondary sex characteristics. The amount and timing of the appearance of the sex hormones seem to significantly influence body build and explain the wide variations of physique evident in teenagers.

Since adolescence is one of the healthiest times of life, accidents are the leading cause of disability and death. Acts of violence, suicide, drug abuse, and automobile accidents are frequently associated with the death of an adolescent.

SOCIAL AND EMOTIONAL DEVELOPMENT

Adolescence is a period of social importance and emotional lability. The life outside the home becomes more important for socialization than the nuclear family. Intense scholastic demands, peer group competition, and sexual conquests make it a period of emotional strain and uncertainty at times.

High school is a time of extreme impact in a young person's life. The relative success in "finding a place" (identity) or failure (diffusion) may have an enduring influence on the remainder of life's experiences.

The freshmen are most variable in size, maturity, and disposition. Girls generally appear more grown up and sophisticated than their male counterparts. By the sophomore year, boys have nearly caught up with girls, but in the meantime girls often have become interested in "older guys," who drive cars and date. Many differences have been resolved by the junior year, and there is considerable tolerance and friendliness among the class. When boys receive their coveted driver's license, they become interested in dating but frequently must ask younger girls because their classmates are dating those older guys. During the senior year the girls often do an abrupt about-face and discover that those "immature" boys that they have been sitting next to in class for 3 years are not so bad after all. However, many are already established in their dating patterns with the sophomore and junior girls and show little interest in their peers.[13]

Parental guidance is extremely useful during adolescence but must be subtle to be appreciated. The id seems to pose a constant threat to the teenager, and it takes much support from within and without to cope with the many urges, both physical and psychological. The superego becomes weaker because there is a lessening of dependency on parents, its original source. The adolescent can make decisions about his own system of values and at times appears to reject everything of which his parents approve. Ultimately, however, he is likely to return to the parental value system.

The school, clubs, parties, teenage music, television, and the telephone dominate the adolescent's life. Often parents and siblings believe that they simply cannot bear another day of the hectic pace. Friends are constantly coming, going, or calling, and often it seems that the whole family adjusts its schedule to meet the needs of teenagers in the home.

The many relationships during the teenage years, however, do not lack purpose. They serve to acquaint the adolescent with social standards within both sexes and prepare him for close relationships of adulthood, including marriage.

DEVELOPMENTAL TASKS

1. Refining peer relationships.
2. Responding to an appropriate sexual role.
3. Accepting one's physique and effectively using the body.

4. Attaining emotional independence.

5. Achieving a sense of economic independence.[4]

The goal of adolescence is the attainment of an *identity* that permits the pursuit of educational and occupational goals and a satisfying marital relationship.

DEVELOPMENTAL HAZARDS

The role of the contemporary adolescent is indeed complex. He is expected to be both a child and adult, with considerable flexibility. The conflicts of the teenage years can lead to consequences that may be viewed as developmental hazards.

Academic failure

In today's world, education is viewed as a necessity that prepares youth for responsible citizenship and creates a nation of informed persons who can serve as leaders and forces of power in a modern society. Therefore, any young man or woman who is not successful in meeting the demands of our educational institutions and who drops out of school at the first opportunity is considered to be launching into adulthood with a serious handicap. It is difficult for the school dropout to obtain employment that is challenging and within his scope of interest and that affords him sufficient earnings to live independently.

The school dropout is a problem in development for several reasons that deserve consideration.

Reasons for teenagers dropping out of school are variable and include financial crisis, health, marriage, inability to make friends or to engage in meaningful activity, pregnancy, and low academic achievement. Family attitudes about education are often cited as at least a contributory cause.

Without a high school diploma it is impossible to get into most colleges or even some vocational schools. Employment opportunities are limited, and financial problems are likely. Perhaps more important are the alterations in the quantity and quality of peer groups relationships, so important to the adolescent. Organized activity such as sports, clubs, and parties may be limited to students, and thus he becomes excluded from his previous sources of relationships and must form few friends. Often these new friends are older, unemployed, and experiencing a similar feeling of being shut out of both school and the adult world. Alcoholism, drug abuse, smoking, illicit sexual relationships, and various forms of delinquency provide amusement, pleasure, and socialization.

Not all persons who leave school become liabilities of society. Some are fortunate in finding meaningful employment that provides adequate social and mental stimulation as well as financial reward. It seems, however, that opportunities for the person who has not completed high school are indeed limited. In addition to coping with the typical developmental adjustments of adolescence, he is facing a number of additional odds imposed by our contemporary society.

Drugs, alcohol, and delinquency

The hazards of adolescence are tragically interrelated. Losing interest in school, facing the stress of unemployment, the boredom of a dull life, and a hunger for companionship and excitement are the forerunners of delinquent acts.

Delinquency takes on many forms, including stealing, vandalism, destructiveness, sexual preoccupation, and risk taking, particularly in speeding automobiles. One of our current problems of grave concern is drug abuse, especially among adolescents and young adults.

Drug *abuse* is the persistent self-administration of a drug without regard to its medical purpose. Drug *dependence* is the continued desire to take the drug to experience its effects or avoid the discomfort associated with not taking it. Drug taking leads to a physiological tolerance, a psychic craving, and in some

42

cases a physical dependence. Although almost any drug can be abused or misused, several have received rather widespread attention: tobacco, alcohol, LSD, marijuana, amphetamines, heroin, and barbiturates.

Teenagers use drugs for the same reasons adults do—to produce certain feelings and moods, to dull or enhance perception, to promote relaxation or the feeling of wellness, and to create an aura of safety and comfort, particularly in social settings.

The teenage years are filled with admixtures of joys, fears, disappointments, frustrations, conflict, anxieties, group pressures, restlessness, and omnipotence. Many persons with a healthy childhood and stable home and family life can resist the temptation of experimentation with drugs. Others, however, are eager to "try something different." Two or three decades ago it was a daring feat to smoke a cigarette or drink a beer with friends before being legally old enough to indulge in such activities. In one way, today's teenagers are the same except that their field of options is considerably more sophisticated. Parent models not only smoke and drink, but they also take drugs to avoid any conceived discomfort. There is almost a belief that life should be chemically controlled, if necessary, to assure a constant state of pleasurable feelings. These and many other arguments or reasons are offered to explain the acceleration of drug abuse in our society, particularly among our youth.

Not many years ago drug abuse was generally confined to the urban areas where derelicts, street gangs, and characters from the underworld mingled for evil purposes. Little concern was widespread then, except perhaps among law enforcement officers. However, there is now considerable interest regarding drug abuse because it reaches into all segments of society and is becoming a compound problem. Law enforcement, dangers to the health and safety of our youth, economics of the habits, and interferences with school and family life are real considerations with far-reaching effects.

Suicide and homicide

Suicide ranks second (after motor vehicle accidents) as the leading cause of death among white teenagers, and homicide leads the list among black teenagers. Suicide among blacks is considerably less likely than among whites of the same age group. Although these topics are usually studied in detail as a part of mental health nursing, they are worthy to note as developmental hazards of young adults.

Emotions and the ability to cope with stress are quite variable in teenagers. The societal pressures are simply too great for some, and they either destroy themselves or others as one way of solving their problems.

The nurse should be cognizant of the risks of suicide and homicide in this developmental period and be alert to signs or symptoms that denote a need for an intervening, helping relationship. Often a verbalized threat or an attempted suicide or homicide precedes the actual event, and such cues should be interpreted as a cry for help from a client with serious problems.

The young adult

SOCIOCULTURAL
IMPLICATIONS

Young adulthood is the first phase of maturity and is characterized by psychosocial phenomena, not by biological growth or changes. This period extends from adolescence to the mid or late thirties and is primarily devoted to the tasks of developing *identity* and achieving *intimacy*. Young adulthood, like adoles-

Foundations of clinical practice

cence, is unique to a society and culture that is relatively sophisticated. In countries where there is poverty, few educational opportunities, and general deprivation, children tend to move abruptly from puberty to full adult roles and responsibilities.

The youthful members of our population—that is, young adults—are biologically mature, and as a rule are in optimal physical and mental condition. However, from this phase on through adulthood, the processes of aging compound. It is clearly apparent why individuals who comprise this age group are in an enviable position.

SOCIAL AND EMOTIONAL DEVELOPMENT

The young adult is obliged to establish his identity, both within himself and in relation to various social roles. "Who am I? How do I fit into my family? My employment? My environment? My community?" These crucial questions must be answered at the same time the individual is searching for intimacy or for a special kind of close relationship with a significant other that is truly satisfactory. Many new acquaintances are encountered within college, employment, and social situations. Each must be experienced and evaluated in an attempt to select those friends who have similar interests, value systems, and needs for contact. Relationships are pursued for mutual satisfaction as well as for ego fulfillment. Human sensitivity and awareness of others tend to heighten, and the ability to commit onself to a long-term bond becomes evident. Engagements, marriage, or a variety of informal arrangements permit more intense development of interpersonal relationships. The larger peer groups of high school days are abandoned for a few close friendships with individuals or couples. Intimate social contacts become very important, and considerable emotional involvement must be expended in their pursuit. Although young adulthood is the traditional time for marriage, it should be noted that there is much variation in readiness of both men and women to enter into a conjugal relationship on a long-term basis. "Kinsey and his associates report that males reach the peak of sexual responsiveness at about nineteen years and that sexual responses then begin a slow but steady decline which continues into old age. Women, however, do not reach the maximum of sexual responsiveness until the middle twenties or even thirties."[4] These observations, coupled with other psychological and social variables, are surely *influential* in the high percentage of failures within the marriages of younger adults.

There is currently a trend for intimate living on an informal basis to test a relationship before entering a legal bond. With more freedom in sexual expression made possible, at least in part, and with widespread use of contraception and legal abortion facilitation, these arrangements are relatively free of the former hazards of unwanted pregnancy and childbearing. It must be noted, however, that acceptance of these informal patterns of intimate living is limited and is strongly influenced by moral and social standards of various communities and societal classes.

Young adulthood is a period where interests such as clubs, work, recreation, and the arts become delimited and more intense. The trend is to abandon superficial or fleeting ideas and devote efforts to fewer but more select endeavors where self-enrichment, not reward, may be attainable. As involvement increases, interests deepen, and ultimately a growing sense of competence evolves, which, of course, contributes to the individual's identity.

2 Client development across the life span

The young adult is particularly concerned about human issues, such as war, peace, poverty, racism, and freedom. Achieving identity means, in part, to synthesize a personal set of values. Since in-depth involvement with others and a desire to communicate openly and intensely are keen at this time, a genuine concern for others is understandable. This is enhanced by caring enough to be involved in action directed toward solution of problems. Young adults seem to assume the burden of society's responsibility for the poor, the handicapped, the oppressed, and the ill. Many volunteer groups are largely staffed by dedicated youth who conscientiously devote much time and energy to human aid programs.

In the late 1960s young adults courageously expressed their convictions through activist movements such as peace marches, antiwar demonstrations, draft-card burning, and campus protests. Many older adults viewed these endeavors as part of a "radical youth" threat to the integrity of society rather than as a concerned and spirited group fighting for a cause. Consequently, some of our older adults have rejected the youth, and failure to engage in joint efforts to achieve mutual understanding has in effect produced alienation and even warring factions at times. For some young adults, it seems important to establish an identity apart from the traditional institutions of society, and this means that either new institutions must be founded or reforms made in the existent ones. This phenomenon may largely account for the "youth versus the establishment" game, which seems to erupt and cause considerable turmoil from time to time within families and communities.

Although the youngest adult (18 to 21) may be physically and socially mature, he is often denied adultlike privileges because of local or state laws, such as buying alcoholic beverages or going to a nightclub. This becomes an awkward circumstance if his social contacts are a year or 2 older. Obtaining a marriage license and car ownership are other situations that may be influenced or curtailed by legislation in some areas. This may be a source of rebellion among youth, since they are expected to be old enough to behave responsibly as adults.

Good grooming, a pleasing personality, the right friends, and special talent serve as a first line of offense in the social arena. Initial impressions are extremely important to young adults.

Lower-class or deprived youths are more likely to enter into early gainful employment or marriage than middle-class youths. They often do not have economic or human support from their nuclear family and thus launch out earlier in hopes of finding security in a new life. On the other hand, those who are fortunate to have a supportive family may take a longer time to prepare for a vocation or select a marriage partner. They do not feel a need to escape.

Social activities of the young adult are interesting, varied, and essentially carefree. Many describe this period as the "best days of life," because a youth can choose to behave as a child or an adult—whichever best fits his mood at the moment.

INTELLECTUAL DEVELOPMENT

Since many youths are still active students, academic pursuits are an important facet of their lives. These pursuits are a means to upward mobility within the adult world, especially economically. Achievement in school is a significant factor in getting the right position or the proper recognition necessary to break the barrier into certain occupational circles.

Foundations of clinical practice

FIG. 2-8
Adult volunteers find satisfaction in performing civic and social responsibilities. (Photo by Florine Rogers, Indianapolis Area Chapter, American Red Cross.)

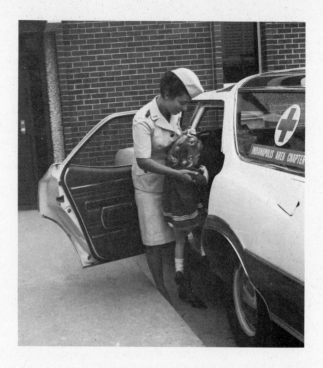

Contrary to many opinions, intellectual ability continues to increase during youth, provided that there is sufficient mental stimulation. Many find themselves a better student because there is a decrease in some of the pressures of high school and home, evident in adolescence. Interests broaden into community and world affairs during this period, further preparing them for the full adult role in society.

DEVELOPMENTAL TASKS

1. Selecting and preparing for a vocation.
2. Preparing for marriage.
3. Developing a civic consciousness.
4. Appreciating socially responsible behavior.
5. Refining a value system.[4]

The exact age at which these tasks are pursued depends on the prevailing ethnocultural phenomena, socioeconomic factors, and individual aspirations (Fig. 2-8).

The middle-aged adult

The fourth to the sixth decade of life is considered to be middle age. It seems to be a point in which individuals begin to focus on what time is left for their living as opposed to what has occurred thus far in their lives. The concept of the "middle years" must be viewed in terms of the quality of earlier experiences as a child, adolescent, and young adult. Essentially, the process of role changes, both in the family and on the job, and decreasing physical vitality seems to dominate this period. Stresses related to "fitting into society" and parenting are reduced. For the first time in several years (even 2 or 3 decades) there is opportunity to deal with self-interests rather than the interests of others. Middle-aged adults may expend considerable time in examining exactly where they are in life and reviewing future plans for maximizing the time left in their span.

Adulthood is a period of *productivity*. Physical, social, emotional, and intellectual growth is essentially mature but profits from proper and consistent stimulation. The body requires a well-balanced diet, sufficient rest, and exercise to maintain itself in optimal condition. Health problems appear with increasing frequency during adult years because of organic disease and stress of many kinds. Cancer, heart disease, and degenerative illnesses are prominent causes of hospitalization and disability. Accidents decline and are infrequently the cause of death.

The years of adulthood have an appealing stability but little freedom before retirement. The primary achievements that one expects to make in one's lifetime are usually accomplished in the adult decades of the thirties, forties, and fifties. The mainstream of society is seemingly held together by the large group of responsible adults going about their daily business of producing goods and engaging in civic, church, club, and other activities. Failure to spend these years as a contributing member of society engaged in generative endeavors causes stagnation and creates a negative state of *self-absorption* rather than self-realization.

There are more middle-aged persons than ever before, and this adult group seems likely to enlarge in subsequent years, since people are living longer.

During these adult years comes the struggle to bridge the generation gap between the young and old and to lend a stable influence to life in our society. For many it is the first time that they can "be themselves" and reveal to others what is truly important in their lives. Their quest for acquiring material goods and status is gradually replaced by enjoying what is already possessed and accepting their role in the community. The middle years are more suited to refining interests rather than pursuing new ones. For some persons, however, this may be an opportune time for exploration of new horizons that had been forsaken earlier in life because of demands of the family or financial and time limitations. Sports, crafts, reading, and political activities are examples of such endeavors.

SOCIAL AND EMOTIONAL DEVELOPMENT

The acceptance of aging tends to come more readily for the nonprofessional, blue-collar members of our society.[1] They start to work early in life, and their self-measure of achievement is primarily job stability, income increments, and good working conditions. There is prevalence of the "work ethic" and a sense of societal responsibility of becoming a mature, contributing citizen.

Highly educated professionals are more reluctant to give up youth and cling tenaciously to a social life and physical attractiveness that they hope will defy the obvious event of becoming old. The professional tends to enjoy less leisure time than the blue-collar worker in today's society. This, of course, has been a recent shift in trends. In order to excel, most professionals must put in long hours beyond the regular 40-hour workweek that is characteristic of business and industry. They must entertain clients, read conscientiously to keep up in their area of interest, and participate in activities and organizations as expected by their peer groups. Success to professionals usually means to distinguish themselves from the mass.

It has been noted that middle-aged adults do not want to be young again—

Foundations of clinical practice

they just want to feel that way. Feeling young is a state of mind as well as a biological phenomenon. It largely comes from viability in roles at home, at work, and in the community. In the middle years, parenting roles are declining as the children become grown and independent. Young aggressive and talented adults are assuming significant roles in the work force, often at the expense of older adults. Organizational, political, and civic leadership positions are taken over by younger individuals with physical and mental energies that surpass those of the more mature adults. The role changes continually remind middle-aged persons that they are growing old and that things are not what they used to be. This potential crisis can be averted, at least in part, by the mature adult's finding new avenues for personal enjoyment and formulating some futuristic goals.

The middle-aged adult who has been a parent must deal with children leaving home and becoming independent. Many become grandparents, too. For women, this time may present the opportunity to pursue a vocation or interest that was set aside while children were growing. Some mothers go back to a career that was interrupted by parenthood. It has been said that this is the era, not of the working mother, but of the working grandmother. Contrary to popular opinion, mothers (and perhaps fathers, too) are glad to have their children grown and independent. The "empty nest" depression is a projection of others, according to recent research, and does not represent the majority of parents' feelings at this time of life.[1]

When children leave home, parents are again faced with relating to each other on a primary basis. Couples must concentrate on their personal relationship more now than at any other point in their marriage. Fortunately, the declining responsibility for children makes this possible. Sexual behavior also receives renewed attention. With the approaching reality of menopause and the male climacteric, sexual functioning may become a real issue. Marriages of 2, 3, or 4 decades often become threatened at this time by a member who feels that extramarital affairs are a way to attest to virility or personal attractiveness and appeal. The divorce rate among couples in the middle years is high, for there is no longer a need to stay together just for "the sake of the children."

The middle years are also a time when attention must be given to parents who are aged and perhaps in declining health. It is often during these years that these parents die, and the increasing awareness of death confronts the middle-aged individual, who himself is aging and facing decreasing physical vigor or chronic health problems. Some adults must care for their aged parents in their own homes or at least assume a major responsibility for their welfare. This kind of burden often strains a marital relationship that may already be facing a crisis because of role changes.

BIOLOGICAL IMPLICATIONS

Adulthood initiates the process of true decline in mental and physical vigor. Chronic illnesses become problematic, and there are day-to-day aggravations of failing vision and hearing, insomnia, stiff joints and muscles, backache, and menopause. Physical attractiveness becomes secondary to maintenance of health despite the appearance of gray hair, wrinkles, and the "middle-age spread." There are naturally occurring losses of vital organ functioning throughout adult life. Cardiovascular, renal, and nervous systems gradually lose their efficiency. Gastrointestinal motility is reduced, and the basal metabolic rate falls. Muscles and bones undergo degenerative changes so that activity potential declines. The period of deep sleep becomes abbreviated, and sexual activity may decrease. These alterations in physiology induce many important changes in life-style and habits of daily living.

OPPORTUNITIES FOR HEALTH COUNSELING

Nurses must be alert to opportunities for health counseling in relation to the middle-aged adult. With reductions in physical vigor and physiological functioning that occur with aging come the problems of balancing dietary intake with a revised activity level in order to prevent obesity. It is not easy to establish new patterns of food intake during a time when stresses of role changes may stimulate "nervous" eating or when a fine meal in an excellent restaurant may induce compensatory feelings of success and esteem. Mature adults tend to maintain eating habits acquired earlier in life. Desserts, alcoholic beverages, snacks in front of the television, and large meals may need to be abandoned and replaced with a dietary plan that ensures adequate nutrition but that guards against high cholesterol and high caloric intake. Certain chronic illnesses such as heart disease, diabetes, or gastrointestinal problems may also enter the picture and influence diet. Food is an important source of satisfaction and enjoyment for persons of all ages, and when its consumption becomes limited for any reason, there is a feeling of discontent and deprivation. Nurses must be prepared to offer guidance in dietary control, specifically addressing the special physical and psychological needs of the middle-aged adult.

Activity needs of the adult also deserve special attention during the middle years to maintain optimal physiological functioning and a sense of well-being. Sedentary persons must be especially counseled regarding ways to engage in healthful exercise appropriate for their unique needs. As circulatory impairment has its gradual onset during this time of life, specific tips should be given for activity that enhances circulation and stimulates normal physiological mechanisms related to the cardiovascular system. Muscles and joints require regular exercise to prevent loss of function and to minimize stiffness and weakness attendant to the aging process. Middle-aged adults need an exercise regimen that is planned for their special needs and that takes into account their health problems or limitations. Obviously, they must be advised that physical fitness programs should be adopted and implemented only after a thorough medical evaluation has been completed.

Alcohol, drug, and tobacco consumption is common among adults. With stresses of these years often comes an increase in their use. Some individuals even develop abuse problems that require specific management. Since excessive smoking has a general deleterious effect on the respiratory and cardiovascular systems, clients should be encouraged to reduce or eliminate the habit. Alcoholism and drug abuse often manifest themselves during the middle years. Tension, worry, depression, and insomnia are characteristically experienced by individuals during these years, and it is easily understood why solutions may be sought through drugs or alcohol. Nurses must be alert to signs of stress and behavior that seem to indicate failure to cope in a healthy manner. They should be prepared to provide counseling, guidance, and referral to appropriate resources if indicated.

With the recent trend toward health maintenance, many individuals take advantage of a routine physical examination and community programs of disease detection, prevention, and treatment. The middle-aged adult should be instructed about particular disease risks for his sex, age, life-style, or predisposition. It is possible to identify risk factors and take precautionary measures to reduce risks by prescriptive adaptations in life-style and health habits.

THE SINGLE ADULT IN THE MIDDLE YEARS

A review of the developmental tasks of the middle-aged adult relates primarily to roles and responsibilities pertinent to marriage and parenthood. Obviously, not all persons in the middle years have a spouse or children who influence their role changes at this time. However, some problems that pertain to the single adult are worthy to note.

According to the U.S. Bureau of Census figures in 1972, approximately one out of five men and women from the ages of 40 to 64 are single.[7] This group does not represent divorced or widowed individuals. It seems that the trend is for this rate to increase, because more people elect not to get married. Many of these single persons (in excess of 40%) live alone, and the majority live in urban areas.[7] The singles can be divided into subgroups: those who are actively seeking a spouse and those who are simply single by choice and plan not to marry. Contrary to stereotypes, most unmarried persons are not carefree. They have many of the same problems as those who are married and more besides.

Many of our social institutions are primarily designed to advantageously accommodate the married couple. For example, airlines have special fares for spouses, there is some tax savings available for joint returns of husbands and wives, and until recently some of the practices of the financial community discriminated against the single individual. Even hospitals restrict visiting in some cases to only the husband or wife of the client. It should be noted, however, that being single does not imply social isolation or starvation from intimacy. Evidence points to the fact that most single persons have close family ties or significant others who are extremely influential in their lives. Nurses should be especially alert to this and should not shut out or impede involvement of any of these persons who might be as emotionally important to the client as a spouse might be.

Single persons have more health problems and tend to succumb to mental illness and suicide more often than their married counterparts.[7] It is unclear why this is the case, but nurses should be aware of this special vulnerability.

In the middle years when problems of aging parents become an emotional and sometimes even a financial drain to the family, it is often the single person who is expected to assume responsibilities for their care and welfare. Reasons for this include the speculation that they have more time, more money, and more energy to assume this role, since they do not have the marriage and child care obligations that other siblings have. This can be a serious problem for single individuals to deal with because they are essentially self-supporting and by necessity assume responsibility for their long-term solvency and living standards. It is a stark reality for many that they will have no children or may have no brothers, sisters, or other relatives to come to their rescue in their own declining years. Nurses should be cognizant of such family dynamics and guard against channeling responsibilities of any type to the single child just because it may seem most expedient or desirable as viewed by other siblings in the family.

The unmarried adult group in our society is growing, and until they are freed of stereotypes so long associated with the unmarried and are afforded equality commonplace to the married adult, nurses must be especially sensitive to their unique needs and characteristics.

DEVELOPMENTAL TASKS

1. Assuming civic and social responsibility.
2. Maintaining an established economic standard of living.
3. Assisting children in their growth and development.
4. Developing leisure time activities.
5. Relating to one's spouse as a person rather than as a role.
6. Accepting and adjusting to physiological changes of the middle years.
7. Responding to and assisting aging parents.[5]

See also the discussion of family tasks in Chapter 3.

DEVELOPMENTAL HAZARDS

Some situations that arise in the adult years can be termed developmental hazards, since they interfere with task achievement. The problems may have their roots in earlier periods of life but become manifest at this time. Others are shared with adolescence and youth, such as drug and alcohol addiction. However, at least three are classically associated with mature adults: alcoholism, divorce, and economic instability or failure to achieve in employment.

For a complete discussion of alcoholism see Chapter 4.

Divorce

Most married couples began their relationship as adolescents or young adults. The decision to marry might have been made for many reasons, but ideally, mutual love was the deciding factor. However, the choice made at that point in life—the early twenties for most couples—affects them for the next half century or actually the rest of their lives. It is not surprising, therefore, that approximately 40% of all marriages end in divorce.

Persons continue to change throughout adulthood, and often enough interests and goals become so diverse that couples face incompatibility in daily living. Some frequently cited causes for divorce include financial insecurity, religious differences, sexual role conflict, and infidelity.

A divorce interrupts the lives of a family, not only of a single member. Often children are faced with a series of adjustments to a one-parent family after a long period of strife in the home. Settlements must be made about mutual property, and the home essentially disintegrates as each spouse goes his separate way. The impact of divorce is far-reaching even in childless marriages. Adjustments to a new mode of single life require much effort for both members of the majority of divorced couples. Teenage marriages are the most likely to fail, since personal values are still in the formative stage. Couples who marry later in life have a better chance for lifelong marital success.

Economic or employment insecurity

Failure of adults, especially men, to sustain themselves economically in employment is essentially a form of failure to achieve. Poor financial management, inferior work performance, a secondary interest in stability of living patterns, and illness are contributory factors. The country's economic trends have also affected the employment status of many individuals. Even college graduates (such as aerospace engineers) can be victims of unemployment or obsolete skilled training as large shifts occur in industrial technology and scientific emphasis. When adults fail to provide adequately for themselves and their families, they are likely to develop a negative self-image, considerable anxiety, and psychological handicaps. Such negative feelings often lead to marital disharmony, family strife, and emotional handicaps that make the individual a "societal cripple" who must depend on others for the necessities of life for himself and his family. In such instances, these persons become a source of problems in the achievement of the family developmental tasks, as well as being unable to proceed normally with their individual goals.

Illness and hospitalization as developmental hazards receive individual attention in subsequent chapters.

The midlife crisis

Some theorists believe that the failure to resolve problems in the transition from young adulthood to mature adulthood is one explanation for a high rate of alcoholism, suicide, divorce, and other problems that characterize midlife. Individuals who lose a feeling of importance about their life role or work are especially vulnerable. Children leaving home, being replaced at work by the younger set, and some physical declining may contribute to the crisis. Midlife is similar to adolescence because of critical changes in identity, sexuality, and role.

The older adult

Later maturity is the period of adulthood that extends approximately from retirement to death. It is called the years of *integrity* by some and the declining years by others who see aging as a period of *despair*. The elderly members of our population represent a heterogeneous and growing section of our society. For those who enjoy good health and financial security, their retirement years can provide contentment when they can enjoy freedom of activity unknown since their youth. For a larger group, unfortunately, aging means illness, hospitalization, loneliness, and living on an insufficient, fixed income, often supplemented by assistance from family members or public sources. To understand and appreciate persons in later maturity, it is necessary to know about their characteristics, needs, and developmental tasks.

Approximately 20 million elderly citizens are found in our present U.S. population. This number will gradually rise throughout subsequent decades; and since women live longer than men, there will be an ever-widening gap between the numbers of men and women over 65 years of age. Current estimates indicate that we can expect to have 28.2 million aged persons in the year 2000 — 10.8 million men and 17.4 million women (Fig. 2-9).[2]

The National Council on Aging estimates that one out of three elderly persons can be considered in the "poverty" category, and approximately one out of five poor people are old. Elderly persons who live in poverty are deprived of the feelings of security and contentment that ideally accompany the later years. They lose a portion of their sense of self-worth and forfeit their independence as contributing citizens in society.

Most retirees live on a fourth of the income that they enjoyed in earlier years. Pensions, Social Security benefits, and local public assistance programs help supplement income from earnings, investments, and other retirement sources.

Many older individuals face a crisis in housing as a result of low income and the limitation of residing close to essential services or transportation. They are not always able to live where they choose but must consider whether or not they can get to the grocery, the pharmacy, the clinic, or the church with ease. Those who are able to drive and can afford a car have more freedom than

2 Client development across the life span

FIG. 2-9
Number of aged and their percent of total population. (From Anderson, Helen C.: Newton's geriatric nursing, ed. 5, St. Louis, 1971, The C.V. Mosby Co.)

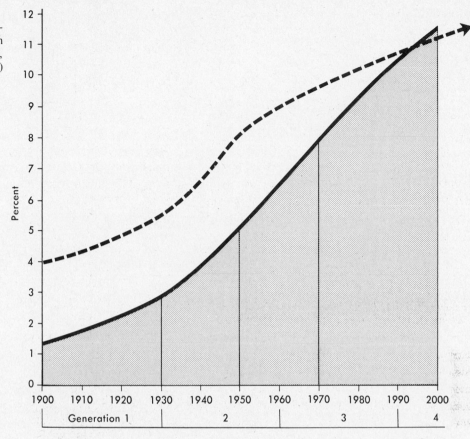

persons who must depend on public transportation. A familiar neighborhood may be more important than modern conveniences to some older persons. Reluctance to leave the security of old friends, trusted shop owners, or known streets may be the most influential factor in selecting a place to live in the later years of maturity.

Elderly persons who cannot be alone because of reasons of failing health or mental alertness may be forced to live in homes for the aged, foster homes, supervised apartments, or similar centers where basic needs are provided along with planned programs of supervised recreation and personal guardianship (Fig. 2-10). Such retirement centers or homes for the aged can be small and intimate, with a homelike atmosphere, or large and impersonal almost like a hotel. They may be supported by public funds, church federations, fraternal groups, or fees paid directly by clients. Often eligibility to enter such a "home" requires one to liquidate his assets and contribute them to the institution for lifetime care.

Another choice of residence for the elderly individual who cannot live alone is the home of a relative, especially a son or daughter. Although many families are delighted with a transient visit from grandparents, long-term or permanent arrangements often interfere with the freedom and life-style of the young families. The household schedule, diet pattern, living space, and center of activity is sometimes dictated by the presence of an elderly person. The television and stereo must be kept low if they have gone to bed, friends must be quiet if they visit in the evening, and total family outings may be forsaken so that someone

FIG. 2-10
These mature adults are spending their retirement years in a modern residential facility.

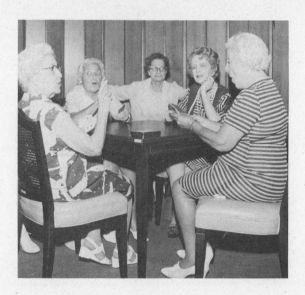

can stay with grandmother or grandfather. Marital stress is not uncommon when parents or parents-in-law enter into the family household. With good intentions, the older member will give unsolicited advice on child rearing or finances or will take sides in family disputes. Sooner or later the tension becomes severe enough to provoke hostility in the family, and feelings are hurt in the confrontation. If the older person is not financially independent, additional problems may be posed when their children must contribute directly to their maintenance in their aging years. For some families with secure finances, adequate space, and intragroup harmony, the additional elderly member is integrated easily into the framework of family life. If the elderly individual's health permits, he can provide valuable assistance in family tasks such as cooking, baby-sitting, household repairs, or lawn work. Each family group must consider its integrity and resources before adding the element of caring for older family members.

Fortunately, today there are a number of alternatives for persons who must deal with aging parents and community agencies and services specifically designed to meet their basic physical and psychosocial needs. The decision on a place for the elderly to live must be made on the basis of the many factors previously discussed and the special needs and desires of the persons immediately involved. In the past it has been considered an obligation to "look after" one's parents in their "old age," but today this obligation can be described as an option. Fewer and fewer elderly persons expect their children to care for them in their homes, realizing how it may adversely affect the life-style of the youngsters and even limit their own independence when required to fit into a new way of living, often too hectic for them. With the succeeding generations' living longer and ideally in a sound state of health, the older person may spend many years after retirement in a new home environment especially selected to meet his personal needs.

The elderly are a highly diverse group. Some are physically or emotionally impaired, and others are well in body and mind. Some want to live alone and maintain their life-style of earlier years; others fear being alone and seek the security of a protective environment. Some are economically independent; others must adjust to poverty-level existence. Some have a great zest for life and its pleasures, but others are content to rock and wait quietly for their imminent death. No single formula can consider all factors in plans to meet the needs of the elderly, but a general knowledge of their developmental tasks will serve as useful guidelines in their care.

DEVELOPMENTAL TASKS

1. Coping with decreasing physical strength and declining health.
2. Adjusting to retirement and a changed financial status.
3. Adjusting to the death of one's spouse.
4. Establishing an affiliation with one's age group.
5. Assuming a new pattern of social and civic responsibilities.
6. Maintaining satisfactory living arrangements.[5]

Coping with death

Man has long recognized that death is the only certain process that occurs in the human life cycle. Death is the most dreaded experience of man, and much of his time and energy has been directed toward finding ways to avoid it for the longest period of time possible or to make it less painful for those who must endure it. Medical science is primarily directed toward prolonging life and has long disregarded its role in dealing with death. Since approximately 80% of all persons die in hospitals, it is important for nurses to understand how individuals cope with impending death of themselves or their loved ones.

Our society is oriented toward life and its pleasures that can be enjoyed in health. The realities of illness, disability, and death are reserved for the elderly who have lived a full measure. One tends to respond with alarm at the thought of death of a child or young adult. Persons in the helping professions such as nursing are stimulated by promoting life. Their reaction to the dying client is too often superficial pity rather than meaningful support in this final stage of the life cycle. When one has an opportunity to share the death process with others, the experience can be one of the richest of his life. Successful coping with the stages of grief and mourning is possible only when one understands the meaning of death and its impact on those left behind, who must reinvest their emotional attachments formerly associated with the deceased individual.

People say, "Death is a sad subject that cannot be freely discussed" and "Death causes pain to those around the dying." So if an individual is facing death, he is too often isolated from the mainstream of life. When a friend or family member becomes infirm or very old, he may be sent to a hospital or a nursing home where he is essentially isolated until he dies.

From early childhood until maturity one gains appreciation of the fact that one speaks cautiously about death because it is an upsetting topic. It is also learned that death is associated with growing old, accidents, disease, and hospitalization. Certain words, such as "cancer" and "heart attack," begin to take on a specific meaning as early as kindergarten and the first grade.

A person who faces death may be more concerned about how others feel about his dying than with his own thoughts. There may be the anxieties about the welfare and security of a family unit if a parent is dying. Others fear death

55

Foundations of clinical practice

because it is a dreadful extension of the loneliness they have faced during their declining years. There are undoubtedly as many responses to the thought of dying as there are people. Various social classes and cultures have evolved accepted ways of dying with dignity. Even a child becomes aware of the rules for dying.

The manner in which an individual faces death depends on his emotional capabilities. Religious faith, ethnic and social backgrounds, and life values all determine the ways in which a person deals with death. The nurse needs considerable information about factors that influence the client's view of death in order to take an active role in helping him cope with his impending cessation of life. An understanding of the various concepts of death, the ways in which different age groups perceive the meaning of death, and the process of grief and mourning is useful.

Death essentially contains the element of nonbeing, and this perception is inconceivable for the average person. It means separation from those he loves. Even though his religious beliefs may include one in an afterlife, he is aware of a temporary isolation while those left behind continue to enjoy the certainty of earthly pleasures. In earlier times before medical advancements did much to relieve pain, persons who had to endure considerable suffering were comforted by the promise of death and heaven as an eternal reward. Modern science has since eliminated much of this suffering by implementing treatments aimed at the reduction of mental as well as physical pain. The constant pace at which steps have been taken to decrease suffering and prolong life has contributed to a lessening of the fear of death and even a denial of its potential by some. Basically, it seems that all human beings can conceive of the death of others, but not of themselves.

Years ago, before the ill and the aged were removed from the family for care, even children were afforded the opportunity to be confronted with death. It is not uncommon in these decades, however, for persons to reach maturity without ever having seriously considered what death means to them. There is value in helping a young child develop his concept of death. As he grows, he can add new experiences that will help him clarify and expand it, such as the death of a grandparent, neighbor, pet, or even a tree. Understanding that all living things must eventually die is the first step in accepting the reality of death. Dealing with this event honestly is highly desirable. Direct and simple answers are most acceptable. No attempt should be made to contrive fables, which the child will later resent as he grows older. Explanations such as ''he has gone to live with Jesus'' or ''your dog is just taking a long sleep'' do little to form realistic and lasting impressions of death. In addition, they may cause the child to lose trust in his source of information and raise doubt about future data on such subjects. Opportunities to see a corpse or attend a funeral should not necessarily be avoided by the young child. These events help make death believable and less mystical. Often what the child imagines is more dreaded than reality. There is no formula for helping persons to develop a reasonable impression of death except to give honest information in terms that the client can understand. The choice of experiences to shape the concept of death must be guided by factors including social custom, religion, ethnic considerations, and family tradition. Adults who attempt to help children with such understandings must have a clearly formulated idea of what death means to them.

2 Client development across the life span

GROWTH AND DEVELOPMENT AND THE MEANING OF DEATH

As soon as a child realizes that he is a separate entity and can differentiate between "me" and "not me," he begins to perceive the possibility of his nonexistence. He poses questions regarding his origin and his ultimate fate. Such reactions occur as early as 3 or 4 years of age. Nightmares at this time often have self-threatening themes that are manifestations of repression and denial of the nonexistence of "me." Play may involve themes of illness and death, for example, cowboys and Indians, doll play, ritualism of funerals, and soldier-war games. At the end of the child's play, even though he has been killed or laid in a coffin, he returns to life again, thus reinforcing his need to refute any thought of permanent annihilation or the threat of separation from his loved ones. As he grows older and attends school, watches television, and interacts with friends and family, he learns the reality of physical destruction as part of death. Watching violent death in movies and news coverage of national events is a reminder that one's body can be destroyed. Associations begin to develop regarding reasons for death and its consequences. For example, one may die or be killed from being bad or disobeying rules. Guilt and punishment become attached to death. Knowing that the process of death results in a destruction or disposal of a body is also added to the child's understanding. Experiences such as attending the burial of a grandparent or seeing the Humane Society pick up for disposal a dead animal that has been run over in the street reinforce the reality of disposition of the body as part of dying. This in itself is a cause for considerable concern to the preschooler. At about age 5 children may perceive death as a manlike creature who steals life away. After the age of 9 or 10 a biological death concept begins to form.

Many young and mature adults spend little time considering their own feelings about death until someone close to them is fatally injured in an accident or dies from illness. Not until middle age when their parents, relatives, and friends begin to die do most persons seriously think about their own death. Each time that an individual experiences the death of someone with whom he can personally identify, he grows in his understanding of the nature of dying and the attendant process of grief and mourning.

GRIEF AND MOURNING

Grief and mourning are emotional responses related to loss or the anticipation of loss. According to Elisabeth Kübler-Ross, they involve a series of five stages: denial and isolation, anger, bargaining, depression, and acceptance.[10] Understanding each of these stages is extremely helpful in assisting others in their responses to death.

Denial and isolation

Denial is the initial response to the knowledge of impending death. "It can't be." This defense is usually temporary and serves to insulate the individual while he has an opportunity to gather additional defenses.

During the stage of denial one may experience a great need to hope for life. Isolation of this hope from the denial portion seems contradictory but permits one to be ambivalent. One can then talk about health and illness and death and immortality as if they were coexistent. Death can be faced while hope is still maintained. This stage, characterized by shock and disbelief that one is not immortal, is usually short lived and paves the way for subsequent coping mechanisms.

Anger

Once impending death has been accepted, one becomes confronted with feelings of injustice. "Why me?" Anger is multifaceted and projected freely onto the environment. The family, physicians, hospital, and nurses may be under attack. Such anger is not too difficult to conceive of when one sees the situation from the dying individual's point of view. His life is interrupted, and his many plans and dreams must be abandoned. Giving up independence and control over his life processes is reason for resentment and anger against everyone, including God. Angry feelings must be accepted as an expression of grief. Even though the client may respond negatively to those he loves and to those who provide his care, they should not abandon him or allow him to face his anger alone. Genuine expressions of concern usually assist in lessening the client's feeling of diffuse hostility.

Bargaining

Bargaining is the third stage of coping with death. It involves a deal with an outside influence (physician, God, nurse, and so forth), exchanging a promise for an extension of life and/or independence—"if I can live to see my daughter graduate from high school, I will be ready to die then" or "if I can go home for one weekend with my family, I will be content to return to the hospital until I die." As far as possible, the client should be granted his special requests. Many such bargainings seem to include some feelings of guilt, often of a religious nature. Although realizing his unworthiness for special favor, the client asks anyway, knowing that the Divine Power is merciful and omnipotent.

Depression

The fourth stage, depression, usually heralds the onset of the inevitable. The loss of integrity is unavoidable. Signs of deterioration are evident, and defense mechanisms used earlier are no longer effective. There is a feeling of sadness, anguish, and a need to cry. One faces the loss of everything and everyone. Crying, although a form of regression, is useful in calling forth essential support from loved ones. Depression is a useful tool in preparing for the loss of a love object, and encouragement is not meaningful during such a state. Permitting a full expression of depression will make it easier for the fifth stage, acceptance.

Acceptance

The final stage is not highly charged with feelings. The individual is quiet and seems rather content. Some have described it as being ready for death. During this period there is a narrowing perspective of interest in the dying person's life. He does not want new stimuli, because he barely has the strength to deal with those already at hand. Quiet visiting without much verbalization seems to be preferred. Being alone with his thoughts seems important as life ends. It is an important time for silence, when one can review his life and contemplate the unknown that lies ahead.

A WORD ABOUT HOPE

Hope may pervade any and all of the stages of the dying process. Only the anticipation of a miracle or scientific breakthrough holds some persons together during the days or weeks before death. The caring staff as well as the family can share in this hope without necessarily promising the prolongation of life.

THE DYING CLIENT'S FAMILY RESPONSES

Families who are close to the dying person also experience the various stages of the dying process. They, too, like the dying client, require understanding and support. Beyond the death of a loved one lie more grief and mourning during a period of restitution. Persons who share the loss of the departed gather together and exchange their feelings of mutual grief. Negative feelings of all types are temporarily repressed, and the positive attributes of the person who died are emphasized. The funeral provides a public acknowledgment that the death is a reality, a chance to eulogize the departed, and the opportunity to reinforce religious beliefs in a future reunion in an afterlife. The comfort provided by the funeral service is a useful tool in helping persons "pay their last respects" and in permitting them to return to their daily lives feeling that they have been dutiful and therefore should be able to enjoy themselves without any guilt or remorse connected with the death.

THE NURSE COPING WITH DEATH

For nurses to be of assistance to clients and their loved ones, they need to understand their own reactions to death and be able to cope with the idea of helping individuals die as well as helping them live.

Since the majority of all persons die in hospitals, often the nurse is the person who must openly discuss, for the first time in the client's life, the subject of death. It is estimated that over half of all mature adults have never seriously considered their dying. Everyone has the right to discuss the topic with someone who cares and understands. The desirable plan is to talk about one's own dying before death is at hand. Persons not labeled "terminal" seem to possess healthier responses to the potential of death than those for whom death is imminent.

Nurses must be aware of their own feelings and needs because they inevitably enter into conversations about death. If they have not accepted the reality of dying, they commonly deny the death process or withdraw from the dying client.

Death, of course, does not always allow for the client or his nurses to be prepared. It may not be anticipated by anyone, or the mode of dying may be unexpected. Merely acknowledging the limitations of medical life-supporting methods may make nurses feel anxious.

The thin line between life and death and the person and the body is often grim reality, difficult to acknowledge and accept. The procedures of dealing with the corpse seem impersonal and in sharp contrast with those used moments before in dealing with the client as a living person. Considerable experience is necessary to work through these responses. Opportunities to share attitudes and feelings with peers, clergy, physicians, and other staff members should be utilized.

Learning the manifestations of grief and mourning and describing and analyzing related incidents may be useful in gaining insight into one's own feelings and needs. To be helpful to clients and their families, the nurse must be prepared to serve as a sounding board for their responses and permit them to express their grief. Allowing them to assist with the physical care of a loved one may be comforting to family members and help them feel like an essential element in the death process. The helpless state of merely standing by is difficult for some relatives to accept.

Death in hospitals can be very lonely for the client and his family who are not blessed with a caring nurse. It is almost a dehumanized process, which at times is controlled by medical procedures and machines that have the capacity to chart the course and even the manner and time of death. If the client is being monitored, infused, ventilated, and so forth, visitation is often limited and seldom private. Nurses and physicians rush around in the environment, checking vital signs, regulating infusions, and adjusting machinery. The client is essentially isolated from those he loves. The family members have no authority in

Foundations of clinical practice

his care and are often treated like unwelcome guests to even their dearest companion at the climax of his life cycle. It is imperative that nurses recognize this seeming atrocity and compensate for it as far as possible by including concern for the family in their care plan for the dying client. If the family cannot be permitted to remain with the dying client at his bedside, they must be regularly informed of his condition.

Although the nurse is concerned for the client's welfare, such concern can seldom approximate the tender feelings of a spouse, father, mother, or child. Care should be exercised not to isolate the client at the hour of his death. Sometimes nurses show obvious ambivalence, which families perceive at the period immediately before death. It is too late to do anything and too early for abandonment. Even clients surely perceive such responses in those caring for them. In some instances the client may be permitted to die at home in the familiar environment of family and friends. Adjustment is often easier and more complete.

Acceptance of death as an inevitable situation by the client and his family helps form the basis for a constructive helping relationship. Care should be taken to keep the encounter at a therapeutic level as opposed to a social level. The nurse's expression of empathy and assurance of caring to the client and his family will mean far more in building a relationship than the sharing of the tragedy of imminent death. The fact should be emphasized that everything feasible will be done to make the client comfortable and that he will receive fine medical management. The family should be cautioned not to abandon the client in a feeling of hopelessness or helplessness. Tearful faces and hushed voices are usually distressing to those already faced with death. It is important, however, to watch for cues that indicate how the family is coping with impending death. They need emotional support as does the client. The problems of the dying come to an end as he expires, but the anxieties and grief of the family live on.

Throughout the nurse-family-client interaction during the death process, the emphasis should be on what can be done for the client rather than what cannot be done. The maintenance of human respect and dignity should always pervade the final stage of life.

DEATH OF A CHILD

The death of a child is always a traumatic event for his family and the staff who have been involved in his care. Regardless of the age or condition of the child, death to a human being who has not had the opportunity for an adult life is considered an insult. People tend to react more aggressively than when faced with the death of an adult who has the strengths and understandings of maturity.

Acute trauma may be a cause of death in childhood, and death, of course, comes quickly. The other category of concern to nurses is the child with a terminal illness that results in a long hospitalization and considerable pain and suffering.

The nurse must learn to deal with the child at his level of understanding and offer the family sympathetic help at the same time. When parents first learn that their child will die, they begin their stages of the grief and mourning process. They deny that their child will die, they become angry with the world that this has happened to them, they bargain for extra time, and finally they are in the midst of a deep depression when the reality of ensuing death becomes unavoidable. Some parents never reach the final stage of acceptance before the actual moment of death. The hope of a miracle seems always present in the care of a dying child. It is far too painful to admit that we can do so many miraculous things with medical science and yet are unable to save a dying child.

When the child is very young, even at the toddler stage, he learns that physicians, nurses, and hospitals mean pain or illness. He recalls the pain caused by some man in a white coat or lady in a white dress sticking his arm with a needle or stitching up his cut. He is unable to separate the caring from the hurting or the helping from the harm. Many children react to hospital personnel with avoidance because merely their white clothing is the threat of an imposition of an outside force that the child cannot control.

Very early the child develops an appreciation that his illness and dying disturb people and that words denoting death are to be avoided, such as "cancer," "tumor," or "leukemia." The significance of a diagnostic term may take on meaning to a child as early as 4 or 5 years of age, because of the conversations of parents or memories of television programs, and he adds the knowledge of these manifestations to his very early fears of the possibility of "me" becoming a "no me." The dying preschool child may devote considerable time to merely contemplating his own destruction. The psychological strength he should be using to live as long as possible may be expended in covering over his fears of annihilation.

The significance of a medical prognosis becomes important to children by the age of 5 to 7. They connect a statement of "6 months to live" with a death sentence and consider it a command. To share this information with the child seems unwise because it may cause him to give up and lose his will to live on. A time prognosis is often inaccurate and may cause a family to mourn the loss of a child too soon or too completely. If the child dies slowly, parents and relatives may have completed the mourning process before actual death occurs. While the child is yet alive, the family may have withdrawn their emotional investment from him. Visits may become merely perfunctory. Their interactions lack genuine involvement. Belongings such as toys and clothes may even be given away, and funeral arrangements made. The child may be essentially dead to the family while still physically alive.

When a child reaches school age, he begins to feel a sense of assuming a certain social role. He sees himself in the protective care of loving parents and enjoys the security of his home. His siblings bring him many hours of pleasure. Facing death means primarily the forfeiting of a happy social role for exchange to an uncertain existence in a strange place. To be told that he is going to live with God in heaven is not a promise of total security to the young child. God in his heaven, regardless of how beautiful adults say it will be, to a child is a stranger in a far-off place where he will be isolated from those whom he knows and loves very much. The school-age child should be allowed to die in the familiar and secure surroundings of his home and family if possible, where the protective and tangible love of his parents can be ever present during his dying.

In late childhood and adolescence when biological death is a reality, the coping mechanisms previously described are brought into play. The dying adolescent should be treated with respect and given all possible opportunities to participate in decisions regarding his care. Although he may deeply resent his dying, he usually participates cooperatively with those who provide him care. The more mature teenager, the young man or woman, can usually allow family members to comfort and to care. Older adolescents die sad, but with honor. On the other hand, the younger adolescent may have too much pride and be too bitter to accept any form of comfort from others and respond to death with defiance in spite of loneliness and fear.

When parents are to be informed that their child will die, they should be told at the same time so that they can be supportive to each other. The integrity of the family unit is essential in times of crisis. For those who live on, sharing the caring for a dying child can be an enriching experience for the family unit. Children who endure the process of dying, surrounded by a treatment team and a family that expresses love, concern, and care, engage in one of life's richest experiences.

DEATH OF THE MATURE AND ELDERLY

The mature adult, although he has lived a relatively full life, also has considerable difficulty facing death. Most have an understanding of the beauty of life and realize that death evokes grief, mourning, and the necessity of emotional reinvestment. They may have experienced the death of many persons, including parents, friends, siblings, and perhaps their spouse.

Mature adults have probably accepted the reality of personal death, and some have made wills and funeral plans. It is imperative that persons who have achieved such an acceptance do not expect the same type of acceptance from younger persons. Anticipation of death is usually reserved for the elderly.

No client can cope completely with his own dying, however, because he possesses the usual weaknesses of human emotion and a mind that cannot fully comprehend the significance of death.

Summary

Human development is directed toward the goal of self-realization from birth to death. As the physical body grows and life becomes a series of encounters with the complex environment, emotions mature, thus contributing to psychological equilibrium.

The urge for man to become what he *can* become is an uncompromising force. All human beings are striving for fulfillment, but the eventual attainment of the goal is dependent on health, environmental experiences, and the integrity of the ego concept.

Some persons need special assistance from parents, teachers, counselors, ministers, physicians, and nurses in their quest. The role of such a helping relationship is to explore attitudes, strengths, and weaknesses as they relate to situations and problems in life. There must be a coordinated effort as each one reaches toward self-realization. The goal can be achieved only when mankind recognizes its interdependence and appreciates growth and development as they relate to understanding and improving the human life experience.[4]

The nurse must possess knowledge regarding the principles of growth and development and be able to participate in physical and developmental assessment processes. An appreciation of major theories related to the subject is also beneficial. Freud, Erikson, Piaget, Levinson, Peck, and Kohlberg are representative of classical theorists of human development, each having made historically important contributions.

It is essential to comprehend the major biological and psychological phenomena in each period of life from infancy through later maturity and to appreciate the importance of the developmental tasks for each.

Numerous problems that can arise at critical periods in the life cycle are termed hazards because they interfere with attainment of developmental tasks. Causative factors include impaired biological equipment, low-quality environment, or certain significant experiences with the physical and social world.

The importance of health care during the prenatal period, the birth process, and the first weeks of life must be appreciated. Many problems of infancy, childhood, and adolescence are closely linked to the quality of home and nurture. Although adult hazards are largely social in origin, they tend to produce far-reaching effects, since adults must set the pace for family life experiences.

Death is the culmination of the life span. The primary role of the nurse in dealing with the dying client, regardless of his age, is to support him and his own healthy coping mechanisms. He and his family should be allowed an opportunity to work through the process of grief and mourning. The nurse can offer sincere understanding and exhibit personal concern in the client's care as well as provide opportunities for the family to continue their loving relationship with the dying and, if feasible, actively include them in selected portions of his care. The nurse should ensure that they are not isolated from him during the climax of his life when he most needs their secure protection and should provide opportunities for visits in privacy if possible. Until death has actually occurred, the dying client should be permitted to maintain his social and emotional attachments. Finally, the nurse should remember that, after death, the family has the restitution and reinvestment period ahead when they may need further support from a professional treatment team.

Table 2-6 and accompanying illustrations describing growth and development from birth through later maturity follow.

TABLE 2-6

Growth and development, birth through adulthood

	Physical development	Sensory-motor development	Speech and adaptive behavior	Personal-social development
Birth to 1 month (neonate)	Weight: 6 to 8 pounds (2.72 to 3.62 kg) at birth; gains 6 ounces (170 gm) a week Length: 18 to 22 inches (45.72 to 55.88 cm); gains 1 inch (2.54 cm) a month Head circumference: 13 to 15 inches (33.02 to 38.10 cm) Face: flat broad nose, fat cheeks, receding chin, eyes with puffy lids Trunk: narrow shoulders, narrow hips, short neck, protruding abdomen, engorged breasts, umbilical stump (which falls off in 6 to 10 days); chest smaller than head Limbs: usually flexed, hands fisted, bowed legs, nails paper thin Skin: covered at birth with lanugo and vernix caseosa	Crying involves whole body; skin flushed, limbs flail about All activity is generalized and diffuse; does not make specific responses to specific stimuli Tactile senses are most highly developed in lips, tongue, cheek Responds to pressure, heat, cold Responds to light and darkness; eye movements are uncoordinated; appears to notice objects in line of vision Responds to sound by increasing activity and staring; resists sour or bitter tastes Lifts head when prone; exhibits crawling movements Reflexes present: Moro, Babinski, tonic neck, rooting, sucking, swallowing, gag and cough, dancing, yawning, sneezing, blinking	Lusty cry when uncomfortable; no tears Character of cry differs with circumstances May make throaty noises	Diminishes activity when face is seen Quiets when spoken to or held Uniqueness and individuality are expressed in posturing while held (such as tenseness, curling up like a kitten) and in response to visual and auditory stimuli Seeks pleasure and immediate satisfaction Sleeps 20 hours a day with unbroken period of about 3 hours
2 months	Cries tears	Lifts both head and chest short distance when prone Head lag is not quite complete when pulled up to sit Holds hands open more Follows object briefly from side to midline Holds toy briefly; does not search when toy is dropped	Crying becomes more differentiated with cause Begins sucking when held in feeding position	Smiles at stimulation Coos Responds to speaking voice Sleeps for longer intervals
3 months	Weight: 12 to 13 pounds (5.44 to 5.89 kg)	Grasp reflex replaced by purposeful grasp Predominately symmetrical posturing with head in midline; faint tonic neck reflex remaining When prone, holds chin and shoulders off firm surface bearing weight on forearms Has improved head control Dancing reflex has been lost Sits, back rounded and knees flexed, when supported	Holds hands in front of face and stares at them Plays with hands and fingers Laughs aloud, gurgles, blows bubbles, coos, chuckles, squeals Reaches for objects but misses Can carry hand or object to mouth at will Hands mostly open Follows dangling toy with eyes from one side to other (180 degrees) Catches sight of object immediately; shows binocular coordination Opens mouth for feeding	Can wait short time for bottle Smiles in response to mother's face Shows pleasure in making sounds Amount of crying reduced Pulls at clothes

Adapted from Watson, Judy: Unpublished paper on growth and development, birth through adolescence, 1966; and Gould, Daniel Levinson, and Vaillant, George: New light on adult life cycles, Time, April 28, 1975, p. 69.

Continued.

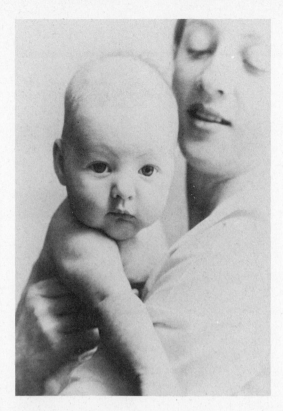

FIG. 2-11
The 2-month old is gaining some head control. (From Phenomena of early development, Columbus, Ohio, Ross Laboratories.)

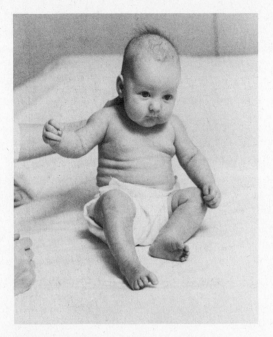

FIG. 2-12
The 3-month-old can sit with support. (From Phenomena of early development, Columbus, Ohio, Ross Laboratories.)

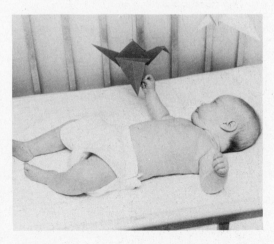

FIG. 2-13
The 3-month-old follows objects with his eyes and reaches for them but misses. (From Phenomena of early development, Columbus, Ohio, Ross Laboratories.)

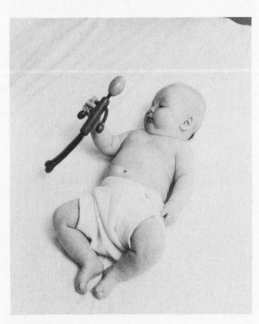

FIG. 2-14
The 4-month-old grasps toys. (From Phenomena of early development, Columbus, Ohio, Ross Laboratories.)

TABLE 2-6

Growth and development, birth through adulthood—cont'd

	Physical development	Sensory-motor development	Speech and adaptive behavior	Personal-social development
4 months	Weight: 13 to 14 pounds (5.89 to 6.35 kg) Drooling indicates appearance of saliva	Posturing is symmetrical Has improved head control when propped in sitting position When prone, lifts head and shoulders at 90-degree angle and looks around Turns from back to side Thumb apposition in graspings Sustains part of his own weight when held standing Pushes with feet if held erect	Laughs aloud, "belly laugh" Watches intently many still and moving objects Reaches out with both hands Can seize toy Shows preference for resting head on one side Brings hands together and plays with them Becomes excited when he sees a toy Coordinates eye and body movement Coos and gurgles when talked to Puts hands in mouth	Sleeps through night without interruption Can anticipate feedings at sight of bottle Shows interest in surroundings Spontaneous social smile; initiates social play Pays attention to human voice Recognizes mother and familiar object
5 months	Weight: birth weight doubled (approximately 15 pounds, or 6.80 kg) Considerable drooling	Rolls from back to stomach Holds back straight when sitting Requires minimal support Stands erect with support Palms or grasps using whole hand Could crawl, but limited by inability to raise abdomen when prone	Reaches out and grasps toy with one hand; approach still inaccurate at times Grasps everything within reach and puts it into mouth Splashes in bathtub Looks to see where toy has gone when he drops it Vocalizes displeasure and joy Babbles vowels; talks to himself when alone Plays with toes Crumples paper	Distinguishes mother from another person May fear strangers
6 months	Gains 1 pound (0.45 kg) a month Grows ½ inch (1.27 cm) a month Lower incisors erupt	Can sit briefly when placed Leans on hands; when prone, bears weight on hands with arms extended, chest and upper abdomen off firm surface Lifts head in anticipation of sitting Rolls from stomach to back, in addition to back to stomach Bears large portion of weight when held in standing position Pulls up to sitting position Puts feet in mouth when supine Grasps with fingers flexed Hitches backward when in sitting position	Holds bottle If he has one toy in hand, drops it and reaches when alternative is offered; may pick up dropped toy Is beginning to show food preferences Cries when provoked Thrashes about Picks up small block using palm or grasp Bangs spoon on table Waves object about Plays contentedly alone Babbles not specific for specific object or people Vocalizes some well-defined syllables Transfers objects from one hand to other	Looks when people enter room Knows strangers Holds out hands to be lifted Begins to act coy Laughs May object to being left alone or having someone take a toy away

Continued.

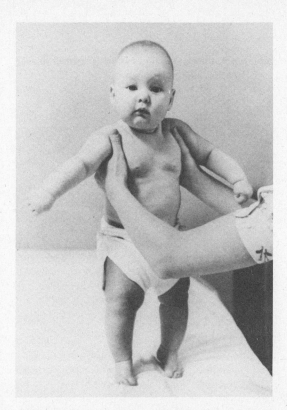

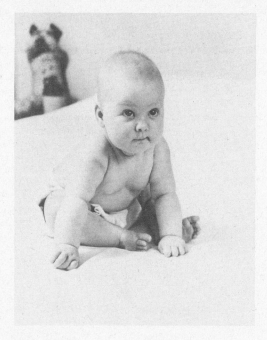

FIG. 2-16
The 5-month-old is acquiring some sitting control. (From The first and second years of life, Columbus, Ohio, Ross Laboratories.)

FIG. 2-15
The 5-month-old can stand erect with support. (From Phenomena of early development, Columbus, Ohio, Ross Laboratories.)

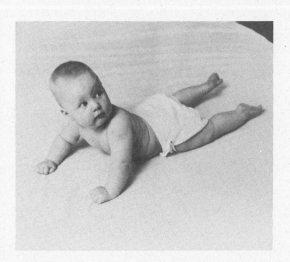

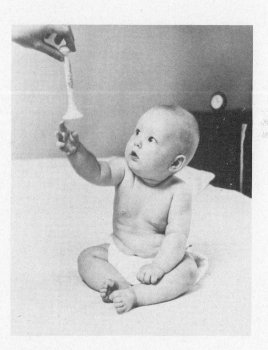

FIG. 2-17
At 6 months the infant can support his weight while prone and lift his chest and upper abdomen off a firm surface. (From The first and second years of life, Columbus, Ohio, Ross Laboratories.)

FIG. 2-18
The 6-month-old reaches for toys. (From The first and second years of life, Columbus, Ohio, Ross Laboratories.)

TABLE 2-6

Growth and development, birth through adulthood—cont'd

	Physical development	Sensory-motor development	Speech and adaptive behavior	Personal-social development
7 months	Maxillary central incisors erupt	Pivots in prone position, bearing weight on one hand Bounces with little hip and knee sag when held in standing position May handle cup fairly well Chews and can take solids Approaches and grasps object with one hand Can sit erect with support for extended periods up to 30 minutes	Is adept at hand-to-hand transfer Inspects objects with eyes, mouth, hands: grasping, feeling, mouthing, looking, withdrawing, contacting, rotating, transferring, banging Crows and squeals Babbles "da, ba" Can feed self cookie Retains first block when second is presented Vocalizes "m-m-m" when crying Purposefully moves toward and reaches out for object he wants	Delights in exercise of new abilities Preoccupied with private enterprise; plays with single toy for extended period Pats mirror image and smiles Responds to name Less concerned with strangers Changes easily from crying to laughing
8 months	Weight: 18 to 19 pounds (8.16 to 8.61 kg) Lateral mandibular incisors erupting	Sits alone steadily Handles toy in each hand Bears weight in legs when supported in standing position Has complete thumb-finger apposition Hand-eye coordination perfected so that random reaching no longer persists; grasps skillfully; holds on to object for longer period of time May begin to crawl or stand	Imitates sounds Helps feed self Reaches persistently for toys out of reach; looks for fallen toy Combines syllables "da da," "ba ba" Can change from prone to sitting position by himself	Responds to "no-no" and displeasure in voice Affection for family group appears Behavior with strangers includes shyness, turning away, hanging head, crying, screaming, refusing to play or accept toy Emotional instability and anxiety manifest Stretches out arms to love adult Likes peekaboo game
9 months	Lateral maxillary incisors erupting	Pulls up to standing position; holds on to furniture; may be able to sit down at will Crawls (abdomen on floor) or creeps on hands and knees Leans forward and recovers balance when sitting Can pick up small objects with thumb-finger apposition	Bangs two toys together Enjoys repetitive activity and words Holds bottle with good hand-to-mouth coordination May show preference for one hand Sounds stand for things to him Likes to drop things in cup or box and recover them	Enjoys mirror Waves bye-bye; plays pat-a-cake Objects strenuously when things are taken away from him Puts arms in front of face to prevent mother from washing Cries when scolded

Continued.

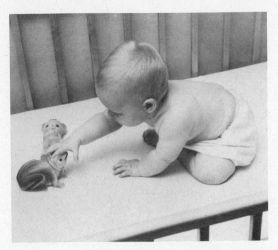

FIG. 2-19
The 7-month-old purposefully explores toys. (From Phenomena of early development, Columbus, Ohio, Ross Laboratories.)

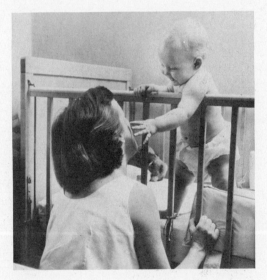

FIG. 2-20
The 9-month-old can pull himself to a standing position. (From Phenomena of early development, Columbus, Ohio, Ross Laboratories.)

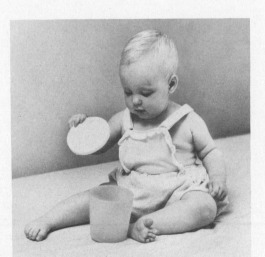

FIG. 2-21
Containers with lids fascinate the 9-month-old. (From The first and second years of life, Columbus, Ohio, Ross Laboratories.)

TABLE 2-6

Growth and development, birth through adulthood—cont'd

	Physical development	Sensory-motor development	Speech and adaptive behavior	Personal-social development
10 months	Slobbering and mouthing begin to decrease	Movement of trunk, arms, hands, legs, feet, and fingers becomes coordinated Changes from sitting to prone and from prone to sitting position Pokes, probes, and plucks objects with index finger and thumb Is beginning crude release Leans from side to side and turns from side to side and turns when sitting without losing balance; cruises well holding on to furniture Crawls up stairs	Matches two objects Says "mama" and "dada" with meaning and one other word Adept in feeding self cookie Shows less oral interest and more digital and visual interest Distinguishes fine detail in objects Paints with index finger Holds own bottle Brings together objects in each hand Cooperates in dressing by holding out arm for sleeve or feet up for socks and shoes	Extends toy to person without releasing it May pull clothes of mother to attract attention Pats and shakes dolls Shows new social interest in home and outside world Imitates gestures, adult voice inflections, facial expressions, sounds Turns head when called by name Is able to play alone for as much as an hour, but enjoys people around May still be shy with strangers Dislikes lying down except to sleep Enjoys repetitive games, such as bye-bye, pat-a-cake, and peekaboo
11 months		Has refined pincer grasp When standing holding on, can lift and replace one foot and alternate May walk with both hands held Stands alone momentarily	Wants to hold spoon when being fed; smears and plays in food Dumps objects out of containers and puts back in Shows interest in simple pictures in books Understands some phrases and the command, "no, no"	Shows more independence; may not like to be held and cuddled Drops objects deliberately so they will be picked up and returned to him Rolls ball toward another person Gives and takes toys in play Repeats performances laughed at Does not like to be left alone, especially in bed
12 months	Birth weight tripled (21 to 22 pounds, or 9.52 to 9.97 kg)	Walks when one hand is held May walk alone Sits down from standing position without help Can pivot while sitting Eats well with fingers Requires help in using spoon	Vocabulary of two or three words besides ma-ma and da-da Finds "hidden" toy Has some memory; may understand "Where's the doggie?" Scribbles with crayon on paper Is able to put peg in round hole Responds to music, loves rhythm Uses expressive jargon to make his wishes known Holds cup to drink when assisted	May kiss on request Enjoys simple tricks or games; laughs at surprises May cry for attention Expresses unmistakable anger, fear, affection, jealousy, anxiety, sympathy Stiffens in resistance Likes to show off for an audience Obeys "no, no" Gives toy on request

Continued.

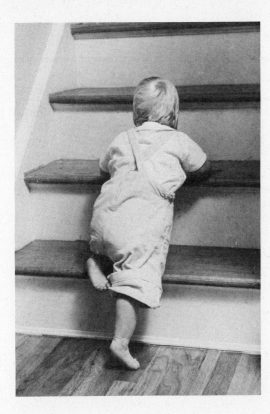

FIG. 2-22
The 10-month-old crawls up stairs. (From Phenomena of early development, Columbus, Ohio, Ross Laboratories.)

FIG. 2-23
The 11-month-old drops objects for others to return to him. (From Phenomena of early development, Columbus, Ohio, Ross Laboratories.)

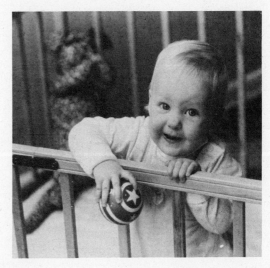

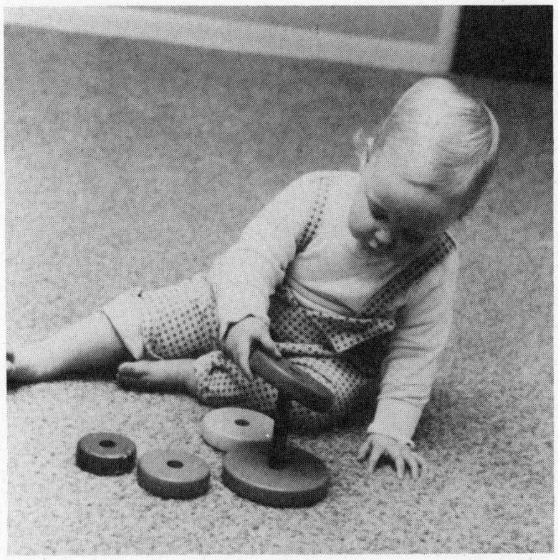

FIG. 2-24
The 12-month-old can put a peg in a round hole. (From Phenomena of early development, Columbus, Ohio, Ross Laboratories.)

TABLE 2-6

Growth and development, birth through adulthood—cont'd

	Physical development	Sensory-motor development	Speech and adaptive behavior	Personal-social development
15 months	First upper and lower molars erupt at 10 to 16 months	Walks alone with feet wide apart for broad base and takes short, flat-footed steps Can get into standing position unassisted Creeps up stairs; walks down holding a hand Holds cup with fingers grasped around it but tips it too soon and spills contents frequently Grasps spoon and scrapes it through a dish Cannot fill spoon well and usually empties it before it reaches the mouth Stacks two blocks Loses balance when standing and throwing or turning corners	Vocabulary includes several words, including names Initiates scribblings Jabbers jargon incessantly Takes off shoes Opens boxes; explores in cabinets and closets Pokes fingers and objects in holes Turn pages in a book, but usually more than one at a time Remembers out-of-sight objects	Pats pictures in books and may kiss animals Says "please" and "thank you" Points out or vocalizes wants Indicates when wet or soiled May give up bottle Throws object in refusal or play; has temper; may choose to disobey Attention is easily diverted
18 months	Abdomen still protrudes Has 12 teeth Can control defecation May control urination during the day Maxillary and mandibular cuspids erupt	May walk backwards Goes upstairs one step at a time, holding on to rail Goes down stairs by creeping backward or by scooting and bumping down on buttocks Feeds self partially; pushes chairs around; seats himself Hurls ball without falling Runs, seldom falling, walks, pulling toy on string Builds tower of three to five blocks Scribbles spontaneously and vigorously Manages cup with little spilling Better use of spoon Smears anything that is wet and soft, including stool	Takes off gloves, socks Unzips clothing Points to nose, eye, hair on request Names some objects; carries out directions, such as "on the chair" Has very short attention span; moves quickly from place to place; explores everything he can get into Bye-bye meaningful now, not just a trick or game Enjoys gathering objects together and frequently tries to carry many objects at once	Shows new awareness of strangers Has frequent tantrums in response to frustration Carries and hugs dolls Shows favoritism for selected toys Copies mother in domestic work such as sweeping Dawdles at mealtime May lie awake and seek attention when put to bed Thumb-sucking reaches peak, especially when sleepy Enjoys solitary play or others' activities May cling to a security object such as a blanket Still self-engrossed Exhibits resistance to change of routine and all sudden transitions
2 years	Weight: 26 to 28 pounds (11.79 to 12.70 kg) Height: 32 to 33 inches (81.22 to 83.82 cm) Teeth: approximately 16; second molars erupt at 20 to 30 months Abdomen protrudes less	Steady gait, walking or running; can pick up object floor without falling; squats easily Can kick ball Goes up and down stairs alone Builds tower of six or seven blocks Drinks well from small glass held in one hand Manages spoon well with little spilling Can string beads	Uses voice tone symbolically Jargon discarded; uses three-word sentences Uses pronouns and readily names familiar objects; refers to self by name; uses verbs; sing-song chanting begins Carries out four directives Pulls on a simple garment Points correctly to seven of ten pictures or items	Fears separation from parents "Flirts" Engages in parallel play Shows pride in independence and accomplishments Pulls people to show them objects Verbalizes toilet needs; consistently uses toilet during waking hours; seldom asks for help Does not know right from wrong

Continued.

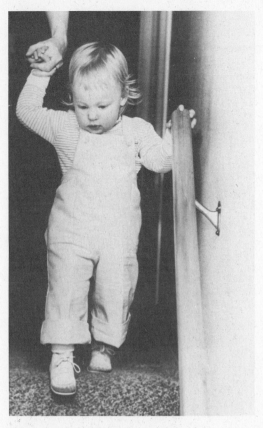

FIG. 2-25
The 15-month-old can walk down stairs with help. (From Phenomena of early development, Columbus, Ohio, Ross Laboratories.)

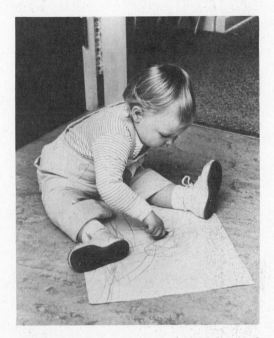

FIG. 2-26
The 15-month-old loves to scribble. (From Phenomena of early development, Columbus, Ohio, Ross Laboratories.)

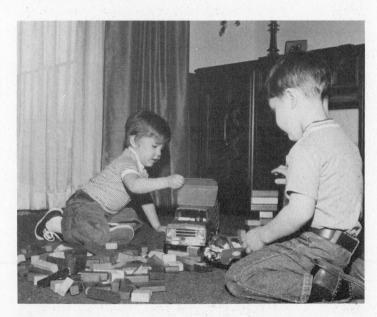

FIG. 2-27
Trucks and blocks are good toy choices for the 2-year-old engaged in parallel play.

TABLE 2-6

Growth and development, birth through adulthood—cont'd

	Physical development	Sensory-motor development	Speech and adaptive behavior	Personal-social development
2 years, cont'd		Imitates vertical and circular strokes with crayon Enjoys gross motor activity, such as running, jumping, climbing, dancing, hand clapping Pushes chair around to climb on it to reach something Begins to know limitations of his power	Turns pages of book one at a time Turns knobs, unscrews lids Repeats things said Washes and dries hands Lines up blocks to make train Cuts with scissors Enjoys simple puzzles Plays with trucks loaded with toys Attention span and memory lengthened Has 300-word vocabulary	Is unable to share possessions easily; knows meaning of "mine" Learns to put toys away Enjoys stories and looking at pictures Mimics parents in play Makes many bedtime demands; has ritual including "security objects" Likes rough play Shows interest in television
2½ years	Has all 20 deciduous teeth	Can jump, walk on tiptoe, and stand on one foot Builds tower of eight blocks Holds pencil in hand, not fist Copies vertical and horizontal lines Likes child's car Can throw a large ball 4 to 5 feet	Repeats two numbers Color sense beginning	Temper tantrums may continue May show interest in genitalia Knows full name
3 years	Height: 37 inches (93.98 cm) Weight: 32 pounds (14.51 kg) Growth begins to slow Nighttime control of bowel and bladder functions	Pedals tricycle Walks up and down stairs, alternating feet Jumps from bottom step Pours fluid from pitcher Hammers pegs into pegboard Builds tower of nine to ten blocks Tries to draw pictures and names them; copies circle Helps dry dishes, dust, set table Feeds self well May brush own teeth Moves with speed and agility	Has vocabulary of 900 words Talks in sentences, often to himself Uses language fluently and confidently Uses plurals in speech Sings simple songs (or television commercials) Knows some nursery rhymes Can repeat three digits Is interested in colors Has conception of time; knows mainly "today" Helps dress himself; can undress himself, unbuttoning side or front buttons Goes to toilet with little assistance Highly imaginative; gives action in picture books Enjoys finer manipulation of play materials Can match simple geometric forms; prefers symmetry Notices missing parts or ken objects and requests parents to "fix" Constantly asks questions: "Why?" What's dat? What cha doin? When, mommy?" Often knows answer Heeds others' thoughts and feelings and expresses own	Knows own sex and some sex differences Plays simple games with others Plays "house" or family games Shares toys Understands taking turns but often impatient Knows own family name Has visual fears of dark or animals Sibling rivalry or jealousy Is still realistic in arranging toys and going to bed Is becoming more manageable by distraction and reason Likes to trade objects Violent rebellions and tantrums less frequent and of shorter duration Father becomes much more important Is friendly and has sense of humor Likes to please parents

Continued.

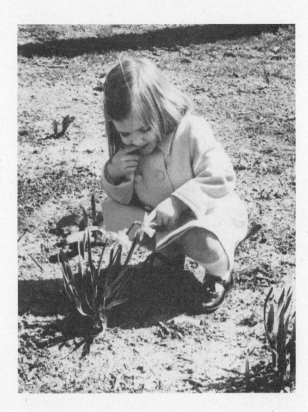

FIG. 2-28
Two-year-olds are fascinated with their environment. (Photo by Florine Rogers, Indianapolis Area Chapter, American National Red Cross.)

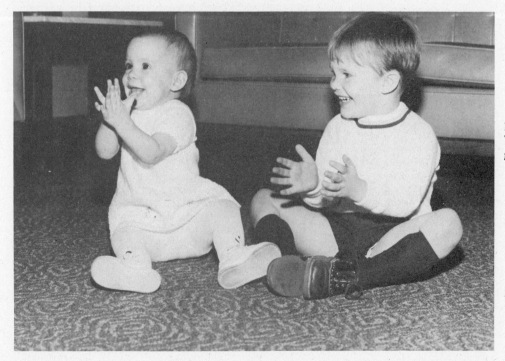

FIG. 2-29
The 3-year-old plays simple games with others.

TABLE 2-6

Growth and development, birth through adulthood—cont'd

	Physical development	Sensory-motor development	Speech and adaptive behavior	Personal-social development
4 years	Birth length doubled Height: 39 to 41 inches (99.16 to 104.14 cm) Weight: 35 to 37 pounds (15.87 to 16.78)	Throws ball overhand Skips clumsily; hops on one leg Copies a square; can cut out pictures Can broad jump and walk a plank Enjoys motor stunts and gross gesturing Can button clothes and lace shoes; distinguishes front	Has vocabulary of 1,500 words or more; may include profanity Has poor space perception Can name one or more colors Can count as high as 3 or 4 Knows which is the longer of two lines Can repeat several numbers in sequence Can go on errands outside of home Perceives analogies; tends to conceptualize and generalize Questioning at its peak; more probing Is beginning to think in consecutive and combinative terms Makes crude comparisons Drawing of man includes head, two limbs, and possibly two eyes Enjoys new activities rather than repeating familiar ones Dramatizes drawings and words Draws first a picture and then names it afterward (often more than one name)	Fact and fiction poorly differentiated Tattles Believes in every detail of Santa Claus Height of Oedipus or Electra complex; boy wants to marry mommy, girl wants to marry daddy Readily relates family tales outside of home Has imaginary companion to whom he projects many of his own feelings and deeds May run away from home Plays cooperatively with larger group of children Games mainly imaginative and of longer duration Is physically and verbally aggressive, selfish, impatient, proud, bossy, dogmatic Uses puns, word play, and clowning to attract attention; tells long stories Is relatively self-reliant in his personal habits Is good at supplying alibis Appraises self and others superficially Likes play with surprises, especially with adults Enjoys television, especially cartoons and commercials
5 years	Height: 43 to 44 inches (109.22 to 111.76 cm) Weight: 40 pounds (18.14 kg)	Can jump rope and roller skate Can run and play games well at same time, such as catch a ball Jumps from three or four steps Can use hammer and hit nail on head Puts toys away neatly May be able to tie shoelaces Skips on alternate feet Can sing relatively well Shows interest and competence in washing dishes Can dance fairly well in time with music "Builds" things out of large boxes Enjoys climbing on jungle gym	Copies triangle Can print first name and possibly other words Can fold paper diagonally Has vocabulary of over 2,000 words Repeats sentences of ten or more syllables Can name at least four colors Asks to have words defined Names days of week Can determine which of two weights is heavier Counts to 10; can add up to sums of 5 Requires less supervision for personal duties than earlier Less imaginative than earlier; interested in actual details	Tells "tall tales" Talks constantly Is interested in the meaning of relatives, such as uncle is mommy's brother Enjoys social contacts and opportunities of kindergarten Dislikes incompleteness; likes to finish what he starts Carries over play projects from one day to the next Play involves acting out concrete situations with familiar people, such as doctor, fireman, mailman, policeman Is dependable, obedient, self-sufficient, helpful in the home, may even look after younger sibling

TABLE 2-6

Growth and development, birth through adulthood—cont'd

	Physical development	Sensory-motor development	Speech and adaptive behavior	Personal-social development
5 years, cont'd		Shows typical hand preference	Seeks to learn physical and social realities Draws fairly complete man, showing differentiation of parts from head to feet Is developing realistic understanding of yesterday and tomorrow An idea in his mind precedes a drawing on paper Questions are fewer and more meaningful; answers to the point Defines objects in terms of use; a ball is to throw; a bike is to ride Begins to collect objects Memory is surprisingly accurate	Remains calm if lost away from home; gives name and address; then entertains self until parents come Is beginning courtesy and tact; sociable Plays with imaginary companions and other children in groups of two to five Enjoys "dress-up" play Has characteristic traits of self-assurance, confidence in others, and conformity Money becomes important—not in itself, but for what it will buy

Continued.

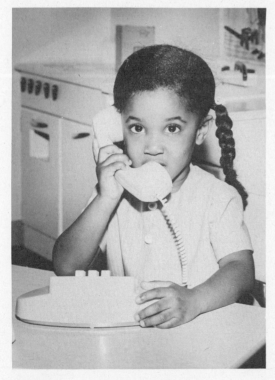

FIG. 2-30
Games of imitation and imagination characterize the 4-year-old's play.

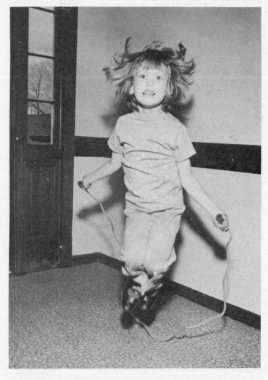

FIG. 2-31
Jumping rope exemplifies the energy and coordination of the 5-year-old.

TABLE 2-6

Growth and development, birth through adulthood—cont'd

	Physical development	Sensory-motor development	Speech and adaptive behavior	Personal-social development
6 years	Height: 44 to 46 inches (111.76 to 116.84 cm) Weight: 45 to 47 pounds (20.41 to 21.31 kg) Sheds central mandibular incisors; 6-year molars erupt Has good appetite Sleeps 12 hours a night Has frequent upper respiratory tract infections	Has improved body balance and control, but is still somewhat clumsy, careless, and restless Play activities are highly physical Uses crayons, pencils, scissors, tape, and glue with skill	Can differentiate between morning and afternoon Knows seasons of the year Religious and death concepts become formed Is involved with fantasy play about church, funerals, Santa Claus, and other highly emotional events Understands right and left Has vocabulary of 2,500 words Can read simple sentences and sound out words Prints letters and numbers Counts by ones, fives, and tens	Loves to have stories read or told to him Fears ghosts, thunder, large animals, and man under bed Tension behavior is common, such as toe-tapping and nail-biting Can bathe and dress with minimal assistance Spilled milk and other mealtime accidents are still common Is interested in sex differences and enjoys babies Father becomes a hero Cannot bear to lose at games and will cheat to win Tattles, bosses, and fights Classroom attention span is short; has trouble sitting still Projects blame on others Has favorite television shows
7 years	Height: 47 to 48 inches (119.38 to 121.92 cm) Weight: 50 to 51 pounds (22.68 to 23.13 kg) Permanent incisors appear and lateral teeth shed Sleeps 10 to 12 hours a night	Play is quieter this year Loves bicycling, swimming, and repeat motor activities	Copies well but has difficulty with spelling Can tell time	Responds well to reason Questions raised often about God and Santa Claus; doubts apparent Takes considerably less help with dressing, bathing, or bedtime Still may take favorite toy to bed Is becoming modest Attention span is longer Play involves male-female roles Alibis replace projected blame Conceptual thinking more apparent
8 years	Height: 48 to 50 inches (121.92 to 127.00 cm) Weight: 57 to 58 pounds (25.85 to 26.30 kg) Lateral teeth erupting Has ravenous appetite; gains weight rapidly Illnesses fewer and less severe	Likes games with gross motor activity and competition More smoothness and noise in games	School work takes on uniformity and neatness; enjoys learning; picks favorite subjects Spatial concepts improve; knows geography of neighborhood; likes trips	Hurries about everything, especially mealtime Does not like to be alone Becomes interested in opposite sex but does not admit it Has "best friends," and secrets become important Enjoys tricks, stunts, and organized sports Develops interest in table games, such as checkers, Monopoly, cards Establishes his collections and swaps with friends

Continued.

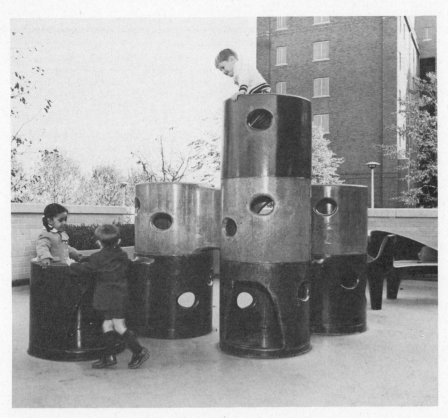

FIG. 2-32
The 6-year-old child enjoys highly physical play and exhibits body balance and control.

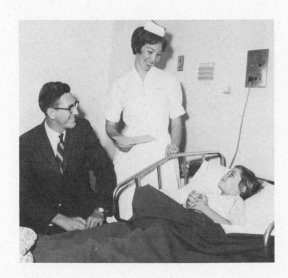

FIG. 2-33
The 7-year-old responds to reasoning.

TABLE 2-6

Growth and development, birth through adulthood—cont'd

	Physical development	Sensory-motor development	Speech and adaptive behavior	Personal-social development
9 years	Height: 52 to 53 inches (132.08 to 134.62 cm) Weight: 62 pounds (28.12 kg) Has excellent appetite Sleeps 10 hours a night	Hand-eye coordination is fully developed Timing and control are more apparent in play Works and plays hard Rests in strange positions	Intellectual capabilities are fairly well defined Puts learning to practical use; reads for information	Completes projects over extended periods of time No longer believes in Santa Claus Has few fears but many worries Likes to please others Is easy to discipline Exercises self-control; is ambitious but realistic Is fairly responsible about his room and possessions Table manners are good, especially when guests are present Is loyal to friends and family Teases friends about "love" and "getting married" Likes clubs with adult leadership Classroom group feeling evolves Is honest and fair; accepts blame; becomes angry if falsely accused
10 years	Height: 54 inches (137.16 cm) Weight: 70 to 71 pounds (31.75 to 32.20 cm) Boys especially are early to bed and to rise; sleep 9 hours Girls may begin to show rounding of hips and softening of the chest	Has greater strength and coorindation in all motor activities	Has broad interests, but is developing special talents Shows interest in social problems, especially cause and effect Can combine time and space concepts Girls are ahead of boys in intellectual development	Suggestions are influential Is happy, casual, relaxed Is full of corny jokes Girls go to bed easier but have trouble falling asleep Likes to spy on opposite sex Becomes lax about hygiene; requires frequent reminders Most know, or learn about intercourse Subordinates own desires for group goals Gets along well with many peers Boys chase girls Play becomes complex Most like singing but boys hate to admit it Good sportsmanship becomes important Hero worships: likes to hear about great men and women Girls are ahead of boys in social maturity

TABLE 2-6

Growth and development, birth through adulthood—cont'd

	Physical development	Sensory-motor development	Speech and adaptive behavior	Personal-social development

11 to 12 years (preadolescence)	Height
	  Boys: 57 inches
	    (144.78 cm)
	  Girls: 56 inches
	    (142.24 cm)
	Weight
	  Boys: 79 to 88 pounds
	    (35.83 to 39.91 kg)
	  Girls: 80 to 92 pounds
	    (36.28 to 41.73 kg)
	Boys are ahead of girls in physical strength and endurance
	Somatic complaints: feet hurt, headache, tired
	Girls may show breast enlargement; some menstruate
	Boys widen, increase in bone size, especially shoulder girdle and ribs; penis and scrotum enlarge
	Has huge appetite, with frequent snacks
		Has excellent athletic skills but tires easily
		Sense of rhythm develops; may learn to dance, but awkwardness is apparent
			Can define abstract terms, such as "justice"
			Understands rationale for hygiene
			Can extract meaning and morals in stories
			Is interested in the how and why of things
			Individuality is expressed in diversion and intellectual pursuits
				Girls giggle; boys "shouldn't cry"
				Is interested in adventure
				Rudeness, devilish unreasonableness
				Wants to postpone bedtime has to be dragged out in the morning
				Helps with household chores after prodding
				Thinks about careers and marriage
				Develops interest in clothes
				Daydreams
				May snuggle up to mother in private
				Family tensions develop over parental nagging
				"Boys against girls" contests are popular
				School is primarily a social experience
				Boys develop interest in girls
				Is strongly influenced by group
				Girls are painfully aware of their appearance
				Is tolerant and diplomatic in social settings

Continued.

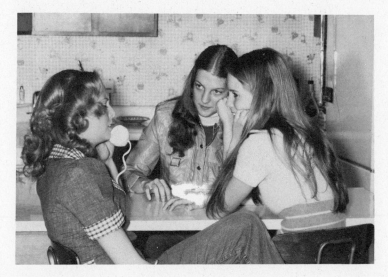

FIG. 2-34
Socialization in adolescence revolves around peer activities. (From Chinn, Peggy L.: Child health maintenance: concepts in family-centered care, ed. 2, St. Louis, 1979, The C.V. Mosby Co.)

TABLE 2-6

Growth and development, birth through adulthood—cont'd

	Physical development	Sensory-motor development	Speech and adaptive behavior	Personal-social development

13 to 14 years (early adolescence)	Height
	  Boys: 5 feet 1 inch to 5 feet 10 inches (154.94 to 177.80 cm)
	  Girls: 5 feet 1 inch to 5 feet 3 inches (154.94 to 160.02 cm)
	Weight
	  Boys: 99 to 122 pounds (44.90 to 55.33 kg)
	  Girls: 103 to 119 pounds (46.72 to 53.97 kg)
	Secondary sex characteristics appear
	Sleep averages 8 to 9 hours a day
	Has excellent appetite, frequent snacks
	May have trouble with obesity or acne
		Sports and dancing are favorite activities
		Mature posturing
		Has increased ease of movement but still has signs of clumsiness
			Is thinking about "the future"
			Analyzes personality of self and others
			Vocabulary is filled with slang and words having special meaning in the peer culture
				Is interested in social problems
				Is friendly, outgoing
				Is interested in appearance
				May want to be alone
				Some masturbate
				Relationships with older siblings improve
				Still argues with younger siblings
				Is independent about schedule of homework and bedtime
				Room is decorated with pennants, sports mementos, emblems, posters
				Assumes household tasks
				May be employed outside home
				Jealously over popularity and privileges
				Sexual interests become more pronounced and open
				Is embarrassed by family in public
				Sports and school clubs are extremely important

15 to 18 years (later adolescence)	Height
	  Boys: 5 feet 10 inches to 6 feet 6 inches (177.80 to 198.12 cm)
	  Girls: 5 feet 3½ inches to 5 feet 10 inches (161.29 to 177.80 cm)
	Weight
	  Boys: 132 to 200 pounds (59.87 to 90.72 kg)
	  Girls: 120 to 150 pounds (54.43 to 68.04 kg)
	Has good appetite; some diet to gain or lose weight
	Boys shave regularly; have good physique; some have acne
	Girls appear mature; have few menstrual problems
	Sleeps late on weekends and during vacations
		Has adult sensory-motor development
		Moves with grace and poise
			College and vocational plans become solidified
			Makes greatest strides toward learning to live in adult society
			Has refined peer group language skills
				Is extroverted; independent in hygiene, clothes purchases
				Many have jobs, drive cars
				Dating is major activity for many
				Can evaluate own emotions
				Jokes, has good humor
				Is highly competitive
				May masturbate
				Experiments with kissing, petting; some engage in intercourse
				Automobile takes on social significance
				Parental relationship improves, especially with mother
				Just "running around" in groups is popular activity
				Eating is important in socialization

19 to 22 years				Leaves family Fantasies about adulthood are abandoned Peers provide structure that family provided earlier Friendships are highly charged with emotions that are seldom shared openly

TABLE 2-6

Growth and development, birth through adulthood—cont'd

	Physical development	Sensory-motor development	Speech and adaptive behavior	Personal-social development
23 to 28 years				Reaching out to others is important Avoids emotional extremes Is devoted to mastering world Acquires mentor who is 8 to 15 years older as patron and supporter Feels need to settle down
29 to 34 years				Life begins to look more painful Self-reflection turns up doubts and raises questions Social life declines Marital satisfaction wanes Spouse may be viewed as obstacle to freedom Infidelity and divorce rise Materialism and crassness are common Struggle between stability and freedom occurs Women strive for generativity
35 to 43 years				Becomes aware that time is running out Explosive, unstable period; values are open to reexamination and change Mentors are abandoned; tendency to want to become "one's own man" Blames parents for unresolved problems Sees this period as last chance to "make it" in career Period ends by trend toward nurturing, teaching and serving younger individuals
44 to 50 years	Physical pursuits decline with decline in energy Chronic illness increases Menopause and male climacteric may occur	Visual and hearing acuity decline		Life settles down Select values and friends get attention Spouse becomes important sympathizer Men find both younger and older women appealing Money becomes less important Children leave home; women may go back to work Increased thinking about death

Continued.

TABLE 2-6

Growth and development, birth through adulthood—cont'd

	Physical development	Sensory-motor development	Speech and adaptive behavior	Personal-social development
50 to 60 years				Feelings are softened Emotionally laden situations are avoided Is preoccupied with everyday things Has little concern for past and future
60 to 70 years	Energy further declines Chronic health problems compound	Increased vision and hearing difficulties		Future seems limited Social contacts decline Friends die; many women are widowed Income may be reduced by retirement adjustments
70 years and over	Physical health may be poor; frailty, disability and invalidism are apparent Activity declines		Mental processes are slowed	Is oriented to past May experience boredom and loneliness

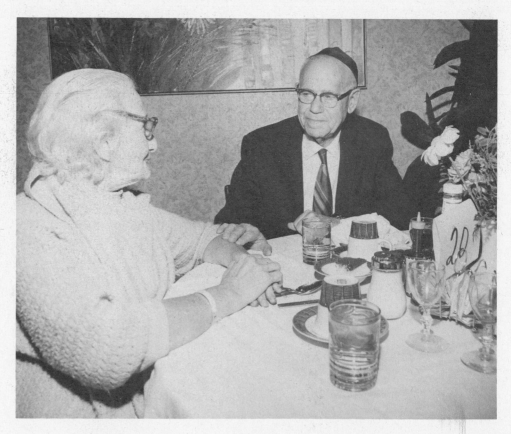

FIG. 2-35
Sharing the contentment of retirement and a secure loving relationship is a rich and beautiful experience for an elderly couple.

References

1. American Medical Association: Quality of life: the middle years, Acton, Mass., 1974, Publishing Sciences Group, Inc.
2. Anderson, Helen C.: Newton's geriatric nursing, ed. 5, St. Louis, 1971, The C.V. Mosby Co.
3. Atchley, Robert C.: The social forces in later life: an introduction to social gerontology, Belmont, Calif., 1972, Wadsworth Publishing Co., Inc.
4. Bernard, Harold W.: Human development in Western culture, ed. 2, Boston, 1966, Allyn & Bacon, Inc.
5. Havighurst, Robert J.: Developmental tasks and education, ed. 3, New York, 1972, David McKay Co., Inc.
6. Kaluger, George, and Kaluger, Meriem Fiar: Human development: the span of life, ed. 2, St. Louis, 1979, The C.V. Mosby Co.
7. Kimmel, Douglas C.: Adulthood and aging, an interdisciplinary development in the first five years of life: a review of recent research, Rockville, Md., 1970, U.S. Public Health Service, Pub. No. 2057.
8. Knobloch, Hilda, and Pasamanick, Benjamin. In Gessell and Amatruda: Developmental diagnosis: the evaluation and management of normal and abnormal neuropsychologic development in infancy and early childhood, ed. 3, New York, Harper & Row, Publishers.
9. Kohlberg, Lawrence: Moral stages and moralization: the cognitive developmental approach. In Lickona, T., editor: Moral development and behavior, New York, 1976, Holt, Rinehart & Winston, Inc.
10. Kübler-Ross, Elisabeth: On death and dying, New York, 1969, Macmillan, Inc.
11. Levinson, Daniel J., and others: The seasons of a man's life, New York, 1978, Alfred A. Knopf, Inc.
12. Piaget, Jean: Six psychological studies, New York, 1968, Random House, Inc.
13. Watson, Judy: Unpublished paper on growth and development, birth through adolescence, 1966.

Additional readings

Alexander, Theron: Human development in an urban age, Englewood Cliffs, N.J., 1973, Prentice-Hall, Inc.

Biehler, Robert: Child development: an introduction, Boston, 1976, Houghton Mifflin Co.

Blewett, Laura J.: To die at home, Am. J. Nurs. **70:**2602-2604, 1970.

Easson, William: The dying child: the management of the child or adolescent who is dying, Springfield, Ill., Charles C Thomas, Publisher.

Goldfogel, Linda: Working with the parent of a dying child, Am. J. Nurs. **70:**1674-1679, 1970.

Gould, Roger, and others: New light on adult life cycles, Time, April 28, 1975, p. 69.

Kübler-Ross, Elisabeth: What is it like to be dying? Am. J. Nurs. **71:**54-61, 1971.

Lichtenberg, Philip, and Norton, Delores G.: Cognitive and mental development in the first five years of life: a review of recent research, Rockville, Md., 1970, U.S. Public Health Service, Pub. No. 2057.

Maxwell, Sister Marie Bernadette: A terminally ill adolescent and her family, Am. J. Nurs. **72:**925-927, 1972.

The middle years (series), Am. J. Nurs. **75:**993-1024, 1975.
   Diekelmann, Nancy: Emotional tasks of the middle adult, pp. 997-1001.
   Diekelmann, Nancy, and Galloway, Karen: A time of change, pp. 994-996.
   Dresen, Sheila E.: The full life, pp. 1008-1011.
   Dresen, Sheila E.: The sexually active middle adult, pp. 1001-1005.
   Galloway, Karen: The change of life, pp. 1006-1011.
   Granquist, Joanne F.: A faculty member reflects, pp. 1022-1024.
   Johnson, Linda: Living sensibly, pp. 1012-1016.
   Owen, Bernice Doyle: Coping with chronic illness, pp. 1016-1018.
   Prock, Valencia N.: The mid-stage woman, pp. 1019-1022.

Neugarten, Bernice: Time, age and the life cycle, Am. J. Psychiatr. **136:**887-893, 1979.

Redl, Frances: The plight of dying patients in the hospitals, Am. J. Nurs. **71:**1988-1990, 1971.

Redl, Frances: Pre-adolescents: what makes them tick? New York, 1968, Child Study Association of America.

Schusler, Clara, and Ashburn, Shirley: The process of human development, a holistic approach, Boston, 1980, Little, Brown & Co.

Senn, Milton J.E., and Solnit, Albert J.: Problems in child behavior and development, Philadelphia, 1968, Lea & Febiger.

Foundations of clinical practice

Stone, L. Joseph, and Church, Joseph: Childhood and adolescence, a psychology of the growing person, ed. 3, New York, 1973, Random House, Inc.

Stone, Virginia: Give the older person time, Am. J. Nurs. **69:**2124-2127, 1969.

Waechter, Eugenia H.: Children's awareness of fatal illness, Am. J. Nurs. **71:**1168-1172, 1971.

Whitehurst, Grover, and Vasta, Ross: Child behavior, Boston, 1977, Houghton Mifflin Co.

3 Role of the family in client development

At birth the overwhelming percentage of human beings become members of a family. A family is the structural unit of society and serves as a nurturing center for the human personality. The physical environment of the home is responsible for facilitating, inhibiting, developing, or modifying inherited behavioral tendencies. The family and the home are the traditional settings for biological reproduction and for maintaining and socializing the human organism.

Types of families

A family must possess the essential characteristics of togetherness in the same household body and of sharing the same value system. There are several basic types of families in today's society.

The *nuclear family* is the most common type of family and is composed of parents and children living in the same immediate environment. The children are usually descendants of the parents, but they may also be adopted or receiving foster care. The majority of nuclear families are considered *patriarchal,* or headed by a man. This concept of a man's being the master of his house has, however, been challenged in recent years by the women's liberation movement, which has given attention to the subject of equality in marriage as well as in the larger society. The movement's emphasis has been focused on giving the woman an integral partnership in the home, not merely the role of subservient housewife and mother.

A nuclear family may be a single-parent family through adoption, the absence of either spouse by marriage failure, death, or prolonged separation. A mother or father assumes total responsibility for both male and female parent roles, sometimes supported by others who contribute to child care.

Unmarried couples of opposite sexes are increasingly becoming apparent in these decades of the new morality. These couples live together, may bear children, and essentially carry out all aspects of family life usually confined to marriage. The relationships are often temporary because of social, financial, or other external pressures but may develop into marriage or at least a stable, rather permanent arrangement.

The *extended family* consists of a nuclear family group plus blood-related relatives sharing common privileges and responsibilities. Grandparents, aunts, uncles, and cousins may compose this type of family.

Matriarchal families are headed by a woman and are usually one-parent groups. They are often associated with the lower socioeconomic segment of society but generally are stable institutions. Uncles of children are often responsible for the masculine role relationships. Illegitimate births, divorces, and extended separations of married couples help foster matriarchal families.

Communes are rare but nevertheless are truly families. Communes are large groups of individuals residing in close proximity and sharing the same value orientation. Members may be of varied ages, but it is not uncommon that all members are of the same generation. Conjugal relationships may or may not exist within the commune. Interdependence typifies the role relationships of such groups. Communes are often founded by individuals choosing to avoid the mainstream of society with its rather fixed pattern of life-style and routine. They seek satisfaction and comfort in the isolation of their "own kind." The Harmonist movement and other similar religious efforts at communal life marked the history of early United States when persons felt the need to escape and seek identity and meaning for life outside the prevailing social order. In the 1970s such groups once again commanded attention as persons groped for security and acceptance in a highly complex and sometimes bewildering societal environment. However, they are declining in popularity and represent an almost insignificant number in our current population.

The *homosexual family* cannot be overlooked as we examine contemporary living patterns. This type of relationship consists of members of the same gender who share a bond of intimacy and interdependence and the anticipation of a long-lasting relationship similar to marriage. The partners in the homosexual family may carry out roles and relationships typical of the heterosexual couple.

There are surely other types of living patterns that could be termed families. The reason for discussing the last two kinds of familial relationships is to demonstrate that the essential meaning and intentions of family life can be achieved in varied ways.

Family roles

Family living has always been associated with definite roles in any given society. Procreation and child rearing, nurturing, and learning are among the essential tasks of any type of family group. Although social, cultural, ethnic, and economic factors have influenced the ways in which these roles have been assumed throughout history, this basic role pattern has remained relatively constant.

PARENTING

Parenthood is an extremely vital role in our society, and yet it is often undertaken with little or no preparation. Traditionally it has been assumed that child rearing ''came naturally'' and that instinct would provide the resources essential for the role of mother or father. It is important to appreciate parenting as an experience for the adults as well as a set of behaviors designed to assist the child's education and welfare.

The assumption of marriage means that two independent adults become interdependent and that their welfare is now a shared concern. When there is knowledge of conception and the anticipation of the birth of a child, each of the partners must relinquish his or her own independence a bit further to accommodate the new family member.

Marital partners are products of unique family backgrounds, customs, and childhood experiences that influence attitudes on child rearing and other responsibilities associated with parenting. Seldom, however, are novice parents able to appreciate the potential impact of their offspring on their personalities and patterns of living. Parenthood is a career—not just a phase of life.

It is beyond the scope of this book to discuss indepth theories and techniques of parenting, but a nurse in any setting must be prepared to appreciate the multiplicity of factors that gives clues to parenting problems as demonstrated in encounters related to nursing care.

PROCREATION AND CHILD REARING

The loving relationships of a stable family provide the ideal place for procreation and child rearing. A child who is conceived through sexual expression of a couple's love is indeed fortunate in the advent of his life. The giving and receiving of love forms the basis for security and *trust,* the infant's first developmental goal. In the companionship and stimulation of the family the infant begins to respond to his parents. He smiles when he is approached and coos, gurgles, and laughs as he learns to interpret their loving care. It is this love found in the warmth and security of his family that will sustain him through the critical periods of his childhood. ''Learning to love is a lifetime achievement. It begins in infancy, flowers in the teens and twenties, bears fruit in the rich full years of childbearing and rearing, and colors and warms the rest of life.''[2]

A family is the link between one generation and the next. The quality of a particular pattern of life is transmitted by the family. Since each unit has its unique characteristics—genetic, physical, religious, racial, ethnic, economic, political, and educational—it is the source of a child's basic value system. The family controls a member's early relationships, and the disciplinary practices encountered in the home shape his concept of what is right. The continuity of companionship and products of associations in the home, whether they be positive or negative, influence each member's character. *The family is the most potent influence during the formative years of early childhood and seems to be the most important determinant of behavior during the life cycle.* ''Behavior tendencies internalized in childhood, in the home, may persist psychologically even when the home has been left far behind in time and space.''[4]

NURTURE

The family is the source of both the physical and emotional nurture, or nourishment, of its members. When a child is born, he must rely on his parents for all basic needs such as food, clothing, and shelter. The home and family life is by design the fundamental purveyor of nurture, since it is the primary and often exclusive environment of the dependent child.

Love is the basis for nurture and the central force that holds family members

Foundations of clinical practice

FIG. 3-1
Family life experience of early childhood provides a foundation for the development of a sense of love and security. (From Sobol, Evelyn G., and Robischon, Paulette: Family nursing: a study guide, ed. 2, St. Louis, 1975, The C. V. Mosby Co.)

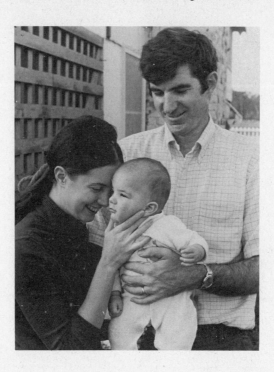

together. Family unity is characterized by understandings that allow each member continued acceptance despite their negative characteristics or shortcomings. In this unique nurturing environment of the family, a member has a ready refuge in the time of distress or danger, loneliness or sadness. For example, a child who is rejected or hurt by his playmates runs home for protection and comfort. A criminal, although despised and alienated from the mainstream of society, is usually not abandoned by parents, spouse, and children, who have an emotional investment in him. A young couple whose marriage fails may each return to their parents for security until certain adjustments are made. A family is the hallmark of the ''unchanging'' in a world characterized by change on every front. Family unity of purpose makes nurture possible, and nurture, in turn, maintains this unity.

The family's role in meeting basic human needs is explored in considerable detail throughout the remainder of this text.

LEARNING   The family is the source of primary learning for its members.

From the first experiences of infancy and throughout childhood and adulthood, individuals learn from experiences within the family unit. Sharing emotions in daily living teaches members the meaning of love, anger, fear, and hostility. How to interpret human expression and acquire meaningful ways to communicate feelings are important learning tasks begun in childhood and built on throughout life.

Understandings and values important to daily living are formulated in the family home. Attitudes and feelings that accompany foods and family mealtime eventually influence a child's pattern of nutrition. The extent to which cleanliness is stressed is an important factor in a child's ultimate health value system. Behavioral coping patterns of family members as they interact are strong determinants of a growing child's mental health development. These are only a few examples to emphasize the strategic role of the family in early childhood learnings important to growth and development.

"One of the primary functions of the family, in almost all parts of the world, is to teach the child the rules and patterns of living of the particular segment of society into which he is born. It may also teach him something about the ways of the wider society in which he may eventually participate. This process is known as acculturation or socialization: raising the child to learn and accept the ways of his particular culture or society."[4] The family, although not the exclusive route of transmitting traditions and conventions necessary for coping with life and work in society, is still the primary determinant in the acquisition of such socialization skills. Poise, politeness, mealtime manners, and exhibiting respect for others are examples of practices parents teach their children so that they may be well accepted by nonfamily associates.

The changing society and the family

Scarcely more than a century ago the family was almost the exclusive institution in society for meeting life's basic needs, for primary social contact, and for learning. In this decade 60% of the U.S. population are not members of nuclear families in their domestic life-style arrangement.

The traditional nuclear family seems to be losing ground as the "nurtural center" for human life. Parents and children spend less time together as a unit today because of the many factors that have changed or influenced life style. Rapid transportation, television, growing educational systems, and social pressures resulting from a fast-moving, complex society have drawn persons away from home for more hours per day. It is not uncommon in American homes to find every member of the family pursuing a unique schedule for meals, recrea-

FIG. 3-2
Children learn traditions and develop social skills in family life experience.

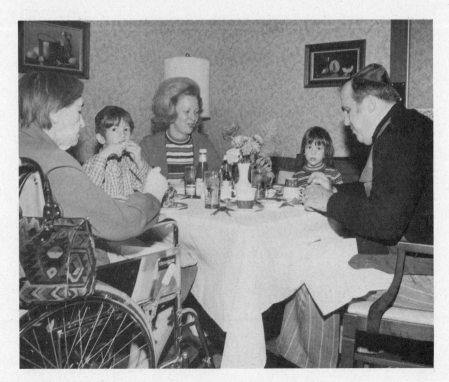

Foundations of clinical practice

tion, and social engagements. Besides school and employment commitments, the Scouts, the PTA, the bowling team, basketball practice, and music lessons demand that the individual family members be with peers outside the household for a significant portion of time each day, leaving less time for interaction as a unit. *"The greater the social heterogeneity to which the family is subjected, the weaker its own internal integration will become."* [1]

Nursery schools, kindergartens, and an elaborate system of elementary and secondary school education have shifted much of the responsibility and influence for learning away from the family. Even educational television vies with parents for a child's learning interests.

Although the family unit has the primary role in assuring that basic needs will be met, it is obvious in our heterogeneous society that some families are not fully able to assume all their roles. The reasons are multiple and include emotional instability of parents, economic plight, confinement of parents outside the home because of employment and illness, and lack of human and material resources. In situations where children do not have the opportunities for meeting their basic physical and psychosocial needs, governmental agencies have chosen to become involved in solving selected problems. Headstart, a preschool program designed to prepare a deprived child for the experiences in the first grade of a regular school system, is one example. School lunch programs, community health clinics, and various welfare benefits are directed toward closing the gap between what the child needs and what the family can or will provide. Throughout each chapter community resources are explored in view of their role in supplementing family resources in promotion and maintenance of healthy family living.

In the view of our contemporary society the family still is the primary unit of influence, but depending on its own integration, it functions with varying degrees of success in meeting its members' basic needs. If individual satisfaction is not achieved within the home and family, members will seek outside resources in the quest for meaning in their lives. Interaction with subgroups that are able to fulfill needs and expectations for love, security, and primary socialization may eventually become a more powerful influence in the members' lives than interaction with their own families. Many authorities believe that the nuclear family is losing influence with its members and that such a decline in family power could have serious consequences on sociocultural development in future generations. Many outside influences will continue to modify the role of the family and the home during this and subsequent decades and will have important implications for human growth and development in our society, but it is anticipated that the central motivation and meaning for life will continue to arise from family orientation.

Family assessment

It is important that nurses understand the factors that are inherent in families that tend to influence their ability to deal with health problems. It is relatively easy, it seems, to identify problems in the family unit (such as absence of a parent, poverty, multiple stresses), but more difficult to identify *strengths*. A family strength is a factor or force that contributes to family unity and solidarity and fosters developmental potential inherent within the family.[3]

3   Role of the family in client development

Research has shown certain family phenomena to be healthy or positive. It is valuable to know what characteristics of family life can thus be considered strengths.

A family home that provides sufficient space for all members' activity and privacy is desirable. When members of the group have specific interdependent roles in carrying out daily tasks (chores) of the household, it is apparent that there is an appreciation for the family life experience. Flexibility in roles is also valuable. The ability of one member to take on the responsibilities of others in their absence is indicative of family integrity. Babysitting by teenagers for their younger siblings so that parents can enjoy an evening away from home together demonstrates an appreciation for the needs of individual family subsystems without compromising family solidarity. Furthermore, such a pattern is exemplary of a developmental experience, particularly valuable to younger members. Sharing responsibility for internal welfare of the unit is to be viewed as a family strength.

The ability of members to communicate openly and honestly with each other is a salient characteristic of a strong family. Listening carefully and with sensitivity is as important as verbalization. Research has shown that it is a definite asset when the family joins its forces in identifying and coping with a problem or stress and when there is consensual decision making.

An emotional support system within the family unit is crucial for its welfare. Ego strength of individual members is strongly influenced by the quality of feedback that they receive from others within the home. Encouragement, praise, and recognition for various efforts is considered a strength. The consistency with which individuals can depend on others is also vital. If the emotional climate changes frequently from warm and loving to cold and hostile or indifferent, it is not feasible to expect that any member would count on family resources for meeting ego needs, and thus outside help would be solicited or the needs would go unmet. If external resources are used with regularity to meet emotional needs of any member, the nurse should note these instances as "significant" since these "outsiders" would also be influential components when establishing a problem-solving framework essential to the management of health problems.

The parenting roles must be an important part of the marriage relationship but not its totality for optimal personal growth of the partners. It is considered highly desirable when each parent pursues his or her own growth-producing relationship or experience to complement those inherent within the family structure. Mothers and fathers whose own personalities and creative potentials are challenged will be better able to stimulate and encourage their children in such directions.

A physically and mentally healthy family tends to be more resistant to negative forces from the outside world that could threaten its equilibrium. Families who have multiple stresses or problems within their structures are considered vulnerable to even further crises. In short, one problem leads to another. Good physical and mental health is an important factor in helping members enjoy and profit from life experiences that promote developmental task achievement. Somatic complaints or problems that can be identified as peculiar to subgroups in the family (such as children or the elderly) should be noted, since they may be indicative of some dysfunctional interaction within the unit. For example, tired, overweight teenagers may point to the need for health instruction that is related to rest, activity, and nutrition. Children who achieve poorly in school may reflect lack of privacy or a disturbing influence at home that impedes their ability to study and concentrate on learning. Nurses should be alert to these indices, since they may be important keys to a problem of the family unit and its life-style.

Strong families tend to engage in growth-producing relationships and experiences as a unit, both at home and in the larger community. The ability of a family to maintain and build significant relationships fosters enrichment of members, individually and collectively. Furthermore, when the family assumes an active position in the church, school, or other community organizations, children learn to appreciate the factors that comprise responsible citizenship. They begin to appreciate the reciprocal nature of giving and receiving, and the rewards of sharing conflicts, satisfactions, and joys. As families reach outside their bounds, both individual and collective strengths can be reinforced, and internal unity, solidarity, and loyalty enhanced. Family integration seems to be

---

FAMILY ASSESSMENT GUIDE

A. Physical environment
1. Does the home provide ample living and play space for all members?
2. Is there privacy potential for all individuals?
3. Are living conditions safe, sanitary, and comfortable?

B. Communication
1. Is there openness and freedom in family communications?
2. Is there evidence of sensitive listening and expression of concern among members?
3. Is decision making a shared responsibility?
4. Are family conflicts and stresses identified and acknowledged?
5. Does it seem or appear that the family has a set of rules that govern communication and interpersonal relationships?

C. Emotional support system
1. Do members express support and concern for each other (such as giving encouragement, praise, or recognition)? Are they close to each other?
2. Is the emotional climate stable? Does it change with the entry or exit of certain individuals?
3. What family member sets the tone of emotions in the household? Are humor and fun acceptable?
4. What member (such as grandparent, minister, social worker, or friend) within the

household, extended family, neighborhood, or community is the resource in times of crisis?

D. Marital relationship
1. Are roles in the marital relationship complementary, supplementary, symmetrical, or parallel?
2. Are marital roles limited to parenting?

E. Physical and mental health status
1. Are there health-related complaints among family members?
2. Are there specific health problems (physical or mental)?
3. Are somatic complaints or problems developmentally related? Infancy? Childhood? Adolescence? Old age?
4. Is there enough rest, activity, and exercise for all members?
5. Are there specific times for privacy and for time together?

F. Growth-producing relationships and experiences
1. Is there evidence of a specific activity or experience (such as camping, mealtime, shopping, church attendance, or sports) that is mutually satisfying to family members?
2. Does the family move outside the family circle to find joys and satisfactions or to meet needs?
3. Do family members exhibit flexibility in filling each other's roles or functioning?
4. Are crises used as growth experiences?

---

strengthened and its traditions and values reinforced when confronted from the outside by disturbing phenomena.

Family strengths are not isolated variables but are dynamic and interrelated, varying with the developmental tasks of the family.[3] Nurses can be more instrumental in helping families if they appreciate the characteristics of a family and recognize whether the involved family members are aware of their own strengths and resources. In addition, a nurse may also be the stimulus who identifies and mobilizes latent or unrecognized potential strengths. The use of a helping relationship in a distributive or episodic health plan depends on the wise use of family strengths. It is imperative, therefore, that practitioners in all settings assess families as well as individual clients in the course of nursing care planning (see family assessment guide on opposite page).

Family development

Because a family is the nucleus of most life experiences, it is important to explore how families begin, grow, and change to satisfy the needs of their members. These specific aspects of the dynamic family role are predictable in their time-order sequence and their effect on an individual member's growth and development. The expected pattern of family development can be defined in terms of family developmental tasks:

> A developmental task is a task which arises at or about a certain period in the life of an individual, successful achievement of which leads to his happiness and to success with later tasks, while failure leads to unhappiness in the individual, disapproval by the society, and difficulty with later tasks.[2]

These tasks originate from human physical maturation, sociocultural environmental forces, self-aspiration, and acquired values. For example, when an individual is physically mature and has acquired sufficient tools for economic stability, he is expected to marry and within a family to rear children. Although developmental tasks seem strongly influenced by culture, they are not an externally imposed obligation but a goal-directed privilege that a person assumes for his or her own development.

Family developmental tasks describe the maintenance roles and dominant goals of the various stages or phases in the family life cycle. They are used as an index to appraise how successfully a given family unit is contributing to a positive societal structure while concurrently meeting the needs of its various members. Obviously, therefore, achievement of family developmental tasks depends on its members' achieving their individual developmental satisfactions.

PHASES AND STAGES
Establishment phase

"The establishment phase of the family life cycle begins with the couple at marriage and continues until they become aware of the fact that the wife is pregnant."[2] When a nuclear family is formed, it consists of a married couple, usually in their early twenties. They extend the interdependent relationship that they have initiated and maintained during their courtship. Through intimate contact in their new home they learn to know each other better and to acquaint themselves with extended family ties. Relatives and in-laws as well as neighbors become a significant part of their newly created social horizons.

Foundations of clinical practice

In young married couples it is not unusual for the husband and wife to face conflicting role responsibilities. These may result from economic stress imposed by the completion of the education of one or both partners or by military service requirements. The husband and wife who must cope with these forces have a real conflict as they divide their attention between study time, military drills, part-time jobs, and the establishment of a meaningful marriage and a home.

Newly married couples find much joy related to establishing their new home. Shopping for furniture and other household articles, using wedding gifts for the first time, and meeting each other's friends bring much pleasure and satisfaction. All these experiences help them know one another better and form a realistic basis for future family building responsibilities.

Family developmental tasks
1. Establishing a home base in a place to call their own.
2. Establishing mutually satisfactory systems for getting and spending money.
3. Establishing mutually acceptable patterns of who does what and who is accountable to whom.
4. Establishing a continuity of mutually satisfying sex relationships.
5. Establishing systems of intellectual and emotional communication.
6. Establishing workable relationships with relatives.
7. Establishing ways of interacting with friends, associates, and community organizations.
8. Facing the possibility of children and planning for their coming.
9. Establishing a workable philosophy of life as a couple.[2]

Expectant phase   ''The expectant phase of the beginning family starts with the awareness that the wife is pregnant and continues until the birth of the first child.''[2] This relatively short time period is filled with a series of reactions determined by the emotional, social, and economic readiness for the child by the couple as individuals and as a unit. During these months they make the necessary preparations for parenthood. The joys of anticipation of a baby, representative of their mutual and intimate love, usually overshadow any ambivalence about the expectant phase.

Family developmental tasks
1. Reorganizing housing arrangements to provide for the expected baby.
2. Developing new patterns for getting and spending income.
3. Evaluating procedures for determining who does what and where authority rests.
4. Adapting patterns of sexual relationships to pregnancy.
5. Expanding communication systems for present and anticipated emotional constellations.
6. Reorienting relationships with relatives.
7. Adapting relationships with friends, associates, and community activities to the realities of pregnancy.
8. Acquiring knowledge about and planning for the specifics of pregnancy, childbirth, and parenthood.
9. Testing and maintaining a workable philosophy of life.[2]

Childbearing stage   ''The child-bearing stage of the family life cycle begins with the birth of the first baby and continues until the firstborn is in pre-school.''[2] It includes the joys of the new life in the home and the conflicts of integrating a new member into an intimate relationship. It is not uncommon for the marriage partners to resent a

FIG. 3-3
Fathers may share responsibility in the care of the child. (Photo by Florine Rogers, Indianapolis Area Chapter, American National Red Cross.)

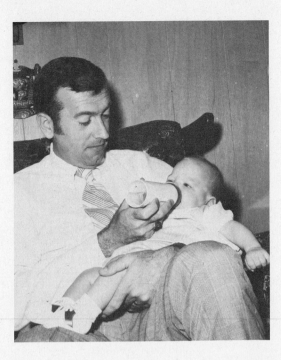

FIG. 3-3
Fathers may share responsibility in the care of the child. (Photo by Florine Rogers, Indianapolis Area Chapter, American National Red Cross.)

division of attention with the child when each has previously enjoyed the exclusive attention of the other.

Accepting the increasing responsibilities of meeting the young child's physical and emotional needs while continuing to build the marriage and home is not easy for parents but affords, in most cases, innumerable satisfactions.

Family developmental tasks
1. Adapting housing arrangements for the life of the little child.
2. Meeting the costs of family living at the childbearing stage.
3. Reworking patterns of responsibility and accountability.
4. Reestablishing mutually satisfying sexual relationships.
5. Refining intellectual and emotional communication systems for childbearing and rearing.
6. Reestablishing working relationships with relatives.
7. Fitting into community life as a young family.
8. Planning for further children in the family.
9. Reworking a suitable philosophy of life as a family.[2]

Preschool stage

The preschool stage includes elements of the childbearing stage and considerations for a family with a child between 2½ and 5 years of age. During this period the possibility exists that a second or third baby will be born before the first has reached school age. The tasks of the preschool stage primarily involve the many considerations associated with the expanding family, especially factors necessary for meeting the basic needs of both child and adult members.

Family developmental tasks
1. Supplying adequate space, facilities, and equipment for the expanding family.
2. Meeting predictable and unexpected costs of family life with small children.
3. Sharing responsibilities within the expanding family.

Foundations of clinical practice

4. Maintaining mutually satisfying sexual relationships and planning for future children.
5. Creating and maintaining effective communications within the family.
6. Cultivating relationships within the extended family.
7. Tapping resources and serving needs outside the family.
8. Facing dilemmas and reworking philosophies of life.[2]

School-age stage

"The stage of the family life cycle characterized by school-age children starts when the first child goes to school, at five to six years of age, and continues until he or she becomes a teenager at thirteen."[2] As the school-age child expands his world to include new friends and activities, the family must often adjust to a hectic schedule. There are school and club activities, friends coming and going, and innumerable family members' projects in various stages of completion. At the same time the family unit attempts to maintain order and integrity and meet its own responsibilities. Parents must learn to find their joys in those of their children and at the same time grow in their relationship as a married couple. The quality of social interplay of a family unit during this stage seems to have considerable bearing on the child's emotional development and his eventual response to the family sphere of influence when he becomes a teenager.

Family developmental tasks

1. Providing the parents' needs for privacy, quiet, and order during the children's vigorous years.
2. Keeping financially afloat while the family nears the flood stage of its needs.
3. Cooperating to get things done.
4. Continuing to satisfy each other as married partners.
5. Elaborating communication systems within the expanding family.
6. Feeling close to relatives in the larger family.
7. Tying in with life outside the family.
8. Testing and retesting family philosophies of life.[2]

Teenage stage

The teenage stage of a family continues from the time the firstborn child is 13 years of age until he departs from the home as a young adult. These years are the most difficult to cope with for many parents. The teenager as an emerging adult is making many of his own decisions and is strongly influenced by his peer group relationships. In many cases the teenager is beginning to seriously contemplate marriage and family living while still caught up in completing his own education. Parents are probably in their forties and are not ready to emancipate their child, although they recognize his growing need for independence. Some parents, in addition, begin to face a decline in their own physical prowess at the same time that they realize their child is fast becoming more involved in his private world than in that of the family.

Family developmental tasks

1. Providing facilities for widely different needs.
2. Working out money matters in the family with teenagers.
3. Sharing responsibilities of family living.
4. Putting the marriage relationship in focus.
5. Bridging the communication gap.
6. Keeping in touch with relatives.
7. Widening horizons of teenagers and their parents.
8. Coping with the hazards, challenges, and dilemmas of teenagers' fami-

3 Role of the family in client development

Launching stage

lies in ways that preserve the positive values of families through the teen years.[2]

The launching stage is heralded by the event of the firstborn's leaving home for a job, college, military service, or in some cases marriage. Although younger children may still be at home, it is usually traumatic for parents to admit that their child is establishing his own life outside their home. Although they may feel satisfaction in the accomplishments that have brought the child to this point in life, they are ambivalent about his true independence. The launching stage extends until the last child departs from home, leaving the parents alone once again. Obviously the launching of an only child or the last child marks a dramatic point in family life and requires a number of adjustments because habits pursued for perhaps 2 decades are broken. The ease of launching the last child is largely determined by the integrity of the couple's relationship with one another. If they are secure in their prospects of a life continuing with rich experiences, the "empty nest" means the freedom and intimacy they have not exclusively enjoyed since the establishment phase.

Family developmental tasks

1. Meeting costs as launching-center families.
2. Reallocating responsibilities among grown and growing children in the family.
3. Coming to terms with themselves and with each other as husband and wife amid the threats of the launching period.
4. Maintaining open systems of communication within the family and between the family and others.
5. Widening the family circle to include the new relatives by marriage within the extended family.
6. Reconciling conflicting loyalties and philosophies of life.[2]

Middle years

The middle years are quite variable in length but extend from the launching of the last child until retirement or death of one of the spouses. It may be the longest stage of the family life cycle, lasting in many cases 16 or more years. During this time parents have the opportunity to grow closer as a couple while maintaining active social contacts including their children's family. Grandchildren, friends, and possibly their own aged parents become active interests. Steps are taken during these middle years to ensure economic security before the onset of the aging years.

Family developmental tasks

1. Maintaining a pleasant and comfortable home.
2. Assuring security for the later years.
3. Carrying household responsibilities.
4. Drawing closer together as a couple.
5. Maintaining contact with grown children's families.
6. Keeping in touch with brothers' and sisters' families and with aging parents.
7. Participating in community life beyond the family.
8. Reaffirming the values of life that have real meaning.[2]

Aging years

The final stage of the family life cycle begins with the wage-earner's retirement and encompasses the death of one spouse and finally the death of the other. These years are rich and satisfying for many couples but less satisfying for others with economic stress, loneliness, and poor health. Some elderly husbands and wives live together in their family home where their children have been nurtured. Others move to smaller homes, apartments, or specialized housing for the elderly, particularly after the death of a spouse.

The elderly family has a difficult role in our contemporary youth-oriented society. Their physical or mental vigor often does not permit them to cope easily with our public transportation scheme. High speeds on freeways may deprive them of a safe automobile-driving environment, and busy airports are merely a confusing place where they feel lost in the fast movement of younger feet. The quick tempo of today's living has forced many of the elderly into isolation from the mainstream of life.

Since women tend to live longer than men, there are traditionally more widows than widowers. Women can manage household tasks if they enjoy good health, but men find it difficult to be independent and yet maintain a comfortable daily routine. Persons living alone may become listless and disinterested in life unless they have regular social contact and active interests. They may neglect hygiene, nutrition, and exercise, thus inviting health problems and illness.

Children or other family members of the elderly may assume some responsibility for assisting them with their basic needs and making them feel an important part of their lives.

The aging stage of the family life cycle is often a curious mixture of reflecting the past and anticipating the future, which holds at most the blessing of a quiet death. Often a deep sense of faith in joining loved ones in death sustains the elderly as they face the inevitable termination of their place in the family life cycle.

If the elderly couple enjoys economic security and good health, their final stage of the life cycle can be an enriching experience. Grandchildren and great-grandchildren may be a source of many hours of pleasure. Travel and other leisure-time activities may provide a reason for living.

For the fortunate couples who live to grow old together, joy may be immeasurable. Warmth of a most mature love and understanding surrounds them as they face the interlude of death and separation. They leave life with the heritage of their children, who will carry on the family traditions and thus extend their being into all future generations.

Family developmental tasks

1. Finding a satisfying home for the later years.
2. Adjusting to retirement income.
3. Establishing comfortable household routines.
4. Nurturing each other as husband and wife.
5. Facing bereavement and widowhood.
6. Caring for elderly relatives.
7. Maintaining contact with children and grandchildren.
8. Keeping an interest in people outside the family.
9. Finding meanings in life.[2]

Childless couples and the single adult

Although we have explored the development of a typical nuclear family across the life span, it must be recognized that not all persons marry and that not all married couples have children.

3 Role of the family in client development

The changing morals of our society have made it more comfortable for persons to meet their sexual role responsibilities without marriage or childbearing. Some couples are deprived the privilege of childbearing because of sterility or infertility. Others choose to voluntarily limit their reproduction for personal reasons. With increasing concern about overpopulation on planet Earth it has become almost a noble gesture to remain childless and do one's part in population control.

Childbearing is a rich and beautiful experience for some, but it is not a requisite for a meaningful marriage or life experience. Many physically complete and emotionally well-adjusted individuals and couples find joys and satisfaction in life apart from reproduction and child rearing and still participate meaningfully in a family life cycle.

From 1970 to 1975 the number of 25- to 34-year-old adults who had never married increased by 50%, according to U.S. Census Bureau reports. One out of four 20- to 35-year-old adults is single.

The choice to marry or to remain single is more realistic in the 1980s. Social pressures of wedlock have declined, and many young adults who have witnessed the miseries of teenage marriage, high divorce rates, and interpersonal trauma may choose to wait before making a lifelong commitment. Career development has also taken precedence over family life for many adults.

Although single adults may choose to live together without marriage, these individuals comprise only 1% of the total population. Single adults who choose to remain unmarried and who are career oriented are usually contented, productive members of our society.

Summary

Since the family is the nurturing center for human personality, the quality of the relationships in day-to-day life are more important than the number or types of persons composing the constellation.

The three basic roles of the family are (1) procreation and child rearing, (2) nurture, and (3) learning. Life-style is a significant determinant of how these functions are regarded and achieved. Although modern society has changed family living patterns considerably, the home continues to be the greatest influence in a child's life.

Developmental tasks for various phases and stages of family life have been formulated and are useful indices for assessing psychosocial needs of individuals and groups and determining their role expectations. *The family is an arena of interaction where each member is striving to achieve his or her unique developmental tasks concurrently with meeting expectations of family tasks.*

References

1. Berelson, Bernard, and Steiner, Gary: Human behavior, New York, 1964, Harcourt Brace Jovanovich, Inc.
2. Duvall, Evelyn M.: Family development, ed. 4, Philadelphia, 1971, J.B. Lippincott Co.
3. Otto, Herbert A.: A framework for assessing family strengths. In Reinhardt, Adina M., and Quinn, Mildred D., editors: Family-centered community nursing: a sociocultural framework, vol. 1, St. Louis, 1973, The C.V. Mosby Co.
4. Singer, Robert D., and Singer, Anne: Psychological development in children, Philadelphia, 1969, W.B. Saunders Co.

Additional readings

Birdwhistell, Ray I.: The idealized model of the American family, Social Casework, April 1970, pp. 195-198.

Hill, Reuben: Generic features of families under stress. In Parad, Howard, editor: Crisis intervention, New York, 1965, Family Association of America, p. 40.

Kaluger, George, and Kaluger, Meriem Fair: Human development: the span of life, ed. 2, St. Louis, 1979, The C.V. Mosby Co.

Kantor, David, and Lehr, William: Inside the family, San Francisco, 1975, Jossey-Bass, Inc., Publishers.

Lidz, Theodore: The effects of children on marriage. In Rosenbaum, Salo, and Alger, Ian, editors: The marriage relationship: psychoanalytic perspectives, New York, 1968, Bacu Books.

McBride, Angela Barron: Can family life survive? Am. J. Nurs. **75:**1648-1653, 1975.

Nye, F. Ivan, and Bernardo, Felix M.: Emerging conceptual frameworks in family analysis, New York, 1966, Macmillan, Inc.

Schuster, Clara, and Asburn, Shirley: The process of human development: a holistic approach, Boston, 1980, Little, Brown & Co.

Sobol, Evelyn G., and Robischon, Paulette: Family nursing: a study guide, ed. 2, St. Louis, 1975, The C.V. Mosby Co.

4 Environment and health problems

The environment has been defined as the "external conditions and influences affecting the life and development of an organism."[23] It has long been established that the environment plays a significant role in man's health. Emphasis has been placed on the inseparability of man and his environment. Since man and the environment are both open systems, they interact with and subsequently tend to influence each other.[8] For example, man takes solids and liquids from the environment and puts back in the environment solid, liquid, and gaseous waste.[12] Man invents machines that exchange matter and energy with the environment. The environment includes not only aspects related to physical conditions but also all other people with whom one comes in contact. This interrelationship is often responsible for the development of health problems. The purpose of this chapter is to describe the effects of physical and social environments on health. Problems associated with the social environment that will be discussed include: accidents, poisonings, drug abuse, smoking, and alcoholism. Because pollution is a threat to health, three types of pollution are discussed: air, water, and noise.

The social environment

ACCIDENTS

Accidents, or sudden unexpected events that result in individual or collective body harm,[22] are the most important physical threats within the environment. They are the fourth leading cause of death in the United States. Among persons in the 14 to 34 age group, accidents are the leading cause of death.

Essential to comprehending accidents is an understanding of the difference between accident repetitiveness, accident liability, and accident proneness. *Accident repetitiveness* is an observed pattern of behavior that may last for varying periods of time.[15] In the young child, increased motor activity, increased curiosity, impulsiveness, and immature judgment skills are important aspects of repeated accidents. The young child's mind has a single focal orientation. For example, if a ball rolls into the street, a child's only motive is to retrieve it immediately. He may not notice the approaching car. The adult, however, can integrate many factors of an experience. The adult first considers how fast the

103

Foundations of clinical practice

car is approaching and then determines whether he has ample time to recover the ball and return to safety before the car arrives.

Accident liability is expressed in terms of the individual's relation to the environment. In addition to the individual's personality characteristics, liability to accidents results from factors such as exposure to hazards; impaired sensory, motor, and neural functioning; the ability to make judgments in relation to hazards; the degree of experience and training; and exposure to various stresses.[15] An important aspect of the concept of accident liability is how well the individual (that is, the child) adjusts to aspects of his environment, such as his family and his home.

Increased liability to accidents can be readily observed at different stages of development. For example, the elderly individual whose coordination is poor will be less able to preserve his balance when in jeopardy. Illness, physical deformity, and weakness due to illness or medication may be factors responsible for his liability to accidents. Environmental hazards such as those related to careless housekeeping, faulty household devices, and the use of improperly maintained home appliances may also make one more liable to accidents.

These factors in accidents should be viewed as symptoms of maladjustment to the environment and not of accident proneness. Therefore, nurses and other health team members must observe the behavior of individuals and environmental hazards in terms of their inherent potential for causing accidents.

Certain individuals have more accidents than an ordinary person would be expected to have under similar circumstances. Such individuals are considered *accident prone*. Behaviors associated with accident proneness include self-centeredness, hostility, insecurity, guilt, and irresponsibility. Behavioral specialists contend that a close relationship exists between accident proneness and suicidal tendencies because the individual feels a need to risk his safety as a means of offering himself for punishment that he feels he deserves. Frequent accidents may be an indirect call for help from a person who is suffering from a physical or psychological handicap.[15]

Where accidents occur
Accidents occur wherever individuals live, work, or play. Although the home is considered a place of safety and security, most accidents occur in and around the home. Many of these home accidents occur among persons who spend a great part of their time in the home—the very young and very old. A high percentage of accidents in the very young is perhaps related to their increased curiosity, lack of self-control, and uncoordinated physical movements. Also, younger children are not able to recognize danger or move out of its way. The older person's susceptibility to accidents is probably related to the degenerative and aging processes. Physical factors such as a reduction in visual and auditory acuity and instability of gait are possibly responsible.

Age and accidents
Between the ages of 15 and 64, most accidents are due to motor vehicles. Drowning, firearms, machinery, and athletics are also responsible for accidents between the ages of 15 and 24. Special instructions should be given regarding the importance of adhering to safe driving and swimming practices and the proper use of firearms and dangerous tools.

Older persons tend to resent, and frequently resist, giving up their freedom. This may be evidenced by the fact that many older persons insist on smoking in bed, although they are unsteady. Many tend to insist on retaining an upstairs room in spite of the hazards it presents. Some tend to mask their physical and mental deficiencies as long as possible, and as a result accidents are not uncommon among them.

Falls are responsible for the majority of accidents in the 65-and-older age group. The most common cause of falls is missing the last step. Slipping on a waxed floor and tripping over rugs are also responsible for a large percentage of falls. Falls among this age group usually result in a fracture because of the brittleness of the bones.

Fires and burns are the second leading cause of accidents in the older age group. They are mainly due to smoking, matches, and the use of defective electrical appliances. Because of these accidents, safety education should be continued throughout the life span.

PROTECTION FROM ENVIRONMENTAL HAZARDS

The nurse, as well as other health team members, should educate families about accidents, environmental hazards, and methods of prevention and protection. Most authorities contend that *most accidents can be prevented*. In such education, parents must be made aware of patterns of growth and development, typical behavior, and hazards that are likely to occur at various age levels. Precautionary measures should be taken to prevent accidents during these stages (Table 4-1).

Parents must be encouraged to protect their families from hazards in the environment. As soon as children are able to understand the simplest language, parents should begin teaching them how to protect themselves from accidents. Children should be prepared for the time when they will be away from home and must take responsibility for their own safety. They should be taught how to avoid certain accidents. Parents should also teach them by example. Activities must be carried out in a safe manner, and ample instructions should be given on the safe methods of play and work. Creating awareness of certain accidents that are likely to occur can serve as a guideline for instruction.

Since it is almost impossible to prevent healthy, active children from injuring themselves, their activities should not be hampered. Under supervision, they should be allowed to climb, play in water, and observe fire. When accidents occur, parents should be encouraged to capitalize on them, using minor accidents as teaching-learning experiences. Neither gastronomic nor emotional reward should be offered when accidents happen, but the causal relationship should be explained. The axiom that "experience is the best teacher" may equally apply here. Most children are likely to touch a hot iron, fall down a couple of steps, or taste a bitter, nonpoisonous liquid. Parents should allow these things to happen under supervision and follow them by a simple explanation, such as "It was hot, you touched it, and it burned you." The same method can be used when children taste a bitter solution or have other accidents. These experiences facilitate their learning the difference between safe and unsafe practices.

The nurse should also teach families about ways of preventing various types of accidents, such as ingestion of various substances, falls, burns, and cuts. Inexpensive safety devices, such as socket covers, safety catches, or hook latches, are available in department stores. Families should be made aware of these.

Preventing injuries from falls

During the early years children are uncoordinated and not able to care for themselves. Parents therefore have the responsibility of protecting them from hazards that may cause them to fall. For example, an infant should not be left alone in the bath or lying on a table from which he could fall. The sides of the

Foundations of clinical practice

TABLE 4-1

Accident risks and precautions at various age levels

Typical accidents	Normal behavior characteristics	Precautions
First year		
Falls, inhalation or ingestion of foreign objects, poisoning, burns, drowning	After several months of age, can squirm and roll, and later in year creeps and pulls self erect Places anything and everything in mouth Is helpless in water	Do not leave alone on tables, and so forth, where falls can occur Keep crib sides up Keep small objects and harmful substances out of reach Do not leave alone in tub
Second year		
Falls, drowning, motor vehicles, ingestion of poisonous substances, burns	Is able to roam about in erect posture Can go up and down stairs Has great curiosity Puts almost everything in mouth Is helpless in water	Keep screens in windows Place gate at top of stairs Cover unused electrical outlets; keep electric cords out of easy reach Keep in enclosed space when outdoors and not in company of an adult Keep medicines, household poisons, and small sharp objects out of sight and reach Keep handles of pots and pans on stove out of reach and containers of hot foods away from edge of table Protect from water in tub or yard
2 to 4 years		
Falls, drowning, motor vehicles, ingestion of poisonous substances, burns	Is able to open doors Can run and climb Investigates closets and drawers Plays with mechanical gadgets Can throw ball and other objects	Keep doors locked when there is danger of falls Place screen or guards in windows Teach about watching for automobiles in driveways and streets Keep firearms locked up Keep knives and electrical equipment out of reach Teach about risks of throwing sharp objects and about danger of following ball into street
5 to 9 years		
Motor vehicles, bicycle accidents, drowning, burns, firearms	Is daring and adventurous Control over large muscles is more advanced than control over small muscles Has increasing interest in group play; loyalty to group makes him willing to follow suggestions of leaders	Teach techniques and traffic rules for bicycling Encourage skills in swimming Keep firearms locked up except when adult can supervise their use
10 to 14 years		
Motor vehicles, drowning, burns, firearms, falls, bicycle accidents	Organic need for strenuous physical activity Plays in hazardous places (street, railroad tracks, near rivers) unless facilities for supervised, adequate recreation are provided Need for approval of age mates leads to daring or hazardous feats	Teach the rules of pedestrian safety Teach bicycling safety Instruct in safe use of firearms Provide safe and acceptable facilities for recreation and social activities Prepare for automobile driving by good example on part of adults and closely supervised instruction

From Shaffer, Thomas E.: Accident prevention, Pediatr. Clin. North Am. **1:**421-432, 1954.

crib should be latched and in the up position when he is left alone. When the child begins climbing, potential hazards should not be left in his path. At an early age the importance of picking up toys or other objects that obstruct the stairway or walkway should be stressed. Adequate play space should be provided away from the kitchen or laundry room. When it is necessary to carry a baby or young child up and down stairs, one hand should be free to grasp the rail. Gates should be used at the top of stairways, and windows should be securely fastened. All these measures are instrumental in preventing the young child from falling.

Since falls are the primary form of accidents in later maturity, the environment should be made free of those hazards that are responsible for falls. Loose rugs, slippery floors, and cluttered hallways should be minimized. Well-fitted shoes should be provided, the use of handrails along stairways should be encouraged, and the environment should be adequately lighted. The use of low beds also helps reduce injuries from falls, arranging storage space within 6 feet of the floor reduces the need to climb, and substances that are spilled on the floor should be cleaned up immediately. In cases in which dizziness is a major complaint, clients should be encouraged to set a slower pace and possibly rearrange their schedules so that rest periods can be taken. All these precautions should be applied regardless of the environment—whether the home or a health care facility.

Preventing other injuries

Suffocation and strangling are not uncommon in young children. Therefore, plastic bags should be discarded and must never be left in or near the child's sleep or play area. Children also have a tendency to engage in games where "victims" are tied up with ropes, drapery pulls, extension cords, and so forth. Such play could lead to accidental strangulation and must be discouraged.

PLANNING FOR THE CARE OF INJURIES

Because accidents are inevitable, health team members should encourage families to maintain a first-aid box. It should be kept in a place that is easily accessible, yet out of the reach of inquisitive children. All equipment that is likely to be needed in a hurry should be in the box. Dressings for wounds, bandages, scissors, antiseptic solutions, a roll of absorbent cotton, applicators, adhesive tape, safety pins, and aromatic spirits of ammonia are some of the materials that should be on hand.

Programs for prevention

Various organizations have been established with the objective of preventing childhood accidents; among these are the United States Public Health Service, the American Academy of Pediatrics, and the National Safety Council. Various insurance companies have sponsored programs along with these major organizations. National committees have also been established to educate health personnel about the problem, to work with technical groups such as engineers to develop manufacturing standards, and to study and make recommendations regarding safety regulations. Educational materials relating to accident prevention may be obtained from the National Safety Council and the American National Red Cross.

POISONINGS

Poisonings are among the leading causes of death between the ages of 1 and 16. The peak age for poisonings is the toddler stage, between 1 and 3 years.[22] Nearly 1000 deaths occur each year from poisoning, especially in the group under 5 years of age. The intense curiosity of this age group accounts for most of these. Also, children in the course of play often ingest poisonous substances, including a number of substances in everyday use, such as medicines, cleansing agents, sprays, and cosmetics, as well as berries and plants. Among the adolescent group, ingestion of drugs in suicide attempts are increasing.[6]

Health care providers and family members must have adequate knowledge about the harmful effects of these agents, emergency therapy for various poisonings, and strategies for prevention. Only the more common types of poisonings are discussed here: salicylates, corrosive acids and alkalis, and lead poisoning. For a more complete discussion the reader is referred to the references at the end of this chapter.

Foundations of clinical practice

Medications readily available in the home account for a large percentage of accidental poisonings. Acetylsalicylic acid (aspirin) and corrosive acids and alkalis are among the common offenders.

Salicylate ingestion

Aspirin accounts for more than half the poisonings in the home. The sources of salicylate poisoning are threefold: the ingestion of pleasantly flavored tablets by a child who considers them to be candy; the ingestion of oil of wintergreen (methyl salicylate), which is a counterirritant but smells like peppermint; and the overuse of aspirin for common illnesses.[14] Toddlers are more commonly victims than any other age group.

Pathophysiology. Salicylates, except methyl salicylate, are rapidly and well absorbed from the gastrointestinal tract.[2] Elimination is largely by the kidney and may start as early as 10 to 15 minutes after ingestion. Methyl salicylate contains more salicylates than any other type (for example, 5 ml is equivalent to 25 aspirin tablets each containing 325 mg).[2] Because of the methyl radical in methyl salicylate, absorption may be delayed for hours. The physiological processes in salicylate poisoning involve stimulation of the respiratory center, stimulation of metabolism, and increased production of organic acids and accumulation of ketone bodies.

Hyperpnea (rapid deep breathing), often the first symptom to appear, occurs as a result of direct stimulation of the respiratory center. The hyperventilation causes an excessive amount of carbon dioxide to be removed, and a subsequent reduction in the serum Pco_2 and an increase in pH. The kidney attempts to compensate for this change by excreting bicarbonate, sodium, and potassium in order to bring the pH back to normal. As a result a compensatory respiratory alkalosis occurs. At this point the buffering capacity of the extracellular fluid will have decreased,[20] and this decrease may result in the development of respiratory and metabolic acidosis. Acidosis may be caused by a number of factors. As previously mentioned, high concentrations of salicylates depress the respiratory center and cause carbon dioxide retention. Impairment in renal function from dehydration, hypotension, and accumulation of acids, and impairment of carbohydrate metabolism cause acetoacetic, lactic, and pyruvic acids to accumulate.[20] These factors are responsible for the development of the acidotic state.

Salicylates also inhibit prothrombin formation by interfering with vitamin K utilization by the liver,[20] thus causing prolonged clotting time. As a result hemorrhage may occur in many tissues of the body.

Assessment. Overdose of salicylates causes nausea, vomiting (due to gastritis), profuse sweating, extreme thirst, diarrhea, fever (possibly related to increasing metabolism and heat production), drowsiness, blurred vision, and changes in the mental state. The mental changes may be characterized by restlessness, irritability, confusion, excitement, and talkativeness.[20] Other central nervous system effects may progressively occur and result in symptoms such as hallucination, convulsions, and coma.[20]

The diagnosis is based on a report that the client ingested aspirin and on the symptoms. Salicylate levels are obtained to determine the severity of the intoxication. Serum evaluation of BUN, electrolytes, and glucose are also useful. Blood gases are obtained, and an analysis of urine is made.

Planning and implementation. Immediate therapy is essential. The goals of therapy are to decrease absorption, correct the electrolyte imbalance, and eliminate the salicylates in the urine.

ASSESSMENT GUIDE AND POSSIBLE CONSIDERATIONS FOR CLIENT WHO HAS INGESTED POISONS

Assessments	Possible considerations	Assessments	Possible considerations
1. Respiratory assessment		4. Assessments related to sensory function	
a. Are respirations depressed?	Barbiturates, sedatives, hypnotics	a. Eyes: What is the condition of the pupils? Are they dilated?	Cocaine, atropine, amphetamines, antihistamines, nicotine (late effect)
b. Is the client experiencing dyspnea? Hyperpnea?	Salicylates	Are they pinpoint?	Nicotine (early effect), opiates, physostigmine
c. Is the client coughing?	Indication that client possibly aspirated		
d. Is cyanosis present?	Kerosene, cyanide, nitrites, aniline compounds	b. Integument: is the skin flushed or pink?	Carbon monoxide
e. What signs of hypoxia are evident? Restlessness? Confusion?	Barbiturates, sedatives, hypnotics	5. Gastrointestinal assessments	
2. Circulatory assessments		a. Is the client vomiting?	Acids, alkalis, metallic compounds, organic phosphorus
a. What are the vital signs?		b. Is the client having diarrhea?	Same as above
b. Is the blood pressure decreased?	Barbiturates, sedatives, hypnotics	c. Is abdominal pain a presenting symptom?	Acids, alkalis, metallic compounds
c. Is bradycardia present?	Organic phosphorus	d. Are there burns about the mouth, lip, or tongue?	Caustic alkalis
3. Central nervous system assessments		e. Is there a characteristic breath odor (such as gasoline)?	Turpentine, arsenic, cyanide, wintergreen, phosphorus
a. Is the client confused?	Organic phosphorus	6. Urinary assessments	
b. Is the client comatose?	Organic phosphorus, central nervous system depressants	a. Are changes noted in urine?	
		b. Presence of albuminuria?	Mercury
c. Is the client having seizures?	Organic phosphorus, central nervous system stimulants, strychnine, camphor	7. Musculoskeletal assessments	
		a. Is trismus being experienced?	Phenothiazides
		b. Is opisthotonus present?	Phenothiazides

General principles of implementation for poisons

Whenever poisons are ingested, some form of therapy should be started immediately. Except for lavage, therapy to prevent absorption may be started in the home. Supportive therapy is primarily carried out in the hospital or other health care facilities. Since measures to prevent absorption may be started at home, they are discussed first.

Preventing absorption. To prevent absorption, several measures may be used. These include measures to induce vomiting, gastric lavage, and antidotes. Emesis is generally preferred over lavage because it facilitates the removal of substances from the small intestines; as a result, more of the unabsorbed substance is returned. Second, if the client does not cooperate, it is difficult to introduce a nasogastric or oral gastric tube for lavage.

Inducing emesis. Most poisons have an immediate emetic effect. If emesis does not occur spontaneously, vomiting should be induced, provided no contraindication exists. Contraindications to emesis include the ingestion of strong acids and alkalis, strychnine, petroleum products, and (though controversial) hydrocarbons. Ingestion of these substances may be evidenced by burns around the lips and mouth. Also, emesis should not be induced in the semiconscious, unconscious, or convulsing client or in one whose gag reflex is absent. The induction of emesis is contraindicated in the former because of the danger of

Foundations of clinical practice

reexposing the epithelial tissue to harmful agents and in the latter because of the danger of aspiration.

To induce emesis, several approaches may be employed. Fluids (such as water or milk) may be given. One glass of water for the child and as many as four glasses of water are recommended for the adult. This should be followed by *stimulating the gag reflex* with a finger or a blunt object.

Other emetics include syrup of ipecac and apomorphine hydrochloride. Syrup of ipecac acts both centrally on the vomiting center and locally within the gastrointestinal tract to induce emesis.[3] For a child or an adult, 15 to 30 ml of the syrup should be given orally. This method should be followed by large amounts (two or three glasses) of water, milk or whatever fluid the client will drink. (Water is often recommended because the vomitus may be examined more easily.) Following this, physical movement (such as bouncing a young child on the knee, or ambulation of an older child, adolescent, or adult) should be encouraged. Activity (such as motion from walking) plus a full stomach increase the rapidity of action of the ipecac syrup. If vomiting does not occur within 15 to 20 minutes, the dose of ipecac may be repeated once. If vomiting does not occur after the second dose (that is, within a 20-minute period) the physician, poison control center, or emergency facility should be contacted again.[2,3]

Syrup of ipecac is inexpensive and may be purchased without a prescription. It may be beneficial to inform families, especially those with small children, to keep the drug on hand in the home. When instructions about this drug are given, the difference between the syrup form and fluid extract elixir should be stressed. The latter is toxic. Ipecac also contains an alkaloid that, when absorbed, can cause cardiac irregularities.

Consumers should be strongly encouraged to read the label on the syrup very closely. The label warns that syrup of ipecac not be used if strychnine or corrosives (such as lye or strong acids) have been ingested. Since clients may not know whether a substance is a corrosive, is highly toxic, or is petroleum, they should be instructed not to hesitate to consult a physician, poison control center, or emergency facility.

Apomorphine, a respiratory depressant, produces vomiting through stimulation of the chemoreceptor trigger zone in the medulla. It is generally administered subcutaneously; however, in critically poisoned clients it may be given intravenously. It is therefore administered in a health care facility. After the drug is given, the client should ingest large quantities of fluids. Vomiting usually occurs as early as 5 minutes after administration. The drug is contraindicated if respirations are depressed or labored or if poisoning is due to a respiratory depressant. When apomorphine is used, an antagonist such as naloxone hydrochloride (Narcan) or nalorphine hydrochloride (Nalline) should be readily available.

When emesis is induced, care must be maintained to prevent aspiration. Small children should be held by their feet, with the head downward. Older clients should be encouraged to remain in a position in which the head is lowered. All vomitus should be saved for analysis. Care should be taken to keep the initial and subsequent vomitus separated. Specimens should be sent to the laboratory for analysis as soon as possible to facilitate identifying the poison and commencing other forms of therapy.

Performing gastric lavage. Another means of removing poisonous substances is gastric lavage. This method is preferred in instances where emesis is contraindicated (seizures, absent gag reflex, unconsciousness). Because of the possibility of esophageal or gastric perforation, lavage is contraindicated in clients who have ingested caustic substances. A gastric tube with large holes is passed through the oral or nasal route. The oral route is preferred for infants and young children because it is easier to pass the tube and is less traumatic. The nasal route is preferred for clients past the preschool period. Before the tube is passed, any foreign objects or dentures should be removed from the mouth. The passage of gastric tubes is discussed in Chapter 17.

Several guidelines should be adhered to when gastric lavage is employed to remove poisonous substances.

1. Instill at least 50 ml of fluid at one time. It has been suggested that large tubes have approximately 25 ml of dead space to fill; therefore, the use of less than 50 ml is inadequate. Ideal amounts to be used per washing are 10 ml/kg for the child and 300 ml for the adult.[25]
2. Avoid excessive force while instilling the fluid. Forceful instillation may cause gastric contents to be passed into the small intestines.
3. After initial instillation, fluids should be warmed to maintain body temperature.
4. Prevent aspiration from reflex vomiting by placing the client on his left side with his head lower than his hips.
5. Continue lavage until returns are clear.

Although tap water is often used for lavage, isotonic saline is preferred because it will not deplete electrolytes. Depending on the nature of the poison, a number of other substances may also be used for dilution and neutralization: tannic acid, potassium permanganate, milk, sodium bicarbonate, calcium salt, and activated charcoal.

Providing antidotes. Antidotes are administered to render the poison inert and to change its physical nature, thus preventing systemic absorption. Activated charcoal is a commonly used antidote, since a large number of poisons are absorbed by it and since there are no known contraindications. Some common drugs absorbed by charcoal include alcohol, amphetamines, atropine, barbiturates, ipecac, salicylates, and sulfonamides. Charcoal inactivates and absorbs ipecac; therefore, it should be administered after emesis.[25]

Currently the use of a universal antidote such as burned toast, milk of magnesia, or tannic acid is discouraged because tannic acid is hepatotoxic and because the other agents are not considered to be very effective.

Providing supportive therapy. Supportive measures are employed to maintain the client's vital functions and to make the client as comfortable as possible. Such measures are essential because often poisons may adversely affect respiratory and circulatory systems and may interfere with the ability of the liver and kidney to eliminate poisonous products. Failure to maintain functioning of the vital organs will cause death; therefore, it is imperative that measures be taken to maintain these functions.

When a client is seen at a health care facility, detailed assessments must be made of all vital organ systems. Depending on the client's pulmonary status, it may be necessary to employ some form of tracheal intubation to maintain adequate ventilation and to administer vasopressors to increase blood pressure. Immediate intubation is indicated in instances where the respiratory status is markedly depressed. Assisted ventilation may be necessary. Fluids may be administered intravenously, and it may be necessary to insert a central venous pressure catheter.

Nursing measures (such as frequent position change and removal of tracheobronchial secretions) must be implemented to prevent pulmonary complications. Periodic determinations may be made of blood and urine. Finally, vital signs, level of awareness, pupillary reaction, urinary output, electrolyte status, blood gases, and fluid balances must be carefully monitored to facilitate early detection of other potential complications.

Facilitating elimination of substances. Facilitating elimination of substances from the system is another aspect of supportive therapy. This objective may be accomplished by any one of three methods: cathartics, forced diuresis, or dialysis.

Cathartics are useful in rapidly removing toxic substances through the gastrointestinal tract and subsequently decreasing absorption of the substance. Common drugs that may be used for this purpose are magnesium sulfate and magnesium citrate.

A number of toxic substances are eliminated, partially or totally, by the kidney without being metabolized. In such instances, *diuresis* may be necessary to facilitate more rapid removal from the system. Alkalizing agents (such as sodium bicarbonate and sodium lactate) may be administered systemically in conjunction with a diuretic such as acetazolamide (Diamox). The value of such a combination is that it alkalinizes the urine and prevents the toxic materials from being reabsorbed by the renal tubules. As a result, excretion of the substances is increased. Fluids are usually administered intravenously. It is important to monitor fluid intake and output and electrolyte balance very closely, and it may be necessary to anchor an indwelling catheter.

Peritoneal *dialysis* or hemodialysis may be indicated, especially if a near-lethal dose was ingested, if an excessive amount of the agent was ingested, or if the lethal dose is not known. The use of dialysis spares the normal pathways (such as liver and kidneys) for elimination of toxic agents. For nursing measures related to dialysis, see Chapter 19.

Preventing injuries from poisons

Children learn by exploring their environment. Hand-to-mouth activity and curiosity are important elements of a child's exploration and are frequently responsible for accidental ingestion of hazardous substances (Fig. 4-1).

Medications, polishes, detergents, and other dangerous products should be kept out of the reach of children and away from food. Medicines should be locked in a medicine cabinet high enough to prevent the child from entering it. Before any medication is administered, an adult should read the instructions carefully to ensure that it is the correct one. Immediately after use, the medication should be replaced in the cabinet, rather than left on the table or bedside stand. As soon as the period for specific prescriptions is fulfilled, any remaining medication should be discarded. Children should not be told that medicine is candy, nor should the giving of medication be made a game, since this practice often invites trouble. Poison labels should be placed on all dangerous medications, including aspirin (Fig. 4-2).

Poisons should be stored only in their original containers and kept well out of reach. Soft drink bottles should never be used to store bleaches or detergents, because this practice only serves to tempt small children.

4   Environment and health problems

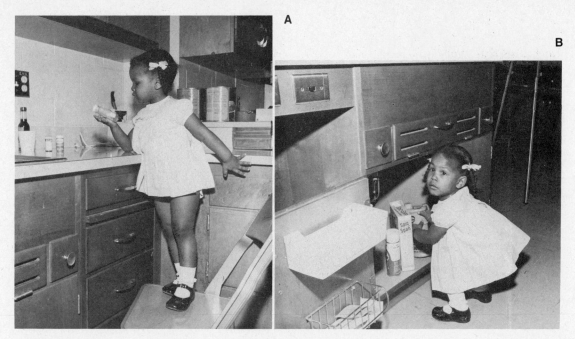

FIG. 4-1
A, Medications should not be stored on the counter tops but should be stored properly in a medicine cabinet, well out of reach of the inquisitive child. **B,** Detergents should not be stored where the toddler can easily get to them.

Lead poisoning

Lead poisoning may be considered an environmental hazard in children and an occupational hazard in adults. In children it frequently occurs between the ages of 1 and 3, especially in those who live in old, poorly maintained housing where lead-containing paints have been widely used. This age period is critical because hand-to-mouth activity is great and is essential in the child's exploration. The problem, however, is not restricted to deteriorating surroundings or to childhood, as is discussed later.

The main source of lead poisoning in children consists of the flakes and chips of woodwork and loose plaster of old houses that contain layers of lead-pigmented paints. Lead-painted toys and furniture (such as cribs) are also sources of lead poisoning. One report indicated printed media (newspaper, magazines) as a source of lead poisoning; pages containing greens and yellows were most heavily laden with lead.[17] Adults, too, may acquire lead poisoning through ingestion. Water that has passed through lead pipes and improperly glazed earthenware pottery are occasional sources.[7] Poisoning from the latter usually occurs after the individual drinks acidic liquids such as fruit juices and colas or eats foods (such as fruits or pickles) that have been stored in lead-glazed pottery. The acids tend to draw lead out of the glaze into solution. Poisoning from improperly glazed dishware accounts for some cases of lead poisoning in adults in the middle and upper classes.

The primary source of lead poisoning in adults is dust vapor. Lead particles in the ambient air from the exhausts of gasoline engines, fumes from industrial plants (such as battery plants), and ashes of painted wood are examples of lead poisoning through dust vapor. Lead poisoning has been reported in the "back to the city" movers who inhale the dust from old houses while in the process of

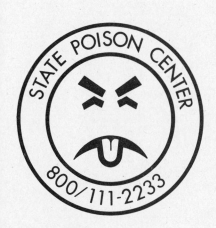

FIG. 4-2
Mr. Yuk: the poison label.

115

renovation.[21] Most of these houses are characteristically old and contain lead-based paints.

Assessment. When a child eats or chews paint chips, or the adult inhales or ingests the lead products, the lead is absorbed from the gastrointestinal tract, passed to the liver, and excreted back into the duodenum through the bile; some of it is reabsorbed and some of it is excreted in the feces. As the process continues, the body continually absorbs the lead until a danger level is reached; the individual may then have a number of symptoms. At first they may be vague, insidious and nonspecific. For example, the child may tend to be more irritable and play less actively. Constipation or diarrhea may develop. Because of the vagueness of the symptoms, parents may not seek medical help.

As the condition becomes progressively worse, the child may lose newly acquired skills; vomiting, anorexia, abdominal pain, hyperirritability, clumsiness and anemia may be manifested. The mechanisms responsible for the anemia are twofold. Lead salts coat the red blood cells and subsequently damage their membranes, with a resultant increase in red blood cell hemolysis. Lead is also thought to affect the hematopoietic system by inhibiting the biosynthesis of heme and the utilization of iron in red blood cells.[21]

Lead encephalopathy, a more severe form of lead poisoning, may occur after repetitive ingestion of small quantities over a 3-month period. Nervous system involvement, affecting either the brain or peripheral nerves, is evidenced by symptoms of gross ataxia, progressive changes in the level of consciousness, and seizures. Individuals who develop coma or seizures suffer irreversible brain damage. Mental retardation, cerebral palsy, blindness, learning defects, behavioral problems, and kidney disease may be consequences of lead poisoning.

In addition to the symptoms, various other parameters are used for diagnosis. In children, x-ray studies are used in determining increased density of the epiphyseal ends of the bone. Increased density is due to the deposit of lead in these sites. Hematological tests (such as complete blood count, hematocrit, morphology of red cells, peripheral smears, and lead analysis of urine and blood) are useful.

The *erythrocyte protoporphyrin* (EP) *determination,* obtained from a finger stick, reflects increased protoporphyrin concentration in the erythroid cells of the bone marrow. Since protoporphyrin is a heme metabolite, it accumulates in the blood when heme synthesis is inhibited by lead. EP determination is considered superior to testing blood lead because it reflects the biological effect of lead in the hematopoietic system.[21]

Planning and implementation. Therapy is designed to facilitate the excretion of the lead. If the metal has been recently ingested, a saline cathartic may be administered to flush the lead from the intestinal tract and to reduce absorption.

Lead is present in three places in the body: blood, soft tissue, and bone. Chelation rids lead mainly from soft tissue and blood and from bone if the lead is loosely bound to it. Lead that is firmly bound is not released and may not be for 1 or 2 decades.[7] Chelation therapy, a process of deleading by the use of drugs, is usually started when the lead level is 60 μg/dl (normal is 0 to 39 μg/dl of blood). Drugs such as dimercaprol (BAL) and calcium disodium edetate (CaEDTA) are common. Lead replaces the calcium and binds as a highly stable chelate; this process changes the lead, allowing it to be excreted by the kidney and gastrointestinal tract. The administration of these drugs demands close monitoring in an acute care setting, since a massive increase in serum lead can be produced as it becomes mobilized from storage places such as the bone.[16]

Penicillamine is sometimes used when other forms of therapy do not return blood levels to normal. The use of this drug requires weekly monitoring of white cell count, and urinalysis.[19]

Renal damage may result from the use of chelation therapy; therefore, renal function must be assessed frequently. Daily blood analysis to determine lead concentration, electrolyte balance, BUN and calcium levels, and hematocrit values is done. A daily urinalysis is also obtained, with urine collected in lead-free containers. The nurse must see that the client drinks ample fluid (for example, 200 ml every hour) to maintain proper urinary excretion of lead. A careful record should be kept of intake and output. the presence of anuria should be reported to the physician, and the client should be carefully observed for the development of dysrhythmias.

In addition, fluids may be administered intravenously to maintain an adequate urine flow. Mannitol and corticosteroids may be administered to relieve increased intracranial pressure, if this is present.

Strategies for prevention. One of the biggest elements in reducing lead poisoning is prevention. Nurses have a leading role in educating the public about the hazards of lead. Literature can be distributed to make the public aware of the hazards and sources of lead poisoning. The community should be made aware of the symptoms of lead poisoning and be encouraged to seek medical help when any of these symptoms are evident. Some states have banned paints containing more than 1% lead from use on interior surfaces. However, if such paints are found in stores, clients should be discouraged from using these on interior surfaces, toys, and furniture. They should carefully read warning labels on paints before purchasing them.

Periodic mass screening has been recommended by the Surgeon General for children 1 to 6 years old who live in old, poorly maintained housing.

When it is necessary to burn or scrape lead-based paints, it should be done when children are not present. This rule is important because a fine dust that is readily absorbed is created from burning and scraping. It is also advisable to contain work in one area, use adequate ventilation, clear the area, and wash (for example, shower) after each work session.

In instances where some doubt exists as to the type of pottery, the Food and Drug Administration recommends that it be used only for decorative purposes. Children should not be permitted to chew newspapers, comics, or magazines, since small amounts may be swallowed; nor should they be permitted to make spit balls. A spit ball that is approximately 25 cm and weighs about 140 mg could contain as much as 1.4 μg of lead. This prohibition is important, since the daily intake from all sources has been proposed as 300 μg.[18] The World Health Organization set the maximum safe daily intake of lead for children 1 to 3 years of age to be 5 μg/kg of body weight. Once lead poisoning is diagnosed, families should be encouraged to continue follow-up care.

DRUGS   Drugs include any substance that is used to alter the physical or mental function of the human body.[22] They are used for several reasons: to produce certain feelings and moods, to dull or enhance perception, to promote relaxation or the

Foundations of clinical practice

feeling of wellness, and to create an aura of safety and comfort, particularly in social settings.

The teenage years are filled with admixtures of joys, fears, disappointments, frustrations, conflict, anxieties, group pressures, restlessness, and omnipotence. Many persons with a healthy childhood and stable home and family life can resist the temptation of experimentation with drugs. Others, however, are eager to "try something different." Two or three decades ago it was a daring feat to smoke a cigarette or drink a beer with friends before being legally old enough to indulge in such activities. In one way, today's teenagers are the same except that their field of options is considerably more sophisticated. Parent models not only smoke and drink but also take drugs to avoid any conceived discomfort. There is almost a belief that life should be chemically controlled, if necessary, to ensure a constant state of pleasurable feelings. These and many other arguments or reasons are offered to explain the acceleration of drug abuse in our society, particularly among our youth.

Not many years ago drug abuse was generally confined to the urban areas where derelicts, street gangs, and characters from the underworld mingled for evil purposes. Little concern was widespread then, except perhaps among law enforcement officers. However, there is now considerable interest regarding drug abuse because it reaches into all segments of society and is becoming a complex problem. This problem is particularly increasing among the adolescent population and among young adults. Increasing attention is being given to the extent of the problem in elementary and secondary schools. Law enforcement, dangers to the health and safety of our youth, economics of the habits, and interferences with school and family life are real considerations with far-reaching effects.

Drug abuse is the persistent self-administration of a drug without regard to its medical purpose. *Drug dependence* is the continued desire to take the drug to experience its effects or avoid the discomfort associated with not taking it. Drug taking leads to a physiological tolerance, a psychic craving, and in some cases a physical dependence. Although almost any drug can be abused or misused, several have received rather widespread attention: tobacco, alcohol, LSD, marijuana, amphetamines, heroin, and barbiturates.

Drug addiction is a by-product of abuse and refers to the physiological dependence of an individual on a drug that requires increasingly larger or more potent dosages to achieve similar effects. Drug addiction is probably more psychological than physiological, however. Most drug addicts have personality disorders in conjunction with their drug problems. Addicts tend to withdraw from society and create their own world through the use of drugs.

The addict personality

The following traits are believed to be characteristic of the hard-core heroin addict:

1. He lacks a value system or a superego. He is sly, dishonest, and he cheats and lies. He is hedonistic, lives from moment to moment, and is unable to stand pain.
2. He has a poor sense of self. He must have instant gratification. He is unable to deal with the world in a realistic way or to meet goals.
3. He generally has impaired emotional relationships.
4. He has little ability to get help.
5. He cannot relate to authority.

118

4 Environment and health problems

Traditional types of therapy, such as psychoanalysis, do not work with addicts. Instead, one must deal with attitudes.[1]

The addict is more likely to eventually succumb to the habit than to be cured. More than 90% of all true addicts who have attempted to undergo curative treatment have returned to drug abuse.

Nursing implementation

One form of therapy, which involves the use of methadone (a synthetic narcotic) as a replacement for heroin, is gaining popularity. This substance negates the effects of heroin but meets the addict's physical need for the drug. Although methadone is addictive, it costs pennies as opposed to many dollars—perhaps $200 or more per day—for the heroin habit. It is expected to reduce the number of crimes committed to obtain money for supporting the expensive heroin addiction. Methadone treatment centers also provide counseling and employment services in hopes that some stable elements can be created in the addict's life.

Clients who have a problem of drug addiction must admit their need for help and present themselves for treatment. It is difficult or even impossible to help an addict who does not want to change. A desire for "the cure" is the first realistic step of therapeutic care.

Psychological withdrawal must accompany physical withdrawal from addicting drugs. Treatment centers and health care facilities must direct programs toward both. A period of confinement is usually necessary to achieve control of withdrawal symptoms and to limit the availability of drugs. The role of the nurse in such settings may include promoting client safety, participating in therapeutic group programs, observing for behavioral cues, recording appropriate data, and serving as an external superego for the client.

The drug abuser as a medical-surgical client

If a known addict is hospitalized for psychiatric treatment of his condition, nurses should be alert to drug reactions and signs and symptoms of withdrawal. However, the expanding number of persons who use certain agents regularly and thus have become dependent physically or psychologically has made it commonplace for nurses to encounter such clients in a variety of health care settings for the management of medical-surgical problems. It is therefore important that nurses be alert to the following physical and behavioral cues related to illicit drug use:

1. Poor general body appearance because of neglect of hygiene, nutrition, and exercise.
2. Reddened, watery eyes; widely dilated or constricted pupils.
3. Lack of coordination of motor and sensory activities.
4. Loss of usual alertness; disinterest in activities, drowsiness.
5. Needle marks, scars, inflamed lesions along course of superficial veins.
6. Labile emotions: hysterical crying or laughing, delusions, hallucinations.
7. Paranoid behavioral tendencies.
8. Appetite extremes; no interest in food or unusual cravings for sweets and liquids.

If an addict is admitted to an acute care setting for treatment of a medical problem, several responses may occur. If he is deprived of his usual drug, he may exhibit agitated behavior, emotional instability, or anxiety. Physical withdrawal signs and symptoms may be present (Table 4-3). If he still has access to

119

TABLE 4-3

Comparison of selected effects of commonly abused drugs

Drug category	Physical dependence	Characteristics of intoxication	Characteristics of withdrawal	"Flashback" symptoms	Masking of symptoms of illness or injury during intoxication
Opiates	Marked	Analgesia with or without depressed sensorium; pinpoint pupils (tolerance does not develop to this action); patient may be alert and appear normal; respiratory depression with overdose	Rhinorrhea, lacrimation, and dilated, reactive pupils, followed by gastrointestinal disturbances, low back pain, and waves of gooseflesh; convulsions not a feature unless heroin samples were adulterated with barbiturates	Not reported	An important feature of opiate intoxication, due to analgesic action with or without depressed sensorium
Barbiturates	Marked	Patient may appear normal with usual dose, but narrow margin between dose needed to prevent withdrawal symptoms and toxic dose is often exceeded and patient appears "drunk," with drowsiness, ataxia, slurred speech, and nystagmus on lateral gaze; pupil size and reaction normal; respiratory depression with overdose	Agitation, tremulousness, insomnia, gastrointestinal disturbances, hyperpyrexia, blepharoclonus (clonic blink reflex), acute brain syndrome, major convulsive seizures	Not reported	Only in presence of depressed sensorium or after onset of acute brain syndrome
Nonbarbiturate sedatives Glutethimide (Doriden)	Marked	Pupils dilated and reactive to light; coma and respiratory depression prolonged; sudden apnea and laryngeal spasm common	Similar to barbiturate withdrawal syndrome, with agitation, gastrointestinal disturbances, hyperpyrexia, and major convulsive seizures	Not reported	Same as in barbiturate intoxication
Antianxiety agents* ("minor tranquilizers")	Marked	Progressive depression of sensorium as with barbiturates; pupil size and reaction normal; respiratory depression with overdose	Similar to barbiturate withdrawal syndrome, with danger of major convulsive seizures	Not reported	Same as in barbiturate intoxication
Ethanol	Marked	Depressed sensorium, acute or chronic brain syndrome, odor on breath, pupil size and reaction normal	Similar to barbiturate withdrawal syndrome, but with less likelihood of convulsive seizures	Not reported	Same as in barbiturate intoxication
Amphetamines	Mild to absent	Agitation, with paranoid thought disturbance in high doses; acute organic brain syndrome after prolonged use; pupils dilated and reactive; tachycardia, elevated blood pressure, with possibility of hypertensive crisis and CVA; possibility of convulsive seizures	Lethargy, somnolence, dysphoria, and possibility of suicidal depression; brain syndrome may persist for many weeks	Infrequently reported	Drug-induced euphoria or acute brain syndrome may interfere with awareness of symptoms of illness or may remove incentive to report symptoms of illness

From Goth, Andres: Medical pharmacology, ed. 10, St. Louis, 1981, The C.V. Mosby Co.; modified from Dimijian, G.G.: Drug Ther. **1:**7, 1971.

*Meprobamate (Equanil), chlordiazepoxide (Librium), diazepam (Valium), ethchlorvynol (Placidyl), and ethinamate (Valmid).

TABLE 4-3

Comparison of selected effects of commonly abused drugs—cont'd

Drug category	Physical depen-dence	Characteristics of intoxication	Characteristics of withdrawal	"Flash-back" symptoms	Masking of symptoms of illness or injury during intoxication
Cocaine	Absent	Paranoid thought disturbance in high doses, with dangerous delusions of persecution and omnipotence; tachycardia; respiratory depression with overdose	Similar to amphetamine withdrawal	Not reported	Same as in amphetamine intoxication
Marijuana	Absent	Milder preparations: drowsy, euphoric state with frequent inappropriate laughter and disturbance in perception of time or space (occasional acute psychotic reaction reported); stronger preparations such as hashish: frequent hallucinations or psychotic reaction; pupils normal, conjunctivas injected (marijuana preparations frequently adulterated with LSD, tryptamines, or heroin)	No specific withdrawal symptoms	Infrequently reported	Uncommon with milder preparations; stronger preparations may interfere in same manner as psychotomimetic agents
Psychotomimetics LSD, STP, tryptamines, mescaline, morning glory seeds	Absent	Unpredictable disturbance in ego function, manifested by extreme lability of affect and chaotic disruption of thought, with danger of uncontrolled behavioral disturbance; pupils dilated and reactive to light	No specific withdrawal symptoms; symptomatology may persist for indefinite period after discontinuance of drug	Commonly reported as late as 1 year after last dose	Affective response or psychotic thought disturbance may remove awareness of, or incentive to report, symptoms of illness
Phencyclidine	Unknown	Disinhibition, agitation, confusion, chaotic thought disturbance, unpredictable behavior, hypertension, meiosis, respiratory collapse, cardiovascular collapse, death	No specific withdrawal symptoms	Occasionally reported	Same as in LSD intoxication
Anticholinergic agents	Absent	Nonpsychotropic effects such as tachycardia, decreased salivary secretion, urinary retention, and dilated, nonreactive pupils plus depressed sensorium, confusion, disorientation, hallucinations, and delusional thinking	No specific withdrawal symptoms; mydriasis may persist for several days	Not reported	Pain may not be reported as a result of depression of sensorium, acute brain syndrome, or acute psychotic reaction
Inhalants*	Unknown	Depressed sensorium, hallucinations; acute brain syndrome; odor on breath; patient often with glassy-eyed appearance	No specific withdrawal symptoms	Infrequently reported	Same as in anticholinergic intoxication

*The term "inhalant" is used to designate a variety of gases and highly volatile organic liquids, including the aromatic glues, paint thinners, gasoline, some anesthetic agents, and amyl nitrite. The term excludes liquids sprayed into the nasopharynx (droplet transport required) and substances that must be ignited before inhalation (such as marijuana).

Foundations of clinical practice

his supply of a given agent and combines it with other drugs given for his current somatic complaints, toxic or untoward synergistic reactions may occur. Combining certain potent agents unknowingly could even result in death, not to mention the confusion in diagnosis and management that would confront the medical team. All nursing personnel must be alert to the possession or ingestion of unprescribed medications and the indications of drug abuse.

Clients being treated for neurological or sensory disorders pose unique problems, since many drugs can cause unusual behavior, altered perception, bizarre complaints, visual impairment, and loss of coordination often associated with brain or spinal cord disease. It is also important to note that addicted clients pose a threat to their own safety because their judgment is frequently impaired, which could result in accidents or willful, self-inflicted injury.

Nurses and others who work with clients in neighborhood health centers, industry, schools, and hospitals should assess everyone encountered as a potential abuser of drugs.

Parents should always consider the possibility of their child's experimenting with drugs and should be alert to attendant signs and symptoms. Most communities, especially in urban areas, have many services to aid families who must cope with the hazards of drug abuse and addiction.

Acute drug overdose by ingestion

Unconscious individual. The nurse should suspect drug overdose in any client who is unconscious from an unknown cause. The first priority in management is to ensure that there is a patent airway and adequate ventilation. If resuscitation is required, consideration should be given to insertion of a cuffed endotracheal tube to guard against gastric aspiration. Oxygen, intravenous fluids, and cardiopulmonary resuscitation may also be required. While these measures are being taken, the history of the ingestion can be elicited or validated from others, if possible. For some drugs, there is a specific antidote that can be employed. However, valuable time should not be lost in search for antidotes or in identification of the ingested substance.

Other considerations. Most central nervous system depressant drugs cause the client to be hypothermic. A hyperthermia blanket or other mode of providing external warmth should be provided.

Elimination of certain drugs may be enhanced by osmotic diuresis and dialysis. Amphetamines, salicylates, barbiturates, lithium, sulfonamides, and penicillin are examples of agents that are eliminated by diuresis with concurrent control of urine pH.

All drug overdose ingestions should be assessed thoroughly and followed up systematically. No management should be considered complete until referral has been made for psychiatric counseling.

Acute drug overdose follows the same treatment principles as ingestion of any poisonous substance:

1. Ensure airway and ventilation.
2. Do initial physical assessment and data gathering.
3. Remove substance from stomach to prevent absorption, and hasten its elimination by diuresis or dialysis, or rapid propulsion through the bowel.
4. Protect the client during the intoxicated state.
5. Initiate psychiatric referral.

4 Environment and health problems

SMOKING AND HEALTH

The correlation between smoking and health has been well documented. The nurse should use every possible opportunity to instruct smokers about the hazards of smoking. Facts from the Surgeon General's Advisory Committee Report on Smoking can be used as a guide for teaching. This report indicates that (1) a close relationship exists between cigarette smoking and the development of emphysema, lung cancer, and coronary heart disease; (2) cigarette smoking is the most important cause of chronic bronchitis, increasing the risk of dying from chronic bronchitis; (3) a correlation exists between smoking and mortality and morbidity—mortality and morbidity increase with the number of cigarettes smoked; and (4) cigarette smoking affects pulmonary function and cardiovascular physiology to the extent that the cleansing mechanism is hampered. For example, smoking alters or destroys the cilia and increases the number of goblet cells, and the bronchial mucous glands hypertrophy. As a result, the individual's ability to expectorate secretions and irritants is decreased.

Cigarette smoking is also thought to cause an impairment in ventilatory function, which affects the diffusion of air into the arterial blood.

Many individuals smoke regardless of their health problems or warnings from health care personnel about the effect that smoking has on health. In fact, smoking has increased among the female population during the past decade.[26] One of the reasons documented for this increasing trend is stress. Smoking is thought to serve as a means of relieving external stress, such as stress from the dual role of homemaker and income producer and dissatisfaction with lower-paying, less-satisfying jobs than men have.[26] The incidence of smoking among teenage girls between 12 and 18 has also increased and is higher than that among teenage boys. As a result of increased smoking, the rate of lung cancer among women has increased.

The pattern of smoking among men has been associated with their socioeconomic status. Men in higher income and educational levels smoke less as compared with men in lower groups.[26] The trend for men in the middle and upper socioeconomic levels is toward giving up smoking.

Effect on nonsmokers

The effect of smoking on the nonsmoker has been well documented. For example, it can cause eye irritation, nasal discomfort, coughs, and headaches. Children, particularly those with asthma, are sensitive to tobacco smoke. Therefore, smoking around children with asthma may aggravate their asthmatic symptoms or directly trigger asthma attacks. Respiratory illnesses have been reported to occur twice as often in children whose parents smoke as in those whose parents do not smoke.

There are two kinds of smoke that enter the environment: *sidestream* smoke, which enters the air directly from the burning end, and *mainstream* smoke, which is pulled through the mouthpiece as the smoker inhales or puffs. The nonsmoker is exposed to the former. According to the American Lung Association, concentrations of noxious substances (tar, nicotine, benzyprene, carbon monoxide, and cadmium) are higher in sidestream smoke than in mainstream smoke, which perhaps accounts for the harmful and irritating effects to the nonsmoker.

Because of documentation of these effects, a bill of rights for the nonsmoker was signed and adopted by the National Interagency on Smoking and Health in January, 1974. This bill declares three basic rights of the nonsmoker. *The right to breathe clean air* gives the nonsmoker the right to breathe air free from

123

harmful and irritating tobacco smoke. In instances where there is conflict, the right to breathe clean air supersedes the right to smoke. *The right to speak out* gives the nonsmoker the right to firmly but politely express this discomfort and reaction to the smoke. It also guarantees his right to voice objection if the smoker lights up without obtaining permission. *The right to act* gives the nonsmoker the right to take action through legislative channels, social pressure, or any other legitimate means.

Effect on pregnancy

Smoking also has an effect on pregnancy. Facts have been established by the American Lung Association that smoking retards fetal growth and increases the risks of spontaneous abortion and premature births. The mortality of babies born of smoking mothers is higher than those born of nonsmoking mothers. The pregnant woman who smokes two packs of cigarettes per day blocks off 40% of the baby's oxygen. Nicotine may cause narrowing of the placental blood vessels and thus decreases the supply of oxygen to the unborn baby.

Antismoking clinics

Antismoking clinics have been established, using the same concept as Alcoholics Anonymous. The nurse should be aware of the objectives and locations of these clinics so the client can be referred if questions are raised as to how to stop smoking. Pamphlets are available from the American Cancer Society, and a number of books have been written that give instructions on how the individual can stop smoking.

ALCOHOLISM

Alcoholism is a chronic disease or behavior disorder that is manifested by the use of alcohol beyond what is socially acceptable in the client's community and that interferes with the client's health and interpersonal relationships.[4,9] Alcoholism is a common health problem and is discussed here as it relates to impairment of nutrition. The nurse is referred to other texts for more complete discussion.

The cause of alcoholism is not known, and the end result of alcohol abuse is a multifaceted problem with physiological, psychological, and sociological consequences interrelated. Several theories have been offered and behavioral models proposed to explain the causes of alcoholism. A nutritional theory postulates that the alcoholic person craves alcohol in order to compensate for nutritional deficiencies. An endocrine theory states there is an endocrine imbalance driving the individual to drink. Other theories maintain that the disease is influenced by heredity or behavioral disorders caused by emotional immaturity, anxiety in social relationships, low tolerance for frustration, poor self-esteem, perfectionism, and compulsiveness.

Alcoholism has become a major health problem in the United States involving over 3 million individuals and is a factor in about 10% of all deaths.[13] There is an increased incidence of alcoholism in men, but the number of alcoholic women is increasing. Though alcoholism is primarily a disease of adults, greater numbers of adolescent alcoholics are being diagnosed and treated. There is also increased incidence of alcoholism in cultural or ethnic groups in which drinking is an accepted norm of behavior. The impact of the disease is further evidenced by the number of hospital admissions related to alcohol abuse, such as automobile accidents and cirrhosis. Those at risk are individuals with a family history of alcoholism or a family history of total abstinence, who spent a childhood in an unstable family environment, who were the last child of a large family or were in the last half of a large family, or who are heavy smokers.

The nurse may have several opportunities to assess the client's response to alcohol. The nurse can use the nursing history and physical assessment skills to obtain data about the client and his drinking habits. The nurse may also assess the client when he is intoxicated, observe the effects of chronic alcohol use on the client's health, or determine signs of withdrawal.

Alcohol produces central nervous system depression. When the client is *intoxicated* the nurse may note that the client has a false sense of well-being. Sensations may be distorted, and the ability to speak and write may be impaired. The client has disturbances in coordination and may have difficulty walking, driving, or judging distances. Because alcohol depresses the medulla, the client may have respiratory depression, shock, or even respiratory arrest.

Chronic alcohol abuse affects all body systems. The nurse should observe these effects on the client's general health. There may be muscle wasting and peripheral neuropathy. The heart may be enlarged, and impairment of nutrition, such as anemia, can be noted. Most significant are the effects of alcohol on the liver, such as hepatitis or cirrhosis. Personality changes and decreased involvement in interpersonal relationships are other effects of chronic alcohol abuse.

Withdrawal symptoms are caused by a reduction or cessation of alcohol intake, when the cells that are no longer under depressant effects become active and produce physiological symptoms of withdrawal. The symptoms may be mild or severe. Mild withdrawal symptoms include tremors and nervousness, which occur 3 to 36 hours after drinking. The client may have insomnia, tachycardia, increased blood pressure, agitation, anxiety or nausea, and vomiting. More serious symptoms of withdrawal are seizures, delirium tremens, and hallucinations.

Chronic alcohol ingestion results in an elevated seizure threshold, followed by a period of lowered seizure threshold. This factor, combined with an altered electrolyte status and a lowered blood glucose level, is likely to produce seizures, even when some alcohol is still being consumed. Withdrawal seizures are usually grand mal and occur 7 to 48 hours after alcohol withdrawal.

Gross motor tremors (delirium tremens) are punctuated with agitation, altered sensory perception (auditory and visual), and grand mal seizures. Delirium tremens and its accompanying manifestations begin 72 hours after withdrawal and continue for several days in many instances. *This is a serious condition that carries a 10% to 15% mortality,* probably because of cardiorespiratory dysfunction and vasomotor collapse. Auditory or visual hallucinations, indicative of a metabolic state of the brain, may be noted, along with a clouded sensorium.

A nursing care plan is developed for the individual client, depending on the state of the client and the reason for contact with health personnel. The short-term nursing objective is to help the client manage withdrawal. Long-term objectives may include plans for detoxification and rehabilitation.

Managing acute withdrawal

The client who is withdrawing from alcohol use should be sedated and given fluid and electrolyte solutions to prevent dehydration. Barbiturates, sedatives, or tranquilizers may be used when the client is agitated. Because these drugs depress the central nervous system, their use should be tapered off gradually. The nurse should offer the client fluids, orally if possible. Magnesium sulfate may be given, as hypomagnesemia may aggravate withdrawal symptoms. When tolerated by the client, full nutritional support with vitamin supplementation as needed is offered.

125

TABLE 4-4

Summary of environmental aspects of physical factors

Physical factor	Sources	Populations exposed	Effects	Ease of control
Ionizing radiation (high-energy particles and electromagnetic radiation)	Natural sources Medical diagnosis and treatment Nuclear energy Consumer products	Whole population Special and occupational groups	Tissue injury Genetic effects Cancer	Can be partially controlled; medical exposures can be reduced
Ultraviolet rays	Sun, sun lamps Welder's arcs Industrial and medical applications	Whole population (sun) Special and occupational groups	Skin cancer "Aging" of skin Eye and skin "burns" Photosensitization Effects on biosphere	Relatively easy to shield or avoid for man, but not for the biosphere
Visible light	Sun, artificial lighting, lasers Communications, industrial and medical applications	Whole population (sun) Special and occupational groups	Retinal burns, photosensitization Effects on circadion rhythms	Relatively easy to shield or to keep confined (lasers)
Infrared radiation Environmental heat and humidity Cold	Sun, summer heat, winter cold, cold water, heat lamps Industrial sources	Whole population (sun, summer heat and winter cold) Special and occupational groups	Thermal stress death in susceptible individuals (elderly, very young, and those with cardiovascular disease) Infrared damage to eyes (cataracts) Cold stress, hypothermia in susceptible individuals (inadequately clad, very young, elderly, and those with cardiovascular disease)	Difficult to control "heat island" of cities Cost of climate control
Microwaves Radio frequencies	Radar and other communications Ovens; industrial and medical applications	Potentially large proportion of population	Thermal effects at high power levels Affects heart pacemakers and metal prosthetic devices Possible behavioral effects at low levels	Difficult where not directional beams Need for inspection of and tight ovens
Magnetic and electrostatic fields	Power lines Fusion power Industrial and research laboratories	Small occupational groups	Behavioral and psychological effects reported	Relatively easy to keep potentially exposed population out of area
Extremely low radio frequencies	Electric power Communications systems	Relatively small occupational groups	Possible central nervous system effects Electrical shock	Not necessary Distance a protective factor
Noise	Occupational sources community and home Transportation (airports, highways)	Special occupational groups, urban populations	Hearing loss Psychological reactions Effects on performance, general welfare, and health	Occupational control costly Difficult for community noise Need to design quieter homes; zoning Control for major noise sources
Vibration	Occupational sources Transportation	Occupational groups Truck and large machine operations	Peripheral vascular disease Neuromuscular effects Motion sickness Behavioral effects	Difficult for certain sources Others can build in isolation
Ultrasonics	Occupational medical diagnosis and treatment	Occupational groups and patients	Potential molecular, cellular, and organ effects	Possible to control energy or to shield

Modified from National Institutes of Health: Human health and the environment: some research needs, Washington, D.C., 1977, U.S. Department of Health and Human Services.

TABLE 4-4

Summary of environmental aspects of physical factors—cont'd

Physical factor	Sources	Populations exposed	Effects	Ease of control
Low barometric pressure	Altitudes over 1300 m Air transportation	Large populations at high altitudes Special recreational groups Aircraft passengers and personnel	Hypoxia, congenital malformation, fetal wastage, synergistic with other factors High-altitude pulmonary edema Cardiovascular symptoms	No real control in general environment Can control cabin pressures in aircraft
High barometric pressure	Underwater operations especially at 2 to 60 atmospheres absolute	Occupational and recreational divers	Bends, oxygen toxicity Nitrogen narcosis Osteonecrosis	Special gas mixtures Controlled ascents and decompression Careful training Special undersea housing

Rehabilitation   In order for rehabilitation to be successful, the client must wish to stop drinking and seek help. Rehabilitation may be accomplished through formal or informal programs as an individual, as a member of a group, or with the family. Many communities have specialized detoxification programs or rehabilitation centers. Alcoholics Anonymous for the client and Al-Anon for the family are resources available in most communities. The nurse may coordinate the use of these services and facilitate client referral.

The physical environment

Air, water, and noise pollution are three sources of pollution among a long list. A complete listing of additional physical factors that affect health can be found in Table 4-4.

AIR POLLUTION   Air pollutants have been identified as one of the most important sources of chemical hazards. Tons of toxic materials are given off yearly from factories, dumps, incinerators, and engines. These pollutants include carbon dioxides, nitrogen oxides, hydrocarbons, and particulates.

Two basic types of air pollutants have been identified: the photochemical haze commonly known as smog (smoke and fog) and particulate matter (such as tiny particles of dust, dirt, smoke, and ash).[22,23] Smog results from the oxidation of hydrocarbons and nitrogen oxide. Photochemical haze causes irritation of the eyes, nose, and throat, but does not seriously affect health. Particulate matter, on the other hand, is more dangerous and results from imperfect combustion of fuel waste (coal, gas, and oil) and other substances. As a result, gases such as carbon monoxide, sulfur dioxide, and nitrogen oxides are released into the air. These pollutants affect various body systems. For example, carbon monoxide (which is colorless, odorless, and poisonous) impairs transport of oxygen to the tissues. It passes through the respiratory system unchanged and combines with the hemoglobin of red blood cells. Because it has an affinity for hemoglobin 210 times greater than that of oxygen, it displaces oxygen, thus causing a decrease in the oxygen content of the blood. Since the heart receives a large proportion of oxygen, which is delivered via the blood, the heart muscle is vastly affected by carbon monoxide. Individuals with a decreased blood supply to the heart, as with angina, will likely have a decrease in exercise capacity. An alveolar concentration of carbon monoxide of 0.1% is deadly.[11] Symptoms such as dizziness, headache, and fatigue may be evident if lesser amounts are inhaled. It may affect the central nervous system by slowing reaction time.

Sulfur dioxide causes irritation to the respiratory tract and subsequent lung damage. The severity of the response depends on the percentage of fumes and vapors in the air.[23]

The harmful effects of air pollution on health have also been explained on the basis of *temperature inversions*. An inversion occurs when a layer of warm air traps the polluted layer of air closest to the ground. This trapping effect prevents the pollutants from rising into the atmosphere and results in a high level of pollution in the ambient air. During periods of inversion illnesses and deaths increase, particularly among individuals with heart and lung diseases.[22]

During periods of inversion, clients, especially those in the older age group with heart and lung diseases, are encouraged to stay indoors and to curtail even routine household activities such as cleaning. Windows should be kept closed, and air conditioners, which recirculate room air, should be used. If ventilation is needed for the home, it should be done after dark or very early in the morning, since pollution levels tend to peak during the hours of bright sunlight.[22]

WATER POLLUTION

In addition to air as a form of pollution, hazards of water have been identified, including phosphates, toxins, acids, and mineral particles. These pollutants contaminate the water and cause damage to health directly through drinking the polluted water or indirectly through eating food, particularly fish, poisoned through the food chain.[27]

Some viral and bacterial diseases have been associated with polluted water. However, at present, these diseases occur sporadically, for example, after disasters such as floods and earthquakes and when the water supply is affected.

NOISE POLLUTION

The problem of excessive noise is nationwide (Figs. 4-3 to 4-5). In fact, excessive noise has become such a health hazard that every nurse should be aware of its effects. Several psychosocial and physiological effects have been documented. The psychosocial effects are that it is annoying, disrupts sleep or relaxa-

FIG. 4-3
Typical outdoor sound measured on a quiet suburban street. (From Protective noise levels, Washington, D.C., 1978, United States Environmental Protection Agency.)

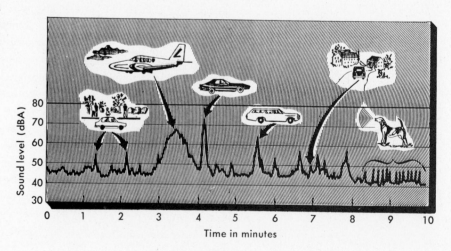

128

4   Environment and health problems

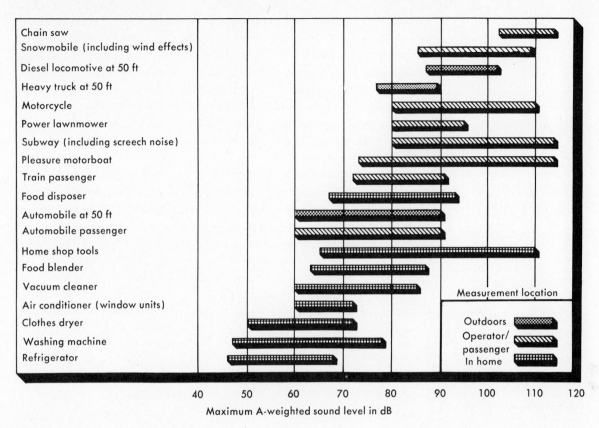

Maximum A-weighted sound level in dB

FIG. 4-4
Typical range of common sounds. (From Protective noise levels, Washington, D.C., 1978, United States Environmental Protection Agency.)

FIG. 4-5
Outdoor day-night average sound levels in decibels, measured at various locations (From Protective noise levels, Washington, D.C., 1978, United States Environmental Protection Agency.)

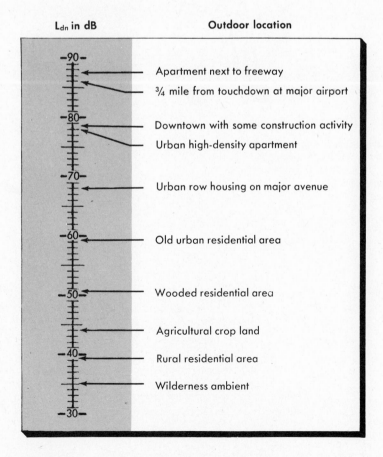

Foundations of clinical practice

tion, and interrupts conversation and thought patterns. Noise can also startle. In addition, it can interfere with job performance and safety. The physiological effects that have been reported include increasing heart and respiratory rates and muscular activity. However, each of these has been demonstrated to disappear even if the noise continues. Changes that have been shown to have a more sustained effect include constriction of small vessels (for example, of the extremities), which in some individuals causes paleness and sensory disturbance (Fig. 4-6).[5] Nausea and pain have been reported, especially when the exposure is severe. A most dreaded effect is that exposure to excessive noise can produce hearing loss. The exact mechanism of how noise produces hearing loss has not been determined. However, it is thought that excessive noise levels cause the hair cells within the inner ear to be overstimulated, resulting in degeneration of the organ of Corti (Fig. 4-7). When this happens, some sound waves are no longer converted into nerve impulses to the brain, and a hearing impairment results.

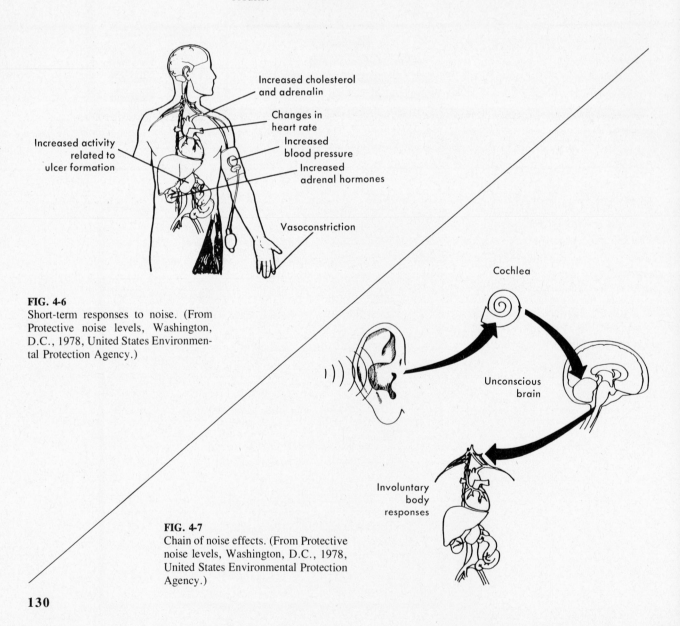

FIG. 4-6
Short-term responses to noise. (From Protective noise levels, Washington, D.C., 1978, United States Environmental Protection Agency.)

FIG. 4-7
Chain of noise effects. (From Protective noise levels, Washington, D.C., 1978, United States Environmental Protection Agency.)

130

Noise-induced hearing loss is thought to be related to three factors: (1) the overall level of noise, (2) the frequency range of noise, and (3) duration of exposure and individual susceptibility.[5] Exposure to noise levels below 85 db usually does not affect hearing. However, exposure to moderate noises for short periods of time may produce temporary threshold shifts. This means that hearing returns to normal levels after a period of rest from hazardous noise. Exposure to 85 to 95 db of sound for several hours a day can lead to progressive or permanent hearing loss. Exposure to more than 100 db for an extended time can damage hearing, and levels above 120 db may cause damage even if one is exposed for only a short period. Usually exposure to sounds within this range causes immediate discomfort, whereas sounds over 130 db produce severe pain.

People with noise-induced hearing loss can hear speech, but not clearly. They tend not to hear high-frequency consonants such as *sh* or *ch*. Hearing impaired by noise exposure does not return to normal even after long periods away from the noise.

Individuals who are affected are usually not aware of the changes until the noise exposure has been of sufficient severity and duration to affect speech frequency range. This is an important reason for encouraging clients to protect their hearing as much as possible.

Summary

The social and physical environments have a vast effect on individuals throughout the life span. Some of the sources of environmental health problems include accidents, poisonings, drug abuse, smoking, and alcoholism, as well as air, water, and noise pollution. The results are varied and include physical as well as psychosocial effects.

References

1. American National Red Cross: Session on drug abuse (instructor's guide), ARC Pub. No. 1679, Washington, D.C., 1970, American National Red Cross.
2. Arena, Jay M.: Poisoning: toxicology, symptoms, treatments, Springfield, Ill., 1974, Charles C Thomas, Publisher.
3. Bottenfield, Gerald, and Cohen, Sanford N.: Therapeutics in pediatric emergency room, Pediatr. Clin. North Am. **26:**867-881, 1979.
4. Burkhalter, Pamela: Nursing care of the alcoholic and drug abuser, New York, 1975, McGraw-Hill Book Co.
5. Burns, William: Noise and man, Philadelphia, 1969, J.B. Lippincott Co.
6. Cahn, Carolyn: Care of the poisoned child, Crit. Care Q. **3:**55-61, June 1980.
7. Chishom, J. Julian, and Maloney, Lucy Ranes: Lead poisoning: man made epidemic, Urban Health **3:**34-35, Dec. 1975.
8. Cook, Rosa Lee: Health environment responsibility arousal, Focus **7:**28-31, Nov./Dec. 1970.
9. Davidson, Sharon: The assessment of alcoholism, Fam. Comm. Health **1:**1, 1979.
10. Dreisbach, Robert H.: Handbook of poisoning, ed. 8, Los Altos, Cal., 1974, Lange Medical Publications.
11. Guyton, Arthur: Textbook of medical physiology, ed. 5, Philadelphia, 1976, W.B. Saunders Co.
12. Hanlon, John Joseph, and Pickett, George E.: Public health: administration and practice, ed. 7, St. Louis, 1979, The C.V. Mosby Co.
13. Healthy people: the Surgeon General's report on health promotion and disease prevention, Washington, D.C., 1979, U.S. Department of Health, Education, and Welfare.
14. Henderson, John: Treatment of poisoning: Emergency medical guide, ed. 2, New York, 1969, McGraw-Hill Book Co.

15. Husband, Peter: The accident prone child, Practitioner **211:**334-335, 1973.
16. Iannaccone, Susane: Intoxication of the central nervous system—lead. In Hoekelman, Robert A., and others: Principles of pediatrics: health care of the young, New York, 1978, McGraw-Hill Book Co.
17. Joselow, Morris M., and Bogden, John D.: Lead content of printed media—warning: spitballs may be hazardous to your health, Am. J. Public Health **64:**238-240, 1974.
18. King, B.C.: Maximum daily intake of lead without excessive lead burden in children, Am. J. Dis. Child. **122:**337-340, 1971.
19. Klein, R.: Lead poisoning, Adv. Pediatr. **24:**103-132, 1977.
20. Koch-Weser, Jan: Poisons—general considerations and principles of management. In Isselbacher, Kurt, Adams, Raymond, Braunwald, Eugene, Petersdorf, Robert, and Wilson, Jean, editors: Harrison's principles of internal medicine, ed. 9, New York, 1980, McGraw-Hill Book Co.
21. Lead poisoning where you least expect it, Emerg: Med. **12:**24-34, Apr. 30, 1980.
22. Marshall, Carter L., and Pearson, David: Dynamics of health and disease, New York, 1972, Appleton-Century-Crofts.
23. Murray, Ruth Beckmann, and Zenter, Judith Proctor: Nursing assessment and health promotion through the life span, ed. 2, Englewood Cliffs, N.J., 1979, Prentice-Hall, Inc.
24. Nolph, Georgia B.: Poisonings: immediate care of the acutely ill and injured, St. Louis, 1974, The C.V. Mosby Co.
25. Rumack, Barry H.: Management of acute poisoning, revised, unpublished paper, 1975.
26. Stellman, Steven D., and Stellman, Jeanne M.: Women's occupations, smoking, and cancer and other diseases, CA **31:**29-40, Jan./Feb. 1981.
27. Waldbott, George L.: Health effects of environmental pollutants, St. Louis, 1973, The C.V. Mosby Co.

Additional readings

Bahra, Robert J.: The potential for suicide, Am. J. Nurs. **75:**1782-1788, 1975.

Delbridge, Patricia M.: Identifying the suicidal person in the community, Can. Nurs. **70:**14-17, Nov. 1974.

Diran, Margaret O'Keefe: You can prevent suicide, Nurs. '76 **6:**60-64, 1976.

Dube, Shiv K., and Pierog, Sophie H., editors: Immediate care of the sick and injured child, St. Louis, 1978, The C.V. Mosby Co.

Golub, Sharon: Noise, the underrated health hazard, RN **32:**40-45, May 1969.

Kottmeier, Peter K.: What the pediatrician should know about pediatric trauma, Current Probl. Pediatr. **6:**4-54, June, 1976.

Krombert, Carol J., and Proctor, Judith Betz: Evaluation of a day program methadone maintenance, Am. J. Nurs. **70:**2575-2577, 1970.

Kryler, K.D.: Non-auditory effects of environmental noise, Am. J. Public Health **62:**389-398, 1972.

Lubin, David: Electrical safety, Hospitals **43:**57-60, Dec. 1, 1969.

Metz, Virginia, and Henenson, Irwin B.: Management of drug overdose in the adult, J. Emer. Nurs. **1:**8-11, Nov.-Dec. 1975.

Miller, James D.: Effects of noise on people, J. Acoust. Soc. Am. **56:**729, 1974.

Olson, Robert J.: Index of suspicion, screening for child abusers, Am. J. Nurs. **76:**108-110, 1976.

Preventing lead poisoning in young children, J. Pediatr. **93:**709-720, 1978.

Rogers, Martha E.: Theoretical basis of nursing, Philadelphia, 1970, F.A. Davis Co.

Stephenson, Hugh E., editor: Immediate care of the acutely ill and injured, ed. 2, St. Louis, 1978, The C.V. Mosby Co.

Taylor, Susan D.: Addicts as patients, Nurs. Outlook **13:**41-44, Nov. 1975.

U.S. Department of Health, Education, and Welfare: Human health and the environment: Some research needs, The Department.

U.S. Environmental Protection Agency: Protective noise levels, Washington, D.C., Nov. 1978, Office of Noise Abatement and Control.

5 Health and health problems

Health and illness (or health problems) are positions on a continuum that reflect man's adaptation to his internal and external environments. Health and illness are defined objectively and subjectively by individuals, communities, cultural groups, and societies, and behaviors are elicited to make positions on the continuum optimal. The purpose of this chapter is to describe the health-illness continuum, identify determinants of health and illness, describe health and illness behaviors, and discuss modes of adaptation and coping. The nurse and client identify positions of health and illness in order to formulate plans for health maintenance or restoration or for prevention of health problems. The nurse must, therefore, be sensitive to individual, cultural, and societal perceptions of health and illness and behaviors associated with these states.

Health-illness continuum

Health and illness are dynamic positions on a continuum that includes states of high-level wellness, health, precursors for illness, illness, and severe illness (Fig. 5-1). An individual may experience any of these states across the life span, and movement on the continuum may be dynamic in either direction as individuals adapt to optimal levels of health.

FIG. 5-1
The health-illness continuum.

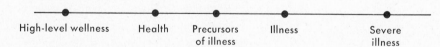

High-level wellness   Health   Precursors of illness   Illness   Severe illness

HEALTH AND HIGH-LEVEL WELLNESS

Descriptions of health and high-level wellness focus on the individual, environment, culture, and universal nature of humans and differ according to the perceptions of the individual or group defining health. Several definitions, however, provide a framework for describing health and high-level wellness.

Man is an open system in dynamic interaction with his environment, constantly seeking growth and equilibrium. Health, from this viewpoint, is a purposeful, adaptive response, physically, mentally, emotionally, and socially, to external stimuli in order to maintain stability and comfort.[11] Positive integra-

133

tion and adaptation, known as health, allows man to perform to his highest capability relatively free of discomfort or disability.[4]

Health as an integrative response of holistic man is underscored in the classic definition of health from the World Health Organization, which describes health as a state of physical, mental, and social well-being, not merely as the absence of disease or infirmity. Healthy individuals, therefore, are physically and mentally well in both the social and personal environments.

Health may also be described from a religious or moral viewpoint. For some individuals and cultures health is a reward for past or present behavior. Health is seen as external to individual and environmental influences and denotes man's spiritual relationships with universal environments.

Health can also be viewed as a dynamic movement toward high-level wellness. High-level wellness for the individual is defined as an integrated method of functioning that is oriented toward maximizing the potential of which the individual is capable within the environment where he is functioning. This classic definition by Dr. Halbert Dunn views health on a continuum, with wellness being a dynamic state of change.[6] Such a concept is oriented toward positive characteristics (assets) of clients, not their limitations.

High-level wellness can be achieved only when there is an integration and satisfaction of the basic needs. The challenge of this concept is that it must be applied to everyday living by both individuals and groups. This concept does not expect an optimal level of wellness, but a progression toward a higher level of functioning that takes into account mental health as well as physical and social health.

PRECURSORS TO ILLNESS: RISK AND VULNERABILITY

Midpoint on the health-illness continuum is a position in which biological, environmental, and behavioral stressors impinge on the individual and the likelihood of movement from health and wellness to illness or severe illness increases. Risk and vulnerability are two concepts that explain this phenomenon.

Risk

Risk refers to the likelihood that a health problem will occur. Risk factors include inherited biological, environmental, or behavioral stressors. *Inherited risks* are those determined by biological characteristics of age, sex, family history, or genetic endowment that have predictable consequences for illness. Hemophilia and sickle cell disease are examples of risk due to genetic endowment; chronic diseases such as diabetes mellitus may be attributed to biological factors of age, sex, or family history. *Environmental risks* are physical, social, and economic stressors such as air pollution, water contamination, noise, radiation, traffic congestion, poor housing conditions, dangerous occupations, poor education, and low income. *Behavioral risks* are those related to health behavior or habits such as smoking, drinking, poor dietary patterns, lack of exercise or sleep, and low values for health practices of self-examination and health appraisals.

The practice of prospective health care is directed toward identifying individuals at risk for health problems and helping them change the movement on the health-illness continuum toward health at the earliest indication of health deviation. Risk can be identified for each individual and the individual described as (1) not at risk; (2) having risk attributed to age or environment; (3) having precursors present; (4) having signs of health problems present, but observable only to the health professional; (5) having signs of health problems present and observable to the individual; or (6) being and possibly moving toward severe illness or even death.[7]

The nurse has a significant role in risk identification. One tool is the Health Hazard Appraisal.[7] This assessment guide elicits data about (1) a client's present health status, (2) habits of daily living (such as smoking, stress, exercise, and the wearing of seat belts in automobiles), and (3) factors in hereditary and familial tendencies as derived from the health history. These data are processed, and risks to health and life are calculated. Finally, and most important, a regimen to reduce risks is prescribed for the individual, which will increase his chances for surviving the next 10-year period of life. Risk management strategies are discussed where appropriate throughout the text.

TABLE 5-1

Social Readjustment Rating Scale

Rank	Life event	Mean value
1	Death of spouse	100
2	Divorce	73
3	Marital separation	65
4	Jail term	63
5	Death of close family member	63
6	Personal injury or illness	53
7	Marriage	50
8	Fired at work	47
9	Marital reconciliation	45
10	Retirement	45
11	Change in health of family member	44
12	Pregnancy	40
13	Sex difficulties	39
14	Gain of new family member	39
15	Business readjustment	39
16	Change in financial state	38
17	Death of close friend	37
18	Change to different line of work	36
19	Change in number of arguments with spouse	35
20	Mortgage over $10,000	31
21	Foreclosure of mortgage or loan	30
22	Change in responsibilities at work	29
23	Son or daughter leaving home	29
24	Trouble with in-laws	29
25	Outstanding personal achievement	28
26	Wife begin or stop work	26
27	Begin or end school	26
28	Change in living conditions	25
29	Revision of personal habits	24
30	Trouble with boss	23
31	Change in work hours or conditions	20
32	Change in residence	20
33	Change in schools	20
34	Change in recreation	19
35	Change in church activities	19
36	Change in social activities	18
37	Mortgage or loan less than $10,000	17
38	Change in sleeping habits	16
39	Change in number of family get-togethers	15
40	Change in eating habits	15
41	Vacation	13
42	Christmas	12
43	Minor violations of the law	11

From Holmes, T., and Rahe, R.: The social readjustment rating scale, J. Psychosom. Res. **11**:213, 1967. Reprinted with permission of Pergamon Press, Ltd.

Vulnerability

Vulnerability refers to a concept of predisposition to crises. Longitudinal studies of children have demonstrated that certain factors contribute to making individuals at "high risk" for succumbing to stress. Children with birth trauma, firstborn children, and those with environmental deprivation tend to have characteristic problems in systematically coping with threatening circumstances. Other precursors to vulnerability involve marital disharmony of parents, alcoholism of parents, frequent moving of residences, childhood illness, or death of a sibling or pet. It is helpful for nurses to have some historical data on a client's earlier life experiences with stress, his modes of coping and adaptation, and the resources that are selected for help. All family associates should be assessed, too, since the combined strength of all members is essential for successful management of situational and maturational crises.

Recent research focuses on change as a stressor increasing vulnerability to health problems.[5] The Social Readjustment Rating Scale developed by Holmes and Rahe lists and rates representative life change events; an individual's score can be used to predict his vulnerability to illness (Table 5-1).[8]

ILLNESS

The positions of illness and severe illness are subsequent to precursors of illness on the health-illness continuum. In an open-system view of man, illness is the failure of one's adaptation to internal and external environments. Failure can be described in terms of social, mental, emotional, or physical adaptation or as failure of function and adjustment of the organism as a whole or of any parts. Adaptation failures can also be described for disturbances in growth or development across the life span.

Disease or health problems are more objective descriptors of illness; classic definitions of disease include absence of health or change of structure or function of the mind or body. Generalized responses to abnormal functioning may be described as disease and legitimized by the society, culture, or health professionals.

Illness exists in a cultural milieu and may be perceived as punishment for thoughts or behavior. Cultural definitions of illness may also include illness behaviors and grant permission for illness.

Determinants of health and illness

The health-illness continuum resides in a context of the dynamic interaction of man and his environment (Fig. 5-2). Determinants of health and illness, therefore, can be identified for each.

HEREDITY AND LIFE-STYLE

Heredity and life-style are two determinants of health or illness. Heredity provides the nonmodifiable factors of age, sex, race, genetic endowment, and family history as a foundation for health. Life-style, on the other hand, includes factors modifiable by choice. These may include health-related behaviors of hygiene, exercise, rest, substance abuse, nutrition, immunizations, self-examination, use of safety belts, and periodic visits to health professionals.

ENVIRONMENT

As discussed in Chapter 4, man's social and physical environment can facilitate or obstruct opportunities for growth and development. The impact of the environment on health is recently recognized, and research data are demonstrating relationships of factors such as education, occupation, economic status, sanitation facilities, noise, population density, housing, disease control, environmental stress, and nutrition to individual and community health.[9]

Perceptions of health and illness

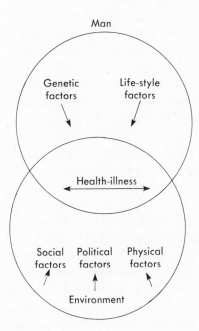

FIG. 5-2
Man, environment, and the health-illness continuum.

Individuals, society or culture, and health professionals can perceive health and illness as subjective states. Although the perceptions of each may be different, health care is facilitated when definitions are congruent. It is important, therefore, for the nurse to identify who is defining health and health problems, and where power for decision making resides.

Any definition of health or illness must incorporate the idea that health is a dynamic phenomenon, that it is a product of the integration of biopsychosocial factors, and that it must be viewed on a continuum.[2] The determination of how clients see themselves as well or sick is a summation of earlier life experiences and learning. For example, an adult with well-controlled diabetes can perceive himself as healthy or unhealthy, depending on his orientation. For some individuals being sick means not feeling well; for others it means not being able to go to work or carry out daily activities.

Since man is an open system, stress affecting any one system can cause another to change. For example, a physical stressor such as pain can produce tension in interpersonal relationships. Marital or job conflicts may contribute to formation of a peptic ulcer. Severe electrolyte imbalance can create mental confusion. The nurse must consider all variables operant for clients in order to adequately evaluate the impact of stressors on their health status.

Health and illness can also be described by the culture or society. Behaviors that are illness related in one group may be indicative of health in another. Cultural health traditions are firmly rooted, and the nurse must be aware of the meanings of health and illness to each individual as defined by his culture.[1] Of particular significance to health care in the United States are the unique perceptions of blacks, Chicanos, American Indians, and Asians.

The way health and illness are defined by health care professionals may diverge from the way they are described by an individual or culture. Individuals' perceptions tend to be more diffuse and comprehensive, whereas those of health care professionals tend to focus on objective data and describe signs that fit a pathophysiological disease causation model. The nurse must, therefore, obtain a nursing history that reflects subjective data and descriptions of health problems as perceived by the client.

Health and illness behavior

Health or illness behaviors are those actions an individual engages in to maintain health or cope with illness. These behaviors are influenced by the individual's family and peers and tend to reflect the values of his culture or dominant society. Several theoretical frameworks explain or predict health or illness behavior, and the nurse can use these to help clients maintain or restore health.

HEALTH BEHAVIOR

Health behavior refers to the activity an individual engages in to maintain health, prevent disease, or treat health problems. It is a response to health when no symptoms of illness are evident. Behaviors may include maintenance activities

137

of proper exercise, nutrition, and rest or prevention of disease by obtaining immunizations or fluoridating teeth. If health problems are identified, the individual with high motivation for health behavior seeks health care services and complies with health instructions.[14]

One model used to explain or predict health behaviors is the Health Belief Model.[12] This model postulates that health behavior depends on the individual's perception of susceptibility to a health problem and his perceived seriousness of the problem; the decision to act is influenced by modifying factors such as health instruction, advice from peers or professionals, age, sex, race, ethnicity, socioeconomic class, and knowledge about disease. The model identifies relationships of perceptions, modifying factors, and action and demonstrates that the likelihood of health behaviors occurring depends on the perceived benefits of action minus the barriers to action.

Nurses motivating clients toward health behaviors must identify the client's perception of the health problem and the modifying factors in order to predict the likelihood of favorable health behavior. Compliance with health instruction is facilitated by reducing barriers and rewarding positive health behaviors.

ILLNESS BEHAVIOR

Illness behaviors are responses to abnormal body signals.[10] Responses may include (1) monitoring body signals, (2) taking action to deal with the signals, and (3) using health care facilities.

Cognitive and affective changes may motivate clients to acknowledge illness and seek health care services. In one model the assumption of the "sick role" is described in five stages: the client (1) experiences symptoms; (2) decides he is ill and needs health care; (3) seeks health care services to validate diagnosis and obtain treatment; (4) assumes a dependent-patient role during treatment, in which responsibility and control are delegated to a health care professional; and (5) during recovery, relinquishes the sick role for rehabilitation.[13] The nurse may interact with the client at any stage of illness behavior, and the role of the nurses changes from supportive to facilitative in concert with changes in the client's illness behavior.

Adaptation and coping

Physiological and psychological responses to changes in the health-illness continuum occur as man seeks to allocate energies to achieve a steady state. Methods of adaptation and coping facilitate the client's attempts to maintain health and achieve high-level wellness.

The steady state is that state existing when energy is allocated in such a way that man is freed to actualize himself according to his nature, maintained by effective and efficient activities of the regulatory processes at all behavioral levels. Essentially, this means that man has internal constancy and is in harmony with his environment.[2] In order for a true steady state to exist, there must be a unified effort of all autonomic physiochemical behaviors and voluntary self-regulating behaviors.

Because every person is unique, a steady state for each individual will be different. All persons are genetically endowed with specific potentials for coping with stress and illness, and all have experienced different life situations that influence their ability to tolerate and deal with stress and illness. Furthermore,

5   Health and health problems

since all human beings possess highly individualized energy levels, some deal with stressful circumstances more successfully than others before becoming vulnerable to instability. Therefore, the conditions that cause illness in one client may not cause illness in another, or at least with the same degree of severity. Nurses who assess persons should consider four factors: (1) nature of the stressor, (2) number of stressors to be coped with simultaneously, (3) duration of exposure to the stressor, and (4) past experiences with a comparable stressor. The combination of data regarding these will provide valuable information about the client's position on the health-illness continuum.

GENERAL ADAPTATION SYNDROME

There are certain physiological responses to an anxiety-provoking situation. This physically oriented adaptation to stress has been carefully researched and has been identified as the body's general adaptation syndrome.

When any human organism *perceives* a threat to its well-being, whether actual or not, *stress* develops. This stress will manifest itself by changes in physiological and psychosocial functioning (Fig. 5-3). The first response to stress is the stage of *alarm*. A threat has been perceived, and the nervous and endocrine systems have been notified of the emergency. The second stage is called *resistance*. At this point nerves and glands are aiding body tissue in resisting stress. The final stage is *exhaustion,* when tissues surrender to stress. For example, in the development of a bedsore, or decubitus ulcer, the client first experiences local pain and discomfort, which serves to alert the nurse as well as the body tissue to take action to relieve the pressure and venous stasis. In the resistance stage, as the body attempts to cope with the ischemic area, it is engorged with blood and appears warm and red. But if relief is not obtained for several more hours, the tissues are forced to surrender, and necrosis and ulceration follow. Such physiological adaptation takes place in the development of any physical illness, but in some it is a more clearly defined phenomenon. Infection is an example of a process that follows a precise adaptation formula. As microbes enter the skin, they trigger an alarm that sets up the inflammatory response. Additional blood and tissue fluid are transported to the area to fight the invading organisms, and the tissue changes to wall off the affected area to confine the threatening microbes. However, if they are too virulent or too great in number, or if the body defenses are limited by poor health or prolonged stress, the tissue

FIG. 5-3
Mechanism of stress adaptation.

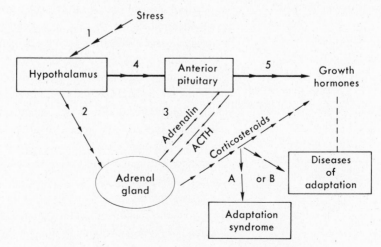

surrenders and a true infection develops, which damages and destroys tissue. This is termed a *local adaptation syndrome*.

In every human adaptive response there seems to be significant involvement of the cardiovascular beds. As the sympathetic nervous system is activated by the perception of a stressful phenomenon (the classic "fight or flight" response), vascular beds all over the body dilate and constrict on cue to stimulate glands and muscles, minimize visceral responses, enhance local blood supplies, and mobilize the body defenses. Long-term stress can be demonstrated clinically by certain conditions called *psychosomatic illnesses*. In these diseases, stress appears to play the primary etiological role and accounts for the symptoms. Among these are migraine headaches, certain collagen disorders such as rheumatoid arthritis, hypertension, allergies, gastrointestinal ulcers, and nervous and mental diseases of many degrees. Pathological findings associated with prolonged stress include adrenal hypertrophy, shrinkage of lymphatic organs, weight loss, alterations in chemical balances, and the appearance of ulcerative areas.

When ordinary physiological adaptations are unsuccessful in protecting tissue, outside invaders are permitted to take over. There is considerable disagreement within the health profession over which conditions are clearly related to stress and may be called psychosomatic illnesses. However, there is nearly universal concurrence that the failure of the body to cope with stress is a factor in all illnesses, whether the stressor agent is of physical or mental origin. At times the line between physical and mental illness is a fine one, and factors can often be interrelated to the degree that clear differentiation is impossible. Some conditions, such as alcoholism, must be managed by both physiological and psychological management principles.

NATURE OF THE CRISIS AND HOW IT IS PERCEIVED

A crisis is a situation or event that disturbs equilibrium because the usual coping behaviors are inadequate in dealing with the problem or are ineffective in resolving the stress that it produces. In simpler terms, a crisis exists when (1) a client views an insurmountable obstacle that he cannot handle with ordinary problem-solving techniques, (2) there is an overwhelming amount of environmental disorganization, or (3) attempts at solutions have been abortive; in short, when coping mechanisms have not been successful.

There are two types of crisis. A *situational* crisis is an external event, such as death of a loved one, disaster, or hospitalization. A *maturational crisis* is an event incurred in the process of psychosocial development, such as puberty, marriage, or menopause. In both types of crises there is an inherent threat to the presentation of self either in concept or role. It is apparent, therefore, that as various family members are faced with problems, the consequences of the problems are interrelated and could even be cumulative. Family members' role changes create losses that compel other members to adapt and compensate. It is this change in role, as opposed to stress, that is actually the precipitating factor in crises. The degree of success in confronting change is the chief determinant of whether individuals and groups deal with crises and grow as a result or succumb to their effects.

Crises involve losses that must be assessed in terms of the type of change they precipitate. For example, pregnancy may affect body image and self-concept. Moving from one city to another creates a revision in the nonhuman environment that demands adjustments to new physical surroundings by those involved. Even changes in beliefs, value systems, and expectations of others can induce crises under certain circumstances.

Perception of crises is based on previous learning, is related to fulfillment of needs, and manifests dominant concerns. Essentially, individuals appraise threats according to personal significance. For example, if a mother is admitted to the hospital for surgery, each member of her family views the situation from his personal viewpoint. A preschool child may feel that his mother has been taken away to punish him. An older child may fear that she will die as a result of her illness. The husband and father may worry more about operating the household and meeting the medical and surgical expenses. Thus each member perceives the same situation in a unique manner. The resultant admixture of guilt, frustration, fear of loss, and anxiety about role functioning and financial obligations creates a crisis within the nuclear family as well as in the injured or ill client's life.

Maturational crises in families
Individuals who have problems in dealing with maturational crises are essentially encountering difficulty in adjusting to a new role. They are unable to incorporate growth and developmental changes into their self-concept; that is, they cannot perceive themselves in a new role. Often their inability to adjust to changes is in part due to a lack of interpersonal resources. Significant others either are unable to be of help in the process of adjustment or refuse to acknowledge that a role change is inevitable. This latter response occurs in part because the role changes of one person force reciprocal changes in the roles of others. All individuals in any family constellation are affected by maturational crises, and these crises directly or indirectly influence how successfully they are managed.

Preventing crises
The nurse can be of value in primary, secondary, and tertiary measures that assist families in surviving crisis periods. *Primary prevention* involves a reduction in conditions that lead to maladaptive functioning. Preparing a young couple for parenting is an example of primary prevention. *Secondary prevention* refers to early recognition of a crisis so that treatment is begun. For example, a woman who is diagnosed early as being depressed about the approach of menopause can be directed to sources of help. *Tertiary prevention* in crisis refers to situations in which there already is decompensation from stress, thus requiring direct assistance from an individual or agency.

COPING MECHANISMS
Coping mechanisms are tools used to deal with anxiety and reduce tension. Their nature and scope vary with developmental experiences, ego composition, and life-style as well as ethnic and cultural patterns. They are highly individualized and often involve employment of mental mechanisms (defense mechanisms).

When faced with a crisis, the human organism directs its behavior toward eliminating the threat by using the least amount of physical energy possible. One of the more popular methods of avoiding threat is by rejection of an idea, or by *denial*. An individual merely refuses to believe or face facts as they exist. Rationalization, sublimation, regression, projection, reaction formation, repression, and identification are other mental defenses often used to deal with the threatening dimensions of injury, illness, and hospitalization. Use of defense mechanisms is measured merely by the extent that they facilitate coping and mastery. It should be noted that successful adaptation does not necessarily require an

Foundations of clinical practice

accurate perception of reality. *When individuals define situations as real, the situations tend to be real in their consequences.*[3]

Successful adaptation requires that the mind and body possess the autonomy, freedom, and integrity necessary for processing data and acting on it. Coping for some individuals would be greatly affected by "paralysis" if their traditional adaptive response involved mobility, such as moving away from a situation. On the other hand, individuals who rely heavily on mental and verbal coping strategies would be nearly helpless if a cerebrovascular accident (stroke) would impair speech and hearing communication and produce mental confusion.

Coping patterns are learned in the course of growth and development. An infant learns to cry in protest to effect a termination of an unwanted stimulus, such as hunger or a wet diaper. A 2-year-old adapts to external threats by a strong "no." Research has confirmed that the relative success or failure of these rudimentary forms of coping is highly correlated with coping in later life.[3] If early crises in life are managed well, it is highly probable that subsequent crises will also be successfully dealt with. However, if maladaptive behavior was used as a coping mechanism, it is likely to be repeatedly used. For example, if one has consistently run away from problems throughout life, it is not reasonable to assume that the individual will voluntarily face unpleasant circumstances and effect the necessary adaptations required for healthy adjustment.

Summary   Health and illness are subjective and objective perceptions on a continuum ranging from high-level wellness to severe illness. Health and illness can be defined from individual, cultural, and environmental perspectives and are perceived uniquely by each. Man seeks constancy in his external and internal environments and to this end uses adaptive behaviors to ensure an optimal position on the health-illness continuum. Nursing care is planned to promote, maintain, and restore health. The role of the nurse in implementing and evaluating health care is discussed in subsequent chapters.

References

1. Branch, Marie, and Paxton, Phyllis, editors: Providing safe nursing care for ethnic people of color, New York, 1976, Appleton-Century-Crofts.
2. Byrne, Marjorie, and Thompson, Lida: Key concepts for the study and practice of nursing, ed. 2, St. Louis, 1978, The C.V. Mosby Co.
3. Coehlo, George, and others, editors: Coping and adaptation, New York, 1974, Basic Books, Inc., Publishers.
4. Cook, Rosa Lee: Health environment responsibility arousal, Focus AACN **7**(6):28-31, 1980.
5. Dohrenwend, Barbara, and Dohrenwend, Bruce, editors: Stressful life events: their nature and effects, New York, 1974, John Wiley & Sons, Inc.
6. Dunn, Halbert: What high-level wellness means, Can. J. Public Health **50:**447-457, 1959.
7. Hall, Jack, and Zwemer, Jack: Prospective medicine, Indianapolis, 1979, Methodist Hospital of Indiana.
8. Holmes, Thomas, and Rahe, Richard: The Social Readjustment Rating Scale, J. Psychosom. Res. **11:**213-218, 1967.
9. Klein, Susan: Class, culture, and health. In Last, John, editor: Maxcy-Rosenau public health and preventive medicine, ed. 11, New York, 1980, Appleton-Century-Crofts.
10. Mechanic, David: Health and illness behavior. In Last, John, editor: Maxcy-Rosenau public health and preventive medicine, ed. 11, New York, 1980, Appleton-Century-Crofts.

11. Murray, Ruth, and Zentner, Judith: Nursing concepts for health promotion, Englewood Cliffs, N.J., 1975, Prentice-Hall, Inc.
12. Rosenstock, Irwin: What research in motivation suggests for public health, Am. J. Public Health **50:**295-302, 1960.
13. Suchman, E.A.: Stages of illness and medical care, J. Health Hum. Behav. **6:**114-128, 1965.
14. Tirrell, Barbara, and Hart, Laura: The relationship of health beliefs and knowledge to exercise compliance in patients after coronary bypass, Heart Lung **9:**487-493, 1980.

Additional readings

Ardell, Donald: High level wellness, Emmaus, Pa., 1977, Rodale Press, Inc.
Bauwens, Eleanor: The anthropology of health, St. Louis, 1978, The C.V. Mosby Co.
Foeta, Jeannette, and Deck, Edith: A sociological treatment for patient care, ed. 2, New York, 1979, John Wiley & Sons, Inc.
Healthy people: the Surgeon General's report on health promotion and disease prevention, Washington, D.C., U.S. Department of Health, Education, and Welfare.
Leininger, Madeline: Transcultural nursing: concepts, theories and practices, New York, 1978, John Wiley & Sons, Inc.
Spector, Rachel: Cultural diversity in health and illness, New York, 1979, Appleton-Century-Crofts.
U.S. Department of Health, Education, and Welfare: Health, United States, 1979, Washington, D.C., The Department.

6 Pathophysiological processes of illness

Health problems have primarily four basic underlying causes: (1) cellular deviation, (2) breaks in body defenses and barriers, (3) physical-chemical insults, or (4) degenerative processes. The multitude of medical and nursing diagnoses encompasses, in most cases, more than one of these pathological processes. For example, a congenital defect of the spinal cord could result in degeneration of the lower extremities if not corrected and could also be accompanied by a local inflammatory process. A tumor displaces surrounding tissues as it grows and interferes with normal cellular processes of adjacent structures. It may eventually lead to obstruction of a hollow organ, such as the bowel, and may ultimately create an inflammatory or even a degenerative process. Nurses should understand these pathophysiological processes and the complicating pathophysiology so that they can assess the effects on clients. Since interventions are directed toward the underlying causes of illness, the pathophysiological processes of illness are an integral part of the data necessary for the nursing process. Medical and nursing intervention is directed toward, and related to, removing the pathological organ or tissue, compensating for the pathological organ or tissue, compensating for the pathophysiology, or helping individuals achieve their own optimal level of health. The purpose of this chapter is to discuss these processes and present a framework for related nursing care. Specific information is presented in subsequent chapters.

Cellular deviation

Illness occurs when there is a deviation in the structure and growth of the cell. The complex structure and function of the cell can be damaged by a variety of influences. When cells are damaged, they may repair themselves, the damage may repeat itself throughout cell reproduction (as in genetic defects), or the cells may die. At this point, a review of the general functioning of the human cell is in order.

6 Pathophysiological processes of illness

CELL STRUCTURE AND FUNCTION

The cell is the basic structural and functional unit of the human body. It is capable of physical and chemical activities that include ingestion and storage of nutrients, protein synthesis, energy production, and reproduction (mitosis). The morphology, or form, of cells differs in various parts of the body, but similar structures are found in all cells, including the cytoplasm and the nucleus; most cells have cell membranes. These structures have components that enable the cell to perform more specific reactions for the organ of which it is a part. The biochemical activities within and among cells enable them to provide the body with energy needed to maintain health.

The cytoplasm contains structures called organelles. These are the mitochondria, lysosomes, endoplasmic reticulum, Golgi complex, centrosomes, and microsomes. Mitochondria are responsible for cell respiration and energy conversion. The lysosomes are part of the digestive system of the cell. The endoplasmic reticulum manufactures protein and contains ribonucleic acid (RNA). The Golgi complex (Golgi apparatus) contributes to the building of carbohydrates and the removal of proteins from the cell. The centrosome is a small body located near the nucleus that is prominent during mitosis (Fig. 6-1).

The major activities of the cell are directed by the nucleus. It determines reactions by the organelles in the cytoplasm and is responsible for cell division and reproduction. A membrane separates the nucleus from the cytoplasm. Inside the nucleus are *chromosomes* and the nucleoli. Deoxyribonucleic acid (DNA), the code for heredity, is a major constituent of the nucleus.

Membranes of the cell surround and contain the cytoplasm and the cell nucleus. This cell wall or membrane is semipermeable and thus allows passage of small molecules. It is well known that cells form *tissues,* that tissues form *organs,* and that organs combine to form the *organism.*

The functioning of the normal cell is complex and can be studied in greater detail. The student is referred to other textbooks.

FIG. 6-1
Normal human cell.

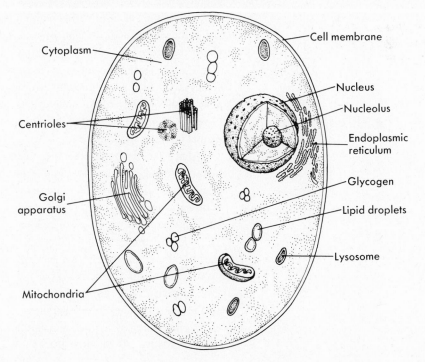

Cytoplasm

Cell membrane

Nucleus

Nucleolus

Centrioles

Endoplasmic reticulum

Glycogen

Golgi apparatus

Lipid droplets

Lysosome

Mitochondria

145

Foundations of clinical practice

Genetic factors determine cell structure and information related to cell growth. DNA is responsible for storing, duplicating, and transmitting information in a given cell. This chemical programs the function of cells in the organism and is found in cells that reproduce as well as those that do not. DNA is visible only with the use of the electron microscope.

The nuclei of cells contain small bodies called *chromosomes*. The *genes* are units or parts of chromosomes that determine the character and activities of cells and transmit inherited traits. Most cells in the human body contain 46 chromosomes, or 23 pairs each. There are 22 pairs of autosomes (meaning any chromosome other than a sex chromosome) and one pair of sex chromosomes. DNA is confined to the chromosomes in the cell nucleus.

CELLULAR DISTURBANCES

Disturbances in cell growth, proliferation, and differentiation are described by the following terms:

aplasia Failure of an organ to grow.

agenesis Absence of an organ. (Both aplasia and agenesis relate to the embryonic development of organs.)

hyperplasia An increase in the *number of cells* in a tissue producing an increase in the size of the tissue or organ (for example, increase in breast tissue during pregnancy).

hypertrophy Individual *cells enlarge;* therefore, organs enlarge. (for example, the increase in size of muscles as a result of weight lifting and exercise).

metaplasia The formation of one type of adult tissue by cells different from them. This is an abnormality of differentiation.

dysplasia Abnormal tissue development.

neoplasia Abnormal cells or a mass of proliferating cells.

GENETIC DEFECTS

Genetic defects result from deviations in the chromosomes and material of human development. The deviations have been attributed to damage to the chemical (enzyme) DNA. Normal growth, development, and heredity depend on adequate ''coding'' of information within the cells. Integration of the genetic material in the uterine and external environment directly affects human development. Genetic defects are heritable variations that occur very rarely.

The physical basis of both heredity and heritable variations is the gene. Genes are located along threadlike chromosomes in the cell nucleus. Cells divide after chromosomes undergo duplication. This division produces an identical set of genes. If there is deviation in a gene at this point, variation occurs and a congenital anomaly is produced.

Many factors contribute to variation, including the intrauterine environment. Optimal chemical and nutritional conditions are needed for normal cell division and growth. When there is a change in some portion of the DNA of a germ cell, *mutation* occurs. This results in altered traits being received by the individual created by the germ cell.

The environment can produce changes in human cells. A virus is capable of causing alteration of genetic materials, such as that seen in the growing fetus exposed to rubella or herpesvirus. Chemical substances such as copper, lead, zinc, and vinyl chloride are known to cause mutation. Radiation exposure can also produce changes in developing and growing human cells.

Abnormality of hereditary material in an individual may be evidenced in numerous ways. Most often the abnormality is not evident until birth. Three well-known examples of inherited diseases are diabetes, hemophilia, and sickle cell anemia. The appearance of a demonstrable trait or characteristic is called *phenotypic*. When one is examining for the presence or absence of a particular trait, it is helpful to review *mendelian* inheritance. Both sickle cell anemia and hemophilia are examples of mendelian inheritance. Some inherited illnesses are not evident until problems arise in childhood or adulthood. Two examples are muscular dystrophy (childhood) and Huntington's chorea (adulthood). One theory of the overall aging process is the "accumulation of genetic error."[3]

There are some inheritable illnesses, such as inborn errors of metabolism, that are less evident. Detection of these problems may require specific laboratory tests. Phenylketonuria (PKU) caused by autosomal recessive genes is an example of an error of metabolism.

Chromosomal disorders represent a great number of defects and illnesses in hospitalized children. When the number of chromosomes is greater or less than the 46 normally found, genetic information is altered. "The chromosomes involved may be one of 22 pairs of autosomes, or the sex chromosome pair (XX in the female and XY in the male). Structural rearrangements also occur that may alter the amount of genetic information without changing chromosome number."[7]

An example of chromosomal abnormality that occurs with some frequency is Down's syndrome, or mongolism. In this abnormality there is an extra chromosome in one pair, resulting in 47 instead of 46. Affected individuals have distinctive physical characteristics. The most common autosomal disorder is trisomy 21. The extra chromosome is located on pair 21 (Fig. 6-2). Genetic studies can determine the exact location of the extra or missing chromosome. Such studies can be done as a diagnostic measure before birth or in the live-born neonate. Whenever there is an affected individual (that is, one with a genetic defect) in a family, counseling regarding future pregnancies should be given.

FIG. 6-2
Autosomal disorder—trisomy 21.

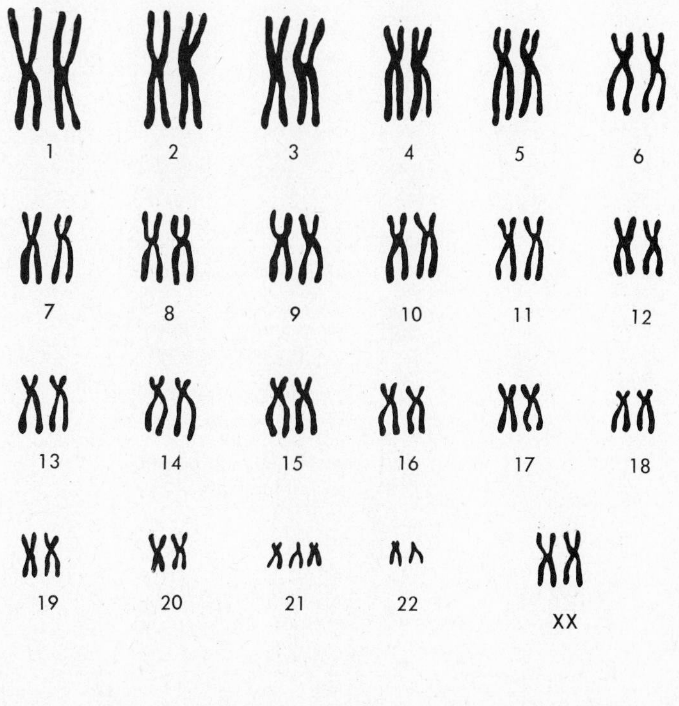

Foundations of clinical practice

Genetic counseling

Genetic counseling is a dialogue between biomedical experts and family members that is focused on the nature of inherited defects and related implications for family planning. Genetic counseling is also appropriate when significant evidence shows that either potential parent has been exposed to environmental hazards that contribute to genetic defects. The nurse plays an active role in the counseling process. Counseling provides an opportunity to clarify misconceptions and offer information regarding the aspects of genetic transmission of disease to offspring. In recent years much information about inherited diseases has been made available to the public through newspaper and magazine articles and radio and television programs. This information, when acquired by family members, may bring added queries regarding inheritance. The informa-

FIG. 6-3
Pedigree chart used in genetic counseling.

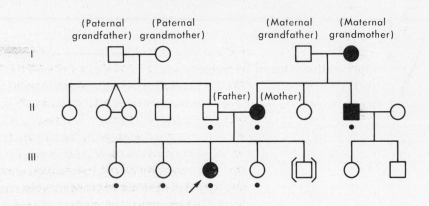

EXAMPLE OF PEDIGREE CHART CONSTRUCTION

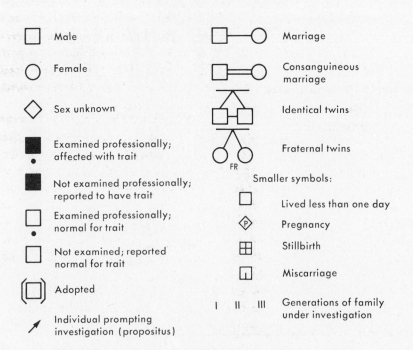

Explanation of symbols

148

tion is often misinterpreted and the facts confused, which leads to fear. The counseling sessions must take into account the psychological status of the family.

The counseling begins with a careful history. Female family members are asked about birth histories, stillbirths, abortions, and miscarriages. The general health status and age of each family member are determined. This information is recorded in a pattern called a *pedigree* (Fig. 6-3). If appropriate, diagnostic tests are performed to determine which member has a transmissible hereditary disorder. The history and diagnostic tests combined help establish a diagnosis and give a basis for prediction of risks. Information is provided to the family by the counseling team with consideration of the family's responses. Such responses may be guilt feelings or denial when knowledge of a transmissible "error" is gained. Genetic counseling often is a "crisis" situation that generates multiple problems. Dealing with these problems may be difficult for the family as a whole or for individual members. Additional follow-up counseling and services may be required. Nurses play an important role in helping families face such crises.

CONGENITAL ANOMALIES

Congenital anomalies are defects in embryological development that become apparent at birth. They may be obvious and gross malformations noted at the time of delivery or subtle abnormalities in germ plasm that may not become evident for several generations to come, at which time they manifest themselves by producing inherited disease traits. Gross structural anomalies often result in death of the fetus during the first trimester of pregnancy. Some defective fetuses, however, survive until the perinatal period, when they must adapt to the new physiological demands necessary for extrauterine life. Many do not adapt successfully and die at this time. Others survive through infancy and childhood because the vital organs are able to cope with the basic needs of the body. It is estimated that about 6% of neonates have some inborn defect.

The overwhelming number of congenital anomalies can be corrected easily through surgical techniques. Others, however, may be quite severe and, in some cases, impossible to alleviate. Some anomalies affect the appearance of the newborn, whereas others interfere with the function of vital organs. It is common for developmental errors to result in both skeletal and organic alterations.

Anomalies have three basic causes: gene mutations, abnormal chromosomes, and adverse intrauterine environment. Some anomalies are suspected to have more than a single contributing cause.

Gene mutations and abnormal chromosomes are a result of phenomena far too complex to be understood completely. Experimentation in genetic surgery, by which specific alterations can be made in the basic composition of the germ cells, is currently in progress. It will undoubtedly be many years before any practical solution for these problems is at hand. However, a considerable amount of information is known regarding factors that adversely affect the development of the fetus in utero. Among these are specific medications, radiation, and maternal rubella (measles). Family histories, clinical observations of clients and their environment, and extensive animal experimentation all contribute to a greater understanding of developmental errors that result in fetal death or congenital anomalies. Heredity studies in which data are collected from blood-related persons have enabled geneticists to trace incidences of certain disorders within one family and compare these to the general population. Monozygotic twin studies have been especially useful in such research. Finally, routine pregnancy histories also yield important data, which can be clues to cause-effect relationship of anomalies.

The entire spectrum of human genetics is a relatively new science and holds the potential for revealing the mysteries surrounding human reproduction and the factors that can alter the products of conception.

Nursing assessment

Nurses may be instrumental in the early detection of congenital anomalies after birth by performing an appraisal. Screening mechanisms are designed to identify life-threatening congenital anomalies so that surgical correction can be performed within the first 48 hours after birth when the neonate is an optimal operative risk. Other health appraisals can be performed during subsequent examinations.

TUMORS

A tumor or neoplasm is a mass of new tissue that persists and grows unrestrained by normal limits of growth. Tumor cells sometimes closely resemble their cells of origin, and at other times there seems to be little similarity. The more a tumor cell differs from a parent cell, the more dangerous it tends to be. These abnormal cells multiply irregularly and perform cellular functions in an erratic way, disturbing body function and even appearance. They usually demand a higher percentage of nutrients and blood than regular cells. Occasionally, the demand for circulation is so great that it cannot be met, and the tumor mass becomes necrotic and sloughs, giving rise to hemorrhage and infection. It should be stressed that tumor cells grow at the expense of other tissue. Tumors may be present in several ways, including masses, nodules, surface growths, ulcers, and hardened tissue areas.

Tumors may be benign or malignant and are classified according to the cells that give rise to their growth (Table 6-1).

Neoplasms have varying effects on the host, as seen in the comparisons that follow:

Benign tumor	Malignant tumor
1. Grows slowly and is often limited in size	1. Grows rapidly and is usually limited in size
2. Is encapsulated	2. Is not encapsulated
3. Does not infiltrate adjacent tissue and remains localized	3. Infiltrates adjacent tissues and spreads to distant ones
4. Reproduces its parent tissues well	4. Does not reproduce its parent tissues well
5. Discloses few and regular mitoses	5. Discloses many and often irregular mitoses
6. Does not recur after removal	6. Tends to recur after removal
7. Does not result in the client's death, except when strategically located	7. Results in client's death by sapping his strength or interfering with vital functions

When neoplastic cells vary greatly from the parent cell, they pose a greater threat. Rapid mitoses and erratic cellular function lead to disturbance in neighboring tissues and to interference in body functions. The neoplastic cells demand a higher percentage of nutrients than normal cells. The body responds in an attempt to maintain balance, but tumor cells do not comply. Their need for oxygen and nutrients comes from the host. Cells are able to take from the neighbor-

TABLE 6-1

Classification of tumors

Site	Benign	Malignant
A. Neoplasms arising from epithelium		
1. Pavement epithelium	Papilloma	Squamous cell carcinoma
		Basal cell carcinoma
		Transitional cell carcinoma
2. Glandular epithelium	Adenoma	Adenocarcinoma
	Cystadenoma	
	Polyp	
B. Neoplasms arising from connective tissues		
1. Fibrous	Fibroma	Fibrosarcoma
2. Embryonic fibrous tissue	Myxoma	Myxosarcoma
3. Fat	Lipoma	Liposarcoma
4. Cartilage	Chondroma	Chondrosarcoma
5. Bone	Osteoma	Osteosarcoma (osteogenic sarcoma)
	Osteochondroma	
6. Synovial membrane	Synovioma	Synovial sarcoma
C. Neoplasms of muscle		
1. Smooth muscle	Leiomyoma	Leiomyosarcoma
2. Striated muscle	Rhabdomyoma	Rhabdomyosarcoma
D. Neoplasms arising in nervous system		
1. Peripheral nerves	Neuroma	Neurogenic sarcoma (neurofibrosarcoma)
	Neurofibroma	
	Neurilemoma	
	(neurinoma)	
2. Sympathetic nervous system	Ganglioneuroma	Neuroblastoma
3. Neuroglia		Glioma
		Retinoblastoma
4. Meninges	Meningioma	
E. Neoplasms of endothelium and structures in which it functions		
1. Blood vessels	Hemangioma	Hemangioendothelioma
		Angiosarcoma
2. Lymph vessels	Lymphangioma	Lymphangiosarcoma
		Lymphangioendothelioma
3. Bone marrow		Multiple myeloma
		Ewing's tumor
		Leukemia
4. Lymphoid tissue		Malignant lymphoma
		Lymphosarcoma
		Reticulum cell sarcoma
F. Pigmented neoplasm (melanocytes, cells producing melanin)	Nevus	Malignant melanoma
G. Neoplasm of trophectoderm (trophoblasts of placental villi)	Hydatidiform mole	Chorionepithelioma (choriocarcinoma)
H. Complex neoplasms occurring in		
1. Ovary	Dermoid cyst	Teratoma
2. Testis		Teratoma
		Choriocarcinoma
3. Kidney		Mixed tumor
4. Salivary glands	Mixed tumor	

Adapted from Smith, Alice Lorraine: Microbiology and pathology, ed. 12, St. Louis, 1980, The C.V. Mosby Co., pp. 612-613.

ing nontumorous tissue. These rapidly multiplying cells can form a vascular supply from normal cells to nourish them.

Tumor growth determines whether it is benign or malignant. If cells grow from their centers and push tissues aside without invading them, they are termed expansive. If the exterior of the cells grows into adjacent tissue, creating death and destruction, they are termed infiltrative. Neoplasms that are expansive are

151

circumscribed, encapsulated, and separated from surrounding tissue. Infiltrative tumors are nonencapsulated and invade surrounding tissue with ease.

Benign neoplasms

The benign neoplasm is primarily a local growth. The cells that make it up are cohesive, and as the mass grows, there is configurational expansion of the mass with a well-defined border. These cells grow in such a manner that they tend to push away normal cells surrounding them. Therefore, the neoplasm becomes encapsulated. It should be remembered that the benign neoplasm is usually encapsulated, grows slowly (as compared with a malignant neoplasm), and may be removed without threat of return.[11]

Papillomas arise from epithelial tissue and are cauliflower-like projections that erupt from skin or mucous membrane. Hard papillomas, or warts, are also called *verruca vulgaris*. *Polyps* are growths that project from the mucous membrane but that do not necessarily arise from the epithelium.

Adenomas are glandular tumors and may be noted in relation to the prostate or breast. If the tumor becomes cystic, it is termed a *cystadenoma*. These latter types are commonly found in the breast and ovary, where glands retain their own secretions that create cysts.

Fibromas are composed of fibrous connective tissue and invade skin and mucous membranes.

Lipomas are large but not serious tumor masses. The buttocks, shoulders, and neck are typical sites. Since lipomas are round and encapsulated, their removal is accomplished with ease.

Myomas are muscle tumors. Frequently they affect smooth muscles, such as the uterus, and are termed *leiomyomas*.

Pigmented nevi (moles) are small, dark spots that occur on the face and neck. They may be covered with coarse hair. Nevi are usually present at birth, grow somewhat, and then become stationary or regress.

Malignant neoplasms

Malignant neoplasms grow more rapidly than benign tumors and tend to expand and invade surrounding tissue. It is difficult to separate malignant neoplasms from their surrounding tissues. The neoplasm has a particular property that makes it truly life threatening. Cells can break away from the parent tumor (the so-called *primary tumor*) and enter the circulation to float elsewhere. When these cells lodge in an area, they obtain a blood supply and commence proliferation at this new location, which is often referred to as the *secondary site*. This process of floating and growing in a new location is called *metastasis*.[11]

Malignant tumors therefore have two main functional qualities: invasion and formation of metastases. Another feature that concerns the pathologist is the change in the nucleus of malignant tumor cells. This enables the pathologist to distinguish between benign and malignant growth when there is a question.

There are various types of malignancies. *Gliomas* arise from the supporting tissue of the central nervous system. The brain and the retina, for example, may be sites for gliomas. *Neuroblastomas* are composed of undeveloped nerve cells and are common only in children. *Malignant melanomas* are associated with pigmented nevi of the skin. It is unknown why moles that are quiescent throughout life suddenly change and become rapidly growing black or brown tumors that metastasize readily and are extremely widespread. Melanomas spread to the lungs, kidneys, and other organs.

Malignant lymphomas are made up of lymphoid cells and occur in the spleen and bowel as well as in lymph nodes themselves. Occasionally, such tumors are termed lymphosarcomas. Other types of malignant tumors are listed in Table 6-1.

Cancer and carcinogenesis. *Cancer* and *carcinoma* are synonymous terms that refer to malignant neoplasms arising from the epithelium. Cancer is basically a change in the cellular function produced by failure in the intracellular enzyme systems. These systems are located mainly in the cytoplasm of the cells. When normal cells change to cancer cells, there is a speeding up of the mitotic (cell division) rate. The nucleus directs the work of cell division. Genetic material in the nucleus of the cell directs enzyme function. Interference with genes that control enzyme activities leading to rapid cell growth causes carcinogenesis.

Carcinogenesis is initiated and promoted by environmental, or exogenous, and internal, or endogenous, agents. These agents may be inhaled or ingested, or they may be related to the climate or to working conditions. For example, workers who come in contact with tar products, oils, and petroleum are more susceptible to skin cancer.[2]

Agents that initiate or cause cancer are termed carcinogens or oncogens. A very slight change in the chemical makeup of a substance may convert it from a noncarcinogenic agent to a carcinogenic agent.

Commonly occurring carcinogens are chemical agents (asbestos, tobacco smoke, dyes, soot, benzene, and arsenic), ultraviolet rays, ionizing radiation, radioactive substances, hormones, viruses, and chronic physical irritations. The genetic constitution of an individual may also contribute to carcinogenesis. According to one author, there is a direct relationship between malignant disease and DNA as well as a relationship between malignancy and autoimmune disease.[3]

Types. Carcinoma may appear as a cauliflower-like growth, an ulcer, or a hardening of tissue. *Squamous cell carcinoma* is typically an aggressive lesion, creating ulcerations in local areas and destroying underlying tissue. Squamous cell carcinoma frequently occurs in the lungs, mouth, cervix, and on the lips.

Basal cell carcinoma is a special type of squamous cell carcinoma that is slower growing and does not create metastasis. It appear on facial regions bordered by the ears, upper lip, and hairline.

Adenocarcinoma refers to glandular (or glandlike structure) cancer. Cells of adenocarcinoma have cytoplasm capable of secretory functions. They are common in the gastrointestinal tract, female breast, uterus, and lungs.

Transitional cell carcinoma is peculiar to cells lining the passages of the urinary tract. The ureters, bladder, renal pelvis, and urethra are potential sites for this malignancy.

Sarcomas are malignant neoplasms arising from connective tissue. They tend to be highly invasive and metastasize rapidly to distant sites early in their course. They are common in youth but are not unlikely to be found in the aged. Sarcomas may occur in any part of the body. A sarcoma is soft, bulky, and has an abundant blood supply. Frequently growth exceeds the available blood supply, giving rise to ulceration and hemorrhage.

Epidemiology. According to present morbidity statistics, one out of four persons in the United States will have cancer. About 805,000 new cases are diagnosed annually.[1] Cancer is the second leading cause of death. Since nurses are frequently in contact with a healthy population and have opportunities to detect early lesions, it is important that they understand factors related to cancer control.

153

Foundations of clinical practice

Early diagnosis and treatment of tumors greatly enhance opportunities for a cure. With certain malignancies statistics indicate that the chances for cure decrease by 16% every month that the tumor goes undetected. Half the number of cancer victims each year could be saved by early diagnosis and treatment.

The American Cancer Society lists the following as important *danger signals of cancer:*

1. Any sore that does not heal
2. A lump or thickening in the breast or elsewhere
3. Unusual bleeding or discharge from a body orifice
4. Any change in a wart or mole
5. Persistent indigestion or difficulty in swallowing
6. Persistent hoarseness or cough
7. Any change in normal bowel habits

It is imperative that nurses instruct clients regarding these "danger signals" and encourage them to have annual physical examinations, to take advantage of opportunities for screening clinics, and to engage in self-examination, such as breast self-examination. Since the cause of cancer is unknown, any factors that seem to increase the probability for cancer should receive special attention. Any form of chronic irritation such as sores that repeatedly heal, break down, and reheal again deserves biopsy. Moles that increase in size and shape can be critical and should be studied. Individuals who smoke or work in high-pollution environments should be advised of their risks. Skin lesions of any type that change deserve treatment. The most common type of cancer is skin cancer. Fortunately, however, it can be cured 90% of the time when detected early. Pap smears for cervical cancer detection, proctosigmoidoscopy for rectal cancer detection, and mammography for breast cancer detection are other simple, rather inexpensive techniques that are available to clients. Well-informed nurses can be extremely influential in guiding individuals to such examinations.

Various types of cancer are often more common in one age group than another; thus health counseling recommendations should be modified on the basis of age and sex, and the major risks considered for each.

Staging. Once diagnosis of malignancy is confirmed, efforts are made to define the tumor by histological and anatomical descriptions. A uniform system of staging is advocated by the International Union Against Cancer (IUAC) and the American Joint Committee for Cancer Staging and End Results Reporting to (1) aid in planning therapy, (2) aid in determining diagnosis, (3) evaluate therapy, (4) facilitate exchange of information about cancer, and (5) aid in investigation.[12] This system of staging tumors is called the TNM system.

The TNM system was developed to identify the extent of the disease. In this system the primary tumor is designated by T, spread to regional nodes as N, and distant metastasis as M. Numbers following each letter refer to the extent of tumor, nodal involvement, or metastasis (Table 6-2).

Some tumors may be classified by the extent of disease at other sites. These schemes may include clinical classification, surgical evaluative classification, or postsurgical treatment classification.

Multimodality intervention. Intervention is planned to remove the tumor or retard its growth with minimal discomfort and functional loss to the client. Therapeutic approaches may be determined by the nature of the tumor, extent of metastasis, and outcomes of various interventions. Surgery, radiation therapy, chemotherapy, and immunotherapy are the most commonly used interventions for malignant tumors. Recent evidence that most cancers produce micrometastasis has encouraged the use of more than one therapeutic approach, either in combination or sequentially. Current advances in cancer therapy are attributed to judicious use of several of these therapeutic modalities.[9]

Surgery. Surgery may be performed to remove tissue for diagnosis and staging. It may also be performed for therapeutic intervention as definitive treatment to remove the tumor or as palliative treatment to either reduce the tumor mass to relieve an obstruction or pain or to reduce the cell mass (cytoreduction) before chemotherapy or radiation therapy.

Since cancer cells can be disseminated by manipulation or implantation, the nurse who prepares the client for surgery or assists the surgeon should be aware of special techniques for preparing the client for surgery. Before surgery the area of tumor involvement should not be vigorously manipulated or scrubbed. Ulcerated lesions should be covered with antiseptic sponges during surgery preparation and then covered with a dry dressing until excised. During surgery any instruments that are in contact with tumor cells (in other words, those used during biopsy, incision, or surgical removal) should be washed and resterilized before being reused for that or other surgeries. Some surgeons may irrigate

TABLE 6-2

TNM categories

Specific criteria related to T categories

	T_1	T_2	T_3	T_4
Depth of invasion				
Solid organs	Confined	Capsule muscle	Bone cartilage	Viscera
Hollow organs	Submucosa	Muscularis	Serosa	
Mobility	Mobile	Partial mobility	Fixed	Fixed and destructive
Neighboring structures	Not invaded	Adjacent (attached)	Surrounding (detached)	Viscera
Surface spread				
Regions (R)	½ to R_1	R_1	$R_1 + R_2$	$R_1 + R_2 + R_3$
Circumference	<⅓	⅓ to ½	>½ to ⅔	>⅔
Size				
Diameter	<2 cm	2 to 4-5 cm	>4-5 cm	>10 cm

Specific criteria related to N categories

	N_1* First	N_2 First	N_3 First	N_4 Second
Station				
Drainage				
Unilateral	Ipsilateral	Ipsilateral	Ipsilateral	Contralateral
Bilateral	Ipsilateral	Contralateral or bilateral	Ipsilateral or contralateral	Distant
Number	Solitary	Multiple	—	—
Size	<2 to 3 cm	>3 cm	>5 cm	>10 cm
Mobility	Mobile	Partial matted muscle invasion	Fixed to vessels, bone, skin	Fixed and destructive

Specific criteria related to M categories

	M_1	M_2	M_3	M_4
Number of metastases	1	>1	Multiple	Multiple
Number of organs	1	1	Multiple	Multiple
Impairments	0	Minimal	Minimal to moderate	Moderate to severe

Adapted from Rubin, Philip, editor: Clinical oncology for medical students and physicians, a multidisciplinary approach, ed. 5, New York, 1978, American Cancer Society, Inc., p. 7

*To distinguish N_0 from N_1, the specific criteria include: *size,* between 1 and 2 cm; *firmness,* soft to hard; *roundness,* ½ to 1 cm.

wounds with tumoricidal agents before closure. Consideration should also be given to spread of cancer cells by vascular routes. Arteries and veins supplying the tumor and surrounding tissue should be ligated before manipulation and removal.

Radiation therapy. Radiation is an electromagnetic radiation from waves of electric energy. The therapeutic uses of radiation include destruction of tissue, remission of tumor growth, and the arresting of tumor growth or palliation of tumor processes. Radiation may be used singly or as an adjunct to other forms of intervention for malignant tumors.

Isotopes, which emit radiation, are synthetic forms of a chemical element. Isotopes, or *nuclides* as they are more generally known, differ from the natural form of the chemical element in the number of neutrons, but they have the same number of protons and emit alpha, beta, and gamma rays. Alpha rays are the shortest and least penetrating; they are stopped by paper. Beta rays are longer and penetrate some tissue; they are deterred by thin metal. Gamma rays are the most potent, penetrate most tissue, and are shielded only by lead.

Each nuclide decays within a known period of time. The time in which one half of the radioactivity diminishes is referred to as the element's *half-life.* One half of the radiation disintegrates in a given time, and the element continues to decay at this rate. Radioactive gold (^{198}Au), for instance, has a half-life of 2.7 days, whereas radioactive cobalt (^{60}Co) has a half-life of 5 years. The effectiveness and danger of each nuclide can be gauged by its known half-life.

The ionizing effect of radiation is cumulative, and body cells respond selectively to it. Ionizing radiation is present in the atmosphere and to a certain extent accumulates in each individual. For this reason caution is used in performing unnecessary diagnostic or therapeutic procedures. The therapeutic effect of radiation therapy is enhanced, however, by the cumulative effect.

Radiation therapy is effective in the treatment of many tumors because it decreases cell division, reduces immune responses, and interferes with cellular supplies of oxygen and nutrition. Cellular reaction to radiation therapy depends on intricate cellular activity. All cells are affected by radiation, but those that are radiated during miotic activity respond most favorably; the more rapidly the cell is dividing, the more susceptible it is to radiation. Furthermore, cells that are in the prophase stage of mitosis, as well as cells that are in highly vascular areas with adequate oxygen saturation, are even more responsive to radiation. Finally, the degree of differentiation influences cellular responses to radiation. Those cells that are immature, embryonic, and nondifferentiated also respond quite favorably to radiation therapy.

Cells that are rapidly dividing are most susceptible to ionizing radiation, but normal body cells are also selectively altered. Blood components, epithelial tissue, and germ cells (gonads) are most affected by radiation, whereas muscles, nerves, and bone tissue are the least affected.

Cellular response is described as *radiosensitive* or *radioresistant,* depending on cellular characteristics responding to radiation. Radiosensitivity is the difference in response to radiation by tumors and normal tissue. Those tissues that are radiosensitive are generally considered favorable for radiation therapy and well tolerated by surrounding normal structures (Table 6-3). A radioresistant tumor requires large doses of radiation with possible damage to surrounding tissue.

Radiation therapy is considered effective if the tumor cells are killed and

TABLE 6-3

Various tumors in decreasing order of relative radiosensitivity based on relatively direct tissue effect (hypoplasia)

Tumors	Relative radiosensitivity	Tissues
Lymphoma, leukemia, seminoma, dysgerminoma, granulosa cell carcinoma	High	Lymphoid, hematopoietic (marrow), spermatogenic epithelium, ovarian follicular epithelium, intestinal epithelium
Squamous cell cancer of the oropharyngeal, esophageal, bladder, skin, and cervical epithelia	Fairly high	Oropharyngeal stratified epithelium, epidermal epithelium, hair follicle epithelium, sebaceous gland epithelium, urinary bladder epithelium, esophageal epithelium, optic lens epithelium, gastric gland epithelium, ureteral epithelium
Vascular and connective tissue elements of all tumors; secondary neovascularization; astrocytomas	Medium	Ordinary interstitial connective tissue, neuroglial tissue (connective tissue of the nervous system), fine vasculature, growing cartilage or bone tissue
Adenocarcinoma of breast epithelia, serous gland epithelium, salivary gland epithelium, hepatic epithelium, renal epithelium, pancreatic epithelium, thyroid epithelium, colon epitheoium; liposarcoma, chondrosarcoma; osteogenic sarcoma	Fairly low	Mature cartilage of bone tissue, mucous or serous gland epithelium, salivary gland epithelium, sweat gland epithelium, nasopharyngeal simple epithelium, pulmonary epithelium, renal epithelium, hepatic epithelium, thyroid epithelium, adrenal epithelium
Rhabdomyosarcoma, leiomyosarcoma; ganglioneurofibrosarcoma	Low	Muscle tissue, neuronal tissue

From Rubin, Philip, editor: Clinical oncology for medical students and physicians, a multidisciplinary approach, ed. 5, New York, 1978, American Cancer Society, Inc.

surrounding tissue remains viable. This is expressed as the *therapeutic ratio,* that is, the relationship of normal tissue to the tumor lethal dose. This varies with each tumor. The goal of radiation therapy then is to achieve an optimal therapeutic ratio.

ADMINISTRATION. Therapeutic doses of radiation may be administered in several ways. Radiation may be given internally in oral, intramuscular, or intravenous forms. A radioactive source may be applied in sealed containers within the tissues (interstitial application) or within a hollow organ (intracavitary application). External uses of radiation are teletherapy (gamma rays from a source at a distance from the client) and external molds (applied in polyethylene molds over the skin of a structure such as the nose).

Megavoltage radiation, such as the linear accelerator, cobalt, or betatron, delivers radiation to deep tissues with less damage to the skin and other tissues, less scatter, and fewer systemic reactions than other methods of teletherapy.

Each mode of administration has a route of elimination in the body, and precautions vary with the dose administered. Radiation that is given internally is excreted from the body by the kidneys in the urine, by the gastrointestinal tract in emesis or feces, and in perspiration. If a therapeutic dose is given to the client, the body wastes are generally flushed in the isolated toilet, and linens are isolated and laundered with special precautions. Implanted sources of radiation may become dislodged and be deposited on the bed, in the bedpan, or on the floor; and the nurse must observe the client, the linens, and the bedpan to be certain none has become lost. The source of radiation, should it be found, is picked up with long-handled forceps and placed in a protective container, and the radiologist is notified.

TISSUE RESPONSE. Most tissue responds when therapeutic doses of radiation are used. The larger the area exposed to radiation, the greater the total effect on the body. The body's reaction to long-term radiation is manifested by local and systemic reactions. The reaction to the therapy is individual and varies with the type, route, and dose of radiation and with the length of therapy.

Tissue response to radiation is also altered by age factors. Children, whose cells are rapidly dividing, are more susceptible to radiation and consequently require lesser amounts. When larger doses are required, caution must be taken to protect the gonads and concern must be given to deleterious effects of radiation therapy on growing bone ends.

Local reactions may include erythema, pigmentation, desquamation, ulceration, epithelial sloughing, blistering, and alopecia. If teletherapy is used, markings, called *ports,* are drawn on the client, indicating where the rays are directed. This marked area of skin is the most irritated and should be cleansed gently with water. When the client bathes, these markings should not be removed. Soap or powders with metal bases are not used, since they potentiate the dose of radiation. The client should also avoid direct sunlight and excessive heat or cold to the area. Tape should not be used on this area, and if dressings must be secured, a hypoallergenic tape is preferred. If there is hair loss on the head, the client may brush his scalp gently and wear a wig to improve appearance until the hair grows again, about 2 months after therapy. The skin should be protected from further irritation. Cortisone cream or lanolin can be used, but the client and nurse should first check with the radiologist. Loose dressing can be applied over the port to prevent chafing. Loose clothing will be more comfortable over this area; elastic and constrictive clothing should be avoided.

Mild *systemic reactions* include anorexia, fatigue, and malaise. Later there may be nausea, vomiting, and small hemorrhages around the mucous membranes. Radiation cystitis may also occur. Certain blood cells are destroyed, and the result may be leukopenia, anemia, and decreased resistance to infection. The client is encouraged to obtain sufficient rest to overcome fatigue. Antiemetics may be given to minimize nausea, and the appetite can be stimulated by small, frequent feedings of easily digested foods. Mouth care is important to soothe irritated areas. Astringent mouthwashes irritate the mucosa, and lemon-glycerine swabs, which are soothing, should be used and followed by an ointment on the lips. Fluids can be encouraged to manage cystitis, and urinary tract anesthetics and antibiotics may be prescribed.

Intermediate and late effects of radiation therapy occur after the course of therapy. *Intermediate effects* are due to injury to slower cell renewal systems and are not permanent. Radiation pneumonitis, pericarditis, myocarditis, hepatitis, nephritis, and paresthesias are examples. These are treated symptomatically. *Late effects* of radiation therapy occur within months or years after therapy and are attributed to radiation dosage effects on surrounding tissue. Fistulas and tissue necrosis or fibrosis may result and should be treated surgically if possible.

A nursing care plan should be developed with each client who is receiving radiation therapy. Table 6-4 illustrates a nursing process for common problems related to the effects of radiation on the individual client.

PROTECTION FROM RADIATION. Protection of the client, health team, and visitors is guided by the principles of time, distance, and shielding. These principles are observed by all personnel in contact with radioactive substances and by clients who are receiving radiation. The radiologist or radiation-detection officer of each hospital determines specific policies related to radiation safety in that hospital. The nurse should contact this person if there is any doubt in planning nursing care.

The known *time* that a radioactive element is emitting rays gives personnel a guide to planning care. When half of the emissions have decayed, the safety for the client and personnel is increased.

Nursing care should be planned so that essential care is given in a minimal amount of time. Different team members may share nursing care so that the time spent with the client is limited. Dosimeters (devices that measure radiation exposure) are worn by personnel who are in daily contact with sources of radiation. The cumulative effects of the exposure are recorded and read every month. When maximal time has been spent near the radioactive source, the person must refrain from working or must seek better protective measures.

TABLE 6-4
Nursing process for clients receiving radiation therapy

Toxic effect or problem	Assessment and analysis	Planning and implementation	Evaluation: expected outcomes
Bone marrow depression Leukopenia	WBC less than 6000/mm³	Maintain asepsis Administer packed WBCs as ordered Instruct client to maintain resistance to infection, practice hygiene, report signs of infection, avoid known sources of infection, use antibiotics and antifungals as ordered	Normal WBC count Absence of infection
Thrombocytopenia	Reduced thrombocyte count Hemorrhage, purpura, ecchymosis	Administer platelets as ordered Avoid invasive procedures Instruct client to prevent bruising and bleeding	Normal thrombocyte count
Erythropenia	Hemoglobin less than 10 g/dl blood Hematocrit less than 30 in females and 35 in males Fatigue, headaches	Administer RBCs as ordered Provide rest Instruct client to obtain rest and avoid fatigue	Normal RBC, hemoglobin, hematocrit
Skin irritation Radiodermatitis Radioepithelitis	Erythema Desquamation Ulceration Pigment changes Telangiectasia	Avoid use of astringents, harsh soaps, and medications on involved area Shave with electric razor Keep area dry—pat, do not rub Avoid irritating clothing Avoid sunlight and heat Instruct client to protect skin as above	Normal integrity of the skin
Alopecia	Hair loss		Hair growth
Gastrointestinal inflammation Nausea, vomiting	Nausea, vomiting, diaphoresis	Administer antiemetics as prescribed Offer small, frequent feedings	Absence or control of nausea and vomiting
Anorexia, weight loss	Decreased appetite, weight loss	Provide high-calorie, high-protein bland foods Oral and parenteral hyperalimentation Mouth care Instruct client to maintain nutrition, control nausea and vomiting, report weight loss	Maintenance of usual weight
Stomatitis, esophagitis, dysphagia	Erythema of mouth and throat, difficulty swallowing Secondary infection	Provide cool, bland foods Use anesthetic mouthwash before meals Instruct client to eat bland, nonirritating foods	Integrity of mucous membranes of mouth and throat
Diarrhea	Frequent stooling, weight loss	High-carbohydrate, low-fat, low-residue diet Force fluids Anticholinergic, antidiarrheal drugs Instruct client to maintain fluid balance, maintain nutrition, and use antidiarrheal drugs	Absence or control of diarrhea

Foundations of clinical practice

The *distance* from the source of radiation reduces the exposure by inverse square of the distance. Thus if the nurse stands 2 feet from the radioactive source, the exposure is reduced to one fourth, and a position of 3 feet from the source reduces the exposure to one ninth. The client is put in a private room to increase the distance from other clients. If he must share a room with others, his bed is arranged so that he is the greatest distance from his roommates. It is advisable for the client's roommates to be past the childbearing age.

The nurse should stand at the farthest distance from the radiation source when assisting the client. When it is unnecessary to be at the client's bedside, the nurse should stand away from the bed. If it is necessary to handle radioactive elements, long-handled forceps are used.

Each type of ray emitted from isotopes is blocked or shielded by specific substances. Gamma rays are most often used for therapeutic intervention and, as previously mentioned, are blocked by lead. For this reason the radioactive material is stored in lead containers, and lead-lined aprons and gloves are used by personnel who are in contact with radioactivity. Radioactive sources that are used as implants in tissues or organs are sealed in applicators to protect non-malignant tissue from radioactive scatter.

Radiation that must be given near the head, neck, or cervical lymph nodes presents certain hazards to the structures of the mouth, and consequently special precautions should be taken. Radiation usually inhibits the protective enamel around the teeth and predisposes it to dental caries. The client should be advised to have fluoride prophylaxis and a dental examination before therapy to prevent tooth decay. Radiation therapy also diminishes salivation, inhibits taste, and increases susceptibility to monilial infections. Mouth care, then, is a vital nursing action to maintain comfort and prevent infection. Toothbrushing, gentle swabbing, antifungal mouthwashes, and lubrication of the lips are appropriate interventions.

Radiation therapy given near the ovaries or testes should be given cautiously. Interestingly, the nearer a woman is to climacteric, the more susceptible she is to becoming sterile. Childbearing function should be considered in treatment plans.

Radiation therapy administered in the area of the eye must be used judiciously. The lens and conjunctiva are susceptible to damage, and the eyes should be shielded with a protective covering.

Chemotherapy. Another approach to managing malignant tumors is the use of chemotherapeutic agents. These agents may be used as adjuncts to surgery or radiation and occasionally as the sole therapeutic modality. Chemotherapy, however, is most often used to induce remissions in some tumor processes, to reduce tumor mass in preparation for other approaches, or to palliate symptoms of advanced disease.

Chemotherapeutic agents may include antineoplastic drugs or hormones. *Antineoplastic drugs* generally interfere with cell growth during various phases of cell division. Classifications include *alkylating agents*—nitrogen mustard, chlorambucil (Leukeran), melphalan (Alkeran), busulfan (Myleran), and cyclophosphamide (Cytoxan); *antimetabolites*—methotrexate (Amethopterin), cytarabine (Cytosar-u), 5-fluorouracil (Fluorouracil), and 6-mercaptopurine; *antibiotics*—dactinomycin (Cosmegen), mithramycin (Mithracin), doxorubicin hydrochloride (Adriamycin), bleomycin sulfate (Blenoxane), and daunorubicin (Cerubidin); *plant alkaloids*—vinblastine sulfate (Velban) and vincristine sulfate (Oncovin). *Hormones* such as ACTH, cortisone, prednisone, estrogens, and androgens may be used to slow cell metabolism and render the hormonal environment of the body less favorable for growth.

Recently, a new chemotherapeutic agent, interferon, a natural glycoprotein, has been heralded with promise in the treatment of cancer.[10] This drug presumably acts by initiating DNA-directed RNA synthesis, resulting in an antiviral effect. The drug may inhibit tumor virus replication or inhibit tumor growth by effects on the immune system. Antitumor effects have been achieved for clients with breast cancer, prostate cancer, multiple myeloma, lymphoma, and ovarian cancer. The drug is administered subcutaneously or intramuscularly and may have side effects of fever, nausea, vomiting, myelosuppression, and local reactions of erythema at the site of injection. Clinical use of the drug remains in investigational stages, and the nurse may be involved in clinical research with this drug.

Common chemotherapeutic agents are listed in Table 6-5.

Chemotherapy is generally more effective when used with small tumor masses and tends to be more effective after surgical removal of the tumor or reduction of tumor mass by radiation therapy. Chemotherapy is more effective in dividing cells and has been described as being *phase specific* (that is more effective during a phase of the cell cycle), *cycle specific* (that is, more effective during cell proliferation as opposed to resting stages), or *cycle nonspecific* (that is, acting independently of cell cycles). Therefore, chemotherapeutic agents may be administered intermittently in high doses during peaks of cellular phases or cycles, allowing for maximal therapeutic effectiveness and better host tolerance.

TABLE 6-5

Cancer chemotherapeutic agents

Name of drug	Mode of action	Indications	Toxic or unwanted reactions
Melphalan (Alkeran)	Alkylating agent	Multiple myeloma Ovarian carcinoma Polycythemia vera Malignant melanoma Testicular seminoma	Bone marrow depression; anemia, neutropenia, thrombocytopenia Nausea and vomiting Possible fetal death and congenital anomalies
Triethylene-thio-phosphoramide (Thiotepa)	Alkylating agent	Hodgkin's disease in breasts and ovaries Malignant lymphomas Bronchogenic carcinoma Intercavity administration for control of malignant effusions	Bone marrow depression: leukemia, thrombocytopenia Mild nausea, vomiting, headache, anorexia
Busulfan (Myleran)	Alkylating agent	Chronic myelogenous leukemia Polycythemia vera	Bone marrow depression: thrombocytopenia Uric acid, neuropathy Nausea, vomiting, diarrhea Skin pigmentation Amenorrhea, testicular atrophy, gynecomastia Fetal death, congenital anomalies Interstitial pulmonary fibrosis Symptoms of adrenal insufficiency: gastrointestinal disturbance, fatigue, weight loss

Continued.

TABLE 6-5

Cancer chemotherapeutic agents—cont'd

Name of drug	Mode of action	Indications	Toxic or unwanted reactions
Cyclophosphamide (Cytoxan)	Alkylating agent	Malignant lymphomas Hodgkin's disease Multiple myeloma Leukemias Neuroblastoma Ovarian, breast, and lung carcinoma Retinoblastoma	Bone marrow depression: leukopenia, thrombocytopenia, anemia Sterile hemorrhagic cystitis, fibrosis of bladder (ample fluid intake and frequent voiding will help prevent) Alopecia, skin and fingernail hyperpigmentation Anorexia, nausea, vomiting, colitis, oral mucosal ulcerations, jaundice Amenorrhea, azoospermia Interstitial pulmonary fibrosis Impaired wound healing
Chlorambucil (Leukeran)	Alkylating agent	Chronic lymphocytic leukemia Malignant lymphomas Hodgkin's disease Ovarian and breast carcinoma	Bone marrow depression: lymphopenia, neutropenia, decreased platelets Gastrointestinal problems
Carmustine (BiCNU)	Alkylating agent	Brain tumors Hodgkin's disease Lung cancer Melanoma Myeloma	Nausea and vomiting Delayed myelosuppression Discoloration of skin (brown) Pain at infusion Pulmonary fibrosis Renal failure
Triazenolamidazole carboxamide, dacarbazine (DTIC-Dome)	Alkylating agent	Malignant melanoma Sarcoma Hodgkin's disease	Nausea and vomiting Hepatotoxicity Myelosuppression Chills, fever, malaise
Mechlorethamine hydrochloride (nitrogen mustard) (Mustargen Hydrochloride)		Polycythemia vera Hodgkin's disease Lung carcinoma Lymphomas	Bone marrow depression: nausea and vomiting Irritating to tissue (prevent extravasation)
5-Fluorouracil (Fluorouracil)	Antimetabolite Interferes with DNA synthesis	Adenocarcinoma of colon, stomach, rectum, pancreas, breast, ovary	Stomatitis, esophagopharyngitis Gastrointestinal bleeding, hemorrhage Vomiting, diarrhea, anorexia Bone marrow depression: thrombocytopenia, leukopenia Photosensitivity: increased pigmentation of skin Alopecia (usually reversible) Dermatitis, epistaxis, euphoria Acute cerebellar syndrome Nail changes
Methotrexate (Amethopterin) *(Leukovoran is antidote)*	Antimetabolite Folic acid antagonist; inhibits reduction of folic acid and interferes with tissue cell reproduction	Choriocarcinoma Lymphosarcoma Carcinoma of cervix, head, and neck Acute lymphocytic leukemia Testicular carcinoma Osteogenic sarcoma	Bone marrow depression: leukopenia, thrombocytopenia, anemia Alopecia Photosensitivity: increased pigmentation of skin, rash, acne Ulcerative stomatitis, diarrhea Oral ulcerations, gastrointestinal ulceration Hepatic toxicity Malaise, fatigue Renal failure, uric acid neuropathy (maintain adequate urinary output) Pleuritis Neurotoxicity: dizziness, headaches, drowsiness, blurred vision, aphasia, paresis Fetal death and/or congenital anomalies Administration of weak organic acids (salicylates) can suppress elimination by kidneys; accumulation leads to toxicity

6 Pathophysiological processes of illness

Additionally, combination of some chemotherapeutic agents may be more effective than use of single drugs without producing additional toxicity.[8]

Chemotherapeutic agents may be administered topically, orally, intramuscularly, intravenously, or by local or regional perfusion. Since circadian rhythms and cellular phases and cycles affect chemotherapeutic effectiveness, complex administration systems have been developed to maximize drug delivery.

ROLE OF THE NURSE. In addition to administering the chemotherapeutic agent as prescribed, instructing the client about the drug, and recording therapeutic effects, the nurse has a major role in assessing and providing intervention for toxic effects of these drugs.

Most drugs have a narrow margin between therapeutic and toxic effects, and the nurse can anticipate several common reactions indicating toxicity. Common toxic effects of antineoplastic drugs are bone marrow depression; gastrointestinal tract inflammation, including anorexia, stomatitis, nausea and vomiting, constipation, and diarrhea; neurotoxicity; hemorrhagic cystitis; and alopecia. Less frequent effects are cardiotoxicity, photosensitivity, local phlebitis, hyperuricemia, and suppression of immune mechanisms. Toxic effects of hormones may include fluid retention, changes in libido, hirsutism, electrolyte imbalance, hypercalcemia, and masculinizing or feminizing effects.

A nursing care plan should be developed for each client, and pertinent data should be shared with the health team. Table 6-6 illustrates a nursing process that can be used in planning care for clients exhibiting common toxic effects of chemotherapeutic agents.

Immunotherapy. Immunotherapy is another treatment modality that is used as an adjunct to surgery, radiation therapy, and chemotherapy. Immunotherapy is based on the premise that tumor cells occur in the body, but in most individuals the immune system destroys these cells as rapidly as they are formed. It is believed that individuals whose immune systems are incompetent are likely to demonstrate clinical evidence of cancer. Improving the immune response in these individuals, then, is the role of immunotherapy in the management of cancer.

TABLE 6-6

Nursing process for clients receiving antineoplastic drugs

Toxic effect or problem	Assessment and analysis	Planning and implementation	Evaluation: expected outcomes
Bone marrow depression			
Leukopenia	Reduced WBC (1000 to 2000/mm³ and less) Decreased resistance to infection: nasal infection, lip ulcers, rectal abscesses	Reverse isolation Life island Maintain asepsis, handwashing Administer packed WBCs as ordered Drug may be discontinued by physician Instruct client to keep away from crowds or individuals with known infections, report signs of infection (fever, swelling, redness) to physician, use hygiene measures (handwashing, bathing) to prevent infection	Normal WBC count Absence of infection

Continued.

163

TABLE 6-6

Nursing process for clients receiving antineoplastic drugs—cont'd

Toxic effect or problem	Assessment and analysis	Planning and implementation	Evaluation: expected outcomes
Thrombocytopenia	Reduced thrombocyte count (20,000 to 100,000/mm³)	Administer platelets as ordered	Normal thrombocyte count
	Petechiae, bleeding from mucous membranes, bruising	Avoid venipuncture, intramuscular injections; use small-gauge needles and apply pressure for 1 to 3 minutes	Absence of bleeding
	Occult blood in stool and urine	Defer invasive diagnostic procedures	
	Cerebral hemorrhage: signs of increased intracranial pressure	Avoid rectal temperatures	
	Hematuria and hemarthroses	Drugs may be discontinued by physician	
		Instruct client to use safety measures to prevent bruising, use soft toothbrush, use electric razors, report tarry stools to physician, carry ID card with blood type and bleeding time	
Erythropenia	Reduced RBCs	Administer packed RBCs as ordered	Normal RBC, hemoglobin
	Reduced hemoglobin	Provide periods of rest	
	Fatigue, headaches, lethargy	Instruct client to plan for periods of rest; obtain diet high in protein, iron, and vitamin C	

Gastrointestinal inflammation

Toxic effect or problem	Assessment and analysis	Planning and implementation	Evaluation: expected outcomes
Anorexia	Lack of appetite	Elemental diet per nasogastric tube; hyperalimentation	Normal appetite and weight
	Poor taste in mouth	Small frequent meals	
	Refusal of foods	Use favorite foods	
		Mouth care before meals	
		Instruct client to maintain nutrition, eat favorite foods	
Stomatitis	Erythema and edema of mucocutaneous junction	Vitamin C	Integrity of mucous membranes maintained; absence of infection
	Dry, burning sensations	Saline mouthwash or hydrogen peroxide irrigations	
	Dysphagia	Viscous lidocaine (Xylocaine) hydrochloride before meals	
	Secondary infection	Antifungal, antibiotic mouthwash	
	Can occur on any mucous membrane (lips, tracheostomy)	Use bland foods and tepid liquids (tea)	
		Instruct client to avoid spicy foods, avoid hot or cold fluids, use mouthwash as prescribed	
Nausea	Feelings of nausea	Cool washcloth	Absence or control of nausea
	Diaphoresis	Position	
	Retching	Carbonated beverages	
		Antiemetics before meals	
		Mouth care	
		Maintain comfortable environment	
		Instruct client to take deep breaths, maintain nutrition	
Vomiting	Reverse peristalsis caused by stimulation of medulla by irritated gastric and intestinal mucosa	Antiemetics, especially before meals	Absence or control of vomiting
		Mouth care	
	Note amount and when occurs	Instruct client to take antiemetics as directed, report to physician	
Constipation	Change in bowel habits	Laxatives	Absence or control of constipation
	Note color, frequency, and consistency of stool	Stool softener	
		Dietary modifications; bulk; fluids	
		Instruct client to maintain diet, use laxatives and stool softeners	

TABLE 6-6

Nursing process for clients receiving antineoplastic drugs—cont'd

Toxic effect or problem	Assessment and analysis	Planning and implementation	Evaluation: expected outcomes
Diarrhea	Change in bowel habits Note color, consistency, and frequency of stool	Diet modification: low roughage, high in constipating foods (cheese, boiled milk) A and D Ointment to excoriated rectal areas Instruct client to maintain fluid balance, use diet, use antidiarrheal agents, report to physician, drink fluids, take antidiarrheal agents	Absence or control of diarrhea
Gastrointestinal bleeding	Black, tarry stools Occult blood in stools	A and D Ointment to excoriated areas Drugs may be discontinued Instruct client to report evidence of bleeding to physician	Absence or control of gastrointestinal bleeding
Inflammatory interferences			
Alopecia	Hair loss on scalp, eyelashes, eyelids, axilla, pubis May be patchy areas of hair growth	Hair loss in blacks can be delayed by braiding hair Comb hair gently Use wigs, turbans, scarves A scalp tourniquet or cap can be used around hairline when administering medication intravenously to reduce circulation to scalp; keep in place 10 to 15 minutes after infusion Instruct client that alopecia may occur up to 3 weeks after drug is administered, hair will usually grow back within 8 weeks	Hair regrowth
Pigmentation	Darker skin color		Avoid sunlight
Exfoliation	Open lesions Flushed skin Temperature elevation	Protect lesions; cover Antibiotic ointment may be prescribed Instruct client to avoid sunlight, practice hygiene measures, protect open areas, report to physician	Absence or management of exfoliation
Rash	Erythema Hyperkeratosis	Use ointments as prescribed Soothing baths Instruct client to report to physician	Absence of rash
Anhidrosis (absence of perspiration)	Dry, warm skin	Gentle bathing Lotions and emollients to skin	
Hyperuricemia	Increased urinary uric acid Intake and output	Force fluids Alkalinize urine Allopurinol Instruct client to take allopurinol as prescribed, 3000 ml of fluids per day	Adequate urinary output maintained Normal uric acid level
Hemorrhagic cystitis	Hematuria Intake and output	Force fluids Antibiotics Instruct client to take 3000 ml of fluids per day, void every 2-3 hours	Adequate urinary output maintained Absence of hematuria or cystitis
Neurotoxicity	Somnolence Paresthesias Tendon reflexes diminished Foot drop Loss of balance, change in gait, ataxia Change in behavior Severe constipation (early) Loss of coordination	Foot board, tennis shoes Protect when ambulating Safety measures Stool softeners, high-roughage diet Instruct client not to drive or use equipment requiring skill and dexterity; most neuropathies are reversible	Control or management of neurotoxic effects

TABLE 6-7
Common immunotherapeutic
agents

Name of drug	Indications	Toxic or unwanted reactions
Bacille Calmette-Guérin (BCG)	Melanoma Cancer of the breast Sarcomas	Local irritation at site of administration Flulike symptoms of malaise, chills, fever, nausea and vomiting
Methanol-extracted residue of BCG (MER)	Lymphosarcoma Melanoma Leukemia	Malaise, fever Inflammation at site of administration
Levamisole	Cancer of the lung, kidney, breast	Nausea, vomiting, diarrhea Agranulocytosis
Corynebacterium parvum (C. parvum)	Cancer of the breast Melanoma	Inflammation at site of administration Nausea, vomiting, chills, fever

Immunotherapy is most effective when the tumor burden is small. For this reason, surgery, radiation therapy, and chemotherapy are used initially to reduce tumor size. Interestingly, these therapies are immunosuppressive, and immunotherapeutic approaches are best used during a rebound period when immunological activity heightens.

Immunotherapy can be active, passive, or nonspecific. *Active immunotherapy* involves the use of specific cancer antigens to stimulate a host-immune response. This is done primarily by intradermal injection of irradiated tumor cells. *Passive immunotherapy* involves injecting antibodies or immunologically active materials or cells. An example is transfusion of immunologically active lymphocytes produced by incubating lymphocytes with the client's own tumor cells. *Nonspecific immunotherapy* involves improving the entire immune system. The most common approach is to inject agents such as bacille Calmette-Guérin (BCG vaccine) or *Corynebacterium parvum*. These agents may be injected directly into metastatic areas or intradermally by the tine technique, heaf gun, or scarification.

Before starting therapy, the client should be tested for immunocompetence by his ability to respond to recall antigen skin testing. Common recall antigens used for skin testing are purified protein derivative (PPD) of tuberculin, histoplasmin, and mumps or tetanus toxoid. These are applied by intradermal injection to the skin of the forearms and observed for erythema and induration at 24- and 48-hour intervals after injection. Induration of greater than 10 mm is positive. Another procedure for testing immunocompetence is the use of a contact-delayed cutaneous hypersensitivity reaction antigen such as dinitrochlorobenzene (DNCB).[9] This solution is applied to the skin (usually the upper thigh) in three doses of 2000 μg, 100 μg, and 25 μg. The solution is applied and blown dry, and the client is instructed to keep the area dry for 48 hours, after which the test is read. Erythema and induration indicate a positive test.

Immunotherapy as a form of cancer therapy is still undergoing clinical trials. It is felt that this modality holds much promise for achieving remissions and cures for cancer.

Commonly used immunotherapeutic agents are listed in Table 6-7.

Breaks in body defenses and barriers

The body is constantly in contact with parasitic microorganisms. Many of these microorganisms are pathogenic or disease producing. As host for these microorganisms, the human body has certain attributes that resist invasion and disease. Physiological barriers prevent entry of pathogens and protect the body from infection, invasion, and disease. The *intact skin* allows very few microorganisms to enter, but the sweat glands and hair follicles may allow pathogens to establish themselves. However, the secretions of these glands have antimicrobial properties and thus can eliminate microorganisms. The skin is commonly referred to as the first line of defense. "Skin resistance may vary with age. In childhood, susceptibility is high to ringworm infection. After puberty, resistance to fungi increases markedly with the increase of saturated fatty acids in sebaceous secretions."[6]

Mucous membranes, which line the various openings of the body provide defense against microorganisms. These membranes secrete substances containing various chemicals that either inhibit growth of microbes or transport them to lymph channels. Membranes in the respiratory tract secrete a viscous substance, mucus, which helps deter entrance of microorganisms. *Cilia,* which drive organisms and foreign particles toward orifices, line the respiratory tract. Coughing and sneezing help expel entrapped matter in the respiratory tract. Bacteria that enter the deeper portions of the lungs are destroyed or inactivated and thus cleared from the bloodstream by *phagocytic activity,* another important defense. Phagocytosis, the reticuloendothelial system, and biochemical tissue constituents all combine to defend the body further against the action of pathogenic microorganisms. Tears contain substances with antimicrobial properties. The gastrointestinal tract defends against microorganisms with the help of saliva and stomach and intestinal secretions. The saliva contains inactivating enzymes; the stomach has highly acidic secretions; and the intestine contains proteolytic enzymes and active macrophages.

"In the adult vagina, an acid pH is maintained by normal lactobacilli that interfere with establishment of yeasts, anaerobes and gram-negative organisms."[6] Once microorganisms pass the skin and mucous membranes, inflammation comes into play.

INFLAMMATION   Inflammation is the body's almost uniform systemic reaction to any insult or injury. It is a pathophysiological response that serves to defend tissue against microorganisms and ready tissue for repair. Classic signs are redness, heat, swelling, pain, and loss of motion. These signs reflect activity at a cellular level. For example, the heat and redness are caused by increased blood flow to the part and local hyperemia. Swelling is primarily due to accumulation of exudate in the tissues. Pain is said to have three contributing factors: one overt factor is pressure of swelling on nerve endings, and two more subtle causes are stretching of tissue richly supplied with nerve endings and the effect of chemicals released during the response on nerve endings.

Inflammation is not the same as infection. Infection may act as an irritant to cause inflammation. In the presence of infection the inflammatory reaction tends to prevent the dissemination of infection. The localization is due to absorption of bacteria and toxins.

Classification   Inflammation may be classified as acute or chronic and local or systemic. In either event the distinction being made is between the early reaction to invasion and the later repair. In chronic inflammation the irritant remains active for a long time, new collagenous fibers develop, and there is an accumulation

Foundations of clinical practice

TABLE 6-8

Sources of inflammation

External	Internal
Microorganisms	Thrombosis
Burns	Neoplasms
Tissue trauma	Infarcted cells
Chemicals	Others, including
	allergy
Organ transplants	

of large numbers of small lymphocytes. An example of chronic inflammation is rheumatoid arthritis.

The cause of inflammation has been reviewed by many authors and scientists. Most agree that the defense response can be initiated by any insult to body tissue. (Table 6-8 gives sources of inflammation.) There is a certain amount of tissue injury in nearly all pathological conditions. (The offending agent is referred to as an irritant.) Therefore, a degree of inflammatory change is seen in the tissues. The suffix -*itis* is added to whatever tissue or organ is involved to indicate inflammatory reaction (for example, gastritis, dermatitis, tonsillitis). Common types of acute inflammation are shown in Table 6-9.

Local inflammation. Local inflammation is characterized by four stages: increased vascular permeability, neutrophil exudation, mononuclear cell exudation, and cellular proliferation and repair.[4]

Increased vascular permeability is the first phase of the inflammatory process. When tissue is exposed to a noxious stimulus, it prepares quickly to defend itself. Capillaries dilate, allowing additional arterial blood to enter the area, which enhances the capacity to cells to overcome damaging agents. As the arterial vessels dilate, the walls become quite permeable, allowing circulating fluid to escape into surrounding tissues. This outpouring fluid contains plasma proteins and fibrinogen. The fibrinogen unites with thrombin to form fibrin. This fibrin plugs spaces between cells in lymphatic channels and those in capillaries to eventually block off the injured area from surrounding tissue. When increased amounts of arterial blood flood the localized area, the erythrocytes become congested and even "clumped," giving the skin a reddened appearance. This process is sometimes also accompanied by a throbbing sensation. Increased vascular permeability may last only a few minutes or may continue for 24 hours.

Histamine, platelets, and kinins are the direct chemical mediators of the initial phase.

The second phase of inflammation begins 30 to 45 minutes after the initial event and peaks in about 8 hours.[4] Neutrophils stick to the blood vessel wall and ultimately penetrate it by squeezing between endothelial cells. These cells phagocytize and destroy microorganisms and release substances that sustain the inflammatory process. The duration of this phase is influenced by several chemical factors. It is lengthy in certain allergic reactions and may continue several days in bacterial inflammation until all invading organisms are destroyed.

Abscess formation may occur when there is a heavy concentration of neutrophils in an area. Fluid contained in abscesses is exudate, highly saturated with neutrophils.

Mononuclear cell exudation is the third phase of the inflammatory process. It begins in the first 4 hours and peaks within the first 24 hours. Little is known regarding the specific mechanisms through which mononuclear cells aid

TABLE 6-9

Types of acute inflammation

Type of inflammation	Characterization	Example
Serous	Serum exudate	Blister
Purulent	Inflammation with suppuration (pus serum)	Abscess
Fibrinous	Fibrin as chief element	Pneumonia
Catarrhal	Mild inflammation of mucous membrane	Head cold

in the inflammatory response. The final stage is cellular proliferation and repair.

Within the first day of injury, fibroblasts are beginning to synthesize DNA in preparation for division, and after 2 or 3 days, fibroblast proliferation peaks. Organ-specific cells such as in the skin and liver may also begin to regenerate.[4] Fibroblasts also produce collagen, which creates a scar. Inflammation may utlimately have one of three results: complete repair with or without scars, abscess formation, or granuloma formation. This last phenomenon occurs when a fibrous capsule (granuloma) forms and envelops the indigestible foreign invader that initially produced the inflammatory response.

Systemic inflammation. When bacterial invaders cannot be successfully localized and destroyed, fever and leukocytosis herald the onset of a systemic inflammatory response.

Fever occurs because endotoxins stimulate the release of endogenous pyrogen into circulation. This protein substance produces fever by acting on the central nervous system. Leukocytosis is usually induced by bacterial infections.

Variables affecting body defenses

The ability of an individual to resist inflammatory agents is influenced by a number of factors. Among these are racial and familial endowment, age, sex, nutritional status, physical exertion, metabolic disorders, and environmental conditions such as temperature and humidity. The inflammatory process is less likely to occur when individuals are in optimal health. Younger persons are more resistive to tissue injury, possibly because of age and because of their nutritional state. Older persons, possibly because of atherosclerosis, are less responsive to changes. An adequate dietary intake, especially of proteins and vitamins, enhances one's resistance to inflammation. It has been demonstrated that cells depleted of proteins and vitamin C are more vulnerable to tissue damage. Blood cells and connective tissue are more easily damaged when vitamin C content is deficient.

Environmental factors such as temperature and humidity cause alterations of the normal physiology of the body and can thus deplete body resources. Poor ventilation is another factor. Failure of the air to circulate results in a buildup of humidity, and as a result, the body has to work harder to cool off. Ultimately, however, the virulence and number of organisms to which an individual is exposed and the resistance of the individual determine the end result of any encounter between the individual and the microorganism.

Nursing considerations

When a client has an inflammatory response, the goal of care should be directed toward preventing further injury. This can be accomplished through adequate rest, maintenance of adequate circulation, removal of inflammatory substances, administration of specific therapies, and provision of emotional support.

Since proper rest enhances the healing process, the nurse should make modifications in the plan of care to ensure that the client has the needed rest. As specific strategies are implemented, consideration should be given to the location and specific source of the inflammation.

All body tissue needs an adequate and continuous supply of nutrients and other substances. On the other hand, the products of tissue metabolism must be removed. As a result, measures must be provided to facilitate this. Such processes can be enhanced with the use of heat. Heat, in either the dry or moist form, facilitates dilation of the blood vessels, which in turn serves as a means of increasing the amount of nutrients to the tissue.

Elevation of the area of involvement, when possible, is another means of increasing nutrition to the involved tissue. This is often helpful, especially if the involved part is an extremity. Regardless of the strategy used, the area of involvement should be assessed closely to determine the adequacy or inadequacy of the circulation.

Specific therapy may be planned to control the agent causing the problem, or therapy may be prescribed to alter the inflammatory response and subsequently prevent damage to the area. Steroids are often prescribed for the latter. Inflammatory debris may be removed by incision and drainage or debridement.

During any illness, clients have a tendency to be apprehensive or fearful, because of either the disease process or therapy. The nurse should therefore keep the client informed of all therapies and related care. The environment should be modified as necessary so that adequate rest is maintained.

IMMUNE SYSTEM

The immune system is a protective body mechanism comprising the thymus, spleen, lymph nodes, gastrointestinal tract, and bone marrow. These organs contribute to development of the immune system at various stages in the individual's life span. The immune system responds to invasion of the body in either a beneficial or a harmful way. The same action that helps the body reject foreign materials such as pathogenic bacteria will reject transplants (for example, kidney) and produce autoimmune disease (for example, collagen disease).

Basically, the immune system defense mechanism is the interaction of antibody with antigen. Antigens are substances capable of inducing synthesis of antibodies. The interaction enables the body to fight or destroy invading bacteria or viruses. The organs in this system all contribute to the development or maturation of lymphocytes, the major white blood cells in the immune response.

Characteristics of antigens and antibodies

Antigens and antibodies are defined in terms of each other. *Antigens* cause antibody formation when the body recognizes them as foreign material. Antigens are proteins, polysaccharides, and nucleic acids. Proteins have a high molecular weight, and polysaccharides and nucleic acids have a low molecular weight. *Haptens* are substances that cannot elicit antibody production alone, but, when they are combined with another molecule, they cause antibody formation.

Antibodies are produced when the individual is exposed initially to an antigen that causes antibody production in low concentrations after a long period. The second time the body is exposed to the same antigen, antibodies are produced in higher concentrations and remain in the circulation for years. Antigen and antibodies react in a lock-and-key fashion. The reactions are called by the following names, depending on the nature of the antigen:

agglutination Visible clumping of particulate antigen resulting from antigen-antibody interaction as in red blood cells.
precipitation Interaction of a soluble antigen with an antibody to form precipitate.
neutralization Reaction of a toxin antigen with a specific antibody or antitoxin.

These reactions may be manifested inside the body or outside the body in diagnostic laboratory tests.

Antibodies are proteins, also known as *immunoglobulins,* and are produced in lymphoid tissues. Five classes of human immunoglobulins have been identified: IgG (gamma G), IgA (gamma A), IgM (gamma M), IgD (gamma D), and IgE (gamma E). The serum of newborns is deficient in most immunoglobulins;

however, *IgG* is present because it is the only immunoglobulin to cross the placenta. IgG comprises the largest part of the immunoglobulins and is present in equal amounts in the plasma and extravascular fluid. It neutralizes toxins and viruses. Since it crosses the placental barrier, it protects the fetus during the early months against a number of infections (diphtheria, tetanus, measles, poliomyelitis, pneumococcal and streptococcal infections). The serum level of IgG has been identified as 12.4 mg/ml.

IgM antibodies are useful in killing gram-negative bacteria. They are not believed to be present in the neonatal period, which possibly accounts for the high susceptibility of infants to gram-negative organisms. IgM has a serum level of 1.2 mg/ml and is found mainly in the intravascular compartments. It has been reported to be the first immunoglobulin to show up in the circulation after initial immunization.

IgA is found in external secretions, such as tears, saliva, and colostrum, and in nasal and bronchial secretions. The presence of large amounts of IgA in colostrum is thought to be responsible for added protection against enteric viruses in the breast-fed infant. The serum concentration level is 3.9 mg/ml.

IgE is responsible for reaginic activity. It is not present in cord blood. This is thought to explain why infants of mothers who have a reagin-mediated allergy (such as hay fever) do not become passively sensitized to the substances to which the mother is allergic.

Immunity   Immunity is gained by the individual either by natural or acquired means. Acquired immunity may be passive or active.

Natural immunity means that an individual is born with the ability to resist certain types of agents. This immunity is not acquired through previous contact with an infectious agent. One type of naturally occurring immunity is *species immunity*. Because of the chemical relationship of the animal tissue and microorganisms, it is not possible to produce most human disease in animals. There have been studies conducted regarding the *genetic* bases of immunity, and the biochemical basis of some genetic immunity has been discovered. Another proposed means of natural immunity is individual resistance. Although the individual has not been previously exposed to an organism, he cannot be infected by that microorganism.

The immune process enables humans to develop *active acquired immunity*. This immunity is obtained by three means. In one method a small amount of weakened or dead bacteria, viruses, or other toxins is introduced into the body in the form of a vaccine (immunization or vaccination). This process prevents the individual from actually having the disease. The vaccine stimulates antibody formation against the specific agent. A second type of active immunity results from an individual actually having the disease. A third type is the subclinical infection. In all three events the individual or host actively produces antibodies, and the host's cells learn to respond to the foreign material. Active immunity develops slowly over a period of days or weeks but tends to persist, usually for years.[6]

Passive acquired immunity differs from active acquired immunity in that it is temporary and antibodies are obtained from some outside source rather than being produced by the body. Although this immunity is temporary, it is available immediately. Passive immunity is of greatest value when an illness is primarily caused by a toxin (for example, tetanus, botulism, or diphtheria).

171

Foundations of clinical practice

An immune serum such as gamma globulin is obtained from a sensitized donor, human or animal, and is injected into a recipient who needs the antibodies to fight a specific disease. Infants are born with a transient immunity to some common infections. This immunity is greatly decreased after 4 months. The infant's immunity is transmitted from the mother through the placenta, and breast milk adds to this immunity. It should be remembered that this is temporary immunity.

Body defense is enhanced by active immunity. Immunizations against certain common childhood diseases are routinely provided in the United States. When antigen and antibodies interact, occasionally harmful and even fatal effects can occur. The body reacts in a certain way when exposed the first time to some substances. It may react differently on the second exposure. *Allergy* is the term used to describe a change in response to exposure. Normally, the individual does not produce antibodies against its own antigens. However, certain diseases (for example, systemic lupus erythematosus and rheumatic fever) are attributed to the immune response of the individual to his own tissue. *Anaphylaxis* and *serum sickness* are examples of harmful results of antigen-antibody interaction. Anaphylaxis is caused by drugs or some other products. It is life threatening, and therefore care should be taken to obtain a careful history before one administers drugs, especially penicillin.

Physical-chemical insults

Physical-chemical insults comprise a broad group of health-related problems, including several unrelated conditions that cause alterations in the body or direct injury to body tissue or organs. These include trauma, obstruction of hollow organs, hernias, thermal disturbances, circulatory disturbances, and alterations in acid-base regulation.

TRAUMA

Trauma is an injury or a wound that affects the continuity of any tissue. Generally, trauma results in a visible effect on the body, pain, and loss of function. Lacerations, incisions, bullet and stab wounds, abrasions, contusions, concussions, and injuries are all classified as trauma.

Complications of trauma encompass several other pathological processes, including inflammation, degeneration, obstruction, and circulatory disturbances.

WOUNDS

A wound is an injury that is often caused by some type of force. Wounds vary in size, depth, and nature. They are frequently sustained by school-age children and adolescents. *Abrasions* are superficial wounds on the skin caused by two surfaces rubbing together. *Contusions* (bruises) result from the rupture of tiny blood vessels caused by a hard fall or blow. A *lacerated wound* is one in which the tissue is torn, resulting in a ragged appearance. An *incised wound* is caused by a sharp object, such as a knife or a piece of broken glass. A *puncture wound* is a small perforation of the skin usually caused by a sharp object such as a nail.

Some wounds are so small that they can be adequately treated by the family with first-aid supplies. However, others may require extensive health care. Therefore, as much as possible, measures should be taken to prevent them. Some of the instructions that should be given follow. Parents should be encouraged to examine toys carefully before purchasing them. Any toy with a sharp edge, or one that can potentially develop a sharp edge, should not be purchased. Sharp objects such as knives and tools must be kept out of the reach of children and should be handled with care when used by adults. Razor blades and broken glass should be disposed of in special containers separate from other household trash. Glassware used by preschool, and possibly school-age, children should be made of break-resistant materials.

Families should be taught the proper care for wounds. Measures must be taken to control bleeding and prevent infection. Hands should be washed thoroughly with soap and water before care for the wound is attempted. The wound should be cleansed with soap and running tap water. After the wound is cleansed and dried, a clean or sterile dressing should be applied. If the wound is tiny, a bandage may suffice. If the wound is severe, pressure must be applied to stop the bleeding, and the client should be seen by a physician immediately. Tetanus prophylaxis is essential when a puncture wound is sustained.

Physiology of wound healing

When a wound occurs, blood fills the space between the edges of the severed tissue and subsequently coagulates to form a clot that facilitates sealing of the area. (Sealing usually occurs within hours after a wound.) An *inflammatory response* characterized by heat, redness, swelling, and pain ensues. White blood cells (such as neutrophils, lymphocytes, and monocytes) appear in the exudate in the wound, and fibrocytes and fibroblasts, which facilitate the formation of fibrils, also appear. The fibrils eventually determine the strength of the healed wound. As the area heals, the inflammatory exudate is resorbed, and phagocytes progressively digest the white blood cells and fibrin. Within a couple of days, endothelial cells follow along the fibrin meshwork, and once the area becomes canalized, blood flows form one margin of the wound to the other. This process may occur within 2 to 3 days.

Within 3 to 4 days, the clot becomes surrounded by vascularized connective tissue, referred to as granulation tissue. Such granulation tissue may be found in small amounts in wounds that heal by primary union, but it is more characteristic of secondary union. Proliferation of fibroblasts continues and produces a cellular scar tissue. On about the fourth or fifth day after an injury occurs, collagen fibers are deposited; these fibers strengthen the wound. Within a couple of weeks, the area has gained as much strength as normal tissue.

Wound healing usually occurs in one of three ways: first intention or primary union, second intention or secondary union; and third intention or tertiary union.

Healing by first intention occurs when tissue injury is minimal (Fig. 6-4, *A*). A common example of a wound that heals in this way is an incised wound made under aseptic conditions. Repair of such injury usually involves bringing the edges of a small area together. During the healing process, a minimal amount of exudate and tissue fluid fills the wound; a small amount of connective tissue forms; and the inflammatory response is minor. After the inflammation subsides, which is usually within a few days, vascularized tissue is formed; circulation across the wound is reestablished; new connective tissue fibrils are formed by the fibroblast; and healing is completed by the growth of epithelial cells from the margins.

Healing by second intention occurs when there is involvement of a large tissue area and in instances when the edges of the wound cannot be joined together (Fig. 6-4, *B*). Repair is not as simple. Characteristically, a large amount

173

of highly vascularized tissue (such as granulation tissue) grows from the margins of the wound to fill the area. Epithelial cells grow over the granulation tissue, and scar formation is evident. Granulation tissue, which is composed of tiny capillaries, gives the wound surface its reddened, granular appearance. Such tissue is thought to be resistant to infection, and as a result it temporarily protects

FIG. 6-4
A, Primary; **B,** secondary; and **C,** tertiary intention wound healing. (From Warner, Carmen G., editor: Emergency care: assessment and intervention, ed. 2, St. Louis, 1978, The C.V. Mosby Co.)

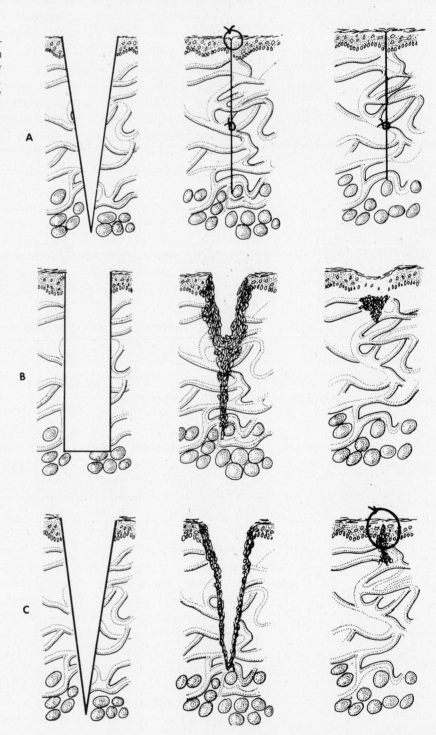

the area against bacteria. Hence, the term "granulation" is frequently used synonymously for healing that occurs by this method.

Since granulation tissue cannot form into a fluid medium, it is often necessary (for example, in abscess formation) to remove the necrotic cells, debris, or exudate from the wound to enhance the healing process. Failure to remove these products results in disfigurement and altered function.

Healing by third intention occurs when a previously sutured area breaks down and necessitates reclosure of the wound (Fig. 6-4, *C*). When healing occurs by this method, the scar formed is larger.

Variables affecting wound healing

A number of variables affect wound healing: age, nutrition, hormonal activity, blood supply, infections, and so forth. Wound healing generally occurs at a faster rate in a young person than in an older person. Adequate nutrition has a positive effect on wound healing; a number of reports have demonstrated the value of high-protein foods.

Ascorbic acid (vitamin C), also an important element in the healing process, is thought to facilitate the formation of collagen. Although the mechanisms are unclear, certain hormones (such as growth hormones, aldosterone, steroids, and sex hormones) tend to depress the healing process. A deficient blood supply and infection also have a negative effect on the reparative process; the former may cause the area to receive inadequate nutrients.

Often in an effort to enhance the healing process, for example, for a client with burns, a diet high in protein, along with whole blood and vitamins, is prescribed.

OBSTRUCTIONS

Obstruction of a hollow organ can affect any part of the body that consists of tubelike structures. Examples are the intestines, biliary tract, respiratory tract, and chambers of the heart. Causes may include congenital anomalies, inflammation, degenerative processes, tumors, and foreign bodies. Obstruction may be partial or complete, and thus it may interfere with the function of a body part or result in total cessation of normal activity. Whenever an organ does not perform its role in body processes, it invariably affects a number of other processes. For example, an obstruction of the common bile duct by a stone may cause distention and inflammation of the gallbladder and interference in liver function as a result of a backflow of bilirubin into the blood, creating jaundice. Furthermore, digestion will be impaired because of the lack of bile. Pathologically, changes in the affected organ proximal to the obstruction consist of (1) accumulation of contents normally transported by the tubes; (2) dilation, thinning, or even rupture of the tubes; (3) degeneration or atrophy and necrosis of the adjacent parenchymatous cells; and (4) secondary inflammation.

HERNIAS

A hernia is a protrusion of an organ, part of an organ, or tissue through an enlarged normal or abnormal opening in the wall containing it. Hernias do not become clinically important until they create anatomical changes in the tissue affected or interfere with normal physiological functioning as a result of ischemia, obstruction, or inflammation.

THERMAL DISTURBANCES

Thermal disturbances are local or systemic reactions caused by externally imposed excessive heat or cold. Burns and frostbite (the most common clinical examples) are discussed in Chapter 15.

Foundations of clinical practice

**CIRCULATORY
DISTURBANCES**

Circulatory disturbances are disorders that affect the quantity and quality of circulating blood and its distribution to various body parts as well as body fluid disturbances. Hemorrhage and shock are the circulatory disturbances of primary concern to nurses.

Hemorrhage

Hemorrhage refers to a large amount of blood loss from a blood vessel. It may be internal and nonvisible, or it may be evident from open wounds or body orifices. Uncontrolled loss of circulating blood volume is always a problem that deserves immediate attention.

The primary role of the blood as a body fluid is to transport chemicals, nutrients, and oxygen to cells (to support life processes) and to carry off cellular waste products for eventual elimination. The loss of circulating blood volume endangers vital organs primarily by depriving them of oxygen. The heart, brain, and kidneys are especially sensitive to hypoxia and may be damaged in a brief period. For example, irreparable brain damage is said to occur in 3 to 5 minutes after the oxygen supply has been interrupted. Any substantial loss of blood from any part of the body will reduce available oxygen to the remainder of the body. Bleeding from a large artery in an arm or leg can result in generalized circulatory failure and hence endanger vital processes and life itself. It is estimated that 50% of circulating blood can be lost before the body's own compensatory mechanisms fail and allow death to result. (These compensatory processes are explored in the discussion of shock.)

Hemorrhage can result from trauma, blood dyscrasias that affect the clotting mechanisms, surgery, disease of the vascular system of various organs, or erosion of tissue that normally protects and confines blood vessels. The hemorrhage may be arterial bleeding that spurts and exhibits a bright red color, or it may be venous, characterized by a dark color and steady oozing from the origin. If the bleeding is occurring internally, the signs and symptoms will be related to oxygen starvation and fluid loss. Among these are apprehension, restlessness, rapid respirations and pulse rate, pallor of mucous membranes, cold and moist skin, thirst, and eventual drop in blood pressure.

If hemorrhage is occurring, it must be controlled and the resultant blood loss compensated for. Hemorrhage from internal organs cannot be stopped except through surgical intervention. The role of the nurse is limited to taking measures that will promote the most efficient use of remaining blood. These measures are discussed as they relate to the care of clients in shock.

Bleeding from the extremities or periphery can be managed by elevation, application of pressure, and application of cold. Elevation of a bleeding part decreases the flow of blood to the area. Pressure occludes the bleeding vessel sources. The occlusion therefore should be attempted between the wound and the heart in arterial bleeding (Fig. 6-5) but distally from the wound in venous bleeding. Pressure may be applied by the open hand or sterile dressings if available. Tourniquets are a last resort. They must be applied tightly enough to interrupt arterial flow and therefore should be applied as close to the wound as possible to minimize tissue damage. The tourniquet should remain in place until medical attention is at hand. The time should always be noted when the application was made so that tissue destruction potential can be assessed. Some attempt should be made to estimate blood loss to help determine replacement therapy. A tourniquet is always a potential cause of severe ischemia and ultimate loss of a limb. It is important that it be viewed as a last resort in controlling hemorrhage and that getting a victim to medical help is a first priority.

176

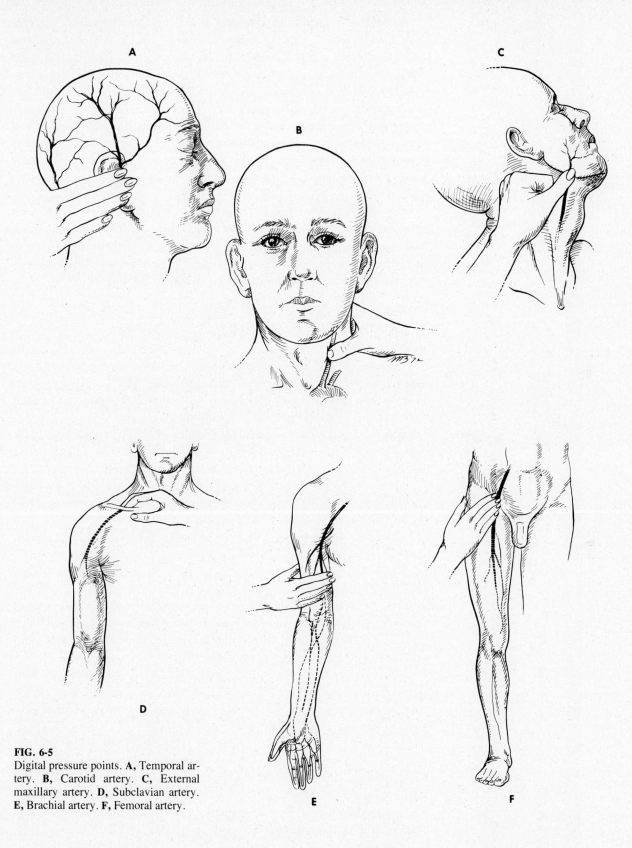

FIG. 6-5
Digital pressure points. **A,** Temporal artery. **B,** Carotid artery. **C,** External maxillary artery. **D,** Subclavian artery. **E,** Brachial artery. **F,** Femoral artery.

Foundations of clinical practice

Emergency personnel may employ military antishock trousers (MAST) compression, or shock pants, to control hemorrhage. This technique involves the application of trousers that can be inflated to force blood from the lower extremities into the vital organ areas, thus increasing cardiac output. They are especially useful in trauma when there is a severe volume deficit. Dramatic improvements in systolic blood pressure have been noted after their application and inflation. Their use, however, is limited to situations in which the cause of shock is determined. They are contraindicated in the presence of, or possibility of, intracranial edema, pulmonary edema, or congestive heart failure, since forcing additional blood to the upper portions of the body would aggravate pathological states.

It is important for nurses to know that shock trousers should be gradually deflated to prevent a sudden reflex drop in blood pressure, even after the client's condition has apparently stabilized. Furthermore, the hypoxic blood that is trapped in the extremities will contribute to a generalized anaerobic metabolic state; thus acidosis should be anticipated and managed during removal of the trousers.

Carotid artery bleeding can be controlled by digital pressure but may cause the client to become unconscious because of a diminished flow of blood to the brain.

Other methods of accomplishing compression include packing a body cavity with dressings and using tubes with inflated balloons, which compress vessels.

Cold and other vasoconstrictors may be employed in superficial bleeding such as occurs in epistaxis or small lacerations.

Shock

Shock is a syndrome in which the circulation or perfusion of blood is inadequate to meet tissue metabolic demands. Under such conditions, cellular anoxia will ensue and ultimately lead to tissue death unless the process is reversed.

Shock can be induced by any state that reduces cardiac output. Primarily such states include (1) a reduction in the volume of circulating fluids and (2) a redistribution of circulatory fluids within the body.

Classification. There are four types of shock: (1) hypovolemic, (2) cardiogenic, (3) distributive, and (4) obstructive.[14]

Hypovolemic shock refers to a state in which the volume contained within the intravascular compartment is inadequate for perfusion of body tissues. This is usually a 15% to 25% reduction of intravascular volume. Causes include hemorrhage, plasma loss caused by burns and inflammation, and electrolyte losses as a result of diarrhea and dehydration. It can also result from fluid extravasation caused by tourniquet application, inflammation, and trauma.

Cardiogenic shock is essentially "pump failure"; that is, the heart is unable to circulate the volume of intravascular fluid as a result of causes such as a cardiac dysrhythmia, heart failure, or myocardial infarction. This type of shock is discussed in detail in Chapter 20.

Distributive shock designates alterations in the distribution of blood volume. It can be manifested by high or normal resistance (increased venous capacitance) resulting from causes such as spinal cord transection, barbiturate intoxication, or ganglionic blockage, or it can be manifested by low resistance (arteriovenous shunt) induced by inflammatory vasodilation or reactive hyperemia. This category includes neurogenic, septic, and vasogenic shock states.

Neurogenic shock is the end result of vasodilation caused by decreased vasomotor tone. Blood volume remains stable, but the increase in the vascular bed causes decreased venous return and ultimately inadequate tissue perfusion. Neurogenic shock can be caused by loss of vasomotor tone at the vasomotor center or peripherally in the blood vessels.

Septic shock is an increasingly common type of shock seen in hospitalized clients. This type is an endotoxic shock, commonly resulting from overwhelming infection, particularly from gram-negative organisms. The cause is unknown, but it may be attributed to the toxins released from the bacteria or to the bacteria themselves.[5] Individuals at risk for septic shock are those with infections, indwelling catheters, peritonitis, burns, surgery, postpartum infection, or septic abortions.

A particular type of vasogenic shock is anaphylactic shock. This is caused by an antigen-antibody reaction and subsequent release of histamine, serotonin, and bradykinin, which causes vasodilation and shift of intravascular fluids.

Obstructive shock is a state in which there is a physical impediment to the mainstream of blood flow. Examples of obstructive shock are pericardial tamponade, pulmonary embolism, dissecting aortic aneurysm, and vena cava compression.

Pathophysiology. The ultimate outcome of inadequate circulation or perfusion of the blood to meet metabolic demands occurs in the cell (Fig. 6-6). Alteration in oxygen distribution to the cell induces anaerobic metabolism and lactic acidosis. Lipoprotein membranes of the lysosomes break down, releasing proteolytic enzymes into the cell and then into the vascular system and stimulating the formation of bradykinin, a potent vasodilator. Histamine, released from mast cells, further interferes with compensatory mechanisms, compounding the shock state.

Compensatory mechanisms and stages. When the body is confronted with a reduction in fluid volume, chemoreceptor reflexes assist in maintaining circulation. Afferent neural discharge from the carotid and aortic bodies is increased, thus aiding vasoconstriction in the periphery. This reflex acts synergistically with carotid and aortic mechanoreceptors.[4] A sympathetic response is stimulated via the medulla's vasomotor center. This sympathetic response causes constriction of precapillary and postcapillary sphincters and increases cardiac output. There is also an adrenal medullary response that increases the amount of circulating catecholamines (epinephrine and norepinephrine), which further aid vasoconstriction by raising central blood pressure and enhancing perfusion to the vital organs. Although blood is diverted from the muscles, skin, bowel, and other areas, circulation to the brain and heart is improved. Coronary and cerebral vessels actually dilate, and veins constrict to raise peripheral resistance.

Additionally, capillary hydrostatic pressure is decreased, and fluid shifts from interstitial to capillary spaces to increase plasma volume and to maintain it at a level for adequate blood pressure, venous return, and cardiac output.

Other adaptive responses also occur during this early phase of shock. Cells are seemingly rendered capable of extracting more oxygen (per unit volume) from blood and are able to maximize utilization of this precious substance. Furthermore, antidiuretic hormone and aldosterone are secreted to assist in replenishing fluid volume. The heart and breathing rates may increase to enhance oxygenation of a limited blood supply and to deliver it expeditiously to the cells.

The human organism is able to compensate for large losses in blood volume,

179

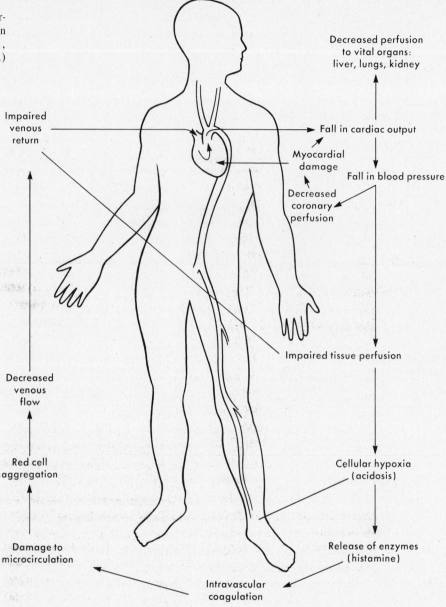

FIG. 6-6
Pathophysiology of shock. (From Hurley, Elaine: Hypovolemic shock. In Current practice in critical care, vol. 1, St. Louis, 1979, The C.V. Mosby Co.)

Impaired venous return

Decreased venous flow

Red cell aggregation

Damage to microcirculation

Fall in cardiac output

Myocardial damage

Decreased coronary perfusion

Fall in blood pressure

Impaired tissue perfusion

Decreased perfusion to vital organs: liver, lungs, kidney

Cellular hypoxia (acidosis)

Release of enzymes (histamine)

Intravascular coagulation

even up to 40%. The determinants of how much blood can be lost are several, including the site of fluid loss, the rate of bleeding during hemorrhage, and the elapse of time. A ruptured aortic aneurysm would cause a profound shock much more quickly than small, severed peripheral vessels that hemorrhage over several hours. Signs and symptoms of shock are clearly evident when losses approach 40% of the total volume. This period during which the body is responding to shock and vital organs are being conserved by compensatory mechanisms is referred to as *reversible shock,* since it responds readily to therapy.

Irreversible shock occurs when prolonged hypoxia causes depression of vital brain centers, which eventually render sympathetic efferent impulses to the cardiovascular system ineffectual; cardiac output and arterial pressure then fall, and progressive cellular anoxia leads to death. The time period between reversible and irreversible shock seems to average about 2 hours.

Prolonged cellular hypoxia leads to anaerobic metabolism, producing higher lactate levels with resultant metabolic acidosis. This metabolic acidosis may be clinically evident before any change in arterial blood pressure is noted. As volume continues to decrease and compensatory mechanisms become ineffective, cardiac filling and output are reduced even further, and tissue perfusion cannot be sustained.

Insufficient cellular oxygenation has direct consequences for organ systems, particularly those with high oxygen requirements. Pulmonary failure results in a syndrome known as shock lung, or adult respiratory distress syndrome. Cerebral edema, renal failure, hepatic failure, and disseminated intravascular coagulation are other outcomes and may be the ultimate cause of death in irreversible shock.

Assessment. Early blood or fluid loss can be noted by the appearance of the client and his behavior. Restlessness, thirst, and generalized anxiety typical of dehydration may be noted long before changes in vital signs. Urinary output is reduced before there is a decline in peripheral resistance. Systolic blood pressure usually does not fall until about 10% of the total circulating volume has been lost. A falling blood pressure, tachycardia, and increased respirations indicate relatively advanced shock. Nail bed compression will denote delayed return of color. There may be ascending cooling of extremities and the development of metabolic acidosis with its characteristic hyperventilation (Table 6-10).

Hemodynamic monitoring can be used to detect cardiovascular changes in incipient stages as well as to evaluate response to therapy. In hypovolemic shock the heart rate increases while the blood pressure and cardiac output decrease. The pulmonary artery pressure and pulmonary capillary wedge pressure also decrease owing to loss of intravascular fluid. An arterial line may be inserted for continuous monitoring of the blood pressure. Hemodynamic changes in cardiogenic shock differ because of the increased vascular resistance. Cardiac output is low, but the pulmonary artery, pulmonary artery wedge pressure, and left ventricular end diastolic pressure are usually elevated.

Planning and implementation. The goal of therapeutic shock management is to increase oxygen consumption by cells, not merely to restore normal blood pressure. Five factors are to be considered: (1) arterial blood pressure must be maintained; (2) blood volume must be supplemented; (3) blood flow must be ensured; (4) oxygen consumption must be increased; and (5) calories and nutrients must be provided for cellular metabolism.[13] These factors are interrelated and interdependent in influencing cellular perfusion and oxygen consumption. Some specific nursing responsibilities that affect hemodynamics are considered here.

Positioning. The bed should be flat to reduce resistance created by a dependent position. Some authorities recommend a shock position (Trendelenburg position), in which the head is lower than the legs to favor the trunk's blood supply. However, this may increase respiratory effort, since the abdominal organs push up against the diaphragm. The heart is required to exert more force to pump blood against gravity for kidney perfusion. Venous return from the head is also impeded. Others, however, advocate the use of a modified Trendelenburg position in which only the legs are elevated. This position overcomes some of the difficulties associated with the full Trendelenburg position but does not take

TABLE 6-10

Identification of degree or severity of shock

Test or sign		Normal or average	Degree of shock		
			Preshock state to mild shock	Moderate	Moderately severe to severe
Sensorium	Orientation	Well-oriented Time/place/person	Oriented	Fairly well oriented	May be confused and disoriented
	Enunciation	Distinct	Normal—slurred words	Somewhat slowed and few slurred words	Slow and slurred to monosyllabic utterances and groans
	Content	Appropriate, structured sentences	Sentences normal	Slow sentences or phrases and words	Often incoherent
Pupils	Size	Equal (2 to 4 mm)	Normal	Normal	Normal to dilating or dilated
	Constriction with light	Rapid	Rapid	Rapid	Slow or nonreactive
Pulse	Rate	60 to 100/min	100 to 120/min	120 to 150/min	Maximal
	Amplitude	Full	Full amplitude to slight decrease	Variable: mild decrease	Thready
Blood pressure (mm Hg)	Systolic	120 to 145	Normal or slightly low	Decreased—often 40 to 50 mm Hg below usual BP	Less than 80 to unobtainable
	Diastolic	60 to 90	Normal or slightly low	Decreased, but less so than systolic	40 to 50 to unobtainable
	Pulse pressure	40 to 70	30 to 40	20 to 30	Less than 20
Jugular vein filling	Patient flat	Fills to anterior border of sternocleidomastoid muscle	Normal to trace of filling	Trace to no filling	No filling
			May be full in septic shock or grossly distended in cardiogenic shock		
Urinary output via catheter	ml/min	0.6 to 1.5	0.6 to 0.8	0.4 to 0.6	0.3 or less
	ml/10 min	6 to 15	6 to 8	4 to 6	3 or less
Tilt test— rapid lying to sitting position	Pulse	Transient increase	Increased	Rapid	Already maximal
	Blood pressure	Less than 10 mm decrease	10 to 25 mm decrease	25 to 50 mm decrease	Marked decrease to unobtainable
	Symptoms	No "light-headedness"	No light-headedness	Light-headedness	Unable to sit up
	Therapeutic, if whole blood loss	—	Probably do not transfuse	Transfuse!	Transfuse!
	Est. blood loss	—	To 750 ml	1000 to 1250 ml	1500 to 1750 ml or more
	Est. % blood volume loss	—	15%	20 to 25%	More than 30 to 35%
Capillary blanching test	Blanching of forehead skin with thumb pressure	Return of circulation in 1.25 to 1.5 sec	1.25 to 1.5 sec	More than 1.5 sec	Pallor before and after test
			Note: With hypercapnia, there may be almost instantaneous return		
Central venous pressure (CVP)		Normal (3 to 12 cm of saline	Normal	Low	Extremely low
			May be normal (unusual) or elevated (common) in cardiogenic shock May be elevated (unusual) in hypovolemia with secondary congestive heart failure; give monitored fluid challenge		
Pulmonary wedge pressure	Normal (4 to 12 torr)		Same as CVP		

From Cain, Harvey D.: Flint's Emergency treatment and management, ed. 6, Philadelphia, 1981, W.B. Saunders Co.

full advantage of the force of gravity for enhancing arterial blood flow to the brain and stimulating venous return from the trunk and lower extremities. Many authorities believe that if the body cannot correct its hemodynamic state by reflex mechanisms while the client is in a flat position, the body will not be able to do so in a full or modified Trendelenburg position either.

Intravenous fluids. An intravenous infusion should be started at the first indication of shock. If rapid hypotension occurs and peripheral veins collapse, a venesection may be necessary. Colloidal substances or plasma expanders are useful to increase both volume and colloidal osmotic holding power of the vascular channels. Red blood cells may also be given to enhance the oxygen-carrying power of the blood. The intravenous route is an essential mechanism for supplementing blood volume, supplying calories and nutrients, and introducing pharmacological agents useful in managing shock.

Pharmacological agents. Adrenergic drugs may be employed to assist the toning mechanisms inherent in the cardiovascular system, but they must be selected to preserve microcirculation as well. Major actions include (1) increasing the rate and contractility of the heart and (2) increasing the peripheral resistance, which in effect raises arterial blood pressure, causing a reflex bradycardia. Commonly used adrenergic shock agents include levarterenol bitartrate (Levophed), phenylephrine hydrochloride (Neo-Synephrine), isoproterenol hydrochloride (Isuprel), epinephrine (Adrenalin), metaraminol bitartrate (Aramine), methoxamine hydrochloride (Vasoxyl), phentolamine (Regitine), propranolol hydrochloride (Inderal), and dopamine hydrochloride.

Steroids are also useful in improving microcirculation in low flow states such as shock. They decrease peripheral resistance, aid myocardial contractility, and enhance the conversion of lactate to glucose.

Methylprednisolone sodium succinate (Solu-Medrol) is a steroid agent typically used in shock.

It is imperative to understand that the goal of therapy in shock is to increase tissue perfusion, not merely to raise blood pressure. The success of clinical efforts is measured by how effectively metabolic acidosis is reversed in low perfusion states, by the adequacy of urinary output, and by the eventual correction of the hypotension.

Oxygen is also a pharmacological agent that is essential to administer in shock, since hypoxia and resultant anaerobic metabolism contribute to metabolic acidosis.

Clinical monitoring. Tubular necrosis and reduced glomerular filtration from inadequate blood pressure can seriously damage renal function. Urinary output must be monitored carefully during and after shock for oliguria and other indications of renal impairment that could be imposed by the shock state. If the client does not have an indwelling catheter, one should be inserted. Output for infants and children should be maintained at 10 to 20 ml/hour; for adults 30 to 50 ml/hour; and for the elderly 20 to 30 ml/hour. When blood is administered, a posttransfusion specimen should be sent to the laboratory for analysis. Intake and output as well as vital signs should be recorded on a regular basis. The skin will be cool and moist in the shock state because of peripheral vasoconstriction. The client should be kept warm with light covers but not so many that he will perspire and lose additional fluids. Both elevated temperature and chills increase metabolism and the subsequent need for oxygen.

**ACID-BASE
REGULATION**

The degree of acidity or alkalinity of body fluids directly influences normal functioning of cells and tissues. Water is the chief constituent of body fluids. It contains electrolytes and other components. Body fluids are found in the intracellular and extracellular spaces and are separated by the walls of the blood vessels and membranes of the cells. These tissues are semipermeable; thus there is a continuous interchange of large volumes of fluids between extracellular and intracellular compartments.

Body fluids contain mixtures of weak acids and their salts, which resist or *buffer* changes in hydrogen ion (H^+), which is produced in normal metabolism. This ion, a unit of positive electricity, is gained or lost by substances to form bases or acids. An acid is an H^+ donor and a base is an H^+ acceptor. In health, the concentration of the H^+ is low; thus fluids react on the slightly alkaline side of neutrality. In many illnesses, pathological changes can occur that increase or decrease the level of H^+ concentration. If compensatory mechanisms are ineffective or the changes are not reversed, acid-base imbalance can lead to death.

Regulation of the H^+ concentration is performed primarily by the lungs and kidneys. When there is excess of the H^+, *acidosis* results. Two examples of H^+ excess are decreased excretion of acids by the body (renal failure) and decreased excretion of carbon dioxide (pulmonary emphysema). H^+ deficits result in *alkalosis* when, for example, there is an increased excretion of carbon dioxide (hyperventilation) or increased excretion of acid (vomiting). The concentration of hydrogen ions in the body fluids indicates their reaction and is expressed as pH. The pH of water is 7, which represents electroneutrality. This is the reference point for ionic concentration of other solutions. Therefore, a shift toward a pH below 7 indicates increased H^+ concentration and acidosis. Decreased concentration of H^+ gives a higher pH and indicates alkalosis.

It is extremely important that the H^+ concentration be maintained within normal limits. The regulation of acid-base balance depends on four principal factors: (1) buffer systems; (2) excretion of acid or base by the kidneys; (3) excretion of CO_2 by the lungs; and (4) manufacture of NH_3 in the renal tubules, which combines with hydrogen ions to form NH_4.[2]

Buffer systems serve to reduce excess acids or bases by minimizing change in the H^+ concentration. The "buffering" action is one of "soaking up" or absorbing protons whenever the H^+ tend to increase or liberating protons whenever the H^+ tends to decrease. Buffer systems are in the blood plasma (that is, bicarbonate/carbonic acid, phosphate system, and plasma proteins), in the red blood cells, and in the extracellular fluids and tissues.

The lungs excrete CO_2 in the event of excessive release of CO_2. When conditions are such that an alkaline substance is in the blood, the respiratory center is depressed, giving off less CO_2 and more carbonic acid to equalize sodium bicarbonate. When CO_2 elimination is altered, the concentration of carbonic acid in body fluids in changed, and this affects acid-base regulation.

The kidneys help maintain acid-base regulation by varying quantities of base (H^+ and NH_4) when needed to maintain a normal level and balance of H^+. Tubular cells help maintain and restore concentration of bicarbonate ions in the blood and other extracellular fluids at normal levels. Essentially, H^+ is secreted into the renal tubule in exchange for sodium. The sodium is then returned to the body.

In summary, acid-base regulation is mediated by the lungs and kidneys. The relationship among the pH, the bicarbonate ion, and carbonic acid reflects the dynamic homeostatic state of the internal environment in maintaining acid-base balance. The H^+ is the determining factor in acidity or alkalinity of solutions. When the H^+ content deviates from normal, compensatory mechanisms that involve physical and chemical buffers come into play. Specific health problems related to acid-base imbalance are discussed when appropriate in subsequent chapters.

Degenerative processes

Degeneration of body tissue is a result of an inadequate supply of nutritive materials or stimulation. It affects vitality as well as physiological function and refers to a reduction in size after reaching normal proportions. Degeneration is a manifestation of all disease processes to some extent. Causes include absence of physical and neural stimulation, pressure and ischemia, inability to obtain or utilize nutrients, and certain physical agents such as thermal stimuli or radioactivity.

Factors that influence the development of degeneration include the nature and intensity of the injurious agent, the duration of exposure, and the condition of the cell at the time of exposure.

Absence of physical and neural stimulation to an organ or extremity over an extended period of time results in atrophy of the body part and concurrent loss of size and strength. This is a common occurrence in the aging process but also frequently accompanies long-term disuse of a limb as a result of a serious fracture, musculoskeletal disease, or paralysis. Active and passive exercises to the extent permissible, as well as electrical stimuli, can prevent such unfortunate sequelae in some instances, even if the client is confined to a bed for an extended period of time. Body parts tend to degenerate simply from lack of use. The adrenal cortex atrophies during long-term cortisone therapy, for example, because it is not being stimulated by neurogenic mechanisms inherent when it is serving its usual critical function. The body tends to channel its supportive efforts to parts that have vital and contributory roles in the life process.

Pressure and *ischemia* are also responsible for degeneration. Pressure ultimately results in ischemia, but not all ischemia results from pressure. An individual with poor peripheral circulation over an extended period of time loses tissue vitality in the regions affected. If ischemia or inadequate blood flow is present for a sufficient period of time for irreversible tissue damage to occur, a body part may become necrotic, or die. An *infarct* is one type of tissue death in which a local area of cells dies as a result of interrupted blood supply. If a clot (thrombus) blocks one coronary artery, which is responsible for nourishing a specific area of the myocardium, that portion of the myocardium will degenerate and die unless the ischemic process has been a gradual one allowing for the establishment of collateral circulation. Such a phenomenon is termed an *infarction.* *Gangrene* is a term used to denote the death of a large area of tissue such as a foot, leg, or portion of the bowel.

Tumors and edema from any cause can create direct compression on surrounding tissue and provoke ischemia. Hydrocephalus, or excessive fluid in the intracranial space, also interferes with normal circulatory mechanisms. Since the cranium is an expandable space in the young child, considerable fluid can collect before severe damage results. However, in the adult whose cranium is a totally confined bony space, pressure from edema can quickly impair circulation and result in degeneration of brain tissue.

Organs with a rich blood supply (such as the heart and kidneys) are extremely susceptible to ischemia, as are organs with poor collateral circulation. Initially, tissues respond to reduced blood supply by limiting their metabolic activity. If the blood supply is sufficient to maintain the cells with limited function, collateral circulation develops to bring additional nutrients to the area. However, sudden interruption of arterial blood to an extensive portion of any one vital organ can result in death of the tissue. Metabolic alterations and cellular activity impairment both precede the ultimate outcome of degeneration.

Nursing has a vital role in preventing ischemia: to recognize it in its early stages and to take measures to increase blood flow to vital areas.

The nurse should be especially alert to the following signs of ischemia: (1) pain, (2) edema, (3) numbness, (4) tingling, (5) bluish discoloration, (6) coolness, and (7) inability to move the part. Special care should be taken to observe for these in clients who are undernourished or elderly, have impaired sensory nerve supply, have casts and bandages, or are unconscious or generally edematous, since they are the most likely victims of complications resulting from pressure and ischemia.

Pressure on susceptible tissue should be avoided by taking specific measures such as alternating positions of the trunk and extremities for a client undergoing prolonged bed rest. Heels, ankles, the sacrum, and ears are frequently affected by pressure, with resulting ischemia and ulceration. Air mattresses, waterbeds, flotation pads, and many other devices have been used to reduce prolonged pressure on any body prominence. Keeping tissue clean, dry, well nourished, and stimulated seems to be useful in combating degeneration from pressure. Edema should be controlled to the extent possible by physical and pharmacological means, and circulation should be stimulated by activity.

Inability to obtain and utilize nutrients is usually due to inadequate circulation to a cell rather than the absence of essential nutrients in the bloodstream or failure of a cell to metabolize them. However, there are conditions of the gastrointestinal and endocrine systems that contribute to the problem. For example, malabsorption of food in the small intestine may cause a general starvation and degeneration of the entire body because cells simply do not have nutrients presented to them, although circulation is normal. Deficiency or absence of cellular enzymes and absorption by tissue of poisons and toxic chemicals can also prevent utilization of certain nutrients, and ultimately the cell dies. Such conditions affecting nutrition are covered in later chapters.

Physical agents such as heat, cold, and radiation can damage tissue structures and initiate a degenerative course. A prolonged or intense exposure to the elements can actually destroy the cell or provoke irreversible structural changes such as fibrosis. Heat and cold generally are encountered in amounts that seem to affect primary circulation rather than create direct cellular destruction.

The numerous diseases of metabolism and connective tissue (collagen) that are considered degenerative in nature will be examined in subsequent chapters as they interfere with basic human needs.

6 Pathophysiological processes of illness

Some pathologists consider degenerative processes to include other problems related to abnormal growth of tissue mass. Among these are the following:

1. Aplasia: failure to develop sufficient tissue because growing tissue is destroyed by an injurious agent
2. Hypoplasia: amount of tissue insufficient to meet functional requirements
3. Hypertrophy: increase in volume of parenchymal functioning tissue, usually the result of responding to increased physiological demands
4. Hyperplasia: increase in number of cells, especially in bone marrow
5. Metaplasia: tissue changes from one type to another to adjust to new demands (such as mucous membrane changing to squamous epithelium to compensate for tracheostomy)
6. Obesity: excessive accumulation of adipose tissue
7. Emaciation: wasting away of body tissue, especially adipose tissue

Degenerative processes are obviously a part of every disease as a primary or secondary factor. They are closely related to other basic pathological processes including congenital anomalies, inflammation, tumors, and physical disturbances. Not uncommonly, several entities occur together, and often it is difficult for experts to find the initial disease process.

Summary

The fundamental pathophysiological bases of health problems are cellular deviation, breaks in body defenses and barriers, physical-chemical insults, and degenerative processes. Whenever deviations in cell structure occur, the cell may be damaged and disease may result. Among the factors that may alter cellular growth are genetic defects, congenital anomalies, tumors, and carcinogenesis. Alterations may occur in the body defenses and barriers, including the mucous membrane, skin, cilia, and phagocytic activity. These body defenses may be protected against microorganisms by the inflammatory process. Such a process is initiated by any insult to body tissue and ends with some type of tissue repair (for example, wound healing). The immune system also protects the body by responding to the invasion of the body in either a beneficial or a harmful way. Immunity affords one an opportunity to resist certain types of agents.

Other phenomena that may have an effect on illness include physical-chemical insults such as trauma, wounds, obstructions, hernias, thermal disturbances, circulatory disturbances (hemorrhage and shock), and acid-base regulations, as well as degenerative processes. Since coping with health and injuries requires knowledge of the underlying reasons for the absence of homeodynamics, the nurse must understand the mechanisms of each of these. The nursing process is influenced by the interrelatedness of pathological phenomena. Approaches such as genetic counseling, recognition of signs and symptoms of inflammation, and awareness of the manifestations of tissue repair and other homeodynamic states are essential to the care of clients who manifest these pathophysiological problems.

187

References

1. American Cancer Society: Cancer 1981, facts and figures, New York, 1981, American Cancer Society.
2. Boyd, W.: A textbook of pathology: structure and function in disease, Philadelphia, 1976, Lea & Febiger.
3. Burnet, F.: Immunology, aging, and cancer, San Francisco, 1976, W.H. Freeman & Co., Publishers.
4. Frolich, Edward, editor: Pathophysiology: altered regulatory mechanisms in disease, Philadelphia, 1972, J.B. Lippincott Co.
5. Groër, Maureen E., and Shekleton, Maureen E.: Basic pathophysiology: a conceptual approach, St. Louis, 1979, The C.V. Mosby Co.
6. Jawetz, E., Melnick, J.L., and Adelberg, E.A.: Review of medical microbiology, Los Altos, California, 1980, Lange Medical Publications.
7. Kaye, R., Osk, F., and Barness, L., editors: Core textbook of pediatrics, Philadelphia, 1978, J.B. Lippincott Co.
8. Marino, Elizabeth, and LeBlanc, Donna: Cancer chemotherapy, Nurs. '75 **75**(11):22-23, 1975.
9. Marino, Lisa: Cancer nursing, St. Louis, 1981, The C.V. Mosby Co.
10. McAdams, Constance: Inferferon: the penicillin of the future? Am. J. Nurs. **80:**714-718, 1980.
11. Price, S., and Wilson, L.: Pathophysiology: clinical concepts of disease process, New York, 1978, McGraw-Hill Book Co.
12. Rubin, Philip, editor: Clinical oncology for medical students and physicians: a multidisciplinary approach, ed. 5, New York, 1978, American Cancer Society.
13. Shoemaker, William C.: Hemodynamic and oxygen-transport patterns of common shock syndromes. Proceedings of a symposium on recent research developments and current clinical practice in shock, Kalamazoo, Mich., 1975, The Upjohn Co.
14. Weil, Max Harry, and Shubin, Herbert: Proposed reclassification of shock states with special reference to distributive defects, Adv. Exp. Med. Biol. **23**(10):13-23, 1971.

Additional readings

American Joint Committee for Cancer Staging and End Reporting, American Cancer Society: Manual for staging cancer 1978, New York, 1978, Whiting Press.

Beland, Irene: Clinical nursing: pathophysiological and psychosocial approaches, ed. 3, New York, 1975, Macmillan, Inc.

Bierman, Charles, and Pearlman, D.S., editors: Allergic diseases of infancy, childhood, and adolescence, Philadelphia, 1978, W.B. Saunders Co.

Budassi, Susan A., and Barber, Janet M.: Emergency nursing: principles and practice, St. Louis, 1981, The C.V. Mosby Co.

Collins, R.D.: Illustrated manual of fluid and electrolyte disorders, Philadelphia, 1976, J.B. Lippincott Co.

Hedlin, A.: The immune system, Can. Nurse **75**(7):28-30, 1979.

Hurley, Elaine: Hypovolemic shock. In Current practice in critical care, vol. 1, St. Louis, 1979, The C.V. Mosby Co.

Kruse, Louise C., Reese, Jean L., and Hart, Laura K.: Cancer: pathophysiology, etiology, management: selected readings, St. Louis, 1979, The C.V. Mosby Co.

Kellogg, Carolyn J., and Sullivan, Barbara P., editors: Current perspectives in oncologic nursing, vol. 2, St. Louis, 1978, The C.V. Mosby Co.

Kintzel, Kay, editor: Advanced concepts in clinical nursing, Philadelphia, 1977, J.B. Lippincott Co.

Meakins, J.: Body's response to infection, AORN J. **22**(1):37-44, 1975.

7 Nursing: process and models for client care

Nursing is a dynamic activity occurring when an agent (nurse) uses its power to aid or manipulate another agent (client) in relation to the client's health status.[20] Nursing practice includes the diagnosis and treatment of human responses to actual or potential health problems. Nursing can further be described by the process that is used; models and theories that explain, predict, or validate nursing actions; the context or health care delivery system in which nursing occurs; and mechanisms used to ensure quality nursing care. The purpose of this chapter is to explore these facets of nursing as they relate to the client, his environment, and his health state.

Nursing process

The nursing process is a method by which nursing care can be determined, planned, provided, and evaluated. The nursing process is a systematic, scientific problem-solving method used by the nurse and client to identify problems, plan solutions, implement care, and evaluate outcomes.[14,25]

The nursing process can be described according to several distinct stages, each of which requires cognitive, affective, or psychomotor activities on the part of the nurse, client, or both. Some nurses use a five-stage nursing process model that includes assessment, analysis, planning, implementation, and evaluation.[15] Others prefer a four-stage model in which analysis (nursing diagnosis) is a component of assessment and the four steps are assessment, planning, implementation, and evaluation.[14,25] Although other nursing process models have been proposed, the five-stage nursing process is used in this text. Regardless of the process used, it is not the number of steps that is significant, but that the process is based on scientific knowledge and applicable to nursing.[24]

The nursing process, as a dynamic interaction of the client and nurse, can be separated into stages for descriptive purposes, but in fact the activities in-

FIG. 7-1
Nursing process is a dynamic interaction between nurse and client.

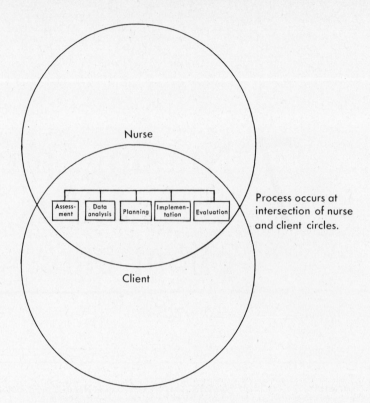

Nurse

Assess-ment | Data analysis | Planning | Implemen-tation | Evaluation

Process occurs at intersection of nurse and client circles.

Client

volved during one stage are interrelated with the others and may occur concurrently (Fig. 7-1). The nursing process, then, is an open system with interrelated parts sharing inputs, outputs, and feedback mechanisms.

ASSESSMENT: DATA COLLECTION

The assessment stage of the nursing process includes systematic data collection. Assessment is a collaborative process involving the nurse, client (individual, family, group, or community), and other health team members.

Nursing history

Data collection is a systematic way to obtain objective and subjective information about the client in terms of his current and past health. The nursing history includes biographical data, information obtained from the health, developmental, social, and psychological histories, the physical assessment, and, if available, data from diagnostic assessment.

Data may be obtained by observation, interview, and physical assessment skills of inspection, palpation, percussion, and auscultation. Several variables may determine the type and amount of data collected. The present status of the client often determines the nature of data collection. In emergencies, for example, clients may be unable to provide information, and the nurse may depend on bystanders or family for an accounting of the recent health history. Furthermore, in this situation a detailed nursing history is inappropriate. Other variables include age of client, reason for obtaining health care services, and availability of previous health information about the client (for example, records and charts).

Systematic data collection facilitates formulation of a problem list, and the nurse should develop one organized approach to gathering data.[5,13] Most nursing service departments have developed tools to help the nurse gather appropriate data (Figs. 7-2 and 7-3). Tools may be developed for specific client populations and focus attention on the unique needs of clients with special nursing

CHILD'S NAME _____ BIRTH DATE _____

We want to make your child as comfortable and happy as possible. If we know about his or her nickname, favorite friends, pets, food preferences and, above all, normal pattern of living, we can help your child feel more at home. Won't you please help by telling us about your child.

Nickname _____ Parent's name _____

Address and phone number _____ Child's religion _____ Baptized _____

Names and ages of your other children _____ Does your child need help with dressing _____

Washing face _____ Combing hair _____ Brushing teeth _____ Has your child been in a hospital before _____

Does the child know why he or she is being admitted to the hospital _____

Does your child seem to make friends with unfamiliar grownups easily _____

EATING HABITS

Is your child breast fed _____ Uses bottle _____ Spoon _____ Cup _____ Feeds self alone _____

Feeds self with help _____ If on a schedule, at what hours _____ What is his present formula _____

_____ What fruit juices does your child drink _____

_____ From bottle _____ From cup _____ Is your child allergic to any foods _____

What foods does your child especially like _____

or dislike _____ Are there any other feeding routines or

aids that we should know about _____

ELIMINATION

Is your child toilet trained for bowel movement _____ For urination _____ For how long _____ Does your child wear diapers _____ Does your child use a toilet

chair or toilet _____ What is word used for urination _____ Bowel movement _____ Is child taken to toilet at night _____ If so, at what time _____

SLEEPING HABITS

Is your child a heavy sleeper _____ When is bedtime _____ Are naps taken _____ If so, at what time _____

Does your child sleep alone _____ Crib _____ Bed with sides _____ Adult bed _____ Does your child climb out of bed _____

Describe any special bedtime routine, e.g., having prayers heard, taking teddy bear or doll to bed, use of night light, etc. _____

PLAY

Has your child a favorite toy _____ Did you bring it along _____ Any favorite games _____

Is the child used to playing alone _____ With other children _____ With grownups _____

Does your child have a pet at home _____ What is it _____ What is its name _____

SCHOOL

Does your child attend nursery school _____ Grade school _____ Name of school _____

Grade _____ Name of best friend(s) _____

Name of favorite teacher _____ List any special interests (hobbies,

favorite books, favorite TV, radio programs, etc.) _____

Is there anything else about your child that you feel we should know to make his or her hospital stay as pleasant as possible? _____

FIG. 7-2
Nursing assessment form for children. (Courtesy Ross Laboratories, Columbus, Ohio.)

FOR USE IN PLANNING NURSING CARE. NOT INTENDED TO REPLACE MEDICAL HISTORY AND PHYSICAL.

A. NURSING ADMITTING HISTORY
1. Reason for hospitalization _____

2. Chief complaint _____

3. General observations: Alert ____ Stuporous ____ Drowsy ____ Coma ____ Other _____
4. Past medical history:
   a. Medical _____
   b. Surgical _____
   c. Past education or instruction: Diabetes ____ Cardiac Rehab. ____ Ostomy _____
       Pulmonary Rehab. ____ Other _____
   d. Activities of normal daily living: Check appropriate level.
       I — Independent   A — Assistance Needed   C — Complete dependence
       Bathing ____ Hygiene ____ Eating ____ Mouth Care ____ Dressing ____ Locomotion ____
   e. Allergies or sensitivities: Include type of reaction.
       (1) Medications _____
       (2) Food _____
       (3) Allergy band on: Yes _____
   f. Medications (Include anticoagulants, hormones, thyroid, and hypoglycemics):
       Those taken at home _____
5. Family history: Diabetes — Hypertension — Cancer — Heart — T.B. — Anemia —
   Sickle cell disease/Trait — Other _____
6. Habits:
   Smokes: Yes ____ No ____ How much _____
   Alcoholic drinks: Yes ____ No ____ How much _____
   Exercise: Yes ____ No ____ How much _____
   Sleep: # Hours ____ Normal bedtime ____ Sleep aids (meds, radio, etc.) _____
   Dietary: Special diet _____ Likes _____
             Dislikes _____ Daily fluid intake _____
7. Psycho-social history:
   a. Expectation of this hospitalization _____
   b. Behavior indicative of mental/emotional status:
       Alert _____ Cooperative _____ Flat affect _____ Sad _____
       Anxious _____ Demanding _____ Guarded _____ Talkative _____
       Apprehensive _____ Depressed _____ Hyperactive _____ Trustful _____
       Calm _____ Distrustful _____ Mentally slow _____ Withdrawn _____
       Other
   c. Occupation: Present _____ Past _____ Working Hours _____
   d. Special interests and hobbies _____
8. Safety factors:
   Over 65 _____ Hx of falls _____ Nocturia _____
   Language barrier _____ Obese _____ Incontinent _____
   Senile _____ Smokes _____ X-ray prep. _____
   Confused _____ Dec. sensation _____ Sleeping pills _____
   Mentally retarded _____ Loss of balance _____ Anticoagulants/Cuts _____
   Emotional instability _____ Seizures _____ Allergy _____
   Overly independent _____ Vision/hearing prob. _____ Hypotension _____
9. Discharge planning:
   a. # of children ____ Age range ____ Role in family ____ # in household ____
   b. Plan for discharge (independent/need assistance). If assistance needed, send
       social service consult (date _____).

Date _____ Time _____ Signature _____
Informant if other than patient _____

Admitting nursing assessment

A

Winona
Memorial Hospital
3232 North Meridian Street
Indianapolis, Indiana 46208

IMPRINT

FIG. 7-3
Admitting nursing assessment form for adults. (Courtesy cooperative efforts of
the nursing staff, Winona Memorial Hospital, Indianapolis, Ind.)

B. NURSING HISTORY
(Circle = + response)
1. INTEGUMENTARY
(Do you have or have you had problems with?)
1. Eczema
2. Psoriasis
3. Dry Oily skin

Comments:_____

2. SENSORY
(Do you have or have you had problems with?)
1. Ears: Hard of hearing   R/L
   Dizziness, ringing in ears
2. Eyes: Vision   R/L
   Blurring, spots, double vision
3. Nose: Bleeding, post-nasal drip,
   obstruction

3. CARDIOVASCULAR RESPIRATORY
(Do you have or have you had?)
1. Heart disease
2. Chest pain (describe)_____

3. Hypertension, Phlebitis
4. S.O.B. (exert/non-exert) # Pillows
5. Lung disease _____
6. Colds frequent/infrequent
7. Chronic cough   Yes/No
   If yes, describe _____

Comments:_____

4. GASTROINTESTINAL
(Do you have or have you had?)
1. Problems with: Swallowing, heartburn/
   indigestion, Hiatal hernia, N&V, gas,
   Abd. pain, recent wt. gain/loss, constipation, diarrhea, abnormal stool
   color, rectal pain/bleeding, distention
   Comments:_____

5. GENITOURINARY
(Do you have or have you had?)
1. Problems with frequency (day x_____,
   night x_____)
   Urgency, pain, burning, difficulty
   starting stream, incontinence, retention, bloody urine, infection, prostate problems
2. Breasts Lumps R/L, Drainage, pain,
   tenderness
   Breasts: Self exam Yes/No
   Do you desire instruction? Yes/No
3. Menses: L.M.P.   Interval
   Comments:_____
   Last pap test _____
   Vaginal discharge, itching

6. MUSCULOSKELETAL NEUROLOGICAL
(Do you have or have you had?)
1. Problems with: Joint pain or swelling, aches, muscle cramps, numbness,
   tremors, seizures, weakness, paralysis, fractures, amputations.
   Dizziness/Loss of balance. Fainting/
   Blackout spells.
   Comments:_____

NURSING OBSERVATION/ASSESSMENT
1. General hygiene:_____

2. Problems:_____

3. Hydration:_____
   Skin turgor_____
   Mucous membranes _____
Comments:_____

OBSERVATION/ASSESSMENT
1. Ears_____
2. Eyes_____
3. Nose_____
Comments:_____

OBSERVATION/ASSESSMENT
1. Pulse—Radial rate____ Regularity____ Quality____
   Other____
2. Extremities—Edema_____
   Color_____ Warm/Cold_____
Comments:_____

3. Respirations—Rate____ Depth____ Pattern____
   If abnormalities in above, assess breath
   sounds & describe.
Comments:_____

OBSERVATION/ASSESSMENT
1. If problems, describe: _____

2. Bowel habits: Last B.M.____ Normal freq.____
   Time of day ____ Aids (laxatives, fluids, etc.)
_____

OBSERVATION/ASSESSMENT
1. If problems, describe:_____

OBSERVATION/ASSESSMENT
1. If problems, describe:_____

2. R/L handed
3. Gait: Not observed, normal, abnormal.
   Describe:_____

Date _____ Time_____Signature _____
Informant if other than patient _____

FIG. 7-3, cont'd
Admitting nursing assessment form for adults.

B

diagnoses related to age, developmental status, or health problem. These assessment tools are described where appropriate throughout the text.

Biographical data. At the outset of assessment certain biographical data must be obtained from the client. These include name, address, sex, and, if relevant, marital status, parity, and occupation. Other biographical data may be required by the specific health care agency. Examples are social security number, insurance policy number, agency file number, and source of referral. This information may be obtained from the client, family member, or significant other at the initial contact or before admission to the health care agency.

Health history. The health history is used to ascertain the client's perception of his health problem and the onset, duration, precipitating factors and recent course of the problem. Other information is obtained about usual habits and previous health problems.

Developmental history. A developmental history is obtained to estimate the client's developmental status as compared with norms. Physical, sexual, emotional, social, and family development should be noted in this history.

Social history. The social history includes information about the client's social environment. Factors such as religion, occupation, culture, ethnicity, economic status, educational background, and family affiliations impinge on the client's life and health and provide useful information for problem identification and subsequent nursing care planning.

Psychological history. Information about the client's mental status, coping mechanisms, and emotional assets and limitations can be used to determine the client's physical and mental well-being. Information about the client's current stresses as well as those incurred during the past year may help the nurse and client identify or predict health problems.

Physical assessment. Physical assessment is the final component of a nursing history and is used to obtain additional information about the client's health status. Physical assessment is facilitated by a systematic approach that usually includes observation of the client's general appearance followed by appropriate use and sequence of data gathering by inspection, palpation, percussion, and auscultation of each body system. These skills are explained in detail in texts on physical assessment[1,7,13,21] and are discussed in relation to common health problems in subsequent chapters.

Adaptations of the nursing history. The nursing history can be modified for the unique needs of the client, and the nurse must adapt data-gathering skills as appropriate. Neonates, infants, and young children and older adults constitute two groups that particularly require adaptations of data-gathering techniques and physical assessment procedures.

Neonates, infants, and children. The nursing history for children requires special data collection, several types of direct observations, some technical procedures, and thorough analyses of the data collected. A history includes "(1) present illness, (2) mother's health during the pregnancy, (3) events of labor and delivery, (4) condition of the child in the neonatal period, (5) growth and development, (6) immunizations, (7) diet and feeding history, (8) previous diseases and whether residual defects occurred, (9) previous operations or hospitalizations, (10) child's mental level, (11) child's emotional adjustments, and (12) family history."[11]

Since young clients often cannot describe their symptoms, objective findings

FIG. 7-5

FIG. 7-4

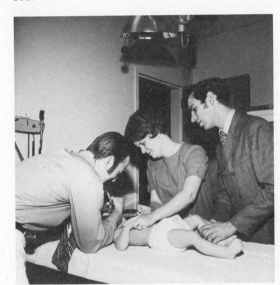

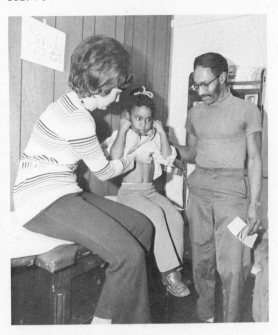

FIG. 7-4   Nurse examines child while parents are nearby for support.

FIG. 7-5   Routine health assessment can be a learning experience for the young child. Note that the nurse is permitting the girl to become familiar with the stethoscope.

must be relied on heavily. As children approach school age, the examination is usually easier to accomplish.

During the physical examination is an excellent time to observe parent-child interaction and to establish rapport with the family.

Very young children and those of 4 or 5 and over seldom present critical problems during examination unless they are unusually dependent. They should be permitted to remain near parents during the observations as much as possible. Often it is helpful if they sit on their parent's lap, stand close to them, or are held by them during certain procedures.

Young children should never be swept immediately from their parent's arms and placed on an examining table. They should be allowed to remain with them to the extent permitted during the initial phases of history taking and observation.

When the child must be removed to the table, having the mother or father close by is usually some comfort to the child, and often the parents can be of assistance. Some children prefer to be in direct view of the examiner; others respond best when they can avoid seeing him, such as being held facing the parent (Fig. 7-4).

If struggling and crying become excessive, a restraining device may be indicated. Occasionally the parents may be asked to leave the room if they seem to be aggravating the situation.

The modesty of both the child and his parents should be respected. Underclothing should be removed only when necessary and replaced as soon as possible. Unusual modesty, however, should be noted, since it may be a clue to a behavioral disturbance.

Nurses find that they usually gain more cooperation from the child if he is acquainted with the tools used in the examination and is allowed to manipulate them or relate them to a familiar object. Often, giving the child a simple object such as a tongue depressor or Band-Aid may divert his interests, at least momentarily, while a specific observation is made (Fig. 7-5).

Once data have been collected, the information must be interpreted according to norms for the client's age. Vital signs and physical findings abnormal in adults, for example, are often normal in children.

Older adults. Since older adults may move more slowly and may have diminished sensory acuity, more time should be allotted for history taking and physical assessment. The additional measures of providing a warm, quiet environment and a comfortable examination room and table designed for safety facilitate the examination.

Interpretation of physical assessment findings should be congruent with the client's age. Older adults are often viewed in the broad group of ''adults,'' even though recent research has revealed that normal ranges for vital signs and physical activity are different in older adults.

Diagnostic assessment

Data obtained from diagnostic examinations such as x-ray examinations, electrocardiogram, blood and urine tests, and other biochemical assays may be added to the data from the nursing history. Diagnostic assessments may be obtained before the nursing history and can be incorporated in the nursing diagnosis. Diagnostic assessments may also be made while the client is receiving health care services and can be used to plan and evaluate nursing care.

DATA ANALYSIS

When relevant data are collected within an appropriate amount of time, they are classified and compared with norms established for the client's developmental, social, psychological, and physical status. Drawing on knowledge from biological and social sciences the nurse, with the client, identifies nursing problems.

Nursing problems may be identified as a problem list or as a list of nursing diagnoses. Nursing *problems* are descriptive interpretations of the categories concerning a given situation, that is, the client's problems and needs, which may be derived from Maslow's hierarchy. A nursing *diagnosis* is a diagnostic category used to determine therapy.[9] The diagnosis identifies existing or potentential health problems that nurses are qualified and licensed to treat.[17] The diagnostic category comprises (1) description of the problem (category label), (2) cause of the problem (etiology), and (3) defining characteristics (symptoms). Nursing diagnoses facilitate descriptions of problems for which nurses can intervene within the scope of nursing practice. A list of accepted nursing diagnoses, which undergoes periodic revision, provides a common basis for communicating about nursing problems; examples are given on p. 197.

The nurse analyzes data to identify either nursing problems or nursing diagnoses. The decision as to which system to use often is determined by the health care agency in which the nurse practices because the interpretation of problem or diagnosis must be consistent for those planning nursing care.

Nursing problems (diagnoses) can be further designated as actual or potential. An *actual* problem is one that currently exists and is identifiable by the nurse

**LIST OF NURSING DIAGNOSES ACCEPTED AT THE
FOURTH NATIONAL CONFERENCE**

Airway clearance, ineffective
Bowel elimination, alterations in: constipation
Bowel elimination, alterations in: diarrhea
Bowel elimination, alterations in: incontinence
Breathing patterns, ineffective
Cardiac output, alterations in: decreased
Comfort, alterations in: pain
Communication, impaired verbal
Coping, ineffective individual
Coping, ineffective family: compromised
Coping, ineffective family: disabling
Coping, family: potential for growth
Diversional activity, deficit
Fear
Fluid volume deficit, actual
Fluid volume deficit, potential
Gas exchange, impaired
Grieving, anticipatory
Grieving, dysfunctional
Home maintenance management, impaired
Injury, potential for
Knowledge deficit (specify)
Mobility, impaired physical

Noncompliance (specify)
Nutrition, alterations in: less than body requirements
Nutrition, alterations in: more than body requirements
Nutrition, alterations in: potential for more than body requirements
Parenting, alterations in: actual
Parenting, alterations in: potential
Rape-trauma syndrome
Self-care deficit (specify level: feeding, bathing/hygiene, dressing/grooming, toileting
Self-concept, disturbance in
Sensory perceptual alterations
Sexual dysfunction
Skin integrity, impairment of: actual
Skin integrity, impairment of: potential
Sleep pattern disturbance
Spiritual distress (distress of the human spirit)
Thought processes, alterations in
Tissue perfusion, alteration in
Urinary elimination, alteration in patterns
Violence, potential for

Diagnoses "accepted" without defining characteristics (therefore, unacceptable, but to be listed separately, as diagnoses to be developed [TBD])

Cognitive dissonance   TBD
Family dynamics, alterations in   TBD
Fluid volume, alterations in, excess: potential for   TBD
Memory deficit   TBD
Rest-activity pattern, ineffective   TBD
Role disturbance   TBD
Social isolation   TBD

From Kim, M.: Classification of nursing diagnoses: proceedings from the fourth National Conference, 1980. Used with permission of McGraw-Hill Book Co.

and client. A *potential* problem, on the other hand, is a problem likely to occur in the future based on data currently collected. A client with a tumor obstructing the airway, for example, has an *actual* problem of airway clearance, whereas the client who is soon to undergo surgery has the *potential* for a problem with airway clearance.

Data collection and analysis form an ongoing process. As plans are formulated, implemented, and evaluated, the client's status changes and provides continual input for revision of the problem list.

Recording data   Data collected from the nursing history must be recorded concisely. In addition to providing an organized presentation of information for data analysis and planning, the data become a part of the client's legal record. Each health care agency develops tools to facilitate recording and retrieval of significant information.

One example of a systematic recording system incorporating problem-solving processes is the *problem-oriented system* (POS) or problem-oriented record (POR). The problem-oriented system was devised by Dr. Lawrence

197

Foundations of clinical practice

Weed. It has at least three salient characteristics: (1) organization of data around problems, not persons or sources; (2) preservation of a system of logic as well as data; and (3) facilitation of the audit of care on a concurrent as well as retrospective basis. The elements of the system are (1) data base, (2) problem list, (3) plans, and (4) progress notes.

The *data base* encompasses all health problems that exist for the client, not merely the problem under current consideration or the problem that is episodic. It includes the chief complaint; a description of the present illness; past family, social, and medical history; a review of systems; physical examination findings; and results of selected laboratory tests and x-ray examinations. The nursing history and assessment are extremely valuable parts of this data base.

The *problem list* is a "table of contents" for the record, and each actual or potential problem is given a number and a title as it is entered with a notation of the date of onset. The problem may be a medical diagnosis (such as diabetes), a nursing diagnosis (such as alterations in nutrition), a sign or symptom, a physiological finding, or an abnormal test result.

The *problem-oriented plans* are titled and numbered to correspond with the problem list and, again, traverse all disciplines that are providing care. They include plans for diagnosis, treatment, instruction, and ruling out of irrelevant data.

Progress notes are also titled and numbered, and an identical format is recommended for all disciplines. Dr. Weed advocates a system that he calls "SOAPing," since the key factors are subjective, objective, assessment, and plan. *Subjective data* are noted in regard to what the client says or feels, that is, his complaint. *Objective elements* are such pieces of information as laboratory reports or other data that are derived or supported by outside sources. The *assessment* is what the recorder thinks is going on based on the previous subjective and objective data. It is an analysis in the sense of relevant information. The *plan* consists of what is being done to resolve the problem. It envelops orders for the diagnostic regimen, referral, nursing care measures, and client instruction. The client's response to all aspects of care or to the related experiences is incorporated into this section of the recording.

Progress notes constructed in this way promote openness of thinking, invite comments, action, and criticism from other practitioners, and encourage dialogue among them. The logic of the care providers can be examined and the rationale for specific measures clarified. Interdisciplinary recording promotes teamwork and serves as an incentive for demonstrating a high quality of care. The problem-oriented progress notes are written in relation to the stated problem and are linked to action. Data are not recorded unless they are related to a problem or linked to action. As the data base expands through new tests and observation, relationships among multiple variables are explored and attempts made to correlate them with eventual solution of the problem.

The impact of the problem-oriented system on client care will relate primarily to ensuring continuity and comprehensiveness of a health care record that will in turn effect a continuous and comprehensive approach to the management of the client and his health care.

Other record systems may incorporate other systematic recording tools and use of flow sheets to demonstrate sequences of care. In some settings information is recorded by computer for easy access and retrieval of data.

7   Nursing: process and models for client care

PLANNING

The planning stage of the nursing process involves three steps: (1) determining priorities of nursing problems or diagnoses, (2) setting goals and objectives with specific client outcome criteria to deal with the problem, and (3) designing methods for implementation. Plans are usually made with the client and family. In certain instances, however, plans may exist in the form of a protocol or actions designed for specific emergencies. During a sudden, unexpected cardiopulmonary arrest, for example, the nurse is not able to plan with the client, nor is it practical to do so.

Placing problems or nursing diagnoses in order of priority is the first step of planning. It is imperative that the client and family assist in the determination of the priority of problems. The nurse and client often do not agree on the significance of problems, and conflicts that make formulation and implementation of plans difficult should be resolved at this stage in planning.

Goals are broad expectations and may pertain to promotion of health, prevention of health problems, or restoration to optimal levels of health or rehabilitation. *Objectives* are more specific and can be stated in terms of client *expected outcomes* for changes in behavior, attitude, or knowledge. An objective contains a subject, observable behavior, condition, and criterion (criteria).[2] For example, the client, Mrs. A. (subject), will walk (behavior) using crutches (condition) 20 feet (criterion). The more specific the objective, the more specific the change is likely to be and the more easily evaluated. Goals and objectives should be realistic and obtainable within the limits of the resources of the client, the nurse, and the health care agency.

As a final step in planning, methods are designed to help the client reach the goal(s) for each problem or diagnosis. The nursing action can be written as a prescription (nursing order) to avoid misconception about the nursing actions to be employed.[2] Nursing orders include nursing action, recipient, object, and frequency. For example, walk (nursing action) with Mrs. A. (recipient) according to the care plan (object) three times daily (frequency).

Since plans are developed for specific and current problems, the nurse must be receptive to changes in other stages of the nursing process. More data may be obtained by assessment, for example, and the problem list revised, or it may not be possible to implement the plans. A final determination of the effectiveness of the plan is made during the evaluation stage of the nursing process; and, depending on information collected at this time, the plan may be discontinued, continued, or revised.

IMPLEMENTATION

In the implementation phase of the nursing process, the nursing orders are used to achieve the planned goals and objectives. The orders are carried out in the interpersonal relationship between the nurse and client (individual, family, group, community) and require intellectual, interpersonal, and technical skills.[25]

Although the plans for nursing action are developed by a professional nurse and the client, they may be carried out by other nurses, other health team members, the client, or the client's family. If the plan is clearly written, implementation will be more specific, more goal directed, and more purposeful. Nursing actions used to implement the plan may include activities such as counseling, teaching, providing comfort measures, coordinating, referring, using therapeutic communication skills, and carrying out medical orders.

The nurse's actions can be described as *independent* if they are initiated

Foundations of clinical practice

by the nurse from the scope of nursing practice, such as turning a patient. Nursing actions are described as *dependent* if they are initiated by a physician to be implemented by the nurse, for example, administering medications.

The implementation stage is complete when the nursing actions are accomplished. The actions should be recorded to ensure communication and continuity and to fulfill legal responsibilities and accountability for the care plan.

EVALUATION

The final step of the nursing process is determination of the *expected outcomes* of the client's behavior. The criteria stated in the objectives in the planning phase of the process are used as criteria of evaluation. The clearly written objectives direct the nurse to specific evaluation. Evaluation is a feedback loop of the nursing process as the nurse seeks to determine the success of the plan and process. Evaluation includes an appraisal of the extent to which client outcomes were achieved for each problem. The nurse may determine that (1) the problem is resolved when client outcomes are achieved; (2) the problem is being resolved, and the plan should therefore continue; (3) no resolution is evident, and assessing, planning, and implementing should be reviewed and altered if needed; or (4) a new problem is evident or assumes priority.[25]

The nursing care plan is revised according to the outcomes determined by evaluation. Since evaluation provides input to assessment, planning, and implementation, actions of the nurse and client during one or all of these stages may require modification.

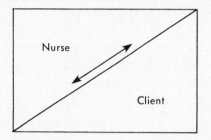

FIG. 7-6
Nursing process is a shared experience of nurse and client, but locus of control varies throughout the relationship.

Participation of the nurse and client in the nursing process depends on the locus of control for decision making about the client's physical or psychological status (Fig. 7-6). In acute emergencies, for example, it may be appropriate for the nurse to make decisions with little or no input from the client. In many instances decision making may be shared as the client is able to exert more control over his health care and can perform certain activities of daily living. In this role the nurse exchanges information with the client and collaborates in formulating goals and objectives. In some instances changes in health behavior can be facilitated by specific contracts between the nurse and client. These contracts specify client outcomes and time periods and serve as guidelines for health-related activities. At other times the client may be able to manage his health care needs independently, and the role of the nurse is supportive. Frequently the involvement of the nurse and client in the nursing process changes over time as the client moves from dependence to independence, and the nursing process is modified to accommodate these changes.

The nursing process is a dynamic relationship of the nurse and client used to identify and solve actual and potential health problems. The process can be used to identify and solve problems of an acute and temporary nature or to plan solutions to problems for which goals are long term and immediate resolution of the problem is not expected. The process can, furthermore, be used in any health care setting and with a variety of nursing care delivery systems.

Nursing models and theories

As with all scientific disciplines, conceptual models and theories can be developed to demonstrate interrelatedness of concepts and explain, predict, or validate actions or events. Nursing as an evolving scientific discipline is developing conceptual models and theories to explain the phenomenon of nursing.

Controversy exists as to differentiation of a conceptual model and theory, and often the terms are used interchangeably. One author attempts to clarify the issue and provides a framework for analyzing and evaluating conceptual models in nursing.[6] A *conceptual model* (conceptual framework) is a set of concepts arranged into a meaningful configuration that depicts connections between the concepts. Conceptual models in nursing are used to describe the interrelatedness of four concepts—man, environment, health, and nursing. Several such nursing models have been developed and are currently being tested in nursing practice.[16,18,19]

A *theory,* on the other hand, is a set of interrelated concepts, definitions, and propositions that presents a systematic view of phenomena by specifying relationships among variables.[15] A nursing theory describes or explains the phenomenon of nursing and evolves (1) from concepts of nursing that view man, environment, health, and nursing as sets of interrelated propositions and (2) from definitions that specify relations among the variables.[6,15,20] Many nurse researchers believe that current models provide foundations for theory building, and as models are tested in clinical practice, nursing theories can be formulated and validated.

Nursing models and theories provide guides for nursing practice, research, and curriculum development. The nurse may wish to use one or more models or parts of models that are suitable for a particular practice setting. A self-care model, an adaptation model, and a life process model, are summarized in this text, although the nurse may choose or develop others.

DOROTHEA OREM: A SELF-CARE MODEL

Self-care, according to Orem, is the "practice of activities that individuals personally initiate and perform on their own behalf to maintain life, health and well being."[16] Self-care, then, is a requirement and attribute of man.

Illness occurs, according to Orem's model, when self-care is not maintained. Health problems can be viewed as a deficit between the ability to provide self-care (or with infants and young children, dependent care) and self-care demand. When demands for self-care exceed abilities, a deficit occurs and the individual is a potential nursing client.

The nurse and client enter a relationship when self-care deficits are identified and clients want and can benefit from nursing care because they have health-related or health-derived limitations that cause them to be unable to provide self-care or dependent care. The nursing systems are described by the locus of control and may be wholly compensatory when the nurse compensates for the client's inability, partially compensatory when the client performs some activities and the nurse assists with others, or supportive-educative when the client performs activities with guidance from the nurse.

SISTER CALLISTA ROY: AN ADAPTATION MODEL

Roy's theory emphasizes the role of the nurse in facilitating man's adaptation to change in his external or internal environment.[19] Roy believes man is a biopsychosocial whole, an open system in interaction with the environment. Man copes with environmental change through adaptation.

Health is viewed on a continuum: death, extremely poor health, poor health, normal health, good health, high-level wellness, and peak wellness. Man continually adapts to maintain positive health.

Man adapts in four modes: (1) physiological needs, (2) self-concept, (3) role function, and (4) interdependence. The goal of nursing is to promote the adaptive modes through nursing activities of assessing adaptive problems, planning, and implementing.

MARTHA ROGERS: A LIFE PROCESS MODEL

Rogers views man as a unitary whole continuously exchanging matter and energy with the environment.[18] Rogers' assumptions about man include (1) man is a unified whole; (2) the individual and environment are continuously exchanging matter and energy; (3) life processes of man evolve irreversibly and unidirectionally along a space-time continuum; (4) pattern and organization reflect man's wholeness and allow self-regulation, rhythmicity, and dynamism; and (5) man is characterized by the capability for abstraction, imagery, language and thought, sensation, and emotion.

These five assumptions are incorporated in Rogers' main theme, homeodynamics. Homeodynamics is composed of three principles: complementarity, resonancy, and helicy. The principle of complementarity describes the relationship of man and environment as a continuous, mutual, and simultaneous interaction process. Resonancy is the identification of the human and the environmental field by wave patterns that continuously change from lower-frequency, longer waves to higher-frequency, shorter waves. The principle of helicy describes the nature and direction of change in human and envionmental fields.

The goal of nursing, according to Rogers' model, is to promote a harmonious interaction of man and environment so that man can reach the highest possible level of health. The nursing process is used to assess the client and intervene to repattern man and the environment for the development of total human potential.

Health care delivery systems

Although some nurses practice independently, most nursing care is provided in the context of a health care agency and complex health care delivery systems. The philosophy, purpose, and organizational structure of the system provide direction for the health care service and may focus on wellness and health maintenance (primary health care), prevention of disease (secondary health care), treatment of health problems, or rehabilitation and supportive care (tertiary health care).

TYPES OF HEALTH CARE DELIVERY SYSTEMS

A health care delivery system may provide a variety of health care services, and the client may receive these services from one or more agencies. The nurse may be a referral agent as the client moves from one department or agency to another as his health care needs change.

Wellness centers and health maintenance organizations

Historically, medical and nursing care has been essentially *episodic,* dealing with a specific illness or crisis and directed toward effecting a cure or an improvement. Since the advent of the concept of health promotion and maintenance (*distributive* care), more energy has been directed toward maintenance of health. Wellness centers are designed to assist clients in maintaining health and offer educational programs such as childbirth education classes, parenting classes, healthy nutrition classes, or heart saver classes. Health maintenance organizations (HMOs) emphasize the regular care of individuals to identify and manage health care problems in incipient stages and provide education for health maintenance.

Community health agencies

Agencies whose primary purpose is prevention of disease provide services for clients at risk for illness. The nurse in these agencies may assist clients in planning to manage risk for disease and protect the client from potential disease. Examples are immunization programs, risk counseling programs, and epidemic management programs.

Hospitals and ambulatory services

Hospitals are traditional centers for providing care to clients with health problems. Although clients may have health problems, few actually require institutional treatment. Certain medical, surgical, and mental illnesses can be managed with medication and other therapies available in a system of extended services. Hospital outpatient departments, physicians' offices, and health clinics are examples of ambulatory services. Such facilities can offer programs for persons of all ages, including family health maintenance, screening for physical and mental illness, mother-child health supervision, family planning, and personal counseling.

In urban areas, particularly in the inner city, health clinics have been established to "take care to the people." These centers may be located in abandoned stores, church basements, schools, or vacant houses and are staffed by a team of professional health workers and lay volunteers from the community. They may manage minor illnesses and injuries and provide family-centered health supervision. Some neighborhood clinics are "satellites" of hospitals and provide supporting diagnostic, therapeutic, and rehabilitative services. Other examples are satellite services that extend the scope of hospital care are mobile intensive care units, dialysis units, surgery centers, and extended care facilities.

Rehabilitative and supportive services

Health care services may be provided in the hospital, community, or client's home, with the primary focus of care directed toward rehabilitation of the client to optimal health or to support the client dying of terminal illness. Home health care agencies, rehabilitation centers, substance abuse rehabilitation programs, and long-term care facilities are examples of health care systems that are designed to assist the client in returning to his optimal level of health.

The United States has recently become interested in the establishment of hospices (shelters or homes) devoted to the specialized management of the dying. The concept of the hospice was popularized in European countries in past decades, particularly to meet the needs of those clients with terminal cancer. The emphasis of hospice care is to achieve comfort rather than to cure. The grouping of individuals with a common problem (facing death) allows them to engage in mutual sharing and support not usually possible among the heterogeneous population in the typical hospital setting. An extension of hospice services may include home care services, hospice teams in the hospital, or palliative care units located in the hospital.[23]

ORGANIZATION AND LOCATION OF HEALTH CARE DELIVERY SYSTEMS

Health care systems may serve client populations at national, regional, and local levels. Recent emphasis has centered on structuring health care services to consolidate resources and expedite client access to the system. Health care services, therefore, may be specialized and located strategically to best serve the population. Systems must also be designed to manage victims of emergencies or disasters. The nurse may be involved in planning the organization of such facilities as well as be an integral component of implementing health care in these settings.

203

Foundations of clinical practice

Health care systems, to ensure comprehensive health care for entire populations, can be organized for health promotion, maintenance, restoration, and rehabilitation. These services may be described as primary, secondary, or tertiary systems. Primary health care services are directed toward health promotion and maintenance. They are usually the point of entry into the health care system. Family practice physicians, neighborhood clinics, ambulatory care services, emergency departments, and health maintenance organizations are examples. Secondary health care services serve clients with specific health problems requiring restorative care. Community hospitals and physician specialists are examples. Tertiary health care facilities are used for complicated health problems. Referral hospitals, specialized health care centers, and rehabilitation centers are considered tertiary health care facilities.

Regionalization

Persons in rural areas and small towns remote from metropolitan centers rely primarily on the family physician and the local hospital for their health care. Available facilities may be grossly inadequate, with many gaps in resources. On the other hand, some urban areas have several sophisticated care centers that duplicate services and overlap in purpose.

In the mid 1960s it was recognized that major illnesses such as heart disease, cancer, and stroke could be dealt with more effectively by grouping certain facility and manpower resources. Legislation was enacted to establish regional medical programs, whose primary purpose was to foster innovation in techniques, health manpower utilization, and other related resources for the improvement of care. Through cooperative arrangements the efforts of individual physicians, allied personnel, hospitals, and other agencies are potentiated above and beyond what they could achieve independently. Regional medical programs consider local resources, needs, and existing patterns of practice and referrals. There is also an integral relationship with other groups interested in similar goals in comprehensive health planning. Regionalization in care delivery is a definitive step toward improved health for all citizens, with greater efficiency, effectiveness, and equity.

Emergency health care services

In the past decade there has been an upsurge of interest in developing an effective system of emergency health services, especially in urban centers. Hospital emergency departments have been supplemented by decentralized mobile emergency health care providers such as emergency medical technicians (EMTs) and emergency paramedics. The concept of the mobile intensive care unit, which takes advanced life-support services to the client in the community, has been realized. Victims of severe illness and trauma are stabilized on the scene before being transferred to a hospital emergency department for more definitive care. Emergency paramedics are skilled in such areas as cardiac monitoring, defibrillation, endotracheal intubation, fluid and drug therapy, and other techniques that are considered essential in the assessment and management of life-threatening crises. Communication and biomedical monitoring are transmitted to a supervising base station hospital, which serves as a source of validation and medical orders. Such a system has extended the realm of field emergency care beyond first aid to a highly sophisticated mode of definitive management.

Disaster services

''A disaster is an occurrence such as hurricane, tornado, storm, flood, high water, wind-driven water, tidal wave, earthquake, draught, blizzard, pestilence, famine, fire, explosion, building collapse, transportation wreck of any other situation that causes human suffering or that creates human needs that the victim cannot alleviate without assistance.''[4] Nurses are key persons in such a crisis because they are equipped with skills and understandings essential for meeting basic human needs and for responding to specialized problems imposed by illness and injury. It is important for nurses to understand the elements of a disaster and how they affect clients and the community.

Types of disasters. Disasters are natural or man made. A natural disaster is a violence of Nature's elements and is related to weather and other geophysical conditions. Man-made disasters include thermonuclear war, fires, plane crashes, and civil disorders. Although each of these disasters is unique in its causation, they have in common their *suddenness in onset* and a series of stages before and after the impact itself.

Stages of disaster. A few disasters occur without even a moment's warning, but usually there is at least a brief period in which can be seen actual evidence of impending crisis.

When situations occur that have the potential of creating a crisis but do not show actual conditions of peril, the period is termed the *threat stage.* Heavy, prolonged rains may be expected to cause the hazard of flooding, or a storm at sea must be watched closely because it may move inland to result in hurricane conditions. However, if the fact is known that a major dam has broken, unleashing an already swollen river, or that the hurricane is a mere hundred miles away and moving toward the coast, the period is termed the *warning stage.* It is more specific than the first stage of threat and almost assures the reality of disaster. The time from these stages to the *impact stage,* when the disaster is manifest full blown, may vary from a few moments to hours or days, depending on the nature of the crisis. The final stage of disaster is *recovery,* when the assessment of the disaster effects is made, the injured are rescued, and rehabilitation of people and their lives is begun. This last stage can also last from a few days to a few years, depending on the scope and effects of the disaster.

Each community struck by a disaster will have similar problems that will affect the ability to get aid to individuals. Homes and other buildings, including perhaps hospitals, will be destroyed. Many persons will be seriously injured or killed. Families may be separated, and persons may be missing or may be trapped and awaiting rescue. Water, electrical power, and telephones may be disrupted. Traffic congestion is probable where streets are blocked with debris. Regardless of the preparation for disaster, there are few opportunities to safeguard against all these perils.

Planning for disaster. Most large communities and some smaller ones have plans for coping with disaster, using resources of the American National Red Cross, Civil Defense, police and fire departments, and local health care facilities. Volunteers supplement the work of these agencies, and nurses are frequently key members of the disaster team.

Community disaster planning is a complex process of assessing the probability of certain types of calamities. A coastal town must be ready for hurricanes. A city with many oil refineries must anticipate fires and explosions. Areas that have been subject to frequent earthquakes, blizzards, or tornadoes must stand prepared to face such crises again.

Disaster planning involves taking an inventory of human and material resources that can be mobilized. Specific steps are outlined to be followed in

Foundations of clinical practice

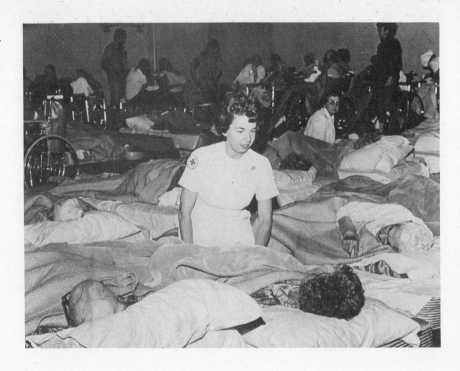

certain eventualities. Everyone on the team, whether he be a regular staff member of an agency or a community volunteer, has a clear-cut guideline to follow and a specific role to assume in given circumstances. Although nurses usually care for the ill or injured, they may assume other roles such as setting up an emergency aid station or portable hospital, planning for immediate needs of families (casework), managing a shelter, or assisting in radiological decontamination of the environment and supplies (Fig. 7-7).

Nature of disaster casualties. The kinds of problems that disaster victims face will be many and varied and will largely depend on the type of catastrophe. For example, fires and explosions are likely to yield large numbers of casualties with thermal or chemical burns and asphyxiation. Hurricanes, tornadoes, and mass transportation crashes, however, would probably create contusions, lacerations, fractures, penetrating wounds, and shock. Floods pose the potential threat of widespread communicable disease resulting from contamination of local water supplies. Furthermore, the victims of any disaster are likely to include expectant mothers, children, adults with chronic illness, and the elderly. It is apparent that the nurse must be prepared to deal with multiple and complex problems.

Role of the nurse in disaster. "Disaster nursing is the adaptation of professional nursing skills in recognizing and meeting the medical, nursing, and emotional needs evolving from a disaster situation."[10]

All nurses should receive specific preparations for coping with disasters so that they can manage their own families during such a crisis and function as useful members of the community team. The Red Cross chapters in many local communities offer courses in general disaster preparedness and specific functions such as shelter management, psychological reactions to disaster, and management principles of disaster nursing, including emergency care of the victims and

206

family casework. Other agencies may also offer educational preparation of a similar nature.

Sorting casualties. One role of a nurse may be to manage many victims with innumerable injuries and to establish priorities of care after the impact period. The guiding principle must be to organize services to benefit the greatest number of people.

In peacetime disasters all persons are likely to receive prompt attention because of the highly sophisticated communication, transportation, and health care delivery system. In a short period of time it is possible to transport casualties out of the affected area to distant cities for treatment. However, in the case of a national crisis such as a thermonuclear war, only those clients having a good possibility for survival would be given vigorous care, since conservation of time, supplies, and personnel is the prime consideration.

When the nurse encounters large numbers of disaster victims, they must be sorted and assigned priorities for care. One sorting procedure assigns victims to the following four major groups:

1. Minimal treatment. Require first aid or minor surgery only. In a national disaster many such clients would probably receive care first so that they could perform useful functioning in aiding others.
2. Antishock treatment. Injuries are severe enough to cause shock, and victims can be transported easily after antishock therapy. Burns, fractures, and severe lacerations are examples.
3. Major treatment. Require rapid emergency surgical intervention or else can be maintained by supportive therapy for later care, up to 12 hours or more. Cases in which waiting would be potentially more dangerous than transporting should be evacuated to other centers by the most rapid method possible, probably by plane. Chest and abdominal injuries, certain neurological problems, and compound fractures may be included in this category.
4. Highly specialized treatment. Require sophisticated management available only in research centers and can withstand transportation. The majority of such injuries would monopolize much time, supplies, and manpower while others with a better chance of survival might be awaiting treatment. Burns of large area (30% to 40% of the body), severe head injuries, and multiple injuries fall into this category. In a disaster such as a thermonuclear war, this group of casualties would probably receive little or no care, since they could not survive without supportive care over a long period of time.

Since persons with acute injuries often have rapid improvements or declines, the principles of triage take this factor into account, and provisions for reassessment and regrouping are an integral part of the sorting process.

Intervention. Nursing intervention in disaster involves a number of steps in the preimpact as well as the postimpact period. Although it is impossible to discuss all of the types of problems that might be encountered by the nurse, several important principles are recognized that are worthy of note.

Some disasters can be prevented by careful planning for emergencies. A flood may occur, with only waterfront homes destroyed. However, if steps are not taken to prevent the spread of communicable disease within the shelters, a

Foundations of clinical practice

secondary disaster epidemic of typhoid could occur that might be far more life threatening than the original emergency. Casualties should be minimized by good planning in the preimpact period and by steps taken to prevent additional casualties after impact. Although skilled rescue teams are usually at hand, the nurse may be involved in freeing trapped victims or finding missing persons. Usually, however, the primary roles are giving definitive first aid and emergency care and evacuating selected casualties to other care resources. Knowledge necessary for such a broad role can be gained best by specialized preparation in the community the nurse serves, since guidelines and details vary considerably from one locale to another. One of the most important responsibilities of a nurse in disaster, however, relates to helping affected families reconstruct their lives after a major crisis experience.

Managing psychological responses in disaster. In every stage of a disaster there are highly individualized responses, but a nurse can be prepared to cope with these by understanding the application of some basic psychological principles.

The preimpact period can be useful for some persons because they are able to mobilize their resources and take definitive, appropriate action. Others, however, when threatened by an impending crisis, become totally helpless and ineffective. It is usually advisable to direct the latter group with firmness. Assign definite tasks and offer reassurance that the impending crisis can be lessened by specific preparatory activities at hand.

At the actual point of impact, despite considerable drilling and preparation, there will be undoubtedly confusion, anxiety reactions, and a prevailing feeling of helplessness and hopelessness. However, with sound support from well-organized activities, this period is brief, and persons return quickly to a functional pattern of behavior. During this time of confusion responsible action can save lives, minimize suffering, and prevent secondary crisis.

Delayed postimpact responses are possible, occurring when the real danger is past. Panic, although rare, can occur. Any individual who seems panic stricken should be isolated from others, since this response is highly contagious in a confined group. Rumors can best be controlled by providing information if it is available. If real truths are known, they are usually less awesome than contrived fears, and intragroup trust becomes more firmly established. Explain to victims how they will be cared for and the plans for assuring their safety. This fosters a feeling of security and lessens the need for useless worrying. Other postimpact responses include overactive responses and conversion hysteria. These latter two problems can best be managed by firm direction and specific work assignments appropriate to a person's state of functioning.

The basic principles of dealing with the behavior of persons in disaster are not unlike those useful for any client facing a crisis.

Avoid judgmental attitudes about behavior and accept everyone's right to his own feelings. Since everyone's response to a crisis varies because of his or her previous life experiences, a wide range of behavior can be expected. All behavior is purposeful, and at any given moment it is the best response that a given client is capable of. Avoid pity and oversolicitousness, since they tend to increase feelings of helplessness. Never offer such statements as "you shouldn't feel that way." Remember that one has no choice but to feel exactly as he does at that time.

All persons in a disaster are likely to have some actual or felt limitations that must be accepted. Visible limitations such as burns and fractures are easy to accept, but clients who are emotionally injured are harder to cope with. Often these impairments are more obscure than physical ones and can be easily overlooked. It is seemingly more difficult to be supportive to persons with psychological injuries than to those who are shattered with visible wounds. The nurse is likely to need some support also after disaster impact and must depend on colleagues for this.

Occasionally behavior problems require definitive treatment such as assigning others to restrain a troublesome, overactive victim. Group sessions or individual conference may be tried to overcome some of the problems. The elderly and small children tend to pose the most difficult behavioral disturbances and need to be placed in quiet surroundings with as much supervision as possible. Sedatives to calm victims should be a last resort because they impair both physical and emotional functioning to some degree. It is important that all disaster victims be as alert as possible in the stage after impact so that they are not liabilities to their fellow survivors.

HEALTH CARE SYSTEMS AND THE LOCAL, STATE, AND FEDERAL GOVERNMENTS

Individual and family resources may be supplemented by assistance from social welfare agencies, health insurance, or several other means available to them through local, state, or federal governmental groups.

There are numerous programs for children, the handicapped, widows, orphans, veterans, and welfare recipients. The elderly also are the targets of many health care legislative endeavors. Recently, however, governmental concerns have gone beyond these specialized groups, and attention is being sharply focused on the health needs of *all* citizens.

Emphasis of state and federal programs has evolved from treating special health problems to a broader approach aimed at a healthy society through education and maintenance services. Health is now considered as the right of all people, not a privilege reserved for some.

State and federal responsibilities presently include the following:

1. Financial grants for direct service to people
2. Research related to prevention, control, incidence, morbidity, and mortality of health problems as they affect various age groups (both physical and mental)
3. Health education
4. Controlling organizational structure of health care services
5. Study of international health as it potentially relates to the United States
6. Regulation of movement of goods and persons to control certain diseases
7. Provision of personnel for consultation
8. Development of standards related to health care delivery

Agencies include Public Health Service, Food and Drug Administration, and Children's Bureau of the Department of Health and Human Services, Bureau of Indian Affairs and Bureau of Mines of the Department of the Interior, and the Veterans Administration.

The National Health Planning and Resources Development Act (PL 93-641) directs the federal, state, and local governments to coordinate and plan health care services, manpower, and facilities. At the federal level, advisory groups recommend national health policy to the secretary of the Department of Health and Human Services. State groups are responsible for developing statewide plans, but the immediate responsibility for planning rests with local health systems agencies that serve geographical districts within the state. Health systems agencies are responsible for developing health systems plans, with emphasis on primary care and health education.

Quality assurance in nursing

Responsibility and accountability for the quality of nursing care are vested in the nurses involved in nursing care. Quality assurance in nursing involves determining standards of care, peer review (evaluation of care by other nurses), and correction of deficiencies.

While the evaluation component of the nursing process is used to provide feedback about outcomes of care for an individual client, quality assurance programs can be designed to monitor nursing care given to groups of clients. A quality assurance program is an evaluative system comprising a variety of tools used to measure the quality of nursing care.[8] The tools for such programs may be used already by the nurse and can include client history forms, nursing rounds, problem-oriented charting and nursing care plans, and systematic client feedback adapted to focus on the quality of care provided.

A quality assurance program can be instituted in the nursing department in any health care delivery system. The program is not dependent on the size of the agency, client population, number of nurses, or staffing patterns used. Quality assurance programs can be instituted by the nurses involved in nursing care or may be headed by a person or department designated to assume responsibility for the program in a given agency.

A MODEL FOR QUALITY ASSURANCE

A model for quality assurance programs in nursing has been used as a framework for establishing standards, evaluating care, and changing behavior of the organization and nurses to provide quality nursing care (Fig. 7-8). The model, suggested by Norma Lang, includes the following five steps for problem-solving[3]: (1) formation of values for client care, (2) establishment of standards and criteria for nursing care, (3) assessment of the discrepancy between the standards of care and the current level of nursing practice, (4) selection and implementation of alternatives for changing nursing practice, and (5) actual improvement in practice. The process is cyclical, and as change occurs, new values may be established, and the process begins again.

NURSING AUDIT

Quality nursing care for groups of clients can be judged by nursing audit or appraisal of care according to preestablished standards and criteria. The audit may be *internal,* performed by nurses involved in the care, or *external,* performed by a committee of peers not involved in the nursing care being reviewed. Audits may be done *concurrently,* while care is being given; *retrospectively,* after care is given; or *prospectively,* before admission of the client to the nursing service. Audits may be used to measure the outcome, process, or structure of nursing, and a quality assurance program may involve use of one or all of these

FIG. 7-8
Quality assurance model. (From Davidson, Sharon, editor: P.S.R.O.: utilization and audit in patient care, St. Louis, 1976, The C.V. Mosby Co. Courtesy Norma Lang, Ph.D.)

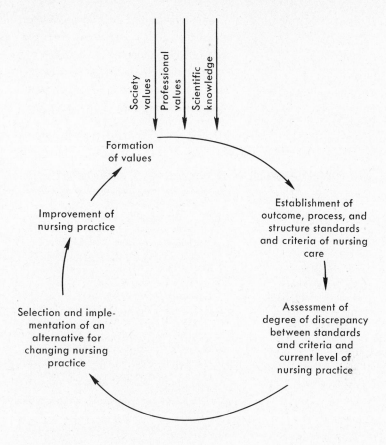

types of audit. *Outcome* audits focus on the client and measure end results of care. *Process* audits deal with the nature and sequence of events in delivery of care. The visible behavior of the nurse as well as the intangible process of decision making can be evaluated. *Structure* audits examine the physical and organizational characteristics of the health care system; physical plant, administrative process, staff qualifications, communication channels, and financial resources, for example, can be reviewed using a structure audit.

The standards and criteria established for audit form a basis for care plans. The standards can be written for clients with specific medical or nursing diagnoses or for clients in specialized settings, and they assist the nurse in planning, implementing, and evaluating care.[12,22]

Summary

Nursing is a dynamic interaction of the nurse and client to help the client maintain wellness or achieve his optimal level of health. The nursing process provides a deliberate problem-solving mechanism for the nurse and client to assess and identify problems, plan solutions, implement care, and evaluate changes in the client's health status that occur during the nurse-client relationship. Conceptual models and theories provide a framework in which the relationship between man, environment, health, and nursing can be understood, validated, or predicted. The nurse may use one or more models for nursing practice. Nursing practice

Foundations of clinical practice

occurs in a health care delivery system, and the nurse must recognize the impact of philosophy, purpose, and organizational structure of the health care agency to facilitate nursing care within the system. Nursing care is planned and deliberate, and the nurse has responsibility and accountability for the quality of nursing care. Quality assurance programs can be instituted to evaluate care and ensure optimal nursing care within the context of the dynamic nurse-client interaction.

References

1. Bates, Barbara: A guide to physical examination, Philadelphia, 1974, J.B. Lippincott Co.
2. Becknell, Helen, and Smith, Dorothy: System of nursing practice: a clinical nursing tool, Philadelphia, 1975, F.A. Davis Co.
3. Davidson, Sharon, editor: P.S.R.O.: utilization and audit in patient care, St. Louis, 1976, The C.V. Mosby Co.
4. Definition of disaster, Washington, D.C., 1975, American National Red Cross.
5. Dossey, Barbara: Perfecting your skills for systematic patient assessments, Nursing '79 **9**(2):42-45, 1979.
6. Fawcett, Jacqueline: A framework for analysis and evaluation of conceptual models of nursing, Nurs. Educ. **5**(6):10-14, 1980.
7. Fowkes, William C., and Hunn, Virginia K.: Clinical assessment for the nurse practitioner, St. Louis, 1973, The C.V. Mosby Co.
8. Froebe, Doris, and Bain, R. Joyce: Quality assurance programs and controls in nursing, St. Louis, 1976, The C.V. Mosby Co.
9. Gebbie, K.M., and Lavin, M.A., editors: Classification of nursing diagnosis: Proceedings of the first National Conference held in St. Louis, October 1-5, 1973, St. Louis, 1975, The C.V. Mosby Co.
10. Guidelines and procedures, disaster nursing services, Washington, D.C., 1974, American National Red Cross.
11. Hughes, James G.: Synopsis of pediatrics, ed. 5, St. Louis, 1980, The C.V. Mosby Co.
12. Johanson, Brenda, and others: Standards for critical care, St. Louis, 1981, The C.V. Mosby Co.
13. Malasanos, Lois, and others: Health assessment, ed. 2, St. Louis, 1981, The C.V. Mosby Co.
14. Marriner, Ann: The nursing process: a scientific approach to nursing, ed. 2, St. Louis, 1979, The C.V. Mosby Co.
15. The Nursing Theories Conference Group, Julia B. George, Chairperson: Nursing theories—the base for professional practice, Englewood Cliffs, N.J., 1980, Prentice-Hall, Inc.
16. Orem, Dorothea, editor: Concept formalization in nursing: process and product, ed. 2, Boston, 1979, Little, Brown & Co.
17. Price, Mary: Nursing diagnosis: making a concept come alive, Am. J. Nurs. **80**:668-671, 1980.
18. Rogers, Martha: Introduction to the theoretical basis of nursing, Philadelphia, 1970, F.A. Davis Co.
19. Roy, Sister Callista: Introduction to nursing: an adaptation model, Englewood Cliffs, N.J., 1976, Prentice-Hall, Inc.
20. Stevens, Barbara: Nursing theory, analysis, application, evaluation, Boston, 1979, Little, Brown & Co.
21. Thompson, June, and Bowers, Arden C.: Clinical manual of health assessment, St. Louis, 1980, The C.V. Mosby Co.
22. Tucker, Susan, and others: Patient care standards, ed. 2, St. Louis, 1980, The C.V. Mosby Co.
23. Wald, Florence, and others: The hospice movement as health care reform, Nurs. Outlook **28:**173-178, 1980.
24. Walker, Lorraine, and Nicholson, Ruth: Criteria for evaluating nursing process models, Nurs. Educ. **5**(5):8-9, 1980.
25. Yura, Helen, and Walsh, Mary: The nursing process: assessing, planning, implementing, evaluating, ed. 3, New York, 1978, Appleton-Century-Crofts.

Additional readings

Byrne, Marjorie, and Thompson, Lida: Key concepts for the study and practice of nursing, ed. 2, St. Louis, 1978, The C.V. Mosby Co.

Campbell, Claire: Nursing diagnosis and intervention in nursing practice, New York, 1978, John Wiley & Sons, Inc.

Ceske, Karen: Accountability—the essence of primary nursing, Am. J. Nurs. **79:**891-894, 1979.

Davidson, Sharon, and others: Nursing care evaluation: concurrent and retrospective review criteria, St. Louis, 1977, The C.V. Mosby Co.

Dobibal, Shirley: Hospice: enabling a patient to die at home, Am. J. Nurs. **80:**1448-1451, 1980.

Douglass, Laura, and Bevis, Em Olivia: Nursing management and leadership in action, ed. 3, St. Louis, 1979, The C.V. Mosby Co.

Gordon, M.: The concept of nursing diagnosis, Nurs. Clin. North Am. **14:**487-495, September 1979.

Hargreaves, Anne: Coping with disaster, Am. J. Nurs. **80:**683, 1980.

Little, Dolores, and Carnovalli, Doris: Nursing care planning, Philadelphia, 1969, J.B. Lippincott Co.

McFarlane, Judith: Pediatric assessment and intervention, Nurs. '74 **4**(12):66-68, 1974.

Newman, Margaret: Theory development in nursing, Philadelphia, 1979, F.A. Davis Co.

Redman, Barbara: The process of patient teaching in nursing, ed. 4, St. Louis, 1980, The C.V. Mosby Co.

Wolley, F. Ross, and others: Problem-oriented nursing, New York, 1974, Springer Publishing Co., Inc.

8 Nursing and the hospitalized client

Hospitalization

The client with actual or potential health problems that cannot be managed at other health care facilities may be admitted to the hospital for diagnosis and/or treatment of his problem. It is estimated that more than 37 million individuals are admitted to the hospital each year for an average stay of 7.6 days.[10]

Hospitalization is a disruption of the life-style of the client and his family. The client's reaction and coping strengths often depend on his age, his developmental stage, family support, and the reason for hospitalization. The nurse must identify these variables and plan with the client to facilitate adaptation to this stress and provide care that assists the client in attaining his own optimal level of health. The purpose of this chapter is to explore the impact of hospitalization on the client at critical stages of the life span and describe nursing actions that can be used to provide safety in the hospital environment, promote sleep and rest, prevent or manage sensory deprivation, relieve pain, recognize changes in body image, facilitate administration of medications and intravenous fluids, and prepare the client for diagnostic tests or surgery.

THE HOSPITALIZED INFANT AND CHILD

The effect of hospitalization on the child and his family will be primarily determined by the growth and development of the family and the individual client. *The age of a hospitalized child is the single most important factor that influences nursing care.* Recognition of this fact has led most institutions to plan their nursing units in relation to age groups as opposed to medical or nursing diagnosis. The total management during the hospitalization must be designed with consideration of the child's unique needs based on his chronological age, developmental stage, and previous life experiences. An infant who has just learned that mother is the most important person in his life will be affected by separation from her. A preschool child who has developed a sense of security with his home and family may regress to an earlier stage of development when placed with strangers and an unfamiliar physical environment. An active school-age child

214

Planning for hospitalization

will find confinement difficult at the time in his life when activity and peers command his primary attention.

Unless an illness or accident results in precipitous hospitalization, a preparatory period is valuable in helping both parents and their children to face this rather traumatic experience. The illness, impending surgery, separation, and even financial concerns contribute to the prehospitalization anxiety. Children are often sensitive to the parents' concerns, and this compounds their own fears. Frank discussions with one's spouse, the physician, a nurse, or another parent who has undergone the experience may help relieve many fears and doubts. In some communities, PTA groups, Scouts, school classes, and individual families are periodically invited to an open house and tours of the pediatric hospital so that they can become acquainted with the environment at a time when they are free from personal involvement with an impending hospitalization.

A child over 2 or 3 years of age should be told a day or so in advance that he will be going to the hospital. Depending on his age and his ability to comprehend the idea, explain the reason for the admission and what may be expected to occur. Promises that may not be able to be kept should not be made, such as "I will stay with you all the time," "It will not hurt," or "You will feel better when your operation is over." Honesty and a matter-of-fact approach are most advisable. Lengthy descriptions of unpleasant aspects should be avoided. It is wise to explain the necessity of certain procedures as they relate to making him well. Describing the type of room that he will sleep in, the appearance of the nurses and physicians in uniforms and surgical attire, the way meals will be served, or the daily routine and schedule may make the experience sound like an adventure as opposed to a horrible ordeal. The child should be told that he must go to the hospital to get well because it has special people and machines that the home does not have. The child must be reassured by feeling that the parents know about and approve what will be happening to him in the hospital and that he will be coming home again when he is well enough to leave the special people and machines behind.

Although explanation of the hospital environment and regimen may be of limited value for the very young child, it should not be omitted. Some children believe that being sent away from home to this strange place may be a form of punishment. Such notions may be, at least in part, alleviated by preparatory explanations. There are a few good picture-story books directed toward helping youngsters understand the hospital experience. These are especially valuable for some children because they can refer to the book as often as needed to reinforce the idea that the hospital is a special place and that he will meet many interesting new friends there. Not uncommonly, the preschooler will have fantasies about hospitalization because of early preconceptions about needles, blood, cutting open the body, pain, and death. For some children, the tours, books, films, explanations, and other information or reassurance may not make them feel less frightened about their impending hospitalization.

The older child, who usually has greater coping abilities, may profit from a more prolonged period of preparation in which feelings can be worked through. School-age children as well as some preschoolers may be helped by playing nurse or doctor, using play kits and dolls in which anxiety-provoking incidents can be somewhat controlled at will by the child himself. The idea of play therapy can be greatly expanded once familiarity with the hospital is attained.

215

Foundations of clinical practice

Admission to the hospital

The nurse who helps admit the infant or child to the hospital should be aware that the entire family is involved and that parents and siblings should not be managed as intruders into the nurse's private domain. Although there are the inevitable hospital rules and regulations, they should not be used as control mechanisms to keep parents uninvolved. It is important to remember that the anxiety of separation encompasses the child and his family and that separation from familiar people, things, and activities is threatening for a client of any age.

Although some hospitals admit the child and his parents to a nurse, rather than a room or a unit, there are still 16 hours a day when this nurse will not be available to the client and his family.

Careful planning on the first few days of hospitalization should ensure that both parents and children are introduced to personnel who will provide care for the 24-hour day (Fig. 8-1). Orientation can also be provided concerning the physical aspects of the unit.

The family should be oriented to the unit environment. Parents' lounges, toilet facilities, dining areas, and the playroom areas should be pointed out. The rules of the hospital should be explained in terms of their rationale, not merely dictated as "policy." For example, if gowning and masking are required, the procedure should be demonstrated in terms of principles, and parents should be given an opportunity to practice the technique under supervision of the nurse. To see nurses and parents working together in this manner is encouraging to the child and provides a good opportunity for health teaching. If emergency or special equipment is at the bedside, it should be explained, and parents should be instructed about its use and how to call for the nurse if the need for help arises.

A favorite toy can be brought to the hospital so the youngster will have something familiar with him. Parents can be encouraged to leave one of their belongings, such as a comb, mirror, or notebook and pencil, so that the child is reassured that they will return—if only because they have left something behind that they need. Most hospitals welcome a child by presenting him with a small toy from the playroom or "treasure chest," which becomes special because the giving of gifts is universally understood by all ages as an expression of friendship, love, and commitment.

On admission, the nurse should ascertain how much the parents and the child understand about the health problem or the nature of hospitalization. A nursing history should include factors about eating habits, elimination, sleeping habits, play, and school, as well as family life experiences. This initial data gathering is extremely important, especially if the parents are not permitted to remain with the child.

Parents must understand that separation should always involve honesty. Leaving the child should not be accomplished by "slipping out" during a nap or going out of the room for an errand and simply not returning. These may cause the child to lie awake, anxiously awaiting their return, and may even result in his doubting everything that has been told him about hospitalization. Nurses know that separation anxiety is felt by parents as keenly as children and that circumventing honesty in severing contacts only compounds the negative feelings for both. Crying when parents leave is a natural form of expressing grief and the pain of loss. The lack of crying and the appearance of submission and resignation can be an unhealthy response and should alert the nurse to observe subsequent parent-child relationships.

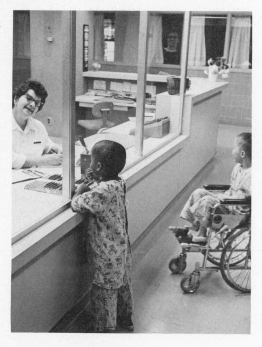

FIG. 8-1
Young client meets unit secretary as he is admitted to the nursing unit.

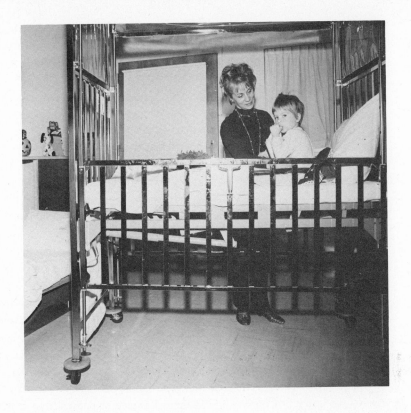

When the separation is accomplished, there will be undoubtedly crying or remorse, and the nurse must be prepared to offer comfort to the youngster to reassure him that he is among friends. Diversion to the playroom or bedside recreation may be of value.

Visiting and rooming-in
Since most hospitals have recognized the hazards of trauma related to separation of parents and children, they have liberalized visiting policies and even established rooming-in plans for parents to stay overnight with the child and participate actively in his care (Fig. 8-2).

Toddlers and preschool children especially benefit from the presence of mother or father. Negativism, regression, and evasion are lessened by the presence of parents, and long-term negative effects of hospitalization can be significantly minimized.

The parents' presence is not all that is necessary, but care must be exercised to foster the parent-child role and relationships. If there are several siblings, a decision must be made about balancing time between the home responsibilities and the hospitalized child. The nurse should encourage parents to participate in the care of the child to the extent permitted by his needs, such as feeding and bathing.

Parents are knowingly hesitant to relinquish the primary care of the child and entrust him to strangers, and they are frustrated by hospitalization because they often have no control over the situation. This may explain why some parents seem to be hypercritical of the personnel and the care that they are providing for their child. It is not an uncommon situation for parents to withdraw from the child hospitalized on a long-term basis, since they are overshadowed by other adults who are nurturing the child to health through skillful care that they themselves are inadequately prepared to provide. They feel left out when the hospital becomes home for the child. Competition for the child may seem to exist as the nurse becomes a substitute authority or mother-surrogate in the hospital. Children may upset their parents by showing preference for a member of the hospital staff and may at times almost deny the presence of their parents. Perhaps the child is expressing some hostility because the parents brought him to the hospital and forced a separation from his home and loved ones. Nurses must realize that they should supplement the parental role and not supplant it and that making a conscientious effort to keep the parent-child relationship in its proper and rightful perspective will be mutually beneficial.

Nurses can offer tips to parents about their visiting, such as talking about their experiences together. The child can relate what has happened at the hospital, and the parents can tell the child about his home, his brothers and sisters, and pets. It is appropriate to allow the child to express feelings of anger, fear, or protest, but parents should be cautioned not to convey to the child that the physicians or nurses are treating him badly. The nurse ought to observe parent-child relationships during visits and be present for answering questions or giving feedback. Through this kind of helpfulness and concern, families develop a better feeling about hospitals, health workers, and the helping relationship.

The diversions of television and telephones for older children keep them in touch with familiar people and circumstances and serve to lessen feelings of loneliness and helplessness.

Psychological impact of the hospital experience

The most adverse responses from separation occur in the child 18 months to 4 years of age. After this time they seem to cope better with stress. The young school-age child is primarily occupied with generalized anxiety about his illness, hospitalization, or pain.

For nurses and physicians diagnostic procedures, pain, fear, and deprivation have become routine. However, to a child these factors may produce considerable anxiety. Such things as delaying breakfast for blood tests, going to and from a dark x-ray room with strange and monstrous machines, or getting an enema are hardly routine to any child. Everything that is done to make a hospital experience less traumatic to a child cannot compensate for the mysterious and frightening separation from his home and family, not to mention his inability to even predict what will happen next.

Children tend to become sick people, not simply people with sick parts. The whole body is ill rather than a single limb or organ. Pain and unexpected responses create a sense of uncertainty and fear, which may eventually make the child feel less secure if not less worthy. Some children feel that their identity has been sacrified to their illness and that they have become a ''heart patient'' or an ''asthmatic,'' as opposed to a child with a heart condition or a child with asthma.

The basic needs of the child must be carried on in the hospital despite the alterations imposed by hospitalization. Children need activity, and when they are confined and forced to be quiet, they feel repressed. Times for noisy fun should be provided as well as times for rest. When injuries make it impossible for the child to leave his bed, other forms of expression should be sought, such as singing, shouting, and writing. Continuing to repress self-expression may thwart emotional development, result in a lack of spontaneity of expression, and limit the child's resourcefulness as well as intellectual development.

Older school-age children should be permitted to organize peer groups, a natural outlet for this age group. Adult supervision will be necessary, however, to keep their activities in check.

School-age children may be well enough to continue their education on an uninterrupted basis. This may be done through closed-circuit telephone and television, bedside tutors, or hospital classrooms.

THE HOSPITALIZED ADOLESCENT

The adolescent is a unique individual, neither a child nor an adult, and the design of hospital facilities frequently ignores his special needs. Many hospitals have only pediatric units for children and medical-surgical units for adults, and the adolescent must be admitted to one. Selection of roommates close to the adolescent's age can often be used to overcome age barriers if the adolescent cannot be assigned to an adolescent unit.

The nursing care plan can be developed from a foundation of understanding developmental tasks of adolescence, including increasing independence, adjusting to sexuality and body image, and selecting a career. Hospitalization at this time disrupts such tasks, and the nurse should be sensitive to the adolescent's needs at this time.

THE HOSPITALIZED ADULT

When adults enter the hospital, they have many of the same anxieties that the child possesses, but they express them in different ways. Separation from the family for adults means they will temporarily be unable to meet their role expectations of earning a living or providing care for small children, a spouse, or even elderly parents, which are essential to identity and self-esteem. Furthermore, illness or injury denotes a failure of the body and a loss of positive body image. Although hospitalization and income protection insurance may help reduce some financial concerns of a hospital stay, these other factors must be considered.

If a parent has anticipated being away from home and has planned for child care, the maintenance of household tasks, and income to meet family needs while he is out of the home, he still faces a certain threat to his integrity. It seems that hospitalization tends to mean giving up his adult privileges of independence and self-determination. Action-oriented, productive living is curtailed with the physical and social limitations imposed by hospitalization. Suddenly he is thrust backward into a childlike state where others plan for his care and decide when and what he eats, at what time he can see his friends, his bedtime hour, and even whether or not he can manage his own elimination needs. This return to a dependency stage is truly difficult for most adults and may account for the negative behavior expressed during their stay. Professional staff should recognize that maladaptive behaviors of clients (such as refusing treatments) may merely be expressions of independence when clients perceive only dependence. In addition, spouses or others who feel helpless in their supporting roles may seem to be demanding of nurses. However, if the nurse considers the needs of the client and is aware of his feelings, much can be done to reduce these responses. In these instances it is valuable for the staff members to validate their observations of behaviors, share interpretations, and formulate a consistent plan to deal with them on a unique basis. It is easy for personnel to stereotype patterns of behavior unless they are keenly aware of all the factors that influence individualized coping and adaptation patterns.

The nurse should be aware of how the institution and its staff can provide a support system for the client. It is important to allow privacy and personal time

Foundations of clinical practice

for independent, autonomous behaviors. Nursing activities should be planned to permit the client to fully use visiting hours for interacting with significant others. Since communication is probably the most effective way to deal with stress, it is important to keep all channels open and to encourage verbalization of anxieties, concerns, and feelings.

Adults should be permitted to determine their care routine to the extent their illness and disability allow. Unfortunately, in most hospitals a definite routine has been determined by departmental schedules or staffing, and little flexibility is possible. However, the nurse who is client oriented will constantly be reminded that each adult has his own life-style—when he awakes or retires, what he prefers to eat, or when he showers and shaves—and must take into account the nature of his socialization and activity pattern. These factors should be elicited in the nursing assessment on admission and incorporated into the plan of care.

The ideal admission routine includes a thorough orientation to the physical environment of the hospital and an introduction to staff members who will assist in the care. Since the admission procedure will do much in forming the client's impression of the hospital and the attitudes of personnel caring for him, it should not be carried out solely by the admitting department. Although there is usually a prescribed routine for getting the client to his room, obtaining admission laboratory tests, recording vital signs, and safeguarding possessions such as clothing, jewelry, or dentures, these should not be the extent of staff responsibilities. Details about the unit, special hospital services, and the plan of care should be offered, perhaps during the initial nursing assessment. A booklet left at the bedside explaining the hospital's services is no substitute for personal orientation. At best such a booklet is reinforcement for the nursing introduction to the hospital experience.

Family members should be included if possible in this initial orientation, since they often have the same questions as the client himself: "How do I call for the nurse, talk with the doctor, or change the position of the bed?" or "Where is the coffee shop, the lounge, the chapel?" Attentive relatives can be an asset in the client's care if they understand the nature of the hospitalization routine.

If a client shares a room with one or more persons, the nurse should introduce them and offer a simple explanation about their reason for hospitalization or the status of their management; for example, "Mrs. Dunn has been here since last Sunday. She had surgery and will be going home in a few days." This indicates to the incoming client that the nurse is aware of the person's management status and sets some parameters for initial conversation. If either is hard of hearing or has poor vision or motor deprivation, the nurse may also find it appropriate to explain this: "Mr. Jackson was in an automobile accident and was severely injured. He cannot talk but will be able to hear your conversation with others."

THE HOSPITALIZED OLDER ADULT

When an elderly person is removed from familiar surroundings and admitted to a hospital or other care facility, he is likely to become upset or even confused. Excessive worry about what is going to happen is common.

Diminished sensory input may contribute to confusion. There may be impairments in vision, hearing, and memory for recent events, which result in the client's inability to connect the series of circumstances that have led him to his current surroundings. Physicians and nurses as well as family members should continually reinforce the client's realization of where he is, to whom he is talking, and what is happening to him.

Blind, deaf, or paralyzed persons may rely heavily on the sense of touch to know that someone is present to help. Touching expresses warmth and reinforces a sense of security and trust essential in the nurse-client relationship.

Not all older people have circulatory disorders, arthritis, or poor mental functioning. However, these are some physical changes characteristic of many elderly clients. The adaptive processes of the central nervous system decrease, allowing some reduction in the mechanisms for maintaining homeodynamic balances. Hypothermia is common, and additional warmth must be provided to compensate for the inefficiency of regulatory mechanisms and the reduced blood supply in muscular areas normally well supplied. Kidneys are also less efficient, and genitourinary problems are to be anticipated. Joint and skin changes occur because of alterations in mineral metabolism, solubility of collagen fibers, and muscle weakening. There may be stiffening of areas such as the rib cage, which causes difficulty in breathing. The vertebral column and shoulder girdle relax, creating a stooped posture. Smell is less acute, and loss of teeth is likely. These factors coupled with a decrease in digestive juices and gastrointestinal motility produce constipation, malnourishment, decreased fluid intake, and an increase in the desire for sweets. The examples are cited only to emphasize the necessity for nurses to be cognizant of these unique features of the aging process. The primary goal of care is to combat disease and maintain optimal mental and motor functioning appropriate to the client's age and health status.

New stimuli, both environmental and social, should be minimized. The client should be moved from room to room as little as possible. The personnel caring for him to be a consistent group who understand his special needs and desires.

Reality orientation can be fostered by simple measures such as providing window views that permit the client to know the weather, see the sunrise and sunset, and remind him of the outside world. Familiar clothes, personal items from home such as photographs and other belongings, and a clock and calendar also contribute to his awareness of reality.

The elderly client should be addressed by his proper name, not by "Grandma" or "Grandpa." When it is feasible, he should be up and ambulating and interacting with others. Dressing and grooming himself are also desirable to promote reality orientation and maintain his sense of dignity.

Families should be encouraged to visit and be honest with the client about his business concerns or personal interests. Learning secondhand that his furniture has been sold or his apartment rented does not necessarily reassure him but makes him feel that he cannot even trust those closest to him. Furthermore, such acts seem to emphasize the transient nature of his worldly concerns. In short, he may feel that his relatives would like to wind up the details of his life as quickly as possible. Nurses need to alert families to the possible effects of gestures that are done in good faith but that may be misinterpreted.

The elderly client needs time—time to think, to act for himself, and to make decisions. Research has shown that there is a positive correlation between the brain alpha cycle duration and reaction time. The alpha rhythm functions like a clock in organizing behavior in the cerebral cortex. In aging such organization

TABLE 8-1

Physical classification

1. a. Capable of unlimited and unsupervised activity
   b. Fully ambulatory; able to go about the city independently in safety
   c. Has no physical condition requiring medical supervision or closeness to emergency medical care
   d. No evidence of heart disease in any form
   e. No evidence of prior cancer except cured skin cancer
   f. No complaints except those that cannot be related to any known disease entity
2. a. Capable of moderate activity; ambulatory without supervision for activities in his own home or immediate vicinity
   b. Can manage without help for personal care and otherwise requires minimal supervision
   c. Physical condition may require medical supervision, but frequent or special treatment or closeness to medical or nursing care not required
   d. May have had a previous illness that has left no residuals, for example, healed myocardial infarction without angina or ECG abnormalities other than healed infarctions, cancer with no evidence of recurrence, or mild diabetes (diet-controlled)
3. a. Limited capabilities
   b. Dependent on others for bed-making and baths and general supervision of activities
   c. May or may not need a walking aid (cane) but can carry on routine activities without additional personal service
   d. Generally requires escort on the outside
   e. May require periodic medical care; availability of emergency medical or nursing care desirable
   f. Has moderate incapacities, such as angina, arthritis that does not require confinement to a wheelchair, chronic respiratory disease, or diabetes requiring medication
4. a. Limited capabilities requiring assistance for personal care and daily living activities
   b. Must be in a protected environment because of need for general nursing supervision
   c. Closeness to emergency medical care desirable
   d. Requires frequent medical care
   e. Is practically housebound
   f. Angina or intermittent heart disease limits physical capacities, arthritis prevents ambulation, and there are severe hearing or visual impairments, but still has the capacity to be independent for daily activities after orientation
5. a. Chronically ill and confined to the vicinity of own room
   b. Requires a large amount of personal service and constant supervision
   c. Should be near own dining and toilet area and have a nurse on call at all times
   d. Physical condition requires 24-hour nursing care or intensive medical treatment
6. a. Requires intensive medical and nursing care
   b. Has infectious or contagious disease

Adapted from Brown, M., editor: Readings in gerontology, ed. 2, St. Louis, 1978, The C.V. Mosby Co., p. 48.

and timing tend to take longer. If signals (input) arrive too rapidly, they must wait to be handled in turn, that is, until the circuits are free. When elderly persons are confronted with complex input, their response may be one of confusion. Instructions or information should be given in small units, and simple tasks (rather than tasks regarding coordination of many details) should be assigned. Demonstrations enhance explanations, and they are usually helpful in facilitating comprehension. If one prepares the client to focus on the task before presentation, he will have additional time to prepare his response. The nurse should express patience and permit the elderly extra time to organize performances. One should speak slowly and listen attentively, exhibiting a genuine interest in what the older client is saying. If the nurse follows these guidelines, communication will be considerably more meaningful and mutually satisfying.

A nursing assessment is vital to the care of the elderly so that special problems, needs, and concerns can be approached systematically. Tables 8-1 to 8-3 are examples of guidelines for assessing clients in regard to physical health and functional capabilities.

Table 8-1 is designed to rate the client on a six-point physical classification scale, which determines the type of care or supervision that he requires. Categories range from independence and health (rating 1) to dependence and illness, which requires hospitalization and specialized care (rating 6).

Table 8-2 is a rating scale for activities of daily living (ADL). Ratings from 0 to 6 are possible, since one point is given for each functional category in which the client is independent. For example, 0 scores essentially imply the need for

TABLE 8-2

Physical self-maintenance scale

Activity	Score
Toilet	
1. Cares for self at toilet completely; no incontinence	1
2. Needs to be reminded or needs help to clean self, or has rare (weekly at most) accidents	0
3. Soils or wets bed while asleep more than once a week	0
4. Soils or wets bed while awake more than once a week	0
5. Has no control of bowels or bladder	0
Feeding	
1. Eats without assistance	1
2. Eats with minor assistance at mealtimes, with help in preparing food or in cleaning up after meals	0
3. Feeds self with moderate assistance and is untidy	0
4. Requires extensive assistance for all meals	0
5. Does not feed self at all and resists efforts of others to feed him	0
Dressing	
1. Dresses, undresses, and selects clothes from own wardrobe	1
2. Dresses and undresses self with minor assistance	0
3. Needs moderate assistance in dressing or selecting clothes	0
4. Needs major assistance in dressing but cooperates with efforts of others to help	0
5. Completely unable to dress self and resists efforts of others to help	0
Grooming	
1. Always dresses neatly and is well groomed, without assistance	1
2. Grooms self adequately, with occasional minor assistance, as in shaving	0
3. Needs moderate and regular assistance or supervision in grooming	0
4. Needs total grooming care but can remain well groomed after help from others	0
5. Actively negates all efforts of others to maintain grooming	0
Physical ambulation	
1. Goes about grounds or city	1
2. Ambulates within residence or about one block distance	0
3. Ambulates with assistance of (check one): *a* ( ) another person, *b* ( ) railing, *c* ( ) cane, *d* ( ) walker, or *e* ( ) wheelchair: 1 ___ gets in and out without help, or 2 ___ needs help in getting in and out	0
4. Sits unsupported in chair or wheelchair but cannot propel self without help	0
5. Bedridden more than half the time	0
Bathing	
1. Bathes self (tub, shower, sponge bath) without help	1
2. Bathes self, with help in getting in and out of tub	0
3. Washes face and hands only, but cannot bathe rest of body	0
4. Does not wash self but is cooperative with those who bathe him	0
5. Does not try to wash self and resists efforts to keep him clean	0

Adapted from Brown, M., editor: Readings in gerontology, ed. 2, St. Louis, 1978, The C.V. Mosby Co., p. 49.

closely supervised institutional care; a 2 to 6 score would make it possible for the individual to be placed in a selected home for the aged, depending on the type of services available.

Table 8-3 assesses "instrumental activities" relative to social life, such as shopping, using transportation services, and handling finances. Each of the eight categories is graduated with several possible levels of functioning, and one point is given if the client attains a minimum level or higher. Tasks highly specific to a given sex role are not included in the scoring for the opposite sex, for example, cooking.

The mental status questionnaire (Table 8-4) is a series of 10 simple items that assist in discriminating between severe and moderate impairment. The examiner, using direct interaction, can compensate for sensory deficits, attention

Foundations of clinical practice

spans, and motivation in ways not possible when using most standardized mental tests. Error scores from 0 to 10 indicate the degree of dysfunction caused by probable chronic brain syndrome (CBS). (It has been discovered that most neuroses and normal aging do not affect the scores.) The list is designed to determine a minimum level of competency but not to differentiate between average and superior mental functioning.

Many agencies and institutions have similar rating scales to assess elderly clients, and the nurse needs to become familiar with using and interpreting such instruments.

TABLE 8-3

Scale for instrumental activities of daily living

	Male score	Female score
Ability to use telephone		
1. Operates telephone on own initiative; looks up and dials numbers	1	1
2. Dials a few well-known numbers	1	1
3. Answers telephone but does not dial	1	1
4. Does not use telephone at all	0	0
Shopping		
1. Takes care of all shopping needs independently	1	1
2. Shops independently for small purchases	0	0
3. Needs to be accompanied on any shopping trip	0	0
4. Completely unable to shop	0	0
Food preparation		
1. Plans, prepares, and serves adequate meals independently		1
2. Prepares adequate meals if supplied with ingredients		0
3. Heats and serves prepared meals, or prepares meals but does not maintain adequate diet		0
4. Needs to have meals prepared and served		0
Housekeeping		
1. Maintains house alone or with occasional assistance for heavy work		1
2. Performs light daily tasks such as dish-washing and bed-making		1
3. Performs light daily tasks but cannot maintain acceptable level of cleanliness		1
4. Needs help with all home maintenance tasks		1
5. Does not participate in any housekeeping tasks		0
Laundry		
1. Does personal laundry completely		1
2. Launders small items; rinses socks, stockings, and so forth		1
3. Needs all laundry done by others		0
Mode of transportation		
1. Travels independently on public transportation or drives own car	1	1
2. Arranges own travel via taxi but does not otherwise use public transportation	1	1
3. Travels on public transportation when assisted or accompanied by another	0	1
4. Travels only in taxi or automobile, with assistance of another	0	0
5. Does not travel at all	0	0
Responsibility for own medication		
1. Is responsible for taking medication in correct dosages at correct time	1	1
2. Takes responsibility if medication is prepared in advance in separate dosages	0	0
3. Is not capable of dispensing own medication	0	0
Ability to handle finances		
1. Manages financial matters independently (budgets, writes checks, pays rent and bills, goes to bank); collects and keeps track of income	1	1
2. Manages day-to-day purchases, but needs help with banking, major purchases, and so forth	1	1
3. Incapable of handling money	0	0

Adapted from Brown, M., editor: Readings in gerontology, ed. 2, St. Louis, 1978, The C.V. Mosby Co., p. 50.

TABLE 8-4

Mental status questionnaire

1. Where are we now? (Correct name of place)
2. Where is this place? (Correct city)
3. What is today's date? (Day of month)
4. What month is it?
5. What year is it?
6. How old are you?
7. When is your birthday? (Month)
8. What year were you born?
9. Who is President of the United States?
10. Who was President before him?
    Scores: 0-2 CBS absent or mild
       3-8 CBS moderate
       9-10 CBS severe

Adapted from Brown, M., editor: Readings in gerontology, ed. 2, St. Louis, 1978, The C.V. Mosby Co., p. 52.

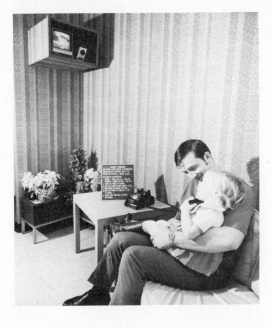

FIG. 8-3

Special communications network allows the child and mother to maintain visual and auditory contact during hospitalization. (Courtesy Methodist Hospital of Indiana, Inc., Indianapolis.)

FAMILY INTEGRITY DURING HOSPITALIZATION

The family who has any member hospitalized is bound to exhibit some disorganization. Nurses and other health team members should use every available means to keep the family unit in touch. Although small children cannot visit their parents or siblings, they can in some instances call or visit through systems such as Visit Vision, which permits both auditory and visual contact through a television-telephone hookup (Fig. 8-3).

  Hospitalization is a crisis that affects the entire family and not just the client himself. Nurses must take special care to preserve as much family integrity as possible.

Nursing care planning for the hospitalized client

Nursing care plans should ensure the client's safety in the hospital environment, promote sleep and rest, prevent sensory deprivation, include proper administration of medications and intravenous fluids, prepare the client for diagnostic tests, and extend care to the client during the preoperative, intraoperative, and postoperative stages. The plans are determined by the client's age and developmental stage and must be varied appropriately.

ENVIRONMENTAL SAFETY

The hospitalized client is subject to injury from falls, ingestion of medications or harmful objects, burns, fires, and electrical accidents. The nurse has the responsibility for maintaining an environment in which these injuries are prevented.

  The environment should be suited to the age and development of the client; therefore, clients may be assigned rooms according to age groups.

  Most children's hospitals are designed to minimize hazards in the environment, which is unfamiliar to the client and thus a more likely setting for accidents. Beds, stairs, bathrooms, chairs, and shelves are scaled to the size and ability of various age groups. Dishes are usually break-resistant, straws are strong but flexible, and plastic containers should replace glass ones when possible. The temperature of water available from the tap in a child's room or the shower is carefully controlled to avoid accidental scalding. Unused electrical outlets should be covered. Nurses should point these precautions out to parents, since they can also serve as a useful educational tool. Toys and games should be chosen with safety considered. Sharp projections, glass, or removable parts small enough to swallow are hazardous for younger age groups.

Physical restraints may be necessary for the very young child, especially during specialized procedures. Elbow, wrist, and ankle restraints, crib nets, jacket restraints, and mummy restraints are commonly used types (Figs. 8-4 and 8-5). When any restraint is used, its purpose should be explained to the parent and to the child if he is old enough to comprehend. Special observations are required whenever certain restraining devices are employed, to guard against circulatory impairment and skin irritation. This is especially true when restraints are used on extremities. The nurse must use judgment in the application of restraints and should be reminded that they are not substitutes for observing the child frequently. Any restraint should be regularly evaluated and should be re-

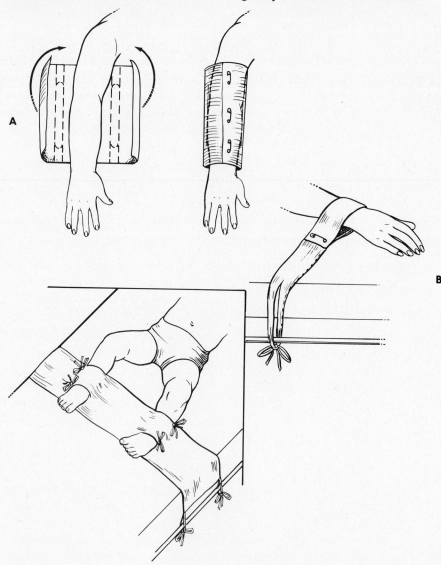

FIG. 8-4
Extremity restraints. **A,** Elbow restraint. **B,** Extremity-to-bed restraint. **C,** Extremities-to-bed restraint.

moved frequently for skin care. Padding some restraints may be indicated to prevent abrasions. Whenever the child is in a highchair or wheelchair or on a cart or an examining table, he should be restrained securely.

The environment for the adult and older client should be suited to their needs. Equipment should be placed where it does not obstruct movement of the client, the nurse, and other personnel. Cords should not be dangling on the floor. Unconscious adults should be protected and restrained if necessary. Older clients are particularly vulnerable to falls and should be assisted when ambulating and restrained as necessary.

Falls

In hospitals the majority of accidents result from clients falling out of a bed or chair or slipping and falling while ambulating. Many of these accidents can be prevented, and the nurse must plan preventive measures according to the age and health status of the client.

For the child the crib should always be latched and kept in the up position when he is left unattended. For the older child and adult the electrical bed should be kept in the low position except when the client is receiving nursing care. Side

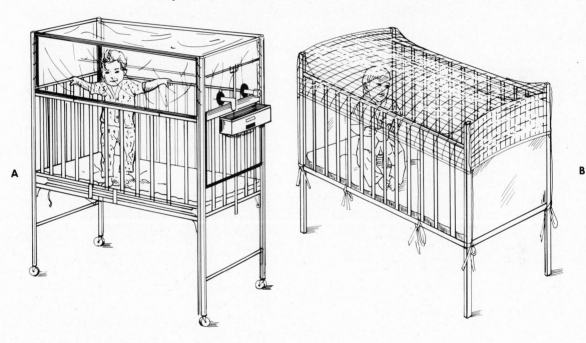

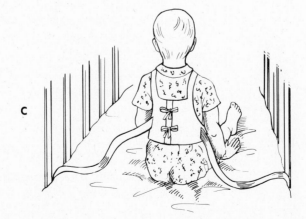

FIG. 8-5
Crib restraining devices. **A,** Crib with see-through plastic dome. **B,** Crib net. **C,** Jacket restraint. Note that jacket is secured to bed frame, not to the rails.

rails should be used. When clients are being assisted for transfer, such as to a stretcher, the stretcher should be locked securely. Beds also should be kept locked.

Assistance should be given to the ambulatory client as often as necessary to prevent falls. Clients should be assisted in and out of wheelchairs, or special instructions should be given for locking wheelchairs and for getting out of them without falling. The client with visual impairment or one who is unsteady should always be assisted when allowed to rise. If it is necessary for a client to use assistive walking devices (crutches or walkers), they should have rubber tips to prevent the client from slipping and falling.

Bathrooms and hallways should be well lighted. Any liquid spilled on the floor should be wiped up immediately. Small, unsecured scatter rugs or other objects such as toys should be removed from the environment. It may be necessary to place protective gates at doorways or at the top of stairways to keep the small child from wandering about or falling.

Ingestion of harmful substances

Accidents may also result from ingestion of medications and other harmful objects. Medication should not be kept at the bedside or within easy reach of inquisitive children. Medication cabinets, particularly on the pediatric unit, should be kept locked. Harmful objects (safety pins, needles, breakable objects) should be kept out of the reach of small children and disoriented clients.

Burns

Burns sustained in the hospital can usually be prevented. The temperature of bath water and hot-water bottles should always be tested before use. The temperature should not exceed the degree of heat required for a specific treatment. Commercial heat packs or pads should be properly regulated before the client is permitted to use them. The nurse should follow all established policies regarding the use of heat lamps and must be knowledgeable about instances in which modifications must be made. For example, the young child, the elderly client, and the seriously ill client are more susceptible to burns. The skin at the extremes of age is thin and less resistant to heat as compared with the older child, adolescent, and young or middle-aged adult. The seriously ill client may not react normally to stimuli; therefore, less protection is afforded.

When it is necessary to defibrillate a client, special precautions must be taken to prevent burns (see Chapter 20).

Fires

Fires are another source of accidents. Clients should be encouraged to smoke only in those areas designated for smoking. No-smoking signs should be displayed prominently in areas where smoking is not permitted. All exits should be kept clear and free from clutter. The nurse should be well informed about specific management responsibilities in case a fire should occur. Although details about fire policies differ, there are many similarities as to basic rules to follow in case of fire. When a fire is discovered in the hospital, clinic, or other health facility, the nurse or individual discovering the fire should intervene by doing five basic things: (1) removing clients from immediate danger, (2) sounding the fire alarm, (3) notifying the fire department, (4) containing or extinguishing the fire, and (5) performing special duties and continuing evacuation. These steps may be carried out simultaneously, provided enough people are available.

Removing clients from immediate danger. *In any fire the first priority should be to preserve the life of clients.* Clients who are in immediate danger, whether by smoke, heat, or flame should be removed as quickly and efficiently as possible. Ambulatory clients may be directed to a place of safety. Bedridden clients may be removed by a number of methods. The method utilized should be the one that seems most appropriate for the situation. A brief discussion of different methods of removing clients from a place of danger follows.

1. *Knee-drop, blanket-drag method.* This method is useful in removing heavy clients and may be accomplished by one person. A blanket is thrown on the floor. The nurse drops the knee closest to the client's feet and places one arm under and around the client's shoulders and the other around his legs. The client

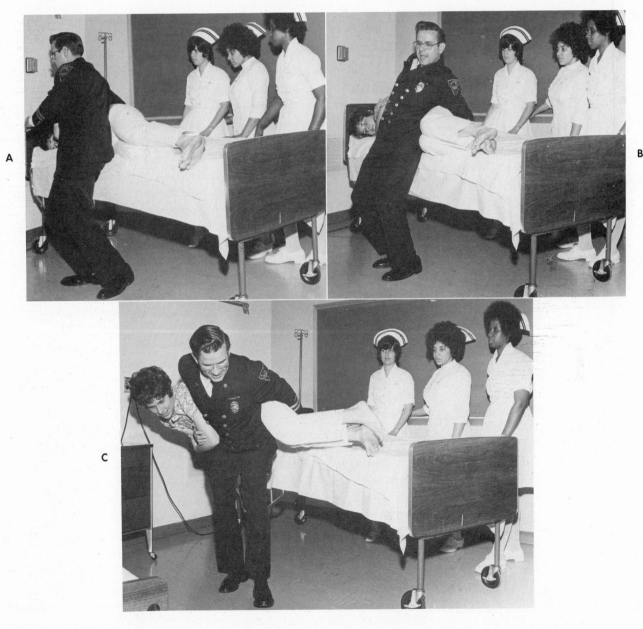

FIG. 8-6
Fireman demonstrates to nursing students the hip-carrying method of removing a client from danger. **A,** Fireman grasps the client and rolls her to the edge of the bed, standing toward the center of the bed. **B,** He places his back against the client and grasps her under the knees. **C,** Fireman carries the client to a place of safety. Note that fireman's back is bent.

is then pulled toward the edge of the bed so that he slides down toward the floor on the blanket. The raised knee prevents the client from hitting his head. The nurse quickly stands, grasps each end of the blanket, and drags the client to safety.

2. *Hip-carry method* (Fig. 8-6). This method can also be utilized by one person. Proper body mechanics are essential. The nurse reaches across the client, grasps his wrist, and pulls and rolls him to the edge of the bed. The client should be on his side, and the nurse's body should be close to the bed to prevent the client from falling. The nurse stands at the center of the client's body, turns, and places the back against the client. One foot should be placed in front of the other so that body weight will be evenly distributed. One arm is placed over the client's body and around his axilla; the other is placed over his body and under his knees. The client should be held firmly, and the nurse's back should be bent while taking the client to a place of safety. To release the client, the nurse places him against a wall and releases his legs first. The nurse then turns, bends slowly, and places the client's upper trunk safely on the floor.

3. *Pack-strap carry method*. The nurse faces the client with back toward the foot of the bed. The client's wrists are grasped, and he is pulled to a sitting position. Both wrists are then held with the left hand, and the right hand is placed behind the client's knees. He is then pulled toward the front of the bed, a move that should leave him sitting on the edge. Next, the nurse's back is placed against the client's chest, and the client's arms are pulled over the shoulders and crossed over the nurse's chest. The nurse's feet should be apart, with one slightly in front of the other to distribute the weight evenly. The nurse pushes out and down while holding the client's wrists firmly; the client is pulled off the bed onto the nurse's back and taken to a place of safety. There the nurse leans, gently falls on the knees, and releases the client slowly to the floor.

4. *Two-person carry with chair*. One person grasps and lifts the front legs of the chair, while another grasps the rear legs. Care must be taken to prevent injury by strapping the client to the chair.

5. *Two-person carry with rolled bedding*. One person stands near the client's head, and the other stands on the opposite side near the feet. The linen is pulled out and rolled toward the client. Each person grasps a roll of bedding on each side of the client, signals, and simultaneously lifts the client and lowers him toward the floor. The bedding is slightly raised, and the client is dragged to safety.

Sounding the alarm. Once clients in immediate danger are safe, the alarm should be sounded by following the directions on the alarm box. All nurses should be familiar with the alarm system in their place of employment.

Notifying the fire department. The fire department should be notified by telephone or by using the nearest alarm box. Many institutions have systems that automatically detect fires, sound an alarm, and transmit a signal to the fire department headquarters. In others it is the telephone operator's responsibility to notify the fire department.

Containing or extinguishing the fire. The fire should be extinguished as quickly as possible by utilizing the most feasible means. Openings leading to the fire should be closed off to prevent the spread of fire. Doors and windows should be closed. Cracks and openings should be stuffed with wet materials to contain the fire. All employees should know where fire extinguishers are located and how

TABLE 8-5

Extinguishers

Type	Class of fire		
	A	**B**	**C**
Soda-acid	x		
Pressurized water	x		
Foam		x	x
Carbon dioxide		x	x
Dry chemical		x	x
ABC	x	x	x

to operate them. Such knowledge is invaluable during a fire. Extinguishers can be hand-carried or dragged if they are too large. The instructions for handling and use should be studied and practiced frequently before they are actually needed.

In order to facilitate extinguishing fires, nurses should be aware of conditions necessary for producing a fire:

1. There must be *fuel* or a substance that mimics fuel.
2. The temperature of the fuel must be raised to the point where it will unite with oxygen *(kindling temperature)*.
3. There must by *oxygen* within the environment.

The nurse must also be familiar with the three classes of fire:

1. Class A: fires in combustible materials such as paper, linen, rags, and wood. These require quenching with varying quantities of water or solutions containing large amounts of water, which reduces the temperature below the kindling temperature.
2. Class B: fires in flammable liquids such as grease or oil, paint, and varnish. These require smothering to exclude the oxygen. Water should not be used, because it tends to spread the flame rather than smother it.
3. Class C: fires in electrical equipment. Nonconducting extinguishing agents are required. Fires in motors or switchboards are examples. The power supply should be turned off.

Since the type of extinguisher used depends on the class of fire, Table 8-5 is included for a general outline. To decrease confusion in trying to remember specific classes of fires, many institutions use the triple-combination (ABC) extinguishers that are effective on all types of fires.

Performing special duties and continuing evacuation. Duties are assigned to available personnel. These should be established well before a fire actually happens. Such duties may include turning off oxygen or utilities, directing traffic, and rechecking rooms. Generally, it is necessary to evacuate only those clients in immediate danger.

Electrical accidents

Electrical accidents in the hospital are not uncommon and can occur whenever an individual becomes a conductor of alternating current. This may happen because of carelessness, faulty equipment, or ignorance about electrical safety. The widespread use of electrical equipment for diagnosis, maintenance, and therapy may also be related to the frequency of electrical accidents.

Injuries resulting from electricity may cover a wide spectrum, ranging from a tingling sensation to electrocution, depending on the amount of voltage available to propel electrons through the body, the path it takes, and the resistance it encounters. Electric current moves according to Ohm's law.*

Whatever effect occurs depends on one of two methods: (1) interruption of neural conduction (normal rhythmic cardiac and respiratory impulses from the medulla) at the same time the protoplasmic elements become ionized, producing injury or destruction to the cells, or (2) transformation of electrical energy into heat-producing burns.

Generally, the tissues of the body are good conductors of electricity and, when placed in the path of an electrical current, transmit the current to some

---

*Ohm's law equates the amount of current (I) (measured in amperes) to voltage (E) in the circuit (measured in volts) divided by resistance (R) of the circuit (measured in ohms) ($I = E/R$).

point of exit on contact with the ground. Because the skin is the most susceptible to electrical energy, injuries that occur are produced at the skin sites of entry and exit. Once the current enters the body, it tends to flow in all directions but may cause little or no damage. The principle that permits this effect is related to the size of the surface area. With a large surface area, such as the skin, the energy load is dispersed, and as a result the generation of heat to a given cell is lowered.

Resistance offered by parts of the body varies under different conditions. For example, the resistance of wet hands and feet to electric current is very low, whereas the resistance from dry skin is very high. Thick skin is more resistant than thin skin. Even when the resistance of the body is high, a large amount of electricity can be forced through it if the voltage is high. Lower voltages may also cause an accident if conditions are unfavorable, such as the touching of a bare wire while the hands are wet. The passage of even a small quantity of current directly into chambers of the heart may cause fibrillation.

The use of defective electrical equipment such as food warmers, floor polishers, electric beds, vaporizers, or suction pumps (especially in the vicinity of a defective radio or television set, oxygen or vacuum outlets, or similar equipment) enhances "macroshock," a form of shock that occurs when the body, particularly the limbs and trunk, becomes a conductor of electricity through contact. Nurses should be aware of such hazards and report any potential hazards to the hospital electricians promptly before using the equipment. It is particularly important to have all electrical appliances that the client has brought from home to the care facility inspected by the staff electricians before allowing them to be used in the environment. Most client care facilities have a routine maintenance program directed toward eliminating electrical hazards such as those described.

Leakage current and grounding. *Leakage current,* a form of nonuseful, unwanted current present in the chassis or frame of electrical equipment, cannot be perceived by touch but is perceptible with the use of specialized equipment. Microamperes ranging from 20 to 2000 have been measured in television sets, electric beds, bottle warmers, monitors, suctioning machines, hypothermia machines, and hemodialysis machines.[11] Leakage current from power cords is thought to be approximately 1 μamps for each foot of cord. Therefore, it is recommended that extension cords or cords longer than 10 feet not be used. *Grounding,* a conduction system, is an added safety precaution that is provided through the green wire, commonly referred to as the "third wire" in a cord or external ground wire. This system diverts the current. Failure to divert it would possibly result in the current's being picked up from the frame or chassis of the equipment. The importance of utilizing grounds cannot be overemphasized.

Ground equalization. The utilization of more than one piece of electrical equipment on one client at the same time can be responsible for causing an electrical accident. The client with a cardiac pacemaker who is attached to the monitor is a common example. The source of the hazard is within the ground system of the electrical distribution system and is caused by a difference in the voltage potentials of two grounding points. As a result of the difference, a current may be driven to the body of the client, provided the body is between the two potentials. The currents may be high enough to cause fibrillation. This hazard is usually prevented by using one "multiple-receptacle" outlet rather than attaching the client at two different points. Such a system is designed to equalize all grounding points and is referred to as an *equalizer ground bus* (EGB). (EGB wire should be no. 0.)

In assisting with defibrillation, personnel must be careful not to touch the client or bed during the procedure to avoid having their bodies pick up the current.

Preventing electrical accidents. Nurses have an important role in instructing individuals within the hospital and other health care facilities about factors relating to electrical safety. The following are some of the pointers that should be stressed:

1. Check the integrity of all electrical equipment (plugs, cords, outlets, machines) before using it.
2. Refrain from using defective electrical equipment (loose plugs, frayed cords, worn insulations, plugs and cords that are warm to touch).
3. Use only equipment that can be grounded with a three-pronged plug. Radios and electrical devices such as toothbrushes and shavers have two-pronged plugs and should not be permitted in client care areas.
4. Use short power cords. Long cords and extension cords are hazardous and should not be used.
5. Unplug all electrical equipment when it is not in use.
6. Use only properly insulated electrical equipment.
7. Refrain from overloading receptacles (using multiple-outlet adapters to one unit, and so forth).
8. Refrain from using cheaters (three-pronged to two-pronged adapters).
9. Refrain from handling electrical equipment with wet hands or feet, since water is a conductor of electricity.
10. Place electrical cords where they can be readily seen, rather than under rugs or furniture.
11. Do not remove a plug from a socket by pulling on the cord. Always grip the plug shell to remove the plug.
12. If an electrical device is dropped, have it checked before using it.

In the home it is not uncommon for individuals to use electrical devices while in the bathtub or shower. This is an unsafe practice that should be discouraged.

As a provider of health care the nurse must also encourage periodic inspection of electrical equipment by an electrician. Such tests should include inspecting the integrity of the outlet system for polarity and grounding, the grounding system in the cords, and the EGB. It has been suggested that the best time to inspect equipment is just before it is connected for use; however, this may not be ideal, particularly in critical care areas. Even so, it may serve to decrease accidents.

A number of testing devices are presently available that can be easily used by nurses and other health care personnel. The equipment is lightweight, inexpensive, and simple to use. These devices are equipped with visual and/or audio alarm systems to indicate whether or not the equipment functions properly. Examples of such test systems are (1) the circuit tester, which lights up when plugged into the electrical outlet and indicates the conditions of polarity and grounding; (2) the biomedical electric field probe, which gives off an instant alarm like a siren to indicate the leakage current of specific equipment; and

Foundations of clinical practice

(3) the EGB tester, which gives off both an intermittent tone and flashing light to indicate differences in ground potential.

All health care personnel should strive to promote electrical safety by being informed about the use of electrical equipment and some of its potential hazards. The nurse particularly should use every available opportunity to teach electrical safety and encourage regular inspection of electrical equipment.

SLEEP THEORY AND PLANNING

During sleep, responses to environmental stimuli are diminished to ensure psychological and physiological recovery from fatigue. Sleep is believed to restore focused attention, improve learning ability and memory, preserve emotional integrity and social adaptation, and restore catecholamine mechanisms. Metabolism slows and anabolic activity is dominant during sleep.

Sleep occurs in an orderly pattern, as demonstrated by research using the electroencephalogram (EEG), electromyogram (EMG), and electrooculogram (EOG).[7-9,12] There are four stages of progressively deeper sleep, or non–rapid eye movement (NREM) sleep, which are followed by a period of rapid eye movement (REM) sleep. The cycle is repeated every 80 to 120 minutes in a pattern that varies with the individual throughout the life span.

Stages of sleep

Stage one sleep is entered only from wakefulness. Muscles are in a state of tonus, and the person is alert to environmental stimuli (sensory stimuli of noise, heat, odors, pain), proprioceptive stimuli (such as a full bladder), or emotional stimuli (tension, worries, fears). This stage of sleep lasts about 10 minutes.

During *stage two* sleep, the muscles begin to relax and cerebral activity diminishes. Sensory stimuli receive less response, and the intensity of response becomes lower. There is a hierarchy of diminishing sensory perceptions, with hearing the last sense perceived before falling asleep.

Stage three sleep follows within a few minutes. The muscles become more relaxed, the skin is flushed and warmer, and the person sweats. Metabolism slows by 10% to 20%, lowering body temperature, pulse, respirations, and blood pressure. The Pco_2 may increase and the Po_2 decrease because of hypoventilation secondary to depression of respiratory center activity. Gastrointestinal activity increases to facilitate cellular metabolism, and blood vessels dilate to provide exchange of metabolites for cellular restoration.

Within 30 minutes the person is in *stage four* sleep. Eye movements are minimal, and the muscles are very relaxed. Stage four is a deep sleep, and only very strong stimuli rouse the sleeper. During this stage children may be unresponsive to stimuli from a full bladder, and bed-wetting may occur. This sleep is also the time of increased growth hormone release. Stage four sleep appears to be necessary for physical restoration; the amount of time spent in this stage increases after physical exhaustion.

REM sleep occurs within 10 to 30 minutes after stage four sleep. The muscles are relaxed, but there is rapid movement of the eyes. The sympathetic nervous system is dominant, and pulse, respirations, and blood pressure rise. There is increased output of adrenal hormones, and the demand for oxygen accelerates. There may be head banging, penile erections, or teeth grinding at this time. Some researchers believe that anginal chest pain, myocardial infarction, and dysrhythmias may occur at this time.[9] There may also be convulsions if the client has a neurological disequilibrium such as epilepsy. Since gastric secretions increase, clients with gastric ulcers may experience abdominal pain. Dreams are intense; if awakened, a person may remember the dream vividly. This period of sleep appears to be necessary for psychological renewal or for sorting and retrieving information and experiences from former periods of wakefulness. REM sleep lasts about 20 minutes. The person then returns to stage two sleep, and the cycle is repeated.

Sleep throughout the life span

The time spent sleeping varies inversely with age, and the nurse must be aware of the differences of sleep in developmental stages in order to plan nursing care. The amount of time spent in REM sleep is also age related and is significant in planning care for hospitalized clients.

Neonates spend most of their time sleeping; 16 to 18 hours of sleep is normal in a 24-hour cycle. Fifty percent of this is REM sleep, and the neonate may be observed having dreams and moving in bed. Growth and development are rapid at this time, and there is a great need for rest. The neonate usually falls asleep after needs for food, oxygen, elimination, and sexual comfort have been met. Crying after these needs have been met may indicate that the need for sleep is dominant.

Infants require progressively less sleep. When the infant is 3 months old, he sleeps about 16 hours a day. By the time he is 1 year old, he usually needs about 14 hours. This sleep is obtained from several sleep periods, which are often determined by the family routine. The smaller stomach and bladder capacity often rouse the infant and determine the shortness or frequency of sleep patterns. Most infants are able to sleep through the night without a feeding when they are 6 to 10 weeks old.

Preschool-age children need 11 to 14 hours of sleep, some of which may be obtained from one or two naps during the day. Sleep may be difficult when the child is more interested in play activities. Young children are very dependent on their parents and may feel that sleep is a threat to that relationship. Frightening dreams related to the child's active imagination may also occur at this age, and fears of monsters and ghosts can make sleep unpleasant.

School-age children begin to establish regular habits of sleep and require 9 to 12 hours a night. Afternoon naps are not usually needed unless indicated by the child. Difficulty in falling asleep may be normal at this age, and a certain amount of independence in determining sleep needs should be offered to the older school-age child.

Adults usually require about 8 hours of sleep, and the amount of REM time is about 25% of total sleep. Sleep is a necessary health habit, and each adult should be aware of how much sleep he needs to function effectively.

Older adults require 6 hours of sleep or less. Because there is less REM and stage four sleep, sleep may be intermittent and easily interrupted. Stage four sleep usually occurs before midnight. Arteriosclerosis can contribute to frequent awakening. Some older persons fear dying in their sleep and may be hesitant in going to sleep.

The amount of time required for sleep does not change with further aging, but the pattern of sleeping may be erratic. Several theories have been advanced to explain this change in sleep pattern.[8] One explanation relates to inadequate amounts of L-tryptophan in the diet, or inefficient absorption or utilization. L-Tryptophan is a precursor to serotonin, a neurotransmitter believed to induce sleep. Others attribute change in sleep patterns to an imbalance of acetylcholine and cholinesterase. Acetylcholine acts to keep the individual awake; cholinesterase decreases sleep for prolonged periods. Many older persons have frequent naps, and adequate sleep time is probably obtained from napping and dozing.

Planning for sleep

Hospitalized clients require adequate sleep for physical and mental restoration. Stresses of hospitalization and health problems contribute to the necessity for sleep. The nurse can plan with the client to follow routines that consider his age and his needs for sleep, and arrange an appropriate environment.

An atmosphere that is conducive to sleep can be created by meeting basic needs and controlling environmental stimuli. Most persons fall asleep when other needs have been met. The client should not be hungry before he goes to sleep; a glass of milk or snack can be given. The bladder should be emptied before sleep, and diapers changed on infants. The linens should be tight, and the client should be in a comfortable position, free of pain and tension. A back rub may assist the client in relaxing, and pain medication can be offered if needed. A sense of security should be established, particularly if the person is in a new environment. The hospitalized client should be informed of routine noises outside his room, and the call bell should be within reach.

As many stimuli as possible should be eliminated. The room should be darkened and quiet. A temperature of 70° F with a humidity of 60% is comfortable for most people. Blankets can be added or removed as needed. Extraneous noise should be eliminated. If the client is in a critical care setting, alarms from monitors should be silenced if possible and monotonous noises reduced. Nurses' stations are often sources of noise, and care should be taken to limit noise and activity.

Neonates should be placed in bed on their side or stomach after eating to prevent aspiration of vomited feedings. Pillows are not used until the neonate is able to turn over. Infants and children usually sleep in a crib or bed with side rails. In the hospital it is particularly important that the bed be a safe environment, since the child is in unfamiliar surroundings and may attempt to get out of bed. Toys should be removed from the bed to prevent injury during sleep.

Planning bedtime for infants and children centers around their need for sleep. Bedtime in the hospital can be made easier if the parents or nurse use a calm approach. Subtle diversion from active play to quieter activities such as reading or listening to records prepares the child for approaching bedtime (Fig. 8-7). When given a fair warning that bedtime is near, the child will usually cooperate. Rituals of bedtime preparation are important to some children and should be followed. One child may take his bath, brush his teeth, read a story, and go to bed with his favorite stuffed toy. This routine is particularly important when the child is away from his own home. If the child gets out of bed or cries out from fright, the parent or nurse should reassure the child and tuck him back in bed quietly. Getting the child out of bed to rock him or punishing him only increases stimulation and disrupts sleep.

The environment is also new for adolescents and adults, and they may become confused. Side rails should be used at night, and restraints employed if necessary. The bed should be put in the low position to prevent injury if the client should need to get out of bed. The bathroom should be lighted so that the client can easily find it. Adolescents and adults have greater independence in determining their sleep needs. The amount of sleep varies, and the time may be governed by employment schedules; if the client worked at night, he may have difficulty adjusting to the rigid daytime routine of the hospital. Sleep needs should be met so that the client is rested and alert on rising.

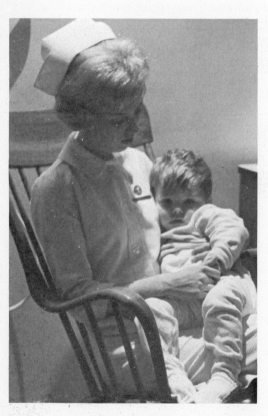

FIG. 8-7
A quiet, dimmed room and being rocked by the nurse make going to bed in a strange environment easier. (Courtesy Methodist Hospital of Indiana, Inc., Indianapolis.)

8 Nursing and the hospitalized client

Planning sleep for older adults can be modified for sporadic napping and dozing. Rest periods may be provided more frequently during a 24-hour period. Older adults may become confused when lights are turned out, and safety is of utmost concern. Side rails should be used, along with restraints if necessary. A light may be left on in the room, and the nurse can periodically check to anticipate elimination needs and assist the client in getting out of bed.

Sleeplessness

Many clients have difficulty sleeping in strange environments. The client may be experiencing anxiety, pain, loneliness, isolation, or other changes in his sleep routine that make sleeping difficult. Sleeplessness is further aggravated by hospital routines of taking vital signs or performing procedures when the client is sleeping.

The nurse can plan with the client to prevent or minimize sleeplessness. Strategies may include modifying activity and diet and minimizing disruptions. Physical activity 4 to 5 hours before sleep increases stage four sleep, and if possible increased physical activity should be arranged for this time. Activity 2 to 3 hours before sleep, however, makes falling asleep difficult; a quiet, restful time before sleeping is preferred. Milk, which contains L-tryptophan, has been known to induce sleep; caffeine, on the other hand, is a stimulant, and tea, coffee, soft drinks, and chocolate containing caffeine should be withheld.

The nurse should plan for each client to have at least 90 minutes of uninterrupted sleep so that a sleep cycle can be completed. Each time the client is awakened he must start the sleep cycle from stage one and consequently may never reach stage four or REM sleep if awakened for hourly vital signs or procedures. The nurse can observe the client's sleep patterns and wait until REM sleep is completed before awakening the client.

Drugs to induce sleep are available but interfere with REM sleep and can be habit forming. Sedatives, hypnotics, tranquilizers, alcohol, and antidepressants shorten the time spent in REM sleep. When the person stops taking these drugs, the amount of REM time increases for several nights to compensate for the lost sleep. This rebound phenomenon is particularly crucial to clients with coronary heart disease or myocardial infarction, since the increased time spent in REM sleep after REM deprivation may precipitate another infarction. If the drugs are used, they should be withdrawn slowly to prevent the wakefulness, restlessness, and anxiety that may be associated with withdrawal. Regular sleep habits, satisfaction of basic needs, and an environment conducive to sleep are more helpful in promoting sleep than the use of drugs.

Sleep deprivation

Individuals who do not sleep through all four stages and REM sleep or who do not obtain an adequate amount of sleep may experience the effects of sleep deprivation. The client may become confused, have a shortened attention span, or become psychotic. Clients in critical care settings or postsurgical recovery units are particularly vulnerable to sleep deprivation and the so-called ICU psychosis, or postoperative psychosis. The hazard of sleep deprivation is compounded by REM rebound, which occurs when the client finally has an opportunity to sleep and more time is spent in REM sleep. The sympathetic activity of REM sleep increases vital signs and oxygen demand, predisposing the client to further risks of dysrhythmias and hypoxia.

The nurse can plan to avert sleep deprivation by ensuring prolonged sleep of at least 90 to 120 minutes. If the client is sleeping, priority may be given to this need and other procedures delayed until the client is awake.

237

SENSORY DEPRIVATION

Sensory deprivation is a state in which environmental stimulation is significantly altered. Several aspects of this phenomenon have been identified: (1) sensory deprivation, or complete reduction of sensory input; (2) perceptual deprivation, or alterations in the patterns of stimulation; (3) monotony, characterized by absence of change within the environment; and (4) sensory overload, or increase in the amount of intensity of stimuli. The phenomenon is thought to occur because the reticulum-activating system is not stimulated or is stimulated minimally. This system, with connections between the higher and lower brain centers, plays a part in alerting and arousing the body. The nurse can assess the client for evidence of sensory deprivation and the environment for sources of sensory overload, deprivation, or monotony.

Sensory deprivation in hospitalized clients can be attributed to several sources. The most common example is the client with sensory losses of hearing or vision. These losses may have occurred before the hospitalization or resulted from medical or surgical intervention. Other causes may be immobilization or physical or social isolation.

When individuals are deprived of environmental stimulation, a number of emotions may be experienced. Fear and anxiety, irritability, annoyance, restlessness, agitation, somatic complaints, mood changes, and depression are not uncommon. Perceptual defects causing changes in color perception, alteration in the size and contour of objects, delusions, distorted thinking, and loss of ability to concentrate have also been reported. In extreme cases the individual may have visual and auditory hallucinations. These symptoms are thought to become more serious as the length of time of reduced stimulation increases. However, less serious symptoms may occur as early as 2 to 3 hours. Regardless of their nature, the symptoms are more likely to occur at night.

Although these behaviors have been reported under experimental conditions, they may also be observed in any client in which the amount of sensory stimulation is reduced for a given time. For example, the client who undergoes eye surgery that is followed by bilateral patching of the eyes experiences deprivation because of decreased visual input; the hearing-impaired client, because of reduced auditory stimulation. The immobilized or isolated client who has limited interaction with his environment may experience sensory deprivation. Both may exhibit symptoms because of the monotonous environment and decreased interpersonal contacts. The elderly client is also prone to sensory deprivation. The use of hypnotics may alter stimulation to the reticulum-activating system and cause the client to be confused and possibly disoriented. This occurs as a result of perceptual deprivation. Pain, especially severe pain, is also thought to be responsible for some clients' experiencing perceptual deprivation.

The physical environment may provide sources for potential monotony or sensory overload. Certain environments are unique because of an absence of stimuli. The client may be isolated in a private room, without a window and with a closed door. Restraints, side rails, isolettes, or crib tops may restrict the field of activity and vision. Visitors may be restricted or otherwise unable to visit the client. Monotony in the environment is noted by limited visual fields, continuous dull noises, and similar tactile and kinesthetic stimuli imposed by a position of confinement to bed. Nursing units and critical care settings can also be overloaded with stimuli. Monitors, equipment, personnel, noise, and continuous light bombard the client who is usually confined to bed in one position. The variety of stimuli is compounded by frequency and intensity, as the client is continuously monitored and various personnel perform procedures.

The nurse, family and client can plan to prevent or manage the various facets of sensory deprivation by providing sensory input appropriate to the client's needs. Goals may include reducing sensory stimulation, providing sensory stimulation, or varying sensory stimulation.

Reducing sensory stimulation

The client experiencing sensory overload is responding to an increased number of multisensory experiences or an increased intensity of stimuli. After the variety and amount of stimulation have been identified, it is possible to limit the sources. These may include noise, light, tactile stimulation, or a variety of unfamiliar persons and objects in the environment. The nurse can plan to simplify the environment and organize care so that minimal inputs are provided. Simple environmental manipulation may include turning off lights, restricting visitors and health care personnel, turning off televisions, and limiting noise. Explanations of procedures and activities reduce confusion and hallucinations. Helping the client focus on one activity at a time may improve concentration.

Providing sensory stimulation

Clients isolated from familiar surroundings and family often require contact with familiar objects to prevent feelings of isolation and sensory deprivation. Family members should be encouraged to visit the client. Calendars, clocks, photographs, and familiar objects may be added to the hospital room to facilitate orientation to time and place. Television, newspapers, radios, records, books, and games maintain contact with current events. If possible the client's environment can be expanded by moving the bed to a playroom, client's lounge, or nurses' station, where additional stimuli of noise, people, and scenery can be provided.

Studies on sensory deprivation have demonstrated the importance of providing sensory stimulation during the critical period of the child's development. Failure to provide stimulation may result in irreversible damage. This is particularly significant for the multiply handicapped child, who must be given as much of the same kind of social contact as the normal child, with consideration for his unique sensory deficits.

Consistency is also important. This assists the client in interpreting the environment. These approaches are particularly imperative for the client with perceptual or emotional problems or the client with brain dysfunction. For the *blind and mentally retarded* individual, attempts must be made to provide an environment that is warm and stable and has a mild amount of variety. Stability is the key to caring for the *brain-damaged* client. Routines and environmental stimulation should not vary too much. A stable background of the same room, similar music, and consistent handling by parents, nurses, and other health personnel is recommended. The *blind and emotionally retarded* individual should have the opportunity to physically explore different situations through tactile, auditory, and kinesthetic modalities. For the *blind and deaf* client, tactile communications are very important.

Varying sensory stimulation

Perceptual monotony is common to clients who are in critical care units or who are confined to bed for long periods. Continuous stimulation from noises or from tactile, kinesthetic, or proprioceptive senses contributes to monotony. Sensory input can be varied by reducing monotonous stimuli or replacing them with different stimuli. Monotonous noises from monitors, ventilators, or other equipment should be limited when possible and interspersed with conversation,

Foundations of clinical practice

light, or other stimuli. The client should be touched and turned frequently to provide social orientation and changes of tactile and kinesthetic stimuli.

PAIN

Pain is an elusive phenomenon experienced by many hospitalized clients. Some persons view pain as a gift from God and accept it freely because there is a divine reason for suffering. Others cannot cope with discomfort and develop considerable hostility. "Why must I suffer so much?" Their behavior is filled with anger and resentment. Clients who must learn to live with the pain of a chronic illness make certain adjustments to it and accept it as a way of life.

Despite its destructive power, pain is useful in sending out to the cerebral cortex the message that something is wrong. The amount of pain experienced, though, gives no true indication of the seriousness or the amount of tissue damage. It is a valuable defense mechanism when the normal functioning or integrity of the body is threatened from internal or external sources. There is always danger when one's neurological structures have been impaired to the degree that they cannot perceive or respond to pain. However, research has shown that satisfactory biological adjustment is possible even if one cannot experience pain. Individuals who have the rare congenital absence of the sense of pain learn to adjust to the environment in the same manner as those who have had pain pathways surgically interrupted. An alarm reaction may be triggered by any stimulus if that particular stimulus has been previously associated with injuries, dangers, or other threatening circumstances. In fact, the bulk of such reactions involved in everyday experience are initiated by nonpainful stimuli. Essentially, pain is an important accessory warning of imminent tissue damage.

Theories of pain

There are three major theories of the psychophysiology of pain: (1) specificity, (2) pattern, and (3) gate control. Although none is entirely acceptable in view of recent research, each contains a rationale for current modes of pain management that is clinically applicable to nursing care.

Specificity theory. Proponents of this theory maintain that a complex of free nerve endings in body tissues generates pain impulses that are carried by specialized fibers (A-delta and C fibers) of the peripheral nervous system to the pain center in the thalamus via the lateral spinothalamic tract. There is no evidence thus far that any receptor fiber units exist *exclusively* for receiving and transmitting pain. There have been findings, however, that substantiate that select fibers respond only under special conditions, such as when skin is damaged, but their behavior does not show a consistent relationship between a stimulus and response. For example, noxious chemical and thermal stimuli do not cause the fibers to fire. They also are influenced considerably by threshold, adaptation, temperature, and other variables that complicate physiological rationale. This specificity theory seems far too simple to explain the complexities that have been observed in the study of the physiological and psychological aspects of pain.

Pattern theory. Several subtheories are combined to form the pattern theory, which associates a stimulus intensity to a central summation mechanism. Networks of large cutaneous fibers supposedly comprise a touch system, and other smaller fibers accumulate their input and transmit a pattern to the brain, where it is interpreted as pain. A related idea proposes that ordinarily an input-controlling mechanism functions that prevents accumulation of sensation-producing pain, and when this system fails, pain is experienced. Although there are several variations to the pattern theory, none possesses the capacity for explaining or integrating all clinical phenomena associated with pain.

Gate control theory. The most popular thinking about pain, which accepts in part tenets of both the specificity and pattern theories, is the gate control theory. This theory maintains that there is a specialized system (gate control) that modulates sensory input before evoking perception and response to the stimuli. Three spinal cord mechanisms play integral roles in this phenomenon.

1. Substantia gelatinosa (modulates afferent patterns before reaching transmission [T] cells of the dorsal horn)
2. Afferent dorsal column fibers that project to the brain, activate brain processes, and by way of descending fibers influence modulating properties of the gate control system
3. Central transmission (T) cells in the dorsal horn that are responsible for ultimate perception and response

The integrated functioning of these three mechanisms explains that when the modulated output of the T cells reaches a critical level, pain is felt.

Recent research has yielded new insight into pain mechanisms, but much remains unexplained. The behavior of the dorsal horn is not completely known because of limitations in methodology related to physiological study of such cells. The variations in actions of large versus small nerve fibers are still tentative, and much is still unexplored regarding changes in membrane potential during depolarization and repolarization. The physiology of T cells also is still in the rudimentary stages of understanding. However, it is known that there are cutaneous zones where stimuli converge, interact, and are controlled (facilitated or inhibited) before perceptions and responses are affected.

Pain and tension

Pain is intricately related to tension. When clients are tense, they are more perceptive to annoyances, and painful responses are more likely to be interpreted and expressed. Discomfort, a minor degree of pain, can often be relieved by nursing measures to promote relaxation. Headache is a classic example of pain that results from tension. Many analgesic medications are enhanced if they are combined with a muscle relaxant.

Threshold and tolerance

Pain is often described in terms of threshold and tolerance. The pain *threshold* refers to the intensity of a stimulus required to cause an individual to experience pain. *Tolerance* of pain is the point at which the individual reacts to the pain with verbal or other responses. No matter what the basic mechanism of the pain is, threshold is essentially the same. Carefully controlled studies have revealed no significant variations in pain threshold among women and men of any group, but considerable variations in their responses to the same painful stimuli.

Psychological, social, and cultural forces seem to affect some of the responses to pain. A multiplicity of ethnic and cultural learnings account for the wide variations in the actual response and expression of pain. For example, blacks and American Indians fail to react to noxious stimuli of intensity great enough to induce a reaction of discomfort in the average white person. Jewish clients tend to have excessive anxiety and worry about pain. Italians speak of it often but do not make an automatic association with illness. Irishmen tend to suffer alone and quietly. Researchers have found that attitudes about pain and reactions to it are acquired by individual members of an ethnocultural society and are derived from earliest childhood experiences in a primary family relationship. Although these may be superficially altered throughout later life by new learn-

Foundations of clinical practice

ings and social contacts, at a time of crisis, especially illness, the individual reverts to his earlier concepts of pain and reacts accordingly.

Types of pain   Intensity and duration of pain are two factors that influence description of pain as acute, chronic, or intractable. *Acute pain* is usually temporary and relieved by analgesia. Examples are trauma, surgery, or headache. *Chronic pain* is of longer duration and generally unresponsive to treatment.

In certain acute injuries and in some chronic illnesses the client may experience pain of such degree and duration that he becomes possessed solely by his agony. He lives from hour to hour focusing on pain, temporary relief, and the knowledge that the pain will return again, perhaps more terrifying than what is now experienced. This type of pain is in sharp contrast to that which follows surgery or minor injury, where improvement is gradual and complete freedom from pain is expected after a few days. Clients with pain as their primary nursing problem become exhausted from their constant bouts with one crisis after another. They face a helplessness and hopelessness that they alone can feel. They may actually express a desire for their life to end so that their suffering might be relieved. Families of such a client may share their wish for "the end."

Pain that cannot be successfully relieved by ordinary methods is called *intractable pain*. In situations where there is great pain of long duration, surgery may be indicated for relief. Certain pain-coordinating pathways are destroyed or divided, or other barriers to pain perception are created.

Referred pain occurs in an area other than that of the origin of pain impulses. Referred pain is usually precipitated by a disturbance in pain pathways.

Assessment   The expression of pain is highly individualized, and signs and symptoms vary with age and the ability to express it. When children are observed, the source of pain is sometimes difficult to determine because their responses may be generalized rather than specific. Adults may withhold or exaggerate their reaction to painful stimuli according to those present in their environment. If a portion of the body was previously damaged, resulting in loss or impairment of all sensation, pain in that region or part may be recognized as actually a very positive sign of recovery, and if it occurs, it is likely to be perceived quite vividly. Management of clients with any injury or illness is seriously complicated when they are unable to perceive, to interpret, or to express pain.

Although most clients will convey to the nurse that they are experiencing pain, there are others who will not verbalize the problem. The nurse should know how to recognize certain signs, symptoms, or behavioral mechanisms known to be indicative of pain.

Assessing infants and children. An infant expresses pain by crying louder and more sharply than normal for him. He may draw up his legs or double up the body to indicate torso pain. An older child may seem fretful and engage in random movement. Until the child can verbalize his complaint, someone else must interpret and manage his discomfort. It is helpful to look for simple explanations first, such as gastric dilatation, cold, wet diapers, hunger, or an open diaper pin, before assuming that medical intervention is indicated.

Older children seem to be distracted by pain and engage in random motion. They may groan or cry, hold their heads, pull their ears, or appear to be tense. They are often unable to localize their pain, especially if there is no obvious "hurt" such as cut or abrasion. As children grow older, they feel that they should react less to pain. Parents and nurses reinforce their feeling through comments.

"You're a big boy now. Big boys don't cry." Older children, especially, feel they should be strong and brave and not complain about hurting. Knowing that children have difficulty perceiving, interpreting, and expressing pain, the nurse should know objective physical signs that can indicate pain.

Superficial pain is often accompanied by a sympathetic response pattern. The peripheral blood flow is reduced and is sent to the vascular beds of large muscles. The blood pressure, pulse, and respirations increase, and the pupils may be dilated.

Pain from the viscera or other deep regions of the body is accompanied by decreased blood pressure, pulse, and respirations and an increase in visceral blood flow. Nausea, vomiting, and generalized weakness are not uncommon. Other signs of pain include increased perspiration, changes in body temperature, and muscle spasms.

Assessing adults. Adult responses to pain are usually more refined than those of children. They verbalize their perception of pain and can interpret its origin and its possible cause. Most adult clients see pain as a real threat to their safety and security, and thus its expression is likely to be highly tinged with anxiety and tension.

Nurses should know how to recognize the signs and symptoms of adult pain and not rely solely on the client's ability to verbalize it. A client may appear pale, perspiring, or restless and be twisting, turning, walking, or clenching his teeth. Facial grimaces are common. He may moan, groan, cry, or scream. One of the first indications of considerable discomfort may be that the client withdraws from people, interrupts his communications, or becomes abrupt in social mannerisms. If adults are hostile about their pain or want to displace part of their discomfort on others, they may curse, complain loudly, talk incessantly about their agony, or ask for help. If the pain has been anticipated, such as that after surgery, reactions are usually less than they would be if pain were not expected.

Data analysis   In both adults and children the nurse can note intensity, duration, and location of the pain. These data are essential to formulating nursing diagnoses such as alterations in comfort.

Planning and implementation   The nurse and client can plan to manage pain with a variety of interventions. These may include administering analgesics, biofeedback and relaxation, electrical stimulation, or use of comfort measures such as repositioning, massage, distraction, or promoting bowel or bladder elimination.

Nurses should not attempt to judge whether or not the client is in "real pain" because it is well known that much of his pain is determined by unique experiences of a biosocial orientation and may not depend on an objective set of circumstances. If a client states that he is in pain, then he should be cared for accordingly.

A careful analysis of an individual client's pain cycle and his response to medication and other modes of intervention should be done, however, because valuable intrinsic clues may be gathered. Does pain always occur during or after a visit by a certain person? Does it occur after a specific activity? Does pain occur at bedtime? How is the pain expressed or described? How quickly is relief obtained by a particular agent?

Nurses caring for those in pain should be observant, take time to care in other ways than merely giving medications, and constantly remind themselves that only the person who has the pain can truly evaluate it as a total physical and emotional experience. Pain perception, interpretation, and coping methods must be intimately shared by nurses and their clients.

Pharmacological intervention. Analgesics are drugs that relieve pain by action on the central nervous system. They interfere with the transmission of painful stimuli from peripheral areas or alter perception at the cerebral level. The choice and use of analgesics depend on the site, quality, nature, and intensity of pain.

Narcotics alter the emotional component of a painful experience. Pain is still perceived but not as an unbearable experience. In fact, a genuine sense of well-being may be evident. Nurses should understand the various potencies, onset and duration of action, side effects, and addiction potential of narcotics that they administer. It is important to note that pain sometimes requires a potent analgesic, and the fear of addiction should not impede the use of a narcotic drug.

Milder analgesics that possess antipyretic and antiinflammatory actions as well as analgesia are widely used. They are thought to prevent mediation of painful stimuli by chemical action at the site. Although these agents are not addicting, some do possess potentially dangerous side effects and, like all medications, should be managed judiciously if given over an extended period of time.

Biofeedback and relaxation. Biofeedback is useful in the management of specific types of pain, especially chronic pain. Biofeedback incorporates attaching a monitoring device to the client that emits a continuous visual or audible signal whenever there are brainwave changes. Such signaled changes, when the client becomes aware of them, may be used to gain an appreciation of parameters that influence physiological states. These data can be used later by the client to control such parameters and consequently to control unwanted functions that are associated with them.

Alpha wave training has been used to manage chronic pain. For instance, when one is relaxed, alpha waves are predominant and indicate a peaceful state. When clients are given a monitoring device that transmits a signal to them when they have increased their alpha wave activity through self-mediated tactics, they are given feedback that can be employed to further control a given parameter. In summary, the concentration on this restful state distracts the clients from pain, promotes relaxation, and essentially gives them control over their pain. Persons can also be trained to control muscle spasm and tension, and the technique has been very beneficial for the treatment of migraine headaches.

Electrical stimulation. Electrical stimulation can relieve pain by blocking pain impulses through stimulating the gating mechanism. An electrical charge is delivered through surface electrodes, causing a buzzing sensation directly over a painful area or adjacent to a peripheral nerve pathway. (The technique can also be accomplished by percutaneous stimulation that employs implanted needles.) After initial controlled clinical experience with the device, the client selects the amount of current to be delivered to a given site for relief. A dorsal column stimulator is an example of a useful application of electricity for pain management.

Hypnosis. Hypnosis (or hypnotic conditioning) can be a useful adjunct in pain management and reduction of tension. It is thought that its success results from the blocking of afferent pain impulses and the inhibition of higher cortical centers; therefore, pain is not perceived consciously. Some theorists also believe that sensory threshold may be raised or a degree of amnesia produced. Hypnosis is used in conjunction with other modes of pain management and is not used alone.

Other approaches. There are certain chemical and surgical approaches that are useful in the control of periodic, low-intensity pain that is unpleasant or unacceptable to the client. Such intractable episodes of pain are virtually impossible to relieve by ordinary means. Intractable pain is usually the result of nervous system dysfunction, carcinoma, ischemia, and selected degenerative disorders. The two most common surgical procedures are cordotomy and rhizotomy.

Cordotomy is a surgical procedure in which the fibers of the lateral spinothalamic tract are divided to avoid transmission of impulses related to pain and temperature to a selected portion of the body. It is usually accomplished by a laminectomy. The spinous processes and laminae directly above the cordotomy site are removed, and the dura mater is incised to permit cutting of the appropriate tract. Before conclusion of the surgical process, the client is usually awakened to assess the adequacy of results, and if necessary the division is enlarged.

A cordotomy may also be accomplished percutaneously in clients too ill for a laminectomy, which requires an anesthetic. Spinal needles are inserted into the anterolateral tract, and the tract is coagulated using diathermy. Cordotomy is used most often for pain relief in the trunk and legs.

Complications of the procedure include weakness of the affected side because of pyramidal tract damage, transient urinary retention, and sexual impotence. Paralysis may result, too, but this is considered a rare complication.

Rhizotomy is a division of anterior or posterior spinal nerve roots between the ganglion and the cord for abolition of related pain-producing sensory modalities. The procedure is accomplished with a laminectomy. Anterior (motor) rhizotomy is reserved for paraplegic and quadriplegic clients who have painful spasm or paralyzed extremities because of mass flexor reflexes. Posterior (sensory) rhizotomy eliminates pain in a designated area, but at the expense of the loss of all motor functioning. Because there is extensive overlapping of dermatome segments, considerable sectioning must be done in adjacent areas to ensure relief of pain.

The most successful rhizotomies seem to be those used in managing malignancies of the head and neck and in the treatment of tic douloureux (see Chapter 10).

Nerve blocks involve the injection of a local anesthetic, such as lidocaine (Xylocaine) or procaine (Novocain), or alcohol, close to nerve trunks to relieve the discomfort related to inflammations and spasms associated with the nerve injury. Alcohol may be used to treat the painful spasms that occur with conditions such as multiple sclerosis, but because alcohol destroys nerve fibers, it is used primarily for peripheral blocks.

Neurectomy is the division of cranial or peripheral nerves in order to eliminate localized pain, especially pain resulting from vascular occlusions in the lower extremities. A *sympathectomy* is a surgical procedure that interrupts afferent pathways in the sympathetic portion of the nervous system. Sympathectomy eliminates vasospasm, and this enhances peripheral blood supply.

There are also some neurosurgical procedures directed at modifying the affective component of pain. Among these are *lobotomy* and *thalamotomy*. The latter is the most successful, it seems, but it is still reserved for terminally ill clients because it alters the personality. Thalamotomy involves the implantation of electrodes via burr holes into the thalamic nuclei. After correct placement is assured, the area is stimulated and thermocoagulated to accomplish the destruction of tissue specifically responsible for pain perception.

Acupuncture is a process that incorporates the insertion of needles into selected body sites to relieve forces that cause disease and pain. Acupuncture is of Asian origin but has recently gained the attention of the Western world. Ancient Chinese believed that there are two life forces called *yin* and *yang* and that disharmony of these forces caused disease and pain. Needle insertion at specific points helps the two forces reestablish harmony, thus relieving uncomfortable symptoms. It is greatly disputed whether the basis for acupuncture's effectiveness is organic or psychological. However, when one considers referred pain to distant sites, it is logical to assume that stimulation at one site could create an effect at another. The search to find the key to this ancient but promising mode of relieving pain is ongoing.

LOSS OR ALTERATION OF A BODY PART

Clients who face loss or alteration of a body part, whether it be a part of the musculoskeletal system, viscera, or neurosensory mechanism, must adjust to a new body image incorporating the particular loss or alteration. The ability of a person to adapt to a new physical image depends on his own inherited capacities for adjustment accumulated through previous life experiences and is undoubtedly much affected by his environment at the times before and immediately after such a loss or alteration.

Throughout the process of growth and development, humans develop a feeling about their bodies, called a *body image*. This image, which is integrally related to self-concept, is formulated from actual visual and tactile experiences that indicate the appearance of the body and its ability to function, from internalized psychological processes and sociological factors or reactions of others about the body, and from attitudes toward the body derived from experiences, perceptions, comparisons, and identifications with bodies of others. Thus the self-concept is made up of psychological, sociocultural, physiological, and physical perceptions.

When one loses the use of a limb through paralysis or amputation or encounters a critical neurosensory loss such as blindness, he is termed *disabled* by many. However, the extent to which his handicap impairs his work productivity or socialization processes is largely the result of his own feeling of self-worth.

Any change in body image imposed by a loss or alteration of a body part requires that the individual adapt to a new body image that incorporates the change. If one has a limb amputated or loses movement and sensation in an extremity, he must reestablish a new picture of himself, incorporating the negative value into his self-concept. Nurses should be cautious, however, during this process of adjusting to a new body image. One must refrain from referring to a paralyzed extremity as the "bad arm" or "bad leg" or to the functionally intact part as the "good arm" or "good leg." Any part that is innately attached to the core of the human body is viewed as an asset by the client, and it is intolerable for him to hear others judge some integral part of him as "bad," hence, useless and undesirable. Words such as *affected* or *unaffected* are suggested as alternate terms to differentiate parts of the injured or ill body.

Strategies for coping with loss or alteration of a body part are discussed where appropriate throughout the text.

246

**ADMINISTRATION OF
MEDICATION, INTRAVENOUS
FLUIDS, AND BLOOD**
Administration of medication

Hospitalized clients frequently receive medication, intravenous fluids, and blood. Special strategies for administration of these may be necessary, since the client's age and developmental skills require adaptations to procedures.

Administration to infants and children. The administration of medications to infants and children is an extremely important nursing procedure. It is essential that dosages be accurately calculated, measured, and administered. Children's responses and tolerances to medications vary considerably and are dependent to a large extent on body mass and physiological maturity.

Age and body weight have a definite relationship to (1) the quantity of fluid available to dilute and transport the drug and (2) the mass of target body tissues to which the drug is distributed. *The greater the relative concentration of a drug in fluid or tissue, the more potent its effect will be.* This fact, along with factors such as general physical condition and immaturity of certain physiological mechanisms in very young children (for example, the inefficiency of the kidneys and liver in detoxifying and excreting drugs), makes it necessary to be extra cautious in administering medications to very young and debilitated clients.

Pediatric doses are often calculated on the basis of body surface, using established formulas. Although the physician is responsible for this initial determination, the nurse should check the prescription to validate that it is within the usual limits before administering. Many pediatricians rely on data established by pharmaceutical companies that supply the various drugs, realizing that their recommendations for dosage have been carefully established for the specific agent by clinical experimentation. Pediatric dosage formulas are, at best, merely guidelines.

Three common formulas are used for calculating doses for infants and children. Clark's rule is based on body weight:

$$\frac{\text{Weight in pounds} \times \text{Adult dose}}{150} = \text{Child's approximate dose}$$

Fried's rule for infant dosage is based on age:

$$\frac{\text{Age in months} \times \text{Adult dose}}{150} = \text{Infant's approximate dose}$$

Clark's rule for child's dosage is also based on age:

$$\frac{\text{Age in years} \times \text{Adult dose}}{\text{Age} + 12} = \text{Child's approximate dose}$$

Many authorities believe that calculations based on body surface, however, are generally more reliable than those using age or weight for dose determination (see Fig. 16-2). There are several published tables that may be employed to verify safe and effective therapeutic levels for clients with various physical characteristics.

Nurses must realize that administering medications to children requires special understanding about how the recipient perceives the total experience of illness or hospitalization. The manner in which the child is approached and dealt with in this one element of care helps formulate attitudes about nurses and medications in general, which may affect all other elements of care. A trusting relationship will facilitate the administration of drugs, and a calm but assertive manner is usually advisable. The nurse should convey to the child that he must take his medicine, but coaxing and bargaining should be avoided. Explanations and instructions about the importance of the medication are advisable if the client is capable of understanding them. The young client should be permitted to express his feelings before and after administration is accomplished and should be praised for cooperation. Play therapy may be a beneficial adjunct in eliciting trust and alleviating fear about medications, particularly injections.

The administration of medications to children is a complicated responsibility and should not be assumed alone by the inexperienced nurse. A great many agencies require the validation of dosage by two registered nurses before certain preparations, such as narcotics, cardiotonics, insulin, or vasopressors, are given. Whenever a question of dosage arises, another nurse or the physician should be consulted before administration. Since children are often unable to perceive side effects or communicate them, they may fail to readily exhibit characteristic signs of overdosage. The nurse must be alert to such adverse responses and report them at once, since the physiological mechanisms of the young client are generally less capable of making adjustments in crises.

Oral route. Although parenteral medications have a more predictable pattern of therapeutic value, oral medications, especially flavored liquids, are preferred because they are more easily administered with a cup, spoon, straw, or calibrated medicine dropper.

Oral dosages of liquid preparations should always be measured by a recognized standard measure. Minute doses may require utilization of a tuberculin syringe to ensure accuracy. Small quantities may be mixed with glucose and water to facilitate administration and to ensure a volume large enough for accurate dispensing. It is not advisable to disguise medicine in a child's favorite food, since it may alienate him from both the food and the medicine. Similarly, milk and formula should not be used as vehicles for drugs. In addition to certain preparations making milk products unpalatable, the efficacy of the drug may also be altered. Furthermore, if only a portion of a feeding is accomplished, there is uncertainty about the amount of drug actually ingested.

The head and shoulders of a child should be elevated before oral administration of medication is attempted. Infants reflexly swallow liquids that are placed well back on their tongue, but older children may be more resistant to taking medicine. The nurse should allow the child time to take the preparation slowly. Forcing a young client to take too large a quantity at once or holding his nose or mouth shut to force swallowing communicates hostility from the nurse rather than a helping, comforting attitude. More important, however, is that such injudicious practices may lead to gagging, choking, spitting, or even aspiration.

Oral medicines may be self-administered under supervision if the child is old enough to feed himself. This practice seems to reduce the threat inherent in the imposition of outside force to accomplish the therapeutic procedure and increases the child's sense of responsibility related to his health care.

Parenteral route. Parenteral routes are the most reliable but offer a number of problems in administration. For example, there is the trauma of the needle puncture, the chance of a local reaction, or in the case of some, the risk of sciatic nerve palsy.

Injections are extremely anxiety provoking for most children; the nurse should be prepared to carry out the procedure quickly after explanations are completed. Occasionally, a second person must be at hand to assist the nurse in positioning, supporting, or restraining the child.

8 Nursing and the hospitalized client

The site of injection varies with the age and size of the child and his muscle mass. The thigh is the preferred site for the very young client. The buttocks and deltoid areas are reserved for older children with considerable muscle development. Preferred sites for intramuscular injections are noted in Fig. 8-8; no more than 1 ml of solution should be injected in one site if the muscle mass is small (infants, young children).

FIG. 8-8
A, Method of bracing a child for an injection. Note that stability is achieved by (1) positioning the client near the edge of the bed, thus bracing him against the nurse's body and (2) firmly fixing the left arm on the bed surface while holding it securely against the child. **B** to **E,** Common sites for injections, with emphasis on important anatomical landmarks. **B,** Dorsal-gluteal. **C,** Ventral-gluteal. **D,** Vastus lateralis. **E,** Anterior thigh and deltoid sites.

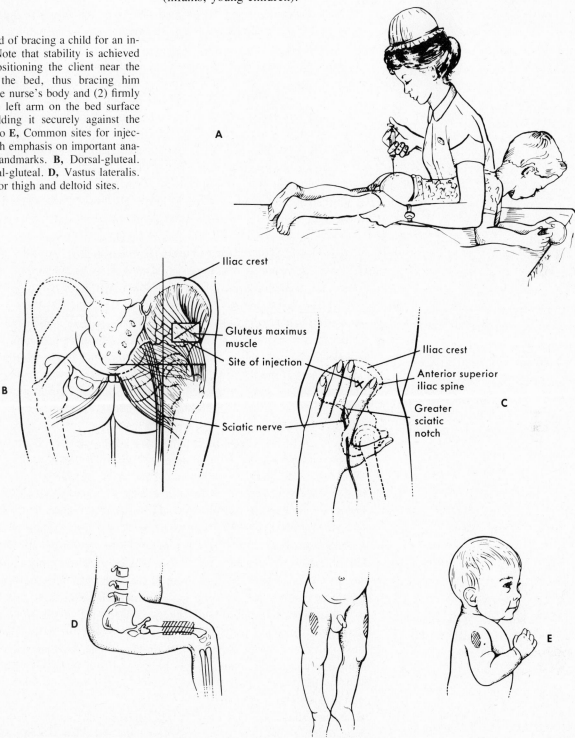

249

Foundations of clinical practice

Administration to older adults. Older adults require special consideration when medications are administered.[2] In aging, changes in physiology can affect the absorption, distribution, metabolism, and excretion of drugs. Generally speaking, these processes are slower and less efficient with advanced age; therefore, it should be recognized that clinical results of drug therapy will be variable and there may be delayed absorption and reduced peak levels of drugs.

Gastrointestinal absorption of medications is influenced by digestive enzymes, gastrointestinal motility, intestinal blood flow, and the number of absorbing cells that are operant. All these factors may be reduced with aging, and thus it is nearly impossible to determine the amount of medication that will actually reach the target cells. Circulation not only affects the distribution of the drug but influences metabolism and excretion as well, especially if the liver and kidneys are essentially involved. Liver enzyme activity is decreased, causing a prolonged half-life of certain drugs, with concomitant increase of plasma levels. Fat distribution, fluid compartment capacity, and protein-binding potential change with advancing age and affect how the agent is localized and metabolized, too. Loss of efficiency of cellular processes in the liver and kidneys may impair detoxification and excretion of drugs, resulting in serious accumulations within certain body tissues and unpredictable levels of therapy.

Nurses should be aware of the normal biological changes that accompany aging and be prepared to make adjustments in nursing care practices. For example, most elderly clients tend to be dehydrated; thus cellular drug levels become concentrated, inviting toxicity. It is imperative that fluids be given freely with medications and throughout the day.

Enteric-coated drugs should *not* be crushed to ease administration, since such agents are pharmacologically compounded to be absorbed in the intestine's alkaline media, not the acid media of the stomach. This erroneous practice creates chemical irritation to the delicate lining of the stomach and additionally affects the drug's solubility, ionization, and ultimate rate of absorption. If the client cannot swallow enteric-coated preparations, another form of the drug should be obtained.

Certain drugs, such as barbiturates and adrenergic blocking agents, often become concentrated in body fat since they are lipid-soluble agents. This fact, of course, affects the drug's duration of action. Since percentages of body fat increase substantially in aging (40% to 50%), there may be serious problems in controlling the activity duration of lipid-soluble medications.

Protein-binding capacities decrease with aging, too, because of a decrease in the amount and quality of plasma protein. Therefore, drugs may not be bound on a predictable basis (making them inactive until released from binding); thus there is more *free* active drug present in the body than with a younger adult. Again, the concerns for adverse drug accumulations and toxicity are valid.

Metabolism is responsible for limiting a drug's activity and preparing it for elimination. Since liver cells and kidneys lose efficiency in aging, drug metabolism and excretion may be altered, permitting higher cellular and circulating levels to remain in the body. It may be judicious for clinicians who prescribe drugs for the elderly to systematically reduce drug dosages from those typically employed for younger adults.

Nurses should be alert to preventing and detecting adverse drug reactions in the older persons. Some of the earliest signs and symptoms of toxicity may be behavior changes and alterations in the level of mental functioning. Fatigue, restlessness, irritability, headache, dizziness, stupor, confusion, and weakness may be indicative of a problem and should not be ignored as a typical "senile" response of the aged. Toxic compounds penetrate the blood-brain barrier more easily in the older client, and thus the brain is less capable of defending itself against noxious overdoses. This fact, coupled with less efficient cerebral blood flow and metabolism, renders the brain of the elderly especially vulnerable to toxic insults. Unfortunately, for some clients, mental symptoms are managed by even another drug, thus compounding the problem and in some cases actually inducing "iatrogenic senility."

Nurses should assist in the maintenance of a drug profile for all clients so that there is a visible guideline indicating the type, dose, and administration schedule of every agent, both prescribed and over-the-counter medications. If clients self-medicate, counseling and guidance are crucial so that there is clarity regarding all factors of drug therapy that are pertinent to them. Nurses should remember that most older adults are managing multiple health problems and may be consuming a multiplicity of agents at any one time. It is therefore essential to be knowledgeable about iatrogenic and adverse reactions of drugs and about the signs and symptoms of overdose and toxicity complications.

Disease caused by drug interactions. An increasing number of serious clinical disorders have been attributed to the adverse interaction of two or more drugs in the body. The wise use of many potent agents for management of complex problems, clients going to more than one physician or pharmacist, or self-medication without medical supervision are common causes of *drug interactions. Iatrogenic* disease (abnormal states caused by inadvertent, erroneous treatment by a physician) may also occur. Considerable research is being done regarding how one medication can enhance or interfere with another. Utilization of computer recall of drug interactions is being studied as a practical means of cross-checking every client's medications and their potential interactions. Individual record cards in a central data bank may soon be a reality to monitor possible interactions or unintentional duplication in therapy.

There are numerous ways in which drugs can enhance or interfere with one another. Some drugs create electrolyte imbalances that alter expected actions, and others interfere with the urinary excretion of another agent. Occasionally enzymatic inhibitory responses occur, altering the normal metabolism of agents given concurrently. Remaining interaction phenomena involve photodynamic reactions, tissue displacement, and interactions with hormones, food items, and environmental contaminants.

Nurses should be aware of drug interactions and know that an important part of every nursing assessment is consideration of any and all medications that the client may take. *Age* is a factor, since the very young and the very old have decreased ability to metabolize or excrete drugs. *Body temperature* is an important element because pyrexia increases biochemical reactions of a multiple and unpredictable nature. Certain *illnesses* and *altered nutritional states* tend to affect metabolism and increase sensitivity to drugs. Even *obesity* can change the distribution and effect of selected agents. Although nurses do not prescribe therapy, they are expected to assume responsibility in the administration of agents, which necessitates some awareness of drug interactions and biological factors that influence response to various medicines.

Foundations of clinical practice

Alcohol potentiates many drugs, including ataractics, barbiturates, and antihistamines. Barbiturates inhibit antihistamines, anticoagulants, hypnotics, phenytoin (Dilantin), and steroids but enhance monoamine oxidase (MAO) inhibitors. Antacids interfere with many agents, including tetracyclines, sulfonamides, penicillin G, nitrofurantoin (Furadantin), nalidixic acid (NegGram), and anticoagulants. The actions of MAO inhibitors can drastically alter blood pressure in the presence of other drugs and even foods such as selected cheeses and wines. Thiazide diuretics potentiate the action of digitalis and muscle relaxants because they induce hypokalemia; in the presence of phenothiazines, they may produce shock. Steroids should always be considered *contraindicated* in the presence of live viral vaccines. They also create adrenal insufficiency and must not be suddenly withdrawn for surgery or substitute-drug therapy, since the body could not immediately cope physiologically with stress.

Obviously this is not an exhaustive account of the effect of selected drugs on each other but merely provides examples of why it is important for clients to be carefully taught about combining various agents in a self-administered regimen, especially nonprescription items. Persons who keep partially used medications from a previous illness, those who go from physician to physician, and those not under careful medical supervision are likely to be victims of drug interactions.

Intravenous additives in various combinations may induce serious drug interactions. Great care should be exercised in mixing all fluids. Since some agents change chemically as soon as they come in contact with another, nurses must watch for precipitates or changes in the characteristics of fluids. If any appear, the infusion should be discarded, and the physician or pharmacist consulted. Caution must be used in following additive instructions provided with the drugs by their respective manufacturers.

Administration of intravenous fluids

Intravenous fluids may be used to replace fluid loss or to administer electrolytes, medication, or blood. As with any procedure, before the infusion is initiated, the client should be made comfortable, and the rationale for the therapy should be explained. It is important to be thorough enough with details that the recipient knows what is to be expected. For example, the limitations imposed by the infusion, such as restriction of activity and the importance of positioning, should be understood so that cooperative behavior of the client can be obtained. Since many, especially the elderly, seem to believe that "feeding through the veins" is a procedure reserved for dire illness or used as a last-resort measure, care should be exercised to explain the purpose and value of this therapy.

An infusion must be ordered by the physician, but the actual procedure may be started by a nurse, a fluid therapy team, or by the physician who ordered it. The usual routine for any medication order should be adhered to. Caution should be used in regard to the condition of the fluid and container. The fluid must be clear and free from any visible foreign material, and the seal must be examined to note its condition. If any question exists regarding the condition of the fluid or the sterility of the infusion set, they should not be used. The label should be compared with the order, for accuracy, and the client identified before the procedure is initiated. If medications or electrolytes are added, the container should be labeled to indicate the name and amount of additives. *There is no margin for error in infusion, since the fluid and medications are directly introduced into the bloodstream and their effects are immediate.* Allergies to antibiotics or sensitivities to any foreign substances should provoke due concern and attendant scrutiny.

The infused fluid is selected based on its composition as a therapeutic agent and a vehicle for transporting pharmaceuticals (Table 8-6).

Before the infusion is begun, it is desirable for the client to be weighed and placed on an intake-and-output regimen. If the client does not have an indwelling catheter, output must be collected and measured or estimated. Linen or diapers may be weighed to evaluate fluid losses for incontinent persons.

TABLE 8-6
Composition of commonly used intravenous solutions

Solution	Properties (mEq/L)						Per liter		Common uses and precautions
	pH	Na$^+$	K$^+$	Ca^{++}	Cl$^-$	HCl$_3^-$	Cal	g CHO	
Dextrose in water									Provides calories and water without
2.5%	3.5 to 6.5						100	25	electrolytes
5.0%							200	50	
10.0%							400	100	Used in hydration
20.0%							800	200	Concentrated solutions should be
50.0%							2.000	500	administered only through a
									large-bore catheter
Saline									
Half normal 0.45%	4.5 to 7.0	77			77				Hypotonic solutions provide excess
Isotonic 0.9%		154			154				of free water
Hypertonic 3.0%		513			513				Hypertonic solutions treat Na$^+$
5.0%		855			855				deficits, especially those related
									to renal insufficiency
Dextrose in saline									
2.5% in 0.45%		77			77		100	25	Provides calories and electrolytes to
5.0% in 0.45%		77			77		200	50	prevent protein substances from
2.5% in 0.9%		154			154		100	25	being used to provide energy
5.0% in 0.9%		154			154		200	50	
Ringer's lactate (Hartmann's solution)	6.0 to 7.5	130	4	3	112	28	9		Increases interstitial fluid pressure and maintains volume during surgery and in shock
									May cause pulmonary edema
									Use blood filter
Plasma		135 to 150	3.5 to 5.0		98 to 106	22 to 30			Same osmolality as blood
									Will not produce electrolyte changes
									Used in hypovolemic shock and for exchange transfusions in hepatic coma
									May cause hepatitis
									Use blood filter
Dextran	4.0 to 5.0								Osmotically active
									Used in shock management to expand volume
									Decrease blood viscosity
									Increase peripheral flow
									May cause pulmonary edema from acute volume overloading or renal tubule obstruction
									Use blood filter
Normal human serum albumin									Markedly hypertonic
									Used to treat edema states
									May cause pulmonary edema or gastrointestinal bleeding by rapidly increasing central venous pressure
									Use blood filter

Foundations of clinical practice

Selecting site for infusion. The infusion site is selected by the location and condition of veins, the purpose of the infusion, the expected duration of therapy, and the comfort of the client. If possible, an easily visible vein that is large and straight is preferred. It is desirable to avoid, for example, the right hand or arm if the client is right-handed. The antecubital fossa or wrist sites are not used if other locations are feasible, since these areas would create the necessity of immobilizing the arm in order to prevent extravasation or kinking of the catheter. Lower extremities are used as a last resort, since they tend to produce more complications, especially thrombi and pulmonary emboli, than the upper extremities. It is also more difficult to expose lower extremity sites for continuous observations. Mobility is an important consideration if the therapy is prolonged, since inability to move joints may create pain and stiffness. The ideal site in infants is a superficial scalp vein. The umbilical vein may be another valuable infusion point for neonates during the first 2 or 3 days of life.

If sclerosing or irritating drugs are to be administered or if the solution is hypertonic, it is important to select a large vein with sufficient volume to rapidly dilute the substances being infused, thus lessening local trauma.

Large central veins are chosen for hyperalimentation or for measuring the central venous pressure (CVP). The basilic, subclavian, and jugular veins are frequently employed for central venous catheterization.

Selecting infusion apparatus. There are four basic types of needles and catheters for intravenous infusions: (1) the metal needle, including scalp vein (butterfly) needles; (2) metal needles with mounted plastic catheter (angiocatheter); (3) an inlying catheter for surgical entry into the vein, such as venesection or cutdown; and (4) the intracatheter, a plastic catheter threaded through a needle.

A butterfly is useful for short-term therapy in small veins. Angiocatheters and intracatheters are preferred if mobility is desired or if therapy is expected to be of long duration. Large-bore devices are used if blood or colloids are to be administered. Venesections with inlying catheters (sutured in place) are reserved for clients who are having surgery or intensive care, usually when regular venipunctures are unsuccessful because of shock and collapsed peripheral veins.

Venipuncture technique. The nurse should explain the procedure to the client and ensure comfort during the venipuncture (Fig. 8-9). The fluid and additives should be checked against the orders, and labels should be prepared. It is the nurse's responsibility to assist in site selection, to position the extremity, and to apply immobilization devices, even if the actual venipuncture is accomplished by a technician.

The site is aseptically prepared. Cold or rapidly evaporating substances (such as alcohol) should be avoided; they cause local vasoconstriction because of the skin's reaction to the temperature change induced by the evaporation.

The vein can be distended for entry in several ways. The most frequently employed device is a tourniquet. Heat applications above and below the site, allowing the extremity to hang in a dependent position, or light slapping of the area will enhance dilation. Clients should be instructed to "make a fist" and to repeatedly open and close their hand until vein entry is accomplished. (Some clinicians use a local anesthesia wheal of a substance such as 1% lidocaine [Xylocaine] hydrochloride to reduce the pain of venipuncture.)

The tubing should be flushed and all air eliminated from the line before the

FIG. 8-9
Venipuncture with a steel needle. **A,** Tension of the thumb distal to the site of venipuncture stretches the skin and stabilizes the vein. The nurse inserts the needle, attached to a syringe, through the skin adjacent to the vein and, **B,** holds the needle at a little less than a 45-degree angle for penetration of the skin. When the needle enters the vein, the bevel is rotated to prevent puncture of the posterior wall of the vessel. **C,** The needle and syringe are lowered nearly parallel to the skin for advancement into the vein. (From Dison, Norma: Clinical nursing techniques, ed. 4, St. Louis, 1979, The C.V. Mosby Co.)

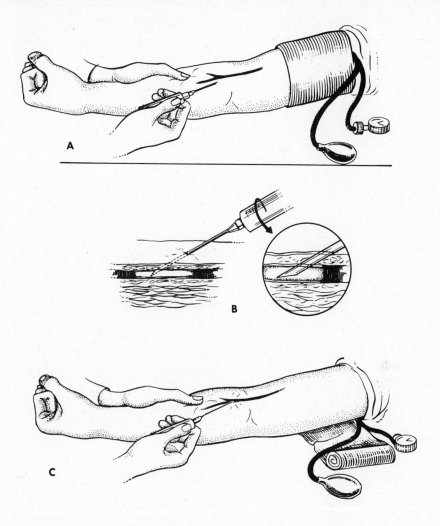

puncture is made since, as soon as the vein is entered, the tourniquet must be released and the infusion tubing attached. As soon as a patent flow is ensured, all connections in the tubing and needle or catheter device should be secured with tape. The type and size of the needle should be noted on the tape. The site of entry should be cleansed and dressed with a small sterile gauze square. It is not essential or desirable to place large, bulky dressings over the site. Such dressings impede observation and may obscure problems such as fluid leakage or bleeding. If an arm board is required, it must be applied securely but not in a way to impede circulation or obstruct view of the venipuncture site (Fig. 8-10). Undue motion can result in the needle's puncturing the wall of the vein and creating infiltration and phlebitis. Any accompanying restraint is applied to the board and not directly to the extremity, since it could impede flow. Since solu-

FIG. 8-10
Arm board used to stabilize venipuncture. (From Budassi, Susan, and Barber, Janet: Emergency nursing: principles and practice, St. Louis, 1981, The C.V. Mosby Co.)

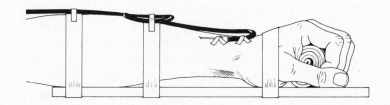

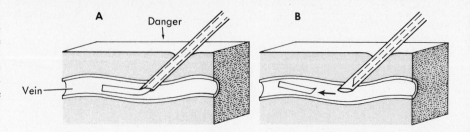

tions infuse by gravity, the container must be positioned at a height sufficient to maintain a steady flow.

Preventing local complications, especially phlebitis, is an important consideration. Besides careful technique in initiation of the infusion, some institutions insist that daily inspection, cleansing, and redressing of the site be done to reduce the possibility of local inflammation. Intravenous solutions, especially glucose, tend to serve as a culture medium; and when they have been opened for a prolonged period of time, they become a potential source of organism growth. Extended therapy regimens are also responsible for some inflammatory responses. It is advisable to change the tubing and the infusion fluid containers at 24-hour intervals and even the site in some instances.

Termination of infusions should include five essential steps: (1) stop the solution flow by clamping the tubing, (2) remove tape and splinting or restraining devices, (3) hold a sterile, dry sponge over the needle site and withdraw the needle, moving it parallel to the skin to avoid puncture trauma, (4) apply pressure, but do not massage the area until any bleeding or fluid seepage has stopped, and (5) record the amount absorbed and the time and reason for termination.

Special caution should be exercised when removing an intracatheter. The needle and the catheter must be removed as a unit. Merely grasping the needle may sever the intracatheter, releasing a portion of the plastic into circulation. Obviously this would be a life-threatening complication (Fig. 8-11).

Special points in nursing management

Heparin lock. The heparin lock is a valuable device for the intermittent administration of intravenous drugs. Previously, these periodic dosages required a keep-open intravenous infusion, which restricted the client's mobility. The heparin lock, a simple method of ensuring a patent intravenous route, was developed to circumvent problems associated with long-term infusions, which were often maintained solely to keep open an intravenous route for medication administration.

The heparin lock (Fig. 8-12) consists of a 19- to 21-gauge scalp vein needle attached to 3- or 4-inch tubing that ends with a rubber diaphragm instead of an infusion tubing connector. Because the diaphragm seals after each injection, the route is maintained for future use merely by keeping the line filled with a heparinized solution.

The site of choice for a heparin lock is the forearm, since it permits maximum client mobility without a splint or armboard. The area is prepared with a surgical scrub, and a tourniquet is applied. A 25-gauge needle is placed into the diaphragm to permit blood to enter the line during vein entry. Venipuncture is accomplished in the usual manner. When blood appears in the tubing, the tourniquet is released, and the wings of the scalp vein are secured to the skin. A hep-

FIG. 8-12
Heparin lock. (Courtesy Abbott Laboratories.)

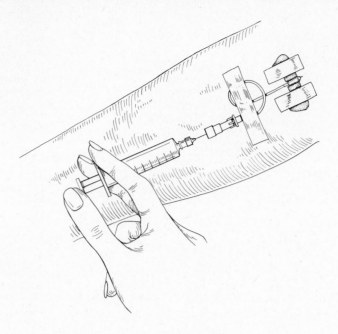

arinized solution is then injected into the diaphragm until all blood is displaced, and then the needle is removed. A small sterile dressing is applied, and the tubing is secured with tape.

After the intravenous drugs are injected (or diluted and infused), the line is refilled with the heparinized solution. The lock may usually be left in place up to 2 weeks without local complications developing. No bleeding tendencies are expected, since the total volume of heparin is so small. However, the presence of the lock must be considered when clotting studies are interpreted.

The client should be instructed to keep the dressing dry over the site and to protect it from external pressure or trauma. The lock must be inspected frequently to ascertain that hematoma, phlebitis, and infiltration are not occurring.

It is important to treat the heparin lock with the same respect as other intravenous infusions to prevent complications that are associated with the administration of intravenous fluids and medications.

Intravenous fluid filters. Intravenous fluid filters may be employed proximal to the venipuncture site to trap particulate matter that could be present in the infusing fluid. Small particles may develop from a variety of sources, such as (1) incompletely dissolved drugs, (2) crystals or precipitates from drug admixtures, (3) glass from ampules, and (4) rubber, plastic, or glass particles from the infusion apparatus. It is desirable that such matter be prevented from entering the bloodstream. Furthermore, some devices have membrane filters capable of trapping microorganisms. However, since pore size is so small, a pump may be necessary to propel intravenous fluid through the filter membrane (Fig. 8-13).

Blood, emulsions, suspensions, and blood fractions must bypass the filter by a Y tube, since they would clog the filter. Most fluid therapy apparatus are designed to facilitate this adaptation with ease.

Intravenous fluid filters must be primed during the tube-flushing routine before administration. The presence of a filter should not alter flow rate unless it becomes clogged with particulate matter. In these instances, it should be re-

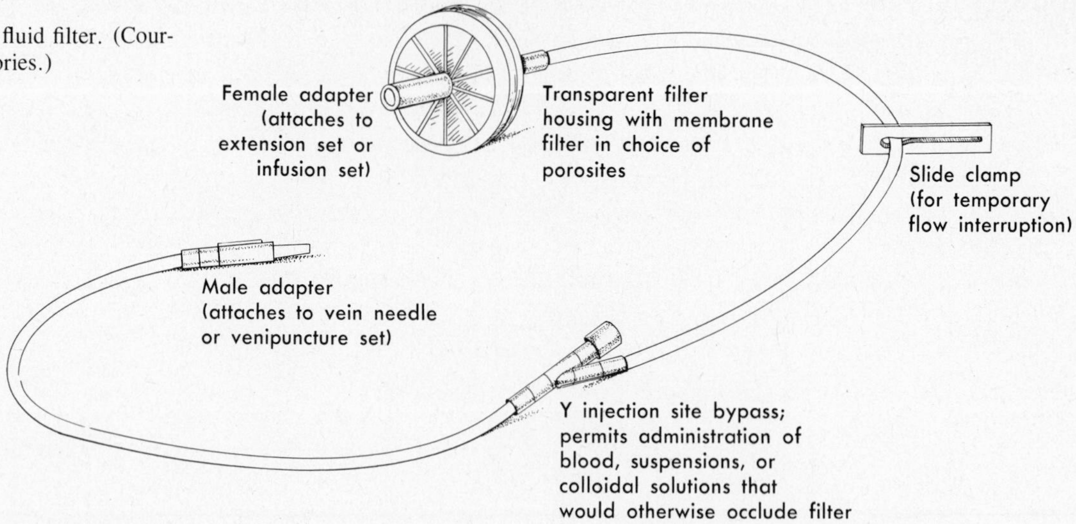

FIG. 8-13
Typical intravenous fluid filter. (Courtesy Abbott Laboratories.)

Female adapter
(attaches to
extension set or
infusion set)

Transparent filter
housing with membrane
filter in choice of
porosites

Slide clamp
(for temporary
flow interruption)

Male adapter
(attaches to vein needle
or venipuncture set)

Y injection site bypass;
permits administration of
blood, suspensions, or
colloidal solutions that
would otherwise occlude filter

moved and replaced promptly. Priming should be repeated after replacement to ensure that all air is expelled from the line. If air does enter the line and accumulate on the filter surface, it will block fluid flow. This air may be aspirated from the line through the medication port or rubber diaphragm in the tubing. However, it is recommended that not more than 2 ml be aspirated at any time, since excessive aspiration would create a reflux of blood at the underside of the filter, which would obstruct flow by clogging the membrane.

The use of intravenous fluid filters may be governed by institutional policy guidelines or may be the prerogative of the nurse or technician initiating fluid therapy. Generally, they should be used if (1) additives to infusions are obtained from glass ampules, (2) frequent use is made of medication ports or rubber diaphragms to gain access to the line, and (3) there is considerable potential of infusion phlebitis or accidental introduction of bacterial contaminants. Administration of certain drugs may also make the use of a filter an important consideration in fluid therapy. For example, cephalothin (Keflin) undergoes certain chemical changes if the pH of the infusion fluid is low (such as 5.0 for 5% dextrose in water), and an insoluble substance is produced. If a filter is used to trap this insoluble material, it must be checked frequently, since it will eventually become clogged.

Most manufacturers of intravenous fluid filters recommend that they be changed every 24 hours, even if they are functioning properly.

Flow rate. The flow rate must be determined when the infusion is initiated and then must be monitored carefully. It is one of the most important considerations in safe fluid therapy.

The physician generally orders the flow rate, but if he or she does not, the range is usually 30 to 60 drops per minute (2 to 4 ml), depending on the type of fluid mixture, the age and condition of the client, the purpose of the procedure, and the intended duration of therapy.

Flow rate depends on the size of needle or catheter, the type of intravenous apparatus (standard or microdrip), the vertical distance of solution from the venipuncture site, the viscosity of the fluid, and the venous pressure of the client.

Size of needle or catheter. The bore size of the needle or catheter will influence the rate of flow. Large ones are capable of more rapid delivery of fluids than small ones and are less likely to become obstructed by particulate matter.

Type of intravenous apparatus. Standard apparatus can deliver up to 50 to 60 ml per minute. Macrodrip devices deliver 10 to 15 ml per minute, depending on the manufacturer.) It is essential that the nurse read package inserts, which convey such information, and make calculations accordingly.

Vertical distance of solution from venipuncture site. The greater the vertical distance between the solution and venipuncture site, the faster the flow rate will be. If the client's bed is raised or if the solution container is lowered, the rate will decrease. If the client's bed is lowered or if the solution container is raised, the rate will increase.

Viscosity of fluid. Viscous solutions such as blood tend to flow less rapidly than regular intravenous fluids. Drops are also larger with increased viscosity. Thus most blood drop regulators are calculated at 10 drops per ml.

Venous pressure of client. A client does not maintain a constant venous pressure. Any factor that influences venous pressure to increase or decrease will cause an inverse flow rate change. For example, if a client coughs, sneezes, rolls over, sits up, or cries, the venous pressure will increase and the flow rate will decrease. This is especially important to consider when caring for agitated children whose crying significantly increases their peripheral resistance and venous pressure and thus slows their infusion. If the nurse increases the flow rate during such an episode, it must be reduced once the child is quieted and relaxed.

Keep-open rates. Keep-open rates are sometimes indicated to maintain an intravenous line but keep infused fluid to a minimum. A keep-open infusion should not be regulated to a rate less than 10 ml per hour, since slower rates are not sufficient to counteract venous pressure. Consequently, flow direction may be reversed, with blood entering the needle or catheter and tubing and eventually clotting and stopping the infusion.

Monitoring the rate should be a continuous concern of nurses. In the first hour of therapy, it is desirable to recheck the flow every 15 minutes until it is ascertained that it is well regulated. If so, hourly monitoring may suffice.

Adjustments of flow rate. Parenteral fluid therapy is usually ordered for a specific amount in a designated time period—number of drops per minute or milliliters per hour. One formula for calculating rates is as follows:

$$\text{Drops/min} = \frac{\text{Volume infused} \times \text{Drops/ml}}{\text{Total infusion time (min)}}$$

Standard intravenous sets are usually calibrated at 10 to 15 drops per ml, microdrip sets at 50 to 60 drops per ml, and blood sets at 10 drops per ml.

Various manufacturers have developed infusion pumps and other apparatus for controlled fluid and medication administration that utilizes a secondary, auxiliary container, or reservoir for pediatric clients or others who require precise delivery and monitoring. A predetermined amount is introduced into the auxiliary unit, and the primary source is clamped off to prevent accidental acceleration of the infusion within a specified time period. This reservoir technique is also useful for introducing medications intravenously, especially those whose effect is enhanced by, or dependent on, timed administration or whose potency is lost when they are diluted for prolonged periods of time in the larger primary container (Fig. 8-14).

If a primary infusion flask contains more fluid than is ordered, all in excess of the prescribed amount should always be discarded *before* the initiation of the infusion in order to prevent accidental overdosage. Nurses must not rely on their intention to discontinue the infusion after the correct amount has been absorbed.

After the rate is calculated and established, adjustments may be required to maintain the schedule. If the infusion is considerably behind schedule (whether or not it includes medications), any appreciable alteration of rate should be done judiciously to avoid circulatory overload or untoward reactions of potent drugs. For example, it is better for an infusion that contains potassium to be running 2 hours behind time than to speed it up, thus administering the delayed dose in a few minutes just to be on time with the fluids. Such considerations are extremely important for clients with cardiovascular or pulmonary dysfunction, those with renal disease, or the elderly. Children are especially prone to complications caused by rapid infusion of fluids. Responses may include seizures as well as pulmonary edema. Injudicious acceleration of fluids can also defeat the purpose of the therapy. To illustrate, if an infusion containing glucose is given so rapidly that metabolic processes are not complete, the glucose accumulates in the blood, increases osmolality, and acts as a diuretic.

Complications. If flow rate is difficult to maintain and seems to be influenced by minor changes in position, the nurse should examine the site and make certain that no complicating factors are evident that are interfering with the vein patency or infusion apparatus. A special problem can occur, called *infiltration,* which results in the fluid flowing subcutaneously rather than intravenously.

Infiltration can be recognized by visual and physical phenomena. If the tissues surrounding the site are swollen or the flow rate is difficult to maintain, the fluid may be meeting direct tissue resistance. If the infusion is indeed in the vein, lowering the bottle below the level of the bed causes venous blood to appear in the tubing. The presence of such a "flashback reaction" is not always assurance that the needle is in the vein, however. The level of the needle may be partially within the vein but also puncturing the posterior wall of the vessel. Blood will flash on negative pressure, but edema will increase as soon as the flow is resumed, because of the partial infiltration. To confirm infiltration, apply a tourniquet proximal to the injection site tightly enough to restrict venous flow. If the infusion continues to drip, extravasation is definite. Because of the variety of highly irritating medications added to infusions, infiltration can invite necrosis of tissues as well as deprive the client of the fluids and additives ordered for therapy. Frequently the site is traumatized to the degree that it cannot be used for subsequent venipunctures.

An infiltrated infusion should be discontinued at once, and the nurse should remove the needle from the site rather than merely turning off the flow. The infusion must be restarted in a new site anyhow, so that there is no reason for the foreign body to remain in contact with the already traumatized tissue, thus giving phlebitis or a thrombus an opportunity for development.

If the flow stops or slows considerably but there is no evidence of infiltration, the setup should be checked for constricting mechanisms that might impede the flow. If no external cause can be noted for obstruction, such as a restraining device, an occluding clot within the vein should be suspected. Only a physician

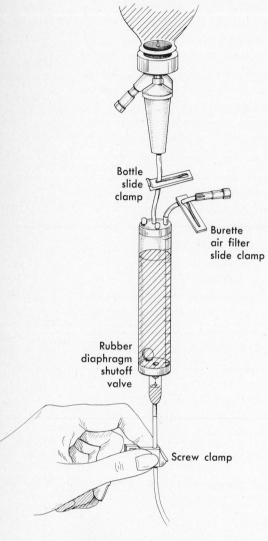

Bottle slide clamp

Burette air filter slide clamp

Rubber diaphragm shutoff valve

Screw clamp

FIG. 8-14
Controlled fluid administration set.

or a highly skilled nurse should tamper with the needles, since the clot could be dislodged and an embolism could enter pulmonary circulation. The needle can sometimes be cleared by aspirating and irrigating with normal saline, but this must be done with considerable caution because of the attendant risks of embolus and vein injury.

Phlebitis, a local inflammatory process, is characterized by a reddened line that follows the course of the vein. Edema sometimes accompanies the phenomenon. The area is warm and painful for the client. A thrombus may contribute to the local reaction process. When phlebitis is discovered, it demands that the infusion be removed from the site and nursing measures to reduce inflammatory responses be instituted. Alternating moist cold and heat compresses relieves pain and inflammation.

Pyrogenic reactions, which are systemic and characterized by fever, chills, nausea, vomiting, headache, backache, and malaise, may occur from solutions

FIG. 8-15

Attachment of a secondary container of additive solution, including drugs. **A,** The secondary container of additive solution is suspended; its tubing is cleared of air; and its clamp is closed. After the injection site is cleansed with antiseptic, the needle on the tubing from the secondary container is inserted into the injection site on the primary tubing. The container of primary solution is suspended lower than the container of additive solution with a special hanger. The rate of flow is adjusted by the clamp on the primary tubing. **B,** Closed valve showing direction of flow. When the tubing from the additive solution is attached, tapping the injection site on the tubing lightly helps ensure that the backcheck valve is seated properly. The higher pressure of the secondary solution forces the valve closed until all of the additive solution has been administered. **C,** Open valve showing direction of flow. When the additive solution has been administered, the equalization of pressure in the containers allows the valve to open, allowing the solution from the primary container to flow. (From Dison, Norma: Clinical nursing techniques, ed. 4, St. Louis, 1979, The C.V. Mosby Co.)

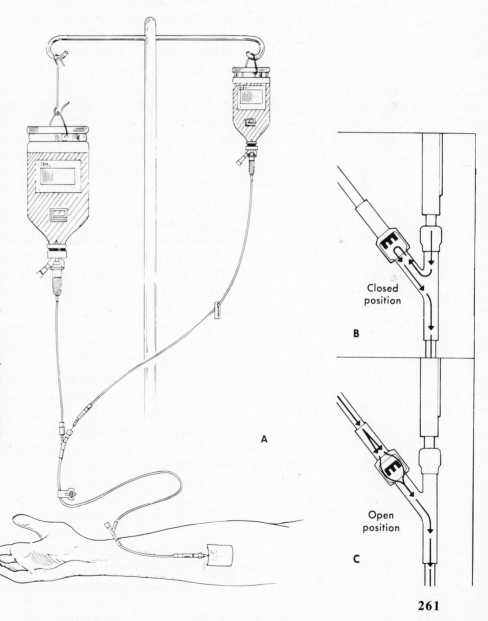

that contain contaminants. These signs and symptoms occur within 30 minutes of initiation of the infusion. Such adverse conditions can be guarded against by checking the solution before and during administration for any particles or cloudiness. If a pyrogenic response is suspected, the infusion must be terminated at once, but the container contents reserved for culture and other laboratory study. Vital signs are monitored, and the physician is notified.

Pyrogenic reactions occur often in conjunction with prolonged keep-open therapy or an intravenous additive program where a diluent or unused portion of an additive is saved for later use. Any opened medication should be discarded and not reserved for future parenteral fluid therapy. Tandem fluid sets (Y-tubing hookups and piggybacks, Fig. 8-15) are likely offenders, and equipment must be changed frequently, as often as every 24 hours.

Air embolism is usually a complication of fluid or blood administered under pressure, allowing air to enter the tubing. The amount of air sufficient to cause air embolism has not been established. A negative intravenous pressure may allow the air to enter the bloodstream, such as when the extremity receiving the infusion is elevated above the level of the heart. If a fluid container should empty completely and a second bottle be started, the trapped air may be forced into circulation. To avoid this, the following steps should be taken: (1) clamp off the tubing with a hemostat proximal to the infusion needle; (2) hang the replacement fluid container; (3) using aseptic technique, insert a needle and syringe into the rubber hub of the tubing; (4) withdraw the trapped air as the clamp is removed; and (5) readjust the flow.

Any Y-tube setup in which more than one solution is run at one time can be a source of air embolism. If either container empties, it becomes a source of air in the other's flow, since atmospheric pressure is greater in the open tubing to the empty container than below the tubing clamp of the infusing side. Air bubbles thus are aspirated into the venous circulation. Only one solution should be run at a time, and if simultaneous flow is ordered, close observation is imperative. Tubing must be clamped off completely before the container empties in any infusion setup, for maximum safety. *Air embolism is a hazard whenever two vented sets infuse through a common needle or when a pump is used.*

If a "cutdown" or venesection has been performed, the stopcock outlets not in use must be occluded completely, or air can enter the vein through the opening. When the administration set is changed, the client should always be placed in a horizontal position.

An air embolism can be recognized by an inrush of air, sudden vascular collapse characterized by hypotension, weak rapid pulse, cyanosis, rapid elevation of the CVP, and loss of consciousness. The nurse should stop the infusion and turn the client onto his left side with his head down, which will permit air to rise in the right atrium and prevent it from entering the pulmonary artery. Administration of oxygen is begun at once, and the physician is notified.

Circulatory overload and *shock* can occur from too rapid flow. Headache, engorged neck veins, apprehension, elevation in blood pressure, dyspnea, chest pain, chills, and tachycardia are manifestations of the complication. If this occurs, measures should be taken at once to combat shock. The infusion should be slowed but the established route left open for administration of antishock therapy. Allowing the client to sit up may lessen dyspnea caused by pulmonary edema. Circulatory overload can be prevented most easily by maintaining a judicious and consistent flow rate appropriate to the functional status of the cardiovascular and renal systems.

Allergic reactions to drugs can occur, especially when antibiotic and protein substances are infused. Anaphylaxis should always be an anticipated complication.

Alcohol infusions are potential problems because of their intoxication syndrome and irritant properties. Infiltration of this substance is often followed by necrosis and sloughing of affected tissue.

Solutions for infusions should be warm or at least room temperature. Cold fluids cause local venospasm, retarded infusion, pain, and potential infiltration. Warm packs applied to the site are useful in managing such reactions.

Speed shock, although not common, can occur when a foreign substance is rapidly administered by the intravenous route. Direct introduction of some substances into the circulation permits plasma concentrations to reach toxic proportions within seconds. This adverse phenomenon is especially damaging to the organs rich in blood supply, such as the heart, kidneys, and brain. Loss of consciousness, shock, and cardiac arrest may herald the onset of this reaction. The most important preventive measure again is judicious regulation of the infusion rate. Utilization of controlled-volume sets are recommended for potent drugs or guarding against accidental administration of a large fluid volume over a short period of time. This is especially true in dealing with a child. Some hospitals require that a hemostat be placed at the bedside of all clients receiving infusions in case the plastic or metal clamp breaks or malfunctions.

Clients receiving any intravenous infusion must be observed and notations made periodically regarding their appearance, behavior, vital signs, output, infusion site, weight, and response to therapy. Although intravenous fluids are a common nursing responsibility, they should never be considered routine. Potential adverse reactions should be well understood, and measures for their prevention and management explicitly outlined for implementation in an emergency. Although modern equipment and sophisticated mechanical devices have been made to cope with infusions and increase administration safety, there is no substitution for continuous client observations and an analytical approach by the nursing staff.

Other considerations: age and general physical condition of client. A *child* receiving an infusion may not be old enough to comprehend the nature of the procedure and may be fretful and irritable. If a nurse or parent can remain with the child, it will ensure more comfort to the client and help maintain a safe, effective administration. An infant may be quieted with a pacifier. Older children need an explanation of the infusion process and must understand the behaviors expected of them in relation to it. Occasionally sedatives may be given to reduce hyperactivity and to quiet the child, since crying tends to increase resistance in the vein and thus to impede the flow.

A scalp vein may be used (especially for infants) to avoid a venesection or cutdown. A short 25-gauge needle is placed in a superficial vein on the scalp. Since the needle is easy to dislodge, adhesive tape must be used to secure it in place (Fig. 8-16). Parents should understand why the site is chosen, since it could be frightening to enter the room and see a needle in their child's head. Scalp-vein infusions may infiltrate, and this could go unnoticed because of the tape and even hair that may occlude direct visualization of the area. Usually the site is changed

Foundations of clinical practice

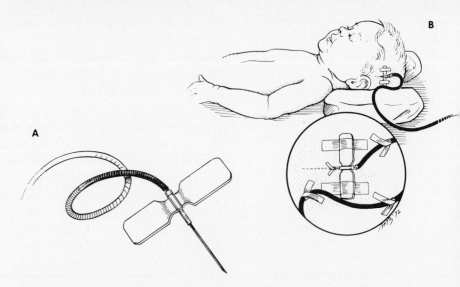

FIG. 8-16
A, Scalp-vein needle with winged tabs that provide a flexible grasping point for insertion. **B,** Scalp-vein needle in position. Note the sandbags, which extend to the shoulders, for immobilization of the head during the infusion. (Elbow restraints may also be indicated.) Limited tape is used to ensure adequate visualization of the infusion site.

every 48 to 72 hours if fluids need to be continued, so that phlebitis can be prevented.

If possible, activity needs of the child should be met. Sitting up for quiet play can often be planned in relation to the infusion. It is usually safe to pick up and hold an infant with a secured scalp-vein infusion, without causing infiltration or displacement of the needle.

Controlled volume infusion sets or pumps are used for all pediatric fluid therapy.

When the *older adult* receives an intravenous infusion, complications are to be anticipated because of the poor condition of the cardiovascular, pulmonary, and renal systems. Phlebitis, hematoma, infiltration, and circulatory overload can occur. The last complication can be avoided by precise monitoring of flow rate and vital signs. If signs of overload appear, the infusion should be terminated at once and measures taken to prevent or correct profound pulmonary edema.

Ambulation should be encouraged while the client is receiving an infusion unless other physical considerations contraindicate this. Activity improves cardiovascular tone and stimulates hormones responsible for renal efficiency.

Even during the infusion, unless it is contraindicated, oral intake of food and fluid should be maintained. This keeps the client interested in food, tones the gastrointestinal system, and maintains the buccal cavity in a normal state. Complete oral intake should be resumed at the earliest feasible time.

Administration of blood

Blood transfusion, while basically similar to an intravenous infusion, is modified in certain respects. The blood is packaged in units that contain 500 ml each. The bag or bottle containing the blood should be carefully labeled. A blood administration set should be used to infuse blood. This contains a filter and a large (10 drops per ml) flow regulator (Fig. 8-17). An 18-gauge needle should be used to accommodate the viscosity of the blood. The blood should be refrigerated until ready for use but administered at room temperature to prevent chilling the client. Blood that has been out of refrigeration for more than 1 hour before use should not be used, however.

Blood used for transfusion is usually obtained from a donor who volunteers or is paid to donate blood. Local regulations vary, but it is encouraged that blood be voluntarily donated through community blood bank programs. This gives

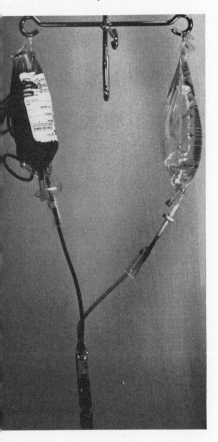

FIG. 8-17
Blood is transfused through a special administration set to remove particulate matter. Note flask of normal saline for infusion before and after administration of blood. (From Ellis, Patricia, and Billings, Diane: Cardiopulmonary resuscitation: procedures for basic and advanced life support, St. Louis, 1979, The C.V. Mosby Co.)

some assurance that the donor is free of diseases that can be transmitted by blood routes such as serum hepatitis, which is the most common disease transmitted in this manner. The individual who receives the transfusion is known as the recipient.

To prevent reactions that can occur from incompatible donor and recipient bloods, a type and cross match must be done before each transfusion. In this procedure, samples of the donor and recipient blood are used to identify the blood type of each. A cross match, or mixing of the two bloods, is performed next to verify that the bloods are compatible and will not agglutinate.

In instances of severe blood loss, blood can be transfused rapidly with the use of a blood transfer pack around the unit of blood in a plastic container. The transfer pack is inflated to create the pressure for infusion. Infiltration of blood and emboli are dangers of administering blood in this manner, and great care should be taken if it is necessary to use this approach to blood administration.

The nurse may have the responsibility for administering the blood and should use utmost caution in following the hospital procedure. The following guide may be used:

1. Check and double-check the donor blood according to hospital policy. Verify the completion of typing and cross-match procedures. Keep the blood chilled until needed.
2. Identify the client.
3. Assess vital signs before starting the infusion.
4. Start an infusion of normal saline and run the saline through the tubing before infusing the blood. Dextrose in water may cause clotting and should not be used.
5. Stay with the client for the first 15 minutes to observe untoward reactions. Run the first 50 ml slowly, about 15 to 30 minutes.
6. Observe the flow rate: adults, 20 drops per minute; children, 10 to 15 drops per minute. Clients with circulatory disturbance or heart disease and infants and children should have blood infused at a slower rate.
7. Mix the infusion gently two or three times during the transfusion to prevent packed cells from entering the bloodstream first.
8. Do not add medications to the blood transfusions.
9. Observe and record intake and output (record by milliliter or weight).
10. When the transfusion is absorbed, run saline through the tubing.
11. Chart the vital signs and the amount of blood infused.

With each transfusion there is danger of a *transfusion reaction* (Table 8-7). For this reason the nurse must observe the client for the first 15 to 30 minutes and discontinue the transfusion if there is any indication of a transfusion reaction. If a blood transfusion reaction does occur, the blood and tubing should be returned to the laboratory for analysis. A urine specimen should be obtained from the client and an intravenous solution kept infusing.

A *hemolytic reaction* may occur if the donor's blood is incompatible with the client's blood. In this case donor blood is agglutinated by the recipient's serum. The agglutinated cells block capillary flow, and when dissolved by macrophages, the product of hemolysis releases hemoglobin, which appears in the plasma and urine. The free-floating hemoglobin can obstruct renal tubules and cause renal failure. The client has pain in the lumbar region, nausea and vomiting, tightness in the chest, a drop in blood pressure and rise in pulse rate, a decreased urine

TABLE 8-7
Transfusion reactions

Reaction	Cause	Prevention	Assessment	Planning and implementation	Evaluation
Hemolytic	Blood incompatibility	Type and cross match; infuse first 50 ml slowly	Fever, chills, dyspnea, tachypnea, lumbar pain, fever, oliguria, hematuria, tightness in chest; collect blood and urine samples	Discontinue immediately; fatality may occur after 100 ml infused	After stopping infusion the nurse monitors vital signs and evaluates client's response to cessation of blood administration
Allergic	Antibody reaction to allergens	Screen donors for allergy; antihistamines before transfusion	*Mild:* chills, hives, wheezing, vertigo, angioneurotic edema, itching *Severe:* dyspnea, bronchospasm	*Mild:* slow infusion; give antihistamine as ordered *Severe:* stop infusion; epinephrine may be ordered	
Pyrogenic	Bacterial pyrogens in blood	Screen donors; use aseptic technique in administration	Fever, chills, nausea, lumbar pain	Stop infusion	
Hypothermic	Infusing chilled blood	Give at room temperature; use warming coils for rapid infusion	Chills	Slow infusion; cover client	
Circulatory overload	Infusion of large amounts of blood especially to clients with cardiac disease or extremes of age	Infuse slowly; check drip rate frequently	Rales, cough, dyspnea, cyanosis, pulmonary edema, increased CVP	Stop infusion; treat pulmonary edema; apply rotating tourniquets	
Air embolism	Entry of air in vein	Use proper infusion technique; avoid giving under pressure; check connections to tubings; avoid Y tubes; use filter; use plastic containers	Chest pain, dyspnea, hypotension, venous distention	Stop infusion; position on left side; give oxygen; embolectomy may be performed	
Hypocalcemic	Precipitate from ACD	Use blood immediately	Numbness, tingling in extremities	Stop infusion; give calcium as ordered	
Hyperkalemic	Hemolysis of red blood cells releases potassium	Use blood immediately	Nausea, vomiting, muscle weakness, bradycardia	Stop infusion	

8 Nursing and the hospitalized client

output, and hematuria. If more than 100 ml of incompatible blood is infused, death may occur. The nurse should discontinue the transfusion on observation of these symptoms and notify the physician.

An *allergic reaction* results when the client is allergic to antibodies in the donor's blood. In a *mild allergic reaction,* the client experiences hives, edema, and wheezing. Often an antihistamine may be given before the transfusion to prevent this reaction. If the reaction occurs, the nurse should slow the infusion rate and administer an antihistamine, if ordered. *Severe allergic reactions* are manifested by dyspnea and bronchospasm and are serious consequences of a transfusion. The transfusion should be stopped at once. Epinephrine may be ordered to reverse the allergic response.

If there is bacterial contamination of the blood, the client may have a *pyrogenic reaction,* causing chills, fever, headache, nausea, vomiting, and diarrhea. The transfusion should be discontinued and the blood returned to the laboratory for inspection.

Circulatory overloading may occur when large amounts of blood have been transfused or when the infusion has been done rapidly, particularly in older adults with cardiac disease. The left ventricle is unable to pump a large volume, and there may be dyspnea, cough, rales, cyanosis, increased CVP, and ultimately pulmonary edema and cardiac arrest. The transfusion should be stopped and interventions for pulmonary edema instituted. It is especially important to monitor infusion rates so that circulatory overload does not occur.

Transfusing cold blood can precipitate a *hypothermic reaction* in which the client experiences chills and in extreme instances death. Warming coils can be used when large volumes of blood must be transfused rapidly.

Air embolism is a hazard during any intravenous infusion, and great care must be used to prevent air entry in the system. Use of a filter and avoidance of giving blood under pressure can help prevent embolism.

Electrolyte imbalances may result from changes in donor blood that has preservatives or has been improperly stored. Hypocalcemia occurs when calcium levels are depleted by acid citrate dextrose and blood preservative. Assessments of numbness or tingling indicate hypocalcemia. When blood is stored for several days, red blood cells break down, releasing potassium. Hyperkalemia is dangerous for clients with cardiac or renal disease, and the nurse should report signs of nausea, vomiting, muscle weakness, and slowing pulse.

PREPARATION FOR DIAGNOSTIC TESTS

Diagnostic tests are inevitably performed on hospitalized clients. The tests may be the primary reason for hospitalization, or they may be used to obtain information before medical or surgical interventions or gather data to evaluate therapeutic interventions. Diagnostic tests may be noninvasive, such as an x-ray examination or collection of a urine specimen, or invasive, requiring an incision or entry into a body cavity, such as a biopsy or collection of a blood specimen. Regardless of the purpose or nature of the test, the nurse can prepare clients for the test by explaining the test and instructing them as to their role during and after the test. Explanations and instructions must be appropriate to the client's needs and level of understanding, and special precautions and procedures may be instituted for infants and children as well as older adults.

Infants and children

In certain diagnostic tests and related procedures the nurse must be prepared to position the child with special restraints. Among these are venipunctures,

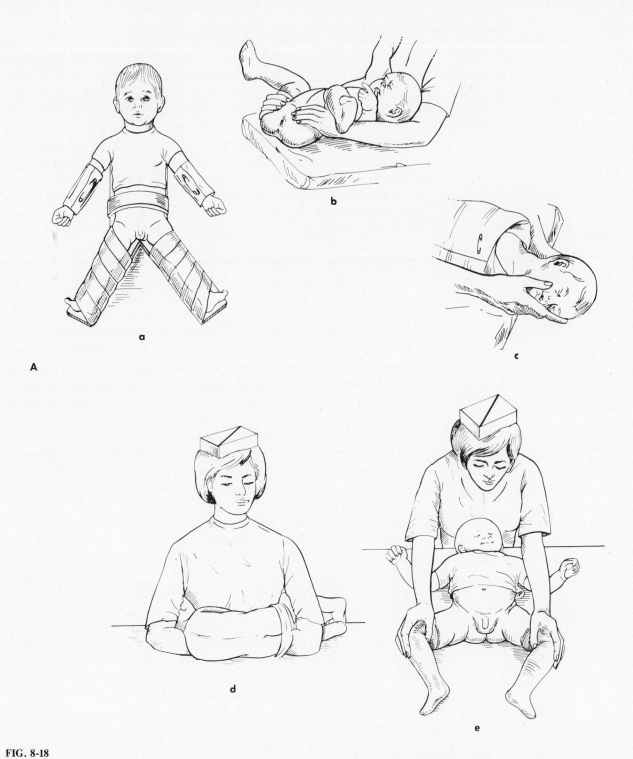

FIG. 8-18

A, Procedural restraints. **a,** Y board (circumcision, exchange transfusion, and so forth); **b,** thigh flexion-abduction (perineal or rectal procedures); **c,** mummy (procedures involving head and neck); **d,** knee-neck flexion (lumbar puncture); **e,** frog position (femoral venipuncture).

lumbar punctures, injections, and instillation of eyedrops (Fig. 8-18). These positions have varied modifications and applicability.

Diagnostic studies involving x-ray films or surgery require special preparation, both psychological and physical. The child who is old enough for vivid imagination views x-ray pictures and surgery as extremely mysterious. Often a simple explanation is that taking an x-ray film is like taking a picture or that surgery is "going to sleep and letting the doctor fix the hurt." A visit to a recovery room where the child can see the equipment to be used may allay some fears but may create others. Play therapy and storybooks may be useful in preparing the child for diagnostic tests.

Collection of urine specimens may be a routine part of a hospitalization for infants. (See Fig. 8-19 for examples of collection devices.) Stool specimens can usually be retrieved from a diaper or bedpan and transferred to a specimen container by a tongue depressor.

Preparation for diagnostic tests or surgery may at times require several factors such as obtaining specimens, giving enemas, or withholding meals. The nurse should be aware that infants and young children tolerate hypoglycemia and dehydration poorly and that close observation is necessary to detect such complications.

Older adults   Physical and metabolic changes in the older adult may necessitate modification of diagnostic tests and procedures. The older adult may have arthritis, for example, and positioning for tests may be uncomfortable. Decreased mobility and slower response time should therefore be considered and the client made as comfortable as possible. Older individuals are more susceptible to dehydration, and the effects of withholding liquids or food for diagnostic tests are soon evident. The client should be well hydrated before the test, and the test performed as quickly as possible so that fluid intake can be resumed. Decreased metabolic rates may alter laboratory values; this must be considered when any tests of metabolic or biochemical activity are evaluated.

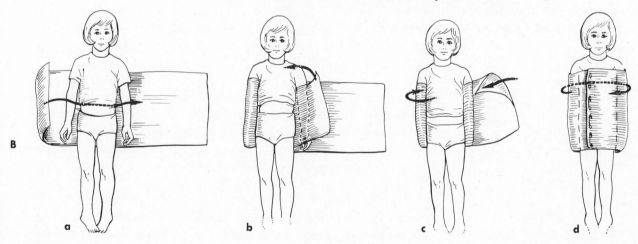

FIG. 8-18, cont'd
B, Body restraint, useful for procedures involving the head or perineum of a young child. **a,** Position the child supine on the treatment table covered with a sheet folded lengthwise, which extends from the axilla to the thighs. Arrange the positioning so that one third of the sheet extends from one side and two thirds from the opposite side. **b,** The shorter side of the sheet is brought (1) anterior to the proximal arm, (2) posterior to the trunk, and (3) anterior to the distal arm. The remaining length is carried posterior to the trunk. **c,** The remaining two thirds is brought (1) anterior to the extremities and then (2) on around the body until the length is exhausted. **d,** Completed restraint secured with safety pins.

FIG. 8-19
Pediatric urine collection. **A,** Disposable urine collector in place. Note the adhesive plate shown in detail. **B,** Test-tube method of collecting a specimen from a male child. **C,** Apparatus for a 24-hour collection.

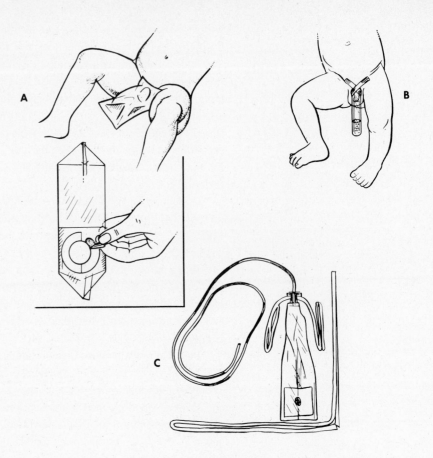

PLANNING FOR SURGERY: PREOPERATIVE, INTRAOPERATIVE, AND POSTOPERATIVE NURSING CARE

Preoperative nursing care

Nearly 50% of clients admitted to community hospitals have surgical interventions.[10] These may be done to diagnose (biopsy, explorative surgery), repair an injury, remove a diseased organ or tissue, or improve cosmetic appearance. Regardless of the purpose of the surgery or the type of surgery performed, the nurse can formulate a care plan that ensures continuity during the preoperative, intraoperative, and postoperative phases of the surgical experience.

The preoperative phase begins when the client is informed that surgery is necessary and ends as the client is admitted to the surgery unit. Nursing care at this time involves assessing the client's risk for surgery, planning for instruction and physical preparation, and evaluating the client's preparedness for surgery.

A nursing history is obtained when the client is admitted to the hospital. While obtaining baseline data and information about the client's usual health and habits, the nurse can assess the client's risk for surgery.

Several factors are considered risks for surgery, and a system to describe the client's risk may be used. Of primary consideration is the client's *age*. Neonates, infants, and older adults, for example, do not tolerate anesthesia and surgery. Neonates and infants have immature physiological coping resources; their resistance to infection is minimal, neuroendocrine responses are not developed, and nutritional reserves of fat and glycogen are not available. The reserves of the older adult may also be depleted, and physiological slowing of oxygen exchange, cardiac output, gastrointestinal motility, and immune system responses compound the assault incurred by surgery.

The client's *nutritional status* may also affect the tolerance for surgery. Clients who are malnourished or dehydrated or who have electrolyte imbalances do not have reserves for fasting required for anesthesia and prolonged surgery. Clients who are obese are also at risk. Obesity places excess demands on the cardiovascular, pulmonary, and renal systems, delays incisional healing, and contributes to problems of ambulation and increasing mobility during the postoperative course.

Concomitant health problems predispose the client to surgical risk. Heart disease, chronic obstructive pulmonary disease, renal failure, diabetes, and infection are examples.

Anxiety may also interfere with preparedness for surgery.[16] Clients who are extremely anxious or who have had prolonged stress may stimulate neuroendocrine responses and deplete coping strengths.

The nurse can also ascertain if the client has been using any *medications* that may interact with proposed surgical interventions. These may include steroids, diuretics, anticoagulants, antibiotics, antidepressants, and phenothiazine drugs. Often these drugs must be discontinued several days before surgery.

Analysis of the data helps the nurse, client, and health team plan surgical approaches. If risk factors are discovered during the nursing history, the surgery may be postponed until the problem can be modified. Alternative surgical approaches or palliative surgery may be performed until the client is better able to tolerate surgery.

The nurse, client, and family can plan for optimal preparedness for surgery. Objectives may include that the client and family will (1) have knowledge about the preoperative, intraoperative, and postoperative course; (2) practice procedures employed during postoperative recovery; (3) demonstrate reduced anxiety about surgery; and (4) be physically prepared for the specific surgery. Nursing research has demonstrated that clients who receive preoperative instruction have shorter postoperative recovery with fewer complications.[6,14]

Preoperative instruction. The nurse can collaborate with the surgeon to explain the purpose and nature of the surgery, including the size and location of the incision, change in body function that may occur as a result of the surgery, and the time and length of surgery. To obtain informed consent the surgeon must also explain attendant risks and alternative interventions. The nurse can be present during this explanation to follow up and reinforce this information.

Information should be offered at the level of the client's comprehension. Instruction can be facilitated by instructional media developed by the surgeon, nurse, and/or surgical team. These may include written instructions, filmstrips or videotapes depicting preoperative and intraoperative care and the places they occur, storybooks for children, role play with dolls, and tours of the facilities. Instructions may be given individually or in groups.

Instruction should be appropriate to the age of the client. Children's fears and fantasies are relieved by simple explanations. Instruction should be given close to the day of surgery, relevant to child's concept of time. Storybooks and role playing with dolls are particularly effective with young children. Adolescents are concerned about body image and peer acceptance. Emphasis on what the client will look like and be able to do are important aspects of preoperative instruction for adolescents. Adults require direct information, with time to make plans for family and job. Older adults may require shorter, more frequent expla-

Foundations of clinical practice

nations so the information can be processed. If instructional media are used, it is important to validate that the client can see and hear them.

Preoperative practice. Instruction should also include an opportunity to practice or imagine any changes that will occur as a result of the surgery or during the postoperative course. The nurse must be sensitive to the client's anxiety and evaluate the client's response to instruction while this information is being presented. Many clients do not wish to know, are yet in denial, or cannot cope with future-oriented instructions. Basic information should include, however, where the client will be after surgery, if other than his or her own room (ICU, cardiac recovery, and so forth); limits of activity; pain management; feeding schedules; what and when he can eat; and elimination patterns if altered by use of equipment such as intravenous catheters, monitors, nasogastric tubes, indwelling catheters, or drains. The client should be instructed on how to take deep breaths and cough to expectorate retained pulmonary secretions. If other exercises are to be done after surgery or if special turning techniques will be used, the client may wish to practice these as well. The family should be included in these explanations, and their role in the recovery can assist the client.

Preoperative anxiety. Clients facing surgery often demonstrate anxiety and fear about the procedure. The anxiety and fear may be related to fear of the unknown, fear of being anesthetized, or fear of being out of control. Other factors may include fears of disfigurement, changes in body image, pain, disability, death, or changes in family and social or economic status. Anxiety and fear may be manifested in a variety of ways, and the nurse can assist clients in identifying anxiety and in marshalling coping resources to deal with it. Anxiety may be relieved by instruction, demonstration, and anticipatory rehearsal of the surgical event. The nurse can facilitate anxiety management with use of therapeutic communication skills appropriate to the needs and age of the individual client.

Physical preparation for surgery. Clients who are having surgery must be in optimal health to withstand additional stress. Special procedures, diets, or medications may, therefore, be used several days before surgery to prepare the client for a specific type of surgery. These are discussed in detail in subsequent chapters but may include use of enemas, bladder catheterization, nasogastric or gastrointestinal intubation, surgical scrubs, douches, diets, and medications.

Diagnostic and laboratory tests are performed several days before surgery to obtain baseline data. These may include chest x-ray examination, ECG, urinalysis, complete blood count, and a type and cross match for blood transfusions.

On the day of surgery, final preparations are made. The client is usually restricted from fluids and foods for 6 to 8 hours before surgery to prevent vomiting and potential aspiration during anesthesia. An intravenous catheter may be used to provide fluid replacement to prevent dehydration. Vital sign measurements are obtained to provide baseline data and validate optimal health before surgery.

The client should void as close to going to surgery as possible. Bladder trauma is averted if the bladder is empty; a catheter may be used if abdominal or urinary tract surgery is to be performed.

The client can be made as comfortable as possible. A hospital gown is used; hairpins and wigs must be removed and a surgical cap used for asepsis. Nail polish should be removed so that nail beds can be inspected. Unless contraindi-

SURGICAL CHECKLIST

		Vital signs		Date/time
Client's name				
Room number		T		
Surgeon		P		
Surgical procedure		R		
		BP		

		Date/time
Laboratory data		
CBC		
Urine		
Type and cross match		

	Date/time	Comments
Intraoperative nursing plan explained		
Operative permit signed		
NPO since _____		
Makeup and nail polish removed		
Jewelry removed		
Prostheses removed		
Premedication administered		

cated by the surgery, prostheses must be removed before the time the client is transported to surgery.

Preoperative medication is used to ensure a relaxed client and to reduce gastrointestinal secretions. Anticholinergic drugs such as atropine are used to dry up gastrointestinal secretions, and a narcotic or tranquilizer such as meperidine (Demerol) or diazepam (Valium) is used to achieve relaxation. These drugs are given 30 to 60 minutes before surgery; once they are administered, the client should remain in bed with the side rails in place. A darkened room and minimal stimulation from family, visitors, and nursing personnel facilitate preoperative relaxation.

Evaluation. Continuity of nursing care can be promoted by communication of the care plan to the nurses in surgery. A checklist or care plan evaluation can be used to evaluate the client's response to preoperative care and should accompany the client as he is admitted to surgery. This information, which is an evaluation of the preoperative care plan, becomes the initial component of the care plan developed during surgery.

Intraoperative nursing care

Postanesthetic recovery is an extension of the intraoperative period. Since the effects of anesthetic agents persist in the immediate postanesthetic period and since these clients may potentially develop complications, the nurse must monitor the client frequently and systematically. From the assessments that are made of the client—the data obtained from the anesthesiologist as well as from the client's record—the nurse can devise a plan of care.

Foundations of clinical practice

When the client arrives in the postanesthetic room, the nurse should receive a complete report from the anesthesiologist. Although this information can be obtained from the client's record, a verbal report from the anesthesiologist gives the nurse an opportunity to obtain clarification of aspects that might be unclear. The data that should be included in the report follows:[13]

1. Client's name
2. Type of operation
3. Vital signs, including baseline and intraoperative blood pressure, pulse, and respiratory rates
4. Anesthetic regimen, including the preanesthetic medications, anesthetic used for induction and maintenance, anesthetic technique, whether or not a muscle relaxant was used, and if the effects have been reversed
5. Fluid status, including estimated fluid loss and replacement
6. Intraoperative complications (for example, hypotension, hemorrhage, or cardiac arrest)

The client may be fully awake or in any one of the stages of anesthesia. Therefore, once the initial data are obtained, the nurse should proceed to make detailed assessments of the client. These assessments should be made (and documented) at frequent intervals. An evaluation of the trends of these assessments, a comparison of these in relation to the client's norms, and an evaluation of baseline data (for example, on admission, preoperatively, and intraoperatively) are essential. This information is useful both in determining the state of the client and as a basis for determining when the client can be transferred from postanesthetic recovery.

Although most clients follow a normal recovery course, the nurse should also be cognizant of potential complications that may occur in the immediate period following surgery. These complications, along with signs indicative of them and nursing strategies, can be found in Table 8-8. Any complication that develops must be handled appropriately and expeditiously.

Stages of anesthesia and their nursing implications in the immediate postsurgical period. The physiological changes produced by anesthetic agents are described in stages.

Stage I is the stage of analgesia. During this stage, the client can be aroused easily, because consciousness is not lost. However, after awakening, the client quickly falls back to sleep. The client's sensation to pain is not absent, and the pain threshold is not altered, but the client's reaction to pain is altered.

Stage II is the stage of delirium or excitement. Varied behaviors can be observed during this stage, for example, excitement or involuntary activity, both of which may be slight or marked. Any form of stimulation has the potential to cause the client to become hard to control. Increased muscle tone, irregular respirations, and rapid eye movements are characteristic. The pupils may be normal or dilated, and retching or vomiting may occur. This stage is short lived.

Stage III, the stage of surgical anesthesia, commences when breathing becomes regular and ends with cessation of spontaneous respiration, which results from a high concentration of the anesthetic agent in the central nervous system. Four planes characterize stage III. The first plane, characterized by loss of reflexes, is the lightest plane; plane 4 is the deepest and is characterized by completely dilated and unresponsive pupils and absence of reflexes in the eye or airway.

ESSENTIAL ASSESSMENTS IN THE IMMEDIATE POSTSURGERY PERIOD

Assess:
Respiratory status—breathing pattern, respiratory rate and rhythm; color
Cardiovascular status—blood pressure, pulse rate, and rhythm
Neurological status—level of consciousness, response to stimuli, reactions or behavior (restless, excitable), reflex activity
Muscular status—response to simple instructions (squeeze my hand, move your arm, move your lips, and so forth), voluntary movement of extremities
Renal status—urinary output, color of urine

Assess for the presence of:
Airway—oral or nasal
Oxygen—route, liter flow
Intravenous fluid—type, flow rate
Drains or tubes—type, proper functioning
Dressing and/or perineal pad—drainage (amount, color); whether dry and intact

TABLE 8-8

Potential complications or problems immediately after surgery

Complications or problems	Signs indicative of complications	Possible strategies
Respiratory		

1. Airway obstruction caused by
  a. Relaxation of tongue on posterior pharyngeal wall as result of anesthetic or muscle relaxant[1]
	Snoring (for example, indicative of partial obstruction)
	Nasal flaring
	Retractions
	Use of accessory muscle
		Goal is to maintain a patent airway
		  Hyperextend head
		  Elevate mandible at its angle
		  Insert oral or nasal airway
		Consult with respiratory therapist or anesthesiologist
		Hyperinflate lungs with oxygen
		Apply positive pressure breathing
		Prepare for intubation

b. Foreign bodies (for example, packings, loose teeth, clots) c. Excessive secretions (for example, mucus) may be caused by tracheal or bronchial irritants, artificial airways, inhalation, or anesthesia	Noisy breathing, rales, rhonchi	Encourage coughing if gag reflex has returned Suction secretions if not relieved by coughing Auscultate anterior and posterior chest
2. Laryngospasms, from reflex contraction of pharyngeal muscles, may also be precipitated by irritants and foreign bodies (more common in children than adults)[3,15]	High-pitched crowing sound Labored breathing	Hyperextend head Administer oxygen Apply positive pressure breathing Consult with anesthesiologist, who may prescribe muscle relaxant or reintubation
3. Laryngeal edema may be caused by endotracheal tubes, fluid overload, allergies, surgical incision around neck	High-pitched crowing sound	Administer oxygen Consult with anesthesiologist, who may prescribe steroids, antihistamine, or reintubation
4. Bronchospasm may be caused by residual effects of drugs or preexisting disease, such as asthma or bronchitis	Wheezing sound—may be detected on auscultation of chest	Notify physician, who may prescribe bronchodilators or humidified oxygen via intermittent positive pressure breathing
5. Hypoventilation may be a result of residual curarization, respiratory center depression, diaphragmatic splinting caused by pain, or tight dressings		Encourage coughing and deep breathing
Circulatory		
1. Hypotension and shock may occur as a result of residual effect of premedication anesthesia and neuromuscular blockers,[4] unreplaced blood loss and/or continuous blood loss,[5] motion, change of position, dysrrhythmias, hypoxia, metabolic acidosis, or electrolyte imbalance	Decreased blood pressure, tachycardia, increased respiratory rate, decreased LOA, cool moist skin, and decreased urinary output (low CVP reading)	Raise legs to increase venous return Increase rate of intravenous fluid Administer oxygen Notify physician and anticipate that the following medications may be prescribed: vasoconstrictors, steroids, volume expanders, whole blood, albumin, solutions of crystalloid, bicarbonates if metabolic acidosis is present As a *preventive* measure, move client slowly and gently during position changes and during preparation for transport
2. Hypertension may occur as a result of hypercardia, hypoxia, hypervolemia, pain,[5] residual effects of vasopressors, or shivering	Elevated blood pressure	Administer oxygen Decrease intravenous fluid rate Notify physician, who may prescribe antihypertensive medication or diuretic drugs Administer medications for pain as needed
3. Dysrhythmias may result from metabolic disturbances, hypoxia, decreased blood volume, stress, anesthesia, or cardiac disease (premature ventricular contraction caused by hypokalemia is considered a common dysrhythmia in the postoperative period)	Irregular apical rate (make frequent assessments of apical and radial pulse rates for regularity and quality; evaluate electrolyte readings)	Administer oxygen Notify physician, who may prescribe antidysrythmic drugs, either as a bolus or continuous drip Provide care in a calm manner
4. Venous stasis often occurs as a result of relaxation of peripheral vessels because of muscle relaxants or spinal anesthesia		As preventive measures, prevent flexion and extension of lower extremities; turn from side to side, if not contraindicated and if vital signs are stable; obtain order for elastic stockings

Continued.

TABLE 8-8

Potential complications or problems immediately after surgery—cont'd

Complications or problems	Signs indicative of complications	Possible strategies
Cardiac		
1. Cardiac arrest may be caused by respiratory arrest secondary to airway obstruction or cessation of cardiac activity	Unresponsiveness Absence of pulse and respirations	Promptly initiate cardiopulmonary resuscitation utilizing the ABC steps (see Chapter 20 for a complete discussion)
2. Hemorrhage may be a result of poor hemostasis or coagulation defect[5]	Changes in vital signs (for example, decreasing blood pressure, increasing pulse and respiratory rates, apprehension, and paleness) Overt bleeding from incision site	See discussion of strategies included under hypotension and shock
Gastrointestinal		
1. Nausea		Administer medications for nausea as soon as client's condition warrants
2. Vomiting may occur as a result of an ileus or gas in the stomach or by diffusion and accumulation of anesthetic gases into the bowel[13]; preanesthetic narcotics and motion may also cause vomiting (a complication of vomiting is aspiration)	Aspiration may be evidenced by signs of oxygen need (for example, difficulty in breathing, rapid pulse, or color change)	Measures should be directed toward prevention—when changing position, move client slowly; administer medications for nausea To prevent complications of aspiration, lower client's head, if possible; position on side and turn head to side; suction secretions as necessary; anticipate reintubation and administration of humidified oxygen
Renal		
1. Oliguria usually occurs as a result of decreased cardiac output, and decreased renal pressure and perfusion[5]	Decreased output (for example, less than 20 ml/hour in adult client) Should have a minimum of 30 ml clear yellow urine/hour (accurately measure fluid intake and output)	Maintain fluid at correct rate Accurately measure fluid output Notify physician when output decreases Anticipate that physician will likely order fluids for volume replacement or medications for heart failure depending on cause
Neurological		
1. Hypothermia may be a result of exposure to long hours of surgical procedures (particularly surgery of the thoracic or abdominal cavity), while normal compensatory mechanisms are depressed[5]; shivering is associated with an increase in oxygen consumption	Bradycardia, hypotension, and subnormal temperature As temperature approaches normal, client will shiver	Make frequent assessments of temperature Provide adequate warmth to decrease oxygen consumption Plan measures to prevent injury Pad side rails with pillows Keep side rails up Maintain oxygen supply

During *stage IV,* the respirations cease from concentration of the anesthetic in the central nervous system. The subsequent result is circulatory collapse. This stage occurs because of error.[5] Emergency measures (for example, discontinuance of the agent or manual ventilation with high-flow oxygen) must be implemented promptly.

The recovery period varies according to the anesthetic used (Table 8-9). During recovery from anesthesia, the client experiences the same stages as during induction. The difference in the recovery period is that the stages occur in reverse order.

Stage IV is rarely, if ever, experienced.

During *stage III,* reflexes return in reverse order of their disappearance.

Stage II is characterized by delirium and excitement. The client is aware of his surroundings and can hear what is being said. Nursing objectives should be

TABLE 8-9

Agents used for inhalation anesthesia

Anesthetic agent	Induction rate	Recovery rate	Postanesthesia concerns
Cyclopropane* (trimethylene)	Rapid	Rapid	Hypotension, depressed respiratory rate, nausea, vomiting, ventricular arrhythmias
Ether† (diethyl oxide)	Slow	Slow	Copious secretions, nausea, vomiting
Ethyl chloride†	Rapid	Rapid	Muscle spasms, arrhythmias, hepatotoxicity
Ethylene*	Rapid	Rapid	Prolonged wound seepage, prolonged clotting time
Halothane†	Rapid	Rapid	Shallow, quiet respirations; shivering; hepatotoxicity
Methoxyflurane†	Moderate	Moderate	High urine output syndrome (decrease concentrating by distal tubules, excessive thirst), hepatotoxicity
Nitrous oxide* (nitrous monoxide)	Rapid	Rapid	Short-term euphoria
Trichloroethylene† (trichlorethene)	Rapid	Rapid	Tachypnea, bradycardia, ventricular arrhythmias
Vinyl ether† (divinyl oxide)	Rapid	Rapid	Copious secretions, nephrotoxicity, hepatotoxicity

From Johns, Marjorie P.: Pharmacodynamics and patient care, St. Louis, 1974, The C. V. Mosby Co.
*Gas.
†Liquid with volatile vapor.

developed to prevent deleterious effects on the client. Possible objectives should be to maintain a quiet environment, eliminate stimuli that may potentially cause excitement, and promote safety. For example, nurses should refrain from talking loudly or excessively. Care should be taken as to what is said and done in the client's presence. Care should be taken to try not to drop objects, slam doors shut, or bang into things. Side rails should be kept up, and someone should constantly be with the client.

The nurse should also evaluate possible causes for excitement and restlessness. Other characteristics of this stage—pain, a distended bladder,[13] an uncomfortable position, and hypoxia—may precipitate the excitement. Therefore, the nurse should check oxygen flow, bladder distention, position, and so forth.

Stage I, characterized by alteration in reaction to pain, makes it essential for the nurse to communicate with the client during assessment procedures. The client can hear but will readily go back to sleep. The client's request for pain medication must be carefully evaluated. The client may ask to be relieved of the pain and immediately return to sleep after making the request. Therefore, the nurse should assess and carefully evaluate the extent of recovery from the anesthetic. For example, has the client recovered enough to warrant medication? How long does the client remain awake after making the request? Does the client immediately go back to sleep? What is the client's respiratory rate? Is the rate at a level that would make it safe to administer the medication?

Pain medications, therefore, should be administered as needed, but cautiously. Narcotics, which are generally prescribed, have a tendency to lower arterial blood pressure. The pharmacological action may be a result of factors such as depression of the vasomotor center, dilation of peripheral blood vessels, or reduction in skeletal muscle tone.[4] Therefore, small doses are safest. It is not an uncommon practice for pain medications to be given in incremental doses in the immediate postoperative period. When administered, they should be documented, with the type, dosage, and route specified. Follow-up assessments should be made of the client's response to the same.

Psychological support to the client and family. As the nurse makes assessments and provides aspects of physical care, emotional support must also be pro-

Foundations of clinical practice

vided. Emotional support involves communicating with the client by giving explanations about nursing care, answering questions, and listening to complaints. All conversations should be carried out in a calm, reassuring manner.

While the client remains in the recovery room, family members must not be forgotten. The physician usually converses with the family after the surgery. However, if the client's stay in the recovery room is extensive, continued emotional support should be provided to the family, for example, informing them of the client's progress and the expected time that the client will remain in postanesthetic recovery.

Dismissal of the client from the recovery room. The criteria used for dismissing a client from the postanesthetic recovery suite varies from facility to facility and includes the reason for admission.[4] For example, clients seen on an outclient basis are kept until they can ambulate without dizziness and until nausea ceases. If spinal anesthesia has been administered, clients are kept in the recovery room until the anesthesia recedes and the vital signs are stable. Although the ultimate decision of when to dismiss a client from the recovery area rests with the physician, some guidelines for dismissal have been developed (Table 8-10). These criteria take into consideration five physiological parameters: activity, respiration, circulation, consciousness, and color. The highest score that can be achieved is 10 and the lowest 0. The final score and a set of guidelines are useful in helping determine when the client can be safely discharged.[1]

In preparation for dismissal of the client, the nurse in the postanesthetic room notifies the nurse on the client's unit. A complete summary of the client's state should be communicated to the receiving nurse. Information such as that received from the anesthesiologist should be given; for example, the client's name; type of surgery; anesthesia; medication; vital signs; fluid status, including intravenous fluid in progress, amount received, and output; drainage (color,

---

TABLE 8-10
Postanesthesia recovery score

Score	Criteria
Activity	
2	Able to move 4 extremities voluntarily or on command
1	Able to move 2 extremities voluntarily or on command
0	Able to move 0 extremities voluntarily or on command
Respiration	
2	Able to breathe deeply and cough freely
1	Dyspnea or limited breathing
0	Apneic
Circulation	
2	BP is ± 20% of preanesthetic level
1	BP is ± 20-50% of preanesthetic level
0	BP is ± 50% of preanesthetic level
Consciousness	
2	Fully awake
1	Arousable on calling
0	Not responding
Color	
2	Pink
1	Pale, dusky, blotchy, jaundiced
0	Cyanotic

From Aldrete, J. Antonio, and Kroulik, Diane: A postanesthesia recovery score, Anesth. Analg. **49**:926, 1970.

Postoperative nursing care

amount, and tubes); and any problems noted during the intraoperative period.

The postoperative phase of nursing care begins when the client returns from the recovery room (or surgery suite) to the nursing unit and ends when the client is discharged. The focus of the nursing care plan may change from supportive to facilitative as the client moves toward recovery.

Immediately after the client returns to the nursing unit it is imperative to assess the client in order to make nursing diagnoses and identify priority problems. The nursing history and care plan established before and during surgery and postanesthestic recovery from the basis of postoperative nursing care planning.

A systematic assessment of the client as he is admitted to the postoperative unit is useful in obtaining data about the client and identifying actual or potential postoperative problems. Priorities should be given to the client's respiratory status, circulatory status, and level of consciousness but may vary according to the age of the client, nature of the surgery, and type of anesthesia used. These are discussed as appropriate in specific chapters throughout the text.

Plans can be developed concurrently and implemented to prevent or manage nursing problems. Evaluation is ongoing as the client responds to postoperative nursing care.

Nursing problems related to the surgery are most likely to occur within 48 hours after surgery. The nurse must, therefore, assess the client frequently during this time. Vital signs and other assessments should be made every 15 minutes for the first hour after surgery, every 30 minutes for the next 2 hours, hourly for 4 hours, and every 4 hours thereafter, or as the client's status warrants. A graphic record may be used to plot changes in vital signs and development of the care plan.

The *respiratory tract* must remain patent at all times. The nurse can count respirations, identify rhythm and depth, and listen to breath sounds to determine airway adequacy. Potential problems of airway obstruction, hypoxia, atelectasis, or hypostatic pneumonia can be prevented or managed by frequent change of position, instructing the client to take deep breaths, and institution of respiratory therapy such as intermittent positive pressure breathing or incentive spirometry.

Alterations in *cardiac output* are assessed by counting the apical and peripheral pulses, taking the blood pressure, inspecting the client for color, and palpating extremities for warmth and moisture. The vital signs can be compared with preoperative values to detect changes. Common problems of circulation may include shock, dysrhythmias, or thrombophlebitis. Shock can be detected in incipient stages by changes in the client's vital signs, noted by an increase in heart rate and a decrease in blood pressure. Shock can be managed by fluid and blood replacement and vasopressor drugs. Dysrhythmias present potential problems of pump failure or cardiac arrest and must be treated when detected. Facilities for basic and advanced cardiac life support must, therefore, be readily accessible to clients recovering from surgery. Thrombophlebitis may be prevented by early ambulation, passive and active exercises, use of antiembolic stockings, and low-dose heparin therapy.

The *level of consciousness* is affected by the type of surgery, anesthesia, use of medication, pain, or sensory and sleep deprivation. The nurse should determine the client's level of consciousness as he continues to recover from anesthesia. Orientation to person, place, and time as well as pupil and motor responses can be used to judge alertness. Problems of consciousness may relate to surgery or the type of anesthesia used. Clients with surgery for removal of a brain tumor, for example, may have impaired levels of consciousness for several days, and the nurse must continuously monitor the client for changes in vital signs and levels of consciousness. Orientation to person, place, and time is facilitated by providing appropriate verbal, visual, and tactile stimulation to the client, such as telling the client where he is, showing the client visual cues of place, time of day, and so forth, and encouraging the client to change his position in bed.

Pain affects each client in unique ways, and the nurse should determine the location, intensity, and type of pain, changes in vital signs, and subjective and objective data from the client's perception of the pain, as well as the effects of medication, positioning, and exercise on the pain. Incisional pain should be distinguished from other pain. Incisional pain tends to be most intense for 48 hours after surgery and gradually subsides. Pain relief may be obtained by narcotics or analgesics, change of position, and manipulation of environmental stimuli.

Skin integrity at the site of the incision must be inspected regularly. The nurse can observe the color, odor, and amount of drainage and examine the suture line for evidence of infection, such as redness or purulent drainage. The nurse can also note the presence of drains and record the amount and color of drainage. Wound infections are prevented by asepsis during dressing changes. In some instances antibiotics may be used prophylactically. Wound infections are generally not evident until the third to sixth day and may be treated with antibiotic dressings or wet to dry soaks to debride the incision and foster healing.

Wound *evisceration,* protrusion of the intestines through an abdominal incision (Fig. 8-20, *A*), and *dehiscence,* separation of the sutures (Fig. 8-20, *B*), are rare complications. If the abdominal organs do eviscerate, the nurse can cover them with a moist, sterile dressing and notify the surgeon. No attempt should be made to reposition eviscerated organs. Wound dehiscence should likewise be reported to the surgeon and the incision repaired.

Bleeding from the wound is noticed as bright red blood at the incision site. Increases in bleeding can be noted by circling the area on the dressing with a pen and noting the time and amount of enlargement of the area. Large amounts of bleeding accompanied by changes in vital signs may indicate hemorrhage and should be reported to the surgeon immediately.

The potential for *impaired nutrition* is evident in clients who have had general anesthesia and of course for clients who have had abdominal or gastrointestinal surgery. The nurse should auscultate the abdomen for the presence of bowel sounds. Potential problems that may occur during the first 48 hours are abdominal distension, paralytic ileus, or obstruction. Drains such as a nasogastric tube or gastrointestinal tube may be used for several days after surgery until peristalsis returns. These tubes provide outlets for air, gas, and fluids and are used to prevent distension or obstruction. *Nausea* and *vomiting* may be caused by anesthesia, pain, obstruction, or medication, and the nurse can determine their cause and administer antiemetic drugs as necessary. Most clients receive nothing by mouth after surgery until the gag reflex returns, and depending on the type of surgery, they may not be taking anything by mouth for several more

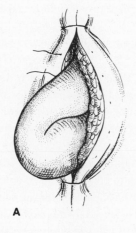

A

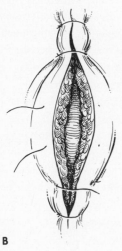

B

FIG. 8-20
A, Wound evisceration. **B,** Wound dehiscence.

days. Nutritional support may be provided by alternative routes such as intravenous feedings or nasogastric or gastrostomy feedings.

Spasms of the diaphragm may cause *hiccoughs*. These can be managed by deep breathing or tranquilizers such as chlorpromazine (Thorazine).

Urinary elimination is monitored by urine output. Unless the client has a catheter or has experienced urinary tract surgery, he should be able to void within 6 to 8 hours after surgery. Since the first voiding signals adequacy of urinary tract function, the nurse should measure the amount of urine output, note color and odor, and record the time. If the client is unable to void in a reasonable time period, the nurse should initiate actions to assist the client. These may include ambulation, running water, and pouring water over the perineum. Catheterization should be considered only if these measures fail and the client's bladder is distended. Urinary output for clients with indwelling catheters should be monitored during the first few hours, as urine outputs of less than 30 to 40 ml may signal shock or dehydration and should be reported to the surgeon. Total urine output for the first 24 hours may be as low as 500 ml, however, because of restriction of fluids, fluids lost from drainage, and insensible losses from respiration and diaphoresis.

Bowel elimination often does not occur until the third or fourth day after surgery, since fluids and food may be restricted and peristalsis may be slowed from anesthesia or immobility. The nurse should note the time, color, and amount of the first stool after surgery. Bulk in the diet, fluids, exercise, stool softeners, or laxatives may be used to promote elimination. Clients who have had gastrointestinal or rectal surgery may have difficulty passing the first stool, and the nurse can plan to prevent constipation and pain by encouraging fluids and if necessary using stool softeners, laxatives, cathartics, and analgesics.

Attention to the client's *comfort* after surgery should be included in the care plan. The nurse can determine the comfort level while making priority assessments and plan to make clients comfortable as soon as possible. Clients may wish to brush their teeth and wash their face after surgery. Dentures and other prostheses should be replaced as soon as possible.

Immobility after surgery may be imposed by the nature of the surgery or by the client's tolerance to pain and activity. Active and passive range-of-motion exercise of all uninvolved joints should be instituted immediately after surgery. Early exercise and ambulation are necessary to prevent the cardiac and extracardiac hazards of immobility.

Rest and sleep are essential to recuperation, and time should be provided for both. Sleep deprivation enhances confusion, pain, and immobility and can be prevented by planning periods of uninterrupted sleep.

The client's *family* can be included in the postoperative plan. The nurse can assess family dynamics and assist the family in providing support to the client during recovery from surgery.

PREPARATION FOR DISCHARGE

Recovering from surgery and gaining strength, the client becomes better able to manage his own care. At this time the nurse, client, and family plan for increasing independence, and responsibility for care shifts to the client and family. The nurse can assess the client's readiness to assume this responsibility as well as his need for information appropriate to continued care. Specific knowledge is determined by the client's activity, medications, diet, and changes in body

Foundations of clinical practice

image or body function created by surgery, and the nurse can facilitate instruction about these.

A coordinated preoperative, intraoperative, and postoperative nursing care plan facilitates the client's adaptation to the stress incurred by hospitalization and surgery. The dynamic interaction of the nurse and client is evidenced as the client progresses from independence at admission, dependence intraoperatively, to regaining independence and new levels of wellness at discharge. Continuity of care is further enhanced by referrals to a community health agency or follow-up visits in a clinic or physician's office. The nurse can then evaluate terminal effectiveness of the care plan as the client reintegrates the surgical experience and obtains his optimal level of wellness.

Summary

The nurse has a significant relationship with the hospitalized client and his family, which may change as the client is variously capable of making decisions and assuming responsibility for care. The nurse must assess the impact of hospitalization on the client, particularly as it relates to the client's age and developmental stage, and develop plans accordingly. Nursing care planning for the hospitalized client may also involve ensuring a safe environment, providing opportunities for sleep and rest, preventing and managing sensory deprivation, relieving pain, helping clients cope with loss or alteration of a body part, administering medications and intravenous fluids, or preparing clients for diagnostic tests or surgery. The client's adaptation to hospitalization and subsequent return to optimal health can be influenced by nurses attentive to the related problems.

References

1. Aldrete, J. Antonio, and Kroulik, Diane: A postanesthesia recovery score, Anesth. Analg. **49:**924-933, 1970.
2. Allen, Marcia: Drug therapy in the elderly, Am. J. Nurs. **80:**1474-1475, 1980.
3. Beal, J.M., and others: Intensive and recovery room care, New York, 1969, Macmillan, Inc.
4. Drippes, Robert D., and others: Introduction to anesthesia: the principles of safe practice, ed. 5, Philadelphia, 1977, W.B. Saunders Co.
5. Flor, Remigio: Postanesthesia recovery room and postoperative complications. In Lichtiger, Monte, and Moya, Frank: Introduction to the practice of anesthesia, ed. 2, New York, 1978, Harper & Row Publishers, Inc.
6. Gruendemann, Barbara, and others: The surgical patient: behavioral concepts for the operating room nurse, ed. 2, St. Louis, 1977, The C.V. Mosby Co.
7. Hartman, Ernest L.: The functions of sleep, New Haven, Conn., 1973, Yale University Press.
8. Hayter, Jean: The rhythm of sleep, Am. J. Nurs. **80:**457-461, 1980.
9. Hemenway, Judith: Sleep and the cardiac patient, Heart Lung **9:**453-463, 1980.
10. Hospital statistics, Chicago, 1979, American Hospital Association.
11. Luban, David: Electrical safety, Hospitals **43:**57-60, 1969.
12. Luce, Gay Gaer: Body time, New York, 1971, Pantheon Books, Inc.
13. Quimby, Charles W.: Anesthesiology: a manual of concept and management, ed. 2, New York, 1979, Appleton-Century-Crofts.
14. Schrankel, Dawn: Pre-operative teaching, Superv. Nurse **9**(5):82-90, 1978.
15. Steward, David J.: Manual of pediatric anesthesia, Edinburgh, 1979, Churchill Livingstone.
16. Totas, Mary: The emotional stress of the pre-operative patient, J. Am. Assoc. Nurs. Anesth. **2:**27-30, 1978.

Additional readings

Bassler, Sandra: The origins and development of biological rhythms, Nurs. Clin. North Am. **11:**575-582, 1976.

Beland, Irene L.: Clinical nursing: pathophysiological and psychosocial approaches, ed. 2, New York, 1970, Macmillan, Inc.

Croushore, Theresa M.: Postoperative assessment: the key to avoiding the most common nursing mistakes, Nurs. '79 **9**(4):47-5, 1979.

Downs, Florence S.: Bed rest and sensory disturbances, Am. J. Nurs. **74:**434-438, 1974.

Foss, Grace: Sleep, drugs, and dreams, Am. J. Nurs. **71:**2316-2330, 1971.

Geolot, Denise, and McKinney, Nancy: Administering parenteral drugs, Am. J. Nurs. **75:**788-793, 1975.

Lanuza, Dorothy: Circadian rhythms of mental efficiency and performance, Nurs. Clin. North Am. **11:**583-594, 1976.

Larke, Georgia: Perioperative charting: OR nursing on display, AORN J. **31:**194-198, 1980.

Lindenmuth, Jane, and others: Sensory overload, Am. J. Nurs. **80:**1456-1458, 1980.

Lichtiger, Monte, and Moya, Frank: Introduction to the practice of anesthesia, ed. 2, New York, 1978, Harper & Row, Publishers, Inc.

Matheny, Norma, and Snively, William: Perioperative fluids and electrolytes, Am. J. Nurs. **78:**840-845, 1978.

Meth, Irving: Electrical safety in the hospital, Am. J. Nurs. **80:**1344-1348, 1980.

Natalini, John: The human body as a biological clock, Am. J. Nurs. **77:**1130-1132, 1977.

Ordronneau, Noreen: Helping patients in the radiology department, Am. J. Nurs. **80:**1312-1313, 1980.

Tom, Cheryl: Nursing assessment of biological rhythms, Nurs. Clin. North Am. **11:**621-630, 1976.

Zelechowski, Gina: Helping your patient sleep: planning instead of pills, Nurs. '77 **7**(5):62-65, 1977.

PART TWO

NURSING PROCESS FOR COMMON HEALTH PROBLEMS

NURSING PROCESS

for clients with common health problems of the

9 Endocrine system

Assessment

Data analysis

Planning

Implementation

Evaluation

Common health problems affecting the endocrine system may occur across the life span. These problems occur either from a deficiency, excess, or disturbance in the secretion of hormones. The endocrine system is essential in maintaining and regulating vital functions of the body such as stress, growth and development, homeostasis, reproduction, and energy metabolism; and is closely interrelated with other systems, specifically the central nervous system. Because of the close interrelation, physiological activity is subject to more than one regulating mechanism. Subsequently a disturbance in one mechanism is likely to incur a disturbance in others. Therefore the health problems affecting the endocrine system can be reflected in altered function of various organ systems, and the symptoms will reflect an increase or decrease in the regulatory process.

Health problems that result from a deficiency in a specific hormone usually result from destruction of the gland, neoplasm, infection, autoimmunity, vascular interference, or from inadequate stimulation; whereas problems related to an excessive amount of a hormone result from tumors, hyperplasia, or hypertrophy. This chapter deals with common health problems of five of the seven glands in the endocrine system: the pituitary, thyroid, parathyroid, adrenal glands, and pancreas. This information can be used as a nursing care plan is developed for clients experiencing health problems of the endocrine system. Common problems of the ovaries and testes will be discussed in Chapter 12. The reader is referred to specialized texts for information related to less common endocrine problems.

Overview of the endocrine system

The endocrine system, closely related to and in conjunction with the nervous system, regulates body functions. The endocrine system is composed of endocrine glands (pituitary, thyroid, parathyroid, adrenal, pancreatic islet, ovarian, and testicular) that secrete a variety of hormones into the circulation. *Hormones* are instrumental in stimulating the activity of specific target tissues, maintaining homeostasis, and regulating enzymatic activity. The manner in which hormones exert their effect on target tissue and cells depend on the structural nature of the hormone. For example, thyroxine, parathormone, tropic hormones of the pituitary (except TSH and gonadotropins), vasopressin, insulin, glucagon, and epinephrine are protein hormones.[28] These hormones act first by interacting with the cell membrane, which contains the adenyl cyclase system. To activate this system the hormones must first bind to specific receptors in the cell membrane. Once activated, adenyl cyclase converts adenosine triphosphate (ATP) into cyclic AMP, which becomes the secondary messenger. This messenger then moves to other structures within the cells and changes the rate of protein synthesis in that cell.[8,11,28]

The second mechanism of hormonal action is through steroid hormones. Adrenocortical hormones and hormones produced by the gonads are in this category. These hormones work inside the cell by binding with protein in the cytoplasm of the cell. From there it migrates into the nucleus, where RNA synthesis is initiated or accelerated.[8,11] Thyroid-stimulating hormones and gonadotropin hormones are glycoprotein.

Hormones regulate their own production through a feedback system (a negative feedback system). In negative feedback, increase in the concentration of a specific hormone inhibits the release of that hormone; whereas a decrease in the concentration stimulates the secretion of the hormone. These hormones have an effect in all body cells.

PITUITARY GLAND

The pituitary (hypophysis) gland secretes several hormones and exerts some effects on the functions of other endocrine glands. It is influenced by activity of

TABLE 9-1

Anterior and middle pituitary hormones

Hormone	Target gland	Functions
Somatotropin (growth hormone, STH, GH)	No specific target organ	Stimulates growth of bone and cartilage[8] through protein synthesis; regulates carbohydrate, lipid, and protein metabolism
Thyrotropin (thyroid-stimulating hormone [TSH])	Thyroid	Stimulates secretion and release of thyroxine (T_4), triiodothyronine (T_3), and thyrocalcitonin from thyroid gland; controls rate of metabolic processes of the body
Adrenocorticotropin (corticotropin, ACTH)	Adrenal cortex	Stimulates production and release of adrenal corticoids
Prolactin (mammatropic hormone [MH]); lactotropic hormone (LGH); luteotropic (LTH)	Mammary glands	Stimulates production of breast milk; maintains corpus luteum and progesterone secretion
Gonadotropic hormones		
Follicle-stimulating hormone (FSH)	Ovaries, testes	Stimulates follicular maturation in females; stimulates development of spermatic tubules and spermatogenesis
Luteinizing hormone (LH); interstitial cell–stimulating hormone (ICSH)	Ovaries, testes	Stimulates development and function of corpus luteum in female; stimulates interstitial cells to secrete testosterone
Melanocyte-stimulating hormones (alpha and beta MSH)[24]	Skin cells	Stimulates melanocytes resulting in increased pigmentation of skin

the central nervous system. As a result, fluctuations of hormones are readily noted in response to sensory stimuli and emotional changes.

The pituitary gland consists of three lobes: *anterior, middle,* and *posterior.* The anterior (adenohypophysis) and middle (intermediate) lobes communicate with the hypothalamus through the portal circulation, a network of vessels.[20] Control of the secretions of the anterior pituitary involves the central nervous system, whereas the mechanisms essential to the immediate regulation of the anterior pituitary hormones is in the hypothalamus and are referred to as releasing factors,[20] or releasing hormones. They include corticotropin releasing factor (CRF), luteinizing hormones releasing factor (LH-RF), thyroid-stimulating hormone releasing factor (TSH-RF), growth hormone releasing factor (GH-RF), and follicle-stimulating hormones releasing factor (FSH-RF). Inhibiting factors (IF) have also been demonstrated to be discharged from the hypothalamus and restrain the secretion and release of the anterior pituitary hormone prolactin inhibiting factor (P-IF) or luteotropic hormone inhibiting factor (LTH-IF).[20]

The *anterior pituitary* secretes several hormones by specific target endocrine glands. A list of these hormones, their target organs, and functions can be found in Table 9-1.

The *intermediate* or middle lobe secretes one hormone, the melanocyte-stimulating hormone (Table 9-1).

The *posterior pituitary* (neurohypophysis) is an extension of neural tissue and contains nerve fibers that originate in the hypothalamus. The posterior lobe is mainly involved with regulation of fluid balance (Table 9-2).

THYROID GLAND

The thyroid gland consists of two lobes and is connected by an isthmus that overlies the area of the tracheal cartilage.[14] It produces several hormones, including *thyroxine* (T_4), which comprises 90% of the body hormones,[31] *triiodothyronine,* which is transported mainly in plasma bound to plasma protein and acts to regulate the rate of cellular metabolism, and *calcitonin,* which lowers serum calcium levels by increasing bone deposition.

Protein and iodine are necessary for the synthesis of these hormones. In addition, their production requires the activation of the thyrotropin-releasing hormone (TRH), which in turn stimulates secretion of thyroid-stimulating hormone (TSH). A balance of these hormones is maintained by a negative feedback system in which a low serum thyroxine level stimulates the pituitary to produce TSH, whereas a high level inhibits its production.

PARATHYROID GLAND

The parathyroid gland, consisting of four glands situated on the posterior surface of the thyroid, secretes parathyroid hormone (PTH), which functions to regulate

TABLE 9-2
Posterior pituitary hormones

Hormone	Target gland	Functions
Vasopressin (antidiuretic hormone, ADH)	Distal, convoluted tubules and collecting duct of kidneys	Stimulates reabsorption of water by distal tubules
Oxytocin (pitocin)	Uterus, mammary glands	Stimulates uterine contractions; facilitates migration of sperm by stimulating fallopian tubal contractions[27]; stimulates release of milk during postpartum lactation[24]; promotes release of prolactin

calcium and phosphorus metabolism. The hormone maintains a normal level of calcium in the blood through its effect on three target organs: bones, kidneys, and the gastrointestinal tract. The hormone acts on target cells through the adenyl cyclase-cAMP system.

The skeleton is considered the most important of these target sites, because PTH promotes bone resorption and liberates calcium and phosphorus. The hormone acts on the renal tubules to increase tubular reabsorption of calcium and to decrease the proximal tubule reabsorption of phosphorus. The hormone also promotes excretion of phosphate in the urine, subsequently lowering the serum phosphate level. PTH in the gastrointestinal tract enhances the absorption of calcium from the tract.

An adequate amount of protein in the diet is essential for the production of parathormone. The serum level of calcium, through a negative feedback system, controls parathyroid activity. For example, an increase in the blood calcium inhibits secretion of parathormone; while a decrease stimulates its production.[8,25] A rise in serum phosphate also stimulates parathyroid activity.

ADRENAL GLANDS The adrenal glands consist of the cortex and medulla. The medulla, an extension of the sympathetic nervous system, produces two hormones, epinephrine and norepinephrine. These hormones function in acute stress situations to prepare

TABLE 9-3

Physiological effects of epinephrine and norepinephrine[17]

Tissue	Epinephrine	Norepinephrine
Cardiovascular system	Constricts cutaneous and renal arterioles	Strongly stimulates contraction of certain blood vessels; constricts arterioles and venules by acting at alpha-adrenergic receptors to increase peripheral vascular resistance and venous tone
	Produces vasodilation in coronary, lung, and skeletal tissue	
	Increases cardiac output and rate	
	Increases systolic blood pressure	
	No change or decrease of diastolic blood pressure	Markedly increases blood pressure because of increased peripheral resistance
	Increases metabolic rate	
	Increases coagulability of blood	Moderately increases pulse rate
Respiratory system	Increases rate and depth of respiration	Same effect
	Dilates bronchi	
Central nervous system	Marked excitatory effect	
	Increases awareness to environment	
	Facilitates reflex responses	
Muscles		
Skeleton	Prolongs contraction; increases force of contraction; produces rapid glycogenolysis; increases blood supply	
Gastrointestinal tract	Contracts relaxed ileocecal sphincter	Same effect
Bladder	Contracts relaxed sphincter	
Spleen	Contracts spleen and shunts red blood cells into circulation	
Eye	Stimulates iris and dilates pupils	
Pilomotor muscles of hair follicles	Stimulates movement of hair	
Liver	Stimulates lipolysis of adipose tissue and leads to insulin resistance	
	Inhibits insulin secretion, thus facilitating lipolysis and glycogenolysis	
	Simulates glucagon secretion	
Adipose tissue	Releases free fatty acids	Same effect
Other body tissues	Increases metabolism and oxygen consumption mainly from increased skeletal use	Same effect

From Krueger, Judith A., and Ray, Janis C.: Endocrine problems in nursing: a physiological approach, St. Louis, 1976, The C.V. Mosby Co., p. 70.

the individual for heightened physical activity ("flight or fight"). See Table 9-3 for comparative effects of these hormones.

The hormones produced by the cortex include glucocorticoid (cortisol), mineralocorticoid (aldosterone), and sex hormones. The glucocorticoids have several functions, including effecting glucose, protein, and fat metabolism; water and electrolyte balance; and inhibition of the inflammatory processes. They are also essential in adjusting to stress. The production of glucocorticoids is stimulated by the adrenocorticotropic hormone (ACTH), which is produced by the pituitary. A balance of the glucocorticoids is maintained by a negative feedback mechanism.

Mineralocorticoids primarily function to maintain extracellular volume, electrolyte balance, and blood pressure. These hormones increase the tubular reabsorption of sodium while promoting the excretion of potassium. The production of mineralocorticoids is controlled by the blood volume—a decrease in volume stimulates secretion and an increase inhibits secretion.

PANCREAS

The pancreas produces two endocrine hormones, insulin and glucagon (in addition to those concerned with the digestion of nutrients), which are synthesized in the islets of Langerhans by alpha and beta cells. These hormones influence glucose metabolism. Insulin promotes the use of glucose for the synthesis and storage of glycogen and fat and for the production of energy. Glucagon is produced by the alpha cells of the pancreas. It produces a hyperglycemic effect on the body, which is caused by glycogenolysis and gluconeogenesis in the liver. Glucagon is also essential for energy metabolism.

OVARIES AND TESTES

The testes in males and the ovaries in females are sources of sex hormones. These hormones are essential in fertility and for sexual development. The sex hormones, androgens and estrogens, primarily function in reproduction. In addition, they are involved in stimulation of anabolic processes. Estrogen increases sodium retention. See Chapter 12 for further discussion.

Assessment
NURSING HISTORY

The nursing history should include information about the client's health, development, social, and psychological states.

This history can be obtained during the initial contact with the client. The information should be analyzed and used as a basis for formulating a nursing diagnosis, and subsequently used for developing an individualized plan of care for the client.

Health history

The health history is an essential part of the nursing history. Important data can be obtained about the client using interviewing skills. The health history should include information about growth and development; sexual function; hair growth; changes in skin; temperature intolerance; emotional state; and changes in energy, nutrition, thought or intellectual function, and voice and urinary patterns. For example: When did secondary sex characteristics develop? Has the development of excessive hair growth been noted? Have changes been noted in the texture and pigmentation of skin? Does the client usually feel hotter or colder when in an environment with others? Does the client often feel uncomfortable (warm or cold) when others feel comfortable? Does the client experience periods of nervousness? Moist or cool extremities? To what does the client attribute these changes? Has the client noticed changes in his or her activity state? Does the client have energy to spare, or does he or she have only enough energy to carry out routine daily activities? Does the client feel sluggish and easily fatigued? Has the client noted any change in appetite? Have any changes been noted in weight? Does the client drink excessive amounts of liquids? Is the client excessively thirsty most of the time? Have changes been noted in the client's thought pattern? Does the client urinate excessively? Has the client noticed changes in his or her voice pattern? Has there been a decrease in libido?

It is always helpful to find out about the extent and duration of each of these. In addition, it will also be helpful to obtain information about past medical history, therapy, and prior surgery. For example, the nurse should inquire as to whether the client currently takes medications (steroids, insulin) or has particularly received steroid drugs within the past year. If so, the specific type of medication should be identified.

Developmental history

In this section no attempt is made to discuss development specifically as it relates to each stage. Rather, the influence that certain endocrine hormones have on growth development is discussed.

The endocrine system is instrumental in the control of skeletal growth and bodily development. The anabolic hormones, essential to promotion of growth, play an important role and are influential during a particular period.[21] The growth hormone is important, although it is not exactly clear as to when its secretion commences, its length of activity, or whether it is important during the adult years. It is thought to play only a small role during the early developmental years as evidenced by the fact that dwarfs grow normally up to 2 to 4 years.[21] During the remainder of childhood, linear growth increases but plays a minimal role in bone maturation. At the time of puberty and adolescence, sex hormones overshadow the effects of the growth hormones.

Thyroxine also has an effect on growth. Its effect on growth is predominant during the first few years of life. Its absence, however, evidences changes in growth at any stage of development, for example, a decline is noted. It exerts its influence on bone maturation rather than linear growth.

During puberty and adolescence a rapid growth spurt is observed. Such rapid growth is caused by testicular androgens in males and adrenal and ovarian androgens in females.[21] Estrogens have a lesser effect. Cortisol excess inhibits growth because of its antianabolic effect, and the fact that it inhibits the release of growth hormone. The effect of insulin on growth has been documented in animals, that is, it is growth promoting.

When the epiphyses fuse with the diaphyses of the long bones, linear growth stops. Androgens accelerate the process. Estrogens play a small part in females. After the epiphyses close, normal influence ceases.

Social history

When taking the client's social history, the nurse should obtain data about the client's age, sex, education, life-style, and occupation. Such information is valuable to the development of an individualized plan of care.

Psychological history

Obtaining information about the client's behavior, coping behaviors, and the family's reactions or responses to problems is useful. The nurse should determine how these behaviors and reactions affect the client's ability to adjust to health problems of the endocrine system. This information can form the basis for a nursing care plan.

Physical assessment

Physical assessment skills that are useful in evaluating the endocrine system are *inspection* and *palpation*.

The nurse should observe the client for height; weight; body stature; distribution of fat muscle mass; muscle wasting; and the presence of striae, hair growth and distribution, and pigmentation of the skin. The eyes should be observed for bulging, and the neck for surgery scars or swelling.

Normally the thyroid gland cannot be palpated. However, in the presence of a health problem the nurse can detect changes in the size, shape, and symmetry of the gland, and the presence of lumps or nodules through palpation. These changes may be indicative of a thyroid problem. The thyroid gland should be palpated, with special attention given to the size, shape, symmetry, tenderness, and possible growths.

DIAGNOSTIC ASSESSMENT

Diagnostic tests for endocrine function are numerous, and many of the tests involve the use of blood samples. The nurse has the responsibility of preparing the client for the test and providing the necessary support during the test. Tests will be discussed in relation to the specific glands of the endocrine system.

Assessment of pituitary function

Hematological studies. Several hematological studies may be used to assess pituitary function. Since the pituitary is interrelated with the function of other endocrine glands, the reader is referred to specific tests under each gland.

Radiological studies. Anterior, posterior, and lateral x-ray studies of the skull are made to detect enlargement of the pituitary gland, calcification, increased intracranial pressure, and erosion in the sella.[7] Asymmetry, demineralization, and changes in the contour are indicative of sellar disease.

Pneumoencephalography may be used in endocrine problems to determine the extent of a pituitary tumor.

Assessment of thyroid function

The following tests are commonly used to diagnose problems of the thyroid gland: hematological, radiological, metabolic, and reflex studies.

Hematological studies. *Protein-bound iodine* (PBI) is a measure of the amount of iodine bound to circulating protein that, in the normal state, is primarily all thyroxine iodine. A blood sample is obtained and analyzed for iodine. A normal value is 4 to 8 μg/100 ml of blood.[8] Iodine, which is necessary to form thyroid hormones, is normally bound to serum proteins. A change from normal indicates hyperactivity or hypoactivity of the thyroid. Estrogens, mercurial diuretics, iodine dyes, vitamin pills, and cough medicines that contain iodine will elevate the PBI and should therefore be discontinued several weeks before the test.[8]

Serum thyroxine (T_4 test) is a measure of thyroxine in the circulation. The normal range is 4 to 10 μg/100 ml.

The T_3 *erythrocyte uptake* test is used to determine the amount of triiodothyronine (T_3) absorbed by the red blood cells. Normally these hormones are bound to plasma proteins, but if there is additional hormonal production, the red blood cells absorb the excess. A blood specimen is obtained, and a measured amount of radioactive T_3 is added. The amount of T_3 that binds to the red blood cells is then measured. Estrogens and anticoagulants interfere with this test and should be discontinued several weeks before examination. Impaired liver function may also interfere with normal determinations. In normal values, 11% to 19% bind to erythrocytes.

The amount of circulating (free) thyroxine (T_4) can be determined by adding ^{131}I-T_4 to a given blood sample (known as the free T_4 test). Unbound T_4 may be recovered and the radioactivity counted.

293

Nursing process for common health problems

The *triiodothyronine (T3) suppression test* measures the activity of the thyroid by suppressing pituitary stimulation. A baseline of iodine normally present in the thyroid is determined by a radioactive iodine uptake (RAIU) test. The client is given a fast-acting thyroid hormone, T3, for 8 days to suppress pituitary thyrotropin (thyroid-stimulating hormone). At this time, iodine level is measured again. Normally the additional thyroid hormone will reduce thyroid-stimulating hormone from the pituitary, and iodine uptake is reduced. Uptake is not suppressed in an overactive thyroid gland because the gland is functioning independently of pituitary stimulation.

The *triiodothyronine (T3) concentration test* measures the serum concentration of triiodothyronine by radioimmunoassay.

The *thyroid-stimulating hormone* (TSH) *test* measures activity of the thyroid gland. It is performed after an RAIU test, and TSH is administered intramuscularly for a specified number of days. The RAIU is repeated. Normal glands respond with an increase of 5% or more uptake of ^{131}I.

Radiological studies. The *radioactive iodine* (^{131}I) *uptake* (RAIU) test measures the affinity of the thyroid gland for radioactive iodine. Normal values are 15% to 40%. The client should not eat or drink for six to eight hours before the test. He is given a tracer dose of ^{131}I in a solution or capsule. After ingesting the ^{131}I, the client may eat and drink. Twenty-four hours later a scintillation scanner is used to measure the amount of ^{131}I absorbed by the thyroid. Excessive accumulation of ^{131}I indicates hyperactivity of the gland, whereas minimal accumulation indicates a hypoactive thyroid gland. The test is affected by any change in the iodine content of the body as might occur from ingesting iodides or use of radiographic dyes.

The *thyroid scan* (scintillation scan) test is similar to the RAIU test and is used to visualize the thyroid gland and identify physiological problems within the gland. It is valuable in evaluating solitary nodules. After the radioactive solution or capsule is swallowed, a scintillation scanner is used to record areas of uptake.

Thyroid activity can also be measured by urinary excretion of an oral diagnostic dose of radioactive iodine. Urine specimens are saved for 24 hours, and the amount of iodine excreted is measured. Hyperactivity of the thyroid gland is indicated by excessive urinary loss of ^{131}I. In normal values, 40% to 80% of the ^{131}I is excreted within 24 hours.

Metabolic studies. The *basal metabolic rate* (BMR) is a measurement of the amount of oxygen needed for basal cellular activity. The client is given an explanation of the equipment and what is expected of him so that he will remain relaxed during the test. The client fasts for 12 hours and should have 8 to 10 hours of sleep. This rest is necessary to obtain a basal measurement of oxygen needs. If the test is performed in a physician's office or in a clinic, another person should bring the client to the office so that he does not exert himself. If the test is performed in the hospital, the client should remain in bed until the test is completed. The instrument for measuring the BMR is brought to the client's bedside. A clamp is put over his nose while he breathes through a mouthpiece that records oxygen consumption. The oxygen consumption is compared with normal values for the client's age, sex, and body size. Oxygen utilization above or below the normal values indicates disturbance of thyroid activity. Normal values would be -20% to $+20\%$ of predetermined normals.

Reflex studies. *Reflex time measurement* (kinemometry) measures the reflex time in the ankle jerk following tapping of the Achilles tendon. The reflex is fast in hyperthyroidism and slow in hypothyroidism.

Assessment of parathyroid function

Hematological studies. Serial laboratory determinations and urinary determinations of serum calcium, phosphorous, and alkaline phosphatase are common tests of parathyroid function.

Serum calcium is a measurement of the amount of ionized and nonionized calcium in the serum. Normal range is from 9 to 11 mg/100 ml of serum.

Serum phosphorus is a measurement of the amount of inorganic phosphate in the serum. The normal range is 3 to 4 mg/100 ml.

Serum alkaline phosphatase is a measurement of the amount of alkaline phosphatase in the serum.

Urinary studies. *Urinary calcium* is a measurement of the amount of calcium excreted in a 24-hour urine specimen following the administration of a calcium-deprived diet. A diet low in calcium is administered 3 to 6 days before the test. The normal range of calcium excreted in 24 hours is 75 to 175 mg.

Tubular reabsorption of phosphate (TRP) is a measurement of the amount of phosphate excreted in the urine in a 24-hour period, and a calculation of tubular reabsorption of phosphate. Measurements of the serum phosphate are also made. The normal range is from 82% to 97%. In hyperthyroidism the value is lower.

The *Ellsworth-Howard test* is a measurement of urinary phosphate at hourly intervals for three to five hours following the intravenous administration of parathyroid extract. The normal response is a fivefold to sixfold increase in the urinary phosphate. The individual with parathyroidism shows a tenfold increase.

Assessment of adrenal cortex function

Diagnostic tests used to evaluate adrenocortical function give a determination of the hormone levels in the blood and the excretion of hormones in urine.

Hematological levels of steroids. The *cortisol level* is a test used to evaluate adrenocortical function by measuring the cortisol levels in the blood at a specified time of day, usually morning and evening to coincide with the diurnal pattern. The time of day is significant to the results. It is sometimes preferred that the specimen be obtained around 8 PM when the level is nearing its lowest point. The normal range for an 8 AM sample is 9 to 24 mg/100 ml; and 3 to 12 mg/100 for a 4 PM sample.[35]

Aldosterone level is a measurement of the level of aldosterone in blood. In addition to variations occurring during the day, other factors that affect aldosterone levels (increase) include increased potassium intake, sodium restriction, and the upright position. Normal values range from 1 to 5 mg/100 ml.

Testosterone level is a measurement of the level of testosterone. There is little variation in testosterone levels during the day, although the morning value may be slightly higher. Variations may be noted in females according to the phase of the menstrual cycle (being higher in the luteal than the follicular phase).[35] The normal range is 0.3 to 1 mg/100 ml in men, and 0.01 to 0.1 mg/100 ml in women.

Urinary levels. Twenty-four-hour urine tests for 17-hydroxycorticosteroid (17-OHCS), 17-ketosteroids (17-KS), or 17-ketogenic steroids (17-KGS) are useful in evaluating adrenocortical function. They involve the analysis of the specimen for specific metabolites. The 17-hydroxycorticosteroids tests include cortisol, cortisone, tetrahydrocortisol, tetrahydrocortisone, and 11-deoxycortisol. The 17-ketogenic steroids tests include cortols, cortolones, and pregnone-triol.[35] The normal values for 17-hydroxycorticoids are 2 to 10 mg/24 hours; for 17-ketosteroids, 7 to 25 mg/24 hours for men and 4 to 15 mg/24 hours for women; and for 17-ketogenic steroids, 5 to 23 mg/24 hours for men and 3 to 15 mg/24 hours for women. Elevated levels of 17-KS are indicative of hyperadrenalism, and elevation of 17-hydroxycorticosteroids is indicative of adrenogenital tumors. It is essential that the urine specimen be collected in its entirety for the entire period of time.

Stimulation tests are tests used to evaluate secretory reserve. They are useful in detecting problems related to hypofunction.

The *glucocorticoid stimulation test* measures changes in adrenocortical function produced by the administration of ACTH. Before the test and before ACTH is administered, control levels of hydrocortisone are determined. ACTH is then administered either intramuscularly, intravenously over an 8-hour period,[8,35] or intramuscularly as a long-acting ACTH. For the intramuscular method, baseline hydrocortisone assay is taken at 8 AM, synthetic ACTH is administered, and blood is taken 1 hour later. An increase in plasma hydrocortisone indicates normal adrenocortical function.

In the 8-hour intravenous method, ACTH is added to 500 mg sodium chloride and is infused over an exact 1-hour period beginning at 8 AM on 2 successive days. A 24-hour urine specimen is collected and analyzed for creatinine, 17-ketosteroids, 17-hydroxycorticosteroids, and 17-ketogenic steroids.[8,35] Plasma hydrocortisone may also be evaluated.

One of the *mineralocorticoid stimulation tests* is the aldosterone stimulation test, which measures the secretion or excretion rates of aldosterone following specified protocols such as sodium restriction, diuretic administration, upright position, or venesection.[35]

Suppression tests are useful in detecting problems related to hyperfunction.

The *glucocorticoid suppression test* involves the administration of dexamethasone at specified intervals for a period of two successive days while urine is collected for creatinine over a 24-hour period.

The *mineralocorticoid suppression test* involves sodium chloride loading either with a saline infusion, oral salt, or desoxycorticosterone acetate (DoCA) to expand the extracellular volume. The normal response would be a decrease in renin release, a decrease in plasma renin activity, and a decrease in aldosterone secretion or excretion.[35]

Assessment of adrenal medulla function

The function of the adrenal medulla can be determined by the assay of catecholamines in the urine: the vanillylmandelic acid test is one such test.

The *vanillylmandelic acid* (VMA) *test* is a 24-hour urine test that determines urinary excretion of vanillylmandelic acid, an end product of catecholamine metabolism. The normal range is less than 7 mg/day[25] (the usual normal range is from 1 gm to 5 mg). A range higher than the normal is indicative of pheochromocytoma. Several factors alter test results, such as certain foods (coffee, tea, bananas, vanilla-containing food, and chocolate),[25] drugs (aspirin),[29] and stress. These foods and drugs should be withheld for a period of time before the test, for example, at least 24 hours or 3 days, and through the completion of the test. Care is planned to avoid stress factors during the test.

Assessment of pancreatic function

Numerous tests are useful in screening for diabetes as well as assessing its control. Hematological and urine studies are primarily used. Measurements of plasma concentrations rather than whole blood are preferred, because they are not affected by the hematocrit and more clearly reflect physiological glucose values. Elevations of plasma glucose (after an overnight fast) above 125 to 140 mg/100 ml are considered diagnostic for diabetes mellitus.

Hematological studies. *Fasting blood sugar* (FBS) *levels* is a measurement of the glucose in the blood during a fasting state. The normal range of blood sugar for the fasting client is 60 to 100 mg/100 ml (Somogyi method) and 8 to 120 mg/100 ml (Folin and Wu's method). In the client who is unable to regulate plasma glucose, the fasting range will show either an increase or decrease.

The *2-hour postprandial blood sugar test* is a test that determines the ability of an individual to dispose of a glucose load. A blood sugar measurement is made 2 hours after ingestion of a predetermined amount of carbohydrate, usually 100 gm of glucose. A disturbance in the glucose regulating mechanism is present if the glucose levels remain high after 2 hours. Normally the glucose should return to normal within this time. This test is frequently used to monitor insulin therapy.

The *oral glucose tolerance test* (OGTT) may be used to confirm a diagnosis when the blood test is borderline.[23] The client should have normal activity and diet containing at least 150 mg carbohydrate for 3 days before the test. Recent illness, thiazide diuretics, steroids, salicylates, oral contraceptives, or hormones alter metabolism, can confuse the results of the test, and should be discontinued 2 weeks before the test.

Immediately before the test the client should receive nothing by mouth for 10 to 12 hours. Some institutions, however, permit the client to drink water. After fasting baseline specimens of blood and urine are obtained, a known amount of glucose, based on body weight, is given. The glucose is usually given in a palatable oral form, but if the client becomes nauseated, it can be given intravenously. If the client vomits, the test should be discontinued. Blood and urine specimens are taken at 30 minutes and 1, 2, and 3 hours after the ingestion of the glucose. Some physicians may order a 5-hour glucose tolerance test, in which case specimens are also obtained at the fourth and fifth hours.

During the test the client should remain in bed so that the amount of glucose used by the body is measured at basal levels. The client should not smoke or ingest any food or medications until the test is completed.[23]

Very little urine is necessary for urinalysis, and the client is encouraged to void at the proper time. After the second specimen is obtained, the client may drink water to facilitate voiding.

The blood and urine are analyzed for the presence of glucose. Normally the blood glucose level rises to 150 mg/100 ml within 30 minutes of ingesting glucose and returns to fasting levels (60 to 120 mg/100 ml) in two hours. No glucose should appear in the urine. Ranges vary with each laboratory, and thresholds vary with age. Blood levels can increase 10 mg/100 ml for each decade after 50. Blood levels that rise to 210 mg/100 ml in 2 hours are considered diagnostic for diabetes mellitus.

Glycosylated hemoglobins (hemoglobin A), elevated in individuals with diabetes mellitus, may be measured in the blood. The measurement is of limited use in diagnosis, because elevations may also occur in healthy individuals. The assay may be used, however, to monitor glycemic control with diet and insulin, and is often used to determine compliance with therapy.

Data analysis

After obtaining the essential information about the client, the nurse should compare the data with norms appropriate to the client's age, sex, and developmental level. Consideration should be given to social and psychological data, because the information is analyzed in preparation for the formulation of nursing diagnoses. Potential or actual diagnoses may include alterations in cardiac output, alterations in comfort, fear, potential for injury, alterations in nutrition, disturbance in self-concept, impairment of skin integrity, disturbance in sleep pattern, alterations in thought processes, alterations in urinary elimination, ineffective coping, noncompliance, knowledge deficit, and fluid volume deficit.

Planning

PLANNING FOR HEALTH PROMOTION

Although individuals are increasingly becoming more informed about health problems that affect the regulatory mechanisms, nurses must continue to provide instructions to clients regarding prevention and care. For example, providing instructions about the importance of using iodized salt, controlling the weight, and seeking health care when problems develop should be part of the instructions related to the promotion of health.

PLANNING FOR HEALTH MAINTENANCE AND RESTORATION

The nurse has an important role in the care of the client with disease of the endocrine system. Much of the care that is planned can be based on symptoms that are commonly experienced, including weakness, changes in appearance, and emotional instability, and the therapy used in treatment of the problems.

One consideration is to modify the environment (physical and emotional) to minimize the problems that are so frequently experienced by these clients. (Information regarding diet should include its relationship to life-style, family support, and so on.)

Many clients with endocrine problems must take drugs on a long-term basis. Corticosteroids and insulin are two of these. Because of the long-term use and self-administration of such drugs, nurses must fully inform the client about the drugs and their safe administration.

Steroid therapy

One such class of drugs is the steroids. All steroids have some metabolic, mineralocorticoid, and sex hormone activities that overlap, but each has its dominant role.

Pharmacological considerations. Administration of cortisol or related synthetic derivatives will result in inhibition of ACTH secretion and thus the diminution of endogenous cortisol production and release. The degree of suppression will depend on the potency and quantity of the agent and the nature and duration of the therapy regimen. There is a high correlation between the length of the exogenous administration and the length of time to recover normal ACTH responsiveness.

Synthetic derivatives of cortisol and cortisone have fewer and less severe side effects than the natural substances. Sodium and water retention is less marked without concurrent loss of antiinflammatory effects. They are also more slowly metabolized by the liver, producing improved tissue distribution and stability. The therapeutic activities continue for a longer period than their measurable presence in the circulation.

Water-soluble corticosteroid esters are often given parenterally in medical emergencies because of their rapid and profound effect with relatively minor attendant hazards. Therapy of this nature, however, is usually limited to 1 or 2 days to avoid side effects and alteration of hypothalamus-pituitary-adrenal responsiveness. A primary problem in short-term, high-dose steroid administration is peptic ulceration. Parenteral steroids may be infused over a prolonged period as replacement therapy for clients who are dependent on exogenous steroids (such as those with Addison's disease) or during surgery or other crises that alter their usual physiological functioning.

Injectable suspensions of steroids may be given intramuscularly and have the advantage of prolonging duration of action (up to a week in some cases).

When steroid therapy for a prolonged period of time is planned, normal steroid levels must be assessed to establish the level of dosage necessary for pharmacological effects. Glucose tolerance tests, 24-hour urine specimens, and gastrointestinal x-ray films are usually ordered for 1 or more days before initial administration, along with several other laboratory studies, to rule out illnesses such as ulcers, diabetes, or tuberculosis that may be aggravated by therapy.

Psychological changes are to be anticipated during therapy and may include mood elevations or frank euphoria. On withdrawal, the client usually has a psychic letdown and often plunges into depression. Sometimes this depression is linked to the exacerbation of discomfort that may occur with withdrawal of symptomatic control. For example, the person with arthritis may feel increased joint pain and general discomfort because of swelling and inflammation of joints.

Problems in long-term therapy include growth retardation, obesity, gastritis, osteoporosis, hypertension, renal calculi, and adrenal atrophy. Some of these are inherent but may be minimized by following some well-known guidelines.

Local administration of any steroid prevents systemic absorption but maximizes desired effects at the site of application. Oral administration is likely to produce gastric ulceration but has the advantage of ease of client self-medication. Sublingual dosage is useful in allergic conditions such as asthma because it reaches pulmonary circulation quite rapidly, has long-lasting effects, and requires only small doses.

Consideration must be given to the *timing* of administration of steroids. Considerable research has been done to relate steroid administration to the normal circadian rhythm. It is recommended that the drug be given to enhance the normal cycle—giving higher doses in the morning and tapering to lower ones in the afternoon. Giving the last dose at, or about, the evening mealtime seems to reduce the side effects of restlessness and insomnia. On the other hand, if it is important to maintain a specific blood level (such as in the management of adrenocortical suppression), the dose should be given close to midnight. (There is marked increase in pituitary-adrenal activity at about 2 AM in the circadian cycle.)

The therapeutic effects last longer than metabolic effects. Administration of double the daily dose every other day seems to produce desired therapeutic effects while reducing side effects and maintaining the hypothalamus-pituitary-adrenal reserve. This pattern also assists in the transition that accompanies withdrawal from corticosteroids. Often, such an every-other-day program has the added benefit of reminding the client that treatment is palliative rather than curative, since the day without therapy may be a time of exacerbation of uncomfortable symptoms. Teaching is especially important with this type of therapy so that the client clearly understands the rationale of the administration procedure.

Nursing process for common health problems

Assessment. Nurses should have knowledge of which clients are currently being managed by steroid therapy. This, of course, requires that nurses know the many names of medications that fall into this category. Even though the preparation is listed with medications, an indication should also be entered on the nursing assessment form and in the nursing care plan that the client *has been* receiving steroids within the past year *or* that he *is* currently receiving such therapy. This knowledge is essential for observing him for complications, preventing complications, and making the staff aware of side effects. Such information is also vital for managing the care of clients who will be subjected to major stresses such as surgery.

Steroid therapy results in suppression of the normal hypothalamus-pituitary-adrenal response mechanism to stress, and if therapy is suddenly withdrawn, the client is not prepared physiologically to cope with crises. Common stresses besides those of an emotional nature include drastic changes in temperature (internal and external), infections, fluid and electrolyte imbalances, and tissue trauma. Even though several months may have passed since the client received systemic steroids, the physician must be aware of this in order to prevent an adrenal crisis related to suppressed endocrine responses to stress.

Acute adrenal crises can be recognized by restlessness, weakness, falling blood pressure, headache, dehydration, and gastrointestinal disturbances such as nausea, vomiting, and diarrhea. If such a shocklike state occurs, it is likely that a temporary dose may be given to ensure the body's ability to cope with stress in a sudden crisis (such as surgery).

Intravenous administration of steroids requires careful monitoring and precise adherence to schedules and flow rates. No interruption in therapy can be tolerated. For example, it is especially important that the nurse recognize infiltration or other problems in regulating flow. Special apparatus to provide mechanical control of the rate may be used, such as the microdrip setup or the infusion pump.

Some physicians require several laboratory studies to determine physiological steroid levels during or after withdrawal to assess the body's inherent mechanism for responding to crises. Especially early after withdrawal the nurse should be alert to weakness, easy exhaustion, and lethargy because these symptoms are indicative of low tolerance to stress.

There are several important considerations in routine nursing assessment for clients currently receiving therapeutic doses of steroids. Side effects from steroid therapy result from dosages congruous with pharmacological rather than physiological doses and are outlined in Table 9-4.

Planning and implementation. Nurses must understand the objectives and hazards related to steroid therapy and be knowledgeable enough about the therapeutic regimen to interpret it to clients.

An important aspect of therapeutic programs is to cope with side effects and minimize their occurrence.

Cushing's disease–like adiposity characterized by truncal obesity, a moon face, and a "buffalo hump" (fat pad just below the back of the neck) can be expected in prolonged and high-dose therapy. Weight gain and sodium retention can be minimized by a low-sodium diet and caloric restrictions.

Since steroids stimulate the appetites of most clients, caloric reduction is difficult to achieve. Foods high in potassium can be employed to reduce the adverse effects of potassium depletion. Dietary restrictions may be complicated, however, in the presence of a negative nitrogen balance, which calls for a high-carbohydrate, high-protein diet. A diabetic diet regimen may be recommended for some clients to prevent steroid-induced diabetes mellitus.

Increased calcium and phosphorus output, which contributes to osteoporosis and even pathological fractures, may be managed by a high-calorie, high-protein diet and activity patterns that encourage regular physical exercise. It seems that calcium has an affinity for active tissue and that sedentary clients are actually encouraging calcium deficits from bones. If the person is confined to bed, range-of-motion exercises are recommended, and measures are taken to prevent pathological fractures from injury.

Wound healing is slow for those on steroid therapy, and this affords an additional incentive to protect the client from any form of tissue trauma.

Gastrointestinal ulceration occurs because of an increase in acidity induced from the stressor effect of the drug. It is advantageous to give the medication with an antacid or with food to minimize mucosal irritation. Nurses should also teach the client to test his stools or emesis for blood and to report any evidence of gastrointestinal bleeding. An ulcer-bland diet and anticholinergic drugs may be useful, too.

The teaching plan should always stress that if the drug is not retained (for example, if it is expelled in emesis) or omitted for any reason, the physician should be notified.

Blood pressure, intake and output, and other clinical measurements are useful in evaluating side effects, but unless coupled with broader observations and laboratory studies, they are of limited usefulness. Daily weights are frequently ordered.

Stress in day-to-day activity cannot always be controlled but should be

TABLE 9-4

Steroid therapy: a nursing guide

Steroids	Normal physiological role	Side effects
Glucocorticoids	Stimulated by pituitary ACTH acting on adrenal cortex; assists in coping with stress	Loss of ability to cope with physiological stress
Short-acting preparation: half-life less than 12 hours	Inhibits peripheral tissue protein synthesis; converts proteins to glucose	Increased fat deposits due to muscle protein destruction
Hydrocortisone		
Cortisone	Increases hepatic gluconeogenesis	Insulin antagonism, steroid diabetes
Intermediate-acting preparations: half-life between 12-36 hours	Suppresses inflammatory responses (inhibits scar formation, blocks allergic responses, decreases lymphatic tissue, reduces exudation)	Exacerbation of inflammations, masking of infections, depression of antibody production
Prednisone		
Prednisolone	Reduces intestinal absorption of calcium and alters behavior of growth hormones	Osteoporosis, growth retardation, renal calculi
Methylprednisolone		
Triamcinolone		
Long-acting preparations: half-life greater than 48 hours		
Paramethasone		
Betamethasone		
Dexamethasone		
Mineralocorticoids	Secreted in response to decreased blood volume; works with ADH to maintain fluid volume equilibrium	Polydipsia, polyuria
Aldosterone		
Desoxycortone acetate		
	Retains water and sodium	Weight gain, edema, hypertension
	Promotes potassium excretion	Muscle weakness, fatigue, alkalosis

considered in planning care. Some physicians even teach their clients to adjust their dosages in stages of unusual stress.

Clients on steroids are not only more susceptible to infections because of decreased amounts of lymphocytes, but the drug also tends to mask symptoms (by its antiinflammatory effects) that commonly denote infection. Fever, redness, pain, and edema, which are cardinal signs of an inflammatory response, are usually not noticeable. All clients should be protected from known infection hazards, and added attention should be given to observing for inflammatory responses such as thrombophlebitis or decubitus ulcers.

Children who are on prolonged steroid therapy are especially susceptible to the mood swings congruent with the drug. When these psychological reactions are coupled with the growth retardation, weight gain, acne and other skin changes, and hirsutism related to the therapeutic regimen, they often make for a real nursing challenge in coping with behavioral responses to negative body images.

Clients of all ages should carry identification with the following information: name, physician's name and telephone number, steroid medication, and emergency instructions. These data may be lifesaving in an accident or undiagnosed medical emergency. Employers, schoolteachers, and babysitters must know what to do in an emergency.

Steroids and their implications should be discussed openly with the client and his family. It is one form of drug therapy that must be clearly understood, and the nurse has an important role in the teaching plan.

Insulin therapy. See discussion of insulin therapy in this chapter.

Implementation

COMMON HEALTH PROBLEMS THAT OCCUR ACROSS THE LIFE SPAN

Anterior pituitary

Problems associated with abnormal function of the pituitary gland include those with hormone deficit or excess.

Hypopituitarism. Hypopituitarism results from a deficiency of one or more pituitary hormones. This state may occur as a result of the effects of disease in the hypothalamic centers that control release of pituitary hormones, or from problems directly involving the pituitary gland.[12] For example, trauma, tumors, or a disease such as sarcoidosis may decrease the pituitary hormone secretions that are primarily controlled by the releasing factors. Damage or destruction of the pituitary gland by infarction (for example, Sheehan's syndrome that occurs in the postpartum period) may also be responsible. The presence of a tumor may invade or compress the gland and result in a reduction in blood flow from the hypothalmic-hypophyseal portal system and interfere with the delivery of the releasing factor.

The symptoms produced in hypopituitarism vary and depend on the specific hormones that are lost. For example, loss of gonadotropin causes hypogonadism, deficient growth hormone causes dwarfism in children, decreased thyroid-stimulating hormone produces hypothyroidism, and lack of ACTH causes adrenocortical insufficiency. (See discussion of hypothyroidism and adrenal insufficiency in this chapter.)

Dwarfism. Dwarfism, resulting from lack of growth hormone, is characterized by a retardation in growth within the first year of life, in spite of the infant being of normal size at birth.[12] The child with dwarfism tends to be chubby and lacks muscular development, and puberty is delayed. The injection of growth hormone intramuscularly is considered successful if started before epiphyseal closure.[12] A protocol for administration of the hormone has been developed, according to Hershman, by the National Pituitary Agency.

Hypogonadism. Children with hypogonadism do not enter normal puberty. In the female the breasts fail to develop, pubic and axillary hair do not develop, and amenorrhea is common. The male has a small phallus and testes, and body hair is sparse.

Acquired hypogonadism in adults may also occur and result in amenorrhea, breast atrophy, and loss of pubic hair in women. In men it causes atrophy of the testes, decrease in body hair, decrease in libido, and impotence. Therapy involves replacement of the missing hormones.

Hyperpituitarism. Hyperpituitarism refers to an abnormal overproduction of one or more of the pituitary hormones.[12] This overproduction is most commonly caused by hormone production by functioning pituitary tumors. Two distinct disturbances of the growth hormone have been widely accepted— gigantism and acromegaly. The only difference in these disorders is the age of onset.

Gigantism. Gigantism results from a sustained hypersecretion of the growth hormone in the child (for example, before puberty). It starts when the bones can grow longitudinally, and subsequently results in a generalized overgrowth of skeleton and soft tissue. As a result, a marked increase is noted in height and size.

Acromegaly. Acromegaly is a condition that results from a sustained hypersecretion of the growth hormone in the adult.

Pathophysiology. Acromegaly occurs after epiphyseal closure.[25] The bones grow wider and thicker. As a result, the extremities are characteristically enlarged. The lower jaw tends to lengthen, and the bridge of the nose becomes broader. The soft tissue of the hand and feet enlarge and take on a coarse appearance.

Assessment. The client may complain of oily skin, excessive sweating, which results from hypertrophy of the sweat, and sebaceous glands.[12] Thickening of the voice, due to thickening of the vocal cords, may occur. Pressure on the visual pathway from the tumor may produce visual impairments. Headaches may also be noted, and examination usually reveals visceromegaly (especially of the heart and kidney).

A diagnosis is generally established on the basis of changes in physical appearance, demonstration of a tumor on x-ray films of the skull, and x-ray films of the structures such as the jaw, sinuses, hands, and feet.

Because glucose normally suppresses growth hormone secretion, a glucose tolerance test may be ordered. In most clients with acromegaly the growth hormone level does not decrease.[22] Cerebral angiography or pneumoencephalography may be ordered to determine the extent of the tumor, particularly if surgery is anticipated.

> *Data analysis*
> *Data analysis may reveal nursing diagnoses of disturbance in self-concept and alterations in comfort.*

Planning and implementation. Either radiation therapy or surgery may be used as forms of therapy. The surgical procedure that may be used is a transphenoid hypophysectomy. With this technique, function of the posterior pituitary is maintained.[25] If either the disease or the treatment result in hypofunction of the anterior pituitary, appropriate substitution therapy (for example, corticosteroids, thyroid androgens, estrogens) may be indicated.[22,25] A craniotomy may sometimes be performed, but may result in posterior pituitary dysfunction.[25]

Pituitary tumor Pituitary tumors account for approximately 10% of all cranial tumors.[22] The most common pituitary tumor is the *chromophobe adenoma,* which may not cause an endocrine deficiency, but may produce symptoms associated with a space-occupying lesion. Such symptoms may vary, depending on the size or location of the tumor. For example, they may compress the optic nerve, hypothalamus, or other nervous structures.

 Assessment. Headache, which is common, can be attributed to stretching of the dura mater from distension of the adenoma. If the optic chiasma is compressed, visual problems may develop (for example, hemianopsia and other visual problems such as blurring of vision, impaired visual acuity, and photophobia). Pressure on the hypothalamus may cause sleep disturbance, disturbances in temperature regulation, loss of appetite, and alterations in levels of consciousness.[12,22]

Varied tests may be used to evaluate the client. Among these are roentgenograms of the skull, ophthalmologic examination, pneumoencephalogram, and carotid angiogram.

> **Data analysis**
> *Data analysis may reveal nursing diagnoses of disturbance in self-concept, disturbance in sleep patterns, and alterations in comfort.*

 Planning and implementation. Therapy for pituitary tumors generally involves surgery or irradiation. Surgery may be delayed in some instances, especially if the tumor is small and localized, during which time hormonal replacement therapy may be instituted.[22] Rapid deterioration of vision and brain compression usually dictate the need for resection surgery.

Radiation therapy is useful in that it is often associated with tumor regression and relief of signs and symptoms. Therapy is prescribed in doses that destroy the diseased area but produce no harmful effect on normal pituitary tissue and surrounding nervous structures.[22] Techniques that have been used and that are still considered experimental include cryohypophysectomy, proton-beam irradiation, and radioactive implants.

Pituitary apoplexy (hemorrhage into a tumor) may develop in clients with a pituitary tumor. It is thought to be caused by sudden enlargement of the tumor, usually from hemorrhage necrosis within this tumor. It is speculated that the spontaneous hemorrhage may be the result of rapid enlargement of the adenoma with infarction, or rupture of the fine-walled vessels in the tumor. It has also been observed following radiation therapy. The symptoms develop suddenly and are characterized by severe headaches, visual impairment (for example, diplopia, blindness) altered mentation, hypotension, and shock.[22]

The sudden appearance of these symptoms dictates the need for emergency therapy. Among the emergency measures that may be employed include surgical aspiration of the sella turcica, use of corticosteroids to correct secondary adrenal deficiency and decrease cerebral edema, and supportive measures.

Diabetes insipidus

Diabetes insipidus is a condition in which there is an absolute or partial deficiency of AVP (ADH). Because of the deficiency, the kidneys are not able to conserve free water, and the consequence is excessive diuresis. As a result, the client drinks copious amounts of water.

Assessment. Diabetes insipidus is rare and is characterized by excessive diuresis and subsequent polydipsia. The urine, which is pale and dilute, generally has a specific gravity that is usually below 1.010, unless the client is dehydrated. [8] The client may lose as much as 15 to 29 liters of urine per day. [7] Consequently, signs of dehydration become evident (for example, dry skin, constipation, intense thirst). The deprivation of water does not alter the diuresis. The diagnosis is based on the presenting symptoms, a low specific gravity of urine, and urinary osmolality below the plasma level.

Planning and implementation. Therapy is planned to correct the underlying cause (for example, intracranial problems). Vasopressin is used as replacement therapy, which is continued throughout life. Vasopressin via intramuscular injection or by nasal insufflation is also sometimes used.

COMMON PROBLEMS OF THE THYROID GLAND

Diseases of the thyroid gland involve an insufficient production of the thyroid hormone (hypothyroidism), excessive production (hyperthyroidism), or an enlargement of the gland (goiter).

Hypothyroidism

Hypothyroidism is a disease that occurs as a result of insufficient synthesis of thyroid hormone. The causes of this insufficiency are many: biochemical defects, absence or destruction of thyroid tissue,[34] and anterior pituitary insufficiency.[8] Iatrogenic factors such as antithyroid drugs, surgery, thiocyanates, paraaminosalicylic acid, and iodides may also be responsible.[34]

Hypothyroidism affects both sexes across the life span, but women in the 30 to 60 age group are more commonly affected. In infants, hypothyroidism is referred to as cretinism; in children and adolescents, juvenile hypothyroidism; in adults, myxedema.

Cretinism. Cretinism, often referred to as congenital hypothyroidism, results from an inadequate output of thyroid hormone during uterine and neonatal life.[28] The thyroid hormone is essential during embryonic life for the development and growth of many tissues, especially brain tissue.[8] Retardation will occur if this hormone is not present during fetal development.

Assessment. Symptoms associated with hypothyroidism result from decreased metabolism. In the infant, lethargy, constipation, feeding problems, weight loss, broad nose, a hoarse cry (which is thought to be caused by the thick tongue), dry thick skin, and hypothermia are evident. The fontanels may be late to close. As the infant ages, symptoms may be evidenced in slowed growth and development. For example, linear growth development may be retarded as evidenced in shortness of stature and short hands and feet. There is also late appearance of teeth. The infant may learn to crawl, sit, or stand at a slower rate. Decrease in physical activity is also often noted. Mental retardation may be present. It is generally considered that infants who must be awakened for feeding and who cry infrequently should be suspected of having hypothyroidism.[14]

Several screening procedures have been developed for the purpose of detecting cretinism in the neonatal period.[8] Cord blood or heel pad blood spots on filter paper are examined for thyroxine (or TSH). A measurement of T_3 in cord blood has also been developed. X-ray examination of bone development and closure of fontanels also is helpful in the establishment of a diagnosis of cretinism.

> ### Data analysis
> *Data analysis may reveal nursing diagnoses such as sleep pattern disturbance and alterations in thought process.*

Planning and implementation. Hormone replacement therapy, the primary form of treatment, is begun as early as possible to prevent brain damage. The dosage is generally high in relation to the infant's size. It is also often necessary for adjustments to be made in drug dosage as the infant grows. It has been documented that by age 3 or 4 the child may be taking the adult dose.[8,10] Therapy, which is continued throughout life, improves the retardation. Parameters that are used to determine adequacy of therapy in the child are growth curve, bone age, and serum T_3 and TSH levels.[14] For a further discussion of thyroid therapy, see planning and implementation section following myxedema.

Juvenile hypothyroidism. Juvenile hypothyroidism (acquired hypothyroidism) occurs when a previously normal child or adolescent develops thyroid deficiency.[14,24] More commonly the thyroid deficiency may be caused by mild genetic enzyme defects, autoimmune thyroiditis,[8] medications used in treating hyperthyroidism (for example, ^{131}I), or following thyroidectomy. Retardation of growth is evident, and there may be a delay in sexual maturation. Irregularities of the menstrual cycle are common.

Myxedema. Myxedema occurs as a result of the conditions discussed under juvenile hypothyroidism. As with all forms of hypothyroidism, deficiency of the hormone decreases metabolism of all body cells.

Assessment. Symptoms such as fatigue, reduced tolerance to cold (for example, the client may complain of being cold regardless of the room or environmental temperature), constipation (from decreased motility of the gastrointestinal tract), weight gain (from fluid retention), hoarseness, dyspnea, and menorrhagia are common.

As the problem worsens, a slowness is noted in intellectual function, for example, the client may more and more find it difficult to concentrate and may have memory lapses. Anorexia, weight gain, changes in speech (which might be evidenced as thick, hoarse and slurred), increased dryness of the hair and skin, and thick, brittle nails are common.

The diagnosis of hypothyroidism is based on clinical symptoms, changes in behavior, and slower thyroid activity as indicated by the BMR, PBI, and RAIU studies. Serum studies of TSH, T_4, and T_3 are also obtained to assist in diagnosis. Serum TSH, which is increased, is the most sensitive indicator.[28]

> ### Data analysis
> *Data analysis may reveal nursing diagnoses of alterations in comfort, disturbance in self-concept, potential impairment in skin integrity, alterations in thought process, alterations in bowel elimination (constipation), potential for injury, and alterations in nutrition.*

Planning and implementation. Therapy is planned to establish a normal thyroid state by administering hormone replacement therapy. Nursing care during diagnosis and early treatment is supportive, both physical and psychological. Commonly prescribed thyroid preparations include thyroid USP (dessicated thyroid or thyroid extract), proloid thyroglobulin (proloid), levothyroxine (synthroid, levoid, levothyroid), liothyronine (Cytomel) and liotrix (Euthroid, Thyrolar). These drugs must be given in gradually increasing doses to prevent the heart from failing under the demands of increased metabolism. The client who is receiving these drugs should be observed for changes in cardiovascular status, since abrupt acceleration in metabolism may cause tachydysrhythmias, angina, and congestive heart failure. Vital signs should be monitored closely. Before administration of the medication, the pulse rate should be assessed. A pulse rate over 120 in the child and 100 in the adult warrants withholding the medication and consulting with the physician regarding the rate. Nervousness, excitability, tremors, tachycardia, and hypertension may be indicative of excessive therapy. The appearance of these should be reported to the physician.

While the client is adjusting to the medications, the nurse should help him understand that the medications must be taken for the rest of his life. Since memory impairment is characteristic and may affect the client's ability to remember instructions, a family member should be included in instruction sessions. It may also be helpful to supplement instructions with printed materials. The client should be instructed to establish the practice of taking the medications about the same time each day as such practice facilitates compliance.

In addition to monitoring cardiovascular effects and the body's response to the medications and giving instructions, the nurse must also observe the client's behavior. Changes in the client's activity are likely. The family and client may be upset over these changes and should understand that they will be reversed. Merely informing them that this is a gradual process, listening, and giving reassurance are supportive strategies. Opportunities should be provided for rest as needed.

Other considerations should be given to the skin temperature, diet, and elimination. Lotions can be used on the dry skin. The environment should be warm, and the client should be protected from chilling. A high-protein low-calorie diet with roughage is used to meet needs for nutrition and to prevent constipation. Laxatives are sometimes prescribed to facilitate adequate elimination.

Evaluation. The evaluation component of the nursing process is continuous. The nursing care plan is individualized and depends on the stage of development when the problem is identified.

EXPECTED OUTCOMES

The client and/or family can:
1. Describe hypothyroidism.
2. State plans for following the therapeutic plan, including those for medications, exercise, diet, stress, and self-care.
3. State use, time, dosage, route, and side effects of prescribed therapy.
4. State the importance of long-term therapy.
5. State strategies for compliance to therapy.
6. Demonstrate ability to accurately monitor pulse rate.

Nursing process for common health problems

7. State signs indicative of cardiovascular changes.
8. State signs indicative of immediate health care.
9. State plans for follow-up care.

Hyperthyroidism

Hyperthyroidism (thyrotoxicosis) is a hypermetabolic state that occurs as a result of excessive production of T_4 or T_3 or both.[14] This excessive release of the hormone usually results from a goiter or hyperfunctioning nodule.[25] It occurs more commonly in women than in men, and is rare in children.[15] Hyperthyroidism is of several types. Graves' disease, which is one of the most common, will be discussed.

Graves' disease (Basedows' disease) is a form of hyperthyroidism associated with thyroidal and extrathyroidal manifestation, for example, a diffusely hyperplastic goiter, infiltrative ophthalmopathy, and dermopathy.[12] The exact cause of Graves' disease is not known; however, immune factors have been associated with it. This association has been related to the demonstration that an antibody, long-acting thyroid stimulator (LATS), reacts with the thyroid cell surface receptor for TSH.[11] The action of this antibody is thought to be of longer duration than TSH and can be sensitized by lymphocytes of persons with Graves' disease.

Graves' disease occurs most often in the third and fourth decades of life. It is more likely to occur at puberty, following pregnancy, during menopause,[12,31] and after physical trauma.[31]

 Assessment. Symptoms that occur are associated with the triad: thyroidal, ophthalmopathy, and dermopathy. These may appear together or separately.[15]

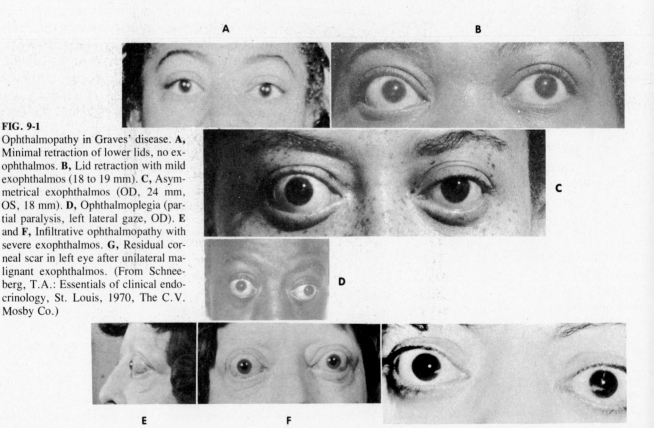

FIG. 9-1
Ophthalmopathy in Graves' disease. **A,** Minimal retraction of lower lids, no exophthalmos. **B,** Lid retraction with mild exophthalmos (18 to 19 mm). **C,** Asymmetrical exophthalmos (OD, 24 mm, OS, 18 mm). **D,** Ophthalmoplegia (partial paralysis, left lateral gaze, OD). **E** and **F,** Infiltrative ophthalmopathy with severe exophthalmos. **G,** Residual corneal scar in left eye after unilateral malignant exophthalmos. (From Schneeberg, T.A.: Essentials of clinical endocrinology, St. Louis, 1970, The C.V. Mosby Co.)

The signs and symptoms related to the thyroid feature generally reflect the rapid metabolism of body cells and increased sensitivity of tissue to catecholamines.[12] Among the commonly experienced complaints are nervousness and intolerance to heat (both of which may not be noticed by the client), diaphoresis, and increased appetite, usually associated with loss of weight. Tremors (for example, fine hand tremors), weakness (associated with catabolism of muscle protein), clumsiness, fatigability, and diarrhea are also commonly experienced. Tachycardia, palpitation, dyspnea (which is thought to be caused by weakness of the intercostal muscle), or increased use of oxygen,[12] and warm, moist skin are usually noted on physical examination. Menstrual changes (for example, oligomenorrhea or amenorrhea) may also occur.

The ophthalmopathy may be mild or severe. Usually ophthalmopathy presents the problem of exophthalmos (proptosis), which is either unilateral or bilateral (Fig. 9-1). Several factors have been documented to cause the exophthalmos infiltration of the retroorbital space with mast cells, lymphocytes, and mucopolysaccharides, and to cause retroorbital muscle edema.[12] Other ophthalmic symptoms that may occur include increased lacrimation, diplopia, and, if severe, vision may be threatened.

Dermopathy is evidenced by thickened shiny skin, particularly over the pretibial aspect of the legs. Hence it is called pretibial myxedema.[8] A diagnosis is based on physical symptoms and results of serum thyroxine, triiodothyronine, and thyroid function tests, specifically PBI, RAIU, and BMR. The results of these parameters are usually elevated.

> **Data analysis**
> *Data analysis may reveal nursing diagnoses of alterations in cardiac output, alterations in comfort, impairment of skin integrity, disturbance in self-concept, potential for injury, and alterations in nutrition.*

Planning and implementation. As a plan of care is developed, consideration should be given to these diagnoses. Adequate rest, comfort, and safety are essential; therefore nursing care should be directed toward this end.

Promoting rest. Rest is essential to conserving the client's strength. The accomplishment of this objective may present a challenge to the nurse because of the client's tendency to be nervous and easily excited. A calm, quiet environment must be maintained, and all stimuli must be kept at a minimum. It may be helpful to plan some form of quiet diversion for the client.

Promoting safety. The weakness, nervousness, and tremors that are experienced make the client prone to accidents. A safe environment must be maintained by removing clutter and breakable items from the environment. If the client desires hot liquids, care must be taken to prevent accidental burns.

Maintaining nutrition. The diet should be high in protein, vitamins, minerals, and adequate in calories to supply the increased body needs. It may be necessary to maintain the nutritional state with frequent feedings. Any foods that act as stimulants should not be permitted the client (for example, coffee, tea).

Promoting comfort. Since heat is so poorly tolerated by many of these clients, a comfortable environmental temperature must be maintained. Clothing should be loose, and it may be helpful to give frequent baths.

Nursing process for common health problems

Supportive therapy. Therapy is planned to reduce the rate of hormone secretion and includes the use of antithyroid drugs, radioactive iodine, and surgery.

Antithyroid drugs. Antithyroid drugs inhibit the synthesis of the thyroid hormone. Commonly prescribed drugs are propylthiouracil (PTU), methimazole (Tapazole), and carbimazole. These drugs are given in divided dosages because of their short duration of action. Clients must be informed of the necessity for long-term therapy, the side effects of the drugs (urticaria, dermatitis, leukopenia, nausea, arthralgia), and the importance of complying with prescribed therapy, including periodic evaluation of serum. Follow-up therapy is essential and should be stressed.

Iodine, which inhibits release of the hormone, possibly by interfering with proteolysis of thyroglobulin,[12] may also be prescribed. Saturated solution of potassium iodide is the commonly used drug in this category.

Finally, a beta receptor blocking drug such as propranolol may be prescribed to control some of the symptoms frequently noted, (for example, tremors, agitation, tachycardia, nervousness).[12]

The use of antithyroid drugs and iodine is likely to result in a dramatic changes in the client's condition. The nurse should, as a result, assess the client closely for signs indicative of a reduction in thyroid activity, for example, the client is likely to be less emotional, less excitable, and calmer, and the pulse rate will decrease. The client's general feelings and symptoms (palpitation and so on) will likely improve.[5] The physician will undoubtedly obtain objective data of the client's response to antithyroid drugs by securing measurements of the BMR and serum thyroxine levels.

Radioactive iodine. Radioactive iodine is more commonly used for clients beyond the childbearing years.[31] It is not a consideration for children because of the risk of carcinoma. A therapeutic dose of the radioactive substance, based on the client's weight, is administered orally. The drug selectively concentrates in the "thyroid follicular cells" and consequently destroys the thyroid tissue.[12] A common complication of this mode of therapy is hypothyroidism. In general, clients have a tendency to associate the use of radioactive therapy with cancer; it is therefore imperative for the nurse to give the client a complete explanation of the medication, its use, and its effects.

Surgery. Surgery, another mode of therapy, is usually elected for clients under 40 years of age.[15] A subtotal thyroidectomy is considered the preferred surgical procedure.

PREOPERATIVE NURSING CARE. Preoperative preparation is directed toward achieving a euthyroid state. This is accomplished with the use of antithyroid drugs. Iodine, in the form of Lugol's solution, is prescribed to decrease the size and vascularity of the thyroid, as well as to promote storage of thyroxine. This solution is unpalatable and should therefore be mixed with fruit juice and administered through a straw.

As the client awaits surgical intervention, information about postoperative expectations (for example, turning, coughing, and deep-breathing exercises) should be provided. Questions should be answered truthfully but calmly, because there is a tendency for many of these clients to panic easily. All conversations with the client should be conducted in a calm manner.

Several comfort measures that relate to the postoperative period should be discussed with the client (for example, how to support the head to prevent strain

310

on the suture line). These activities should be practiced and explanations given as to their importance.

POSTOPERATIVE NURSING CARE. When the client returns from surgery, the objectives of care established for the client will be similar to those noted preoperatively, and with added consideration given to observing and preventing postoperative complications. The position the client maintains is one measure that directly relates to these objectives. A semi-Fowler's position with the head, neck, and shoulder well supported with pillows is desirable. Hyperextension of the neck should be discouraged. Initially on moving or turning the client, the nurse should manually support the client's head. Later, support can be provided by the client. Such practice minimizes stress on the suture line. Excessive talking should not be permitted.

As healing takes place and the sutures are removed, full range of motion of the neck can be encouraged. When the client initially sees the suture line, there may be concern expressed regarding the appearance of the incision. The client should be reassured that the swelling will gradually decrease and the color will return to normal.

In addition to engaging the client in activities to promote comfort and prevent complications (for example, turning, coughing, deep breathing, and leg exercises), the nurse should closely observe the client for development of complications. Potential complications following a thyroidectomy that require emergency care include hemorrhage, recurrent laryngeal palsy, and tetany.[5] Other complications include persistence of hyperthyroidism, postoperative myxedema, and permanent hypothyroidism. Thyroid storm is extremely rare,[8] but because of its emergency nature, it will be mentioned here. Otherwise, only those complications requiring emergency care will be discussed.

Because the thyroid gland is highly vascular, *hemorrhage* is a likely complication and is most common within 12 to 24 hours after surgery.[5] Hemorrhage tends to occur into an enclosed space, and the blood subsequently presses on the internal jugular veins, trachea, and may require a tracheostomy. The nurse should therefore observe the operative site for swelling and for changes in the client's respiratory status. Any complaint of fullness in the incision area warrants close assessment and evaluation. Detection of bleeding can best be ascertained by checking the side and back of the neck. Since internal bleeding and edema may obstruct the airway, a tracheostomy set should be readily available at the bedside.

Damage to the *recurrent laryngeal nerve* may result in the development of *palsy*, which may lead to paralysis of the vocal cords. Therefore listening for changes in the client's voice is essential. The nurse should listen carefully for changes in pitch and tone quality of the voice. Any significant changes may be an indication of damage to the laryngeal nerve. Damage to both cords may cause spastic airway obstruction, requiring a tracheostomy.

Tetany, which is caused by hypocalcemia, occurs as a result of inadvertent removal of the parathyroid during surgery. Signs of impending tetany include numbness and tingling of the nose, ears, fingertips, and toes. Latent tetany may be manifested in the development of *Chvostek's sign* and *Trousseau's sign.* Chvostek's sign is produced by tapping the client's face lightly over the periauricular region, which is the site of the facial nerve.[27] The tap results in marked twitching of the facial muscles, especially those of the corner of the mouth and upper lip. Trousseau's sign is carpopedal spasm, which may be elicited by temporarily impairing the circulation to an extremity either by manual constriction or by applying a sphygmomanometer to the upper arm and maintaining the pressure above systolic levels. This test produces spasms within 3 minutes of compression.[27] The importance of the nurse detecting tetany and consulting the physician when signs initially develop cannot be overemphasized. Progressive development can result in closure of the glottis.

When tetany develops, the physician will plan a regimen to increase the calcium level. Intravenous calcium, usually 10% solution of calcium chloride, is administered intravenously. The solution is highly irritating to the tissue, burns, and may cause tissue sloughing and thrombosis; therefore, care must be maintained during the injection of the medication.

 Evaluation. The evaluation component of the nursing process is continuous. The nursing care plan is individualized and depends on the stage of development when the problem is identified.

EXPECTED OUTCOMES
The client and/or family can:
1. Describe hyperthyroidism.
2. State plans for following therapeutic plan.
3. State plans for health maintenance including medications, how to deal with stress, prevention of infection, maintaining rest, and nutrition.
4. State use, time, dosage, route, and side effects of prescribed medications.
5. Explain importance of long-term therapy.
6. State indications of immediate health care services.
7. State plans for follow-up health care.

Thyroid storm

Thyroid storm (thyroid crisis), commonly experienced in clients with severe hyperthyroidism, may develop spontaneously but usually develops as a result of a condition that overtaxes the overloaded cardiovascular and nervous system.[5] For example, surgery (particularly after subtotal thyroidectomy), infection, anesthesia, and other forms of physical stress (such as postoperative pain) and emotional stress (such as anxiety).[2,5,8] It has also been reported to occur following radiotherapy.[8]

 Assessment. Thyroid storm is characterized by fever, apprehension, restlessness, tachycardia, extreme irritability, vomiting, and diarrhea. Some clients exhibit apathy, stupor, and coma.

> **Data analysis**
> *Data analysis may reveal nursing diagnoses of fear, alteration in nutrition, and sleep pattern disturbances.*

 Planning and implementation. Care is generally planned to prevent this complication by administering antithyroid drugs and iodides, especially before surgery, and by avoiding other forms of stress. Therapy for clients who develop thyroid storm will likely include oxygen; hypothermia or alcohol sponge baths to reduce the temperature; intravenous therapy for fluid and electrolyte replacement; corticosteroid therapy; and the use of sedatives or narcotics, antithyroid drugs, and a beta blocker such as propranolol; and potassium intravenously. Carditonic drugs may be prescribed if heart failure develops.

9 Endocrine system

Discharge instructions. As the client is prepared for discharge from the health care facility, the nurse should inform him of the importance of follow-up care. This is essential for the detection of late complications, especially hypothyroidism. Although most clients produce an adequate supply of thyroid hormone, some develop hypothyroidism, which necessitates the use of thyroid drugs.

Goiter

A goiter, an enlargement of the thyroid gland, may occur in euthyroid, hypothyroid, or hyperthyroid states.[35] Two types of goiters are discussed: nontoxic and toxic.

Nontoxic goiter. Nontoxic goiter (also referred to as colloid, simple, euthyroid) is an enlargement of the thyroid gland that occurs with normal hormone secretion. The mechanisms responsible for causing nontoxic goiter include iodine deficiency, goitrogens, and biochemical defects.[7,28]

Pathophysiology. Regardless of the mechanism involved, the development of a nontoxic goiter is thought to be a reflection of a defect in hormone synthesis in which increased glandular stimulation by TSH has been successful in compensating for the block in hormone formation.[20] Another possibility is that depletion of glandular iodine along with the impaired hormone synthesis increases the responsiveness of thyroid structure and function to basal levels of thyroid stimulation hormone.[15] Subsequently the gland enlarges in an attempt to produce a sufficient amount of hormone.

Nontoxic goiter (for example, one caused by iodine deficiency) is more common in areas where the soil is deficient in iodine and where no preventive measures are taken. They are more common in women and most commonly occur at adolescence[8] and during pregnancy, lactation, and menopause.[8,20] These are considered times of rapid growth or change; as a result, the demands for thyroid hormone and the need for iodine increase concomitantly.

The ingestion of high quantities of goitrogenic substances have also been associated with the development of goiters. These substances interfere with the normal production of thyroid hormone[20] and consequently increase pituitary thyrotropin secretion.[8] As a result, the gland enlarges by a mechanism similar to that discussed under iodine-deficient goiter. A list of goitrogenic substances can be found in Table 9-5.

There are several mechanisms that may cause goiters that are the result of biochemical defects. However, only two are mentioned. One is the result of a defect in iodide trapping. In such instance the thyroid gland cannot concentrate iodide. A second defect is one in which the thyroid traps and concentrates the iodide but has difficulty converting it into iodine.[8] Each of the defects occurs rarely; therefore the reader should refer to specialized texts for a discussion of goiters caused by defects in biochemical mechanisms.

Assessment. Most individuals are asymptomatic[20]; however, symptoms that occur are often the result of an enlarged gland. Some clients complain of a mild discomfort in the neck. As the gland enlarges, the trachea and esophagus may become compressed and produce symptoms such as stridor and dysphagia. Compression of the laryngeal nerve may cause hoarseness or other signs indicative of voice changes.

Physical examination of the thyroid reveals an enlarged thyroid. Laboratory studies show a normal PBI concentration, and usually a normal RAIU. The diagnosis is made after a normal metabolic state is demonstrated.

TABLE 9-5

Goitrogens

Foods	Drugs
Soybeans	Iodine (effect same as thioureas)
Peanuts	
Peaches	Paraaminosalicylic acid
Peas	Salicylates
Strawberries	Sulfonamides
Spinach	Thiocarbamides
Carrots	Thioureas (inhibit oxidation of iodides to iodine)
Cabbage	
Turnips	Thiocyanate or perchlorate (inhibits ability of thyroid to concentrate iodine)
Rutabagas	
Kale	
Radishes	

Nursing process for common health problems

> **Data analysis**
> *Data analysis may reveal nursing diagnoses of ineffective breathing patterns (potential), alterations in comfort, disturbance in self-concept, and sleep pattern disturbance.*

Planning and implementation. Therapy is generally planned to put the thyroid gland at rest. A thyroid hormone is prescribed to suppress TSH and inhibit thyroid function in an effort to shrink the thyroid gland. The therapy is usually prescribed for a specified time period (ranging from 6 to 12 months to 2 years),[20] after which the medication may be discontinued and the client re-evaluated.

Surgery (subtotal thyroidectomy) may be indicated when compression symptoms occur. If the goiter develops as a consequence of insufficient iodine, supplementing the diet with additional iodine is useful. The use of iodized table salt is considered most effective and should be encouraged.

If the goiter occurs as a result of ingestion of a large amount of goitrogenic substances, client instructions can be directed toward prevention. Foods that have been identified as goitrogenic should be discouraged in excessive amounts (for example, soybeans, peanuts, peaches, peas, strawberries, spinach, carrots, cabbage, turnips, rutabaga).[31] The importance of a well-balanced diet and the avoidance of fads and food binges should be stressed.

Toxic nodular goiter. Toxic nodular goiter (Plummer's disease), common in the elderly, often is a consequence of simple goiter of long standing.[8,15] In many instances the exact cause is unknown; however, one common element that has been documented is a reduction in the iodine content of thyroglobulin, which is suggestive of a deficiency of iodine or an impairment in its ability to become incorporated into iodinated amino acids.[15] Two patterns have been demonstrated in regard to the iodine accumulation: (1) iodine accumulates diffusely but in a patchy fashion; and (2) iodine accumulates in one or more discrete nodules.[15]

Assessment. The symptoms are varied. Some clients develop thyrotoxicosis, subsequently resulting in physiological effects on the cardiovascular system. As a result, tachycardia, dysrhythmias, or signs of congestive heart failure may occur. Weakness and anorexia may also be experienced. The diagnosis is established by visual observation and palpation of the thyroid gland. Serum studies of T_3 and T_4 confirm the diagnosis.

> **Data analysis**
> *Data analysis may reveal nursing diagnoses of alterations in cardiac output, alterations in comfort, and sleep pattern disturbances.*

Planning and implementation. Radioactive iodine is most commonly used as a means of treatment. It is not uncommon for radiation therapy to be preceded by antithyroid drugs to bring the client to a euthyroid state.

Neoplasms of the thyroid

The relationship between radiation exposure and the development of thyroid cancer has been explored. Children who have received radiation therapy (for example, to shrink an enlarged thymus or tonsils[8,12] or for acne) in early life are considered to be at a greater risk of developing cancer of the thyroid in late life. The incidence is also higher in individuals who are exposed to radioactive isotopes.

Neoplasms of the thyroid may occur as single masses or nodules. Several types have been identified: papillary, follicular (adenocarcinoma), and anaplastic (undifferentiated).[8]

Papillary tumors, the most common type,[8] account for 70% of all tumors of the thyroid. These are common in the younger age group and peak during the third and fourth decades. The tumor tends to grow slowly and is confined to the neck for a long period of time. However, it may later invade the blood vessels, the regional lymph nodes (cervical or mediastinal), and metastasize to the lung.

Follicular tumors are more common in older age groups, have a peak incidence around age 50,[8] and tend to mimic the function of normal thyroid tissue.[15] The tumor tends to invade blood vessels early and metastasize to bones, lung, brain,[15] and liver.[12]

Anaplastic (undifferentiated) *tumors* occur in the over-50 age group. They grow rapidly and tend to extend rapidly into blood vessels and metastasize to lungs, liver, and bone. They usually are rapidly fatal.[15]

☞   **Assessment.** A painless lump in the neck is often experienced. However, symptoms may not occur until metastasis is evident. For example, the client may have hoarseness, dyspnea, and dysphagia when metastasis has occurred. Bone fractures are common.

Clients may give a history of having received irradiation for thymic or tonsillar enlargement during childhood.

☞

Data analysis
Data analysis may reveal nursing diagnoses of ineffective breathing patterns and fear.

☞   **Planning and implementation.** Surgery (thyroidectomy) is the accepted primary form of therapy. Several weeks after surgery, a radioactive iodine is administered to abate any residual normal thyroid tissue and to demonstrate any functioning metastatic lesions that concentrate the iodine. If further metastasis is seen, a therapeutic dose of ^{131}I is administered. This may be followed with the use of thyroid suppression therapy (for example, levothyroxine), except for brief interruptions for the remainder of the client's life. Suppressive therapy may be interrupted for 3-week periods at yearly intervals; at which time levothyroxine is replaced by liothyronine. This is then withdrawn to permit the rapid resumption of TSH secretion and the stimulation of any functioning tissue.[15] If functioning tissue is found, another therapeutic dose of ^{131}I is administered. This is repeated during ensuing years until the disease is eradicated.

Thyroiditis   Thyroiditis has been classified into subacute (nonsuppurative) and chronic (Hashimoto's) thyroiditis.

Subacute thyroiditis. Subacute thyroiditis is a disease in which the exact cause is not known. However, it commonly occurs in association with viral infections, including mumps, measles, and influenza, and usually follows an upper respiratory tract infection.

Assessment. Symptoms usually occur following an upper respiratory tract infection and include malaise, muscle pain, anorexia, slight fever, and fatigability. Sore throat, hoarseness, tenderness in the area of the thyroid, and pain that may radiate to the ear, lower jaw, or occiput[15] are common.

Laboratory tests are useful in establishing the diagnosis of thyroiditis. Serum studies of the sedimentation rate (which is increased) and PBI (also increased) are useful. The RAIU is decreased. The diagnosis is usually confirmed by needle biopsy.

Data analysis
Data analysis may reveal nursing diagnoses of alteration in comfort and fear.

 Planning and implementation. Although spontaneous remission is common, aspirin or other analgesics, rest, and increased fluid intake may be prescribed to control symptoms. In instances in which the symptoms are more severe, steroid therapy (for example, prednisone) may be prescribed.

Chronic (Hashimoto's) thyroiditis. Chronic (Hashimoto's) thyroiditis is a chronic inflammatory disease of the thyroid for which immunological factors are thought to be responsible.[15] Evidence of the immunological basis is related to increased concentrations of immunoglobulins and of antibodies directed against several components of the thyroid.[15] It is considered to be the most frequently observed thyroid disorder in the United States[12] and occurs almost exclusively in women. It tends to peak in middle life (age 40 to 50) and has a familial tendency. The thyroid gland may be enlarged though not symmetrical. Pain and tenderness are unusual.

 Planning and implementation. Thyroid hormone replacement is the primary form of therapy. It is prescribed so that the thyroid gland will rest (for example, by decreasing TSH stimulation). If symptoms of compression occur, surgery will likely be performed.

COMMON PROBLEMS OF THE PARATHYROID

Hypoparathyroidism

Hypoparathyroidism, a metabolic disorder characterized by hypocalcemia, results from a deficiency of parathyroid hormone production. A deficiency of parathyroid hormone causes calcium to leave the blood, enter the bones, and be excreted in increased amounts. It may be caused by a congenital absence of the parathyroid gland or accidental removal or damage of the gland during surgery of the thyroid, which is considered the most common cause. It may also occur following a parathyroidectomy.[25]

Varied types of hypoparathyroidism have been identified: hereditary, idiopathic, and surgical. Hereditary hypoparathyroidism, occurring during the first year of life, affects boys more than girls. Infants so diagnosed manifest the failure-to-thrive syndrome, may have severe diarrhea, and are susceptible to infection. *Idiopathic hypoparathyroidism* is thought to begin late in life and is usually associated with adrenocortical insufficiency. *Surgical hypoparathyroidism* usually occurs several days after thyroid surgery, but it may not be diagnosed for several months or years. It has been speculated that this may occur because the gland gradually atrophies.

Assessment. The symptoms that occur reflect altered neuromuscular irritability caused by decreased concentration of ionized calcium (for example, paresthesias of the extremities or around the mouth and convulsions). The diagnosis is established on the basis of low calcium values and presenting symptoms.

> **Data analysis**
> *Data analysis may reveal nursing diagnoses of ineffective breathing patterns and alterations in comfort.*

Planning and implementation. Therapy is planned to restore calcium toward normal. Vitamin D and calcium supplements are prescribed to accomplish this and subsequently relieve symptoms of increased muscular irritability. Vitamin D is administered as vitamin D_2 (ergocalciferol) dihydrotachysterol (Hytakerol). Vitamin D has a tendency to accumulate in the system and subsequently cause an increase in calcium and may result in the development of hypercalcemic toxicity.[8] Therefore the nurse should be cognizant of the precautions that should be taken when these preparations are used. Information should be given to the client regarding signs of toxicity and the need for periodic serum calcium determinations. (Some authorities recommend withholding the medication for 1 to 2 weeks when the serum levels of calcium increase.)[10] When administered in liquid form, it should be diluted in fluid (water, juice, or milk) and given after the client has taken food. Forms of calcium that may be prescribed are calcium carbonate, lactate, or gluconate.

As care is provided, consideration should be given to seizure and safety precautions. The side rails should be padded and remain in the up position (see Chapter 10 for care). Listen closely to the client for signs of stridor and hoarseness. The nurse must anticipate that an emergency may develop and keep emergency equipment ready at the bedside (for example, tracheostomy set and injectable calcium gluconate).

Hyperparathyroidism

Primary hyperparathyroidism. Primary hyperparathyroidism is an altered state of calcium, phosphate, and bone metabolism that results from an increased secretion of parathyroid hormone. The excessive concentration of parathormone usually leads to hypercalcemia and hypophosphatemia. Hyperparathyroidism may occur as a result of adenomas, hyperplasia,[8,13,31] or malignancy of the parathyroids.[8,31] Although it may first appear in young children and the elderly, it most often affects women between 35 and 65 years of age and is most common after menopause.[13]

Assessment. The symptoms that occur reflect pathophysiological consequences of increased calcium. Although many organ systems may be affected, renal, skeletal, and gastrointestinal symptoms are most common.

Renal involvement occurs because of a deposit of calcium in the renal tissue; or because of renal stones, which are usually composed of calcium oxalate or calcium phosphate. The increase in calcium interferes with the ability of the kidney to concentrate urine; subsequently, polyuria and polydipsia are experienced. Bone pain, particularly of the back, is commonly experienced. The bones become demineralized, and as demineralization occurs, bones become fragile and the client is prone to develop pathological fractures. A number of other symptoms may also be experienced, including anorexia, nausea, vomiting, muscle weakness, fatigability, and lethargy.

A diagnosis of hyperparathyroidism is based on symptoms presented by the client, results of laboratory tests (for example, serum phosphorus, serum chloride, serum calcium), x-ray studies of the bone, and renal bone biopsy[25] to determine osteoblastic and osteoclastic activity.

> ### Data analysis
> *Data analysis may reveal nursing diagnoses of potential for injury, alteration in urinary elimination pattern, fear, and ineffective coping.*

Planning and implementation. Therapy for hyperparathyroidism depends on the cause. Surgical removal of the hyperplastic tissue is considered the therapy of choice for primary hyperthyroidism. However, in the client who is a poor surgical risk because of age or cardiopulmonary instability, surgery may be delayed. For these clients, sodium phosphate therapy may be prescribed. Phosphate promotes the deposition of calcium into the skeleton.

Intravenous infusion of sodium chloride (as much as 5 liters per day) in conjunction with diuretics is another form of therapy sometimes used. With this regimen it is imperative for the nurse to carefully observe the client's intake and output, as well as observe the client for signs of fluid overload.

As the nurse implements care for the client, care should be taken to prevent added stress on the bone when the client is moved in bed or when assistance is given with ambulation. Consultation with a physical therapist may be useful, especially if the client's mobility is severely limited. The side rails should be padded.

The vital signs, particularly the pulse rate, should be monitored carefully so that any irregularities can be detected. A pulse rate indicative of bradycardia should be reported to the physician.

To further reduce phosphate levels in the blood, foods low in phosphate should be encouraged. High-phosphate foods include milk products, cauliflower, and molasses.

Surgery. In preparation for surgery, consideration must be directed toward providing physical and emotional support to the client. The actual preoperative and postoperative care is similar to that of thyroid surgery. For example, the nurse should inform the client about strategies for preventing postoperative complications (for example, turning, coughing, and deep breathing) as well as strategies essential for comfort.

During the postoperative period the nurse should be alert to potential complications such as hemorrhage, paralysis of the recurrent laryngeal nerve, and tetany. Tetany is characterized by carpopedal spasms and demands immediate care. If severe, intravenous calcium is administered to raise the calcium levels. Oral forms of calcium may be used. A tracheostomy set should be kept at the client's bedside.

As the client's condition improves, he should be encouraged to engage in progressive ambulation activities. These generally are encouraged to promote recalcification of the bones. Weight-bearing activities should be planned. As the client engages in these activities, cardiac status should be monitored closely.

Secondary hyperparathyroidism. Secondary hyperparathyroidism is characterized by excessive production of parathyroid hormone. It may occur in clients with osteomalacia and chronic renal failure. Therapy may be planned to reduce the phosphate level in the blood. Phosphate in the diet is restricted and nonabsorbable antacids are sometimes used in an attempt to reverse calcification. If these measures are effective, the need for surgery will be eliminated.

COMMON PROBLEMS OF THE ADRENAL GLAND

The adrenal cortex synthesizes and secretes four types of adrenocortical hormones: *glucocorticoids, mineralocorticoids, androgens,* and *estrogens.* The glucocorticoid secreted by the adrenal gland is cortisol, and the mineralocorticoid secretion is aldosterone. Deficient or excessive secretion of either may result in disease. Therefore the following discussion focuses on diseases associated with hypofunction and hyperfunction of the adrenal gland.

Hypofunction of the adrenal gland

Adrenocortical hypofunction includes all conditions in which the secretion of the adrenal steroid hormones are below the amount needed for body requirements. Two types have been identified: primary adrenocortical insufficiency and secondary adrenocortical insufficiency.

Primary adrenocortical insufficiency. Primary adrenocortical insufficiency (Addison's disease or glucocorticoid deficiency) is a disease resulting from the lack of adrenocortical hormone. It may result from several factors, including idiopathic atrophy, which is often associated with an autoimmune disorder.[8] The majority of these are related to this factor. The presence of circulating adrenal antibodies help confirm the autoimmune relationship. These antibodies react with antigens in the adrenocortical tissue and produce an inflammatory reaction, which causes a destruction of the adrenal gland. Tuberculosis was, at one time, considered a primary cause of the disease. Hemorrhage may destroy the gland and cause the disease. Although rare, primary adrenocortical insufficiency may occur at any age and with equal frequency among sexes.

 Assessment. Symptoms occur gradually and include fatigue (which at first occurs sporadically but later occurs almost continually), weakness, anorexia, nausea and vomiting, weight loss, increased pigmentation (especially around elbows, knuckles, creases of the hand, and in normally pigmented areas such as the areolae of the nipple), hypotension, and hyperglycemia secondary to loss of minerals and glucocorticoid effect. Personality changes usually manifest as irritability and restlessness. Alterations in the sensory modalities of taste, smell, and hearing[25,35] and a decrease in axillary and pubic hair are common in females. The latter occurs because of adrenal androgen production. The diagnosis is established by measuring plasma cortisol levels in the morning and afternoon.

> *Data analysis*
> *Data analysis may reveal nursing diagnoses of alterations in self-concept, alterations in comfort, fear, and alterations in sensory perceptions.*

 Planning and implementation. Steroid replacement therapy is the primary form of treatment. Cortisone (or hydrocortisone) is administered orally daily and in divided doses. Usually the large dose is given in the morning and the smaller dose in the late afternoon to simulate the normal diurnal adrenal rhythm. The medication should be given with meals, milk, or an antacid to counteract the local effects on the gastric mucosa. The client's response to therapy should be observed closely. Insomnia, irritability, mental excitement, and psychosis may occur after therapy is initiated.[35] The client's weight, pulse rate, and blood pressure should be monitored closely, along with serum potassium and cardiovascular changes. In addition, the nurse should educate the client about the disease, the need for continuous therapy, and his responsibility during stressful situations. The client should be instructed to wear an identification bracelet or necklace indicating the disease so that prompt therapy can be implemented if he should become unconscious for any reason. It is not uncommon for the physician to instruct the client to double the dose of the glucocorticoid for a couple of days after stressful periods,[8] for example, after an upper respiratory or urinary tract infection. Nausea is usually the first symptom of relative adrenal insufficiency.[8] The client should also be informed of the importance of registering with the National Medical Alert System.[35]

The nurse should protect the client from any physical and emotional stress, either of which can precipitate crisis. Vital signs should be monitored closely and significant changes reported to the physician.

 Evaluation. The final stage of the nursing process encourages the nurse and client to make judgments about goal achievement relative to plans for health promotion, maintenance, and restoration.

EXPECTED OUTCOMES

The client and/or family can:
1. Verbalize the relationship between others and the development of complications such as crisis.
2. State the importance of long-term administration of medicine.
3. State use, dose, frequency, time, and side effects of prescribed medications.
4. Verbalize the importance of wearing an emergency identification bracelet.
5. Freely express feelings about the health state.
6. Identify strategies for compliance with therapy.
7. State plans for follow-up care.
8. State signs and symptoms indicative of emergency care.

Secondary adrenocortical insufficiency. Secondary adrenocortical insufficiency results from hypofunction of the pituitary or from prolonged therapeutic administration of glucocorticoids.[25,35] The development of the deficiency following long-term steroid therapy is related to prolonged suppression of the hypothalamic corticotropin-releasing center and occurs because of atrophy of the adrenal gland. Atrophy occurs because of the absence of endogenous ACTH stimulations, which is essential for maintaining the normal size of the gland. As a result, these clients experience two defects: loss of adrenal responsiveness to ACTH and failure of the pituitary gland to release ACTH.[35]

The symptoms experienced by the client are similar to those that occur in primary adrenocortical insufficiency, except for absence of hyperpigmentation.[35] Therapy is also similar.

Adrenal crisis. Adrenal crisis, also referred to as *acute adrenocortical insufficiency* or *addisonian crisis,* reflects an absolute or complete absence of adrenocortical hormone. In clients with no adrenal reserve, it can be precipitated by stress or by withdrawing glucocorticoid substitution therapy.[8]

Assessment. It is characterized by anorexia, nausea, vomiting, weakness, hypotension, dehydration, and shock. It may occur gradually over a period of days if the client is not severely distressed, or it may occur abruptly when an individual undiagnosed suffers from trauma or stressful situations.

 Planning and implementation. Therapy is planned to raise the circulatory adrenocortical hormone at a rapid rate. The client is given a corticosteroid preparation such as hydrocortisone sodium succinate (Solu-Cortef) intravenously. This is followed by rapid infusion of 5% dextrose in normal saline. The corticosteroid preparation is repeated at specified intervals (for example, every 6 hours) for a couple of days. Fluid replacement up to 3 to 4 liters may be prescribed to correct the electrolyte and fluid imbalance caused by the nausea and vomiting.[8] The steroids are gradually reduced to maintenance levels after the crisis is over.

During the crisis the nurse should facilitate restoration of circulation. The client should be kept quiet and comfortable. All care should be implemented by the nurse, including simple activities as brushing the teeth, feeding, and providing other minor activities of daily living. Communication with the client should be minimal. Individuals with any type of infection should not be permitted near the client.

Prevention of adrenal crisis is also essential. The nurse should inform the client that any form of stress (for example, infection, trauma, gastrointestinal upset) should be reported to the physician. If instructions have been given to increase the drugs during these states, then they should be strictly adhered to.

Hyperfunction of the adrenal gland

Cushing's syndrome. Cushing's syndrome (hyperadrenocorticism) is a disorder caused by a sustained overproduction of glucocorticoids by the adrenal gland or from excessive administration of glucocorticoids. Hence the source of the problem is often referred to as being endogenous or exogenous (iatrogenic). The majority of the clients with the syndrome from an endogenous source are found to have bilateral adrenal hyperplasia, which is generally secondary to excessive production of ACTH by the pituitary, which in many clients is caused by pituitary tumors.

Adrenal tumors (for example, adenomas or carcinomas), another endogenous source, often produce more androgens than cortisol.[25] This effect can possibly be related to some of the symptoms noted by the client. Finally, the exogenous source often responsible for the syndrome results from overzealous use of glucocorticoids. Clients with asthma, arthritis, lymphomas, or rheumatic heart disease who receive glucocorticoids as antiinflammatory agents may potentially develop Cushing's syndrome. Cushing's syndrome may occur at any age, but more commonly occurs in women during the third and sixth decades of life.[8]

 Assessment. The signs and symptoms exhibited by these clients are caused by the effects of excessive production of cortisol and androgens. Obesity, the most common symptom,[12] occurs mainly on the face and trunk. Consequently, mooning of the face (for example, extreme rounding of the face) and "buffalo hump" (a deposit of fat on the back and neck) are frequently observed. The deposition of fat in these areas is responsible for the fat changes. In addition, retention of sodium and water gives the client a puffy look. Thinning, especially of the extremities, occurs because of loss of muscular tissue, which occurs as a result of excessive catabolism of protein. Thinning of the skin in other parts of the body may also be observed and result in the appearance of purple striae. The thin skin along with loss of perivascular supporting tissue makes the small vessels of the skin more prone to rupture; as a result, the client has a tendency to bruise easily and develop ecchymoses at the slightest trauma.[25,26,35] Muscle weakness and easy fatigability that are frequently experienced are related to loss of muscle tissue and loss of potassium.

Androgenic effects (from excessive androgens) may be manifested in symptoms such as oligoamenorrhea and hirsutism (especially over the face, body, and upper lip in female clients). Estrogen excess may produce gynecomastia in men.[8,12,25] Decreased libido has also been documented.

Hypertension is thought to occur as a result of an increase in the secretion of mineralocorticoid secretion[12] or weak mineralocorticoid activity. Emotional disorders that are sometimes experienced may range from irritability to depression, confusion, or psychosis.[25,26,35]

The diagnosis of Cushing's syndrome is made on the basis of physical findings and confirmed by measurement of high levels of cortisol in the blood and urine. Other diagnostic procedures, including radiological methods (for example, intravenous pyelogram, skull x-ray films, adrenal venous angiography), are useful in helping to determine the underlying cause of the syndrome. A CAT scan is also useful.

Data analysis
Data analysis may reveal nursing diagnoses of disturbance in self-concept, impairment of skin integrity, and potential for injury.

Planning and implementation. Nursing objectives for the care of the client should consider providing psychological support, preventing infection, promoting safety, and promoting rest.

Providing psychological support. Clients with Cushing's syndrome tend to react emotionally to marked changes in appearance. The nurse should develop a relationship with the client that will facilitate verbalization of feelings and subsequently increase the client's ability to cope with the changes. The nurse should educate the client and family about the disease and help them understand that most of the changes that stem from the condition are reversible.[31]

Preventing infection. Since the mechanisms of inflammation and immune responses are greatly suppressed, these clients are more prone to develop infection. Signs of infection are more likely to be masked. The nurse should therefore carefully assess and evaluate the client's temperature. Exposure to individuals with infections should be avoided.

Promoting safety. Weakness and weakened muscles and bones that result from continued protein catabolism make the client prone to soft-tissue injuries and fractures (for example, from progressive osteoporosis). The client also has a tendency to be clumsy. A protective environment should be established. Environmental hazards should be removed, furniture should be padded, and assistance should be given with ambulation and activities of daily living as needed.

Promoting rest. These clients tend to tire easily and experience difficulty sleeping because of the psychotropic effect of cortisol. Therefore a quiet, relaxing atmosphere should be provided.

9 Endocrine system

Surgical intervention will be based on the cause. A subtotal or total adrenalectomy may be performed to remove an adrenal tumor for carcinoma or for hyperplasia. Such surgery removes the negative feedback control of ACTH production. If a total adrenalectomy is performed, physiological dosages of cortisol are administered. If the problem originates in the pituitary gland a hypophysectomy, cryohypophysectomy, or transphenoid resection may be performed, or radiation may be used or radioactive isotopes implanted. [8]

Aldosteronism. Aldosteronism is a syndrome associated with hypersecretion of aldosterone, the mineralocorticosteroid hormone of the adrenal cortex. Two forms have been identified: primary aldosteronism and secondary aldosteronism. The distinction is based on whether the stimulus for increased secretion comes from the adrenal gland itself or from a source outside the adrenal gland.

Primary aldosteronism. With *primary aldosteronism* (Conn's syndrome), hypersecretion of aldosterone occurs because of a problem within the adrenal gland. A consequence is that aldosterone is no longer under feedback control.

The cause is usually bilateral adrenal hyperplasia or a solitary adrenal adenoma. Aldosterone acts on the distal tubules of the kidney to enhance the reabsorption of sodium. It is at this site where the exchange of potassium or hydrogen ion for reabsorbed sodium takes place. Consequently, electrolyte disturbances (hypokalemia, hypernatremia) and hypertension, which occurs as a result of the increase in sodium reabsorption and increased blood volume, are common.[35] Metabolic alkalosis also occurs in response to the shift of hydrogen ions into the cells to replace potassium and maintain electroneutrality (Fig. 9-2).[11]

Assessment. Paresthesia, fatigue, and muscle weakness are thought to occur as a result of the decrease in potassium. The weakness is most often experienced in the legs and may progressively develop into paralysis. Nocturnal polyuria and late polydipsia occur as a result of an impairment in the ability of the kidney to concentrate urine. Tetany has also been reported to occur, but for unknown reasons.

FIG. 9-2
Effects of increased aldosterone. (From Krueger, T.A.: Endocrine problems in nursing, St. Louis, 1976, The C.V. Mosby Co.)

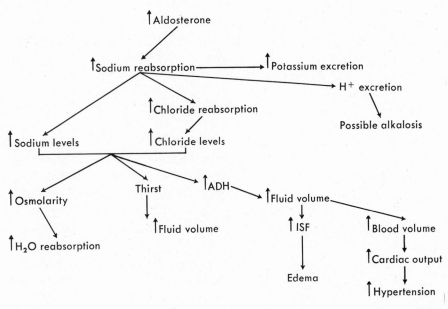

Nursing process for common health problems

The diagnosis of aldosteronism is based on serum and urine measurements of aldosterone (both of which are increased) and measurements of plasma renin (which is low in primary aldosteronism and high in secondary aldosteronism.

> *Data analysis*
> *Data analysis may reveal nursing diagnoses of potential for injury and alterations in comfort.*

Planning and implementation. Nursing care should be directed toward monitoring the client's cardiovascular and electrolyte status. Therapy is directed to its cause. A partial unilateral adrenalectomy is generally performed if the problem is the result of a tumor. If the problem results from hyperplasia, a subtotal or total adrenalectomy is performed. If surgery is not possible, the administration of aldosterone antagonist (Aldactone) may be used to block effects of hormone stress. In preparation for surgery, hypertension and hypokalemia are corrected with the use of a low-sodium diet, antihypertensive medication, and potassium supplements.

Following an adrenalectomy, the client's vital signs should be monitored carefully because of the potential for shock to develop.

Clients who have undergone an adrenalectomy must be followed by a health care professional for the remainder of their lives. They should understand this long before discharge from the hospital.

They should also understand that they may experience hypoaldosteronism for approximately 1 month. During this time period, supplemental salt may be administered daily. (If the hypoaldosteronism is a result of hyperplasia, some recommend bilateral adrenalectomy, whereas others treat it medically.)

Secondary aldosteronism. Secondary aldosteronism represents an increase in aldosterone production in response to a problem outside the adrenal gland. A decrease in afferent arteriolar pressure in the renal glomerulus, causing stimulation of the renin-angiotensin system, is thought to be responsible for the increase.[28,35] Angiotensin stimulates aldosterone production.[28] Secondary aldosteronism is often seen in conditions in which edema is common (for example, congestive heart failure, nephrotic syndrome, cirrhosis) and in conditions in which the renal artery is partially occluded. The occlusion may be caused by atherosclerotic plaques or by fibromuscular hyperplasia.[35]

When aldosteronism occurs in hypertensive clients, it is associated with an overproduction of renin, which may result from a decrease in renal blood flow. Edema is the primary symptom in secondary aldosteronism.

Hypoaldosteronism. Hypoaldosteronism is rare and therefore is not discussed other than to say it has been found to occur following removal of an aldosteronoma, during protracted heparin administration, in complete heart block, and in severe postural hypotension.[8]

Adrenogenital syndrome. Adrenogenital syndrome is a group of disorders that occur when the adrenal androgens (dehydroepiandrosterone and androstenedione, which are converted to testosterone)[8] are produced in excessive amounts. An impairment in the synthesis of cortisol is the cause of the excessive production. Hyperplasia, adenomas or carcinomas, or enzyme defects may be responsible for the adrenal gland increasing its secretion. The latter gives rise to what is referred to as androgenital hyperplasia. Congenital hyperplasia generally does not become manifest until adolescence or early adulthood.[8]

 Assessment. The symptoms that occur are varied and may include virilization of the female to feminization in the male. Virilization is associated with multiple signs of androgen excess (as opposed to hirsutism, which signifies excessive hair growth). Virilization in the female at birth is associated with ambiguous external genitalia (pseudohemaphroditism); in the male it is manifested as premature virilization (isosexual precocity). Macrogenitosomia may be present in the male infant at birth; the clitoris may be enlarged in the female.

In adults, hirsutism, acne, temporary baldness, deepening of the voice, decreased size of the breasts, atrophy of the uterus, amenorrhea, enlargement of the clitoris, and increased heterosexual drive may occur in women,[35] but may be unrecognized in men.

COMMON PROBLEMS OF THE ADRENAL MEDULLA

Pheochromocytoma

Pheochromocytoma is a secretory tumor primarily of the adrenal medulla. However, extrarenal tumors may occur anywhere along the sympathetic chain,[25] including the neck, chest, and urinary bladder.[8] The majority of the tumors are benign, although a small percentage (5%) are malignant.

Pheochromocytomas affect both sexes and all age groups, but most commonly affect young adults[25] in the second to fifth decades. When the tumors occur during childhood, they are usually bilateral and frequently familial.[12]

Pathophysiology. Pheochromocytomas produce large quantities of catecholamines (epinephrine, norepinephrine). One of the effects of catecholamines is that they produce peripheral vasoconstriction; as a result, hypertension is common. Catecholamines enhance glycogenolysis; therefore the client with pheochromocytoma develops a mild form of diabetes.[4] In addition, these substances produce an elevation in cardiac output by producing an increase in the force and rate of myocardial contraction. Therefore a sustained increase in catecholamines causes myocardial irritability, dysrhythmias, cardiomegaly,[26] myocardiopathy, and, subsequently, congestive heart failure. Sustained levels of catecholamines over a period of time may also produce hypovolemia.[4] Such an effect is masked because of the increase in blood pressure. Catecholamines initially constrict "restrictive" and "capacitance" vessels, which in return causes a reduction in blood volume[4] and a subsequent decrease in red blood cell production. (This effect is significant in the postoperative period, as discussed later.)

 Assessment. The effects of both catecholamines may be evident in the client with a pheochromocytoma. The tumor produces a physiological stress response that mimics an individual who is in a state of constant panic.[26] For example, associated with paroxysmal hypertension are symptoms such as attacks of sweating, anxiety, palpitation, and sometimes headache,[25] pallor, angina, nausea, and vomiting[26] (which may last from a few minutes to a few hours and may come and go spontaneously). (Death has been reported to occur during attacks from intracranial hemorrhage, ventricular fibrillation, or heart failure.[25]) In addition, nervousness and tremors occur and reflect the action of catecholamines on the central nervous system. Tachycardia, weakness, fatigue, weight loss (which reflects a hypercatabolic state), nausea, and anorexia are sometimes experienced and reflect gastrointestinal effects of the activities of the sympathetic nervous system.

325

Nursing process for common health problems

A diagnosis is established on the basis of the history, physical examination, and tests such as 24-hour urinary assay of catecholamines (metanephrine, normetanephrine, and VMA), the excretion of which is increased. Plasma catecholamines are also useful. Computerized axial tomography, contrast angiography, x-ray films of the abdomen, and intravenous pyelography are all useful in locating the tumor.

> **Data analysis**
> *Data analysis may reveal nursing diagnoses of alterations in cardiac output, fear, alterations in comfort, potential for injury, and alterations in sensory perception.*

Planning and implementation. The primary form of therapy is removal of the tumor. However, clients who are poor surgical risks (for example, those with functioning metastases) are managed medically with adrenergic blocking agents.

By the same token, those who are good surgical risks are preoperatively prescribed an alpha-adrenergic blocking agent such as phenoxygenzamine, which is long acting, to decrease the blood pressure to normotensive levels. Phentolamine, a shorter-acting alpha blocker may also be prescribed to control severe paroxysms in acute situations.[12] If dysrhythmias occur, propranolol may be used.

When the client receives the adrenergic blocking agents, the client's vital signs, particularly blood pressure and pulse rate, should be monitored closely. It is not uncommon for an order to be written to monitor the blood pressure in the supine and standing positions. Often the dosage of medication is gradually increased until a mild hypotensive state is produced.[4] (The dosage may start at 10 mg three times a day.) After this state is produced, the dosage remains at this level. With adequate therapy, other effects may be noted. The client feels better, dysrhythmias disappear, and changes are noted in serum studies (for example, blood glucose falls to normal levels and hematocrit may fall).[4] These are considered indications of the client's readiness for surgery. Therefore, in addition to monitoring vital signs, the nurse should carefully assess and document all symptoms experienced by the client, as well as test the urine for glucose and acetone at frequent intervals. Episodes of hypertensive attacks should be reported to the physician immediately. It is also essential for the nurse to anticipate the potential nature of these attacks and consult with the physician in regard to desired emergency therapy.

In preparation for surgery and throughout the client's hospitalization, care and therapy are directed toward promoting rest and comfort, promoting safety, monitoring for potential complications, and preparing for surgery.

An environment should be created that is free of physical and emotional stress. Bed rest is usually maintained with the head of the bed elevated. This position takes advantage of the orthostatic drop in blood pressure that is known to occur in some clients. Sedatives are sometimes prescribed to promote rest. The use of stimulants such as coffee and tea should not be included in the diet, and smoking and any other activity that will potentiate the release of catecholamine should be discouraged (for example, palpation of the abdomen, exercise, Valsalva's maneuver).[26]

Because visual disturbances are commonly experienced by these clients, safety strategies should be used (for example, assisting with ambulation). A high-sodium diet may be prescribed to counteract volume depletion.

During the preoperative period the effects of therapy are carefully evaluated. Varied tests are prescribed, especially those that test myocardial function (ECG, x-ray films, stress tests, and so on).

Preoperative nursing care. Once the acute stage is over and the client is ready for surgery, efforts can be directed toward instructing the client about preoperative and postoperative care. Such instructions help prevent postoperative complications (for example, hypostatic pneumonia and phlebitis). For example, turning, coughing, deep breathing, and leg exercises should be demonstrated and their rationale explained. It might also be helpful to inform the client that possibly two intravenous fluids will be administered simultaneously postoperatively, one of which will be to maintain fluid regulation and one for medication. Antihypertensive drugs will be prescribed postoperatively to maintain the blood pressure within a specified range. The administration of such medication requires frequent (every 2 to 5 minutes) assessments of the blood pressure. If the client is informed of this during the preoperative period, it will eliminate unnecessary worry.

All questions and concerns should be answered and dealt with in an honest manner. The nurse should not hesitate to use other health care resources when indicated.

Postoperative nursing care. The care that is planned in the preoperative period should be implemented postoperatively. The client should be encouraged to turn, cough, and breathe deeply every 3 to 4 hours.

The client should be carefully monitored for signs indicative of complications. The adrenal glands are highly vascular, therefore hemorrhage and shock are potential complications. Frequent assessments and evaluation of the vital signs and urinary output are essential.

The prescribed fluid therapy should be maintained and the client carefully evaluated for problems that might be responsible for postoperative hypertension (fluid overload, pain, essential hypertension and so on).

Analgesics should be administered as needed for pain. When such medications are administered, it is essential for the nurse to closely assess the client for the effects of the drug and plan care accordingly.

Discharge instructions. Clients who have had surgery for a pheochromocytoma are usually encouraged to return to normal activities. Corticosteroids will be prescribed if an adrenalectomy has been performed. These are started far in advance of the client's discharge so that adjustments can be made before discharge from the hospital.

 Evaluation. Evaluation of the nursing care plans is an ongoing process.

EXPECTED OUTCOMES

The client and/or family can:
1. Describe pheochromocytoma.
2. State plans for following the therapeutic plan.
3. State plans for health maintenance.
4. Verbalize the importance of long-term drug therapy.
5. State the use, route, time, frequency, and side effects of prescribed drugs.
6. State conditions demanding prompt health care (such as infections, significant changes in blood pressure).
7. Demonstrate the proper technique for monitoring blood pressure.
8. State plans for follow-up health care.

COMMON PROBLEMS OF THE PANCREAS

Diabetes mellitus

Diabetes mellitus is a chronic disease of relative or absolute insulin deficiency characterized by disorders of carbohydrate, protein, and fat metabolism and concomitant atherosclerosis and arteriosclerosis. Early symptoms of the disease are related to metabolic changes, whereas later findings are associated with the vascular defects.

Diabetes mellitus may be classified according to etiopathological factors. Type 1 diabetics are those with absolute insulin deficiency who are insulin-dependent and ketosis prone. They are usually lean and within normal weight range. Clients with type 2 diabetes have reduced insulin receptor activity, delayed insulin release, and are not insulin dependent. These clients are ketosis resistant and tend to be obese. These classifications replace the terms *juvenile onset diabetes* (type 1) and *adult onset* or *maturity onset diabetes* (type 2) in favor of more accurate descriptions of pathophysiological mechanisms.

The cause of diabetes mellitus is not known. Some believe the disease may even represent several distinct entities with the only common factor being hyperglycemia.[33] The mechanisms of insulin deficiency can, however, be described for type 1 and type 2 diabetes. Absolute insulin deficiency (type 1) is caused by destruction of beta cell function. Viral or autoimmune factors may precipitate beta cell destruction as complexes of human leukocyte antigen that predispose beta cells to damage by viral agents such as the cytomegalovirus or coxsackie B, measles, or mumps virus have been identified.[30] Furthermore, individuals with diabetes mellitus frequently are identified as having autoimmune antibodies directed against protein components of the islet cell.

The mechanism of relative insulin deficiency (type 2) appears to be located at the site of insulin transport in muscle, adipose, and liver tissue. There is delayed release of exogenous insulin in relation to carbohydrate load.[33] Relative insulin deficiency also correlates with obesity as the increased numbers of fat cells become less responsive to insulin and the glucose uptake is decreased. With increased carbohydrate ingestion there is hyperglycemia, and the added burden of insulin demand creates the relative insulin deficiency.

Pathophysiology. Regardless of the cause, insulin deficiency produces generally predictable consequences. In the normal state, insulin (formed by the beta cells of the pancreas by the precursor proinsulin) acts to facilitate transport of glucose, some amino acids, and some fatty acids across cell membranes of tissues that are insulin sensitive, namely, liver, skeletal muscle, and adipose tissue. In the liver, glucose is used as glucose or stored as glycogen. In the absence of sufficient insulin, excess glucose accumulates and circulates in the bloodstream (hyperglycemia) and spills into the urine (glucosuria). Muscle cells require insulin to incorporate amino acids into muscle protein. Insulin deficiencies cause withdrawal of amino acids and subsequent increases in serum amino acid levels. Finally, insulin is needed to facilitate transport of glucose into the cells to maintain a balance of lipolysis of stored triglycerides and esterification of fatty acids to triglycerides. In insulin-deprived states there is an increase in release of fatty acids and glycerol.

The interference with glucose transport to liver, muscle, and adipose tissue, and resulting serum elevations of glucose, amino acids, fatty acids, and glycerol, precipitate further metabolic changes. There is hypertonic dehydration as water leaves the cells, osmotic diuresis brought about by glucosuria, and limited tubular reabsorption, causing polyuria and loss of electrolytes, notably sodium

	Risk (%) of being affected by		
	Age 25	Age 45	Age 65
Population at large	0.2-0.3	0.5-0.9	1.8-3.8
1st-degree relative affected Age at onset			
0-24	5-8	5-13	5-17
24-44	1-2	2-3	6-10
45-64	0.2-0.5	0.5-1.5	8-10
65-84	0.2-0.5	1.5-2.0	6-8
2d- or 3d-degree relative affected	Divide above risks by 2		
Two 1st-degree relatives affected Age at onset			
0-44, 0-44	Multiply above risks by 2-4		
0-44, 45-84	Multiply above risks by 1.5-3		
45-84, 45-84	Multiply above risks by 1.5-2		
1st-, 2d-, or 3d-degree relative affected	Multiply above risks by 1.5-2		

From Waife, S.O., editor: Diabetes mellitus, ed. 8, Indianapolis, 1980, Lilly Research Laboratories.

and potassium. Finally, fatty acids break down into ketone bodies, acetoacetic acid, beta-hydrobutyric acid, and acetone, causing a state of ketoacidosis.

There are currently about 5 million diabetics in the United States, and diabetes mellitus is the sixth leading cause of death. Although diabetes is primarily a disease of middle-aged adults with an incidence increasing with age, children and adolescents account for approximately 15% of the diabetic population. The disease is more common in women.

Individuals at risk are those who are overweight, as obesity increases the demand for insulin; and in states of relative insulin deficiency, diabetes can be induced in these individuals. Risk also increases with a family history of the disease, although the significance of genetic influences on the distribution of diabetes has changed with abilities to identify genetic markers. It is believed that in susceptible individuals with leukocytes of a certain type (human leukocyte antigens), an infection with certain agents might predispose to development of insulin-dependent (type 1) diabetes.[33] Table 9-6 shows recent findings of probable risks in relatives. Women delivering babies weighing more than 4 kg are also associated with risk for diabetes mellitus.

Assessment. The clinical evidence of diabetes mellitus is a manifestation of disrupted carbohydrate, protein, and fat metabolism. Unused glucose remaining in the bloodstream is excreted by the kidneys. The excessive glucose in the urine, as much as 120 g of carbohydrate (or 480 calories) lost per day, draws water to dilute the glucose-loaded urine and produces one of the main symptoms of diabetes, polyuria. Frequent urination is reported by older children and adults; enuresis may be noticed in the toilet-trained child.

To prevent dehydration the body compensates with increased thirst (polydipsia). The client loses weight, and hunger (polyphagia) results to offset the weight loss. Weight loss is marked in children. These three cardinal symptoms—polyuria, polydipsia, and polyphagia—signal the onset of clinical diabetes. There may be fatigue, because glucose is unavailable for energy needs. Women may have pruritus vulvae caused by glycosuria, which provides a medium for vaginal infections. Numbness and tingling may be noticed when the peripheral nerves suffer glucose loss. Nervousness, irritability, and personality changes may also be noted.

If faulty metabolism progresses unchecked, reserves of fats are used, and ketones are excreted in the urine in the oxidation process. The resulting metabolic acidosis stimulates the respiratory center to exhale carbon dioxide, and there may be hyperpnea, dehydration, weakness, drowsiness, and coma. The onset of the disease is rapid in clients with type 1 diabetes (usually children) and is often diagnosed when the child is in a state of ketoacidosis. The onset of type 2 diabetes is much less rapid, and the symptoms may go unchecked for some time. In older adults, diabetes may be noted by the presence of concomitant disease such as peripheral neuropathy or dermatological changes.

Diabetic detection. The detection of diabetes mellitus is an important community health commitment, because 25% to 50% of those with diabetes are unknown. In an attempt to discover these unknown diabetic individuals, the American Diabetic Association, in cooperation with local community health officials, sponsors diabetic detection drives. Screening tests using finger-prick blood samples or urinalysis can be used for detection.

> **Data analysis**
> *Data analysis may reveal nursing diagnoses of alterations in nutrition, knowledge deficit, noncompliance, and alterations in self-concept.*

Planning and implementation. The nursing care plan is developed with the client and family to meet the needs of the client, depending on age, stage of growth and development, and type of diabetes.

The client who is diagnosed as having diabetes is faced with a chronic health problem that requires modification of life-style to control the disease. The reaction of the client when hearing the diagnosis may take many forms. The client may be depressed or may fear the complications of diabetes from experiences with diabetic relatives. Parents of children with diabetes may feel guilty. The client will need some time to accept the diagnosis before therapeutic intervention can be discussed. Each client will react individually, and the meaning of the disease will be based on age, life-style, and the things that are important in his life. Acceptance of the diagnosis may come initially or not for several years, and the nurse must assess the client's acceptance of the diabetes before helping him understand his therapeutic plan.

Diabetes mellitus is a chronic disease, and therapeutic management depends on the client assuming responsibility for maintaining a life-style that may include modifications of activity and diet and perhaps use of medication. When the client has worked through his initial feelings, the nurse, with other health team members, can begin to instruct the client about his therapeutic plan. Instruction is best given in a simple progression, and it may be helpful if the same nurse cares for the client during initial instructions. Care plans and assessment guides can be developed to share teaching plans with the health team. Teaching may be done with the client, family, or groups, depending on resources available.

Some clinical settings have special nursing units for individuals with diabetes mellitus. There nurses make assessments and use ongoing intervention and instructional skills. The health team may include a dietitian to assist the nurse, physician, and client in planning diets and instructing the client about required dietary changes.

Therapeutic plan. Glucose, fat, and protein metabolism are regulated by a balance of activity, glucose intake (diet), exogenous insulin, and hormonal activity of epinephrine and glucocorticosteroids (Table 9-7). The objective of therapeutic management is to achieve euglycemia by manipulating these factors. The nurse and client can establish goals for the client to learn about activity, diet, pharmacological therapy (if necessary), and the relationship of hormonal activity to glucose metabolism.

Activity. Activity determines the client's need for nutrition and insulin. Clients who are in periods of growth, such as infants and adolescents, have greater energy requirements than those who are not growing rapidly. Clients with increased metabolism, the younger person, and those who lead an active life need more calories for their metabolic needs. These needs are taken into account before any further planning for diet or medication is done.

Exercise is important to the diabetic. Activity uses up extra calories and does not put a demand on the insulin supply to convert ingested glucose for storage. The client is therefore encouraged to participate in a moderate activity such as walking or bicycling. Exercise is also encouraged if the client is overweight.

The client should obtain the same amount of exercise every day. When diet and medications are used to regulate glucose use, it is particularly important that energy expenditure is stable. The secretary who sits in the office during the week and plays tennis on the weekend, for example, does not have the same daily energy requirements. Exercise and metabolic needs also tend to be seasonal, and if the client is more active during the warmer summer months, he should be aware of this change in activity.

When the client is learning about his activity needs, he should follow a routine in the hospital that is comparable to the activity he has at home. Young children are encouraged to play outside. Adults should be out of bed; some may even make beds and prepare meals in the diet kitchen. Diet and pharmacological therapy are based on the client's activity, and he should attempt to simulate his normal life-style.

Diet. Diet is the second facet of diabetes control. The diet is planned for the

TABLE 9-7

Factors influencing glucose, fat, and protein metabolism

Factor	Glucose		Fat		Protein	
	Hypoglycemia	Hyperglycemia	Hypoacidemia	Hyperacidemia	Decreased amino acids	Increased amino acids
Activity	Increased activity	Decreased activity	Increased activity	Decreased activity	—	—
Diet (glucose intake)	Decreased intake	Increased intake	—	—	—	—
Insulin	Increased insulin	Decreased insulin	Increased insulin	Decreased insulin	Increased insulin	Decreased insulin
Epinephrine	Decreased epinephrine	Increased epinephrine	Decreased epinephrine	Increased epinephrine	Decreased epinephrine	Increased epinephrine
Glucocorticoids	Decreased glucocorticoids	Increased glucocorticoids	Decreased glucocorticoids	Increased glucocorticoids	Decreased glucocorticoids	Increased glucocorticoids

Nursing process for common health problems

ideal weight of the client and to support his individual metabolic needs during activity, growth, and illness. Clients who are underweight or overweight may be on a weight-gaining or weight-reducing diet. The diet is also planned to satisfy cultural and economic food preferences. Often diet control alone is sufficient to regulate carbohydrate metabolism in the type 2 diabetic, and is preferred to chemotherapeutic control.

Physicians vary in emphasis on adherence to a diet. Some believe the diet must be observed strictly to maintain the plasma glucose levels at 60 to 120 mg/100 ml. Others feel the client is following the diet adequately if he does not have any clinical symptoms of diabetes. A third philosophy is that excess glucose levels are permissible as long as no ketones are spilled. In these instances, the diet should be selected from the basic four food groups with avoidance of artificial foodstuffs and excessive sweets. Most physicians, however, follow a dietary pattern in the middle of the extremes.

The diet is calculated to provide the ideal amount of calories for each individual. The caloric content of the diet is more significant than reduction of carbohydrates, because, in fact, higher amounts of glucose do not affect plasma glucose levels.

Since type 1 individuals are often underweight, a high caloric diet may be required to correct the catabolic effects of faulty glucose metabolism. Clients with type 2 diabetes, on the other hand, are usually overweight, and a diet that allows weight loss of about 2 pounds per week can be designed for these individuals.

The diet is then planned for the protein, carbohydrate, and fat content, with protein comprising approximately 20% of the diet, carbohydrates 50%, and fats 30%. The diet, furthermore, in compliance with nutrition recommendations for health, should contain a lower proportion of saturated fats and an increased amount of fiber. The greater amount of fiber, up to 20 g daily, is believed to slow glucose absorption in the intestines and avoid wide variations in plasma glucose concentration.

Once the caloric content and nutrition values are determined, the foods are apportioned in meals. The meal plan for type 2 diabetics includes three meals and a bedtime snack, whereas the plan for type 1 individuals, particularly children, should also include an afternoon snack.

If the physician wishes the diet to be followed closely, the client will need to obtain a food scale and weigh all food to ensure exact servings of all foods. The dietitian can be helpful in demonstrating how to use the scales and prepare foods for serving. If a more liberal food plan is permitted, the food exchange lists recommended by the American Diabetes Association and the American Dietetic Association (Tables 9-8 and 9-9) or the exchange lists for infants (Table 9-10) are used.

This diet plan stresses a well-balanced diet that can be estimated in serving sizes. The exchange lists are devised so that within any one list, the protein, carbohydrate, and fat content of the various foods on this list are similar. Any food from that list can be substituted for another food on the same list. There are six exchange lists, which follow the basic four food groups. A variety of meals can be planned by using the exchange lists, but the client must remember to eat all the prescribed foods at each meal. No meal or no item on the menu is to be omitted or held over until the next meal.

TABLE 9-8

Foods allowed as desired

Diet calorie-free beverage	Celery salt
	Parsley
Coffee	Nutmeg
Tea	Lemon
Bouillon without fat	Mustard
Unsweetened gelatin	Chili powder
	Onion salt or powder
Unsweetened pickles	Horseradish
	Vinegar
Salt and pepper	Mint
Red pepper	Cinnamon
Paprika	Lime
Garlic	

Data from American Diabetes Association, Inc., and the American Dietetic Association, 1976.

Text continued on p. 337.

TABLE 9-9

Food exchange lists

LIST 1: Milk exchanges *(includes nonfat, low-fat, and whole milk)*
One exchange of milk contains 12 g of carbonydrate, 8 g of protein, a trace of fat, and 80 calories.

*This list shows the kinds and amounts of milk or milk products to use for one milk exchange. Those that appear in **bold type** are **nonfat**. Low-fat and whole milk contain saturated fat.*

Product	Measure	Product	Measure
Nonfat fortified milk		Low-fat fortified milk	
Skim or nonfat milk	1 cup	1%-fat fortified milk (omit ½ fat exchange)	1 cup
Powdered (nonfat dry, before adding liquid)	⅓ cup	2%-fat fortified milk (omit 1 fat exchange)	1 cup
Canned, evaporated skim milk	½ cup	Yogurt made from 2%-fat fortified milk	1 cup
Buttermilk made from skim milk	1 cup	(plain, unflavored) (omit 1 fat exchange)	
Yogurt made from skim milk (plain, unflavored)	1 cup	Whole milk (omit 2 fat exchanges)	
		Whole milk	1 cup
		Canned, evaporated whole milk	½ cup
		Buttermilk made from whole milk	1 cup
		Yogurt made from whole milk (plain, unflavored)	1 cup

LIST 2: Vegetable exchanges
One exchange of vegetables contains about 5 g of carbohydrate, 2 g of protein, and 25 calories.

This list shows the kinds of vegetables to use for one vegetable exchange. One exchange is ½ cup.

Asparagus	Carrots	Greens	Mustard	Rhubarb	Tomatoes
Bean sprouts	Cauliflower	Beet	Spinach	Rutabaga	Tomato juice
Beets	Celery	Chards	Turnip	Sauerkraut	Turnips
Broccoli	Cucumbers	Collards	Mushrooms	String beans, green or yellow	Vegetable juice cocktail
Brussels sprouts	Eggplant	Dandelion	Okra	Summer squash	Zucchini
Cabbage	Green pepper	Kale	Onions		

The following raw vegetables may be used as desired.

Chicory	Escarole	Radishes
Chinese cabbage	Lettuce	Watercress
Endive	Parsley	

Starchy vegetables are found in the bread exchange list.

LIST 3. Fruit exchanges
One exchange of fruit contains 10 g of carbohydrate and 40 calories.

This list shows the kinds and amounts of fruits to use for one fruit exchange.

Product	Measure	Product	Measure
Apple	1 small	Mango	½ small
Apple juice	⅓ cup	Melon	
Applesauce, unsweetened	½ cup	Cantaloupe	¼ small
Apricots, fresh	2 medium	Honeydew	⅛ medium
Apricots, dried	4 halves	Watermelon	1 cup
Banana	½ small	Nectarine	1 small
Berries		Orange	1 small
Blackberries	½ cup	Orange juice	½ cup
Blueberries	½ cup	Papaya	¾ cup
Raspberries	½ cup	Peach	1 medium
Strawberries	¾ cup	Pear	1 small
Cherries	10 large	Persimmon, native	1 medium
Cider	⅓ cup	Pineapple	½ cup
Dates	2	Pineapple juice	⅓ cup
Figs, fresh	1	Plums	2 medium
Figs, dried	1	Prunes	2 medium
Grapefruit	½	Prune juice	¼ cup
Grapefruit juice	½ cup	Raisins	2 tablespoons
Grapes	12	Tangerine	1 medium
Grape juice	¼ cup		

Cranberries may be used as desired if no sugar is added.

Adapted from American Diabetes Association, Inc., and the American Dietetic Association, 1976.

Continued.

TABLE 9-9

Food exchange lists—cont'd

LIST 4: Bread exchanges *(includes bread, cereal, and starchy vegetables)*
One exchange of bread contains 15 g of carbohydrate, 2 g of protein, and 70 calories.

This list shows the kinds and amounts of breads, cereals, starchy vegetables, and prepared foods to use for one bread exchange. Those that appear in **bold type** *are low fat.*

Product	Measure	Product	Measure
Bread		Rye wafers, 2 × 3½ inches	3
White (including French and Italian)	1 slice	**Saltines**	6
Whole wheat	1 slice	**Soda, 2½ inches square**	4
Rye or pumpernickel	1 slice	**Dried beans, peas, and lentils**	
Raisin	1 slice	**Beans, peas, lentils (dried and cooked)**	½ cup
Bagel, small	½	**Baked beans, no pork (canned)**	¼ cup
English muffin, small	½	**Starchy vegetables**	
Plain roll, bread	1	**Corn**	⅓ cup
Frankfurter roll	½	**Corn on cob**	1 small
Hamburger bun	½	**Lima beans**	½ cup
Dried bread crumbs	3 tablespoons	**Parsnips**	⅔ cup
Tortilla, 6 inches	1	**Peas, green (canned or frozen)**	½ cup
Cereal		**Potato, white**	1 small
Cooked cereal	½ cup	**Potato, mashed**	½ cup
Puffed cereal, unfrosted	1 cup	**Pumpkin**	¾ cup
Bran flakes	½ cup	**Winter squash, acorn or butternut**	½ cup
Other ready-to-eat unsweetened, un-	¾ cup	**Yam or sweet potato**	¼ cup
puffed cereal		Prepared foods	
Grits, cooked	½ cup	Biscuit, 2 inches diameter (omit 1 fat ex-	1
Rice or barley, cooked	½ cup	change)	
Pasta, cooked	½ cup	Corn bread, 2 × 2 × 1 inches (omit 1 fat	1
Spaghetti, noodles		exchange)	
Macaroni		Corn muffin, 2 inches diameter (omit 1 fat	1
Popcorn (popped, no fat added)	3 cups	exchange)	
Cornmeal, dry	2 tablespoons	Crackers, round butter type (omit 1 fat	5
Flour	2½ tablespoons	exchange)	
Wheat germ	¼ cup	Muffin, plain small (omit 1 fat exchange)	1
Crackers		Potatoes, french fried, 2 to 3½ inches long	8
Arrowroot	3	(omit 1 fat exchange)	
Graham, 2½ inches square	2	Potato or corn chips (omit 2 fat exchanges)	15
Matzoth, 4 × inches	½	Pancake, 5 × ½ inches (omit 1 fat	1
Oyster	20	exchange)	
Pretzels, 3⅛ inches long × ⅛-inch	25	Waffle, 5 × ½ inches (omit 1 fat exchange)	1
diameter			

LIST 5: Meat exchanges
One exchange of lean meat (1 ounce) contains 7 g of protein, 3 g of fat, and 55 calories.

This list shows the kinds and amounts of lean meat and other protein-rich foods to use for one low-fat meat exchange.

Products	Measure	Products	Measure
Beef		Poultry	
Baby beef (very lean), chipped beef, chuck,	1 ounce	Meat (without skin) of chicken, turkey,	1 ounce
flank steak, tenderloin, plate ribs, plate		cornish hen, guinea hen, pheasant	
skirt steak, round, (bottom, top), all cuts		Fish	
rump, spare ribs, tripe		Any fresh or frozen	1 ounce
Lamb		Canned salmon, tuna, mackerel, crab, lob-	¼ cup
Leg, rib, sirloin, loin (roast and chops),	1 ounce	ster	
shank, shoulder		Clams, oysters, scallops, shrimp,	5 pieces or 1 ounce
Pork		sardines (drained)	3
Leg (whole rump, center shank), ham,	1 ounce	Cheese containing less than 5% butterfat	1 ounce
smoked (center slices)		Cottage cheese, dry and 2% butterfat	¼ cup
Veal		Dried beans and peas (omit 1 bread exchange)	½ cup
Leg, loin, rib, shank, shoulder, cutlets	1 ounce		

9 Endocrine system

TABLE 9-9

Food exchange list—cont'd

This list shows the kinds and amounts of medium-fat meat and other protein-rich foods to use for one medium-fat meat exchange. For each exchange of medium-fat meat omit ½ fat exchange.

Product	Measure	Product	Measure
Beef		Liver, heart, kidney, sweetbreads (these are high in cholesterol)	1 ounce
Ground (15% fat), corned beef (canned), rib eye, round (ground commercial)	1 ounce	Cottage cheese, creamed	¼ cup
Pork		Cheese	
Loin (all cuts tenderloin), shoulder arm (picnic), shoulder blade, Boston butt, Canadian bacon, boiled ham	1 ounce	Mozzarella, ricotta, farmer's, neufchatel, parmesan	1 ounce / 3 tablespoons
		Egg (high in cholesterol)	
		Peanut butter (omit 2 additional fat exchanges)	2 tablespoons

This list shows the kinds and amounts of high-fat meat and other protein-rich foods to use for one high-fat meat exchange. For each exchange of high-fat meat omit 1 fat exchange.

Product	Measure	Product	Measure
Beef		Veal	
Brisket, corned beef (brisket), ground beef (more than 20% fat), hamburger (commercial), roasts (rib), steaks (club and rib)	1 ounce	Breast	1 ounce
		Poultry	
Lamb		Capon, duck (domestic), goose	1 ounce
Breast	1 ounce	Cheese	
Pork		Cheddar types	1 ounce
Spare ribs, loin (back ribs), pork (ground), country-style ham, deviled ham	1 ounce	Cold cuts	4½ × 4½ × ⅛−slice
		Frankfurter	1 small

LIST 6: Fat exchanges
One exchange of fat contains 5 g of fat and 45 calories.

This list shows the kinds and amounts of fat-containing foods to use for one fat exchange. To plan a diet low in saturated fat, select only those exchanges that appear in **bold type.** *They are* **polyunsaturated.**

Product	Measure	Product	Measure
Margarine, soft, tub, or stick*	1 teaspoon	Margarine, regular stick	1 teaspoon
Avocado (4 inches diameter)†	⅛	Butter	1 teaspoon
Oil, corn, cottonseed, safflower, soy, sunflower	1 teaspoon	Bacon fat	1 teaspoon
		Bacon, crisp	1 strip
Oil, olive†	1 teaspoon	Cream	
Oil, peanut†	1 teaspoon	Light	2 tablespoons
Olives†	5 small	Heavy	1 tablespoon
Almonds†	10 whole	Sour	2 tablespoons
Pecans†	2 large whole	Cream cheese	1 tablespoon
Peanuts†		French dressing‡	1 tablespoon
Spanish	20 whole	Italian dressing‡	1 tablespoon
Virginia	10 whole	Lard	1 teaspoon
Walnuts	6 small	Mayonnaise‡	1 teaspoon
Nuts, other†	6 small	Salad dressing, mayonnaise type‡	2 teaspoons
		Salt pork	¾-inch cube

*Made with corn, cottonseed, safflower, soy, or sunflower oil only.

†Fat content is primarily monounsaturated.

‡If made with corn, cottonseed, safflower, soy, or sunflower oil, it can be used on fat-modified diet.

TABLE 9-10

Food exchange lists for infants

LIST 1: Milk/formula exchange*

	Protein/g	CHO/g	Fat/g
Whole milk	8	12	10
Similac	3.6	17.0	8.8
Enfamil	3.6	16.8	8.8
SMA	3.6	17.3	8.6
Prosobee	6.0	16.3	8.4
Isomil	4.8	16.3	8.6
2% milk	8	12	5†
Advance	6.7	14.9	4.8†

LIST 2: Bread exchanges for diabetic infants‡

Dry baby rice cereal	5 tablespoons
Baby oatmeal cereal	5 tablespoons
High-protein cereal	9 tablespoons

"Strained" jar = 4.75 oz (135 g)

Strained baby rice cereal with mixed fruit (also count 1 fruit exchange)	1 jar
Baby oatmeal cereal with applesauce and banana	1 jar
High-protein cereal with applesauce and banana	1 jar
Creamed corn	1 jar
Mixed vegetables	1 jar
Sweet potatoes	1 jar

"Junior" jar = 7.75 oz (220 g)

Junior rice with mixed fruit	1 jar
Oatmeal with applesauce and banana	1 jar
Creamed corn	1 jar
Teething biscuits, arrowroot cookies, animal cookies, and pretzels	3

LIST 3: Fruit exchanges for diabetic infants§

Baby apple juice	¾ can (3 oz)
Mixed fruit juice	½ can (2 oz)
Prune-orange juice	⅓ can (1½ oz)

"Baby" can = 4.2 oz

Strained applesauce	½ jar
Bananas	⅓ jar
Peaches	⅓ jar
Plums	¼ jar
Prunes	⅓ jar
Cherry vanilla pudding	½ jar
Chocolate custard	⅓ jar
Dutch apple dessert	⅓ jar

"Strained" jar = 4.75 oz (135 g)

Junior applesauce	⅓ jar
Bananas	¼ jar
Peaches	⅕ jar (5 tbsp)
Pears	⅓ jar (5 tbsp)
Plums	⅕ jar (5 tbsp)
Prunes	⅕ jar (5 tbsp)

"Junior" jar = 7.75 oz (220 g)

LIST 4: Meat exchanges for diabetic infants‖

Strained egg yolk	1 jar
Strained chicken	½ jar
Ham	½ jar
Lamb	½ jar
Beef	½ jar
Pork	½ jar
(Above also must count 1 fat)	

1 jar = 3.33 oz (94 g)

Junior chicken	½ jar
Ham	½ jar
Lamb	½ jar
Beef	½ jar
Pork	½ jar
Meat sticks	½ jar

1 jar = 3.5 oz (99 g)

LIST 5: Vegetable exchanges for diabetic infants¶

Strained carrots	1 jar
Beets	½ jar
Creamed spinach	1 jar
Green beans	1 jar
Squash	1 jar
Peas	1 jar

"Strained" jar = 4.5 oz (128 g)

Junior carrots	½ jar
Creamed spinach	½ jar
Green beans	½ jar
Squash	½ jar

"Junior" jar = 7.5 oz (213 g)

LIST 6: Multiple exchanges for diabetic infants

Strained beef with egg noodles and vegetables	1 jar = ½ bread ½ meat
Cereal and egg yolk	1 jar = ½ bread ½ meat
Chicken and noodles	1 jar = ½ bread ½ meat
Vegetables and chicken	1 jar = ½ bread ½ meat
Macaroni and cheese	1 jar = 1 fruit ½ meat
High meat dinners	1 jar = 1 meat ½ bread

"Strained" jar = 4.5 oz (128 g)

Junior beef with egg noodles	1 jar = 1 bread ½ meat
Cereal and egg yolk	1 jar = 1 bread 1 fat
Chicken and noodles	1 jar = 1 bread ½ meat
Vegetables and chicken	1 jar = 1 bread ½ meat
Macaroni and cheese	1 jar = 1 bread ½ meat

"Junior" jar = 7.5 oz (213 g)

From Kohler, E.: Baby food exchanges and feeding the diabetic infant. Diabetes Care **3:**553-556, 1980. Reproduced with permission from The American Diabetes Association, Inc.

* One 8-oz cup = 160 cal.
† Add 1 fat exchange.
‡ Each item is 1 bread exchange (68 cal).
§ Each item is 1 fruit exchange (40 cal).
‖ Each item is 1 meat exchange (73 cal).
¶ Each item is 1 vegetable B exchange (36 cal).

There are many aids to help the client with his diet. The dietitian or nurse can furnish some of these written guides. The client's menus while in the hospital are also useful aids. He learns what foods he may have and what an average serving looks like. It may be helpful for clients to have recipes for casseroles, desserts, or hors d'euvres that can be made from foods on the exchange lists. Some food distributors will furnish the exchange list proportions of such prepared food items as soups and frozen dinners. Dietetic foods are for sale in most grocery stores, but generally they are expensive and may have more calories than the client is permitted. Clients should be instructed to read labels on all foods to be sure there are no harmful additives. Many foods on the "free" list (see Table 9-8) are helpful in supplementing the diet. The client should be familiar with soft drinks that are essentially calorie free and other food items that may be used in the diet, such as artificial sweeteners for use in preparation of certain desserts and sauces.

When meal planning is discussed with the client, the person who is going to do the cooking should also be present. The nurse can suggest that the food for the family be prepared simply and that gravy, sauces, and side dishes that the diabetic cannot have be added at the table. Diet classes for diabetic individuals and their families are offered in most hospitals, and both groups should be encouraged to attend them.

Food has varied meanings for each client, and the nurse should attempt to understand his feelings as he adjusts to these changes. To children, food can mean love and security. The controlled diet should not be presented as a withdrawal of needed attention, and the parents can plan to give the child extra attention in other ways. To adolescents, eating is a social experience and an important way to be part of the peer group. Asking the adolescent to give up pizza and soft drinks is difficult. The diet can be planned to be flexible so that he can enjoy snacks with his friends. The adolescent assumes much responsibility for his eating habits and needs encouragement, not criticism, when following a diabetic diet. He may eat in the school cafeteria and should be assisted to select appropriate foods. Adults also enjoy food as a social experience, and the cocktail party or dinner in a restaurant presents certain problems. If indicated by the physician, a cocktail can be worked into the diet, and if the client is using exchange lists, he soon learns how to use them when eating in restaurants. Adults have tendencies to skip meals, work past the lunch hour, or have dinner late. The nurse should help them arrange schedules that can accommodate these variances. Older clients may find it difficult to prepare meals and, if living alone, may tend to skip some meals. The community health nurse can be helpful in observing dietary patterns in the home and in suggesting home dietary services that provide daily meals.

Compliance with diet therapy increases if the diet is adapted to the client's life-style. Restrictive diets are often difficult to follow, and eating habits that are ingrained over a lifetime are nearly impossible to change. When the focus of diet instruction is centered on eating foods that are nutritious and acceptable to the client, the diet plan will more likely be followed.

Pharmacological therapy. The third factor in the control of diabetes is the use of drug therapy. Two types of drugs are used: oral hypoglycemic drugs (used by clients who have islet function) and insulin (used when exogenous replacement is required). These drugs are used to maintain euglycemia to prevent or postpone development of microvascular and macrovascular changes associated with hyperglycemia.

337

Nursing process for common health problems

ORAL HYPOGLYCEMIC DRUGS. The sulfonylurea drugs, tolbutamide (Orinase), tolazamide (Tolinase), chlorpropamide (Diabinese), and acetohexamide (Dymelor), are used with type 2 diabetics whose plasma glucose remains elevated in spite of dietary management. The action of sulfonylurea drugs is unclear. Some believe the drug acts to stimulate beta cell production of insulin. Others suggest that these drugs act to reduce hepatic glucose output and thereby reduce blood glucose levels.[1,16]

The side effects of sulfonylureas may include headache and gastric upset. Hypoglycemia can occur, however, if the client does not maintain his diet. Ongoing research has demonstrated an increased number of deaths from cardiovascular disease in individuals using oral hypoglycemic agents, and for this reason it is recommended that these drugs be used only by those who cannot be controlled by diet or cannot or will not use insulin. Since oral hypoglycemic agents seem particularly dangerous to the fetus, the pregnant client is generally maintained on insulin. The agents are usually taken daily (before breakfast) or twice daily (before breakfast and the evening meal).

The sulfonylureas are potentiated by phenylbutazone (Butazolidin), MAO inhibitors, sulfonamides, diphenylhydantoin, anticoagulants, alcohol, and high doses of aspirin. The following drugs inhibit the hypoglycemic effect of the oral hypoglycemia drugs: corticosteroids, oral contraceptives, thiazide diuretics, and furosemide (Lasix).

INSULIN. Clients who have absolute insulin deficiency or relative deficiency during pregnancy or stress may require exogenous sources of insulin. Insulin is obtained from extracts from beef or pork pancreas. Most insulin currently manufactured is a combination of beef and pork insulin, although beef only or pork only insulin is available if the client is allergic to one type.

Insulin in current production is 99% pure (single peak insulin), and the likelihood for skin reactions, lipodystrophy, and allergic reactions is minimized. Clients who have used other insulins previously may experience hypoglycemia after the first dose, because they may be receiving a higher dose of insulin in this purified form of insulin. If hypoglycemia, as noted by headaches, shakiness, or diaphoresis, does occur, the client should report the signs to the nurse or physician and the dose of insulin may need to be lowered.

TABLE 9-11

Lilly insulin preparations used in the United States

Type of insulin	Appearance	Action	Peak activity (hours)	Duration (hours)	Zinc content (mg/100 units)	pH buffer	Protein	
							Type	mg/100 units
Regular crystalline	Clear	Rapid	2-4	5-7	0.01-0.04	7.2	None	—
NPH	Turbid	Intermediate	6-12	24-28	0.01-0.04	Phosphate 7.2	Protamine	0.4
Protamine zinc	Turbid	Prolonged	14-24	36+	0.15-0.25	Phosphate 7.2	Protamine	1-1.5
Semilente	Turbid	Rapid	2-4	12-16	0.14-0.25	Acetate	None	—
Lente	Turbid	Intermediate	6-12	24-28	0.14-0.25	Acetate 7.2	None	—
Ultralente	Turbid	Prolonged	18-24	36+	0.14-0.25	Acetate 7.2	None	—

Waife, S.O., editor: Diabetes mellitus, ed. 8, Indianapolis, 1980, Lilly Research Laboratories.

Newer methods of recombinant DNA research have produced human insulin in *E coli*. The activity of this biosynthetic human insulin is the same as pancreatic human insulin on amino acid analysis, and wide use of this drug is anticipated for the future.[9]

Insulin is dispensed in concentrations of units per millimeter. The most common form of insulin is U100 insulin, that is, 100 units of insulin are contained in each milliliter. For those requiring larger amounts of insulin, a more concentrated form (U500 insulin) containing 500 units of insulin can be obtained. Less concentrated insulins (U40 and U80 insulin) were once commonly used, but because of confusion and resultant dosage errors, the production of these concentrates is limited, and U80 will no longer be produced.

There are several types of insulin with differing peaks and duration of action. They are classified by their time of action as rapid, intermediate, and long-acting (Table 9-11). Each type of insulin is packaged in a different shaped bottle so that the client will be able to distinguish different types if he is using more than one. Black lettering on a white background signifies the U100 concentration, and the bold letters can be used to identify the type.

Insulin is best stored in the refrigerator if kept over a long period of time, but it may be stored at room temperature if used within a few weeks. Insulin is always given at room temperature. Some insulins form a precipitate after standing, and the bottle should be gently rotated to redistribute the contents. The bottle should not be shaken because air bubbles make withdrawal of an accurate dose difficult.

Insulin can be administered by several routes, depending on the individual needs of the client. The most common route is subcutaneous, though insulin can be given intramuscularly or intravenously when rapid lowering of blood glucose is required.

Insulin administered by the subcutaneous route requires the use of special syringes (Fig. 9-3). They are calibrated in units to correspond to the insulin units and have ⅝-inch needles. Uniform use of U100 insulin has eliminated the need to use more than one calibration of syringes, but it is important for the nurse to verify that the syringe is calibrated in units to correspond with the concentration of insulin. There are four commonly used syringes for use with U100 insulin; all are calibrated for U100 insulin use. A 35- or 50-unit syringe is used for doses of less than 35 to 50 units. Each unit marking on this syringe represents 1 unit. The larger markings make withdrawal of smaller amounts of insulin easier and more accurate. Most clients use the 1-ml, U100 syringe. Each unit mark on this syringe is equal to 2 units. For persons who use more than 100 units, a special 2-ml, U100 syringe can be obtained.

The client should be instructed to use the same brand of syringes because "dead space" in syringes varies with manufacturer, and dosage errors can result. However, some syringes are manufactured free of dead space.

In an emergency or disaster, regular syringes may be used, and the units of insulin converted into milliliters, because 100 units of insulin is contained in

FIG. 9-3
U100 Insulin syringe. Each mark on syringe represents 2 units. Forty units of insulin is indicated. (Courtesy Eli Lilly and Co., Indianapolis.)

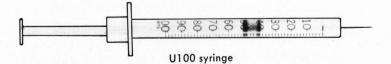

U100 syringe

FIG. 9-4
Nurse instructs client about insulin injection technique.

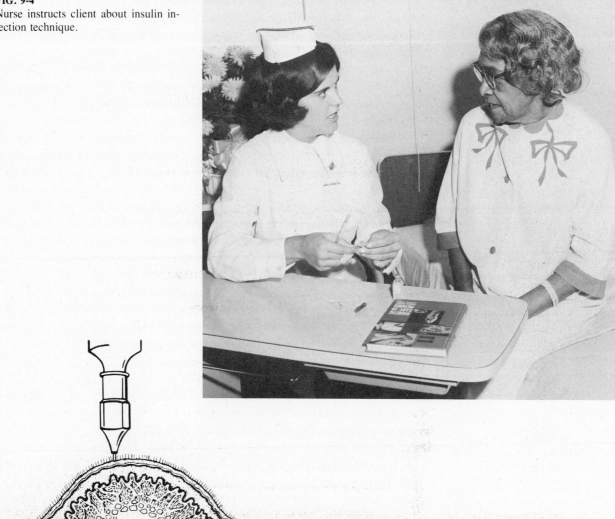

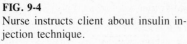

FIG. 9-5
For thin clients, skin is rolled and a ⅝-inch needle is inserted at a 90-degree angle for injection of insulin. (Courtesy Eli Lilly & Co., Indianapolis.)

1 ml. Utmost care should be used when preparing insulin for administration. The insulin doses (units/ml) *must* correspond to the unit scale on the syringe.

The nurse can instruct the client how to administer his own insulin. Instruction is facilitated when the same nurse instructs the client and individualizes instruction for the client's needs (Fig. 9-4). Instruction should include information about injection technique, sites for injection, and care of syringes. There are several techniques that can be used to inject the insulin. The object of each technique is to deposit the insulin directly below the subcutaneous fat. Many recommend that the injection be given at a 90-degree angle, with the skin taut. If the client is thin, it may be necessary to pinch up a roll of skin (Fig. 9-5). Others suggest using a 45-degree angle, with the skin rolled and elevated. In another approach the skin folds are gently pinched and raised off the muscle. The width of this fold is measured to determine needle length, and the injection is made the width of the fold at a 10- to 30-degree angle (Fig. 9-6) into the space created by lifting the skin off the muscle. After the insulin has been injected, the site may be held with an alcohol swab for several seconds.

Insulin can cause local reactions such as localized allergic reaction, generalized reactions, or lipodystrophy. A local reaction can be identified by stinging, induration, or itching at the site of injection. A generalized reaction includes hives and urticaria. These reactions can be treated by giving antihistamines 30 minutes before injection, by desensitizing, or by changing to pure beef or pork insulin. Fewer reactions can be anticipated with the use of the new purified insulins.

Lipodystrophy (Fig. 9-7) may be caused by faulty injection technique, trauma, or injection of refrigerated insulin. Lipodystrophy includes accumulation of fatty masses, whereas in lipoatrophy the fat deposits disappear and excavation of the skin is noted. This latter phenomenon can be treated by injecting single-peak insulin directly into the area, causing fat deposits to fill these sites. The area can be injected from the center outward until the excavation is filled. Initially there will be doughy consistency, but eventually the area will become firm.

To prevent local reaction and lipodystrophy, some suggest that the site of the injection be rotated so that the same area is not used again for at least 30 days. Fig. 9-8 indicates possible injection sites. The client can put his hand at the top of his thigh and top of his knee and any area in between these points may be used. Numbering the sites facilitates a rotation plan whereby no one site is used more often than every 30 days. Giving insulin in the abdomen may be frightening to the client, but when he overcomes his fears, he has another area to use for injection. It is helpful if a family member can learn to give insulin so that the buttocks and arms can be used. The client should keep a chart to remind him to rotate

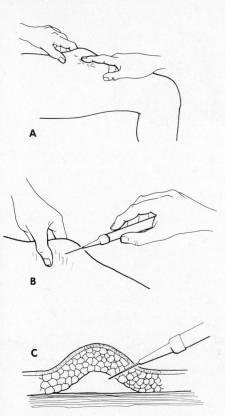

FIG. 9-6
Alternative insulin injection technique. **A,** Lift skin off muscle. **B,** Measure needle length according to width of skinfold. **C,** Inject at 20- to 45-degree angle into space created by lifting skin and fat from muscle.

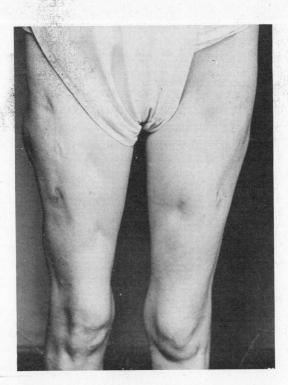

FIG. 9-7
Lipodystrophy can result if client does not use appropriate insulin injection technique. (Courtesy Eli Lilly & Co., Indianapolis.)

FIG. 9-8
Injection sites and rotation.

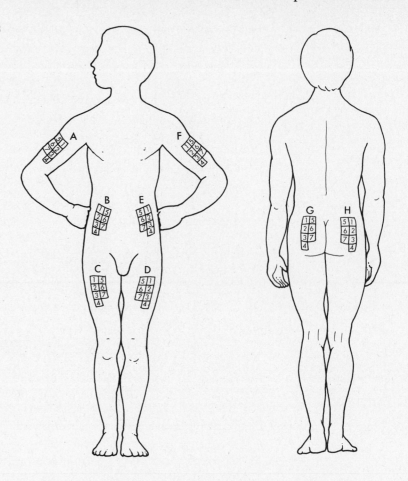

injection sites. A methodical rotation of sites in a clockwise direction is easy to remember.

The site of injection affects insulin absorption and peak glycemic levels. Insulin injected in the abdomen achieves peak concentration rapidly, and when insulin is injected into the anterior thigh, concentration is slowest.[9] Absorption from the arm is intermediate.[32] Insulin injected near a muscle such as the thigh or arm used in heavy exercise is absorbed rapidly, and hypoglycemia is more likely to occur. Persons engaging in vigorous exercises should therefore inject the insulin in the abdomen.[9] Some even recommend using only one anatomic area for injection to avoid unpredictable absorption and peak concentration.[32]

The use of insulin syringes and other equipment will vary with the client's preference, needs, and economic resources. All equipment can be purchased with a prescription at the pharmacy. Glass syringes with stainless steel needles are easier to read, but they must be boiled for 5 minutes at least weekly and stored aseptically. Special syringes can be bought for clients who have vision problems. Syringes with magnified numbers are available, as well as syringes with a preset trigger device, which can be filled only to a fixed point. Disposable syringes are convenient and safe but more expensive. Some clients prefer to buy disposable needles for a glass syringe and boil the syringe weekly. Research has indicated that disposable syringe-needle units can be reused for 3 days without problems of infection, altered insulin dose, or blunt needle.[6] The needle should

FIG. 9-9
Insulin infusion pump. (Courtesy Auto-
Syringe, Inc.)

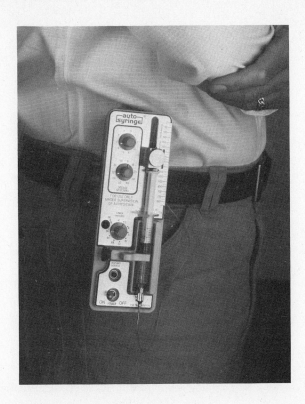

be kept clean and stored safely. Reuse serves to reduce the cost of this equipment.

In specialized health care centers, insulin infusion pumps (Fig. 9-9) are being used to administer insulin subcutaneously or intravenously. The battery-driven pump holds a syringe filled with insulin, which slowly infuses the prescribed dose of insulin. In one method a plastic cannula is attached to the syringe and the distal end attached to a 27-gauge needle inserted into the subcutaneous tissues in the client's abdomen. The sites can be rotated every 24 to 96 hours.[30] Insulin can be administered every 4, 8, 16, or 32 minutes to simulate continuous infusion, and larger doses can be given before meals by pressing an ''instant dose'' button that delivers a larger dose over 1 minute. The pump can be worn on a belt around the client's waist. Continuous infusion by the portable pump provides the client flexibility of meal planning in relation to insulin administration, prevention of fasting hypoglycemia, and more normal maintenance of plasma glucose levels.[9]

Hormonal activity. The fourth factor in controlling plasma glucose levels is the influence of the adrenal gland hormones—epinephrine and the glucocorticosteroids. Increases of circulating blood levels of both of these hormones cause hyperglycemia, and the nurse and client must be aware of situations that precipitate hormone release and learn to adjust activity, diet, and, if insulin dependent, the insulin to compensate for the hyperglycemia. Epinephrine is released from the adrenal medulla and glucocorticosteroids from the adrenal cortex and may be noted during physical trauma, stress, infection, anxiety, anger, fear, or change in life-style. The nurse can help the client identify and anticipate the presence of any one of these situations and instruct the client in stress modification and adaptation of the therapeutic plan.

Nursing process for common health problems

MONITORING GLUCOSURIA, KETONURIA, AND GLYCEMIA. The client can determine the effects of activity, diet, insulin, and hormones on glucose metabolism by testing the urine or blood for glucose. Glucosuria can be monitored by the Clinitest method or with enzymatic indicators. These tests are easy to perform, but many clients find urine testing unpleasant or time consuming, and compliance with daily testing is not always easily achieved. Home monitoring of blood glucose, although requiring a greater expense for equipment, provides for more accurate information about therapeutic control, particularly for the insulin-dependent diabetic, and, because the test need only be done daily or every other day, there may be increased client interest and likelihood of monitoring glycemia.

CLINITEST. Glucose in the urine can be measured qualitatively by Clinitest, a copper reduction assay of glucosuria. The test comes in a kit with a test tube, dropper, and Clinitest tablets. The client is instructed to test his urine before meals and at bedtime or on a schedule given him by his physician. If possible, the urine specimen should be a second-voided specimen so that fresh urine is evaluated rather than urine that has been in the bladder for several hours. If the specimen is obtained from an indwelling catheter, the urine should be obtained from proximal tubing or by aspiration from the catheter. Urine from continuous bladder irrigations should not be used.

The test is made by mixing 5 drops of urine and 10 drops of water and adding 1 Clinitest tablet. The client observes the reaction for color changes. A color chart comes with the kit with which to compare the urine for indications of glucose. The client should use the chart each time for comparisons, since it is not easy to remember each color change.

Color changes can occur rapidly, and any indication of an orange color (indicative of a positive reaction), even though the reaction returns to blue or green (a negative reaction), is recorded as 2%. This phenomenon is known as the "pass through" and may cause the client to misinterpret the results.

When there is 2% glucosuria, the *2-drop Clinitest method* can be used. Two drops of urine, 10 drops of water, and a Clinitest tablet are placed in the test tube; after 15 seconds the reaction is compared with a special color chart that is used only for the 2-drop Clinitest method. Glucosuria up to 5% can thereby be ascertained. Further information can be obtained from the *1-drop Clinitest method* in which 1 drop of urine is added to 11 drops of water and 1 Clinitest tablet. The color chart is interpreted, and results doubled to accommodate the dilution factor. Glucosuria up to 10% can be determined.

The client is advised not to touch the test tube while the reaction is occurring, because it is hot from chemical reaction. The tablets should be kept in a dry, dark place, out of the reach of children. Touching the tablets with the hands adds moisture, and therefore the tablets should be dropped directly into the test tube.

False positive reactions from the Clinitest methods can occur if the client is taking certain drugs such as nalidixic acid (NegGram), cephalexin monohydrate (Keflex), or probenecid (Benemid), cephalothin (Keflin), cephaloridine (Loridine), salicylates, vitamin C, or penicillin. The client should tell his physician if he is taking these drugs.

The client should be instructed to test his urine before meals and at bedtime to monitor the effects of oral hypoglycemic agents or insulin therapy. Specimens tested before breakfast give indications of the effectiveness of intermediate-acting or long-acting insulin given the previous day. Tests of urine samples obtained before lunch indicate the effectiveness of rapid-acting insulins given before breakfast. Testing the urine before the evening meal gives information about intermediate-acting insulins given before breakfast, and the bedtime Clinitest indicates that the insulin being used is sufficient to handle foods eaten during the evening meal. Records of these patterns are helpful to the physician while planning and continuing therapy.

ENZYME INDICATORS. Tape and sticks with enzymatic indicators may also be used to detect glucose in the urine. They provide quantitative measures of glucosuria and are much easier to use. They are helpful on a trip or when the client is away from home. They are also useful when certain drugs invalidate Clinitest determinations. The tape or stick is dipped into urine and compared with special color codes. The hands should be washed before the test to prevent contamination of the sticks. The test tape is invalidated by methyldopa (Aldomet), ascorbic acid, aspirin, levodopa, and dipyrone (Narone). Results should be reported as percentage rather than pluses (+), because confusion in reporting may occur if Clinitest and enzymatic indicators are used alternately.[19]

URINE TESTS FOR ACETONE. The amount of acetone (ketone bodies) being excreted in the urine is a significant indication of body metabolism. Because ketone bodies are excreted when the body is using fats for energy because glucose is unavailable, the test should be done for clients who are ketosis prone, have positive Clinitests, have vomited, are losing weight, are going through growth spurts, are under stress, or are having surgery. Pregnant women should test early-morning urine samples for ketones. The test is made by putting one drop of urine on an Acetest tablet and watching for color changes. A chart comes with the tablets, and the client should use it as a basis of comparison each time he makes the test. Ketostix or Acestix are easier to use, because the client needs only to dip them in urine and observe the paper stick change color. The client should be instructed to record color changes at the exact time indicated by the manufacturer. The results of these tests are recorded along with the Clinitest results. Usually the physician will want to observe the record as an indication of metabolic difficulty.

MONITORING BLOOD GLUCOSE. Blood glucose levels can be monitored by clients at home using a glucose oxidase–impregnated strip (Dextrostrip) that, when exposed to blood from a finger stick, undergoes color changes that can be read on a reflectance meter.[3] Easy access to information about blood glucose levels, more accurate than urine glucose levels, improves insulin regulation for the client who can, if so instructed, adjust doses himself based on information from the blood glucose assay.

To obtain a blood sample, a lancet is used to make a stick in the finger or thumb to obtain a drop of blood. The blood is placed on a reagent strip, washed with water from a squeeze bottle, and read with the meter. The meter should be calibrated before each use.

Metabolic changes related to diabetes

Hypoglycemia, diabetic ketoacidosis, and metabolic complications. Changes in the balance of activity, diet, insulin, and hormone levels, and acute infection may produce dramatic changes in glycemic levels. The client must be aware of the necessity for maintaining a balance and recognize the signs of imbalance. Two significant imbalances are hypoglycemia and diabetic ketoacidosis. Complications of diabetes mellitus can also result from metabolic changes that can precipitate hyperglycemia, hyperosmolar nonketotic coma, and lactic acidosis. Although these complications are rare, the nurse and client must be able to recognize them.

Hypoglycemic reactions. All clients who take insulin or oral hypoglycemic agents face the possibility of having a hypoglycemic reaction (insulin shock or insulin reaction). A hypoglycemic reaction may occur when the client has too much insulin in the body for the available glucose and usually happens because the client has not eaten enough food or has exercised too vigorously and used up too much glucose.

Hypoglycemic reactions are caused by a rapid shift of blood glucose, which triggers the sympathetic nervous system, and by epinephrine release, causing hunger, irritability, sweating, and dilated pupils. Overdosage of insulin because of inaccurate measuring over a period of time will also produce an insulin reaction. This more serious reaction causes hypoglycemia and reduced glycogen stores. The onset is insidious, signaled by headache and weakness, and it may proceed to unconsciousness and seizures (Table 9-12). Nausea, vomiting, diarrhea, or delay in eating after taking insulin may also cause a hypoglycemic reaction. Changing sites of insulin injection to a point where it is more rapidly absorbed may also precipitate hypoglycemia. Certain drugs may increase carbohydrate metabolism and thereby contribute to insulin shock. Propranolol hydrochloride (Inderal) and large doses of salicylates are two such drugs, and the client should advise his physician if he is taking these so that the dosage of insulin can be reduced.

The client should be instructed to recognize certain symptoms that indicate to him that a reaction is imminent. In the hospital most new diabetics experience insulin reactions while they are becoming regulated on insulin. It is a highly individual experience, and no two persons have the same warning symptoms. Generally there is weakness, fatigue, headache, restlessness, yawning, confusion, nervousness, sweating, cold clammy skin, dizziness, hunger, blurred vision, or tachycardia. The reactions are less obvious in children, and they may cry or become moody. Insulin reactions during sleep (usually caused by peak action of long-acting insulins) may be manifested by nightmares, night sweats, crying during sleep, sleep walking, or inability to be aroused. Older individuals may exhibit psychotic behavior, slurred speech, or somnolence. Atherosclerosis may mask the symptoms of hypoglycemia.

The physician may wish to have a blood sample drawn when the client exhibits symptoms of insulin reaction. On diabetic nursing units, the nurse may be the one to obtain this specimen. Examination of the blood reveals hypoglycemia, and there is no glucose in the urine.

The symptoms are reversed if the client takes some food, usually 10 g of a fast-acting sugar such as 3 ounces of soft drink, 4 ounces of orange juice, a candy bar, 5 ml of honey, or five to six Lifesavers. It is not necessary to add sugar to drinks because the sweetened drink may cause nausea or vomiting. If food is not given, the client proceeds to unconsciousness.

When the client is unconscious, it is necessary to give the glucose intravenously or subcutaneously. In the hospital the glucose is given intravenously. At home, the family may be taught to use a syrette of glucagon, which is given subcutaneously or intramuscularly, or in various sublingual preparations such

TABLE 9-12

Differential diagnosis
of diabetic coma
and hypoglycemic reactions

	Diabetic coma	Hypoglycemic reactions	
		Regular insulin	Modified insulin or oral agents
Clinical features			
Onset	Slow — days	Sudden — minutes	Gradual — hours
Causes	Ignorance Neglect of therapy Intercurrent disease or infection	Overdosage Omission or delay of meals Excessive exercise before meals	
Symptoms	Thirst Headache Nausea Vomiting Abdominal pain Dim vision Constipation Dyspnea	"Inward nervousness" Hunger Sweating Weakness Diplopia Blurred vision Paresthesia Psychopathic behavior Stupor Convulsions	Fatigue Headache Nausea Sweating (sometimes absent) Dizziness
Signs	Florid face Air hunger (Kussmaul's respiration) Finally, respiratory paralysis Dehydration (dry skin) Rapid pulse Soft eyeballs Normal of absent reflexes Acetone breath	Pallor Shallow respiration Sweating Normal pulse Eyeballs normal Babinski's reflex often present	Skin may be dry Pulse not characteristic
Chemical features			
Urine glucose	Positive	Usually absent, especially in second voided specimen	
Acetone	Positive	Negative	
Diacetic acid	Positive	Negative	
Blood glucose	>250 mg/100 ml ordinarily	60 mg or less/100 ml	
CO_2 combining power	<20 volumes/100 ml	Usually normal	
Leukocytosis	Present; may be very high		
Response to treatment	Slow	Rapid; occasionally delayed	May be delayed

From Waife, S.O., editor: Diabetes mellitus, ed. 8, Indianapolis, 1980, Lilly Research Laboratories.

as Instant Glucose or Neg React, which can be applied to the mucous membranes of the mouth and act to stimulate release of glucose from the liver. Twenty minutes should be allowed for the client to arouse. When the client is alert, he should be given 3 ounces of a soft drink or 4 ounces of juice. If the reaction occurs near mealtime, this meal can be eaten early.

These reactions are frightening to the client at first, but he soon learns to cope with them. The client is encouraged to keep a source of sugar with him and at his place of business or school for these emergencies, and the employer or teacher should be informed of the possibility of an insulin reaction and be prepared to assist the client. All diabetic individuals should wear a Medic-Alert bracelet or carry a card stating that they are diabetic so that if they are found unconscious, they will receive appropriate assistance.

To prevent exercise-induced hypoglycemia, the client who uses insulin can be instructed by a physician or nurse practitioner to modify diet and insulin dose. If the client anticipates an increase in activity, he may decrease the insulin dose 20% to 25%. If he has already injected his insulin, he can avert a hypoglycemic reaction by taking 20 to 40 g of a carbohydrate such as fruit juice before exercising. Glucosuria can be monitored with blood or urine tests, and, if nonreactive after exertion, more carbohydrates may be needed.

Ketoacidosis. Ketoacidosis occurs when fatty acids are broken down to ketone bodies because of an absolute or relative deficiency of insulin or, rarely, in states of glucagon excess.[18] There is gluconeogenesis and decreased peripheral uptake of sugar. This is followed by urinary glucose loss, osmotic diuresis, and electrolyte depletion. Ketogenic pathways in the liver are activated and, compounded with impaired peripheral metabolism of ketones as a result of decreased insulin, overload the buffer system, and acidosis follows.

Ketoacidosis may be a result of improper attention to the therapeutic plan by eating too much or obtaining insufficient insulin. Ketoacidosis is also precipitated by stress states, particularly infections, acute illness, pregnancy, surgery, or periods of growth. Ketoacidosis is not unusual in children whose metabolic needs are constantly changing.

Symptoms of ketoacidosis are similar to those of diabetes and develop over a period of days or weeks (Table 9-12). There is thirst, hyperglycemia, glucosuria, polyuria, acidemia, listlessness, nausea and vomiting, and headache. As dehydration occurs, there is flushed face, fever, dry skin, parched lips, soft eyeballs, decreased urine output, and hypovolemic shock. Metabolic acidosis is manifested by an air hunger (Kussmaul respirations), which is a compensatory mechanism to blow off carbon dioxide, and a sweet odor to the breath (ketone breath). Sodium and potassium become depleted, and eventually coma and death occur if the process is not reversed.

Laboratory findings reveal hyperglycemia, ketonemia, and acidosis. Serum plasma sugar reaches 300 to 1000 mg/100 ml; urinary glucose is 2% and positive for ketones. The electrolyte loss is difficult to determine if the client is severely dehydrated, but plasma bicarbonate of less than 15 mEq/L and arterial pH of less than 7.25 are indicative of metabolic acidosis. The BUN may be elevated as a result of both increased protein metabolism related to insulin deficiency and decreased glomerular filtration in dehydration.

The person with diabetic acidosis or impending acidosis is hospitalized immediately. If the client is found unconscious by strangers, he may be confused with an alcoholic because of the usual odor to the breath. He should carry identification that indicates he is a diabetic so that he can be managed properly.

Diabetic ketoacidosis is a medical emergency, and the client is usually admitted to an intensive care setting where monitoring facilities are available. Here medical and nursing care is directed toward correcting metabolism and maintaining fluid and electrolyte balance. The goals of nursing care are directed to (1) reducing hyperglycemia, (2) restoring fluid and electrolyte balance, (3) managing dehydration, and (4) reestablishing consciousness. Insulin is administered to lower plasma glucose. Rapid-acting insulin may be given intravenously, intramuscularly, or subcutaneously in amounts sufficient to cause a continuous drop in plasma glucose. Protocols for insulin administration vary. One author prefers a loading dose of 20 units of insulin given intramuscularly or subcutaneously followed by a continuous infusion of 4 to 8 units of insulin, or hourly intramuscular injections of 5 to 10 units of insulin, or hourly subcutaneous injections of 10 to 100 units of insulin.[18]

Those who favor a continuous intravenous infusion of small doses of insulin believe that smaller doses prevent the adverse effects of hypoglycemia, hypokalemia, and cerebral edema caused by rapid drops in serum glucose. To administer insulin in a continuous drip, 200 units of U100 regular insulin is added to 200 ml of 0.9% normal saline and 0.5 g of salt-poor human albumin (to prevent absorption of insulin on glass or plastic tubing) to provide 1 unit/1 ml. Six to ten units of this infusion is given per hour along with an infusion of normal saline. An infusion pump should be used to control infusion rates. When the serum glucose value reaches 250 mg/100 ml, the insulin is stopped, and D_5W is infused at 100 ml/hour.

When insulin is administered, the lowering of the glucose can activate release of other hormones for glycogenolysis and gluconeogenesis such as catecholamines and cortisol, and cause a rebound hyperglycemia known as *Somogyi phenomenon*. This phenomenon often occurs with ketoacidosis and is evidenced by wide fluctuations of plasma glucose concentrations. Insulin doses are reduced and adjusted as necessary to prevent recurring rebound hyperglycemia.

The nurse can evaluate the effect of insulin on lowering serum glucose by monitoring serum glucose levels and clinical indications as the client regains consciousness. When the client is conscious and taking oral fluids, insulin may be administered by subcutaneous routes.

Restoring fluid and electrolyte balance. Electrolyte solutions are given to correct acidosis and electrolyte depletion. Sodium bicarbonate, sodium chloride, and potassium chloride may be used in intravenous solutions. Potassium may not be administered initially, because clients who are dehydrated may have hyperkalemia because of shifts of potassium to extracellular fluid. As dehydration is corrected and potassium returns to intracellular compartments, hypokalemia occurs and can then be treated. The nurse must carefully evaluate potassium shifts and monitor the ECG for effects of potassium on cardiac function.

Managing dehydration. Rehydration is accomplished with isotonic saline. If the client is in shock, plasma expanders can be used. Fluids may be given at a rate of 1 L/hour for adults without cardiac disease, and the nurse must monitor the client for signs of fluid overload and measure hourly urine output. Clients with severe dehydration have dry skin and mucous membranes, and the nurse can use lotions and lubricants to prevent skin breakdown. Thermal regulation of the environment is important to keep the client warm and prevent loss of body heat. Sponge baths may be used for the client with fever and diaphoresis.

Reestablishing consciousness. Clients with diabetic coma are unconscious until metabolic pathways are restored. During this time the nurse should ensure an open airway and prevent hazards of unconsciousness.

Recovery from ketoacidosis is usually favorable, particularly if treated in incipient stages. When the client is responsive, he may be able to recognize the cause of the ketoacidosis, and the nurse may use this opportunity for instruction about compliance with the therapeutic plan and make plans to prevent recurrence.

Hyperglycemic, hyperosmolar, nonketotic coma (HHNK). Hyperosmolar coma is a state of dehydration that can occur in ketosis-resistant diabetic clients, as well as from other causes. Generally the clients are over age 60 and may have an accompanying illness that precipitates hyperglycemia and polyuria. There is reduced glomerular filtration, loss of sodium and water, and ultimately dehydration, particularly of cerebral cells. Polydipsia, polyuria, poor skin turgor, soft eyeballs, seizures, and unconsciousness are clinical indicators. Hyperosmolar coma occurs slowly over a period of time and, unfortunately, may be difficult to recognize.

Intervention is directed at restoring fluid loss. Intravenous infusions of 0.45% saline are given, and small doses of insulin are used to lower blood glucose levels. Potassium is given to reverse hypokalemia. The prognosis is more favorable when the condition is detected early and water replacement is instituted rapidly.

Lactic acidosis. Lactic acidosis is an infrequent complication of diabetes mellitus, which is caused by the production and retention of excessive lactic acid. This state can occur in nondiabetic clients as well. Lactic acidosis usually occurs in instances of tissue hypoxia, and in diabetic clients is believed to be caused by both tissue hypoxia and the inability to convert lactate to pyruvate. There is no hyperglycemia or ketosis. Intervention involves reducing tissue hypoxia and administering sodium bicarbonate to alkalinize the lactic acid. Nursing care should be planned to support the client's adjustment to these metabolic changes.

Concomitant health problems associated with diabetes mellitus. The individual with diabetes mellitus must not only follow a therapeutic plan to maintain metabolic stability but must also cope with the concomitant cardiovascular problems. These cardiovascular changes are believed to occur as the result of thickening of the basement membrane and cause large vessel disease (atherosclerosis) and small vessel disease (arteriosclerosis, microangiopathy). Infection, retinopathy, neuropathy, nephropathy, and increased mortality from ischemic heart diseases are the ultimate consequences of basement membrane thickening.

Controversy as to the relationship of vascular manifestations of diabetes and the degree of therapeutic management is unresolved. It is noted, however, that the vascular changes are related to the age of onset and the duration of the disease, with early onset and increasing duration adversely affecting the client's maintenance of wellness.

Because these changes are likely to occur, the nurse should instruct the client about observing health habits that will minimize vascular impairment.

The client should be instructed about preventing infection and recognizing changes in vision, the peripheral nervous system, and kidney function. Finally, stress states of pregnancy and surgery temporarily alter the diabetic client's therapeutic plan, and certain modifications may be required.

Infections. Clients with diabetes are prone to infection, particularly in distal areas where circulation is poorest. Infection is also a hazard for such individuals because phagocytosis occurs more slowly in diabetic clients and because insulin deficiency is believed to impair granulocyte, lymphocyte, and leukocyte function. Promotion of circulation and prevention of infection are imperative, and the nurse and client must incorporate aspects of hygiene in the daily care plan.

Circulation is promoted by avoiding any constriction of blood vessels as may be caused by round garters, girdles, panty girdles, or tight belts. Prevention of skin infections, particularly in the feet where circulation is the poorest, is also important. The client should take a bath daily and soak his feet (see foot care, at left). The water for a bath or foot soaks should be 95° F (35° C) so that the skin is not burned. After a bath, the feet should be dried carefully, with special attention to the spaces between the toes. Lanolin may be rubbed into dry skin to prevent it from cracking. Nails should be cut straight across to prevent ingrown toenails; a podiatrist may be needed to cut the toenails safely. The client should not attempt to remove corns or calloses or to treat any sores on the feet with irritating medicines. The client should wear clean, white cotton socks to absorb perspiration, and his shoes should fit well. Irritations from rubbing by shoes or slippers that do not fit well cause skin breakdown rapidly in diabetics. This attention to the feet should be given to all diabetics daily. The nurse in the hospital or extended care facility or on a home visit should observe that the client carries out these measures.

Skin infections present a serious threat to health. Gangrene can develop rapidly in an anaerobic environment caused by atherosclerosis. Amputation of the involved part is too often required to inhibit spread of the infection. Prevention of these problems by attention to skin care is preferable.

Attention to feminine hygiene is important in diabetic girls and women, because certain microorganisms thrive on the sugar spilled in the urine. The nurse should instruct the client in measures of feminine cleanliness and suggest she wear cotton underwear to absorb perspiration.

Retinopathy. Retinopathy is a common concomitant of diabetes and is now the leading cause of acquired blindness in adults. There are capillary microaneurysms, and the blood vessels supplying the eye become sclerosed, causing refractive errors, paresis of eye muscles, cataracts, retinal detachment, and ultimately blindness. Therapeutic intervention such as photocoagulation may be used to control the bleeding and resultant retinal detachment.

The client with diabetes is encouraged to have yearly examinations by an ophthalmologist. Glasses are often needed, and changes in the prescription are made frequently.

Neuropathy. Peripheral neuropathy is described by some researchers as being a part of vascular changes causing diminished blood supply to the nerves. Others cite demyelination of nerve sheaths as the basis of neurological changes. In either instance, the client may have numbness and tingling, pain, or paresthesia in the lower extremities. There may be diminished reflexes and reduction in the vibratory senses.

INSTRUCTIONS FOR FOOT CARE

1. Promotion of circulation
   a. Avoid constricting clothing such as girdles, panty girdles, round garters, garters, or tight belts.
   b. Avoid tight-fitting stockings.
   c. Exercise daily.
   d. Massage feet.
2. Daily foot care
   a. Inspect all surfaces for redness, cracking, or infection.
   b. Wash feet daily. Use water at 95° F (35° C); test with bath thermometer. Dry thoroughly and gently.
   c. Apply lanolin to dry areas; *powder between toes* if moist.
   d. Cut toenails straight across. Do not file nails.
   e. Do not use medications on corns or infections.
   f. See a podiatrist for removal of corns, calloses, or blisters.
3. Footwear
   a. Do not go barefoot.
   b. Use clean, white cotton socks; change daily.
   c. Wear properly fitting shoes; alternate pairs daily.
   d. Wear properly fitting, supportive bedroom slippers.

Nursing process for common health problems

The client should be cautioned to be aware of and avoid extremes of heat and cold. The client should also inspect his extremities for injuries, because he may not feel bruises or infections that may be developing.

Damage to the parasympathetic nerves may produce impotence in diabetic men. This disruption to sexual role satisfaction is believed to occur in as many as one half of diabetic men. The impotence may be transitory if the diabetes is out of control, but many well-controlled diabetic men also are impotent. Diabetic juveniles are often sterile. Impotence tends to be permanent, although testosterone may be used to treat impotence. Others may consider implantation of a silicone prosthesis. Some may find that a rubber band used at the base of the penis preserves erection long enough for intromission and intercourse. In any instance, support from the partner is essential to adapting to changes in sexual role satisfaction.

Parasympathetic neuropathy in women may be manifested by interference with orgasm and lack of orgasmic response. Although most women remain fertile in childbearing years, there is increased incidence of stillbirths, spontaneous abortions, and delivery of large babies of diabetic women.

Nephropathy. Decreased blood supply to the kidney produces a syndrome known as Kimmelstiel-Wilson syndrome. There is intracapillary glomerulosclerosis, with resultant renal failure. The client is encouraged to report any dysuria or pyuria. Bladder infections may be more common in diabetic clients perhaps the result of increased protein and glucose in the urine, causing favorable media for bacterial growth, or nerve damage, causing incomplete emptying of the bladder. Bladder infections may cause *pneumaturia,* a bubbly urine caused by a hydrogen gas produced by the action of bacteria on glucose.

Diabetes and pregnancy: the high-risk mother and neonate. Pregnancy places increased demands for carbohydrate metabolism, and the woman with diabetes is presented with certain problems of managing her diabetes during the pregnancy. Changes in activity, diet, and drug therapy are necessitated by the additional stress of the pregnancy.

Diet modifications are made to accommodate fetal nutritional needs. Insulin requirements generally decrease during the first trimester of pregnancy, and if the woman is using oral hypoglycemic agents or insulin, the medication is adjusted accordingly. In the second and third trimesters, insulin requirements increase to one and one-half times the usual requirements. Some suggest using two doses of intermediate-acting insulin and increasing to four doses during the third trimester. Insulin needs then are reduced during the postnatal period. Induction of labor may be suggested by some physicians so that therapeutic plans can be more carefully controlled and neonatal complications averted.

Diabetic women have increased risks of having premature births and neonates with hypocalcemia, hyperbilirubinemia, respiratory distress syndrome, and various congenital anomalies. These risks should be explained to each couple before conception is planned.

Since offspring of diabetic mothers are at risk, special facilities should be available for monitoring the neonate after birth. The main concern after delivery is change in fetal glucose utilization. It is believed that maternal hyperglycemia causes fetal hyperglycemia, with increased production of insulin and storage of maternal glucose in the fetal liver during gestation. This may account for the large polyhydramic babies at birth. After delivery, maternal sources of glucose are removed, yet the neonate's insulin production remains high. The rapid decrease of blood glucose causes brain damage and even death if not reversed immediately.

Serum glucose assessments must be made immediately after birth and on a frequent basis for this high-risk neonate. Epinephrine may be used to decrease insulin reserves, and 10% dextrose may be given intravenously to maintain adequate blood glucose levels. Fluid and electrolyte needs must also be monitored and adjusted as necessary. Anticipating these consequences and maintaining adequate nutrition serve to avoid crises situations during this critical period.

Diabetes and surgery. Individuals with diabetes mellitus who undergo surgical interventions require special management to maintain insulin and glucose balances. Alterations in nutritional needs are incurred by changes in activity and the withholding of food as well as the emotional stress, surgical trauma, and metabolic changes during wound healing. Consequently, it is advisable for the surgery to be scheduled early in the day.

Therapeutic intervention before and immediately after surgery depends on the severity of the diabetes and the extent of surgery. Nutritional requirements are usually met by D_5W or $D_{10}W$ and supplementary insulin. Frequent determinations of blood glucose levels guide insulin administration. Insulin requirements decrease as surgical stress is minimized, and most clients resume their previous therapeutic plan in 4 to 7 days after surgery.

Discharge instructions and continuity of care. Instruction about the therapeutic plan should be incorporated into the life-style of the individual client. Ultimately, he is responsible for his own care, and the nurse should help the client and his family anticipate these needs.

Children under age 5 can take little responsibility for managing their diet or medications and require close supervision from their parents. When the child enters school, the teacher and school nurse should be informed of the child's needs because they will be responsible for his care during school hours. The teacher should learn the indications of impending insulin reaction or acidosis and what to do for the child. If food is served at school, the teacher should also know what foods the child can eat. In spite of limitations, the nurse and teacher should plan to create a normal, healthy environment for classroom participation.

While the older school-age child is assuming independence in other areas of his life, he should be permitted more responsibility for coping with his diabetes. He may be able to give his own insulin and select appropriate foods for his diet. The parents, however, should continue to provide supervision in these areas. Many communities have summer camps for diabetic children, and the school-age child may enjoy such an experience. Sharing common experiences with peers in a supervised environment contributes to maturity.

Full responsibility for the therapeutic plan can be managed by the adolescent. Fluctuations from independence to dependence—a normal adolescent behavior—as well as rapid physical changes make control of diabetes difficult. Parents should help their adolescent cope with these changes and not punish him for lapses in control.

Type 2 diabetes is usually not evident until middle or late adulthood, and the adjustments in life-style that need to be made may be difficult for one who has had no limitations on his activity or diet. The nurse can assist these clients by encouraging them to decide which aspects of their lives are similar to the therapeutic plan and will be possible to follow.

Elderly clients may have added difficulties because of partial or total blindness, and the nurse should seek teaching aids and equipment that will make assuming responsibility for the therapeutic plan easier. Special syringes can be obtained for individuals who have vision problems. Some syringes have preset trigger devices, or the client may be able to place a tape on the syringe to indicate the point to which the insulin should be drawn. Economic factors and concurrent crippling diseases such as stroke, arthritis, or Parkinson's disease may complicate insulin injection. The nurse should plan with these clients for alternatives and resources for obtaining assistance as needed.

It is important that the client with diabetes have continuity of health care. The community health nurse should be contacted before a new diabetic client is dismissed from the hospital to assist with adaptations of the therapeutic plan at home. Often, clients have questions at this time, when they are fully responsible for their own care. The client may be making return visits to a hospital, clinic, or community health center. Communication is essential to ensure continuity of care. The nurse in the school, industry, or nursing home where the client spends much of his time should be aware of the client's needs. Teaching, adaptations of diet, and medications may be necessary to adjust to these activities. The persons with whom the client works should be aware of his diabetes so that they can observe him and know what to do for insulin shock or acidosis.

Diabetes is a chronic health problem that requires changes in the diabetic's life-style. The nurse can be understanding while supporting the client in his adjustment to therapy and help him comply with the therapeutic plan.

 Evaluation. The evaluation component of the nursing process is continuous as the client learns about his health problem and meets objectives for changes in attitude, knowledge, and skills. The nursing care plan is unique for each client and depends on his stage of growth and development.

EXPECTED OUTCOMES

The client and/or family can:
1. Describe diabetes mellitus.
2. State plans for the following therapeutic plan:
    a. Diet (exchange list or weighed diet).
    b. Exercise (daily exercise in moderation).
    c. Medication (insulin, oral hypoglycemic agents): state use, time, dosage, route, and side effects; demonstrate insulin injection technique.
3. Demonstrate ability to monitor glycemia and ketonemia with urinalysis and/or blood analysis.
4. Describe indications of hypoglycemia or impending diabetic ketoacidosis.
5. State plans for health maintenance:
    a. Skin care and foot care.
    b. Activity and rest.
    c. Stress management.
    d. Prevention of infection.
6. Modify the therapeutic plan for age and developmental stage.
7. State indications requiring immediate health care services. Carry identification card or wear identification.
8. State plans for follow-up care and know of community resources for individuals with diabetes mellitus.

Evaluation

Evaluation, the final stage of the nursing process, encourages the nurse and client to make judgments about goal achievement relative to plans for health promotion, maintenance, and restoration for common health problems of the endocrine system. Nursing problems often include ineffective coping, fear, disturbance in self-concept, sleep pattern disturbance, fluid volume deficit, potential for injury, knowledge deficit, alterations in cardiac output, alterations in nutrition, potential impairment of skin integrity, noncompliance, alterations in comfort, alterations in thought processes, and alterations in urinary elimination.

EXPECTED OUTCOMES

The client and/or family can:
1. Recognize the impact the health problem has on various body systems and self-concept.
2. State plans for health maintenance, including balance of activity and rest.
3. State plans for health restoration, including use of medications, diet, and activity restrictions.
4. State indications for health care and/or plans for follow-up care and use of community resources.
5. Use appropriate coping resources.
6. State use, dosage, time, route, and side effects of prescribed medications (for example, replacement therapy).
7. Explain the necessary modifications for dietary intake.
8. Explain ways of altering life-style.

Summary

The care of clients with problems of the endocrine system is based on a thorough knowledge of physiology and pathophysiological conditions affecting the endocrine system. The nursing process commences with the acquisition of data from a number of modes, including the nursing history, which includes data about the client's health, development, social, and psychological states. The physical assessment skills useful in obtaining additional data are *inspection* and *palpation*. A variety of diagnostic tests, specific to the seven glands of the endocrine system, may be performed, including tests for hematological, radiological, metabolic, reflex, and urinary studies. Once the data are obtained from the varied sources, they are analyzed and used in formulating care for clients with problems of the endocrine system.

Health problems that affect the endocrine system, for the most part, may occur any time across the life span. Some of these problems include hypopituitarism (dwarfism, hypogonadism), hyperpituitarism (gigantism, acromegaly), pituitary tumor, pituitary apoplexy, hypothyroidism (cretinism, myxedema), hyperthyroidism (Graves' disease, thyroid storm, goiters, neoplasms, thyroiditis), and hyperparathyroidism (primary and secondary). Common problems of the adrenal gland include hypofunction (primary adrenocortical insufficiency, secondary adrenocortical insufficiency, adrenal crisis), hyperfunction (Cushing's syndrome, aldosteronism—primary and secondary), adrenogenital syndrome, and adrenal medulla problems of which the most common is pheochromocytoma. Diabetes mellitus is another common health problem.

As care is planned and implemented, the process of evaluation is continually used.

355

References

1. Askew, Gail, and Letcher, Kenneth: Oral hypoglycemic agents, Nursing 75 **5**(8):45-50, 1975.
2. Bacon, George E., Spencer, Martha L., and Kelch, Robert P.: Pediatric Endocrinology, Chicago, 1975, Year Book Medical Publishers, Inc.
3. Bernstein, Richard: Blood glucose self-monitoring by diabetic patients: refinements of a procedural technique, Diabetes Care **2**(2):233-236, 1979.
4. Brown, Burnell R. Jr.: Anesthesia on pheochromocytoma. In Brown, Burnell R. Jr., editor: Anesthesia and the patient with endocrine disease, Philadelphia, 1980, F.A. Davis Co.
5. Cope, Oliver: The thyroid glands. In Committee on Pre and Postoperative Care, American College of Surgeons: Manual of preoperative and postoperative care, ed. 2, Philadelphia, 1971, W.B. Saunders Co., pp. 456-480.
6. Crouch, Mary, and others: Reuse of disposable syringe—Needle Units in the Diabetic Patient, Diabetes Care **2**(5):418-420, 1979.
7. Dingman, Joseph F., and Thorn George W.: Diseases of the neurohypophysis. In Harrison's Principles of internal medicine, ed. 9, New York, 1980, McGraw-Hill Book Co.
8. Ezrin, Calvin, Godden, John O., and Volpe, Robert: Systematic endocrinology, ed. 2, Hagerstown, Md., 1979, Harper & Row, Publishers.
9. Galloway, John: Insulin treatment for the early 80s: facts and questions about old and new insulins and their usage, Diabetes Care **3**(5):615-622, 1980.
10. Gellis, Sydney, and Kagan, Benjamin M.: Current pediatric therapy, Philadelphia, 1978, W.B. Saunders Co.
11. Gröer, Maureen, and Shekelton, Maurine E.: Basic pathophysiology: a conceptual approach, St. Louis, 1979, The C.V. Mosby Co.
12. Hershman, Jerome M.: Endocrine pathophysiology: a patient-oriented approach, Philadelphia, 1977, Lea & Febiger.
13. Hoffman, Jeanette T. T., and Newby, Thelma B.: Hypercalcemia in primary hyperparathyroidism, Nurs. Clin. North Am. **15**:469-480, Sept. 1980.
14. Hung, Wellington, August, Gilbert P., and Glasgow, Allen M.: Pediatric Endocrinology, New York, 1978, Medical Examination Publishing Co., Inc.
15. Ingbar, Sidney H., and Woeber, Kenneth A.: Diseases of the thyroid. In Harrison's Principles of internal medicine, ed. 9, New York, 1980, McGraw-Hill Book Co.
16. Keyston, Leonard: Endocrinology and diabetes, New York, 1975, Grune & Stratton.
17. Krueger, Judith A., and Ray, Janis C.: Endocrine problems in nursing: a physiologic approach, St. Louis, 1976, The C.V. Mosby Co., p. 70.
18. Kymer, Joseph: Diabetic ketoacidosis, Crit. Care Q. **3**(2):65-75, 1980.
19. Lundin, Dorothy: Reporting urine test results: switch from + to %, Am. J. Nurs. **78**(5):878-879, 1978.
20. Melby, James C.: Diseases of the pituitary gland. In Keefer, Chester S., and Wilkins, Robert W.: Essentials of clinical practice, Boston, 1970, Little, Brown Co.
21. Montgomery, Desmond A.D.: Medical and surgical endocrinology, Baltimore, 1975, The Williams & Wilkins Co.
22. Nelson, Don H.: Diseases of the anterior lobe of the pituitary gland. In Harrison's Principles of internal medicine, ed. 9, New York, 1980, McGraw-Hill Book Co.
23. O'Connor, Michael: Glucose tolerance test: how you can make it reliable, Nursing '75 **75**:10-11, July 1975.
24. Rimoin, David L., and Schimke, R. Neil: Genetic disorders of the endocrine glands, St. Louis, 1971, The C.V. Mosby Co.
25. Ryan, Will G.: Endocrine disorders: a pathophysiologic approach, ed. 2, Chicago, 1980, Year Book Medical Publishers, Inc.
26. Sanford, Sarah J.: Dysfunction of the adrenal gland: physiologic considerations and nursing problems, Nurs. Clin. North Am. **15**:481-498, September 1980.
27. Schneeberg, Norman G.: Essentials of clinical endocrinology, St. Louis, 1970, The C.V. Mosby Co.
28. Schteingart, David E.: Endocrinology and metabolism. In Price, Sylvia, and Wilson, Lorraine: Pathophysiology, New York, 1978, McGraw-Hill Book Co.
29. Sherwin, Robert, and others: Treatment of juvenile-onset diabetes by subcutaneous infusion of insulin with a portable pump, Diabetes Care **3**(2):301-305, 1980.
30. Shuman, Charles: The new diabetic, An American Family Physician Monograph, April 1979.
31. Spencer, Roberta T.: Patient care in endocrine problems, Philadelphia, 1973, W.B. Saunders Co.
32. The fine points of insulin injection, Emerg. Med. **12**(11):143, June 15, 1980.
33. Waife, S.O., editor: Diabetes mellitus, ed. 8, Indianapolis, 1980, Lilly Research Laboratories.
34. Wake, Madeline M., and Brensinger, John F.: The nurse's role in hypothyroidism, Nurs. Clin. North Am. **15**:453-467, Sept. 1980.
35. Williams, Gordon H., Dluhy, Robert G., and Thorn, George W.: Disease of the adrenal cortex. In Harrison's Principles of internal medicine, ed. 9, New York, 1980, McGraw-Hill.

Additional readings

Coates, Florence, and Fabrykart, Maximillian: An injection technique for preventing skin reactions, Am. J. Nurs. **65**(2):127-128, 1965.

Controlling diabetes mellitus, programmed instruction, Am. J. Nurs. **80**(10):1827-1850, 1980.

Daniel, William A.: Adolescents in health and disease, St. Louis, 1977, The C.V. Mosby Co.

Eliopoulos, Charlotte: Diagnosis and management of diabetes in the elderly, Am. J. Nurs. **78**(5): 884-887, 1978.

Fletcher, H. Patrick: The oral antidiabetic drugs: pro and con, Am. J. Nurs. **76**(04):596-599, 1976.

Fonville, Ann: Teaching patients to rotate injection sites, Am. J. Nurs. **78**(5):880-883, May 1978.

Garofano, Catherine: Deliver facts to help diabetics plan parenthood, Nursing 77 **7**(4):13-16, 1977.

Garofano, Catherine: Travel tips for the peripatetic diabetic, Nursing 77 **7**(8):44-46, 1977.

Gotch, Pamela M.: Teaching patients about adrenal corticosteroids, Am. J. Nurs. **81**:78-81, Jan. 1981.

Guthrie, Diana: Exercise, diets and insulin for children with diabetes, Nursing 77 **7**(2):48-54, 1977.

Guthrie, Diana, and Guthrie, Richard: DKA, breaking a vicious cycle, Nursing 78 **8**(6):55-61, 1978.

Hayter, Jean: Fine points in diabetic care, Am. J. Nurs. **76**(4):594-599, 1976.

Hershman, Jerome M.: Management of endocrine disorders, Philadelphia, 1980, Lea & Febiger.

Hickler, Roger B., and Thorn, George W.: Pheochromocytoma. In Harrison's Principles of internal medicine, ed. 9, New York, 1980, McGraw-Hill Book Co.

Kaufmann, Susan: In diabetic diets, Realism acts results, Nursing 76 **6**(11):75-77, 1976.

Krugman, Saul, and Ward, Robert: Infectious diseases of children and adults, St. Louis, 1973, The C.V. Mosby Co.

McConnell, Edwina: Meeting the special needs of diabetics facing surgery, Nursing 76 **76**(6):30-37, 1976.

McFarlane, Judith, and Hames, Carolyn C.: Children with diabetes: learning self-care in camp, Am. J. Nurs. **73**(8):1362-1365, 1973.

Petrdik, Joan C.: Diabetic peripheral neuropathy, Am. J. Nurs. **76**(11):1794-1797, 1976.

Petrokas, Judith: Common sense guidelines for controlling diabetes during illness, Nursing 77 **7**(12):37-38, 1977.

Schulz, Joyce, and Williams, Marie: Encouragement breeds independence in the blind diabetic, Nursing 76 **6**(12):19-20, 1976.

Schumann, Delores: Assessing the diabetic, Nursing 76 **6**(3):62-67, 1976.

Skillman, Thomas: Diabetic ketoacidosis, Heart Lung **7**(4):594-602, 1978.

Slater, Norma: Insulin reactions vs. ketoacidosis: guidelines for diagnosis and intervention, Am. J. Nurs. **78**(5):875-877, 1978.

Solomon, Barbara L.: The hypothalamus and the pituitary gland: an overview, Nurs. Clin. North Am. **15**:435-451, Sept. 1980.

Thomas, Katherine P.: Diabetes mellitus in elderly persons, Nurs. Clin. North Am. **11**:157-168, 1976.

VanPoole, Mary: Penile prosthesis in impotence AORN J. **22**(2):207-209, Aug. 1975.

Walesky, Mary: Diabetic ketoacidosis, Am. J. Nurs. **78**(5):872-874, 1978.

Wolfe, Lawrence: Insulin: paving the way to a new life, Nursing 77 **7**(11):38-41, 1977.

NURSING PROCESS

for clients with common health problems of the

10 Neurological system

Assessment

Data analysis

Planning

Implementation

Evaluation

The brain, spinal cord, and a complex peripheral nervous system are responsible for a client's ability to relate to his world. Although birth injuries and congenital anomalies account for some dysfunctions, a far greater problem is created by trauma and infections. Accidents related to sports and motor vehicles comprise the overwhelming number of serious injuries to the brain and spinal cord. These are common among adolescents and young adults, in particular. Later in life, cerebrovascular pathological conditions and degenerative phenomena may alter central nervous system activity and lead to motor and sensory deficits, which alter the client's ability to relate both physically and mentally to his environment.

The purpose of this chapter is to present information about assessment modes for the nervous system and parameters for nursing care planning, implementation, and evaluation. Particular emphasis is given to the unconscious client, or one who is paralyzed as the result of trauma or other causes, because nursing care in these instances is indeed complex, involving physical, social, and psychological factors.

Overview of the nervous system

The brain, the spinal cord, and a complex peripheral nervous system are responsible for a client's relating to his world. Although there is considerable protection of the delicate neural structures by bone and fluid barriers, they are subject to the adverse effects of congenital anomalies, inflammatory processes, mechanical and physical disturbances, and degenerative disease. Factors that interfere with the normal functioning of the human nervous system may directly impair the brain or spinal cord or may alter the structures that support, protect, and nourish neural tissue.

The nervous system has two distinct divisions: the sensory and the motor. The latter is perhaps the more important, because it influences all the functions and activities of the body. It is estimated that less than 1% of sensory information is actually used in a specific motor response; the remainder is discarded after intricate processing or stored for future use as memory. For practical purposes, the central nervous system can be considered to have three levels of functioning: (1) the spinal cord, which governs automatic motor responses and reflexes; (2) the lower brain, which controls subconscious responses and vital processes; and (3) the higher brain, which is a vast storage area where memories and reaction patterns reside for recall at will. These three levels are interrelated and interdependent, and factors that interfere with any portion have some effect on others.

The central nervous system comprises the brain and spinal cord. The brain has several divisions.

BRAIN

The largest portion of the brain (seven eighths of the total weight) is the cerebrum. The cortex is the most sophisticated part (Fig. 10-1). The white matter that lies below the cortex has several important tracts of nervous tissue. The cerebrum is divided by the falx cerebri into two hemispheres. The corpus callosum links the two hemispheres, which are largely responsible for motor activity of the contralateral half of the body. Most individuals possess a dominant hemisphere through trained associations over an extended period of time. The cerebral hemispheres are each divided into four lobes named for the overlying bony portions of the skull: the *frontal, parietal, temporal* and *occipital*.

The *diencephalon* is located in the forebrain and is made up of the *thalamus* and *hypothalamus*. The thalamus is a sensory relay center, integrating sensory impulses except for olfaction. Because of the unique anatomical location, it is capable of facilitating or inhibiting motor impulses from the cerebral cortex. Furthermore, it has a certain role in integrating emotional behavior. The thalamus contains the pineal gland in its dorsomedial section. Any malfunction of the thalamus affects the interface of sensory cord pathways and the brainstem with the cerebral cortex.

The hypothalamus regulates renal water flow, body temperature, and certain endocrine and metabolic processes. It, along with the reticular activating systems of the brainstem and thalamus, plays an important role in the state of arousal and also influences the emotions in subtle ways.

The *midbrain* has a critical role in motor coordination and postural reflex patterns. The superior section controls conjugate eye movements and the upward gaze.

The *hindbrain* consists of the cerebellum, pons, medulla oblongata, and

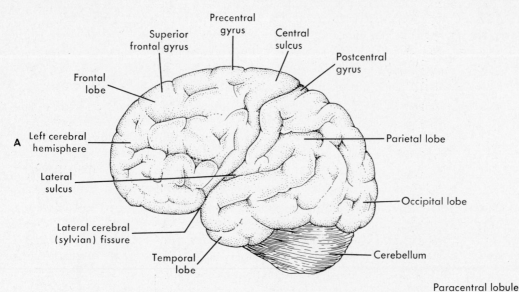

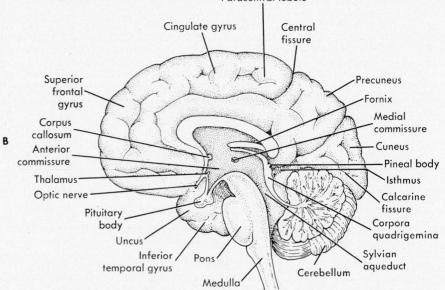

FIG. 10-1
Cerebral cortex: **A,** lateral view; **B,** medial view. (From Budassi, S.A., and Barber, J.M.: Emergency nursing: principals and practice, St. Louis, 1981, The C.V. Mosby Co.)

Fundamental physiological concepts

the reticular formations. The cerebellum controls equilibrium, the integration of voluntary movement, posture, and sense of position. The *pons* functions as a relay station from the medulla to higher centers as well as being a mechanical bridge and a base for the nuclei of cranial nerves. The *medulla oblongata* is continuous with the pons and the spinal cord and possesses a representation of all afferent and efferent tracts of the cord. In addition to controlling certain reflex actions, it also is the regulatory center for cardiac, respiratory, and vasomotor mechanisms.

Reticular formations are interrelated neurons that modify reflex activity of spinal neurons. The formations are sometimes called the *reticular activating system* (RAS), because this is thought to be the center of wakefulness. Severe injury to reticular formations will usually result in unconsciousness.

The brain requires an estimated 15% to 20% of the total circulating blood at all times in order to ensure proper functioning. Any factor that alters blood supply to any cerebral area will affect the functional activity of that area. Other consequences in addition to hypoxia or anoxia stem from metabolic disturbances such as hypoglycemia.

Glucose metabolism supplies most of the energy required for brain tissue. Since this tissue has only minute capabilities for storing glucose, there must be a constant supply of circulating blood to deliver this nutrient, along with the vital element, oxygen. A temporary disturbance in blood supply of even 4 to 6 minutes can result in cellular dysfunction and impairment. It is interesting to note that the brain consumes about 65% of the body's glucose on a daily basis. A failure of this supply can induce neuron failure, seizures, unconsciousness, and death.

Blood vessels within the brain dilate and constrict in response to alterations in pH, $Paco_2$, and Pao_2. Acidosis causes vasodilation; alkalosis causes vasoconstriction. Therapy to reduce intracranial hypertension is therefore largely influenced by respiratory responses. Thus mechanical ventilation becomes a significant factor in controlling brain edema.

The brain and spinal cord are constantly bathed in about 120 ml of cerebrospinal fluid, which is produced, circulated, and reabsorbed on a dynamic basis. Intracranial pressure is largely controlled by changes in this fluid volume.

A *blood-brain barrier* prevents certain substances from passing between the blood and CSF. Water, glucose, and blood gases move freely, for example, but certain steroids, catecholamines, and antibiotics do not. Much therapy is specifically controlled by the selectivity of this anatomical barrier.

A working knowledge of these basic physiological concepts helps the nurse understand the clinical management of many central nervous system problems.

SPINE

The spinal cord integrates the lower portions of the body with the brain and mediates sensation, reflexes, and motor responses to distal parts. If interferences occur at any level of the cord, the functions below the level of injury are damaged. There may or may not be pain at the level of injury.

If the interference is at the cervical spinal level, *quadriplegia* (tetraplegia) may ensue. Because the phrenic nerve arises in the cervical plexus, the diaphragm and respiratory muscles are potentially affected, and breathing may be dysfunctional. A tracheostomy or ventilatory support may be required. If the damage is at the thoracic or lumbar level, there is full use of the upper extremities and no damage to breathing mechanisms; however, the lower extremities and processes of elimination will be impaired. This paralysis of the lower extremities is called *paraplegia*.

Diagnosis of the nature and level of the injury is confirmed by radiography and information gleaned during the history taking and physical examination. Determination of CSF circulatory patterns also lends invaluable diagnostic assistance.

Motor activity is achieved and regulated by five levels of central nervous system functioning: spinomuscular, extrapyramidal, pyramidal (or corticospinal), cerebellar, and psychomotor.

Spinomuscular level

The motor impulses originate in the anterior horn cells of the spinal cord and in the motor nuclei of the brainstem and are transmitted to individual muscles via the myoneural junctions. The anterior horn cell is the final common pathway through which all nervous impulses from higher centers must pass to reach the myoneural junction and influence striated muscle.[6] Pathological conditions re-

Nursing process for common health problems

lated to the anterior horn cells include those entitites that create dysfunction of the neuraxis, the myoneural junction, or the muscle itself. The major characteristic of each is the *loss of motor power* in muscles or groups of muscles supplied by the involved cells or nerves. There is complete paralysis of muscle fibers no longer being stimulated. Voluntary contraction in response to stimulation is lost, and there is weakness in all movements in which the affected muscle is involved. There is a flaccidity (hypotonicity), or loss of tone, in the muscles. If the motor neurons are actually destroyed, atrophy will ensue. Up to 70% or 80% of the original muscle mass may be lost within 3 months, and connective tissue overgrowth replaces the degenerated fibers.[6] Contractions and deformities may be caused by contraction of antagonists whose action is no longer opposed by paralyzed muscles or by atrophy and fibrosis of affected muscles. Electromyographical data demonstrate fibrillations (fine, rapid contractions) that cannot be seen by the naked eye. Some diseases of the motor neuron (such as progressive muscle atrophy) may create fasciculations (spontaneous twitching movements) that can actually be seen and palpated through intact skin. Electrical testing is useful, therefore, to detect degenerative changes before they become obvious. Degeneration usually is evident within 2 weeks after the lesion has been present.[6] Biopsy and chemical assessments of muscle mass will also show histological and biochemical alterations characteristic of degenerative processes. Reflexes in the areas involved will be diminished or absent, but pathological reflexes or abnormal movements will not be found. Vasomotor changes may be detected, and skin, hair, nails, and bones may manifest trophic changes. There will be no sensory changes if the lesion is truly limited to the motor units.[6]

Extrapyramidal level

The extrapyramidal level is a conceptual framework for motor activity, not an anatomical or physiological entity. The existence has been validated chiefly by clinical data of pathological conditions, which are characterized by disturbance of tone, movement, and/or posture. The major nuclear centers of the extrapyramidal level are in the basal ganglia, but there are other closely linked structures of the brainstem concerned with motor integration. Of particular importance are the midbrain and vestibular components essential to regulation of muscle tone, postural and righting reflexes, and facilitation or inhibition of motor responses. The cerebral cortex also must be considered as it relates to motor control. The extrapyramidal level is not an independent neural system or mechanism; it is a group of neural organizations that are not directly concerned with the production of voluntary movements but are closely linked to other levels of the motor system to achieve control of muscular activity.

Pyramidal or corticospinal level

The pyramidal level is one of the several motor fiber systems that converges on the anterior horn cells and hence is only one of the upper motor neuron levels. Its origin is in the motor nuclei of the cerebral cortex. This pyramidal level never functions independently but is closely tied to other mechanisms of motor activity and to incoming sensory impulses.

Cerebellar level

The cerebellar level is more truly a coordinating mechanism than a motor level. It is intimately related to pyramidal and extrapyramidal components of motor function and the brainstem reticular formation.

Psychomotor level

The psychomotor level is chiefly concerned with memory, initiative, and conscious and unconscious control of motor activity.

362

10 Neurological system

These five levels do not act independently, but closely relate in the production of motor behavior essential for the client's activity. Pathological conditions that interfere with activity usually will involve more than one of the levels. Purposeful movements of the human body are initiated and guided by a constant transmission of afferent impulses to the cerebral cortex. Therefore, volitional movement requires interdependence of sensory and motor functions. Sensory deprivation, for example, can affect all motion—volitional, reflex, postural, tonic, and phasic.[6]

Assessment
NURSING HISTORY

The nursing history of a client with a problem of the nervous system provides valuable clues to the present situation and serves as a basis for care planning. The history should include data of the client's health, developmental, social, and psychological states.

Health history

The taking of a health history in older children and adults is particularly useful because it provides an opportunity to observe general appearance, posture, emotional and mental status, speech, and the ability to relate thoughts in an organized way. It also provides an opportunity to observe spontaneous family interaction and behavior, as well as serving as a means of establishing client-nurse rapport.

The nursing history should encompass the client's usual patterns of activity and rest, giving particular attention to limitations. Changes in sensation, motion, or strength of extremities should be noted, along with specific complaints such as pain, weakness, paresthesia, or loss of coordination. The nurse should ask about previous trauma or illness that could be relevant to the current problem and record any medications that are being taken on a regular or intermittent basis.

Because the onset of many neurological problems may be insidious, even remotely associated data should be explored carefully.

It is useful to elicit data about pregnancy, labor pattern, and early neonatal life if the subject or his family can provide these data. Factors such as birth weight, Apgar score, immediate behavior after delivery, vital signs, use of resuscitative measures, oxygen, or incubator, or the presence of any congenital anomalies should be noted. The characteristic growth and development pattern should be recorded and any past illnesses delineated.

Developmental history

Neonate. Although the neurological structures of the neonate are complete, they do not reach their optimum maturation until later childhood. The neonate's head size averages about 14 inches (35 cm) at birth and is characterized by two fontanels, or gaps in bone structure, that permit molding of the head during delivery and allow for expansion of the head structure as growth continues.

Neonatal reflexes reveal important clues to development. Those related to feeding behaviors (rooting, sucking, swallowing, gagging) are usually strong at birth. Other reflexes that are evident at this time are considered "protective" and often are associated with specific environmental stimuli. (See the section later in this chapter for a complete discussion of reflexes.)

Sensitivity to pain and temperature is present in neonates, but may not be well localized. Crying is the usual response to any discomfort. Motor activity is largely involuntary and reflexive, although the neonate is capable of a full range of motion.

363

Nursing process for common health problems

Infant. As the infant grows, certain primitive reflexes disappear and the skull bones fuse, closing the fontanels. The anterior fontanel fills completely within 1 year to 18 months. The posterior fontanel is closed earlier, often within 2 to 3 months. With continued development, the infant learns to grasp objects, sit alone, roll over, crawl, stand alone, and finally walk. Coordination improves by the end of the first year of life as the spinal cord matures. Visceral reflexes are also becoming refined, making toilet training feasible.

Child. The young child can perform most motor activity with a high degree of independence and has highly differentiated sensory responses. Gait and coordination continue to be refined as activity becomes "purposeful." Total continence is usually achieved. Language and emotional and social development are evident, but essentially primitive.

Around school age, neuromuscular structures continue to develop along with skeletal growth, and coordination is sufficient to ensure most simple skill learning. The later school years find the normal child exhibiting fine motor coordination, a sense of rhythm and balance, and finely differentiated social skills.

Adolescent. The adolescent may be nearing adult size, and most neuromuscular functioning and sensory potential has been realized. Although some awkwardness is characteristic during early teen years, the older adolescent is quite poised.

Adult. Adults should possess maximum nervous system function, including motor, sensory, reflexive, and cranial nerve potential.

Older adult. As degenerative characteristics of aging affect the nervous system, several changes occur. The brain shrinks in size and occupies less space within the calvarium. Blood supply may be reduced, resulting in sluggish functioning in motor, sensory, and intellectual spheres. As the bones decalcify and lose their flexibility within the spinal column, motor functioning may be impaired. Furthermore, pain and stiffness are common complaints of the older adult. Finally, as circulatory impairment takes its toll on the peripheral vessels, the related superficial nervous tissue may be subject to deterioration, resulting in loss of sensation, paresthesia, and even limited motion.

Social history

The general appearance, social skills, and modes of interaction reveal much about the client and may provide important clues to neuromuscular status. Sleeping patterns, the use of excessive alcohol or drugs, sensory deprivation, or limiting social circumstances are relevant to a comprehensive assessment. Occupational factors should also be considered, because they may relate to both the cause of the problem and its ultimate management.

Psychological history

The development of neuromuscular functioning is largely influenced by environmental variables such as family interaction and a sense of security with one's surroundings. The usual coping style of the client should be elicited, because it will be useful in evaluating the responses to therapy and undoubtedly helpful in planning subsequent nursing care. A thorough understanding of the individual's life-style and interaction with significant others is imperative.

Physical assessment

The physical assessment skill commonly used for assessing the neurological system is *inspection*. The general appearance of the client should be symmetrical. Any asymmetrical flexion, extension, abduction, or adduction can indicate the presence of nerve injuries, usually from the birth process.

The trunk should be examined for any evidence of spinal abnormalities.

The column should be digitally followed to locate any absence of vertebrae, malalignment, or curvature of the column. Any evidence of swelling or unusual characteristics of the vertebral column may indicate abnormalities.

Examining the child. The nurse who assists the physician in a neurological examination should be cognizant of factors that may affect the findings, such as certain medications (especially sedatives) and the client's being chilled, embarrassed, or frightened. If possible, the examination should be done before feeding, since many responses are diminished after mealtime. The most traumatic elements should be left until last because an agitated child is difficult to assess. Equipment and supplies should be at hand so that delays can be avoided. One of the most important responsibilities of the nurse who assists the physician is to ensure the safety and comfort of the client.

Those who examine the young child must remember that they are dealing with an immature neurological system and that responses may be primitive. Therefore a thorough assessment of growth and development is essential and perhaps the most revealing factor in determining nervous system functioning. Physical problems, sensory deprivation, and social deprivation must also be taken into account.

Important aspects in the examination of the very young child are the suture lines and fontanels. The suture lines should be approximated but not fused, and the fontanels should be neither depressed nor bulging. Depressed fontanels can be an indication of severe dehydration. However, there is some depression of the anterior fontanel when the baby sits up, allowing the cerebrospinal fluid to drain downward by gravity into ventricles. Bulging of fontanels may be caused by increased intracranial pressure. Early closing of the fontanels can cause permanent brain damage because the brain is prevented from

TABLE 10-1

Cranial nerve testing as part of the neurological examination

Nerve	Equipment	Procedure
I. Olfactory	Aromatic substances such as clove oil, tobacco, vanilla, perfume	Clear nasal passages. Ask client to sniff and identify each substance; both nostrils are checked.
II. Optic	Ophthalmoscope, eye chart	Vision and visual field determined; fundus observed for changes in arteries and veins and optic nerve swelling (papilledema).
III. Oculomotor* IV. Trochlear* VI. Abducens*	Penlight	Pupils examined for size, shape, equality, and reaction to light as well as ability to converge; client instructed to follow objects up and down, right and left, and diagonally.
V. Trigeminal	Safety pin, hot and cold substances, cotton wisp	Assessment of sensations of pain, touch, and temperature; corneal reflex checked by wisp of cotton; motor branch evaluated by ability to bite and open mouth against resistance.
VII. Facial	Sugar, salt, vinegar, and bitter substance such as quinine	Anterior two thirds of tongue checked for taste of sweet, salty, sour, and bitter substances; symmetry of face observed; client instructed to raise eyebrows, close eyes, show teeth, smile, and so forth.
VIII. Acoustic	Audiometer, tuning fork	Hearing checked by air and bone conduction.
IX. Glossopharyngeal X. Vagus	Tongue blade	Assessment of response and position of uvula, gag and swallowing reflexes; client speaks and coughs on command (taste on posterior third of the tongue may be checked).
XI. Spinal accessory		Sternocleidomastoid and trapezius muscles checked for strength by rotating head and shrugging shoulders against resistance.
XII. Hypoglossal		Client moves tongue and protrudes it on command; position and any deviation noted.

*Examined together, using same equipment.

growing normally. Late closing or failure to close may be caused by increased intracranial pressure.

Head measurements are routinely done for children to determine the skull growth pattern and to detect the adverse effects of hydrocephalus or premature approximation of sutures.

There may be bumps on the scalp of the infant that are the result of bleeding from the skull's periosteum at birth. Such a swelling is called a *cephalohematoma*. The blood resorbs in a short time without notable consequence. (Cephalohematoma in the older client may indicate a skull fracture or recent trauma to the head.)

Sleeping patterns, interest in surroundings, vigor and persistence of cry, and many other phenomena are useful data sources for the examiner and provide valuable clues about the child's growth and development.

Examining the adult. The intent of the adult neurological assessment is the same as for the child, although it is based less on growth and development indices and relies heavily on historical data, cranial nerve testing, checking of the well-defined reflex patterns appropriate for the mature nervous system, and determining motor and sensory functioning.

Cranial nerve testing. Cranial nerve assessment must be carried out in a precise manner, because the status of individual nerves provides clues for localizing central nervous system dysfunction and for diagnosing systemic disease (Table 10-1). In order to understand the significance of cranial nerve testing as it relates to pathological processes, one must understand the anatomical and physiological relations of the cranial nerves to other structures.

The *olfactory nerve* is a sensory nerve with a single function, that of smell. The loss of impairment of smell (anosmia or hyposmia, respectively) indicates lesions of this first cranial nerve. Since olfaction is related to taste, individuals with anosmia or hyposmia, especially with bilateral nerve involvement may experience an inability to discriminate certain food flavors. Olfactory acuity is thought to be greater before meals and reduced after meals. This diurnal cycle may be an important factor in the regulation of appetite and satiety.

Loss of smell may be congenital or may be associated with the aging process. Trauma, neoplasms, inflammation, and certain toxic agents may produce impairment of olfaction.

The *optic nerve* is a fiber pathway that links the retina to the brain. The actual peripheral optic nerve fibers are in the cellular layers of the retina. Fibers of the optic nerve carry visual impulses and mediate reflex responses to light, accommodation, and other stimuli. The optic nerve is evaluated by determining visual acuity, visual field, and color vision. This second cranial nerve is the singular cranial nerve that can be directly examined.

The ophthalmoscope is an essential tool in complete assessment of the optic nerve. It is used to elicit the red reflex and to scrutinize the optic disk, the macula, the fundus and vessels, and the humors (see Chapter 13). Special skills beyond the scope of this book are essential for using the ophthalmoscope.

Papilledema, or "choked disk," is a significant neurological finding made possible by ophthalmoscopy. Papilledema, usually the result of increased intracranial pressure, is characterized by swelling of the optic nerve head. Mechanical pressure on sheaths of the nerve interferes with lymphatic drainage and venous outflow, thus producing a rise in intravenous pressure. Consequently, the papilla protrudes into the globe of the eye. Progressive papilledema eventually can produce retinal hemorrhage, retinal edema, and optic disk atrophy.

The ocular nerves (oculomotor, trochlear, and abducens nerves) function together in eye movements and thus are examined as a unit. The *oculomotor nerve* (cranial nerve III) is responsible for innervating muscles that control eye movement within its socket. The *trochlear nerve* (cranial nerve IV) innervates the superior oblique muscle on the contralateral side of the nucleus of origin. This muscle depresses the eye, abducts the eyeball, and rotates the abducted globe. The trochlear nerve is the smallest cranial nerve and the only one whose fibers arise from the posterior aspect of the brainstem. The *abducens nerve* (cranial nerve VI) has the longest intracranial course of the cranial nerves. It emerges from the brainstem at the pons-medulla junction and enters the orbit via the superior orbital fissure. It supplies a single muscle, the lateral, or external rectus, which abducts the eye or deviates it laterally. In paralysis of cranial nerve VI, the eyeball is turned medially and cannot be moved laterally. Because of its long intracranial course, cranial nerve VI is frequently involved when there is elevated intracranial pressure, inflammation, or hemorrhage.

The ocular nerves are united and coordinated in the brain for conjugate action so that no isolated action of any eye muscle is ever possible.

They are also connected to nuclei of the vestibular and cochlear portions of cranial nerve VIII, the trigeminal and facial nerves, the spinal accessory nerve, the hypoglossal nerve, the motor nuclei of the upper cervical nerves, and other centers that ensure that head and body movements are correlated with eye movements. Responses to visual, auditory, sensory, vestibular, and other stimuli therefore cause conjugate deviation of the eyes and head.[6]

When ocular nerves are assessed, it is appropriate to consider the pupils, eyelids, extraocular movements, and eye position.

The size of the pupils varies greatly with environmental illumination but is usually from 3 to 4 cm in diameter. At birth they are small and react poorly to light. In childhood, adolescence, and young adulthood, the pupils tend to be perfectly round and measure about 4 cm in diameter. In middle age and in the elderly, they become smaller (3 to 3.5 cm) and are often irregular.

Small or miotic (less than 2 cm) pupils are characteristic of arteriosclerosis, syphilis, alcoholism, drug intoxication, sleep, coma, increased intracranial pressure, and certain brain lesions. Pupils constrict slightly during the expiratory phase of breathing.[6]

Dilation of pupils, mydriasis (more than 5 cm), occurs in conjunction with fear, pain, hyperthyroidism, cerebral anoxia, coma, and certain brain lesions or toxic states induced by drugs. Muscular activity, inspiration, low lighting, and loud noises can also cause dilation. It is imperative for the nurse to determine whether the client is taking any medications, because certain agents greatly influence the size and response of pupils.

Inequality of pupils is called *anisocoria*. Unequal pupils may occur congenitally, as a result of iritis, inner ear disease, or in response to cranial nerve III insult. Unequally dilated or fixed pupils are often seen after cerebrovascular accidents or in association with severe head trauma.

Pupillary reflexes are cardinal aspects of the neurological assessment. Light and accommodation-convergence reflexes are usually evaluated.

Ordinarily pupils constrict when light is focused on the retina and dilate

Nursing process for common health problems

when the light is withdrawn. This phenomenon is termed the *direct light reflex*. Both eyes respond in concert because of anatomical arrangement of fibers (even when light is directed at one retina). This is termed a *consensual light reflex*. Eyes should be tested individually for both the direct and consensual reflexes.

It is best if an indirect light source is used, since a light shown directly into the eye elicits the accommodation-convergence response as well as the light reflex. The light reflex can be tested by the examiner standing behind the client, who has been instructed to gaze at a distant source of light. The examiner then interrupts the source of light by placing hands in front of the client's eyes. The hands are withdrawn alternately to observe direct and consensual reflexes for both eyes.

The *accommodation-convergence reflex* is elicited by having the client shift his gaze to a near object after looking into the distance. This results normally in a lens thickening, convergence of the eyes, and pupillary constriction.

Eyelids should be assessed by having the client open and close his eyes without and against resistance. Any *ptosis* (drooping of the eyelid) should be noted.

Ocular movements and eye position are evaluated by directing the client to gaze (1) laterally, (2) medially, (3) upward and laterally, (4) upward and medially, (5) downward and laterally, (6) downward and medially, (7) directly upward, and (8) directly downward.

Nystagmus is a pathological eye movement that frequently manifests nervous system dysfunction or diseases of the eye and inner ear. Nystagmus is an involuntary trembling or oscillation of the eyeball. This movement may be rhythmic or dysrhythmic. Like other conjugate eye behavior, both eyes move together over the same range. (Unilateral nystagmus, however, does occur.) Differential assessment and determination of the cause of this phenomenon is complicated. The nurse, however, may be asked to make periodic observations and recordings about this abnormal eye movement. See Chapter 13 for other aspects of eye assessment.

The *trigeminal nerve* (cranial nerve V) carries both motor and sensory fibers. It is the largest and most complex cranial nerve, because it connects with cranial nerves III, IV, VI, VII, IX, and X, and with the sympathetic nervous system. The trigeminal nerve nuclei arise from the pons. The clinical assessment of cranial nerve V involves (1) determining the motor power of the muscles of mastication, (2) testing for skin and mucous membrane sensation along its distribution, and (3) observing reflexes, especially the corneal reflex.

To test functions of mastication, the client is instructed to do such things as clench or protrude his jaw, move his jaw from side to side against resistance, and bite down on a tongue blade. The examiner will observe for symmetry, tone, volume, and contour of the related muscles.

Skin and mucous membrane sensory reactions are evaluated along the distribution of cranial nerve V. The conjunctiva, cornea, oral cavity, and nostrils are examined for loss or absence of sensation by using the media of heat, cold, superficial pain, and light touch sensations.

There are several reflexes pertinent to the trigeminal nerve, but the corneal reflex is among the most important for neurological assessments. The client should be instructed to turn his head slightly in the opposite direction while

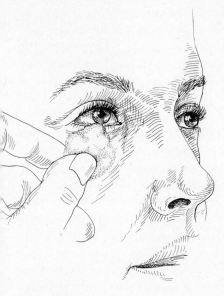

FIG. 10-2
Assessing the corneal reflex.

the examiner approaches from the side and touches the cornea lightly with a moistened wisp of cotton. This maneuvering avoids the visual palpebral blink reflex. The normal response to corneal stimulation is a closing of the ipsilateral eye and the consensual closing of the contralateral eye (Fig. 10-2).

The *facial nerve* (cranial nerve VII) has both motor and sensory functions. Lesions of the facial nerve generally involve motor functioning. Cranial nerve VII innervates the muscles of facial expression and carries parasympathetic secretory fibers to the salivary and lacrimal glands and to the oral and nasal cavities. It also is responsible for taste on the anterior two thirds of the tongue and for general visceral sensation from the salivary glands and nasal and pharyngeal mucosa.

The client is asked to do such things as frown, wrinkle his brow, raise his eyebrows, show his teeth, puff out his cheeks, whistle, and grimace.

Secretory function is evaluated by stimulating the nasolacrimal reflex by an irritating substance (such as ammonia) that will cause tearing, and by placing highly flavored substances on the tongue to produce salivation.

Taste is assessed by using sweet, sour, bitter, and salty substances. Bitter substances should be sampled last, because they leave an unpleasant aftertaste. Loss and diminution of taste are called ageusia and hypogeusia, respectively. Age, excessive smoking, and a coating on the tongue can reduce the ability to taste.

The *acoustic nerve* (cranial nerve VIII) has both a cochlear and a vestibular portion to be tested. Hearing plus equilibrium, coordination, and orientation in space are the two respective functions. See Chapter 14 for detailed methods of evaluating the acoustic nerve. Lesions of cranial nerve VIII may involve one or both portions of the nerve. Tinnitus and deafness result from cochlear dysfunction and from phenomena such as vertigo and nystagmus caused by vestibular dysfunction. Inflammation, edema, trauma, degenerative disease, or mechanical obstructions may contribute to disturbances of this cranial nerve.

The *glossopharyngeal* and *vagus nerves* (cranial nerves IX and X) are tested together, because they innervate muscles of the mouth and throat. Both have motor and automatic branches that arise from the medulla. These nerves are tested by noting the position and response of the uvula when it is stimulated by a tongue blade or cotton applicator. Normally the soft palate elevates and the uvula retracts simultaneously. The client is also asked to speak, cough, and swallow. Taste on the posterior two thirds of the tongue may be checked. Although the vagus nerve has widely distributed functions that affect the heart, lungs, kidneys, and gastrointestinal tract, these facets are seldom evaluated in a routine neurological test.

The *spinal accessory nerve* (cranial nerve XI) is entirely motor in function. It is closely associated with the glossopharyngeal and vagus nerves. The clinical assessment of this nerve is limited to noting the functions of the sternocleidomastoid and trapezius muscles. The client is directed to rotate his head and to shrug and retract his shoulders against resistance. Motor power, tone, contour, symmetry, and volume of muscles are noted.

The *hypoglossal nerve* (cranial nerve XII) is the motor nerve to the tongue. The examination of this nerve consists of evaluating the position of the tongue at rest and in protrusion, its range of movement, and its strength. Weakness, paralysis, deviation, or abnormal movements are noted as the client is instructed to move the tongue in various directions or to press it against his cheek.

Deviation from the midline or protrusion toward one side may indicate paralysis; loss of power or control may suggest degenerative disease; and tremors may arise from organic lesions or may be of psychic origin such as hysteria. Trauma, inflammation, and intracranial hemorrhage may damage the nerve before it leaves the skull.

Modifications for cranial nerve assessments. Cranial nerve testing for children under 2 or 3 years of age is difficult to carry out; however, much data can be gathered by observing the child's movements, his response to pain and other stimuli, and motor reflexes. Elderly individuals often have difficulty understanding instructions of the examiner or communicating their responses, especially in regard to sensory testing. It is imperative that the nurse consider such limitations while performing neurological assessments and when recording qualitative and quantitative results.

Cranial nerve testing can be performed in an abbreviated way, even when the client is comatose. However, the appraisal is usually limited to motor function or reflex phenomena. Oculocephalic and oculovestibular reflex testing are unique to the comatose client and deserve particular explanation.

The oculocephalic reflexes (or oculocephalogyric response) test the gaze (or turning response) of the eyes as the head is briskly rotated or the neck is briskly flexed and extended. If the brainstem is intact, the eyes will move erratically or will remain fixed in the visual field. When the head is rotated to the right, for example, the eyes turn left in the orbits. When the brainstem is not intact, the eyes remain fixed with head rotation. This latter response is termed the *doll's head phenomenon,* or "doll's eyes." This reflex should not be tested after trauma until cervical spine injury has been unequivocally ruled out.

The oculovestibular reflexes (caloric stimulation) test consists of irrigating the external ear canal with 10 ml of cool water while the client's head is elevated 30 degrees. A normally reactive labyrinth will create fast nystagmus directed toward the stimulated ear. With loss of consciousness, the fast compo-

---

MODIFIED CRANIAL NERVE TESTING FOR THE COMATOSE CLIENT

Nerve	Procedure
I. Olfactory	Not tested
II. Optic	Pupillary reflex: direct and consensual
III. Oculomotor	Pupillary reflex: direct and consensual *and* spontaneous or induced medial, superior, or downward eye movements
IV. Trochlear VI. Abducens	Eye movements: spontaneous or oculocephalic reflexes, such as "doll's eyes"
V. Trigeminal	Corneal reflex; supraorbital compression, jaw reflex
VII. Facial	Facial movement or grimace during supraorbital compression or while testing corneal reflex
VIII. Acoustic	Oculocephalic reflex and caloric stimulation
IX. Glossopharyngeal X. Vagus	Gag, cough, carotid sinus reflexes
XI. Spinal accessory	Spontaneous or induced shoulder elevation
XII. Hypoglossal	Tongue movement against examiner's finger

nent of nystagmus disappears so that the eyes will move slowly toward the irrigated ear for 2 or 3 minutes if the brainstem remains intact. The examiner must wait 5 minutes before testing the other ear.

It is also important to test for a corneal reflex and for the presence of lacrimation, because the normal protection of the eye depends on the these phenomena. Response to loud noises, the ability to swallow, and the gag reflex are also valuable clues to neurological status. The presence of salivation or drooling, especially if unilateral, is clinically significant. The list on p. 370 briefly summarizes adaptations and indicates which particular maneuvers are most beneficial for comatose clients.

Reflex testing. Evaluation of reflexes is considered by many clinicians to be the most valuable part of the neurological examination. Reflexes are significant for several reasons. Alterations in the intensity or character of a specific reflex may suggest early and delicate imbalances in the nervous system function. The evaluation of reflex phenomena is also more objective than many other parts of the examination when the client's voluntary cooperation and subjective responses must be relied on to a certain extent. Reflexes are not significantly altered by the subject's attention span, mental status, or intelligence and thus can be tested in infants and small children, and even during altered states of consciousness, including coma. Reflexes provide immediate data on motor and sensory mechanisms and are often used to elicit qualitative and quantitative measurements in preference to the detailed, time-consuming investigation, especially of neurological and musculoskeletal mechanisms.

A reflex is an involuntary action in response to a stimulus. Reflexes depend on (1) intact motor and sensory nerves and on (2) a functional reflex arc. Loss or disturbance in receptors, sensory nerves, intercalated neurons, motor units, efferent nerves, or effector mechanisms will interrupt the reflex arc and cause the loss of the reflex.

Reflexes are checked to determine how well sensory information is being integrated in the brain and spinal column to effect corresponding motor re-

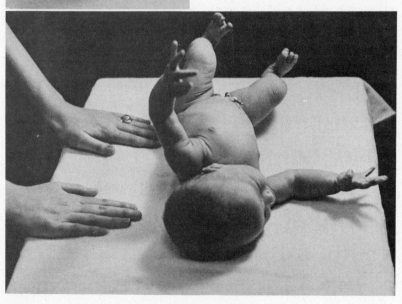

A

B

FIG. 10-3

Moro's reflex. **A,** When an infant is startled, he responds by drawing up his legs and arms and usually by crying. **B,** If the reflex is absent or unilateral, this fact may be indicative of brain damage or birth injuries, especially brachial palsy. Moro's reflex disappears after 1 or 2 months. (Courtesy Mead Johnson Nutritional Division; Evansville, Ind.)

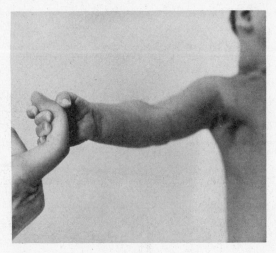

FIG. 10-4
Grasping reflex. This primitive reflex is characterized by the newborn's fingers curling tightly around a cylindrical object, especially adult fingers. It disappears a few days after birth. (Courtesy Mead Johnson Nutritional Division, Evansville, Ind.)

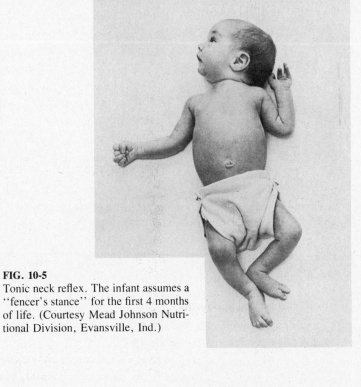

FIG. 10-5
Tonic neck reflex. The infant assumes a "fencer's stance" for the first 4 months of life. (Courtesy Mead Johnson Nutritional Division, Evansville, Ind.)

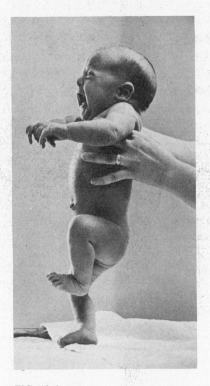

FIG. 10-6
Stepping reflex. When held upright with his feet placed on a flat surface, the infant tends to make stepping or dancing movements. (Courtesy Mead Johnson Nutritional Division, Evansville, Ind.)

sponses. If reflexes are weak, exaggerated, or absent, they may point to serious central nervous lesions.

For standard note-taking regarding description of reflex activity, responses are graded as follows: 0 = absent; + = present but diminished; + + = normal; + + + = increased but not pathological; + + + + = markedly hyperactive. Responses should always be compared bilaterally, because inequality of responses may be as significant as increased or absent reflexes.[6]

Reflex patterns are not consistent across the life span. Immature central nervous system structures of the child under 1½ years of age yield varied responses, depending on the developmental status. Reflex patterns are particularly useful in evaluating the overall physical status of infants and determining gestational age (Figs. 10-3 to 10-7).

There are some reflexes that are normal for the primitive nervous systems of infants but would be considered pathological for adults (Table 10-2). The flexor plantar response (elicited by stroking the lateral aspect of the sole of the foot) causes a curling under of the toes (flexion with adduction) in the normal adult. If dorsiflexion of the great toe and fanning of the remaining toes occur, the condition is termed pathological and is indicative of pyramidal tract disease (Babinski's reflex). Up to 1½ years of age, however, when the central nervous system structures are not fully developed, the latter phenomena occur but are considered nonpathological.

There are many types of reflexes, but only two will be considered because they are most often encountered in the routine neurological examination. These are superficial (cutaneous) reflexes and deep tendon reflexes.

Superficial reflexes are elicited by application of a stimulus to the skin or mucous membrane. Usually a tactile stimulus such as stroking or scratching is

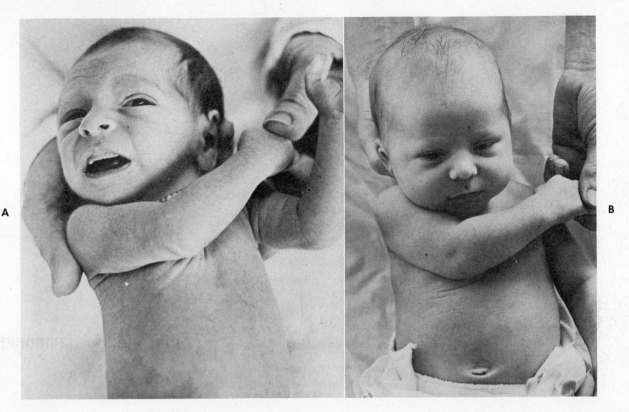

FIG. 10-7
Neck-righting reflex. When an infant's head is turned forcibly to the side, his whole body attempts to turn. This reflex follows the disappearance of the tonic neck reflex and disappears at about 1 year. Note that the full-term infant, **B,** has more resistance to the turning than the premature infant, **A.** (Courtesy Mead Johnson Nutritional Division, Evansville, Ind.)

sufficient to evoke the skin-muscle responses. Superficial reflexes respond more slowly to a stimulus than do deep tendon reflexes, their latent period is longer, and they exhaust readily.[6]

Superficial reflexes depend on upper motor neuron pathways as well as on the reflex arc and thus may be absent in upper and lower motor neuron disorders.

The abdominal, cremasteric, and plantar reflexes are often selected to evaluate skin-muscle responses. The abdominal reflex consists of gently stroking a selected part of the abdomen with a blunt object, which normally causes a homolateral contraction of abdominal muscles and a deviation of the umbilicus toward the area stimulated. The client must be recumbent and relaxed. The

TABLE 10-2
The disappearance of infantile reflexes

Reflex	Time of disappearance
Sucking	Persists throughout infancy; particularly during sleep
Rooting	3 to 4 months while awake; may persist during sleep for 9 to 12 months
Palmar grasp	5 to 6 months
Plantar grasp	9 to 12 months
Moro reflex	4 to 7 months
Stepping	3 to 4 months
Placing	10 to 12 months
Incurvation of trunk	2 to 3 months

From Chinn, P.L.: Child health maintenance, ed. 2, St. Louis, 1979, The C.V. Mosby Co., p. 172.

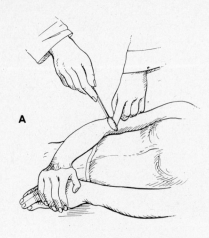

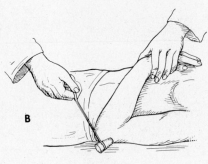

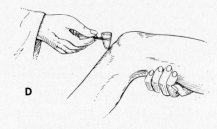

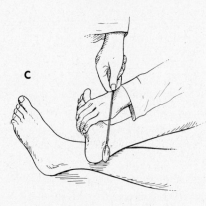

FIG. 10-8
Positions for testing the tendon reflexes: **A,** biceps tendon; **B,** triceps tendon; **C,** Achilles tendon; **D,** patellar tendon. (From Fowkes, W.C. and Hunn, V.K.: Clinical assessment for the nurse practitioner, St. Louis, 1973, The C.V. Mosby Co.)

cremasteric reflex produces muscle contraction with homolateral testicular elevation when skin on the upper, inner aspect of the thigh is stroked. The plantar (or Babinski's) reflex has been previously discussed.

Deep tendon reflexes, or "muscle-stretch" reflexes, are elicited by application of a stimulus to tendons, although bones, joints, and fascia may be tapped for selected responses. A soft rubber percussion hammer is employed to strike the desired area. The client should be as relaxed as possible. The stimulus must be quick and direct, but no harder than necessary to evoke a threshold response. Most deep tendon reflexes can be successfully evaluated with the client in the recumbent as well as in the upright sitting position. The examiner must note the speed and intensity of response, the range of motion, and the duration of the muscle contraction. It is essential to feel as well as see the reflex response for accurate assessment. It is essential to evaluate deep tendon reflexes bilaterally.

Biceps, triceps, ankle (Achilles), and knee (patellar) reflexes are the reflexes most frequently examined, although numerous other sites may be selected (Fig. 10-8). Hypoactivity or absence of deep tendon reflexes may indicate peripheral nerve or anterior horn cell disease and possibly certain cerebellar lesions. Hyperactive deep tendon reflexes are characteristic of pyramidal tract lesions and some psychogenic disorders. Deep reflexes may be increased in early stages of coma but are absent in deep coma, heavy sedation or sleep, and early spinal shock (see discussion later in this chapter).

Determining motor and sensory functioning. Motor function is noted, and muscles are inspected for contractures, atrophy, tremor, tone, and abnormal movements. Muscle groups are checked for strength, and joints are put through the range of motion. Coordination is also assessed in variable ways, such as asking the client to place his finger on his nose or to trace his shin with the heel of the opposite foot and then alternating the procedure. Gait and balance while walking provide valuable clues related to weakness and spasticity of the legs and pelvic girdle. Muscle tone, clonus, and sensory functioning can also be evaluated at this time. Any areas of paresthesia, anesthesia, or other abnormal sensations should receive additional attention.

Meningeal irritation is always a significant factor in neurological disease and may be recognized by such factors as nuchal rigidity, photophobia, unusual sensitivity of muscles, Brudzinski's sign, and Kernig's sign (see discussion later in this chapter).

Ideally, evaluation of motor activity should take place in a warm, comfortable, well-lighted area where the client can be undressed for portions of the examination. Subjects who are alert, keen-minded, and cooperative obviously yield the most reliable data. Pain, discomfort, sedatives or narcotics, alcohol ingestion, tension, fatigue, and apprehension are factors that tend to interfere with the mechanics of the assessment as well as alter results. The assessment of motor functioning involves evaluation of: (1) general body appearance, (2) motor strength and power, (3) muscle tone, (4) muscle volume and contour, (5) coordination, (6) abnormal movements, (7) station and gait, and (8) electrical impulses of muscles. Intricate details of this complex system of assessments are beyond the scope of this text, but general principles and techniques are presented.

Inspection. The client is observed for basic body build and posturing. Absences of parts or abnormalities of the musculoskeletal system are noted.

Muscle masses are visually studied for symmetry and bulk, and comparisons of the left and right sides of the body are made. (It is useful to note at this point whether the client is right- or left-handed.)

Motor strength and power. Motor strength and power relate to the expenditure of energy for exerting or releasing force. Power to change position (kinetic) and force to resist movement (static) are both studied. Impaired strength or power is termed *weakness* or *paresis;* loss of strength is termed *paralysis.*

Fatigability, decreased dexterity and coordination, and abnormalities in speed and range of motion are considered along with power loss or weakness.

The techniques of systematic study of individual muscles and groups of muscles are carried out. All joints are assessed for functioning, and focal losses of power or strength are noted. The following are terms used to define special clinical entities important to the nurse:

monoplegia Paralysis of one extremity
quadriplegia or *tetraplegia* Paralysis of all four extremities
hemiplegia Paralysis of one half of the body
paraplegia Paralysis of legs or lower portion of the body

Muscle tone. Within relaxed muscle there is some tension that holds joints in position, retains posture, and awaits stimuli to contract or relax. The motor centers of the cerebral cortex and basal ganglia, the vestibular apparatus, the cerebellum, and facilitatory and inhibitory centers in the midbrain and brainstem reticular formations all supply impulses that influence tone to the motor nuclei in the spinal cord. Tone is a reflex phenomenon with both afferent and efferent components, and muscles are flaccid when deprived of motor and sensory nerve supplies. Tone can be influenced by interferences in the spinal reflex arc or supraspinal levels that normally inhibit lower reflex centers. Higher centers may also affect tone, at least partially, at a voluntary level. Environmental factors such as heat and cold, respectively, decrease and increase tone.

Assessment of tone can be reliably accomplished only by skilled clinicians with repeated experiences in evaluating the passive movements during relaxation as absence of voluntary control. The major evaluation involves collecting data regarding the *resistance* of *muscles* to *passive manipulation.* Extremity muscles are the areas more frequently assessed.

Palpation may also be done to determine the consistency, turgor, or firmness of muscle mass or to check for the presence of tenderness.

Lost or diminished tone is called *hypotonicity* or *flaccidity,* and pathologically increased tone is called *hypertonicity.*

Muscle volume and contour. Determining muscle volume and contour is essential in the search for *atrophy* (wasting) or *hypertrophy* (increase in mass).

Inspection, palpation, and measurements of selected muscle masses comprise this evaluation. It is usually accomplished during the range-of-motion maneuvers essential for determining motor strength, power, and tone.

Coordination. Skillfully executed motor activity requires the organization of motor, sensory, and synergistic factors, especially the cerebellum, which is thought to be chiefly responsible for coordination. Any interferences related to motor control levels, sensory functioning (especially proprioception), or the vestibular system may alter coordination.

Examinations for coordination include factors of agility, balance, and equilibrium. The test subject may be asked to perform such acts as touching his index finger to his nose successively, completely abducting and extending his arm each time. This *finger-to-nose test* is carried out with eyes opened and closed. Another typical maneuver is the *heel-to-knee-to-toe test,* in which the subject is asked to place the heel of one foot on the knee of the opposite leg and to trace the shin to the great toe. The *Romberg test* is a classic technique to assess equilibratory coordination. The client stands with his feet together and his eyes open and then closed. If the individual is unable to maintain this erect posturing without swaying or lurching, it is referred to as a positive Romberg sign and is indicative of a conductive disturbance of proprioceptive impulses through the spinal cord. The client may also be instructed to hold his extremities in position with his eyes open and then closed, or to repeatedly pronate and supinate his hands.

This battery of coordination tests is an integral part of the neurological examination and is refined and expanded when used other than for initial screening purposes.

Abnormal movements. Abnormal movements, or hyperkinesias, may be noted in any part of the body and are considered as signs or symptoms, not clinical pathological entities.

Tremors are involuntary, rhythmic, purposeless, oscillatory movements that result from alternate contractions of opposing muscle groups. They are classified according to location, rate, amplitude, etiology, rhythmicity, and relationship to rest and movement.

Fasciculations are fine twitching movements that appear with the contraction of a bundle, or fasciculus, of muscle fibers. They are usually not intense enough to cause joint movement and vary greatly in size, intensity, and regularity of occurrence. *Fibrillations* are related to a similar phenomenon but are limited to single muscle fibers or minute groups of fibers.

Myokymic movements are transient, persistent movements that spontaneously affect a few muscle bundles. They are usually limited and do not cause joint motion. They myokymic movements occur in normal individuals after strenuous exercise or in states of extreme fatigue. Occasionally, the associated irritability causes cramping or other pain.

Myoclonic movements are brief, rapid, jerky involuntary contractions of muscles. The most frequently encountered myoclonus occurs in seizure activity (see discussion later in this chapter).

Choreiform movements are involuntary, purposeless, irregular, asymmetrical, and nonrhythmic. They appear during resting states but become exaggerated by activity and tensions. They may involve an extremity, one half of the body, or the entire body. The associated muscles are essentially hypotonic; thus purposeful activity is limited. *Huntington's chorea* is one of the most typical clinical entities when such movements are noted.

Athetoid movements are slower and more sustained than choreiform movements, but their amplitude is larger. They are sometimes referred to as a *mobile spasm.* The movements are characterized by several degrees of flexion, extension, pronation, supination, abduction, and adduction. Athetoid movements are characteristic of certain cerebral palsies of congenital origin and may occur following trauma.

Spasms are reflex contractions of muscles that often result from irritation. Painful tonic spasms are sometimes called cramps or charley horses. Even a hiccough (singultus) is technically classified as a spasm of the diaphragm. A *tic* is a conditioned reflex (or habit spasm) of psychogenic origin. Tics appear suddenly and recur irregularly in response to selected physical or emotional stimuli. Children are more likely to experience tics than adults.

There are many other abnormalities of movement that are subcategories of these just presented, but they are not routinely encountered by nurses, and their clinical significance is questionable. It is useful for the nurse, however, to be able to describe hyperkinesias that are observed, because they are often valuable clues in diagnostic and management strategies of several pathological conditions.

Station and gait. Station is the client's attitude or manner of position, especially standing. Posture, body position, relation of parts, and symmetry are components assessed. The Romberg test (previously described) is the classic maneuver employed to evaluate station. Gait is the act of walking. It is checked with the client's eyes open and closed. The client may be instructed to walk backward, sideways, around chairs, or to follow a line on the floor. Tandem walking (one heel directly in front of the toes of the other foot), heel walking, or toe walking may be performed on command to appraise the client's ability to control motion at will.

It is essential that ataxic gaits be differentiated from difficulties in locomotion that occur as the result of serious weakness from illness or chronic inactivity.

There are typical gaits that are repeatedly found in conjunction with certain disease entities and even occupations (sailor's gait or cowboy's gait).

ASSESSMENT GUIDE FOR MOTOR ABILITY

1. General factors
   a. Is the client warm? Comfortable? Relaxed? Able to cooperate?
   b. What is the general appearance of the client? Body build? Posturing? Do the right and left sides appear symmetrical? Are there absences of parts or abnormalities of parts? Is the individual right- or left-handed?
2. Motor strength and power
   a. Is there any focal loss of motor strength and power when client is assessed by range of motion? Ability to grasp? Resist passive movement?
   b. When the client engages in range of motion, are there abnormalities in speed? Dexterity? Smoothness? Coordination?
   c. Is there fatigability or loss of dexterity when motions are successively repeated?
   d. Is there any paresis or paralysis?
3. Tone, volume, and contour
   a. Do muscles resist passive manipulation?
   b. Is there apparent hypotonicity or hypertonicity?
   c. Do muscle masses feel firm, have normal consistency and turgor?
   d. Is there any tenderness?
   e. Is there atrophy or hypertrophy when muscles are measured and compared bilaterally?
4. Coordination
   a. Can the client successfully accomplish finger-to-nose and heel-to-knee-to-toe tests?
   b. Is there a positive Romberg's sign?
   c. Do movements appear smooth and skillfully executed?

5. Hyperkinesias
   a. Are there any tremors, fasciculations, or myokymic movements? Choreiform movements? Athetoid movements? Spasms? Tics?
   b. What stimuli seem to evoke or exaggerate these abnormal movements?
6. Station and gait
   a. What is the client's posture at rest (standing)? With eyes open? Closed? Does he appear to sway or require support to maintain an upright position?
   b. What is the client's posture at rest (sitting)? With eyes open? Closed? Does he appear to sway or to require support to maintain an upright position?
   c. What is the client's posture at rest (in bed)? Does he appear bilaterally congruent? Can he move his legs and arms? Sit up without assistance?
   d. What is the client's ability to walk without assistance? Does he walk erect? With a wide-based gait? Shuffling gait? Is there any limp? Does he drag one foot? Do arms swing freely while walking? Does he watch his feet?
   c. Can the client turn on command without support? Is a change in pace smoothly accomplished without hesitation? Is walking pace even?
   f. Can the client perform tandem walking? Heel walking? Toe walking?
   g. Does the client have a weakness or infirmities from illness or injury (or chronic inactivity) that could affect gait?

TABLE 10-3

Changes in motor function

	Loss of power	Tone	Atrophy	Fasciculations	Reaction of degeneration
Spinomuscular lesion	Focal and segmental Muscles or muscle groups Complete	Flaccid	Present	May be present	Present
Extrapyramidal lesion	Generalized Movements or extremities Incomplete	Rigid	Absent	Absent	Absent
Pyramidal tract lesion	Generalized Movements or extremities Incomplete	Spastic	Absent	Absent	Absent
Cerebellar lesion	None Ataxia may simulate loss of power	Hypotonic (ataxia)	Absent	Absent	Absent
Psychogenic disorder	Bizarre No true loss of power May simulate any type	Normal or variable Often increased	Absent	Absent	Absent

From DeJong, Russell N.: The neurological examination, ed. 4, Hagerstown, Md., 1979, Harper & Row, Publishers, Inc.

The nurse should be prepared to evaluate the station and gait of all clients, because the ability of an individual to stand, sit, or walk is baseline data for developing a nursing care plan. Furthermore, unsteady stations or walking gaits that are unnoticed could contribute to serious accidents for ambulatory clients. If a client sways to one side when he sits or walks, he will need some support on that side. If he shuffles as he ambulates, scatter rugs or mats might pose a hazard. A systematic assessment guide to station and gait appears as an integral part of the assessment guide for motor ability (see p. 377).

Electrical impulses of muscles. The evaluation of motor activity thus far has been discussed in terms of assessments that involve the subjective interpretations by the examiner. There are, however, three electrodiagnostic tests that are useful in objectively determining the behavioral characteristics of muscles or groups of muscles.

One of the earliest tests of nerve and muscle behavior still in use employs the percutaneous application of current and the measurement of that current level essential for stimulation. Current can be delivered through the motor nerve, or the muscle mass can be excited by direct application of the stimulus.

Electromyography records the electrical activity of the muscle at rest and during activity. Needle electrodes are inserted into muscles that pick up impulses that are then transmitted, amplified, and displayed on an oscilloscope. Response intensity can also be recorded by translating voltage changes that occur into sound waves. Surface electrodes are also used in electromyography but yield less precise data because they cannot isolate single muscle groups.

Nerve conduction velocity combines stimulation and recording techniques. It has the added dimension of determining the velocity or speed of response in relation to the application of the stimulus. The conduction time of nerve fibers can thus be determined. Nerve conduction velocity studies are especially useful in assessing peripheral nerve injuries or disease.

Ataxia	Reflexes	Abnormal movements	Associated movements	Trophic disturbances
Absent	Deep reflexes diminished to absent Superficial reflexes diminished to absent No pyramidal tract responses	None, except for fasciculations	Normal	Present
Absent	Deep reflexes normal or variable Superficial reflexes normal or increased No pyramidal tract responses	Present	Absence of normal associated movements	Absent
Absent	Deep reflexes hyperactive Superficial reflexes diminished to absent Pyramidal tract responses	None	Presence of pathologic associated movements	Usually absent
Present	Deep reflexes diminished or pendular Superficial reflexes normal No pyramidal tract responses	May be present (intention tremor and ataxia)	Normal	Absent
Absent (may simulate ataxia)	Deep reflexes normal or increased (range) Superficial reflexes normal or increased No pyramidal tract responses	May be present	Normal	Absent

The preceding components of motor evaluation can be adapted for routine nursing assessment of all clients. Voluntary control of muscles is essential for safety and security as well as for purposeful activity. It is imperative that the nurse know the motor function capabilities and the limitations of each client in order to plan and implement care (Table 10-3).

DIAGNOSTIC ASSESSMENT

Special diagnostic studies may be performed to supplement the routine neurological examination, but they are usually reserved for clients whose preliminary findings raise suspicions of nervous system involvement. Test categories include (1) lumbar puncture and spinal dynamics, (2) isotope scanning, (3) electroencephalography and echoencephalography, and (4) radiological studies using dye and air contrast media. These tests are summarized in Table 10-4.

Lumbar puncture

Normal cerebrospinal fluid (CSF) is clear and colorless, and it contains almost no white blood cells. In the presence of recent hemorrhage, the fluid may appear pinkish red (xanthochromic). Yellow, orange, or brown discoloration may indicate less recent hemorrhage, often as long as several weeks before the tap. If there is an infectious process occurring, the fluid may appear cloudy or turbid because of an increase in the presence of white blood cells. There is little protein in normal CSF, because it does not cross the blood-brain barrier. However, tumor growth within the central nervous system can be manifest by elevated protein levels. Glucose is a constituent of CSF, and its level depends to a large degree on systemic levels. It is imperative to obtain a blood glucose specimen before performing the lumbar puncture so that glucose levels of blood and CSF may be correlated. Low glucose levels of CSF may indicate an infectious process such as meningitis.

Pre–lumbar puncture care. The nurse should prepare the client for a lumbar puncture by explaining the procedure and making certain that he is as

TABLE 10-4

Common diagnostic studies utilized

Diagnostic test	Procedure	Information obtained	Possible complications	Lesions best demonstrated
Lumbar puncture	Insertion of needle into lumbar subarachnoid space and withdrawal of fluid	Presence of abnormal amounts of cells, and alterations in chemical content of CSF	Herniation of temporal uncus or cerebellar tonsils with compression of brainstem	Meningitis, subarachnoid hemorrhage
Echoencephalography	Transmission of ultrasonic waves coronally through brain and recording of echo at brain-fluid and brain-bone interfaces	Lateral shift of normally midline structures (third ventricle) by mass lesions	None	Lateralized tumors of cerebral hemispheres, subdural and epidural hematoma
Electroencephalography	Application of electrodes to scalp and recording of cortical electrical activity	Abnormal wave forms and seizure discharges from areas irritated or compressed	None	Brain abscess, seizure focus
Isotope scanning	Parenteral injection of a radioactive isotope and counting of radioactivity transmitted through to scalp	Neoplasms, vascular malformations, and abnormal brain tissue taking up more than normal amounts of isotope	Allergic reaction to isotope or its carrier	Meningioma, arteriovenous malformations, highly vascular malignant neoplasms
Computerized axial tomography	Tomograms of head with computer-derived image of structures of different densities	Transverse outlines of ventricular system, fluid and semifluid cavities	Allergic reaction to enhancing drugs, if used	Hydrocephalus, neoplasms, cysts, hematomas, infarcts
Pneumoencephalography	Lumbar puncture and injection of air into subarachnoid space	Outline of subarachnoid cisterns and ventricular system that may be distorted or shifted by mass lesions	Herniation of temporal uncus or cerebellar tonsils with compression of brainstem	Tumors in chiasmic cistern, floor of third ventricle, aqueductal obstructions
Angiography	Insertion of needle into the carotid or vertebral artery in the neck and injection of contrast medium	Opacification of cerebral blood vessels to show vascular anomalies, or neovascularity and displacement by mass lesion	Thromboembolism with cerebral infarction, local hemorrhage with tracheal compression, allergic reaction to contrast media	Vascular anomalies (aneurysm, arteriovenous malformation), subdural and epidural hematoma, vascular neoplasms, especially meningioma
Myelography	Lumbar or cisternal puncture and injection of positive contrast medium or air	Outline of spinal subarachnoid space that may be distorted or blocked by mass lesions in the spinal canal	Spinal arachnoiditis — inflammatory reaction to contrast medium or contaminant	Tumors in the spinal canal, herniated intervertebral disc, avulsion of nerve roots
Discography	Injection of contrast medium into intervertebral disc	Abnormal configuration of disc and leakage of contrast through ruptured annulus fibrosus	Extravasation of contrast into subarachnoid space	Degenerated or ruptured intervertebral disc

From Liechty, Richard D., and Soper, Robert T.: Synopsis of surgery, ed. 4, St. Louis, 1980, The C.V. Mosby Co., p. 513.

comfortable as possible. It is important to obtain baseline vital signs and to ensure that the individual's bowel and bladder are emptied.

The client is positioned on his side with the head and neck flexed and the knees drawn up on the abdomen. It may be helpful to instruct the individual to "try to touch his chin with his knees" or to "curl into a ball." Such positioning separates the dorsal vertebral processes in the lumbar area for needle insertion.

Lumbar puncture and spinal dynamics. After the client is positioned on a firm surface and restrained, if necessary, the puncture site is surgically prepared. It is scrubbed with an antiseptic solution, dried with sterile towels, wiped with an antiseptic solution, and draped. The physician, usually seated for improved

FIG. 10-9
Lumbar puncture. **A,** Client positioned for puncture. **B,** Physician introducing needle and stylet. **C,** Manometric determination of cerebrospinal fluid pressure.

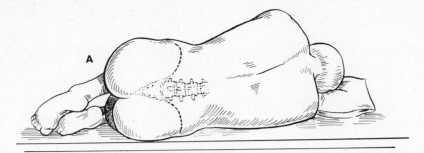

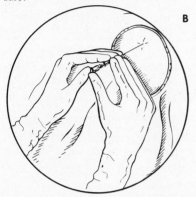

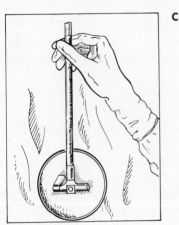

visualization and dexterity, uses a sterile gloved hand to locate the appropriate interspinous space (usually L4-5). A local anesthetic such as 1% lidocaine (Xylocaine) hydrochloride is introduced at the site. A hollow needle with a stylet is slowly inserted. Correct placement of the needle in the subarachnoid space is assured by CSF fluid dripping when the stylet is removed after piercing the dura mater. At this time, the client may note that he has sharp pains shooting down the leg. This phenomenon is caused by the needle coming into contact with dorsal nerve roots and is only a temporary discomfort. However, considerable reassurance is needed to help him relax.

The physician will usually want to record CSF pressure before collecting laboratory specimens. A manometer with a three-way stopcock is attached to the needle (Fig. 10-9). It is essential that the client be relaxed in order to obtain accurate readings, because any increase in thoracic or abdominal pressure causes elevations. Suggesting that the client take deep breaths, straighten his legs, and unflex his neck usually promotes relaxation. The client may also be asked to cough or perform Valsalva's maneuver (see Chapter 13) during spinal dynamics measurements, or the nurse may be instructed to apply abdominal pressure. These measures raise CSF pressure and thus are useful in ensuring manometer patency.

Spinal fluid pressure is recorded at the lowest levels during fluctuations, which occur during respirations. The opening pressure normally ranges from 60 to 180 mm of water. When pressure readings are completed, other tests such as the Queckenstedt test (see below) may be done before the manometer is removed for CSF specimen collection.

In sequence, three or four samples (approximately 3 ml each) are collected in prelabeled and numbered test tubes for laboratory analysis. It is important that the serial collection is done, because any blood associated only with the trauma of the tap would most likely appear in greater quantity in initial CSF and thus not be confused with central nervous system hemorrhage.

The *Queckenstedt test,* also termed a *spinal dynamics test,* is performed to assess the CSF circulation and to determine whether there is any obstruction in the subarachnoid space between the foramen magnum and the needle. With the manometer in place after an initial CSF pressure reading has been made, the neck is compressed, which should raise the fluid level in the tube. When the pressure is relieved, the fluid level should fall quickly to the earlier established level. If a block is present, the fluctuation will be sluggish or absent.

A small sterile dressing may be placed over the site after ascertaining that all CSF leakage has ceased.

Post–lumbar puncture care. Few complications are associated with the procedure, but headache is a frequent complaint. The cause of this phenomenon is unknown but is felt to be linked to CSF hypotension. When CSF is removed, the brain loses some of its "cushion," and traction may affect the meninges and other intracranial structures. The headache is variable and may last for days or weeks in rare instances. However, it usually appears and disappears proximal to the procedure within several hours.

The client is usually instructed to avoid strenuous activity after the puncture to minimize seepage of fluid through the dural wound. Ambulation or sitting in an upright position (formerly advised against after puncture) reportedly does not contribute to the development of a headache. Some neurologists feel that psychogenic influences (expecting a spinal headache) are etiological in most instances if headache does occur. In one study, when a needle was inserted into the subject's lumbar area (but not into the subarachnoid space), nearly half of the subjects who had asked about the potential complication of headaches developed one. However, in the other group who had not inquired about headaches as a complication, just slightly over 10% of the subjects developed one.[13] It is recommended that clients not be preconditioned to expect this postpuncture headache. However, if large amounts of CSF are extracted for that purpose, forcing fluids or administering saline or glucose intravenously may be indicated to restore hemodynamics of the CSF volume.

Rarely, intracranial pressure variations induced by the lumbar puncture can potentiate herniation of the brain and brainstem compression, especially in the presence of intracranial pressure elevations. Most clinicians will defer puncture if papilledema or other signs of elevated intracranial pressure are detected. Following any lumbar puncture, the nurse should observe for any pupillary changes (especially dilation of one or both), decreasing level of consciousness, and changes in motor ability. Vital signs should be monitored and elevations in blood pressure, decreases in pulse rate, or respiratory difficulty promptly reported.

Other complications that may occur are backache (perhaps caused by positioning strain or puncture site irritation), meningitis, subarachnoid hematoma, trauma to disks or spinal nerve roots, or needle breakage.

Cisternal and ventricular punctures

Cisternal puncture is sometimes performed in clients with a suspected subarachnoid blockage or with elevated intracranial pressure, because it decreases the potential danger of herniation and brainstem compression.

The client is positioned in a lateral recumbent position with the head flexed. The head should be shaved up to the external occipital protruberance. Preparation of the site and actual collection of fluid are similar to those for a lumbar puncture. Postpuncture care should emphasize observations of breathing and heart rate, because medullary trauma is the most frequent complication.

A ventricular puncture is indicated in the same situations as cisternal puncture, but it has the added risk of actual entry into the brain tissue. Prepuncture preparation and postpuncture care are congruent with that of ventriculography (see discussion later in this chapter).

Isotope scanning of the brain

Brain scans using radioactive isotopes are useful for initial assessment of intracranial lesions (especially neoplasms) and vascular abnormalities.

After injection of an isotope such as technetium (^{99}Tc), a brain scan can be completed in a few hours. The process of scanning begins at a selected interval

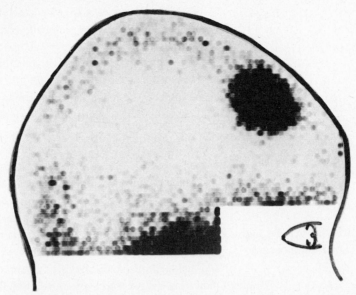

FIG. 10-10
Radioisotopic brain scan. The venous sinuses take up relatively heavy concentrations of isotope, whereas normal brain tissue does not. In this right lateral projection, an area of dense uptake is seen high in the frontal area. The rounded outline suggests a neoplasm. In this case, the lesion proved to be a meningioma. (From Liechty, Richard D., and Soper, Robert T.: Synopsis of surgery, ed. 3, St. Louis, 1976, The C.V. Mosby Co.)

after injection of the isotope substance. Preliminary films may be taken to observe the flow process, which presents an indication of how effectively the vascular system is handling the substance. At intervals of 30 to 60 minutes the brain is filmed and scanned to evaluate the absorption of the isotope (Fig. 10-10). Abnormal tissue takes up more of the isotope than normal tissues do. Sophisticated modern scan equipment gives multidimensional views, including rapid serial presentations of uptake and distribution. Most brain scans are completed in periods of 1 to 4 hours.

Isotope scanning carries a small risk and can be done for ambulatory clients as a primary screening procedure to avoid more complicated and unpleasant tests. However, only angiography or ventriculography can explicitly reveal circulatory patterns of blood or cerebrospinal fluid, respectively.

The CAT scan is a method of brain scanning that uses an x-ray beam and a computer to produce a detailed study of the brain without the use of a radioisotope. This scanning device (produced by Electronics and Musical Instrumentation, Ltd.) is sometimes referred to as an EMI scanner. A complete brain study can be completed in 20 or 30 minutes. The client's head is scanned 180 times at various angles with an x-ray beam, and tissue absorption in contiguous tissue is calculated by computer and displayed as a printout of numerical values and gray-shaded oscilloscopic visualization, which corresponds to tissue density. These data are then recorded on a Polaroid film. Densities with their related computer readouts can be used to differentiate between air, CSF, brain tissue, bone, blood, and calcified lesions. The accuracy and usefulness of the EMI scan is enhanced even further when combined with nuclear medicine scanning. Use of pneumoencephalography is reduced in regional centers where CAT scans are available to physicians (Fig. 10-11).

No special client preparation is necessary except to shampoo hair to remove hair spray. The scan is completed with the client lying on a table in front of a rotating scanning device while a technician observes from a monitor outside the area, making machine adjustments at various intervals. Usually intercom communication is possible, but it is essential that the client does not move while the machine is moving.

Computerized axial tomography (CAT scan)

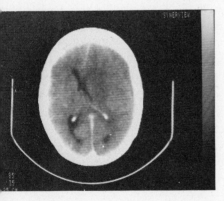

FIG. 10-11
This CT scan, performed with contrast, demonstrates a deformity of the ventricular system with a left to right midline shift secondary to deep cerebral edema. (From Budassi, S.A., and Barber, J.M.: Emergency nursing; principles and practice, St. Louis, 1981, The C.V. Mosby Co.)

Nursing process for common health problems

Nursing care related to a brain scan involves primarily client instruction. It is important to stress the simplicity and lack of discomfort and risk associated with the procedure.

The actual brain scan may involve the injection of an intravenous radioisotope and requires that the client lie quietly on a table or sit in a chair while a cameralike device records the absorption of the isotope. Certain isotopes make tears and saliva radioactive for a few hours; it is therefore important to avoid hand contact with the eyes or mouth accidentally, which could spread the substances and distort the scan. It should be emphasized, however, that the dosage of the isotope is so small that it poses no radiation hazard during or after the scan.

Some radioisotopes require prescan administration of agents that selectively block uptake of the isotope by the thyroid, salivary glands, or kidney, but no other preparation or postscan nursing care is required.

Electroencephalography and echoencephalography

An electroencephalogram (EEG) is a record of electrical activity patterns of the brain, made with scalp electrodes. Like brain scanning, it is without risk and available for nonhospitalized clients. It is useful in localizing seizures and indicating the presence of tumors and inflammatory processes. Electroencephalograms have limited value with young children, because the brain wave activity pattern does not become fully mature until the preadolescent years.

The regimen 1 or 2 days before the EEG is given usually calls for the discontinuance of all tranquilizers, anticonvulsants, and stimulants, including alcohol, because these substances alter brain wave patterns. Dietary restrictions are unnecessary except for omitting tea, coffee, or cola drinks. It is imperative that the test subject understands that regular meal and sleep patterns should be maintained before the EEG is given because hypoglycemia and sleep deprivation also affect brain patterns and may evoke abnormal brain potentials.

The client should be instructed that the actual procedure involves the application of 19 to 21 scalp electrodes. Baseline electrical waves of the brain are recorded at rest. The effects of other factors such as flickering lights, sleep, and hyperventilation on brain activity may be also subsequently recorded.

Although the test is essentially a painless, noninvasive procedure, the individual may feel anxious, because it involves a search for possible pathological conditions of the brain. It is helpful if the nurse fully understands the EEG and can interpret it realistically.

Echoencephalography uses ultrasonic sound waves. A probe is held to the scalp to pick up echoes from various intracranial tissues. The time that elapses before the echoes return is an important factor in assessing structures that can be compared bilaterally (Fig. 10-12). For example, if identical sites are used on both sides of the skull, the time lapse should be the same; deviations probably indicate structural abnormalities within the cranial vault.

The procedure is safe for the client and without discomfort, but it does not point to any underlying rationale for deviations; it merely determines that they exist.

Nurses should advise clients that the electrode paste used in such testing may be removed by one or more regular shampoos. Brushing the hair may also help rid the scalp and hair of paste encrustations.

There is no other specific nursing management related to electroencephalography and echoencephalography. Depending on the established procedure, these tests may take 1 to 2 hours to complete.

FIG. 10-12
Echoencephalography. **A,** Probe is applied in turn to the temporal scalp on each side in a case of left-sided mass, causing shift to the right. **B,** Polaroid print of oscilloscope trace, indicating midline closer to right side of skull. (From Jennett, W. Bryan. In Operative surgery, vol. 14, London, Butterworth & Co., Publisher, Ltd.)

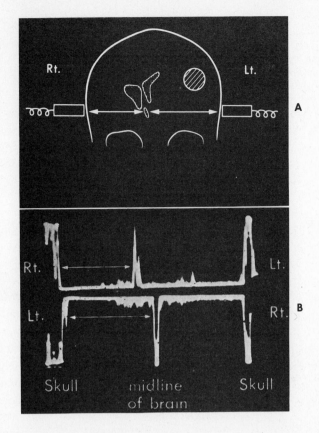

Evoked responses

Evoked responses (ERs) are electrical responses of the brain to an external stimulus, for example, visual or auditory. A computer averaging of evoked responses is a useful adjunct to the conventional EEG in diagnosing certain neurological phenomena. The method is based on the principle that electrical responses to stimuli always occur at the same interval of time after the stimulus is applied; thus related changes in EEG patterns as a result of stimuli can be separated from random background EEG activity caused by spontaneous electrical brain activity (alpha waves).

Visual stimuli such as strobe light flashes and auditory stimuli consisting of a series of clicks are commonly employed for recordings.

ERs are useful in diagnosing multiple sclerosis and localized brain lesions, and as a mode of defining brain death.

Client preparation and test participation are similar to those required for an EEG.

Radiological studies

Radiological studies using dyes and air contrast media are more complicated and involve greater risk and discomfort for the client than other categories of neurological tests, but they afford highly valuable data about nervous system functioning.

Angiography is the method of studying cerebrovascular activity after injection of a radiopaque dye (Fig. 10-13). An *arteriogram* is a similar study but concentrates on the cerebral arteries.

A *pneumoencephalogram* is an air contrast picture of the subarachnoid cisterns and ventricles made possible by the injection of air into the subarachnoid space via a lumbar puncture (Fig. 10-14).

FIG. 10-13
Angiogram showing meningioma. The tumor (outlined by arrows) contains many neovascular channels that, when filled with contrast medium, produce a stain or blush in the angiogram. Malignant gliomas may also show vascular stains, and differentiation is not always possible. (From Liechty, Richard D., and Soper, Robert T.: Synopsis of surgery, ed. 4, St. Louis, 1980, The C.V. Mosby Co.)

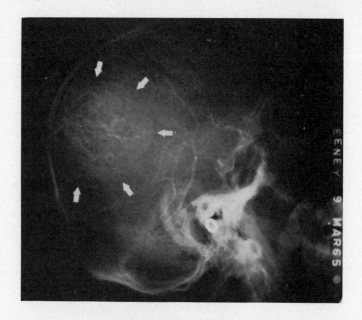

Myelograms are films showing an outline of the subarachnoid space, made with a dye or air contrast media introduced by lumbar or cisternal puncture. This test is useful in locating pathological conditions of the spinal cord.

Discography employs a contrast medium that has been injected into an intervertebral disk to locate abnormal configurations characteristic of damaged intervertebral disks.

The most complicated specific test is the *ventriculogram,* which is a study accomplished by injecting dye or air into the lateral ventricles through burr holes (Fig. 10-15). Distortions and obstructions, usually the result of tumors, are located.

Nursing care. The radiological studies may be done in the x-ray department or the surgical suite of a hospital. The presurgical routine, including a sedative, may be indicated. The frontal portion of the head may be shaved for a ventriculogram. If angiography is contemplated, peripheral pulses should be assessed and marked. If a carotid or vertebral puncture is anticipated, neck circumference should be measured and recorded. A primary responsibility of the nurse is to record baseline neurological data and to explain the nature and rationale of the study to the client.

Following completion of these radiological procedures, nursing care includes those considerations relative to care after a lumbar puncture. The client should be instructed to remain flat and quiet for several hours and frequent assessments made of vital and neurological signs. (Elevation of the bed to a semi-Fowler's position is preferred following ventriculography.) If vomiting occurs, it should be quickly managed by medications because it raises intracranial pressure. Some physicians believe that forcing fluids is important in hastening absorption of contrast media and in replacing CSF volume, thus reducing headache risk.

Since autonomic centers are close to ventricles, they may be irritated by air or contrast media introduced during the procedures. Increased salivation, perspiration, and respiratory secretions may be noted. Chilling, bradycardia, nausea, and vomiting are sometimes observed. Although these signs and symp-

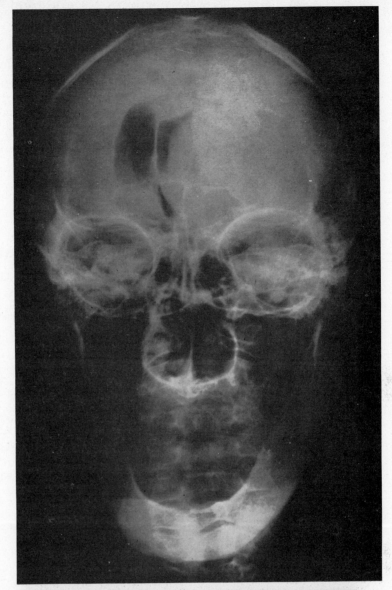

FIG. 10-14
Pneumoencephalogram (abnormal), showing a shift and distortion of the lateral and third ventricles. This was caused by an intracranial tumor. (From Conway-Rutkowski, Barbara Lang: Carini and Owens' Neurological and neurosurgical nursing, ed. 8, St. Louis, 1982, The C.V. Mosby Co.)

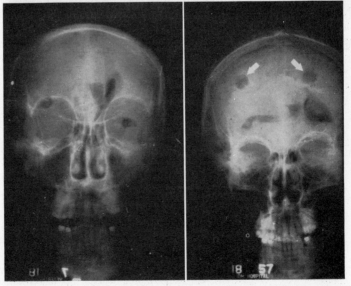

FIG. 10-15
Ventriculogram showing right parietal tumor. Air has been injected into the lateral ventricles through the bilateral parietoccipital burr holes (arrows). The entire ventricular system is shifted to the left by the right-sided mass. (From Liechty, Richard D., and Soper, Robert T.: Synopsis of surgery, ed. 2, St. Louis, 1974, The C.V. Mosby Co.)

toms are transient (subsiding in a few hours), they require skillful nursing management in order to keep the client comfortable.

All environmental stimuli, including bright lights, should be reduced, because most clients experience increased irritability following these procedures.

If headache occurs, management should be accomplished with drugs that are not also antipyretics, because masking fever could prevent early detection of meningitis. Rectal temperatures are recommended for greater accuracy.

Angiography complications (both local and systemic) must be anticipated and minimized by the nursing care management. Vasospasms, cerebral emboli, seizures, hematomas, thrombosis, cardiac dysrhythmias, and allergic reactions to the dye must be considered.

GLASGOW COMA SCALE

The Glasgow coma scale has been designed to quantitatively relate consciousness to motor responses, verbal responses, and eye opening. Coma is defined as no response and no eye opening. Scores of 7 or less on the Glasgow scale qualify as ''coma''; all scores of 9 or more do not qualify as ''coma.'' The examiner determines the *best* response the patient can make to a set of standardized stimuli. Higher points are assigned to responses that indicate increasing degrees of arousal.

1. **Best motor response.** (Examiner determines the *best* response with *either* arm.)
   a. *6 points*. Obeys simple commands. Raises arm on request or holds up specified number of fingers. Releasing a grip (not grasping, which can be reflexive) is also an appropriate test.
   b. *5 points*. Localizes noxious stimuli. Fails to obey commands but can move either arm toward a noxious cutaneous stimulus and eventually contacts it with the hand. The stimulus should be maximal and applied in various locations, i.e., sternum pressure, or trapezius pinch.
   c. *4 points*. Flexion withdrawal. Responds to noxious stimulus with arm flexion but does not localize it with the hand.
   d. *3 points*. Abnormal flexion. Adducts shoulder, flexes and pronates arm, flexes wrist, and makes a fist in response to a noxious stimulus (decorticate rigidity).
   e. *2 points*. Abnormal extension. Adducts and internally rotates shoulder, extends forearm, flexes wrist, and makes a fist in response to a noxious stimulus (decerebrate rigidity).
   f. *1 point*. No motor response. Exclude reasons for no response; for example, insufficient stimulus or spinal cord injury.
2. **Best verbal response.** (Examiner determines the *best* response after arousal. Noxious stimuli are employed if necessary.) Omit this test if the patient is dysphasic, has oral injuries, or is intubated. Place a check mark after other two test category scores after totaling to indicate omission of the verbal response section.
   a. *5 points*. Oriented patient. Can converse and relate who he is, where he is, and the year and month.
   b. *4 points*. Confused patient. Is not fully oriented or demonstrates confusion.
   c. *3 points*. Verbalizes. Does not engage in sustained conversation, but uses intelligible words in an exclamation (curse) or in a disorganized manner which is nonsensical.
   d. *2 points*. Vocalizes. Makes moaning or groaning sounds that are not recognizable words.
   e. *1 point*. No vocalization. Does not make any sound even in response to noxious stimulus.
3. **Eye opening.** (Examiner determines the minimum stimulus that evokes opening of one or both eyes.) If the patient cannot realistically open the eyes because of bandages or lid edema, write ''E'' after the total test score to indicate omission of this component.
   a. *4 points*. Eyes open spontaneously.
   b. *3 points*. Eyes open to speech. Patient opens eyes in response to command or on being called by name.
   c. *2 points*. Eyes open to noxious stimuli.
   d. *1 point*. No eye opening in response to noxious stimuli.

From Teasdale, G., and Jennett, B.: Assessment of coma and impaired consciousness, Lancet **2**:81-84, 1974.

The puncture site should be inspected frequently for a developing hematoma or bleeding. Pulses distal to the puncture must be palpated to detect arterial occlusion. The temperature and color of the extremities should be compared to confirm circulatory adequacy and equality.

A carotid puncture site may be managed with an ice collar, but again, it is essential to visually assess the site frequently. Edema can be detected by serial neck measurements compared with those taken before the angiography. Neck swelling may impair respirations so that the rate and character of breathing is also regularly assessed and recorded.

Femoral sites are often covered with a sandbag for 3 or 4 hours to control bleeding and to prevent hematoma. It should be noted that clients with blood dyscrasias, hypertension, or who have been receiving anticoagulant therapy may need even more scrutiny to prevent complications.

Cerebrovascular accidents and arterial occlusions must be constant concerns of the nurse caring for the client having cerebral angiography.

Level of consciousness

Many factors that interfere with normal functioning of the central nervous system affect the level of consciousness. Consciousness implies that there is a continuous and effective interaction between the cerebral hemispheres and the reticular activating systems of the upper brainstem. Consciousness consists of two components: (1) the content, or total mental functions, and (2) arousal, or the degree of wakefulness. The content is linked to cerebral functioning and arousal to the brainstem. These two factors can vary considerably and independently from nil to a physiological maximum. The level of consciousness is assessed by estimating behaviors. Factors such as alcoholism, psychic withdrawal, and motor paralysis can seriously deter evaluation of both content and arousal components. The scale on p. 388 is one way to grade the levels of consciousness.

Data analysis

After the nurse has collected relevant data about the client, the information is compared with norms appropriate to the client's age, sex, developmental level, and family and social background. The assessment phase of the nursing process ends with analysis of data and the formulation of nursing diagnoses or a problem list. Potential or actual diagnoses may include impaired verbal communication, ineffective coping, fear, grieving, impaired home maintenance management, impaired mobility, self-care deficit, alterations in sensory perceptions, sexual dysfunction, impaired skin integrity, alterations in thought process, disturbance in self-concept, potential for injury, diversional activity deficit, and alteration in bowel elimination.

Planning

PLANNING FOR HEALTH PROMOTION

Dietary factors

A sound program of diet, exercise, risk management, and attention to personal safety is advised throughout life to maintain a healthy nervous system.

Dietary factors that affect the central nervous system are operant during prenatal development and are even more prominent in infancy and early childhood. Because the brain reaches near adult size by age 4, nutrition during these

389

years is an important consideration. Essential fluids and electrolytes, particularly calcium, is required for normal nerve irritability and muscle contractions. Thiamine and niacin are required for the breakdown of glucose and the support of the nervous tissue. Deficiencies may be first noted when peripheral nerves become irritable and fail to function normally. All four basic food groups are required to ensure adequate intake of these essential coenzymes. Vitamin B_6 is another important element that supports nervous system functioning. Deficiencies may be evidenced by nervous irritability and even seizures. Again, attention to the basic food groups alone will ensure the basal vitamin B_6 needs. Finally, Vitamin B_{12} has a significant role in the metabolism of nervous tissue. Deficiencies create poor coordination, and in some cases, even slowed mental functioning. The nurse can reassure clients that a regular diet with recommended daily allowances will meet these fundamental needs for nutrients to support nervous tissue. Anemias, however, including iron-deficiency anemia, must be managed judiciously to ensure that enough oxygen-carrying cells are present for delivery of the required oxygen to the brain.

Exercise

Regular exercise is essential for developing normal neuromuscular control and coordination. When aging occurs, there is a definite need for continual stimulation to prevent degenerative processes. Weight control and regular exercise are vital elements in a program to control atherosclerotic phenomena and thus prevent degenerative cardiovascular disease, which may lead to strokes and their devastating consequences.

Personal safety

Trauma is a leading cause of morbidity in children and young adults and almost invariably involves head and spinal cord injury. Attention to protective headgear when engaging in certain sports and motorcycling could significantly reduce many serious neurological injuries. Back injuries are among the leaders in disabling trauma, too. Good body mechanics, if practiced routinely, could drastically curtail these problems.

Finally, many neurological tragedies are the result of automobile accidents. The use of safety belts on a regular basis has been demonstrated to be a distinct advantage for both the driver and passengers. Health care workers can be instrumental in promoting routine practices that minimize risks of vehicular accidents, such as the wearing of protective helmets and the use of safety belts.

PLANNING FOR HEALTH MAINTENANCE AND RESTORATION: UNCONSCIOUS CLIENT

Nursing care planning for the client with a nervous system problem involves an understanding of basic physiological responses that occur when the brain or spinal cord is insulted by trauma or disease. Because the nurse has a crucial role in monitoring the client's reaction to therapeutic management, a thorough knowledge of the effects of increased intracranial pressure, seizures, syncope, and headache is needed. For clients with altered levels of consciousness or paralysis, specific skills are required for care planning during the acute phase and to promote rehabilitation.

Unconsciousness is a state of depressed cerebral function in which the reaction to stimuli is lost, and any response, if present, is on the reflex level.[4] The depth of unconsciousness varies (for example, from stupor to coma [see Glasgow Coma Scale, p. 388]).

Causes of unconsciousness. Several factors may be responsible for producing an unconscious state. Regardless of the state of unconsciousness, however, the basic mechanism that produces it relates to an interruption of the oxygen and glucose supply as well as an interference with the transmission of neurons.[24] Among the factors that may cause unconsciousness are drugs (alcohol, barbiturates, anesthetics) and drug overdose, which block synaptic transmission; cerebral ischemia (for example, thrombosis, embolism), which decreases oxygen and glucose supply to the brain; space-occupying lesions (tumor, hemorrhage, abscess, cerebral edema), which depress the reticular activating system and increase cerebral resistance; trauma (head injuries such as concussion, contusion, lacerations); electrolyte imbalances (such as sodium and potassium deficiencies), which prevent transmission of neuronal impulses; and diseases or conditions such as uremia, hypoglycemia, diabetes, encephalitis, meningitis, and seizures.

Nursing care is essential to the care of an unconscious client. Such a client is totally dependent on nursing care to maintain him during this state. Therefore nursing care should be planned to meet the following objectives:

- Maintain a patent airway.
- Monitor vital signs and neurological status.
- Maintain integrity of the skin.
- Maintain joint mobility.
- Maintain sensory function.
- Maintain fluid and nutritional status.
- Maintain bowel and bladder function.
- Maintain psychosocial function.

Assessing for and maintaining a patent airway

The highest priority of nursing care is to maintain a patent airway. Relaxation of the muscles of the pharynx, in clients who are semicomatose, permits the lower jaw and tongue to fall backward, and subsequently obstructs the airway.[3] Signs indicative of airway obstruction are noisy breathing and irregular respirations.

An oral airway may be placed in the oral cavity to maintain a patent airway. Suctioning and positioning are other measures to maintain airway patency. The unconscious client cannot get rid of mucus, and therefore the nasopharyngeal and oral secretions may be aspirated as frequently as necessary. Care must be maintained during suctioning to prevent trauma and irritation. Either of these serves only to increase the amount of secretions. For a discussion of the principles of suctioning see Chapter 21.

The client should be turned frequently from the right lateral to the left lateral and the semiprone positions. These positions facilitate drainage of secretions from the oral cavity and prevent the tongue from falling back to obstruct the airway. The supine position should never be used, because it favors aspiration of secretions. If the client wears dentures, these should be removed for the duration of the coma. The nostrils should be kept clean. Any encrustations or discharge should be removed frequently.

Monitoring vital signs and neurological status

Assessments should be made of vital signs and neurological status when the client is admitted. The initial assessments serve as a basis for comparing later assessments.

In assessing the vital signs, the nurse must not only assess the rate of the pulse and respiration but also observe their quality and rhythm so that proper therapy can be implemented before a complication such as increased intracranial pressure occurs (see Fig. 10-47). Therefore, any significant changes should be evaluated and reported to the physician. In the unconscious client, the temperature should be taken rectally. (One exception to this is the client whose disease process involves hemorrhage. In such cases, rectal temperatures are generally contraindicated because of vagal stimulation. Any vagal stimulation may increase the cranial pressure and thus increase the hemorrhage.) The alternative route, axillary, should be used.

In addition to vital signs, neurological assessments ("neuro checks") should be made and include assessment of the level of consciousness, pupillary reaction, motor strength, and sensory function.

In assessing the level of consciousness, the nurse should observe and specifically define the type of stimuli, if any, to which the client responds (for example, verbal or painful stimuli). The client's ability to follow simple commands should be assessed. The client's responses should be recorded as descriptively as possible (see elsewhere in this chapter for a complete discussion of levels of consciousness). Assess whether or not the client is oriented to time, place, or person.

When assessing pupillary reaction, the nurse should observe the size, shape, and equality of the pupils as well as the pupillary reaction to light. To assess the latter, the nurse covers one of the client's eyes, shines a penlight into the other eye, and notes the response. The same is repeated for the opposite eye. Normally, the pupils constrict briskly when exposed to light. This assessment should be made in a darkened room, because this will facilitate observing the reaction.

An assessment should be made of the presence or absence of voluntary movement and the client's handgrip and motor strength. The assessment of the latter is an indication of the function of the descending pathways.[3] The nurse might ask the client to "squeeze my fingers" or "move your leg" and note the client's ability to follow the request.

Maintaining integrity of the skin

Clients with neurological problems have a tendency toward sensory impairment to the skin. As a result, they are more prone to develop decubiti. If the integrity of the client's skin is to be maintained, the nurse must know the factors responsible for producing skin breakdown. Various factors have been identified. Pressure is considered to be the primary factor. Pressure on a particular area causes tissue to be squeezed between the underlying bone and the skin surface. As a result, blood flow to the area is reduced, and if pressure is allowed to continue, tissue damage occurs. Areas that lie over bony prominences—iliac crest, great femoral trochanters, heels, elbows, ears, ischial tuberosities, scapulas, or sacrum—are most often affected. These parts therefore must particularly be protected from pressure.

One factor related to pressure is *intensity,* and it has been demonstrated that low pressures for long periods of time produce more damage than high pressures for short periods.[11] Another factor that should be considered is the *shearing force.* It occurs when the client is in bed with the head of the bed elevated approximately 30 degrees or more or when he sits at a reclining angle in a chair. In either situation he tends to slide downward, and as a result, a great force is exerted through the ischial tuberosities by the entire weight of the trunk, which presses on this small area. Therefore, measures must be included in the care plan that will help relieve pressure and reduce the shearing force.[9]

A regular turning schedule must be established. The client's position should be changed as frequently as necessary. Unless he is comatose, all positions—prone, supine, and lateral—should be used. When the client's position is being changed, care must be taken not to drag him over the sheet, because this practice also causes damage to subcutaneous tissue and ruptures small vessels.

As the client is changed from one position to another, the nurse should observe his skin closely for signs that indicate the formation of a pressure area.[1] Bony prominences must particularly be observed. Ischemia, the first stage of pressure formation, is characterized by blanching. The appearance of this sign indicates the need for more frequent position change. The surrounding area should be massaged, and the client should not be positioned on that area. Other devices such as sheepskin, foam rubber, gel pads, and flotation beds may be instituted during this stage to prevent further damage. In addition to relieving pressure, sheepskin or its synthetic kin tends to absorb moisture from the client's body while the wool promotes warmth and dryness. Air is also thought to circulate through the springy fibers of the sheepskin. Although this has been thought to be the case, nurses should be cognizant that sheepskin causes some clients to perspire; therefore, its usefulness for them would be nil.

The alternating-pressure mattress may also be used to relieve pressure. The CircOlectric bed may be employed to facilitate turning, as well as to stimulate circulation.

The second stage of pressure formation is the stage of hyperemia. Redness and increased temperature to the pressure area are manifestations of this stage. This is the stage in which the sore is actually observed. Cell destruction and hemorrhage have already occurred. Circulation to the area must be increased. In order to accomplish this, the nurse should gently massage around the reddened area in a circular motion each time the client's position is changed. Such action prevents further damage to the skin.

A break in the skin (ulcer) is the last stage to develop.[1] This stage may develop within a day after blanching is observed if measures are not planned to prevent further damage. Therefore, measures must be employed *before* ulceration occurs.

Weight should be distributed evenly over a wide area to alleviate pressure within a given area. Therefore, when changing the client's position, the nurse should avoid point pressure on a particular area. The bed must be free of wrinkles and debris.

Excessive moisture is also responsible for tissue damage. Moisture on the skin may result from urination or from excessive perspiration. Moisture from any source reduces the skin's resistance to other physical factors such as pressure or friction. Urine contains urea, which is decomposed by bacteria and changed to ammonia. The latter is highly irritating and easily produces cell destruction if measures are not taken to keep the skin free of urine. The skin must be kept clean and dry by washing with soap and water as often as necessary. When linen becomes wet, it should be changed promptly. Powder may be spread evenly and sparingly over the buttocks to help absorb moisture. Tissue resistance is lessened when the diet is inadequate in the basic nutritional factors (proteins, carbohydrates, fats, and vitamins). Therefore, the nurse must help the client maintain an adequate diet by providing foods that he can chew and swallow and assist him with his meals as much as necessary to ensure that these foods are eaten.

Maintaining joint mobility   Measures to prevent deformities must be started during the acute period and must be continued throughout the client's hospitalization. These measures include proper positioning, frequent turning, and exercises.

Positioning. Correct positioning is essential in preventing deformities of the extremities. Upper extremity deformities include adduction deformities and internal rotation of the arm, flexion contractures of the elbow, and wrist drop; lower extremity deformities include adduction and external rotation of the hip, flexion contractures of the hip and knee, and foot drop. Both upper and lower deformities can be prevented by maintaining correct positioning. The erect body in correct posture shows the center of gravity of the head, arms, and trunk situated slightly behind the hip joint. When paralysis is present, the force of gravity pulls paralyzed muscles out of position. The nurse must therefore intervene to facilitate maintenance of the body in as near functional position as possible.

Mechanical aids. Mechanical aids should be provided for support, while at the same time maintaining proper position. A *bed board* should be placed under the mattress to provide better skeletal support. Commercial *footboards* are available; however, the nurse may improvise by using a heavy cardboard box or rolled blankets to prevent deformities of the feet. Blankets are thought to be more adjustable to the contour of the feet and can more effectively be used while the client assumes the supine position. Tennis shoes are commonly used in many institutions to prevent foot deformities. *Trochanter rolls* should be provided to prevent outward rotation of the affected hip. Blankets, mattress pads, pillows, and sandbags are frequently used as trochanter rolls. *Hand rolls* are used for the hand to maintain a functional position, thereby preventing flexion contractures of the fingers. These are made by folding two washcloths together in half, rolling them, and securing them with tape. Hand rolls made of soft material are most beneficial for the flaccid hand, whereas a hard cone should be used for the spastic hand.

Basic positions. Three basic positions can be used for the client who must remain in bed: the supine, lateral, and prone positions. Modifications of these positions may be made. For example, the lateral position can be adapted to a half-sidelying, or half-lateral, position. Regardless of the position used, maintenance of correct alignment is essential (Fig. 10-16).

Supine position. When a client assumes the supine position, the body should be in full extension, a position that closely resembles the upright position. A small pillow should be placed under the head to keep the neck in extension. The shoulders and hips should be straight. The feet should be placed firmly against a footboard to prevent foot drop and contraction of the Achilles tendon. The heels should be free from the mattress to alleviate pressure on them. Often ample space can be provided between the mattress and footboard to accomplish this. However, if space is not provided, a small sponge pad or small pillow may be placed under the heels for this purpose. To prevent outward (external) rotation of the affected hip, a trochanter roll should be placed on the side of the extremity extending from the hip to just above the knee (Fig. 10-16, *A*).

A number of positions may be used for the upper extremities. Each position is planned to prevent frozen shoulder or an adduction deformity. The upper extremity should be abducted preferably at right angles to the shoulders. While the arm is in this position, the elbow may be flexed, with the forearm rotated and resting forward, or the arm may be extended over the head, with the forearm resting on a pillow. The wrist should be in a supine position, with the fingers and thumb around a hand roll to maintain the functional position.

Poor venous drainage, possibly from decreased movement and vascular and

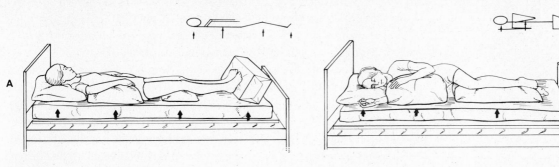

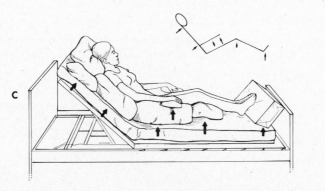

FIG. 10-16
Proper positioning for client in **A,** supine, **B,** sidelying, and **C,** semi-Fowler's positions. Arrows indicate where support should be placed. (Courtesy Metropolitan Life Insurance Co., New York.)

lymphatic stasis, produces swelling and dependent edema. These symptoms can be prevented with proper positioning of the extremities. The distal joints should always be higher than the proximal ones. For example, the forearm and wrist should be placed higher than the elbow.

Lateral position (sidelying). In the lateral position, a full-sized pillow may be used under the head to promote comfort and maintain alignment. The back must be straight. Pillows may be used to support the back and to keep the body in straight alignment. If used, they should be placed lengthwise and firmly from the client's shoulders to midbuttocks. The upper leg should be flexed at the hip or knee. One or more pillows should be placed under the upper leg, extending from the knee to the foot, to prevent internal rotation of the hip. The lower leg should be extended in a straight line with the spine, or it may be flexed at the knee. The feet must also be well supported. Care must be maintained not to permit the top leg to rest directly on the bottom leg. Such a practice may result in damage to the intimal lining of the vessels of the legs, which then becomes a primary source for thrombus formation. The buttocks should be pulled slightly backward so that the body is maintained in straight alignment (Fig. 10-16, *B*).

Several positions may be used for the upper extremities. The top arm can be placed in front of the client and supported with pillows, or it may be placed at the client's side. The lower arm can be placed on a pillow at the head. The wrist should be extended, and a roll placed in the hand.

Prone position. Although the prone position is the only position that permits full extension of the hip, it is seldom used. Its use should be encouraged. When the prone position is used, the feet should be extended over the end of the mattress. A small pillow may be used to free the toes from the mattress if the space between the bed and mattress is not adequate. A small pillow may be placed under the abdomen for support. While this position is maintained, the arms may

395

be placed at the sides or at right angles to the body. Another position that may be used is with the shoulders externally rotated and the opposite arm internally rotated. No pillows should be used under the head for this position.

Range-of-motion exercises. Range-of-motion exercises are performed to provide full movement for all joints of the body. They prevent joint and muscular contractures and thereby facilitate maintenance of joint mobility. These exercises also help maintain muscle tone and improve venous and lymphatic circulation. Exercises for a client with a cerebrovascular accident should be started on the day of admission and continued three or four times a day throughout hospitalization. Each joint should be moved at least four or five times during each exercise period.

Although range-of-motion exercise is an independent nursing function, the nurse should not hesitate to consult the physician if there is even a slight doubt about the advisability for instituting exercises for a client.

Before performing range-of-motion exercises, the nurse must be cognizant of normal movements of the joints and muscles, as follows:

MOVEMENTS OF THE EXTREMITIES

abduction Movement away from center of body.
adduction Movement toward the center of the body.
circumduction Movement of the distal part of a limb in a circle, while the proximal end is fixed.
extension Movement to straighten out joints.
flexion Movement to bend joints.
hyperextension Movement that extends beyond the ordinary range.
inward rotation Movement that turns inward toward the center.
outward rotation Movement that turns outward away from the center.
rotation Movement of the body part around its axis.

MOVEMENTS OF THE UPPER EXTREMITIES

opposition Movement of the thumb toward the little finger.
pronation Turning downward.
supination Turning upward.

MOVEMENTS OF THE FEET

dorsiflexion Movement that bends a joint backward.
plantar flexion Movement that bends a joint forward.
eversion Movement that turns the feet outward.
inversion Movement that turns the feet inward.

The major types of range of motion exercises are passive, active, and active assistance. Regardless of the type of exercise used, the nurse should observe and record the degree of movement, the presence of pain or spasticity, any limitation of movement, and the client's overall tolerance to the activity. The nurse's observations should be recorded as accurately and descriptively as possible.

Passive range-of-motion exercises. Passive range-of-motion exercises are performed by someone other than the client at a time when the client cannot do so himself. When passive exercises are performed, the nurse must follow these basic principles:

1. The client should be placed in correct alignment for the exercises.
2. The client should be instructed to relax.
3. Restrictive clothing should be removed.

4. Exercises should be carried out slowly, gently, and rhythmically while each joint is moved through the client's full range of motion.
5. The joints above and below the joint to be moved must be supported while it is in motion.
6. The belly of the muscle should not be held but should be supported by cupping the muscle above and below the joint.
7. The joint should not be taken beyond the point of resistance or pain. If this is allowed to happen, the exercise becomes a stretching exercise, which requires an order from the physician and should only be performed by a physical therapist. Care must particularly be maintained if the muscles are flaccid.
8. In the moving of an extremity with spastic paralysis, the movement should be performed slowly to prevent spasms. If the muscle becomes spastic during the exercises, the nurse should stop the exercise until the muscle relaxes.
9. Assessments of a client's normal range of motion can be made if the unaffected extremity is exercised first.
10. The nurse should maintain proper body mechanics to avoid unnecessary strain as well as conserve energy.

The exercises of flexion, extension, rotation, abduction, and adduction can be incorporated with the bath. For example, during the bath the nurse can raise and lower the client's head for neck flexion and extension and open and close the paralyzed fingers for flexion and extension. The forearm can be pronated and supinated; the elbow and wrist flexed, extended, abducted, and adducted. The leg can be raised and lowered and moved inward and outward for flexion, extension, abduction, and adduction of the hip joint. It is important that these exercises be carried out not only on the involved extremities but on the uninvolved extremities as well. There have been reports that clients have developed contractures on the uninvolved side because the nurses worked diligently with the affected side but neglect the unaffected side.

Participation from family members must be encouraged. They should be instructed on the rationale for and how to correctly perform range-of-motion exercises (Fig. 10-17).

Active range-of-motion exercises. Active range-of-motion exercises are performed by the client without assistance from other individuals or mechanical means. These exercises are beneficial in maintaining the strength of muscles. As a result, muscular atrophy is prevented. They should be encouraged and carried out under the supervision of the nurse until assurance is given that the client can carry them out alone. He should be encouraged to think about the movement of the joints as the exercises are performed. If the client can adequately carry out normal activities, then a special plan is not necessary.

Active assistance exercises. When these are performed, the client exercises with assistance from himself, another person, or a mechanical device. When the client assists himself, he uses the unaffected extremity to assist in movement of the affected one. The client should be encouraged to perform these as soon as possible. The nurse should observe the client carefully so that assistance can be given as necessary. Pulleys are the devices used for active assistance exercises (Fig. 10-18). Rest periods should be planned after the exercises.

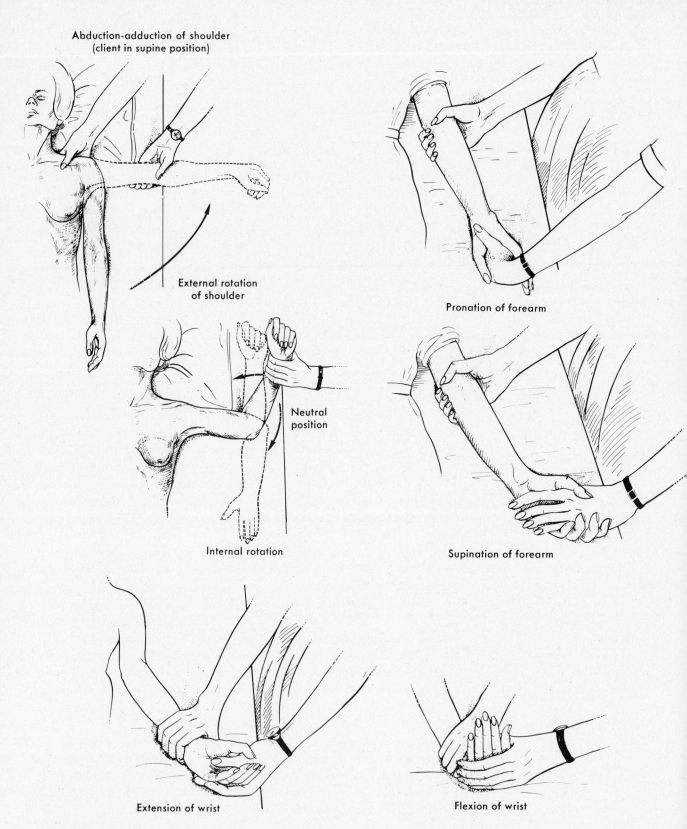

Abduction-adduction of shoulder
(client in supine position)

External rotation
of shoulder

Neutral
position

Internal rotation

Pronation of forearm

Supination of forearm

Extension of wrist

Flexion of wrist

FIG. 10-17
Passive range-of-motion exercises. All joints should be taken through a full range of motion three or four times each day.

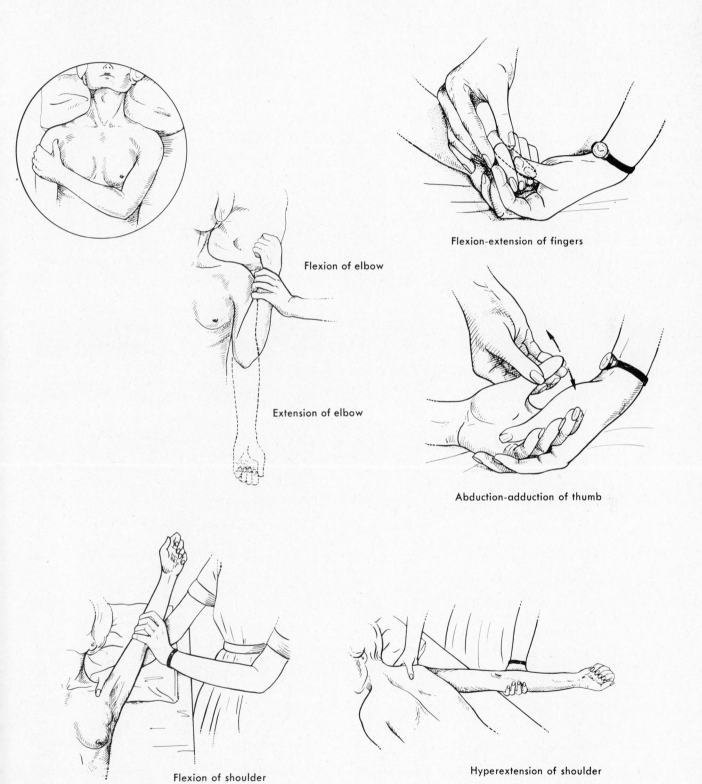

Flexion-extension of fingers

Flexion of elbow

Extension of elbow

Abduction-adduction of thumb

Flexion of shoulder

Hyperextension of shoulder

Continued.

FIG. 10-17, cont'd
Passive range-of-motion exercises.

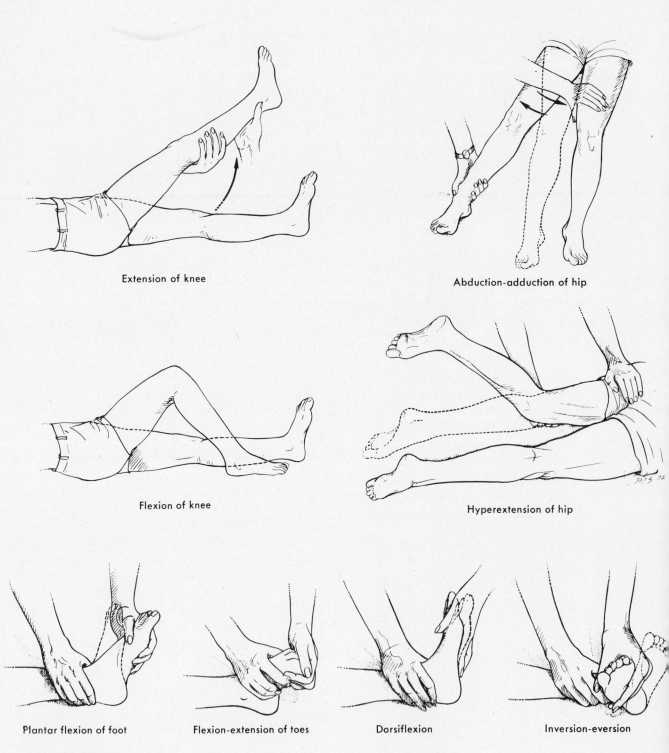

Extension of knee

Abduction-adduction of hip

Flexion of knee

Hyperextension of hip

Plantar flexion of foot

Flexion-extension of toes

Dorsiflexion

Inversion-eversion

FIG. 10-17, cont'd
Passive range-of-motion exercises.

FIG. 10-18
Pulley exercises allow the client to use the uninvolved extremity to assist in movement of the involved shoulder. Note that the glove on the left hand helps the client hold the bar. (From Rusk, Howard A.: Rehabilitation medicine, ed. 4, St. Louis, 1977, The C.V. Mosby Co.)

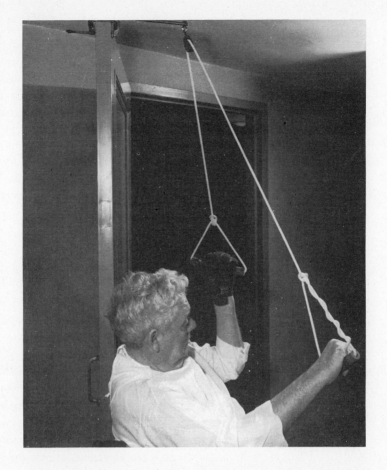

Maintaining sensory function

A client who is unconscious is often not able to close his eyes, or he may lose his blinking reflex, especially if the facial nerve is involved. When normal eye secretions are not spread by blinking, the cornea becomes dry. Absence of the reflex causes the eye to remain opened and may predispose the client to corneal ulcers. The nurse must therefore observe the characteristics of the eye on the affected side and report any changes so that measures can be prescribed to protect the eye. Special ophthalmic solutions may be prescribed for irrigation or instillation three to four times a day. A butterfly gauze may also be used to keep the eye closed.

The sense of *hearing* is the last faculty to be lost in an unconscious client. He may therefore be able to hear although his physical response is nil. Thus the nurse must communicate as though he can hear. Family members must be cautioned about the client's probable hearing ability. The nurse must converse with the client and keep him informed of all aspects of care. Explanations should be kept simple until he is responsive and the nurse is assured he can understand more detailed explanations.

Maintaining fluid and nutritional status

During the unconscious period as much as 3000 ml per day of fluids and electrolytes may be administered intravenously. In prolonged coma, intravenous fluids should be discontinued, and a nasogastric tube inserted for feedings. When gavage feedings are ordered, the nurse must determine the amount and frequency of each feeding. Explanations of the principles of gavage feedings are found in Chapter 17.

Nursing process for common health problems

After the comatose period is over and the gag reflex returns, the client may be given fluids by mouth. Solid foods are gradually added. The importance of the nurse's checking the gag reflex before administering fluids or foods cannot be overemphasized. This test may be made by touching the posterior pharynx with a cotton swab and observing whether or not the client swallows. If the reflex is present, the client should be spoon-fed. Several approaches have been suggested for feeding the client with paralysis of one side of the mouth. Foods may be placed in the unaffected side of the mouth or in the middle of the mouth. The nurse should observe the client closely and use the method that seems most effective.

Oral hygiene should be administered after feeding and every 2 hours during the day to prevent drying of the mucous membrane and parotitis. Parotitis develops from lack of stimulation of the salivary glands. As a result, the ducts of these glands become congested. If the client wears dentures, these should be removed and cleansed at least four times each day, and the mouth rinsed with cold water or with mouthwash before they are replaced. Not only do these measures remove debris, but refreshed oral mucosa may enhance the client's interest in food.

Regardless of the route of fluid administration, accurate records must be kept of intake and output. In addition, keeping records of the client's weight helps determine the degree of fluid balance.

Maintaining bladder and bowel function

The comatose client is generally incontinent of urine and feces. Retention may also occur. The former occurs if there is motor loss; whereas sensory loss results in the latter. An indwelling catheter is prescribed and usually remains until the client regains consciousness. When a catheter is inserted, it is the responsibility of the nurse to plan for maintenance of the catheter. Efforts must be directed toward preventing urinary tract infections by applying principles of asepsis as catheter care is given. The amount and character of the urine must be observed. For a discussion of catheter care and bladder training see Chapter 18.

Since bowel control is not present in the unconscious client, the nurse should observe the client for incontinence, constipation, or impaction. An awareness that diarrhea is an early sign of fecal impaction should alert the nurse to check the client for an impaction. If he does not have a bowel movement for 2 or 3 days or if the stool is hard, nursing measures must be employed to prevent constipation or an impaction. In the comatose client, the rectum may be stimulated at the same time daily unless hemorrhage is the cause of the disease process. In such cases rectal stimulation may increase intracranial pressure and should be avoided. Suppositories or enemas may be prescribed. When the client regains consciousness, other measures such as wetting agents (stool softeners) and mild laxatives may be prescribed. A diet high in bulk and adequate in fluids should be encouraged. The client should be placed on the toilet or commode after breakfast or at the time of his normal schedule. Privacy must be provided. Regardless of the routine followed the basic principle for a successful bowel program is *regularity*. Refer to Chapter 18 for a summary of bowel training.

Maintaining psychosocial function

When a client regains consciousness, varied reactions may be observed. He may be frightened, apprehensive, confused, depressed, and demanding. Inability of the client to recognize his environment, to speak clearly or at all, or to move his arm or leg may provoke added anxiety. He may have intravenous fluids in progress. He may have a catheter in place. He may laugh or cry at inappropriate times. He may be irritated with little provocation and may use profanity. The whole situation may cause him apprehension and embarrassment.

The nurse should assess the state of the client and explain to him in simple terms what happened, the reasons for therapeutic measures, and the basis for his behaviors. He should be oriented to his environment, and as much emotional support as necessary should be given. If he is apprehensive, a quiet, restful environment should be provided to promote a sense of security.

If the client uses profane words, the nurse must accept them without comments or displeasure, because he is not able to inhibit these reactions. Efforts to scold or correct him may only serve to frustrate him more, thus increasing the use of profanity. Therefore situations that evoke this behavior should be avoided as much as possible.

The nurse should also spend time with the family, assessing their reactions to the client's behavior and helping them understand the basis for it. They must be instructed on how to deal with it and the importance of accepting the client as he is.

Implementation

COMMON HEALTH PROBLEMS OF THE NEONATE AND INFANT

Hydrocephalus

Hydrocephalus is a condition characterized by an abnormal accumulation of cerebrospinal fluid (CSF) in the cranial vault. It may be caused by an excessive production or faulty resorption of the fluid, or it may result from an obstruction in the normal circulatory channels.

When cerebrospinal fluid is produced too rapidly, does not circulate freely, or is not resorbed with ease, the excess in its quantity becomes pathological, a condition known as hydrocephalus. The exact type and degree of the consequences depend on the cause of the condition. Sometimes hydrocephalus may be termed noncommunicating (intraventricular) or communicating (extraventricular). *Noncommunicating hydrocephalus* is a partial or complete obstruction between the ventricles and subarachnoid space. It may be caused by an infection, tumor, or maldevelopment of the CSF circulation pathway. *Communicating hydrocephalus* is a defect in absorption of CSF that occurs as a result of a congenital defect such as Arnold-Chiari malformation, meningeal hemorrhage, or adhesions between meninges.[24] Communicating hydrocephalus implies not an interference in circulation but rather an accumulation of fluid because of an inability to diffuse into the venous sinuses by way of the arachnoid villi. The most common type is noncommunicating hydrocephalus, congenital in origin.

 Assessment. The head of the young child has an enlarging space potential because of the nonunion of suture line and the presence of fontanels, thus providing considerable room for expansion within the skull. As the accumulation of fluid causes a rise in intracranial pressure, the sutures separate, allowing the head to enlarge. The child with advanced hydrocephalus has a characteristic appearance, with a large rounded skull, a thin scalp with engorged superficial veins, sparse hair, and a small triangular face. The frontal bone arches down to the root of the nose, the sockets of the eyes are widely separated, and the temples have an overhanging appearance. The fontanels may be bulging and pulsating. The roof of the eye orbit may be depressed, and the eyeballs displaced downward and outward with scleral prominence, referred to by some as "sunset eyes."

Nursing process for common health problems

The infant with hydrocephalus is irritable, anorexic, feeble, and has a high-pitched cry and decreased motor power. Hemiplegia, spastic paraplegia, and absence of deep reflexes may accompany the other clinical manifestations. It is not uncommon for the child to develop motor skills late, especially walking. Although some children with hydrocephalus are retarded, others have normal or above-average intelligence. However, if the disease is allowed to progress and the brain is subjected to severe pressure, retardation is likely to develop concurrent with organic damage.

Hydrocephalus is usually diagnosed by the appearance of the child, the increasing head circumference, neurological signs, and confirmed by ventriculography or CAT scan. Transillumination is helpful in diagnosing communicating hydrocephalus.

Data analysis
Data analysis may reveal nursing diagnoses of sensory perception alterations, impairment of skin integrity, and ineffective family coping.

Planning and implementation. Nursing care is planned to help parents cope, to monitor neurological status, to prevent pulmonary and integumentary complications, and to maintain adequate nutrition. The nurse must help parents cope with the child with hydrocephalus. The stigma of the characteristic appearance associated with the condition cannot be ignored. Because the infant has the usual needs for nurture but must be especially protected and cared for, the health team should provide specific instructions related to management and observations for increased intracranial pressure, particularly if the child is to be cared for in the home.

The child's position must be changed frequently to protect the thin, delicate scalp, which is sensitive to pressure. Foam pillows, gel pads, or water pillows may be useful in distributing weight of the large head. The infant's head and body should be turned at the same time to prevent trauma. The head should always be supported when the child is lifted, carried, or held. Since the child has little or no control of his head position, it is advisable to position him on his side after a feeding, with the head elevated to prevent aspiration if vomiting should occur.

Observations to determine whether there is progression of the condition should be made daily by routine measurements of the head, examination of the sutures and fontanels, and notation of any behavioral changes such as decreasing alertness, vomiting, or seizures. Protection from infections is also important for this weakened child.

If the cranial vault has enlarged to the extent that the upper eyelids are elevated substantially and cannot close completely, the eyes should be protected from dryness and ulceration. Other aspects of care should be determined primarily by the child's age and general physical condition.

When surgical intervention is performed, the general principles of management remain the same. However, added attention should be directed toward caring for the head dressing. The nurse should especially observe for excessive drainage of clear fluid or blood.

Surgery. Surgery is planned to relieve the effects of the obstruction. If a tumor is responsible for the obstruction, then the tumor is removed in order to facilitate normal circulation of cerebrospinal fluid. Shunting procedures, used in instances in which the factor responsible for the hydrocephalus is untreatable, bypass the point of obstruction or malformation. A common procedure that may be performed is a shunt from one lateral ventricle into the internal jugular vein and into the right atrium of the heart or the superior vena cava (Fig. 10-19, *A*). A valve is used to prevent reflux of CSF back to the ventricles. A *ventriculocisternostomy (Torkildsen's operation)* is the procedure used in older children to arrest the progression of hydrocephalus by bypassing the obstruction in noncommunicating hydrocephalus. A burr hole is made in the occipital region, and the shunt is placed between the lateral ventricle and the great cistern (Fig. 10-19, *B*). A preferred and most frequently used alternative procedure is the *ventriculoperitoneal shunt.*

Other alternative procedures include the *lumboureteral shunt,* or the *ventriculoureteral shunt,* in which removal of the kidney is necessary in order to insert the tube into the ureter. Electrolyte imbalance and ascending urinary tract infection frequently accompany the procedure. Lengthening of the tube to accommodate growth is not necessary with the lumboureteral shunt; however, it is required for a ventriculoperitoneal shunt. Spinal and lumbar shunts can cause compression of the spinal nerve roots.

Several medications may be prescribed following surgery: dexamethasone (Decadron) for its antiinflammatory effect (that is, it controls edema and ICP), antibiotics for infection, and anticonvulsants to prevent seizures.

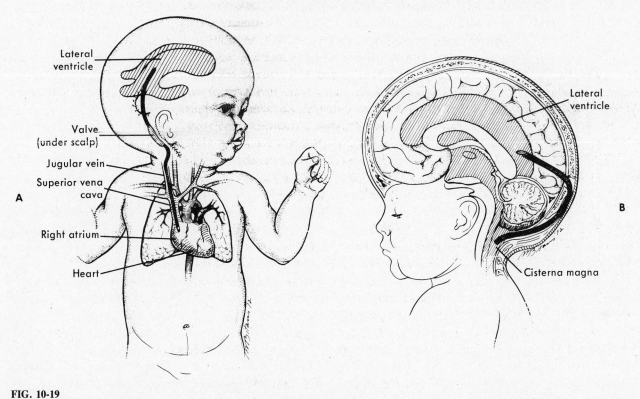

FIG. 10-19
A, Cerebrospinal fluid drained into right atrium for management of hydrocephalus. **B,** Cerebrospinal fluid drained via a ventriculocisternostomy for management of hydrocephalus (Torkildsen's procedure).

405

Postoperative care. Following surgery, care must be directed toward maintaining patency of the shunt, assessing for patency and proper functioning of the pump, preventing infection, and maintaining nutrition.

MAINTAINING PATENCY OF THE SHUNT. Positioning is one measure that is directed toward this end. For 2 to 4 days after the surgery the child is usually kept flat to prevent formation of a subdural hematoma. Rapid removal of CSF causes the cerebral cortex to pull away from the dura, tears veins, and causes blood to slowly collect in the subdural space.[24] Positioning on the operative side is contraindicated because of tenderness and the presence of edema. However, care must be planned to protect the skin, prevent impairment of the integrity of the skin, and prevent pulmonary complications (see earlier discussions in this chapter). When the danger of hematoma formation is over, the child's head can be elevated to promote venous drainage.

ASSESSING FOR PATENCY AND PROPER FUNCTIONING OF THE SHUNT AND FOR INFECTION. The infant must be monitored at regularly scheduled intervals for signs indicative of increased intracranial pressure. Such an increase may be indicative of a malfunctioning pump. Other signs that may indicate shunt failure are resistance on attempting to pump the shunt and failure of the shunt pumping device to refill after being depressed.

If the CSF is shunted into the peritoneum, signs of peritonitis may be apparent (fever, elevated temperature, abdominal tenderness, and vomiting).

PREVENTING INFECTION. The application of principles of medical and surgical asepsis is essential to accomplishing this objective. Signs that may be indicative of infection are local swelling, redness, and tenderness. When an infection occurs, antibiotics are administered intravenously and intraventricularly. Until the infection has subsided, an external shunt is employed. Afterward a new shunt is inserted.

MAINTAINING NUTRITION. The child is able to take a regular diet the first postoperative day. The nurse should closely observe the ability of the child to take the prescribed diet. If there is some neurological damage, difficulty in sucking may be experienced. Because of the electrolyte imbalance (for example, sodium loss from CSF) that may be apparent in the child who has had a ureteral shunt, intravenous sodium replacement may be necessary.

Discharge instructions. A liaison with parents of the child with hydrocephalus should be maintained through use of community resources, especially those that can provide a continuing supportive relationship, such as the Visiting Nurse Association, family physician, or neighborhood health center. Instruction is an ongoing process as the child grows. Parents should be informed of signs of increased intracranial pressure, early signs of infection, or signs indicative of shunt malfunction. Neurological and psychological testing must be performed on a regular basis to evaluate potential of mental and motor development. In cases in which there is severe retardation and motor impairment, institutional care for the child must be considered.

Encephalocele

A meningoencephalocele is the protrusion of meninges and brain, whereas an encephalocele is a protrusion of the cranial contents through the skull. The occipital region is the most common site of protrusion. Signs indicative of the defect depend on the area that is compressed by the tissue. X-ray studies are helpful in establishing the exact location of the defect. Surgery to repair the defect is the form of therapy.

10   Neurological system

Spinal cord abnormalities

Congenital anomalies of the spinal cord are usually caused by a faulty development of the vertebral column, especially nonunion between the laminae of the vertebrae. Spinal cord abnormalities are usually located in the lumbosacral area and may be of any size, ranging from a marble to a large ball. They are frequently associated with other anomalies such as hydrocephalus, Arnold-Chiari malformation, prolapsed anus, clubfoot, cleft lip and palate, and hypospadias.

 Assessment. A simple nonunion is called a *spina bifida occulta*. There is no outward protrusion of the meninges or spinal cord. The condition is often apparent only by a tuft of hair or a dimpling at the site. When the meninges protrude from the site, the malformation is termed a *meningocele*. This bulging, saclike lesion is covered with thin, atrophic, bluish, and ulcerated skin. The lesion contains only cerebrospinal fluid and is transilluminatory. If spinal cord elements also protrude, the malformation is called a *myelomeningocele,* and light will not traverse the lesion. The latter is the more common of the two (Fig. 10-20).

X-ray studies, transillumination, and inspection are the primary diagnostic assessment tools.

Planning and implementation. An uncomplicated spina bifida occulta requires no treatment, and vertebral fusion may occur later in life. However, repair of the other lesions is necessary to prevent damage to the cord or the occurrence of meningitis, which may result from invading organisms or trauma. Surgical correction also improves the cosmetic appearance of the child's body. Early closure (that is, within 24 to 48 hours) is recommended. Today's techniques and care increase the chance of survival. The prognosis depends on other congenital problems and complications.

Preoperative nursing care. Preoperative management of the child with spinal abnormalities such as meningocele and myelomeningocele should encompass (1) protecting the delicate lesion from trauma and infection and (2) making periodic assessments of motor and sensory functioning.

Protection of the lesion. The saclike lesion is delicate and covered only by a thin, parchmentlike membrane. It should be inspected for evidence of irritation, CSF leakage, and infection. The importance of cleanliness is to be em-

FIG. 10-20
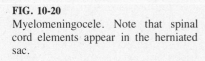
Myelomeningocele. Note that spinal cord elements appear in the herniated sac.

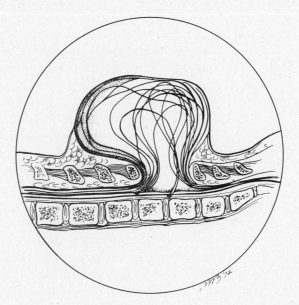

FIG. 10-21
Proper positioning for infant with myelomeningocele.

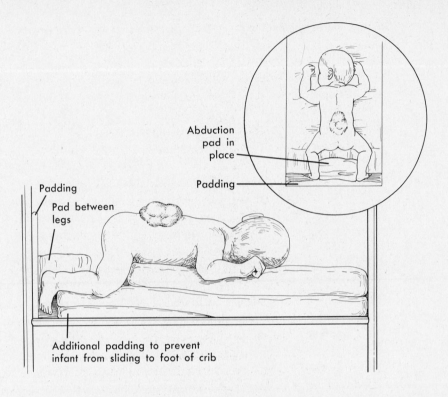

Abduction
pad in
place

Padding

Padding

Pad between
legs

Additional padding to prevent
infant from sliding to foot of crib

phasized, and if there is any sign of infection or leaking of fluid, the lesion should be covered with a dry, sterile dressing or a medicated meningocele dressing. Dressings must be changed frequently to keep the sac free from exudate and to ensure sterility. Positioning is also a valuable tool in protecting the lesion.

Positioning should be directed toward (1) protecting the sac from trauma and contamination and (2) preventing pressure areas of the skin and musculo-skeletal deformities. Some physicians prefer to place the child on his abdomen or in lateral Sims' position (semiprone) with sandbags to maintain the position (Fig. 10-21). The use of the Bradford frame, however, is still a favored method of positioning in some institutions because it prevents any pressure on the mass and exposes it readily for cleansing, dressing, and examination. The Bradford frame suspends the child above the surface of the bed, permitting stool and urine, which may be excreted almost constantly, to be deposited in a receptacle pan below. Diapers or disposable pads are folded under the abdomen and thighs to protect the frame opening and to absorb excess drainage of any urine and fecal contents. (Diapers should not be used in their usual way because they will serve as a wick to carry organisms from excreta upward toward the sac.) Perineal care, including cleansing and protective lubrication, is essential.

When the abdominal position is used (with or without a frame), chest or ankle restraints may be necessary to maintain security for the child. A small rolled pad may be placed under his lower legs to prevent pressure on the toes and foot drop. If paralysis is present or if the abdominal position must be maintained over an extended period of time, special care must be exercised to prevent abrasions or pressure areas on the skin that is in contact with the frame or linens. Water pillows or gel pads may be useful in some instances.

If a sidelying position is used, a diaper placed loosely over the perineal area between the legs may control some excreta, although a waterproof barrier is more desirable, especially if the lesion is draining cerebrospinal fluid. A small pad should be used between the knees and ankles to protect them from pressure. Positioning also may depend on whether there are other anomalies to be considered, such as hip dysplasia.

Assessment of motor and sensory function. Feeding and bath time are excellent periods for observing the motor and sensory status of the child with a spinal cord abnormality. Any significant changes should be reported at once. Observations include responses to handling, movement of extremities, reflexes, bowel and bladder function, and vital signs. Flaccid paralysis, absent reflexes, incontinence, sensory impairment, and spasticity of the lower limbs deserve immediate attention if they have not been previously noted. Since meningoceles communicate with the subarachnoid space, external lesion pressures may cause increased intracranial pressure and alter the level of consciousness. Hydrocephalus (Arnold-Chiari malformation) occurs in a high percentage of children with myelomeningocele and obstructs the flow of cerebrospinal fluid. To detect its development, the head should be measured, and the fontanels examined at least daily. Observation of behavior and vital signs is also important in the discovery of meningeal irritation, a precursor to meningitis. An elevated temperature, hyperirritability, restlessness, nuchal rigidity, and vomiting should be reported to the physician.

Other elements of care. Vesical and rectal sphincter disturbances are commonly associated with the condition and deserve special attention. If the client is likely to have a residual urine volume after voiding, this can be lessened by applying gentle pressure to the bladder, starting at the umbilicus and moving downward to the symphysis pubis (Credé maneuver). Systematic emptying of the bladder in this manner about every 2 hours not only prevents restlessness from distension but also is valuable in avoiding urinary tract infections, which are inevitably associated with residual urine. Fecal impaction can be lessened by administration of a mild laxative and a high-residue diet.

General body skin care deserves attention. The use of ointment on the face, elbows, knees, and buttocks is important to prevent excoriation caused by abrasion from linens.

The child with a spinal abnormality has the same need for attention and affection as other children. Parents and nurses should be encouraged to provide frequent sources of stimulation for the child appropriate for his age level.

Postoperative nursing care. If surgical intervention is performed, the postoperative nursing principles are basically the same as those used preoperatively, with a few exceptions.

Observations in the postoperative period are aimed at detecting shock, meningitis, and increased intracranial pressure. The child is to be positioned on his abdomen (at least until sutures are removed) to prevent the loss of excess cerebrospinal fluid through the wound and to maintain normal fluid pressure in the cranial vault. Feedings should be performed without moving the child during this early postsurgical phase. To facilitate this process, chest restraints may need to be relaxed to permit lateral rotation of the head and trunk. It is important to feed the child slowly, giving him time to expel any air that he may have ingested.

Abdominal distension should be watched for. Since some children seem to void and defecate regularly after feeding, it may be advisable to slightly elevate the head and trunk to prevent gravity soiling of the lesion for a specific period of time. Urinary retention should also be anticipated and managed promptly if it occurs.

Postsurgical respiratory difficulty must always be anticipated. Oxygen and suctioning equipment must be at hand. A heat cradle or incubator may be employed for thermal regulation.

Discharge instructions. The child with a severe spinal abnormality may require special care. He is often cared for in the home setting by parents. Certain developmental goals must be postponed because of the lesion. The child requires considerable attention from the family. The entire household must understand the principles and mode of treatment and be encouraged to share in the regimen. Before discharge from the hospital, family members should not only be instructed about the child's care but also be permitted to participate in it under supervision. In this way, questions can be answered, and any problems encountered may be dealt with before the child is taken home. A community health nurse can be consulted to provide regular guidance and assist in the resolution of care problems.

Supportive, long-range care may include elements of physiotherapy, orthopedic procedures, and bowel and bladder management as well as care of the primary lesion. Activities of daily living should be promoted to the extent permitted by the limiting components of the spinal cord abnormality.

Detection. It is possible to identify infants in utero who are at high risk for spinal cord abnormalities, such as spina bifida, by amniocentesis. Beyond the fourteenth week of pregnancy there is a significant elevation of alpha-fetoprotein (AFP) concentrations in the amniotic fluid surrounding fetuses with neural developmental pathological conditions. Selective abortion is still possible at this time. A less accurate determination of AFP levels can be made using maternal serum levels. Since amniocentesis is still considered a relatively high-risk procedure, mass screening of all early pregnancies is not feasible.

 Evaluation. The evaluation of the nursing plans for the infant with hydrocephalus is ongoing.

EXPECTED OUTCOMES

The family can:
1. Verbalize comfort measures that can be used in the care of the child.
2. Openly express feelings and concerns.
3. Identify signs indicative of emergency health care.
4. Verbalize ways of maintaining a safe environment.
5. Indicate plans for follow-up care and verbalize knowledge of community resources for health care.

COMMON HEALTH PROBLEMS OF THE CHILD AND ADOLESCENT

Cerebral palsy

Cerebral palsy is a neuromuscular disability in which voluntary muscles are poorly controlled because of brain damage. It is the largest single cause of crippling in children, with almost 6 of 1000 births being affected. Although the overwhelming number of cases are present in the neonate, we discuss the condition with childhood disease. It should be recognized that it can have its onset after birth from cerebral trauma, infections, or toxicity that directly affects the brain.

The exact cause of cerebral palsy is unknown and is widely disputed. Some authorities have indicated that it has a hereditary tendency; others firmly deny this possibility. Adverse intrauterine environment before birth seems to be at least one cause. Maternal diabetes, rubella, or toxemia of pregnancy are generally accepted factors. Unrecognized or poorly managed Rh incompatibilities cannot be ignored as a source of brain damage. Birth injuries that can cause intracranial hemorrhage may account for many cerebral palsied children. Prolonged and difficult labor, forceps or breech delivery, precipitous birth, and *asphyxia neonatorum* are the most important causes of brain injury. However, because only a small percentage of infants born under these circumstances actually develop palsies, it must be assumed that unknown factors are contributing to the pathological condition.

Cerebral palsy may be immediately detected at birth, or in less severe cases it may be suspected when the child cannot hold up his head, stand, or walk properly. The neonate with cerebral palsy usually exhibits a feeble cry, general weakness, and difficulty in eating. His body may be noticeably arched, with the head characteristically retracted. The diagnosis is made primarily from overt behavior exhibited in feeding movements and from responses to stimuli. Irritability, lethargy, stiffness, spasticity, or seizures may be noted. In older infants a failure-to-thrive syndrome may be present (see Chapter 17). In toddlers and preschoolers, cerebral palsy may not be identified until signs of mental retardation are present or the child's developmental patterns, particularly walking, are distorted. Children with cerebral palsy have a spastic gait and tend to walk on the toes. The thighs are adducted, the knees rub together, and the legs cross in a scissors gait. The trunk moves laterally as the child walks, and the limbs are rigid and held in extension. The arms may also be involved, with adduction, elbow and finger flexion, and pronation of the forearm. There may be evidence of paresis or even paralysis in some muscle groups, but spasticity is the dominant characteristic.

Up to one half of all children with cerebral palsy are subject to seizures, and approximately one third have some hearing difficulty. Some children with cerebral palsy have a tongue that deviates to one side and is difficult to control. Eating and swallowing are impaired. Excessive salivation and drooling may be present. Grimaces, uncontrolled movements of limbs when attempting to perform a purposeful act, hyperexcitability, and athetoid movements of the fingers and toes may complement the clinical picture of cerebral palsy. Although some severely affected children die soon after birth, others live to adulthood. The primary problems of cerebral palsy are related to interferences with normal growth and development. The affected children are late in learning skills associated with eating, sitting, walking, and talking. Occasionally the involvement of muscles is so severe that deformity is noted.

Assessment. The following are the six types of cerebral palsy: (1) athetosic (characterized by fine involuntary movements that inhibit normal coordination), (2) spastic (with tension and the presence of a stretch reflex in the involved muscles—the most prevalent type of cerebral palsy), (3) tremulous (fine muscular movement with a rhythmic pattern), (4) rigid (resistance in the extensor and flexor muscles), (5) ataxic (characterized by hypotonic muscles, making it difficult to balance and maintain posture), and (6) atonic. Children who have the condition may possess any combination of the six diagnostic characteristics.

Planning and implementation. The care of the child with cerebral palsy is determined primarily by the extent of the lesion and its underlying cause. The

Nursing process for common health problems

goals of both nursing and medical care are directed toward helping the client and his family cope with the disabilities and to preserve and utilize the remainder of the physical and intellectual capacities possessed by the child. Depending on the severity of the condition, care may be provided in the home or in an institutional facility such as a center for retarded children, a nursing home, or an educational center for the handicapped (Fig. 10-22).

Persons who observe a child with cerebral palsy may assume that he is retarded, because of his general appearance, speech patterns, and emotional responses. Parents may be particularly sensitive to these factors and need considerable help in dealing with their feelings and responses toward the child. As with any congenital condition, guilt may be assumed unnecessarily on the part of one or both parents. The reasons for cerebral palsy are not clear-cut, and the vagueness of the etiology should be stressed to parents. This may help eliminate their feelings of direct responsibility for the condition.

Because many cerebral palsied children have some mental retardation, psychological testing should be done at regular developmental intervals to assess the capabilities of the child for coping with day-to-day life problems. One third have normal intelligence, one third are mildly retarded, and a third are moderately or severely retarded.

Most large cities have a day-care facility for special education, training, and management of the cerebral palsied victim. After a rather elaborate period of psychological and physical testing, a planned program is developed for the individual client, based on the assets and limitations of his parents and home environment. Social workers, therapists, teachers, physicians, nurses, psychologists, and nutritionists are some of the team members in such facilities. Programs include family and sibling instruction, guidance, and therapy, all directed toward enhancing the child's physical, social, and emotional environment and

FIG. 10-22
Children in a cerebral palsy clinic are involved in a group project designed according to their learning and activity needs. (Courtesy Cerebral Palsy Clinic, Indiana University Medical Center, Indianapolis.)

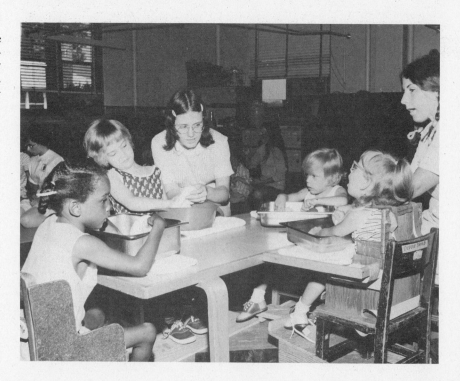

setting realistic goals and expectations for his development and performance. Discipline may be a real problem in some instances, whereas providing opportunities for independence in an atmosphere of safety and security may be paramount in others.

Therapists direct their efforts toward training in coordination, balance, and walking and preventing further deformity or disability. Deformities that affect functional abilities are managed with orthotic devices. These aids are valuable

FIG. 10-23
A, Cerebral palsy ring walker. **B,** Cosmetic polypropylene brace. **C,** Hip action and short leg braces. **D,** Body brace with head sling.

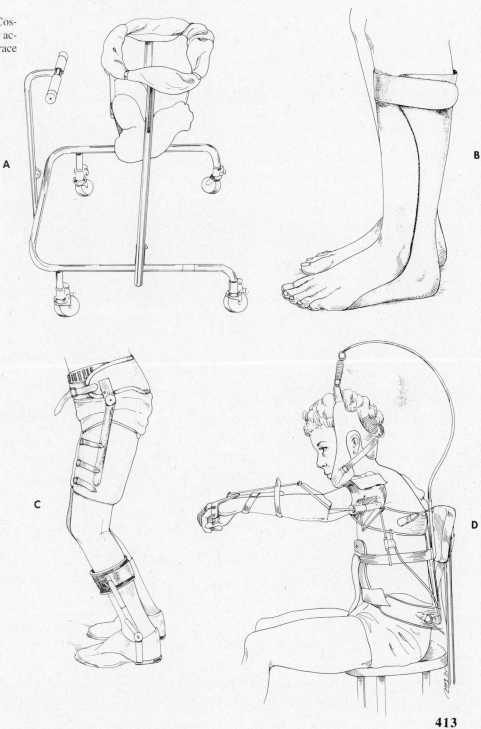

in that they enhance the client's ability to perform (or potentially perform) certain activities; they do not necessarily prevent or correct a deformity.

Devices for ambulation consist of ring walkers useful for aiding in balance achievement (Fig. 10-23, *A*). If the client progresses satisfactorily, he is graduated to a classical pick-up walker, and finally to a crutch or cane.

Individuals with spastic hemiplegia of mild involvement seem to profit from a brace, which provides a stable walking platform (Fig. 10-23, *B*), because their typical deformity is equinovarus, or clubfoot (see Chapter 11). Hip abduction deformities are managed by braces that facilitate hip action (Fig. 10-23, *C*), and the upper extremities (if functional) provide walking balance using crutches.

The severely involved client may need bracing to maintain a sitting position, which enhances interaction with the environment, permits hand use, and facilitates feeding. In some instances, it also aids in ease of transfer (Fig. 10-23, *D*).

Surgical intervention may be used to reduce athetoid movements and to limit rigidity and spasticity.

Occupational therapists help the child perform purposeful activity to help him in daily life activities such as eating, dressing, toileting, and play (Fig. 10-24). As a child grows toward adulthood, vocational educational programs that prepare him to be productive, even a wage-earner, are introduced in appropriate instances.

Nutritionists may assess the child's eating patterns and instruct the parents about dietary requirements. Occupational therapists are helpful in training and instructing the individual client and his family regarding feeding techniques and the development of skills related to chewing and swallowing. Immediately before feeding, *muscle facilitation techniques* are usually employed to enhance chewing and swallowing. Since the tongue of many clients is not in the midline and often is uncontrolled, eating may be difficult because food tends to be pushed out by the protruding tongue rather than being propelled to the back of the throat. Food may need to be placed in the back of the mouth on either side of the tongue toward the cheek with a slight downward pressure of the utensil on the tongue. The head is never tilted backward—this would cause choking. In severe cases, artificial methods of feeding may be necessary. Ample time should be set aside for meals, because feeding or eating may be slow and tedious. Children with cerebral palsy often need high caloric diets to compensate for the nearly constant activity of their extremities in random motion.

Speech and hearing evaluation and therapy may be indicated for some children. Usually these therapists work closely with the teachers, psychologists, and other therapists as well as the parents to ensure a balanced and integrated total management program.

It is not uncommon for children with cerebral palsy to be involved in innumerable accidents caused by their lack of coordination and frequent seizures in some instances. Special protective headgear such as a football-type helmet is sometimes used to prevent head injury. At home and at specialized educational and training facilities, safety and security needs should receive attention.

The child with cerebral palsy may be well enough managed to attend public schools with other children or special educational programs for the handicapped. As he grows older, he can be employed in sheltered workshops such as Goodwill Industries and even in the general population, and be a productive citizen and

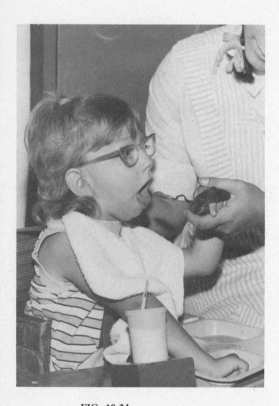

FIG. 10-24
Child with cerebral palsy acquiring the skills of self-feeding with the aid of a teenage volunteer. Note the special devices used for stabilizing the child's position and the eating utensils. (Courtesy Cerebral Palsy Clinic, Indiana University Medical Center, Indianapolis.)

wage-earner. Considerable research efforts are being directed toward the reduction of such birth defects by the National Foundation, National Institute of Neurological Diseases and Blindness, The National Association for Retarded Children and Adults, the Association for the Aid of Crippled Children, and the United Cerebral Palsy Research Foundation.

Minimal brain dysfunction

Minimal brain dysfunction (MBD) is a term used to describe learning and behavioral disorders that occur because of central nervous system malfunctioning. MBD is not mental retardation. In fact, children with the phenomenon are of average or above-average intelligence. The cardinal signs of MBD are hyperkinesis, lack of coordination, short attention span, impulsiveness, thinking and memory disorders, speech and hearing problems, perceptual deficits, and electroencephalographic irregularities. It is estimated that about 5% of all children may have this neurological problem.

FIG. 10-25
A, Aggressive behavior is one manifestation of MBD. **B,** The child with MBD often provokes others.

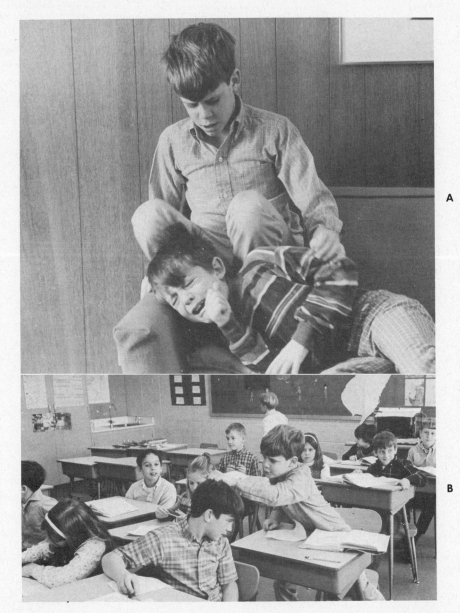

A

B

Nursing process for common health problems

One hypothetical cause of MBD is a delay in brain maturation. The brain is normally formed but is unable to refine and organize its activity into patterns suitable for the child's age and stage of development. The dysfunction may relate to events in pregnancy, neonatal life, or early childhood illness. It seems that both organic and psychogenic phenomena must be considered in assessing etiology (Fig. 10-25, *A*).

Assessment. The child's behavior is often aggressive (Fig. 10-25, *A*). He teases and provokes others (Fig. 10-25, *B*). Hostility and resentment of authority are commonplace, and discipline may be difficult. MBD children have behavioral patterns that tend to alienate others, even parents and siblings. Because of their short attention span, they are underachievers in school. The vicious cycle of dissatisfaction in relationships and accomplishments creates further problems of hostility, aggression, and spontaneous outbursts of negative behaviors. A pediatric neurologist is helpful in diagnosis, because unusual expertise and patience are required to obtain a satisfactory electroencephalogram (EEG), which must be made with the child awake and cooperative. Other impairments that may be noted during the neurological study include inability to coordinate movements and gait, speech disorders, tics and grimaces, and abnormalities in reflexes. Psychological tests are aimed at assessing the child's self-concept, his verbal and performance abilities, and perceptual-visual-motor coordination. Obviously, if diagnosis is delayed, serious learning difficulties become apparent.

Planning and implementation. The goals of therapy are (1) to assist the child in emotional development by reducing frustration and increasing gratification and (2) to maximize educational opportunities for the child during the formative years.

Parents, teachers, nurses (especially school nurses), counselors, psychologists, and others who come in contact with MBD child should be aware of the problem, its causes, and the goals of management. A positive, understanding attitude is essential. Patience and reassurance are two essential elements in guidance.

Routine is especially important in the management of a child with MBD. It not only provides safety and security but helps organize his tumultuous world. Simplify the environment and reduce distractions to the minimum. For example, place his desk against a blank wall so that pictures and other objects do not attract him. Reduce work loads or school assignments into manageable units to be completed one at a time.

Discipline is extremely important for a client with MBD. Rules must be explicit, and rewards and punishments mutually understood. Deal with offenses at the time they occur, not later, and attempt to relate punishment directly to the forbidden or distasteful act. It is important to avoid disciplining for circumstances the MBD child cannot avoid, such as awkwardness, distraction, hyperactivity, or other pathology-related problems. Generosity with rewards seems to be a positive influence in reassuring the child and motivating him toward improved performance. As growth is evident, the MBD child should be permitted to do household tasks or errands to increase his self-confidence and sense of responsibility.

Teachers, siblings, and playmates must be informed about the special needs of the MBD child. Adult supervision is sometimes necessary to reduce frustrations inherent in peer-related activity. Adults in the neighborhood can assist with the problem if they are told about the routine of coping with the affected youngster. Since the MBD child has many special needs that require considerable alteration of the home life-style, parents should plan for occasional outside supervision so that they can spend time with each other. After a short time to release tensions, free from the child's special needs, mothers and fathers are more likely to be able to cope with the problems of MBD and give love freely without interfering with the security of their marital relationship.

Pharmacological therapy is useful in management of MBD. Among drugs often employed are central nervous system stimulants. Methylphenidate (Ritalin) hydrochloride and certain amphetamines seem to be agents of choice. They tend to create a greater awareness of consciousness and thus improve concentration and adaptive behaviors. Anticonvulsants are of questionable value. Barbiturates aggravate most cases. Drugs are used primarily to facilitate management of behavior and must be used judiciously to avoid interference with learning and motor-sensory functioning. They are not a substitute for wise nurture and competent professional therapy.

TABLE 10-5

Five levels of mental retardation with approximate IQ ranges and developmental, educational, and vocational expectations

Level of mental retardation	Approximate IQ range	Preschool (age 0 to 6); maturation and development	School age (6 to 21); training and education	Adults (21 and over); social and vocational adequacy
Profound	Under 25	Gross retardation; minimal capacity for functioning in sensorimotor areas; needs nursing care	Obvious delays in all areas of development; shows basic emotional responses; may respond to skillful training in use of legs, hands, and jaws; needs close supervision	May walk; needs nursing care; has primitive speech; usually benefits from regular physical activity; incapable of self-maintenance
Severe	25 to 40	Marked delay in motor development; little or no communication skill; may respond to training in elementary self-help, such as self-feeding	Usually walks, barring specific disability; has some understanding of speech and some response; can profit from systematic habit training	Can conform to daily routine and repetitive activities; needs continuing direction and supervision in protective environment
Moderate	40 to 55	Noticeable delays in motor development, especially in speech; responds to training in various self-help activities	Usually in "trainable" classes; can learn simple communication, elementary health and safety habits, and simple manual skills; does not progress in functional reading or arithmetic	Can perform simple tasks under sheltered conditions; participates in simple recreation; travels alone in familiar places; usually incapable of self-maintenance
Mild	55 to 70	Often not noticed as retarded by casual observer, but is slower to walk, feed self, and talk than most children	Usually in educable classes; can acquire practical skills and useful reading and arithmetic to a third to sixth grade level with special education; can be guided toward social conformity	Can usually achieve social and vocational skills adequate to self-maintenance; may need occasional guidance and support when under unusual social or economic stress
Borderline	70 to 80	Frequently not detected as slow until kindergarten or first grade; physical development and acquisition of self-help skills only slightly below average or sometimes average	Usually in educable classes or "slow learner" classes; can acquire practical skills and useful academic skills to a seventh or eighth grade level with special education; without special education is likely a dropout; can conform socially	Can achieve social and vocational skills adequate to self-maintenance; needs less guidance than mildly retarded group but may require support under unusual stress; typically in semiskilled, skilled, or service occupations

Modified from chart book: Mental retardation, a national plan for a national problem. The President's Panel on Mental Retardation, Washington, D.C., 1963, U.S. Department of Health, Education, and Welfare; from Hughes, James: Synopsis of pediatrics, ed. 5, St. Louis, 1980, The C.V. Mosby Co.

Nursing process for common health problems

Mental retardation

Mental retardation is a form of cerebral dysfunction characterized by impaired or incomplete mental development.

Assessment. The victim has limited ability to learn and to implement learning. There is a wide range of retardation from borderline to profound (Table 10-5). Research is currently being directed at uncovering some of the mystery of retardation (Fig. 10-26). Some conditions such as Down's syndrome (mongolism) can be recognized at birth and explained in genetic terms. Other congenital problems of metabolism, maldevelopment of the central nervous system, and birth injuries are not well understood.

Planning and implementation. Management problems vary from simple adjustments in the home to institutionalization of the child. Mental retardation, like learning disorders of cerebral palsy and MBD, is rooted in problems of genetics, pregnancy, birth trauma, neonatal life, and childhood illness and injury. Careful assessment of developmental progress is the best tool for discovery of mental retardation and charting a course of therapeutic intervention.

A wide number of educational, vocational, and recreational services are available for the client in any age group who is retarded, especially in urban areas. Most states and many localities have specialized institutions for management of the mentally retarded. Public schools have graded classes in special education planned for the handicapped child of school age. Unique services for adolescents and young adults include puberty counseling, genetic counseling, family planning (especially contraception), psychotherapy, day-care centers, and sheltered workshops where skill training can be accomplished. For the mature adult there are similar services aimed at maintenance of healthful daily living and societal coping.

Down's syndrome (mongolism). Down's syndrome is a chromosomal abnormality that results in mental retardation. The normal human somatic cell

FIG. 10-26
Research efforts are being directed toward revealing new etiological factors related to mental retardation. (Courtesy March of Dimes Birth Defects Foundation.)

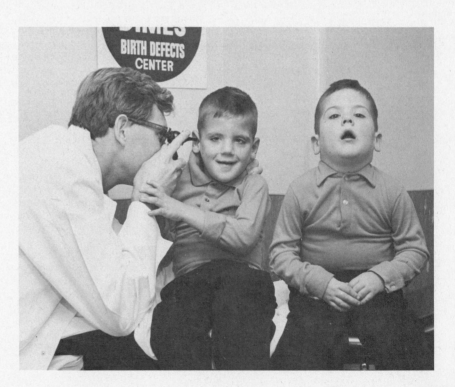

has a chromosome constitution of 44 autosomes (22 pairs) and 2 sex chromosomes. In 1959 a trisomy (triplication) of chromosome 21 was discovered in Down's syndrome. Since that time several other trisomies have been defined, along with their unique developmental results. Down's syndrome occurs in approximately 1 out of 600 births in all races and is worldwide. Advanced maternal age is well linked to the phenomenon. Eighty percent of mothers bearing children with this condition are over 35 years old at the time of the birth.

Assessment. Anomalies of trisomy 21 include a rounded head with flat occiput, enlarged protruding tongue, short nose, slanted eyes, broad and short neck, elastic joints, epicanthal folds, a characteristic single crease on the palm (simian crease), and short, inward-curving fingers. Leukemia and other blood disorders are common in clients with Down's syndrome. About one out of four have a major heart defect, and as a group they are especially susceptible to respiratory infections (Fig. 10-27).

Planning and implementation. Many persons with Down's syndrome can be cared for in their homes quite successfully and managed like a handicapped child with special needs. Genetic counseling for the client and his family, however, is advised as an integral part of the professional helping relationship, although risk of recurrence is relatively low in most types defined in chromosomal analysis. Amniocentesis for prenatal ascertainment of genetic factors is performed in some regions of the country for high-risk pregnancies so that families have the option of therapeutic abortions early in pregnancy, or the family can be reassured, according to the findings. Some genetic specialists believe such a prenatal chromosome analysis should be performed for all pregnant women over 40 years of age.

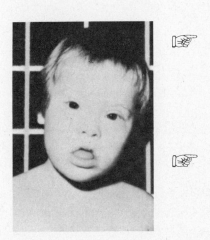

FIG. 10-27
Three-year old girl with Down's syndrome. (From Hughes, James G.: Synopsis of pediatrics, ed. 5, St. Louis, 1980, The C.V. Mosby Co.)

Muscular dystrophy

Muscular dystrophy is an inherited disorder that causes weakness and atrophy of muscles. It affects basically the muscular portion of the spinomuscular level. There is no loss of reflexes until atrophy becomes extensive, but flaccid paralysis is remarkable. Essentially in dystrophic processes (or myopathies) the anterior horn cells and nerve tracts remain intact, but muscle fibers degenerate, often being replaced with connective tissue and fat. There is a loss of contractility, but not excitability.

Muscular dystrophy is usually not apparent in infancy, but as the child grows, his motor development is retarded.

Reye's syndrome

Reye's syndrome is an acute disease that tends to follow an upper respiratory tract (URT) infection in previously healthy children. The exact cause of the syndrome is unknown, although it has been related to viral and toxic agents.[12] Infants and children up to 12 to 15 years of age are generally affected. Both sexes are equally affected, and it tends to occur in white children who live in rural and suburban areas.[12,21] The incidence is higher during the winter months.

Assessment. Characteristically, a previously healthy child develops a mild illness, usually a nonspecific URT infection. One to two days following the URT infection as the child appears to be recovering from the illness, persistent vomiting occurs. Within 2 to 3 days, signs of encephalopathy appear. Symptoms indicative of central nervous system stimulation occur, including irritability, restlessness, hallucinations, delirium, and seizures. The pupils dilate, and spasticity commonly occurs. Hyperventilation is also experienced early in the disease; subsequently respiratory alkalosis is manifest. Respiratory acidosis develops as the disease progresses. In severe cases, the stage of excitement has been followed by decorticate and decerebrate posturing. Symptoms generally progress rapidly, and varied levels of awareness may be experienced. Liver and renal involvement may also occur; but the signs of central nervous system involvement tend to overshadow these. Death from cerebral damage is not uncommon after 3 to 4 days. The laboratory studies usually reveal an increase in serum transaminase, low blood sugars, increased levels of ammonia, and metabolic acidosis.[12]

 Planning and implementation. Since the exact cause of the syndrome has not been identified, supportive care is essential; care is directed toward protecting the brain from irreversible damage and correcting the metabolic disturbance. Varied forms of therapy have been used, including intravenous fluids, which are administered carefully. The volume is based on the output, blood pressure, and osmolarity. Laxatives and enemas are generally prescribed to decrease the ammonia level. Corticosteroids have been used to decrease cerebral edema. Other forms of therapies have been used, but for many, controlled studies have not been performed.

Epilepsy   Epilepsy is a form of idiopathic seizures that are recurrent and may be primary (no known cause) or secondary (caused by infections, trauma, congenital illness, brain tumors, and other disorders that affect the brain). The term *epilepsy* is usually reserved for seizures without a known cause that have their onset between early childhood and young adulthood. Epilepsy is more common in firstborn children, presumably because of birth trauma from a long, difficult labor. It does not alter any other physical or mental processes; thus general health status is not affected. See discussion of seizures later in this chapter.

 Assessment. The client with epilepsy may display automatic behavior such as lip smacking, chewing, pulling on clothes, or rubbing the fingers.[21] An aura may or may not be experienced before a seizure activity.

> **Data analysis**
> *Data analysis may reveal nursing diagnoses of potential for injury, ineffective coping, fear, grieving, knowledge deficit, noncompliance, and disturbance in self-concept.*

Planning and implementation. The most important aspects of care for epilepsy are (1) regular use of an anticonvulsant medication, (2) avoidance of stress and fatigue, and (3) prevention of febrile illnesses. Irregular use of prescribed anticonvulsant medication is the most common cause of seizures in a client diagnosed as having epilepsy. Older children should be given responsibility for managing their own drug therapy to normalize the coping with the condition. They should understand that additional sleep is needed but that normal activity is encouraged. Regularity in bowel elimination is especially important because constipation seems to be related to seizures. Young ladies need to be aware that extra precautions should be taken during menstrual periods because seizures often occur at this time from the added body adjustments to stress. Peer group and family members should understand how to cope with a seizure if it occurs. An identification bracelet or wallet card with notations about epilepsy, drugs, and physician's name is helpful for the client to carry at all times.

Most persons with epilepsy (more than 80%) are well controlled with anticonvulsant medications and can lead normal lives. A few occupations do not permit such persons to be employed because of high accident factors, for example, airline pilots, heavy equipment operators, and construction workers on high-rise buildings. With better education of the public about the illness, it is losing some of its stigma, and affected clients can enjoy a typical life pattern including college, marriage, and rearing children. Most restrictive laws about epileptics' driving or obtaining insurance are being removed in most states for persons under sound medical management for seizure control.

The parent's role in managing epilepsy in a child relates to (1) making sure that he has the proper medication daily, (2) recording seizure episodes systematically, (3) noting reactions to drugs, (4) helping the child structure a healthy balance of activity and rest, and (5) communicating pertinent data of the child's condition to teachers, peers, and other family members.

The hospitalized client with epilepsy. During the initial nursing assessment for any client, historical data regarding seizures should be elicited. When did they begin? How often do they occur? What is the nature of the seizure and the aura if one is experienced? What anticonvulsant medications are regularly taken? If the physician is not aware that the client has epilepsy, the nurse should inform him accordingly. All clients who have a known history of seizures episodes should be placed on seizure precautions as described on p. 496. Nurses must recognize that even the well-managed client, when faced with the additional stresses of illness and hospitalization, may have a seizure although he has not had one for several months or even years.

Nursing care relating to seizure management must include (1) preventing the attack when possible by use of anticonvulsant drugs, (2) promoting safety of the client during and after the attack, (3) respecting his need to rest undisturbed after the seizure, (4) recording careful descriptive observations regarding seizures, and (5) educating clients, families, and others about seizures and their management.

Anticonvulsant drugs include barbiturates (especially phenobarbital), diazepam (Valium), phenytoin (Dilantin), chlordiazepoxide (Librium), primidone (Mysoline), and ACTH and corticosteroids. (The last group is useful primarily in the treatment of seizures relating to infantile cerebral damage.) Hypothermia suppresses electrical discharges in the brain and enhances positive responses to drug therapy and thus is useful for some clients. Experimental stereotaxic surgery is being attempted in some individuals where anticonvulsant therapy has been ineffective and where incapacitation of the involved brain tissue would not alter vital functioning or mental processes. The surgical approach is reserved for seizure patterns that are well localized and confined.

 Evaluation. Evaluation of the nursing plans for the young client with epilepsy is an ongoing component of the nursing process.

EXPECTED OUTCOMES

The client and/or family can:
1. Describe epilepsy, including the basis for the problem.
2. Demonstrate satisfactory adjustments of life-style imposed by epilepsy.
3. State signs and symptoms that indicate progression or regression.
4. State limits of activity.
5. Verbalize the importance of compliance to prescribed therapy including medications.

6. State use, dosage, time, route, and side effects of prescribed medications.
7. State problems requiring health care services.
8. Indicate plans for follow-up care and knowledge of community resources.

COMMON HEALTH PROBLEMS OF THE YOUNG ADULT

Multiple sclerosis

Multiple sclerosis (MS) is a disseminating, degenerative disease characterized by demyelinization of conducting pathways of the central nervous system. The process that impairs and destroys is poorly understood, but it either (1) causes a blockage of nerve impulses to a selected part, bringing about paralysis, or (2) allows the impulse to pass through the damaged pathways in an unusual fashion, creating disturbed functioning of the affected part.

Multiple sclerosis is a particularly important degenerative disease because it affects primarily young adults, especially those in their third decade of life. An afflicted young parent may be prevented from pursuing his or her mode of earning a living or caring for his family in the usual manner. MS is a long-term condition that may last several decades. It creates physical, emotional, and economic problems for a family. Since it is characterized by episodes of remissions and exacerbations, the disease may be gone—sometimes for years—only to return again with more severe symptoms. The causes of the temporary improvements are unknown, but much research effort has been directed toward understanding the causes of these remissions, because this may be a key toward finding a cure. The cause of MS is unknown, although many theories blame enzymatic disease, allergic responses, viruses, infection, and stress factors such as trauma, fatigue, and pregnancy.

MS is neither inherited nor contagious and its prevalence does not seem to be determined by race, gender, ethnicity, occupation, or economic level. It does seem to predominantly occur in cold climate areas, however.

Assessment. The symptoms of MS are related to the area of the nervous system that has been affected. The National Multiple Sclerosis Society lists the following as symptoms that might indicate the presence of the disease:

- Partial or complete paralysis of part of the body
- Numbness in parts of the body
- Double or otherwise defective vision, such as involuntary movement of eyeballs
- Noticeable dragging of one or both feet
- Severe bladder or bowel trouble (loss of control)
- Speech difficulties such as slurring
- Staggering or loss of balance (MS patients erroneously are thought to be intoxicated)
- Extreme weakness or fatigue
- Prickling sensation in parts of the body like pins and needles
- Loss of coordination
- Tremor of hands

It is especially significant for diagnosis if there is an unexplained disappearance of one or more of these symptoms either permanently or temporarily. On occasion, symptoms may disappear for periods of several years and may never return. Diagnosis is based primarily on the presenting symptoms and the history. Autopsy is the only sure way of diagnosing the illness, according to some authorities.

The multiple sclerosis personality. Psychiatric and psychological studies indicate that demonstrable changes in personality and intellect take place in victims of MS. Euphoria and mood swings have been classically associated but tend to be evident only in clients who have cerebral pathological conditions. However, the wide range of manifestations, including emotional lability, depression, and irritability, that may also be evident has given rise to the term *multiple sclerosis personality*. The personality does not predispose the individual to the illness but occurs as a result of the impact of the diagnosis. Receiving a diagnosis of MS means many things. It means being a marginal human being—not sick or well, not an invalid or a healthy productive person, not able to be entirely independent or dependent. It means also that one lives in a world of uncertainty about the nature and progression or disappearance of the unpredictable symptoms. Finally, MS means accepting a certain loss of control over one's body and mind. Acts that were once controlled at will become difficult or impossible to perform, or behavior occurs spontaneously and inappropriately, especially laughing and crying.

Planning and implementation. There is no effective treatment for MS. Experimentally, anticoagulants and steroid therapy directed toward venular thrombosis associated with lesions have been tried, but because of unpredictable remissions, their value is difficult to determine, and the side effects are often severe. As physical and mental impairment become greater, the client becomes increasingly more dependent, and complications ranging from urinary tract infections to decubitus ulcers to contractures are noted. The client should be encouraged to remain as active as possible, while avoiding stress and fatigue. A physical therapy program directed toward the activities of daily living is of some benefit to most clients, since it helps them remain relatively independent. The program should be planned to provide for sufficient rest periodically. Eventually, however, the MS client becomes bedridden and dependent and requires supportive nursing care.

Nurses who work in industry, office, schools, or community health centers are likely to encounter a client with MS. Often the client is experiencing vague symptoms or characteristics of MS but has not sought medical attention and thus needs guidance and referral. Health teaching for all groups, especially young adults, should include the symptoms of MS. Care should be taken to explain that these manifestations are often vague and may indicate a number of conditions other than MS but that they deserve further observation and study.

Known MS clients should be supervised in a well-planned program of daily living. Family members may need help in understanding the rationale of the regimen and in learning meaningful ways to participate in the client's care. They should be referred to the local chapter of the Multiple Sclerosis Society for specialized help in coping with the illness. Many clients eventually must be cared for in nursing homes; so personnel working in such agencies need to understand the client, his illness, and its physical and mental implications in order to participate most meaningfully in the nursing care.

Brain pacing. A "brain pacemaker" is sometimes useful in improving skeletal-motor activity that has been impaired by seizures, stroke, epilepsy, brain injury, and certain degenerative conditions such as multiple sclerosis that affect the inhibitory control mechanisms of the cerebellum.

The pacemaker consists of electrodes that are implanted in the cerebellum

423

via an occipital craniectomy, a radio receiver that is implanted in the chest, and an external transmitter and antenna, which accomplish and control stimulation.

Intermittent cerebellar stimulation helps many clients regain enough muscular coordination and control that they can engage in activities of daily living and in further rehabilitation efforts. Often anticonvulsant medication dosages can be significantly reduced and is often eliminated. Although still in an experimental stage, brain pacing offers considerable hope for selected clients who have neurological pathological conditions that adversely affects muscular control.[14]

National Multiple Sclerosis Society. Considerable attention has been given in recent years to conquering MS, because it affects young adults in the prime of their life and results in many years of declining health. The National Multiple Sclerosis Society is a voluntary organization that helps victims and their families cope with the disease. It maintains research centers, clinics, and local units devoted to providing special services. Counseling, recreation, physical appliances, and rehabilitation supervision are some of its major functions.

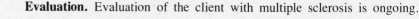 **Evaluation.** Evaluation of the client with multiple sclerosis is ongoing.

EXPECTED OUTCOMES

The client and/or family can:
1. Describe multiple sclerosis, including the neurological deficit and potential for recovery.
2. Demonstrate satisfactory adjustments of life-style imposed by neurological deficits.
3. Strive to maintain a maximum level of activity within limitations imposed by multiple sclerosis.
4. State signs and symptoms indicative of a progression or regression in neurological status.
5. State plans for health maintenance.
6. State use, dosage, time, route, and side effects of any prescribed medications.
7. Verbalize the importance of compliance to prescribed therapy.
8. State plans for follow-up care, and problems requiring health care services.

Myasthenia gravis

Myasthenia gravis is a degenerative neurological disease characterized by a lack of acetylcholine at the myoneural junction, which impairs muscle contractractions. It may occur at any age, although young adults are usually affected. The cause is unknown but it may be (1) a basic lack of acetylcholine production, (2) inability of the motor end plate to use it, or (3) a premature chemical destruction of the agent by acetylcholinesterase before it performs its vital function.

 Assessment. The onset of myasthenia gravis is gradual, with symptoms first noticed when the client is fatigued. Complaints of early symptoms may include difficulty in chewing and swallowing and ptosis. Some speech, vision, and breathing disturbances may be present. Fatigue and stress worsen the symptoms, but rest is usually followed by noted improvement. The client with myasthenia gravis appears sleepy and apathetic because of the bilateral ptosis, and because the muscles around the mouth are weak, a snarling appearance may be manifest. Various changes occur after fatigue and may in severe cases reach aphonia. When the respiratory tract is involved, the cough reflex is impaired, and fluids and mucus cannot be easily expelled.

The diagnosis is confirmed by the medical history and a test employing a short-acting anticholinesterase drug such as edrephonium (Tensilon) chloride. In such a test, a calibrated dose of the drug is administered, and in clients with myasthenia, exhausted muscles will perform normally within a few minutes. The action of the anticholinesterase drug is primarily to inhibit and inactivate acetylcholinesterase (known for its ability to neutralize acetylcholine).

Planning and implementation. Anticholinesterase (cholinergic) drugs are the main agents used in treating the client with myasthenia gravis. The nurse should be thoroughly familiar with their action, side effects, and considerations of dosage regulation.

Administration of cholinergic drugs must be regulated for the individual client and based on his living patterns and physiological needs. It is extremely important that the drug be given on time as ordered so that a safe therapeutic margin can be maintained at all hours of the day. Effects should be carefully noted.

Since overdosage and underdosage occur frequently for some clients, it is imperative that they and their families understand how to adjust the dosage to maintain muscle strength at the optimum and to recognize signs of too little or too much medication.

Too little medication can cause a "myasthenic crisis" as a result of deficient levels of acetylcholine at the myoneural junctions. This situation is evidenced by profound symptoms of the disease and unusual respiratory difficulty.

Too much medication can result in a "cholinergic crisis" caused by an excessive accumulation of acetylcholine at the myoneural junction. This crisis is marked by muscarinic side effects—nausea, diarrhea, abdominal cramping, and hypersecretion of saliva, sweat, tears, and mucus—as well as respiratory difficulties and profound muscle weakness.

Nurses or family members should not attempt to diagnose the cause of the crisis but should recognize that it is a medical emergency requiring the help of a physician. Atropine sulfate is useful in either instance and should be available for parenteral injection.

A family member or neighbor should be alert to check on the client, especially on his waking, and ascertain if he is able to take his medication. If not, parenteral administration supplies should be at hand for immediate use. If a myasthenic client is too helpless to take his drug, he is probably unable to summon help, and thus his needs must be anticipated. He should never be left completely alone or without his drug. Family members should know mouth-to-mouth breathing techniques in case of a respiratory crisis. A medical identification tag may be useful for the victim to wear at all times to alert persons who might attempt to help him regarding his condition and medication.

The client should understand the need for rest and the avoidance of over-exertion and fatigue. The level at which any individual participates in his own care is determined by his response to therapy and his general condition.

Since respiratory mechanisms are impaired, special care should be taken to avoid exposure to infections. Emergency airway and ventilatory equipment should be at hand if a crisis occurs in the breathing mechanism. Suctioning equipment should be at the bedside to help remove secretions or in an emergency to prevent aspiration of food or fluids, because the protective cough and gag reflexes are often impaired.

Nursing process for common health problems

Although myasthenia gravis can be successfully controlled in many cases, it results in rapid death for some victims, primarily from respiratory failure.

Clients and their families may contact the Myasthenia Gravis Foundation Incorporated for assistance in coping with the disease. The organization has three basic objectives: education, aid and treatment of victims, and research. It can help interpret the disease and plan a supportive regimen in conjunction with other health care personnel.

Daily visits, or at least periodic ones, by a community health nurse are desirable for some clients. Nurses in the home can offer instruction, give support to the family, and validate the therapeutic regimen and its consequences. Often their observations may indicate the need for referrrals to other agencies to assist in medical and nursing management or in the socioeconomic problems assessed in the home.

 Evaluation. Evaluation of the nursing care plan for the client with myasthenia gravis is ongoing.

EXPECTED OUTCOMES

The client and/or family can:
1. Describe myasthenia gravis, including the basis for the deficit.
2. Demonstrate satisfactory adjustments of life-style imposed by myasthenia gravis.
3. Maintain a maximum level of activity within limitations imposed by myasthenia gravis.
4. State signs and symptoms indicative of a progression or regression in neurological status.
5. State plans for health maintenance.
6. Exhibit caution in activity in order to facilitate personal safety, which is threatened by various neurological deficits.
7. State use, dose, time, route, and side effects of prescribed medications.
8. Verbalize the importance of compliance to prescribed therapy.
9. State plans for follow-up care and problems requiring health care services.

COMMON HEALTH PROBLEMS OF THE MIDDLE-AGED ADULT
Parkinson's disease

Parkinson's disease, sometimes called "paralysis agitans" or "shaking palsy," is a degenerative disease of the nervous system, characterized by muscular weakness and rigidity, intentional tremor, and an accelerating gait. The cause is unknown, but it is related hypothetically to arteriosclerosis and encephalitis.

Assessment. The client who has the disease has a characteristic appearance and behavior. The face appears expressionless, with the eyebrows raised but the wrinkles smoothed out. Facial muscles are virtually immobile. Eyes seem to be wide open and to stare without blinking. This typical pattern of facial appearance is sometimes referred to as "Parkinson's mask."

The accelerating gait associated with the disease appears also as a classic manifestation. As the victim walks, he inclines forward, and his steps become faster and faster. They begin as slow, short, shuffling steps but may become spontaneous running. This is also termed "festinating gait."

Movements are slow, especially in small muscle groups. A characteristic tremor often develops in the fingers and thumbs, termed "pill rolling." Tremor is usually more severe when the client is at rest, and it seems to disappear during sleep. Speech and writing may also be impaired.

 Planning and implementation. There is no known cure for Parkinson's disease, but there is a fairly well-established medical as well as surgical regimen aimed at controlling symptoms.

Levodopa, or L-dopa, is the drug used in controlling symptoms of Parkinson's disease, especially posture instability, gait disturbances, tremor, and rigidity. It provides a source of dopamine, which seems to be absent in the disorder.

The side effects of L-dopa are numerous and affect all individuals who are using the drug, to some degree. Among these are nausea, anorexia, dizziness, hypotension, anxiety, depression, agitation, hallucinations, delusions, nightmares, and insomnia. Numerous other psychiatric, gastrointestinal, urogenital, neurological, cardiovascular, respiratory, dermatological, musculoskeletal, sensory, and hematopoietic changes can occur to a degree that prohibits the use of the agent. The nurse who cares for a client who is receiving L-dopa must be alert to the drug's side effects and understand the ways in which to control them.

It seems helpful to administer the drug with food to lessen gastrointestinal symptoms of nausea, anorexia, and vomiting. Since the dosage is carefully titrated for each client, it is important to observe the client for noticeable side effects of the drug and signs of overdosage or toxicity. If overdosage is suspected, gastric lavage may need to be instituted, and fluids administered intravenously. Attention should be given to maintaining a patent airway and to cardiac monitoring.

The client should understand as much as possible about his drug and should be made aware that (1) L-dopa is not curative but controls symptoms through an unknown action, (2) only half or two thirds of clients receiving the drug will note an improvement, (3) side effects are to be expected and will undoubtedly be a source of displeasure. The need for close medical supervision must be stressed to the client and his family, because the dosage must be carefully titrated for the individual. Now commonly used, L-dopa is instrumental in controlling symptoms despite its unpleasant side effects.

Other pharmacological agents employed in the management of parkinsonism include analgesics, the belladonna group, antihistamines, and synthetic compounds.

The general nursing care of the client with Parkinson's disease is similar to that of the client with multiple sclerosis.

A variety of surgical procedures have been employed to destroy selected portions of the globus pallidus or its major outflow. Although pallidectomy has been used frequently in the past, the surgery of choice at this time seems to be a stereotaxic thalamotomy. Electrocoagulation or freezing of a precisely located portion of the thalamus has reportedly reduced both tremor and rigidity of limbs. Other factors such as gait and posture disturbances, akinesia, and voice problems are not improved, however. Stereotaxic surgery is usually limited to candidates who experience unilateral symptoms and whose course seems to be progressing slowly. This group accounts for only about one tenth of all parkinsonism victims.

 Evaluation. Evaluation of the client with Parkinson's disease is an ongoing component of the nursing process.

EXPECTED OUTCOMES

The client and/or family can:
1. Describe Parkinson's disease, including the basis for the neurological deficit and potential for recovery.

2. Demonstrate satisfactory adjustments of life-style imposed by Parkinson's disease.
3. Maintain caution in activity in an effort to facilitate personal safety.
4. State signs and symptoms that indicate progression or regression in neurological status.
5. State plans for health maintenance.
6. State use, dose, time, route, and side effects of any prescribed medications.
7. Maintain a maximum level of activity within limitations imposed by Parkinson's disease.
8. Exhibit compliance to prescribed therapy, including medications.
9. State plans for follow-up care and problems requiring health care services.

Tic douloureux (trigeminal neuralgia)

Tic douloureux is a degenerative neurological condition of the trigeminal nerve. It may affect any or all branches of the trigeminal nerve.

Assessment. Symptoms depend on the involved portion of the nerve and may include (1) radiating pain around the eye and forehead; (2) pain of the cheek, upper lip, and nose; or (3) pain in the lower lip and outer border of the tongue on the affected side of the face for the first, second, and third trigeminal nerve branches, respectively. Pain can be triggered by any mechanical or thermal stimulation to the nerve branches, and although the pain is transient, it is excruciating and recurrent. Eating, washing the face, or even a draft can cause the painful phenomenon.

> **Data analysis**
> *Data analysis may reveal nursing diagnoses of alteration in comfort and ineffective coping.*

Planning and implementation. Treatment includes injecting the branches with absolute alcohol to inactivate them or surgically dividing the sensitive routes. Radiofrequency coagulation (via an implanted electrode at the gasserian ganglia and adjacent nerve rootlets) is a refined technique to surgically affect pain control. With the use of a similar principle and addition of a transmitter and antenna, clients can send radiofrequency impulses at will to block the pain of tic douloureux.

After most surgical procedures, however, symptoms of pain are replaced with permanent anesthesia of the areas served by the branches. The affected portion of the face is "woody feeling," and if the first branch is cut, the eye loses its normal sensory reflex protection, and the cornea may be dry and open to damage. Care must be taken to protect the eye from trauma, and moisture must be provided by the use of artificial tears.

Evaluation. The evaluation of the client with tic douloureux is an ongoing process.

EXPECTED OUTCOMES

The client and/or family can:
1. Identify factors that precipitate the pain.
2. State methods of pain control.
3. State the use, action, frequency, route, and side effects of prescribed analgesic medications.
4. Verbalize the different methods of dealing with the problem.
5. State plans for follow-up care.

**COMMON HEALTH
PROBLEMS OF THE
OLDER ADULT**

Cerebrovascular disease

The nerve cells of the brain determine one's reception and interpretation of sensations, as well as bodily movements. To receive and interpret sensations, brain cells must be supplied with a continuous and sufficient supply of oxygen and other nutrients. It is the function of the cerebral vessels to supply the cells of the brain with nutrients and metabolic substrates so that the high energy requirement of the brain is met. The resultant waste products of metabolism are also removed. Any interference with the supply of oxygen to the brain cells for as short a period as 3 minutes may result in cerebral damage or death of the brain cells. When this occurs, cerebrovascular disease exists. Such disease may have an ischemic or hemorrhagic basis. Ischemic problems include transient ischemia attack, thrombosis, and embolism, and cerebral infarction. Hence they are presently being classed as ischemic strokes. Intracerebral hemorrhage, associated with hypertension, and subarachnoid hemorrhage, are the common manifestations of cerebral hemorrhage.

Ischemic strokes. Several types of clinical strokes indicate the chronology of stroke. These include transient ischemic stroke, stroke in evolution, and completed stroke.

Transient ischemic stroke. A transient ischemic attack (TIA) or *transient cerebral ischemia* (TCI) is a focal neurological deficit that lasts from a few seconds to a few hours. The attacks result from a transient interruption of the blood supply and oxygenation to a localized area of the brain. Recovery generally occurs spontaneously and completely within 12 to 24 hours.

A number of factors predispose to TIA: (1) the release of tiny fragments of blood clots, fused platelets, and atheromatous materials from plaques (microaggregates), which occlude small intracranial vessels; (2) a sudden drop in blood pressure, in which case the pressure returns to normal spontaneously or by an increase in collateral circulation; (3) a sudden reduction in cardiac output that occurs with dysrhythmias or heart block; and (4) a temporary compression of the vertebral artery, such as from turning the head.[8] Emboli from the heart and cervical vessels are also considered as possible causes.

 Assessment. The National Stroke Congress has developed a list of signs and symptoms of TIA. The symptoms of these attacks vary according to the area involved. For example, with involvement of the carotid or the middle cerebral artery, the client may have monoplegia or hemiplegia, monoparesthesia or hemiparesthesia, unilateral blindness, disturbance of speech, and confusion; whereas dizziness, numbness, and visual impairment may be experienced if there is involvement of the vertebral basilar system.[7] In addition, headache, lightheadedness, syncope accompanied by pallor and postural slump, fall or "drop attack" without loss of consciousness, transient ataxia, transient dysphasia, and transient disorientation are not uncommon. Seizures (in persons over age 40) and transient cranial palsies may be experienced. The attacks tend to occur when the client is up and around.

> *Data analysis*
> *Data analysis may reveal nursing diagnoses of potential for injury, sensory perception alteration, and fear.*

Nursing process for common health problems

Planning and implementation. All persons who exhibit these symptoms are potential candidates for a stroke. Therefore nurses, especially nurses who visit in the home or work in community health clinics, should be alerted to these symptoms. Clients who experience one, or a combination, of these symptoms should be encouraged to seek medical counsel. Early medical assistance enables the client to receive therapy before a stroke develops. When the client is hospitalized, he should be instructed to inform the nurse of each transient attack. Therapy may be planned to dilate the vessels and thus improve cerebral circulation using carbon dioxide inhalation or vasodilating drugs such as papaverine hydrochloride, or measures to prevent clotting (anticoagulants) may be used. Whenever anticoagulants are prescribed, the nurse should instruct the client and his family about the effect of the medication, particularly emphasizing signs and symptoms that should be reported to health care personnel and those indicative of complications, especially hemorrhage. The client should be informed of the need for follow-up care (for example, prothrombin checks). Certain drugs potentiate the effects of anticoagulants. The client should therefore be instructed not to take any medications without first consulting with the physician. Aspirin, usually taken at least 4 times a day, has been reported to significantly decrease stroke. The effect is that they prevent platelet aggregation.

Other therapies include controlling underlying disease that accelerates the development of atherosclerosis (for example, diabetes, hypertension), discouraging smoking, and encouraging the client to avoid any form of stress. If dietary or activity changes are indicated, the nurse should instruct the client regarding these modifications.

SURGICAL INTERVENTION. Several surgical techniques may be employed to restore normal circulation to the brain: endarterectomy, patch graft angioplasty, and bypass graft. Carotid angiograms confirm the percentage of occlusion and location of the plaque. Clients with generalized arteriosclerosis are not treated surgically. Without complications, these surgical procedures improve cerebral circulation and decrease the possibility of a stroke occurring.

An *endarterectomy,* or removal of the atheromatous plaques, is commonly performed, especially if the plaque is in the internal carotid artery. Following an endarterectomy, the blood pressure should be monitored closely. An adequate blood pressure is necessary to maintain patency of the vessel, and therefore maintain cerebral blood flow. Neurological status (for example, pupils, movement, and handgrip) must be monitored and evaluated.

In another surgical procedure, a *patch graft angioplasty,* the diseased portion of the artery is excised and replaced by synthetic material or a natural artery. Although still in the evaluation stage, extracranial and intracranial shunts are being performed.[25]

Stroke in evolution. Stroke in evolution (evolving or progressing stroke) is an uncommon stroke syndrome characterized by movements of neurological deficit covering a period of hours or a few days.[25] Stenosis or thrombosis of an internal carotid artery in the neck is frequently the cause of this group of symptoms.

Assessment. Characteristically, a stroke in evolution commences with a flurry of TIA, and incomplete deficit may fluctuate for a period of time (a few hours to days), with each succeeding attack being worse, and with more and more incomplete recovery. A CAT scan and a lumbar puncture confirm the diagnosis.

10 Neurological system

> *Data analysis*
> *Data analysis may reveal nursing diagnoses of ineffective airway clearance, alteration in sensory perception, potential for injury, alteration in thought process, and ineffective coping.*

Planning and implementation. Nursing care should be directed toward maintaining an adequate airway and frequent monitoring of neurological status. The vital signs, especially blood pressure and pulse rate, should be monitored closely. Anticoagulant therapy, usually starting with heparin and then warfarin (Coumadin), is one form of therapy.

Completed stroke. A completed stroke is characterized by cessation of progression of neurological difficulty. It occurs when the deficit becomes stabilized. A thrombus or an embolus may be the source of the problem. The pattern of onset provides information about the cause.

Cerebral thrombosis. Cerebral thrombosis is the formation of a clot within an artery of the brain. This clot may either partially or completely occlude the vessel. It accounts for the greatest percentage of all strokes. The vessels more commonly involved are the middle cerebral, basilar, and carotid arteries. Arteriosclerotic changes in the walls of the vessel and/or atherosclerotic plaques, which change the caliber of the vessels, interfere with the free flow of blood. The plaques also extend through the intima of the blood vessels and result in the development of rough surfaces. This slow blood flow and the roughened lining favor stasis and clot formation. For example, platelets, which adhere to the roughened surface, release an enzyme, adenosine diphosphate, which sets the coagulation mechanism in action.[19]

ASSESSMENT. The majority of individuals with a cerebral thrombosis exhibit transient ischemic attacks.[7] Consequently, cerebral thrombosis generally does not develop abruptly. Although cerebral thrombosis may occur at any time, it usually occurs when the client is sleeping. On awakening, the client experiences difficulty in speaking, walking, and remembering. The symptoms may progressively worsen during a 24-hour period. A massive thrombosis may produce an infarction.

> DATA ANALYSIS
> *Data analysis may reveal nursing diagnoses of ineffective airway clearance, ineffective breathing patterns, impaired verbal communications, ineffective individual coping, ineffective family coping, fear, potential for injury, impaired physical mobility, alterations in nutrition, disturbance in self-concept, sensory perceptual alterations, potential impairment of skin integrity, and alteration in thought process.*

PLANNING AND IMPLEMENTATION. Skilled nursing care is essential during the stage in which the client is unconscious. During this time the client is totally dependent on the nurse to meet all of his needs. Inherent within meeting these needs are frequent assessment. The frequency of assessments will depend on the stability of the client's condition. Because of involvement of the vital centers,

431

Nursing process for common health problems

detailed assessments must be made of airway patency, vital signs, level of consciousness, pupillary reactions, motor and sensory ability, and skin color. Additional assessments can be found in the guide below. Other aspects of care, discussed in Chapter 21, should be planned to meet the total needs of the client.

Cerebral embolism. Cerebral embolism occurs when a clot that has formed someplace else in the body is transported, through the vascular system, to the brain. This clot commonly results from fragmentation of mural thrombi in the heart, which frequently complicates diseases of the heart. For example, it is generally associated with rheumatic heart disease, bacterial endocarditis, myocardial infarction, and atrial fibrillation. Emboli may also result from ulcerated atherosclerotic plaques in the carotid and possibly the vertebral arteries.[15]

PATHOPHYSIOLOGY. The embolus usually stops at a bifurcation, or a narrow site of a vessel. Although any part of the brain may be affected, the area of the middle cerebral artery is most frequently involved.[3,7,19]

ASSESSMENT GUIDE FOR THE CLIENT WITH CEREBROVASCULAR DISEASE

Throughout the course of the client's confinement, a number of assessments should be made. Consideration should be given to orientation, communication, social behavior, and interests as well as environmental interest. Physical assessments must also be made.

1. Orientation
   a. What is the client's orientation to time, place, person, individuals within the environment, that is, family or health personnel?
   b. What is the client's awareness of length of illness or hospitalization?
2. Verbal communication
   a. What is the client's ability to speak? Is the speech understandable? Does the client ramble? Is it sensible most of the time? Is it occasionally off the point? Does he speak normally and sensibly?
   b. Is the client able to answer questions? Are answers to questions meaningful or meaningless? Does he sometimes fail to respond?
3. Social behavior and interests
   a. Assess the client's response to others. Does he respond or make contacts with others?
   b. What is his relationship with others? Does he take a social interest in his family? Hospital personnel?
   c. What is his concern about appearance and cleanliness? Is he careless in dress? Unconcerned about cleanliness?
   d. Is he belligerent or unstable?
4. Environmental interests
   a. Is interest shown in things in the environment?
   b. Is he aware of what goes on in the environment?
   c. Does he react normally to things in the environment?
   d. Is he unconcerned about things in his environment?
5. Physical assessment
   a. Does he complain of dizziness? Muscle weakness?
   b. Assess the client's impairment of hearing and visual acuity.
   c. Are his muscles weak or strong?
   d. Are his muscles flaccid or spastic?
   e. Does he have any joint movement?
   f. What is the steadiness of his gait?
   g. Assess his coordination.
   h. Assess his vital signs and perform a neurological assessment.

ASSESSMENT. Strokes from cerebral embolism develop suddenly, within seconds or a minute[7] and without warning. The client suddenly develops focal signs that give an indication of the area of involvement. For example, hemiplegia usually develops, especially if the internal carotid or middle cerebral artery are obstructed. An embolus that passes into one of the middle cerebral artery branches produces problems such as motor aphasia or monoplegia.

> DATA ANALYSIS
> *Data analysis may reveal nursing diagnoses such as those established for cerebral thrombosis, including ineffective breathing patterns, impaired physical mobility, sensory perception alterations, potential for impairment of skin integrity, and alterations in thought process.*

PLANNING AND IMPLEMENTATION. Therapy for cerebral embolism is similar to therapy for cerebral thrombosis. An embolectomy may also be performed, and the client may be placed on long-term anticoagulant therapy.

Cerebral infarction. Cerebral infarction is death of neural parenchyma secondary to inadequate blood supply to the involved area. This usually results from occlusion of the major arterial vessels by thrombosis or embolism, spasm, or from severe stenosis of the arterial supply. As a result, it is more likely to occur when there are atherosclerotic changes in the vessels, particularly the internal carotid and cerebral arteries. Pressure from tumors may also compress the arteries. Vessels may become kinked when the head is turned, resulting in thrombus formation and a vascular occlusion. Polycythemia also enhances the thrombotic tendency by increasing the viscosity of blood, thus resulting in clot formation. Symptoms become manifest as a result of ischemia to the part of the brain supplied by the occluded vessel.

ASSESSMENT. The onset of symptoms is usually abrupt and may occur while the client is sleeping. On awakening, the client may be stuporous. Coma may gradually develop. One complete side of the body is usually affected. The involvement may be in the form of contralateral weakness (hemiparesis) or paralysis (hemiplegia), homonymous hemianopsia (blindness in one half of the visual field), hemisensory loss, and facial weakness as evidenced by a distinct puckering of the involved cheek on expiration. Contralateral involvement indicates that the dominant hemisphere in the brain is affected; that is, the client whose right side is affected has pathological involvement on the left side of the brain. This effect is noted because the motor fibers cross to the opposite side at the medulla. Dysphasia is also common. Recovery is slow. Only partial improvement may be noted in the major manifestations.

If the infarction is massive (over 2 to 3 cm), complete hemispheric involvement, cerebral edema, and a resultant increase in intracranial pressure ensue. The brainstem may be compressed, and death may occur from respiratory failure.

> DATA ANALYSIS
> *Data analysis may reveal nursing diagnoses of ineffective breathing patterns, sensory perception alteration, impaired physical mobility, and impaired verbal communication.*

Nursing process for common health problems

PLANNING AND IMPLEMENTATION. The care planned for the client is similar to that planned for the unconscious client (see discussion earlier in this chapter). Neurological assessments must be monitored closely and at frequent intervals. Vital signs should be monitored and evaluated. Significant changes must be communicated to the physician (for example, slow pulse and respiration, increasing coma). These are indicative of pressure on vital centers.

Intracranial hemorrhage. The majority of strokes resulting from hemorrhages are caused by hypertensive intracerebral hemorrhage or ruptured aneurysm,[7] an arteriovenous anomaly, or intracerebral tumor hemorrhage.

Intracerebral hemorrhage. Intracerebral hemorrhage, or hemorrhage into the substance of the brain, is generally associated with hypertension and arteriovenous anomalies. The blood pressure level may be as high as 160/90 or higher. The sites most frequently affected are (1) the putamen, (2) thalamus, (3) cerebellar hemisphere, and (4) pons and parts of the white matter (for example, frontal lobe).[7]

Pathophysiology. Hemorrhage is often referred to as massive or small. Massive hemorrhages refer to hemorrhages several centimeters in diameter; whereas small is used to refer to those 1 to 2 cm in size. When a hemorrhage occurs, blood extravasates into the tissue. The extravasation of blood from an artery escapes into the adjacent brain tissue and results in displacement and compression of the tissue. A massive hemorrhage may move structures to the opposite side and compress the vital centers. Subsequently, coma and death may occur.

Assessment. The onset of the hemorrhage is usually abrupt and without warning signs. The client may experience headaches, lightheadedness, and a feeling of malaise, but these symptoms are usually no different than usual. The hemorrhage is often associated with activity (for example, usually occurring while the client is up). The signs and symptoms will vary with the site and size of the extravasation, the most common being those associated with putaminal hemorrhage.[7] For example, slurred speech and hemiparesis are experienced. Hemiplegia gradually follows aphasia, and the client may become confused and abruptly or gradually lose consciousness.

The paralysis becomes gradually worse and flaccid. The pulse becomes full and bounding, the blood pressure is elevated, the face is flushed, and the respirations become stentorous. The pupils dilate and become fixed.

A spinal tap (lumbar puncture) is usually performed shortly after the client is admitted to the hospital. The fluid is usually grossly bloody, indicating an abnormal communication within the cerebrospinal fluid system. Nuchal rigidity and other signs of meningeal irritation may occur if blood escapes into the spinal fluid or if a pressure cone is produced from the expanding hemorrhagic lesion. Death may occur within a few hours if the hemorrhage is massive and in 1 to 2 days in less severe cases. A number of clients survive the hemorrhagic attack. In these, improvement may be noted within a couple of days. Residual defects such as aphasia, hemiplegia, and hemianopsia are generally manifested.

Data analysis
Data analysis may reveal nursing diagnoses of sensory perceptual alteration, impaired physical mobility, impaired verbal communication, and ineffective breathing patterns.

Planning and implementation. Therapy is similar to that outlined under cerebral thrombosis. However, there are some measures worthy of reemphasizing. These measures should be planned to reduce physical and mental stress, subsequently preventing increased intracranial pressure. Added stress, whether physical or mental, increases chances of hemorrhage occurring. Therefore the environment must be quiet and visitors limited. Bed rest must be maintained. Observe the client's psychological response to factors such as inadequate sleep and stress. Such factors should be communicated to the physician so therapy can be planned.

In addition to monitoring vital signs and neurological status, the nurse should evaluate these data for signs indicative of increasing intracranial pressure and shock. The temperature should be taken by the axillary route.

Arterial aneurysm. An arterial aneurysm is a sac formed by dilatation of the wall of an artery and filled with blood. The cause is thought to be a combination of congenital and acquired factors. The congenital factor is thought to be a developmental defect in the media and elastica[7] of the vessel usually located at an arterial bifurcation and its branches. Hypertension and atherosclerosis are the acquired factors associated with the development of aneurysms. Arterial aneurysms found in cerebral vessels include mycotic, dissecting, fusiform, and saccular—the latter two are so named because of their shape.

Mycotic aneurysms arise from infected emboli that lodge in the artery and cause arteritis and consequent dilatation of the vessels.[23] The common source of the aneurysms is subacute bacterial endocarditis. These aneurysms occur at the branches of the middle cerebral artery. The vessel may rupture and cause bacterial meningitis. Antibiotics are used before surgery to control the infections.

Dissecting aneurysms are rare and sometimes occur in association with saccular aneurysms.

Fusiform aneurysms are spindle-shaped dilations that occur as a result of arteriosclerosis. Arteriosclerosis tends to destroy the media and elastic membrane, which results in the spindle-shaped dilation of the artery.[23] The arteries involved are the basilar, internal carotids, and vertebral. Rupture is uncommon, though they tend to produce symptoms by compressing, distorting, or destroying adjacent structures. They are inaccessible to a direct surgical approach.

Saccular aneurysms are small dilations that are shaped like beans. The majority are found in the anterior half of the circle of Willis on the internal carotid, its branches, or the anterior communicating artery.[7,23] They are rarely found in children, and most frequently become symptomatic around the fifth decade. Most intracranial aneurysms do not produce symptoms unless they rupture.

Pathophysiology. Hemorrhage from a saccular aneurysm usually occurs in the subarachnoid space. (The circle of Willis lies in the subarachnoid space.) The sudden release of blood under high pressure tends to raise the intracranial pressure or may cause rapid displacement of the brain. The blood tends to irritate the blood vessels and produce a sterile meningitis.[5] Spasms of the vessels may occur and produce ischemia or necrosis.

Assessment. The rupture may occur suddenly in association with physical or emotional stress, or it may occur during normal activities or at rest. The client may complain of a severe generalized headache (bursting in character) and may suddenly become unconscious; or the headache may develop suddenly and the client remains alert; or the client may become unconscious without any symptoms preceeding it.[7] If the hemorrhage is massive, the client goes into a deep coma, respirations become irregular, respiratory arrest and circulating collapse may develop, and death may occur.

In clients experiencing less severe hemorrhage, if consciousness is lost, it may be momentary. However, dizziness, drowsiness, confusion, amnesia, and headache may also occur. Meningeal irritation, characterized by a stiff neck (nuchal rigidity), may persist for a couple of weeks. Compression of the neural tissue by a hematoma may produce focal signs such as weakness, paralysis, seizures, and visual disturbances. The specific focal symptoms will depend on the exact site of involvement. Once the client's condition stabilizes, one of several diagnostic studies may be performed, including carotid and vertebral angiography, computerized axial tomography (CAT), brain scan, and electroencephalogram.

Data analysis
Data analysis may reveal nursing diagnoses of sensory perceptual alteration, impaired physical mobility, and impaired verbal communication.

Planning and implementation. Therapy is planned to prevent and control increased intracranial pressure and to promote cerebrovascular function to prevent complications.

PREVENTING AND CONTROLLING INCREASED INTRACRANIAL PRESSURE. The client is placed on "aneurysm precautions," which include strict bed rest for at least a 3- to 4-week period, with the head raised 15 to 20 degrees.[7] The client's environment should be darkened and quiet. Any form of exertion should be avoided. Excessive movement should be discouraged, and all activities, such as hygiene care and turning, should be done for the client. Turning must be accomplished gently. Sedatives and analgesics (for example, codeine) may be prescribed to promote relaxation and to control the headache. Psychological support should be provided by alleviating anxiety as necessary. The use of morphine is contraindicated because of its depressant effects and its masking of pupillary signs. Frequent neurological assessments must be made and their findings evaluated. Any significant change in the neurological status should be promptly reported to the physician. Antihypertensive drugs may be prescribed for the hypertensive client.

PROMOTING CEREBROVASCULAR FUNCTION. Adequate fluids should be administered. Intravenous fluids should be infused slowly to prevent a rise in the client's blood pressure. A CVP line may be inserted to facilitate close monitoring of fluid therapy. If oral fluids are permitted, they should be given through a straw to avoid having to raise the client's head higher than prescribed. Osmotic diuretics are used to reduce cerebral hydration. Steroids are prescribed to control the cerebral edema. Accurate records must be kept of intake and output.

In an effort to prevent hemorrhage, aminocaproic acid (Amicar), an antifibrinolytic agent is used. This drug reduces recurrent bleeding by inhibiting clot lysis because the drug crosses the blood-brain barrier to the cerebrospinal fluid. Blood levels of the drug should be monitored. Nausea and vomiting are common side effects and are managed with supportive therapy. Additional nursing strategies are directed toward preventing stress and promoting rest and comfort are employed. For example, a close check must also be kept on the client's elimination pattern. A laxative or stool softener may be prescribed to keep the bowels open and thus prevent straining and consequent elevations in intracranial pressure. The client should be observed closely for symptoms of an upper respiratory tract infection. These should be reported to the physician at the onset so that measures can be prescribed to prevent common symptoms such as coughing and sneezing, which raise intracranial pressure. If the client is unconscious, nursing care should be planned to meet all his needs. See section earlier in this chapter for a discussion of care of the unconscious client.

SURGERY. Surgery, another form of management, is generally not planned until the client's condition is well stabilized. Intracranial or extracranial surgical procedures may be performed, and these are sometimes combined. The *intracranial method* is performed on clients who are good surgical risks. For the intracranial method, varied approaches may be used. A craniotomy is performed to expose the aneurysm. (A surgical microscope is generally used, and a temporal, frontotemporal, or suboccipital approach.) Once exposed, a clip may be applied to the neck of the aneurysm, the aneurysm may be resected, or the aneurysmal sac may be wrapped in fascia, muscle, Gelfoam, arterial grafts, or coated with plastic material.[7,23] The plastic makes a firm support around the aneurysm. Another approach, which is useful if the vessel has not ruptured, is to inject a foreign substance into the body of the aneurysm to produce thrombosis. Nursing care is the same as for a client who has had a craniotomy.

The *extracranial method* is performed by occluding one of the arteries supplying the circle of Willis. This may be done suddenly or by compressing gradually with Silverstone clamps. The rationale on which ligation is based is that pressure and pulsation within the aneurysm are reduced, resulting in a thickening of its walls, a reduction in size, and thus a lesser change of rupture. If it is done suddenly, the neurosurgeon ligates the artery. When the artery is occluded gradually, a clamp is inserted around the carotid or vertebral artery on one side of the neck, and the artery gradually occluded over a period of several days by tightening the screw. The clamp is designed so that it can be released if signs of cerebral ischemia develop. The nurse must therefore observe the client frequently for signs of ischemia, such as aphasia, changes in level of consciousness and vital signs, and motor and sensory deficits. The appearance of these symptoms should be reported to the physician immediately.

The client is maintained on complete bed rest and should be positioned so that the function of the screw is not affected. The nurse must also be cognizant of potential complications and work toward preventing them. In addition to signs of ischemia and alterations in levels of consciousness, the client should also be observed for other signs of cerebral edema and increasing intracranial pressure. Other neurological assessments must be carefully evaluated.

Other problems of clients with cerebrovascular disease

The client with aphasia. Aphasia, an impairment in the language ability, is commonly experienced in the client with a cerebrovascular accident, but it may also be experienced in any client with cerebral trauma such as after an automobile accident. The language center is found in the dominant hemisphere, usually the left, of the brain. Therefore any involvement in this hemisphere usually

437

Nursing process for common health problems

results in aphasia. When aphasia occurs, it can present a number of problems. The nurse must therefore be aware of the cause and types of aphasia as well as its nature and manifestations.

Common terms that have been used to describe aphasia are *expressive,* or *motor, aphasia* (inability to initiate ideas through spoken words, written symbols, or gestures), *receptive,* or *sensory, aphasia* (an impairment in perception), and *global aphasia* (combination of both). It should be emphasized that rarely does a true form of expressive or receptive aphasia exist. Usually the client experiences degrees of both. Both may be equally severe, or the defect may be minimal in both expression and perception.

Expressive language. All individuals communicate through various means—gestures, facial expression, writing, and speaking. Therefore even if the client is not able to speak, he may be able to use one of the other means to express himself. The nurse must assess the client to determine the means by which he expresses himself. The following assessment guide may be useful as a plan of care is formulated.

- Can he communicate by speaking, writing, or use of gestures?
- Can he perform in one means of communication, but not another? For example, can he write, but not speak or make gestures?
- Can he mimic speech? If he can, does he mimic words or phrases?
- Can he name objects in the environment?
- Does he use automatic speech? Does he use profanity? Does he say yes or no to all questions or statements?
- Can he recite the days of the week? Months of the year? (serial speech)

Receptive language. Receptive language relates to perception of language. Perception refers to the meaning the brain places on the message it receives. The ability of the client to understand language can be determined through assessing the client's reactions to spoken language (auditory-verbal) or his reactions to printed letters, words, or phrases (visual-verbal). In assessing the client's ability in this area, the nurse should observe the client's ability to perform the following:

- Follow simple directions. For example, will he squeeze your hand when asked? Will he hand you a spoon when requested to do so? Will he point to a glass or comb his hair on request? In assessing the client's ability to understand spoken language, the nurse must avoid the use of gestures. Many clients with receptive impairment can interpret gestures, thereby giving the appearance that they understood what was said when, in essence, they picked up cues from the gesture.
- Follow directions with the use of gestures.
- Follow complicated directions.
- Recognize printed words or phrases.
- Match objects with their names when a series of objects and names are presented simultaneously.

Answers to these and similar questions and observations in these areas will enable the nurse to develop a plan that will be workable for the client.

Levels of speech. Automatic, or emotional, speech, automatic casual speech, and volitional speech are the three levels of speech used by humans.

438

Automatic speech, the most primitive form, involves cursing, singing, and using exclamatory remarks such as "Oh!" or "Ouch!" In aphasia, this form is often the least affected. Casual speech involves simple greetings and responses such as "How are you?" or "It's a nice day" or yes or no. Volitional speech, the highest level of speech, requires thought, concentration, and perception. This level is the first to be affected and the last to return.

Clients with expressive aphasia may retain a slight degree of automatic and casual speech. Therefore it is not unusual to hear the aphasic client curse or yell exclamatory remarks during conversations. They may be able to recite the days of the week, count, answer "yes" or "no" to questions, or greet the nurse and family with "How do you do?" The "How are you today?" question may be answered automatically by "fine," or he may shake his head affirmatively. Therefore the nurse must be aware that simple verbal responses do not necessarily mean that the client understands or is improving. In contrast, they may mean that the client has automatic speech. As a result, the nurse should use performance rather than verbal response as a criterion for understanding.

The care of the aphasic client must be a team effort. The nurse must work closely with the client, his family, and the speech therapist. The nurse can help the client cope with the disability by following the therapist's recommendations and by offering support and encouragement to the client and family.

Because most asphasic clients are hospitalized during the early stage of their illness, nurses must be aware of certain guidelines that will help them manage the client. In caring for the aphasic clients, the nurse must not forget the uniqueness of each client and therefore plan for intervention according to individual needs.

The aphasic client experiences frustrations and misunderstandings either from not being able to express his thoughts, feelings, or desires or from not being able to understand what others say to him. The nurse should decrease the client's frustrations as much as possible by helping him express himself. Only after assessing the client's limitations can the nurse plan an effective means of communication. If the client cannot speak or write, the nurse should use gestures as a form of communication. If he is not able to verbalize, he may be able to identify objects. The nurse may suggest that the client point to what he wants. The nurse may use cards on which pictures of useful objects are placed. Such pictures often help the client perform activities of daily living. The use of any type of visual aid should be reinforced with speech and pantomime to help the client relearn speech. If he can understand simple verbal communication, then the nurse should by all means talk to him.

In verbal communication the nurse and family must speak clearly and distinctly and in short sentences. Slow, quiet tones are usually better understood than loud tones, because the latter serve only to cause more confusion. If the client can understand sentences, one-concept sentences are generally better understood than multiple-concept sentences. If he can understand simple directions, then directions should be simple and uncomplicated. The nurse must refrain from giving more than one direction at one time, especially if it is known that he cannot respond to lengthy directions. If he can understand written language, the nurse and family may write to him. Complex conversations must be avoided. If the client is to communicate effectively, the environment should be relaxed and free of disruptions, because the aphasic clients must be able to concentrate. The conversation should be geared toward immediate needs and surroundings, and concrete objects that can be seen, heard, touched, smelled, and tasted. For example, at mealtime talk about food. Only one individual should engage in conversation with the client at one time.

The aphasic client must be given ample time to express himself and formulate ideas. The nurse or family must not speak for him. Assistance should be given only after several attempts have been made; and the supplied words should be given in "multiple choice" fashion so that the client has an opportunity to choose exactly what he wants or desires. Sometimes it may be necessary to ask the client to give simple directions such as "show it to me" when he is attempting to talk. The nurse might also ask questions that require yes or no answers. However, the yes or no answer must be evaluated, because the client may say "yes" when he means "no" and vice versa. Thus the nurse and family help the client maintain a feeling that he has not lost all his ability to communicate.

In assisting the client with care, the nurse must work in an unhurried manner. This approach enhances the client's ability to find words and formulate ideas and makes him feel that people have time for him.

The aphasic client has a tendency to isolate himself and withdraw. This is one means of protecting himself from a threatening environment. It also relieves him from having to communicate, thus sparing him some frustrations. Not uncommonly, an aphasic client can be observed spending most of his time in bed or covering his head during rest periods. A client should not be permitted to withdraw, nor should he be permitted to become isolated. The nurse should use every available means to prevent this occurrence. He should be included in conversations. The client should be informed of routines, procedures, and current events. Newspapers and magazines should be shared with him. Active participation in games and unit activities should be encouraged. The family should be encouraged to engage in activities with the client. This practice helps stimulate him more. Scheduled times should be allotted to communicate with the client periodically throughout the day. An occupational therapist may be consulted to help plan activities for him.

Being unaware of exactly how much the client can or cannot understand, the family and nurse should refrain from talking about the client in his presence. Facial cues and tones of voice can readily be picked up by the client, and therefore the nurse and family must not display cues that could easily be misinterpreted by the client.

The client with perceptual defects. Clients with central nervous system disorders frequently experience perceptual defects. That is, they fail to integrate and correctly interpret sensory messages from the internal and external environment. They may not be aware of the paralyzed side and may have hemianopsia.

It is not uncommon for the hemiplegic to be unaware of his involved side. This may be evidenced by the fact that the client continually ignores his involved side or things on the involved side. For example, when walking or riding in a wheelchair, the client may continuously bump into objects on his involved side. In locking the wheelchair, he may lock the unaffected side but leave the lock on the affected side unlocked. In dressing himself, he may dress himself on the unaffected side but leave the affected side undressed.

The nurse must plan care so that the client is made aware of the affected side. Several approaches have been suggested. One suggestion is placing the important items on the side of awareness; the other is to instruct the client to take care of items on the affected side. Those who support the first approach suggest placing the call light, nightstand, and other objects on the side of awareness. All other activities such as conversation and care should be carried out on the side of unawareness. This stimulates him to turn his head.

Stimulation must be produced on the involved side. The nurse must continuously remind the client of the involved side either by touch or by asking him to look at the affected side. Statements such as "look to the left," accompanied with a pat on the arm, are helpful. Such reminders not only help to increase awareness but also enable the client to avoid running into objects or people.

Hemianopsia is a visual defect in which blindness occurs in one half of the visual field. When this happens on the nasal half of one eye and the temporal half of the other, homonymous hemianopsia is present. It occurs because the optic tract and radiation beyond the optic chiasma contain fibers from the temporal retina (nasal field) of one eye and the nasal retina (temporal field) of the other. This defect is common in the stroke client. The client sees clearly on one side of the midline but sees nothing on the other side. As a result, problems related to safety are presented.

When this deficit is present, the nurse and family must plan measures that will help the client compensate. It is often necessary to rearrange the total environment. The bedside stand may be changed to the client's unaffected side. At mealtime foods may be placed in the line of the unaffected visual field, and plate guards may be used.

The client should be encouraged to turn his head toward the side of the visual defect. Such practice will enable the client to see, as well as prevent accidents.

Many of these clients also tend to misjudge distances. This may be evident by the fact that they underplace objects. One may note that in an attempt to place a glass on the table, the client dropped it or in trying to pick up a water glass, he knocked it over. To help the client overcome this, he must be assisted in placing objects. In spite of accidents, he must be continually encouraged to perform tasks.

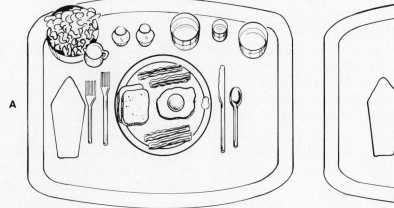
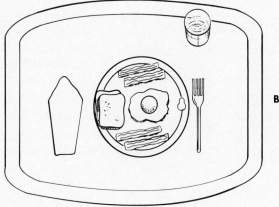

FIG. 10-28

A, Overcrowded tray causes frustration for client who has difficulty making decisions. **B,** Providing tray with minimal foods prevents confusion from having to make choices.

Nursing process for common health problems

Another guiding principle that should be used in caring for the client is *simplicity*. The meal tray should be simply set, and only a minimal number of foods should be placed on the tray at one time (Fig. 10-28). Less confusion is caused if the meal is served in three small courses rather than as a single course. In this way the client does not have to make choices, and as a result, frustration is prevented.

In the care of these clients, they must be allowed to repeat activities as often as necessary, and *consistency* is a must. Some of these clients also have problems understanding left and right. When the client is requested to move his right hand, he may move his left. When this happens, some special plan should be devised to help the client remember right or left. Color codes are useful when the client has this difficulty.

The client's self-concept and image must also be considered as assessments are made of his behavior. The self-concept is made up of how an individual thinks and feels about himself. It is developed over many years through association with significant people in the environment. The self-image is internally and externally developed. An impairment of brain function that results from a stroke may result in alterations in the concept an individual has of himself. The behavioral changes that result from cerebral damage may also threaten the client's security and affect his adjustment to both the physiological and psychological manifestations of the damage. His family and friends may change their concept of the client. This, in turn, may also affect how the client feels about the disability and himself. See Chapter 8 for a complete discussion of body image.

The client's gender, education, value system, and cultural background may influence his reactions and his adjustment to the disability. For example, an active person may have a hard time adjusting to curtailment in physical activity. The inability to use hand or foot may mean that he cannot drive a car or engage in his favorite sport. The breadwinner may become frightened or depressed about the thought of not being able to return to his job or not being able to support his family. The independent person may be resentful of others' having to care for him. The dependent, insecure person may welcome being cared for by someone else. The wife may worry about the care of the family and management of the home. The nurse should find out as much about the client as possible. Information may be obtained from the family about his emotional pattern and life-style. All findings should be taken into consideration as care is planned for the client. The nurse can evaluate the impact of the client's disability on the family. In this way the nurse can possibly help them accept limitations more realistically.

Rehabilitation

Promoting independence. The nurse must constantly encourage self-help. As soon as the comatose period is over, the client should be engaged in self-care activities. These include activities related to personal hygiene, such as combing the hair, brushing the teeth, bathing, self-feeding, and dressing. See Table 10-6 for a list of activities of daily living. He must be encouraged to turn himself from side to side and move about in bed. He must be permitted to carry out all of these activities even if it takes him a long time to do so. As much as possible he must be encouraged to use the affected extremities.

The nurse must use ingenuity and imagination in devising assistive devices so that these tasks can be performed with minimal difficulty. In eating, for example, handles of the utensils should be enlarged by padding with a tongue blade,

TABLE 10-6

Activities of daily living (total activities = 60)

Roll to right, left	Turn pages of book	Open and close window
Sit erect in bed	Wind wristwatch	Pull window shade
Comb or brush hair	Strike match	Work light switches
Brush teeth	Get out of bed and stand up	Push doorbell
Shave or apply make-up	Get into bed and lie down	Work pull-chain light
Wash arms and legs	Stand up from chair	Open and close cabinet lock
Cut meat	Sit down	Turn faucet
Butter bread	Sit down on toilet	Open and close bottle
Drink from glass	Get down on floor	Walk up 15-degree ramp 3 feet
Stir coffee	Get up from floor	Walk down 15-degree ramp 3 feet
Dress	Walk forward 30 feet	Walk up one flight of stairs with handrail
Tie shoelaces	Walk backward 10 feet	Step up curb
Tie necktie	Walk sideways 10 feet	Step down curb
Undress	Open and close door	Cross standard street on green light (in 20 seconds)
Write name and address	Open and close cylinder lock	Get in and out of bus, use turnstile (in 20 seconds)
Fold letter, seal envelope	Open and close icebox door	Get into car
Open envelope, remove letter	Open and close drawers	Get out of car
Open and close safety pin	Open and close padlock with key	Pick up object from floor
Use dial telephone	Open and close door hook	Carry cafeteria tray with dishes

From Gordon, Edward E.: A home program for independently ambulatory patients, New York, 1957, National Multiple Sclerosis Society.

gauze, and tape. Commercial leather devices are also available. Such measures facilitate better manipulation of the utensil. A rocker knife may be used for cutting meat. If coordination is poor, a small juice glass can be handled better than a large one. Plastic glasses with lids through which a straw can be placed are useful for the client who has difficulty in swallowing. The practice of sucking through a straw is particularly helpful because it facilitates redevelopment of both facial and swallowing muscles. Many of these devices may be obtained from commercial supply houses. The handles of toothbrushes and combs can also be enlarged. Electrical appliances such as electric shavers and toothbrushes also facilitate self-care. To help the client write, a paperweight can be used against the sheet of paper while the client attempts to write with the affected extremity. A peg may be attached to a pencil to facilitate writing.

Dressing activities should be included as soon as the client's sitting balance is stable. The least difficult activities should be started first, and the more difficult ones added after mastery of the least difficult ones. Loose-fitting garments (robes and pajamas) should be practiced with first. This should be followed by allowing the client to dress in his own clothing. When the client is helped with dressing activities, the affected extremity should always be placed into the sleeve or pants leg before the unaffected extremity, and the garment should be removed from the unaffected extremity first. Buttonhooks may be used to fasten buttons. The ability of the client to assist with, or carry out, these activities offers ego-support. Independence in one or all of these activities motivates the client to attempt other tasks.

As the client's condition stabilizes, he will be permitted to sit and stand. It is believed that if the client is allowed up within the first 24 to 48 hours after a cerebrovascular accident, he will do much better in rehabilitation than will those who remain in bed for longer periods.[26] Although mobilization should be started early, it must be done gradually with increasing periods out of bed. Initially, as the client is prepared for getting out of bed, he should gradually be elevated. If the client has been in bed for an extended period of time, postural hypotension is not uncommon. As his tolerance indicates, he should be permitted to sit on the side of the bed for a few minutes before the transfer activity is started. During each stage the client's vital signs (blood pressure, pulse, respirations) and color must be assessed. If signs of fainting or shock develop, the client should be placed in the supine position, and his vital signs should be reassessed. Often it is necessary to apply an abdominal binder or elastic stockings to aid circulation. They are particularly useful if postural hypotension is a problem. As these activities are advanced, the nurse must continue to observe principles of correct alignment. When the client is allowed to sit and stand, his sitting and standing balance should be observed. If he leans forward or toward one side, this should be corrected as soon as possible. He should be permitted to practice sitting balance, because adequate balance facilitates transfer. Whenever poor posture is observed, he should be instructed to sit up straight. Assistance should be given if necessary. The nurse may also permit the client to view his posture in a mirror that has been placed in front of him.

Subluxation of the shoulder, or partial dislocation, results from muscle weakness and gravity pull on the arm. Therefore, when the client is permitted to sit in a chair, the affected arm should be supported on a pillow, and when he is allowed up, the arm should be placed in a sling to prevent subluxation. The wrist and hand must be supported in the sling to prevent wrist drop, and the hand should be slightly higher than the elbow to prevent edema. Other nursing measures should be considered when a sling is used. The arm should be taken out of the sling and exercised frequently throughout the day to promote comfort as well as to prevent contractures. The sling should be adjusted to prevent the knot or buckle from pressing against the collar bone or cervical vertebrae. Placing the knot lateral to the vertebrae or placing a piece of foam rubber under the knot relieves pressure.

Later rehabilitation activities. Later rehabilitation activities include more complicated activities such as transfer, bathroom activities, and ambulation. In helping the client accomplish these activities, the nurse must work closely with physical and occupational therapists and follow their recommendations so that confusion for the client can be minimized.

Transfer is the movement of a client from one surface to another, as from bed to wheelchair, wheelchair to commode, and vice versa. Transfer may be either active or passive. In *active transfer,* the client assists with the movement, whereas if the movement must be performed completely by another person or a device, it is termed *passive transfer*.

Persons assisting the client with transfer techniques must be fully aware of the importance of promoting safety. The energy of the client, as well as the energy of the person assisting with the transfer, must be conserved. If proper body mechanics are maintained (straight back, flexed knees, hips and feet apart) and if the nurse has adequate knowledge of transfer techniques, one person can easily transfer the client. In assisting with transfer, the nurse should be familiar with the following pointers:

1. The client should always be moved toward his unaffected side.
2. If the client is transferring to a chair, it should be placed close to the unaffected side.

3. The bed should be low and locked.
4. Brakes on the wheelchair should always be locked during the transfer procedure.
5. If the bed has half-bed rails, these should be in the up position.
6. The footrest and chair arm may be removed to facilitate transfer.
7. The client should wear shoes for support.
8. Always make sure the client sees the surface to which he is to transfer.
9. The person who assists the client with transfer should stand close to him.
10. Assist the client at the waist. Never pull on the affected extremity. The transfer belt may be used for any type of transfer.

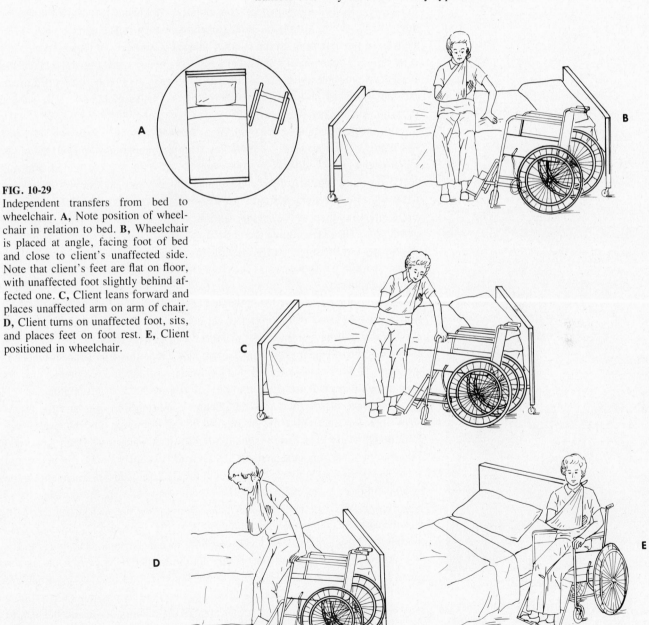

FIG. 10-29
Independent transfers from bed to wheelchair. **A,** Note position of wheelchair in relation to bed. **B,** Wheelchair is placed at angle, facing foot of bed and close to client's unaffected side. Note that client's feet are flat on floor, with unaffected foot slightly behind affected one. **C,** Client leans forward and places unaffected arm on arm of chair. **D,** Client turns on unaffected foot, sits, and places feet on foot rest. **E,** Client positioned in wheelchair.

Nursing process for common health problems

For illustrations of transfer techniques see Fig. 10-29. Readers who are interested in more details about transfer techniques should refer to a text on rehabilitation.

Bathroom activities are generally started after transfer activities have been accomplished. The activities primarily include taking a shower or bath. Certain assistive devices may make the task easier. A soap brush that is attached to a long handle is helpful. A shower hose that fits on the faucet enables the client to shower himself. A bench may be placed in the shower stall or in the bathtub for the bath. A chair draped in a plastic cover and towel also enables the client to sit while showering. Sitting also helps the client conserve his strength. A scrub brush or hand brush that is attached to a suction tip is another useful device.

Safety devices must also be considered. A bath mat with suction tips or safety strips should always be placed in the tub. Side rails should be affixed to the wall of the bathroom. If the client's balance is unsteady, it may be necessary to tie him in a chair. In this and other activities the nurse must give the client the needed support and assist him whenever necessary. At first he may need much assistance, but as physical power increases and balance improves, he should carry out the activity independently.

Ambulation should be encouraged as soon as possible. Previous activities and exercises influence early ambulation. Before ambulation is started, the physical therapist works toward strengthening the affected and unaffected extremities. To accomplish this, the therapist may utilize pulley and bicycle exercises. These are also excellent exercises for flexion and extension of the shoulder and hip joints. Standing and walking activities are important in preparation for ambulation. The occupational therapist also works toward increasing strength by coordination of the upper extremities by engaging the client in activities such as leather working, woodworking, weaving, and other activities that require fine motor coordination.

At first, the client may be ambulated between parallel bars or with two persons. When the latter method is used and if the client is unsteady and weak, it is good practice to have a third person follow with a wheelchair so that the client can be allowed to sit if he becomes too weak. Once this part is accomplished, the client progresses to a walker and/or a cane. Splints and leg braces may be used to facilitate walking if the muscles are too weak to permit ambulation.

Discharge instructions. As the client's condition improves and the previously discussed activities are accomplished, preparation must be started for community living. The family should be allowed to participate in all activities. The occupational therapist and the nurse work toward training for household activities. The exact activities should be individualized and be dependent on the responsibilities of the client in the home environment. For the female client, homemaker activities are the main focus. Preparation for such activities is directed toward teaching the client how best to conserve energy, how to master household activities with one hand, and how to use assistive devices (Fig. 10-30). As often as possible, some of the activities should be carried out in the client's home environment. If this is not possible, the practice environment should be made as nearly like the home environment as possible. Therefore it may be necessary to coordinate activities with the community health nurse who visits the home and reports back to the occupational therapist or nurse.

It must be remembered that many of the activities discussed are carried out

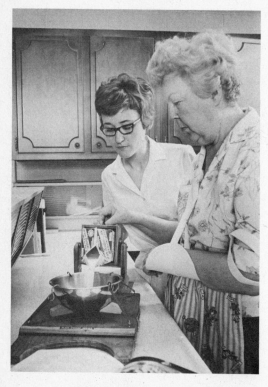

FIG. 10-30
Occupational therapist instructs home-maker in use of assistive device. (Courtesy Crossroads Rehabilitation Center, Inc., Indianapolis.)

simultaneously to facilitate early discharge so that the client can return to the home environment as early as possible.

The family should be allowed to assist with and observe these activities long before the client is discharged. They must be encouraged to foster independence. Allowing the client to go home on weekends as he masters varied activities may be an important step in preparation for discharge. The family should be referred to publications that will help them master various techniques and procedures. The United States Public Health Service publication, *Strike Back at Stroke,* contains simplified drawings and illustrations of many activities such as range of motion, positioning, and transfer. The family of a client with a stroke will possibly find such publications very useful.

In spite of extensive therapy, some clients may not become totally independent. Therefore all clients may not be fortunate enough to go back to their home environment for many reasons. There may not be anyone in the home who can adequately give care, because of age; or because of work schedule, perhaps no one can stay home to care for the client. Some families may feel that an extended care facility can better meet the needs of the client. When the client is discharged to home or an extended care facility, the nurse should always send a care plan with the client, stressing his physical limitations and assets as well as other factors that relate to his individual needs.

Vocational preparation. If the client's physical and psychological status is satisfactory, he may have a vocational evaluation either before or after discharge. The evaluation may be made by a vocational counselor, occupational therapist, or physician. The client who retired before the cerebrovascular accident should have plans made for leisure time activities.

The care of the client with a stroke is a team effort. The nurse must work closely with the client, his family, physician, and several therapists. Goals, both short-term and long-term, must be set. Every possible effort must be made to assist the client in meeting these goals so that he can take care of his own needs.

Evaluation. The last step in the nursing process is evaluation. This is an ongoing component of the process and is used as the client with cerebrovascular disease progresses toward a state of wellness.

EXPECTED OUTCOMES

The client and/or family can:
1. Describe stroke.
2. Demonstrate plans for independence in self-care activities, including self-feeding, bathing, grooming, dressing, and toileting.
3. State limitations of activity and alternative plans for self-care.
4. Demonstrate independence in transfer activities and ambulation.
5. Recognize limitations and accept assistance as needed.
6. Demonstrate satisfactory adjustments to changes in life-style created by the stroke.
7. Demonstrate ability to communicate effectively with appropriate mode (for example, written communication or gestures, if unable to engage in verbal communication).
8. Describe prescribed physical therapy, including the purpose and frequency.
9. State the need for daily exercise.
10. Demonstrate exercises.
11. State plans for health maintenance.
12. State plans for follow-up care and problems requiring health care services.
13. Indicate plans for follow-up care and knowledge of resources for continuity of care.

Nursing process for common health problems

Presenile dementia

Presenile dementia represents a progressive form of mental deterioration. It reflects the mental, social, and emotional capacities of the individual before the onset of the degenerative process. It frequently affects the client during his most productive years, often in the fourth or fifth decade of life.

Pathophysiology. Pathology is questionable, since most brain tissue examined is not remarkable except for the atherosclerosis and other signs of degeneration characteristic of aging. Somatic mutations rather than single cell abnormalities seem to be an etiological factor. An autoimmune response is also related, at least theoretically, and neuronal degeneration may be prompted by virus, radiation, or toxic plant alkaloids. The brain appears to have neurofibrillary tangles, atherosclerotic plaques, and some atrophy.

Assessment. Normal pressure hydrocephalus, Huntington's chorea, and Alzheimer's and Pick's diseases represent the classic picture of presenile dementia.

Normal pressure hydrocephalus (NPH). NPH is a clinical syndrome characterized by ventricular enlargement, resulting in compression of cerebral tissue, although the CSF pressure is normal (less than 180 to 200 mm of water pressure). NPH occurs in adults and is sometimes called occult hydrocephalus, low pressure hydrocephalus, communicating hydrocephalus, or adult hydrocephalus.

The anterior horn cells of the lateral ventricles, the temporal horns, and ultimately the third and fourth ventricles enlarge. It is felt that some phenomena (such as elevated CSF pressure) cause the ventricles to enlarge, thus losing their tensile strength in the walls. Consequently, less pressure is required to keep them expanded. There is obstruction and/or decreased absorption of CSF. Other theories offer additional explanations for etiology. Arachnoid villi may be blocked by red blood cells, for example, after trauma and hemorrhage. Trauma may also cause scarring of the basal cisterns or may result in a superior sagittal sinus thrombosis. White blood cells, which may be increased after bacterial meningitis, may block the arachnoid villi. Occasionally spinal anesthesia has been felt to contribute to a meningeal fibrosis, thus contributing to the development of NPH.

Classic symptoms consist of (1) mental changes, (2) gait disturbances, and (3) urinary incontinence, although many other neurological deficits may occur, including nystagmus, abnormal reflexes, and speech disturbances.

Therapy is surgical and involves one of several shunting procedures similar to those described for congenital hydrocephalus.

Huntington's chorea. Huntington's chorea is an inborn metabolic error that produces choreiform movements and mental deterioration in its victims. It is most frequently encountered in adults but may be seen in children and the elderly. The degenerative changes occur principally in the caudate and lenticular nuclei and in the cerebral cortex.

This chorea has an insidious onset and is characterized by personality changes as well as the classic choreiform movements. Jerky contractions of the face produce grimacing, and contraction of the respiratory muscles, face, lips, and tongue creates speech disturbances, such as hesitating or explosive speech. Gait disorders, especially shuffling, are classic. Finally, mental processes such as thought, attention, judgment, and memory are affected, and long-term mental hospitalization may be imperative.

448

Genetic counseling is imperative for clients with Huntington's chorea, because there is no effective treatment to alter the progressive, degenerative course of the disease.

Alzheimer's and Pick's diseases. Alzheimer's and Pick's diseases are so closely related that little distinguishing data are noted. Alzheimer's disease is not an inborn metabolic error, but Pick's disease is seemingly transmitted by a dominant autosomal mode. Areas of brain atrophy appear in both but in different regions, and there are some histological contrasts. The degenerative course, however, is essentially the same.[18]

Presenile dementias such as Alzheimer's disease frequently go undetected or are viewed as organic brain syndromes. It is thought that one out of five women in geriatric institutions may be affected by such chronic neuropsychiatric disorders. Women are three times more susceptible than men, it seems. Onset is usually between the ages of 45 and 65, with death by age 70.[11] Alzheimer's disease and some other presenile dementias have two distinct phases, the first of which lasts 2 to 4 years. There is memory loss, time disorientation, and reduced sensitivity. Others may interpret these changes to lack of motivation and attention, apathy, or even carelessness.

The second stage lasts for several years. Memory loss continues and aphasia, apraxia, and agnosia may occur. An annoying problem of inability to correctly name familiar objects may be apparent. The individual may say, "Here are your car checks," rather than "your car keys." The client often engages in repetitive movements such as licking the lips or chewing. His appetite may be so great that he may eat someone else's food. He touches everything. The walking gait is wide, but coordinated. Muscle twitching and jerking may be evident. All manifestations seem to worsen with stress.

Terminally, the client becomes debilitated and disinterested in life. Forgetfulness increases, and the client may have seizures. Death follows shortly at this point, perhaps within a year, since there is no satisfactory treatment at this time for the disorder.

Planning and implementation. Presenile dementia is basically managed as a social and behavioral problem requiring a gentle, protective environment where others listen carefully to the client and serve an advocate role in his behalf.[10]

Individuals with presenile dementia are best cared for in familiar surroundings, both environmental and social. They should be encouraged to maintain role functions as long as possible. For instance, women who have been primarily homemakers should continue to cook, bake, clean, and sew as long as they can engage in such activity safely. Family members, however, need to provide supervision from time to time, since the client may have periods of forgetfulness that could result in accidents, such as leaving the stove on or letting the bathtub overflow. Patience is essential in coping with the individual with presenile dementia. It is difficult for loved ones to observe mental deterioration and encounter day-to-day stresses involved in supportive care of the client. Nurses should be certain to plan for family counseling opportunities that provide a forum for information sharing, problem solving, and ventilation of frustrations and anxieties that are certain to accompany living with the individual with progressive presenile dementia.

Evaluation. Evaluation of the client with presenile dementia is ongoing.

EXPECTED OUTCOMES

The client and/or family member can:

1. Describe presenile dementia.
2. Strive to maintain a maximum level of activity within limitations imposed by presenile dementia.
3. State plans for health maintenance and follow-up care.
4. Demonstrate satisfactory adjustments of life-style imposed by presenile dementia.

COMMON HEALTH PROBLEMS THAT OCCUR ACROSS THE LIFE SPAN

Neurological trauma

Although the brain and spinal cord are well protected by bony encasements and the shock-absorbing cerebrospinal fluid, they are subject to injury from both internal and external sources.

As previously mentioned, the cranial vault of the young infant is not a totally confined space. The fontanels and suture lines allow for expansion (as in hydrocephalus). However, in the adult the skull is fused, and the bony structure completely covers the delicate brain. Therefore any factor that occupies space must do so at the expense of the compressed brain tissue. Compression such as this interferes with normal cerebrospinal fluid and blood flow, besides altering the normal functioning of the area involved.

Some of the common causes of internal mechanical injury include space-occupying lesions such as a tumor or hemorrhage or a block in the normal blood supply to a portion of the brain, such as a cerebrovascular accident. External disturbances involve primarily traumatic injuries from severe impact. Auto accidents account for the highest number of mechanical injuries to the central nervous system.

HEAD INJURY

Head injury from trauma is one of the most frequent causes of direct insult to the brain. Auto accidents, severe blows, falls, and firearms are among the leading causes of such damage. Brain damage can occur with or without an accompanying skull fracture. For any accident victim in whom there is even a remote suspicion of head injury, observations should include monitoring of neurological signs for at least 72 hours.

The client with head trauma may be placed in an intensive care unit, because he deserves close attention and his status can change rapidly during a short period.

Types of head injury. Head injuries may be open (communicating with the environment by way of an open wound) or closed (confined within the cranial vault).

Open head injuries: skull fracture. Open head injury means that the skull has been fractured and the dura mater lacerated. Shock and unconsciousness are apparent. Immediate attention must be taken to debride the wound and treat the shock. If bone fragments are driven into the brain, as in a gunshot wound, considerable damage may occur, depending on the area affected. Other complications of open injuries include infection, meningitis, and hemorrhage. Fortunately, however, the skull can withstand much impact before an open injury occurs. Closed injuries are therefore more common problems.

A skull fracture is a break in the continuity of skull bones, which may or may not be accompanied by displacement of fragments. It may be a linear break (without alteration of parts) or comminuted (several linear, fragmented interruptions to skull continuity). Often skull fractures are missed on preliminary examinations because the bone is layered (tabled) and the surface may not be indicative of what is happening immediately under the area (Fig. 10-31).

Basilar skull fractures are usually not detected on x-ray films, since they occur at the very base of the skull. Clinical signs are essential to diagnosis, and there are four that classically indicate this type of fracture.

1. Battle's sign: ecchymosis over mastoid region
2. Hemotympanum: bleeding from ear or visualization of blood behind the eardrum
3. Periorbital ecchymosis: black eyes (occurring without direct eye injury)
4. Rhinorrhea or otorrhea

The basilar skull fracture usually does not involve brain damage and coma, and other neurological deterioration is not a concern. Meningeal irritation and the threat of meningitis from spinal fluid leakage constitute the greatest concerns in emergency management.

The type and extent of the fracture varies with the age of the client, the nature of the offending agent, and the amount of force applied. In neonates the skull may be indented without interrupting the continuity of the bone, and in young children trauma may cause a separation of the sutures. Because of the absence of buttresses and immaturity of the skulls, fractures in infants do not conform to any pattern.

Skull fractures seldom require emergency treatment unless they are severely depressed, thus insulting vital brain centers, or are basilar, potentially irritating the meninges. Depressed skull fractures require that the bone be elevated to relieve pressure on the brain. Ice bags may be used to relieve edema and head-

FIG. 10-31
Types of skull fracture. **A,** Simple. **B,** Depressed. **C,** Hidden.

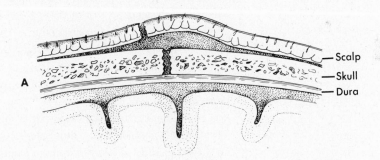

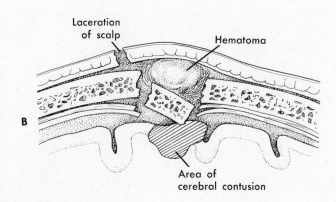

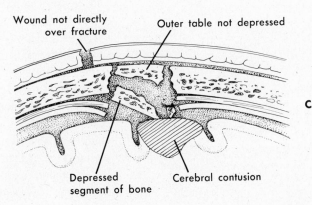

ache. Rest for at least 2 weeks is a typical recommendation until initial healing is complete. Antibiotic therapy is initiated for most basilar fractures to prevent meningitis. If there is CSF leakage, continued observation is essential to ensure that otorrhea or rhinorrhea has ceased.

Closed head injuries. When there is severe impact to the head area, several things may occur, but the initial shock response is called a *concussion*. Concussion is direct neuronal injury with loss of consciousness as its immediate effect. As the brain is set in motion during injury, it creates torsion of the immobile brainstem and interrupts the reticular activating system, thus impairing consciousness. These phenomena may last a few seconds, minutes, or an hour and are usually followed by gradual recovery of alertness and orientation. Concussion is not a benign injury, as once thought where the victim is "knocked out" momentarily but quickly regains consciousness without sequelae. It is now known that concussion can result in long-term disturbances of consciousness followed by residual symptoms.

A *postconcussion syndrome* characterized by headache, dizziness, undue fatigue, loss of insight, inability to concentrate, euphoria, irritability, and insomnia has been identified. This syndrome may persist for weeks without any improvement being evident.

Contusions are localized brain injuries of a most serious nature that involve bruising, hemorrhage, and edema. Like concussion, the impact sets the brain in motion, and as it rakes against the bony internal surfaces of the skull, the delicate tissue is damaged. Two distinct entities, *brainstem contusion* and *cerebral contusion,* must be differentiated to understand clinical management.

Head injuries may produce damage at the actual site of impact or may create damage to a point opposite the actual site of impact. These lesions are termed *coup* and *contrecoup,* respectively.

 Assessment. Concussion is usually diagnosed by history of an alert client who demonstrates a lack of memory for a time segment related to the traumatic event. Other than slight disorientation, perhaps, there are no other abnormalities found in the neurological examination. A concussion always yields an alert individual or one who is progressively awakening from unconsciousness. Any deterioration in level of consciousness is necessarily attributed to possible hematoma.

Brainstem contusion always implies damage to the upper brainstem and the reticular activating systems; thus, the victim is rendered unconscious immediately, and there is little or no improvement for several hours. If an individual is unconscious at once after the trauma and remains so, hematoma can be ruled out since blood could not collect rapidly enough to cause immediate loss of consciousness. However, of course, a client with a brainstem contusion could also have a developing hematoma.

The level of consciousness in brainstem contusion is stuporous at best. Respiration may be abnormal. Pupillary reactions, reflexes, and posturing are bilaterally congruous. This symmetry is characteristic of the typical brainstem contusion. Occasionally, however, lateralization does occur, but there is variability in abnormal findings from time to time. For example, one pupil may dilate, then neither, then both, and so forth.

Cerebral contusion results in dysfunction of a bruised portion of the cerebral hemispheres. Aphasia, for example, may indicate a frontotemporal lobe contu-

TABLE 10-7
Summary of brain injuries

Injury	Neurological findings
Concussion	Immediate interruption of level of consciousness with gradual recovery of alertness and orientation; no abnormal neurological findings
Brainstem contusion	Immediate unconsciousness with no improvement for several hours; symmetrical neurological findings or variable lateralization
Cerebral contusion	Level of consciousness may range from alertness to coma; findings depend on area of brain that is bruised
Intracranial hematoma	Deteriorating level of consciousness with no improvement of neurological status; lateralization of pupillary dilation and paresis

sion; hemiparesis, a frontal contusion; or bizarre, agitated behavior, a temporal lobe contusion. Diagnosis of a cerebral contusion can be accomplished only when a client is alert enough to cooperate in a test of cerebral functioning. Lethargic or stuporous clients may have a cerebral contusion, but one cannot be sure that a hematoma is not existent instead. Only continued observation can rule out hematoma.

If one understands how to differentiate concussion and brainstem contusion, the parameters of diagnosing hematoma should be obvious. A hematoma gradually expands within the skull, creating an increase in intracranial pressure. Lateralization of neurological findings occurs, since hematomas affect only one side of the brain in most instances. An alert client, as mentioned earlier, who has lateralization in findings has a cerebral contusion, not a hematoma (Table 10-7).

 Planning and implementation. The relationship of the brain to metabolic activities and other organ systems must be appreciated and understood in order to plan effectively for nursing care. The primary goal of clinical management is to establish and support optimal conditions under which the brain can recover. It is imperative, therefore, to understand the physiological consequence of head injury in relation to several hemodynamic mechanisms.

Metabolic factors. After head injury, like most other body trauma, there is a marked tendency to retain sodium and water and to lose a considerable amount of nitrogen.

Trauma evokes release of ADH, which contributes to water retention. Urinary output tends to be low and is characterized by a high specific gravity and elevated electrolyte concentrations. Sodium is retained because of stimulation of the hypothalamus, resulting in the release of ACTH and the consequent secretion of aldosterone. Renal hemodynamics also plays an important role in sodium retention. It is interesting to note, however, that there seems to be a lack of correlation between serum sodium levels and the occurrence of sodium retention. Posttrauma hyponatremia is not indicative, necessarily, of body sodium depletion and thus is not managed by therapeutic sodium administration. During these 3 or 4 days that water and sodium are being retained, the nurse should not judge the adequacy of hydration merely from the urinary output.

Increased nitrogen loss is another significant metabolic response to trauma. Inactivity, low nutritional intake, and general physical factors such as age, sex, and state of health seem to influence this phenomenon. Skeletal muscle protein is felt to be the chief source of the nitrogen that is lost. The degree of loss seems to be proportional to the amount of trauma incurred. Since nitrogen balance depends partially on an adequate caloric intake, it is thought that 250 to 300 calories per g of nitrogen with a nitrogen intake of 10 to 15 g per day (62 to 92 g of protein) should be adequate for most clients' nitrogen balance.[2] Hyperalimentation or gavage feedings are useful to increase nutritional efficiency. High protein and high caloric intake may precipitate azotemia or hyperglycemia if fluid balance and insulin requirements are not met.

Cortisol secretion, growth hormone activity, and the production of catecholamines and prolactin are accelerated, probably because of a response mediated by the hypothalamus. Glucose tolerance is present in most brain-injured persons, at least to some degree, for 3 to 5 days after the trauma. Several other intermediary metabolic responses to brain injury are also currently under clinical investigation.

Serotonin levels are generally elevated after the trauma. It is thought that serotonin in the free state produces neurological deficits and contributes to edema formation.[2]

Excessive accumulation of acetylcholine also has been noted following brain injury. Its elevation seems to be significant, because it is capable of influencing synaptic transmission.

Most individuals with brain injury have an arterial pH that is slightly acidotic. Usually respiratory alkalosis develops within the first 24 hours. Urinary excretion of hydrogen ions is elevated soon after injury but decreases progressively. Early after trauma there is essentially a respiratory alkalosis and a metabolic acidosis; however, the former problem may remain obscure until fluids and oxygen are used to combat hypoxia responsible for the metabolic acidosis.

The degree of CSF metabolic acidosis shares a positive correlation with the severity of the head injury. It depends on the production of lactate by the traumatized, hypoxic brain. Researchers believe that CSF lactate levels are perhaps the most reliable method of determining gross brain damage. Head injury victims who have a CSF lactate concentration exceeding 27 mg/100 ml usually do not survive.[2] CSF lactate levels, however, correlate poorly with arterial lactate levels; thus the latter is seldom used to assess brain damage. In metabolic acidosis and alkalosis, the concentration of hydrogen ions may change in opposite directions in the blood and the brain because of the slowness with which fixed acids and bases cross the blood-brain barrier and because of the ease with which molecular carbon dioxide traverses such membranes. "This means that the acid-base environment of the central nerve cells critical in respiratory control may not be altered to the same degree or even in the same direction, as is indicated by measurements made only on circulating blood."[16] Arterial blood sampling is of limited use; therefore, when metabolic activity of the brain is assessed, CSF sampling is preferred.

Respiratory factors. Respiratory complications constitute the most common cause of death in victims of brain injury after 48 hours of survival. Ventilatory failure may be a primary factor in producing death, or it may compound cerebral damage caused by hypoxia or by contributing to vasodilatation, which raises intracranial pressure, further compromising cerebral circulation.

Brain injury, like all trauma, tends to produce hyperventilation in the initial period after injury. High tidal volumes, some increase in respiratory rate, and actual alveolar hyperventilation characterize the clinical picture. The resultant hypocapnia is not altered even by exposure to 100% oxygen, demonstrating that hypoxemia is not the cause of this hyperventilation. Hypoxemia, however, is nearly always present, resulting from impaired ventilation-perfusion relationships associated with increased physiological dead space in the lungs and an acceleration of physiological shunting, that is, alveolar-arterial oxygen tension gradient difference. This increased ventilation-perfusion ratio accounts for hypoxemia despite hyperventilation.

Hyperventilation after head injury seems to result from intense sympathetic stimuli to the lungs, causing pulmonary vasoconstriction, pulmonary hypertension, and edema. The consequent reduction of lung compliance and the pulmonary edema trigger irritant receptors, which reflexively cause hyperpnea and bronchoconstriction.

Cheyne-Stokes respirations, characterized by regular alternating periods of hyperpnea and apnea, occur because of an increased sensitivity of the respiratory mechanism to carbon dioxide and to the occasional episodes of posthyperventilation apnea. Breathing builds from respiration to respiration in a smooth crescendo and then, when a peak is reached, declines in an equally smooth decrescendo. In most instances the hyperpneic phase endures longer than the apneic phase.

Another respiratory pattern that can be evident is "ataxic" respiratory effort, characterized by irregular rate, rhythm, and volume. The cause is thought to be damage to the medulla. It is accompanied by hypoxemia and is an ominous prognostic indicator.[2] Finally, Biot's respirations (totally irregular respiratory activity, both in frequency and volume) may occur in relation to brain injury, especially in conjunction with elevations in intracranial pressure.

Without vigorous respiratory support, hyperventilation, hypocapnia, and alkalosis create progressive pulmonary insufficiency, especially if the client remains unconscious. Alveolar-arterial gradients rise, and oxygen concentrations must be increased. Hypocapnia usually persists, despite assisted ventilation, but metabolic acid-base imbalances replace the mild respiratory alkalosis.

The nurse should appreciate limitations of mechanical ventilation and its effects on the body's own regulatory systems. Mechanical ventilation contributes to water retention, because there is a reduction in pulmonary blood volume and left atrial pressure resulting from positive pressure breathing. A decrease of afferent impulses from the stretch receptors of these structures leads to additional ADH output and thus promotes water retention. This may contribute to body fluid hypotonicity and thus to cerebral edema. Excess water, in turn, creates the tendency for pulmonary failure by the addition of extravascular pulmonary water and an increased alveolar-arterial oxygen gradient.

The importance of preventing and correcting hypoxemia is apparent, because it contributes to further brain damage. Provision of a patent airway, delivery of adequate oxygen concentrations, controlling hypocapnia and its resultant vasospasms, and correcting acid-base imbalances are crucial considerations in the clinical management of a client with head injury.

A cuffed endotracheal tube or tracheostomy may be necessary in an unconscious individual if secretions are copious, if there is an accompanying cervical spine injury that contraindicates hyperextension of the head, or in the event of soft tissue neck injuries that might compress the trachea.

Suctioning must be immediately available. Oral suctioning is preferred until the nature of injury is fully determined because of the proximity of the cerebrum to the nasopharynx.

Cardiovascular factors. Head injury seems to result in a series of consequences that affect cardiovascular functioning, including atypical myocardial activity, pulmonary edema, and vascular pressure alterations.

Cardiac changes include ECG abnormalities such as large T waves (with normal or abnormal polarity), prominent U waves and prolonged QT or QU intervals. These changes are the result of altered autonomic tone on functional variations of ventricular recovery time. Notched T waves, elevated P waves, and sinus dysrhythmias with wandering pacemaker, atrial fibrillation, and ventricular tachycardia also occur.[2]

Myocardial activity changes include increased heart rate and stroke index, reduced stroke work, and a subnormal CVP reading. Intracranial pressure correlates positively with cardiac output and inversely with total peripheral resistance. A transient functional insufficiency of the ventricles seems to be present immediately after head injury. An absence of endogenous sympathetic neural stimuli may be largely responsible for the reduced ventricular contractility.

Head injury sets off a series of hemodynamic consequences that often lead to pulmonary edema. At first there is general systemic vasoconstriction, causing blood to be shunted to the pulmonary vascular bed. Ventricular compliance is lessened, and as intracranial pressure rises, there is an acceleration of venous return and cardiac output, which leads ultimately to rises in systemic and pulmonary vascular pressures. Peripheral resistance may fall, however. With continued physiological stress, there is a rise in peripheral resistance so that the diastolic pressure is great enough to ensure adequate brain perfusion. Left atrial pressure is elevated with a consequent decrease in cardiac output, and eventually pulmonary edema ensues.

Another factor that may add to the production of pulmonary edema is increased arteriovenous shunting in the lung and in the periphery. There is a rise in the volume of acidotic blood returning to the heart. Persistent autonomic stimulation does not permit the heart to relax in diastole, further encouraging failure. Since pulmonary edema and pulmonary shunting relate to intracranial pressure elevations, clinical management should incorporate attention to these phenomena. Cardiac monitoring, central venous or arterial pressures, capillary wedge pressures, and CSF sampling must be considered essential assessment techniques.

Gastrointestinal factors. Gastric ulceration and hemorrhage are not uncommon after head injury, especially after trauma that involves the brainstem or produces decerebrate rigidity. It usually occurs from 3 to 7 days following the injury. Gastric hyperacidity (from vagal stimulation) and hypothalamic activity seem to be largely responsible. Increased output of catecholamines, alterations in gastric blood flow, and accelerated mucus production all have been implicated. Hypothalamic stimulus also excites the anterior hypophysis to increase its adrenal steroid output. This latter factor, coupled with the clinical use of glucocorticoids to control cerebral edema, relates closely, it seems, to ulcerogenesis.

Nurses should be aware of clues to gastric bleeding. Oligemic shock may be a singular clue, especially in children, that bleeding is in progress. Special attention should be paid to clients with decerebrate rigidity, since they seem to be highly susceptible.

Gastric intubation is often employed to reduce hyperacidity as well as to prevent aspiration pneumonitis. Anticholinergic drugs and antacids are also useful. Observation for metabolic alkalosis must be paramount whenever gastric aspiration and antacids are used for extended periods of time.

10   Neurological system

Emergency care of head injuries. The initial observations and data gathering regarding head injuries are essential to diagnosis. The nurse must understand what information to elicit as a first responder "on the scene" and as a member of a hospital emergency department team. (1) What is the level of consciousness? Is it stable? Improving? Deteriorating? (2) Is there lateralization or symmetry of abnormal neurological findings? (3) Are there signs or symptoms of increasing intracranial pressure? (4) Are there contributory factors, such as alcohol ingestion, drug overdose, or accompanying injuries, that could affect neurological findings? No singular assessment is adequate in head injury, because subtle or rapid deterioration can occur while treatment is in progress. The client should not be left unattended for over 15 minutes in the emergency department or x-ray department while skull films are being taken. In fact, most neurologists avoid x-ray studies unless a cervical fracture is suspected or if it is unclear whether the victim is deteriorating, especially if there is lateralization of findings. The goal of most emergency skull films is not to see fractures but to determine if the calcified pineal gland is in the midline or if it has shifted because of an expanding lesion such as a hematoma. Similar data can be obtained from echoencephalography, which uses high-frequency waves to assess whether the brain is in midline or has been shifted by a mass. This can be done easily in the emergency department, but reliability is not perfect. It is most useful for depressed clients with vague history and symptoms.

Seizure precautions are essential in every case of head injury until stabilization is well documented. Because clients often pass through several states of consciousness, they may be noisy and confused at intervals. A sound barrier room is desirable for the mutual welfare of all clients within the area because added stimuli often compound such behavioral problems. As consciousness returns, there is increased motor activity, excitement, and delirium. Clients may pull off clothes or want to wander around. They seem oblivious to their surroundings and often have visual or tactile hallucinations that tend to worsen at night. Restraints are sometimes used on ankles and wrists to guard against client injury or equipment displacement.

It is always important for the nurse to check to see if the client is wearing contact lenses. If so, they must be removed to prevent corneal ulceration (see Chapter 13). If the eyes do not close, they should be protected from drying and ulceration by instilling normal saline or artificial tears.

As treatment of head injury proceeds, the nurse may be responsible for intravenous therapy, ventilatory support, blood sample collection, vital signs monitoring, or the placing of an indwelling catheter. During these contacts with the client the nurse should make continued neurological assessments. Special attention should be given to noting the presence of cerebrospinal fluid or blood draining from the ears or nose, which may be indicative of severe brain injury related to dural tears into air sinuses after facial or nasal fracture. Detecting CSF leakage is important for two reasons: (1) it is significant in diagnosis and management, and (2) it indicates a potential medium for ascending infection and the development of meningitis. A client complaining of a salty taste in the back of the throat or a wet pillow may be presenting clues of CSF leakage. If enough can be collected for analysis, it will test positive for glucose (using Uristix or Dextrostix) if it is CSF. CSF also tends to separate from bloody drainage and outlines itself with a light blue halo ring on the perimeter of the moisture. This is another useful method of detecting CSF and differentiating it from water, blood, and mucus.

If CSF is confirmed, it should be permitted to drain freely onto an absorbent dressing. No attempt should be made to control the drainage by pressure tamponade, since it would restrict the flow and potentially cause a back pressure in the cranium, and it would also permit the cranial vault to communicate with a contaminated surface.

Bleeding scalp wounds, fractures of extremities, and even cerebral contusions are subordinate to expanding intracranial hematoma, which deserves top priority for management. Only cardiorespiratory failure or severe shock takes precedence over hematoma.

Scalp wounds are generally not serious problems in head injury. However, profuse bleeding may need to be controlled by pressure dressings and a circumferential head wrap. Hemostat placement is seldom useful. In some instances when pressure is insufficient to control bleeding, lacerations may need to be sutured. It is sometimes a nursing responsibility to prepare scalp wounds for minor surgery. This involves initial cleansing and exploration of the area, shaving the hair away from the laceration for 1 or 2 inches on all sides, flushing thoroughly with normal saline, and a final 5-minute scrub with an antiseptic soap solution. When the regimen has been accomplished, the laceration should be draped with sterile towels for the surgeon.

Scalp contusions and scalp hematomas usually receive little attention except for perhaps an ice pack, which reduces discomfort. Abrasions should be washed with an antiseptic soap solution and left unbandaged to promote the formation of a normal healing scab (eschar).

Cerebral concussion requires no treatment, except diagnosis and continued observation. Cerebral contusion is similarly managed except that steroids may be employed to control edema formation.

Individuals with brainstem contusion need specific nursing care and constant neurological monitoring. Airway management, ventilatory support, and blood pressure maintenance are critical components of dealing with this stuporous or comatose client. Remember that hypoxia and hypercapnia aggravate brain damage; therefore, it is essential to monitor oxygen flow, respiration, and arterial blood as well as CSF gases to ensure that ventilations are adequate.

Cerebral hematomas are the most serious head injury and involve all nursing care measures appropriate to caring for individuals with increasing intracranial pressure. The victim may be stuporous or comatose and have lateralized neurological findings that indicate active deterioration. Dilation of one pupil, hemiparesis, and decreasing responsiveness may herald a surgical emergency, because downward brain displacement and herniation are probable.

Individuals who are stable with lethargy or light stupor, who have lateralized neurological findings, but who do not have pupillary inequality, need primarily close observation while precise diagnostic work is being completed.

The nurse should be alert to postural changes that characterize brain deterioration. The classic ones are decorticate and decerebrate posturing. Both may be motor responses to painful stimulation as well as indices of cerebral dysfunction.

Decorticate rigidity is a postural attitude that indicates that the cortex of the brain is nonfunctioning. There is marked flexion of the wrists, arms, and digits. Upper extremities are adducted and flexed at the shoulder. Hands are rotated internally. Legs are extended and internally rotated with plantar flexion of the foot. Symptoms may be unilateral or bilateral. Unilateral involvement is particularly characteristic of spastic hemiplegia (Fig. 10-32, *A*).

It is theorized that the stretch reflex is regulated by extrapyramidal fibers descending to the cord from the brainstem rather than being regulated by the pyramidal tract. Extrapyramidal fibers have both suppressor and facilitator effects on the cord. Because suppressor fibers are in close association with pyramidal fibers, lesions that interrupt the pyramidal tract also damage suppressor fibers, thus restricting the activity of the stretch reflex. This influence of facilitory fibers, without the counterbalancing effect of suppressor fibers, is responsible for the resultant spasticity.

Progressive brain lesions may eventually lead to decerebration with its classic posturing (Fig. 10-32, *B*).

Decerebrate rigidity is a postural attitude characteristic of upper brainstem damage. There is rigidity and contraction of all exterior muscles. The legs are extended and the feet plantar flexed. Arms are markedly extended and hyperpronated. Opisthotonous may also be evident along with a clenched jaw and an erect head.

It is theorized that decerebration follows brainstem transection, which releases vestibular nuclei from extrapyramidal control. With the absence of inhibitory effects on the vestibular portion of the reticular formation, there is increased activity of the stretch reflexes of extensor muscles.

Decerebrate posturing is often associated with abnormal respiratory patterns and a grave prognosis. Decerebration lasting more than a week is associated with high mortality and morbidity.

Clients with head injuries may be transported frequently for diagnostic tests, therapy, or surgery. Each is subject to sudden vomiting and possible aspiration, airway obstruction from the tongue falling backward, or excessive secretions. The nurse should accompany the client during transfers in the event that an emergency should arise. Prone or semiprone positions are recommended during transportation; however, one disadvantage is that it impedes observation of the client's status. If it is not feasible to accompany the individuals, technicians and aides should be advised of precautions and specific measures to be taken in the event of seizures, vomiting, or respiratory distress.

FIG. 10-32
A, Position assumed by patient with decorticate rigidity. Note again position in which extremities, especially upper extremities, are held. **B,** Position held by patient with decerebrate rigidity. Note position of arms and legs. Decerebrate rigidity includes other manifestations not seen here. (From Budassi, Susan A., and Barber, Janet M.: Emergency nursing: principles and practice, St. Louis, 1981, The C.V. Mosby Co.)

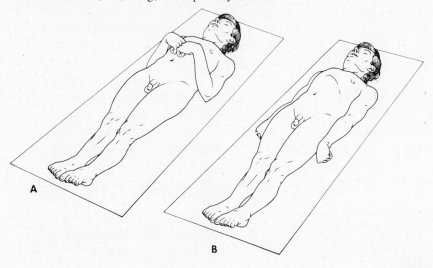

Nursing process for common health problems

Hemorrhage and hematoma from trauma. Hemorrhage may occur in the brain tissue, into the CSF, or into the extradural and subdural spaces. The most commonly occurring hemorrhage is subarachnoid, produced by traumatic tearing of vessels on the superficial surface of the brain (thus allowing blood to pass freely into the subarachnoid space) or by rupture of an aneurysm. Traumatic subarachnoid hemorrhages accompany most severe head injuries and many mild ones.

Extradural (epidural) *hemorrhage* results from the tearing of blood vessels on the outer aspect of the dura mater as the brain is pulled away from the bone at the time of impact or where vessels are broken at a fracture line. The middle meningeal artery and vein complex is the most common location of extradural bleeding. Children under age 10 have a low incidence of extradural hemorrhage because of a greater adherence of dura to bone and a lack of vascular depression in bone.

Extradural hemorrhage is a potential sequela of a fall, a direct blow to the head, or a low velocity impact. Gunshot and other penetrating wounds are among frequent causes, but the highest incidence is related to bicycle accidents.

If an extradural hematoma is recognized, it can be removed by craniotomy with few sequelae. However, if it has been overlooked, because of slow progression (because the dura resists separation from the skull) or because of failure to present symptoms, it can continue to enlarge and create dangerous compression and displacement of the brain.

Subdural hemorrhages are less confined than epidural ones, because their extension is limited only by the tentorium and the falx barriers. They may be *acute* (signs and symptoms occuring within 48 hours of injury), *subacute* (up to 2 weeks after the injury), or *chronic*. Subdural hematomas result from tears of connecting veins between the surface of the brain and the dural sinuses. Accumulation of blood may vary from 30 to 300 ml. Although subdural hemorrhages usually result from trauma, they may be associated with intracranial aneurysm, arteriovenous malformations, tumor masses, or blood dyscrasias. Birth injuries, falls, and auto accidents account for the greatest incidence in infancy and childhood. Stupor and coma in the elderly, in chronic alcoholics, and in clients taking anticoagulant drugs should be suspected to be caused by chronic subdural bleeding.

In acute subdural hemorrhages the primary lesion is blood that clots and later liquefies. Subacute lesions are composed of blood and CSF and tend to be more liquid in nature. In order to appreciate the chronic subdural hematoma, it is essential to recognize the pathophysiology of the subdural hemorrhage lesion.

Clots are tolerated for long period of time, days or weeks, and eventually are liquefied with a concurrent rise in osmotic pressure. Simultaneously, in an effort to absorb the clot, connective tissue proliferates on the dural side, resulting in membrane formation. Since the arachnoid membrane by nature has a limited blood supply, it does not appreciably contribute to absorption. However, because the arachnoid is a semipermeable membrane, the clot expands as CSF and other tissue fluids are drawn into the clot. The lesion therefore enlarges and may result in additional bleeding. Eventually signs and symptoms of increased intracranial pressure ensue. It has been reported that subdural lesions may calcify, thus becoming self-limiting.

Chronic subdural hemorrhages in children may be manifest by vague signs and symptoms exhibited over a considerable time span. Episodic seizures, vomiting, irritability, failure to thrive, fever, hyperactive reflexes, anemia, bulging fontanels, and abnormal fundi may be manifest, but without a history of trauma, they are necessarily associated with a subdural lesion. Signs of child abuse and deliberate trauma may clue the clinician to suspect this chronic process.

Headache, stupor, and hemiparesis may indicate the presence of a chronic subdural hematoma in an adult. It should be stressed that persons should be alerted not to overlook a seemingly minor head injury, since venous bleeding may occur so slowly that signs of damage may not appear for quite a while after the accident and, as a result, may not be associated with the injury.

Assessment. Clients who exhibit stupor or coma or who have a history of head trauma or unrelenting headache must be evaluated for brain hemorrhage or hematoma. Five general areas of data are useful in determining the type of lesion and the direction of the lesion's process: (1) levels of consciousness, (2) respiratory pattern, (3) pupil size and reaction, (4) eye movements and oculovestibular responses, and (5) motor responses from skeletal muscle.

Levels of consciousness. The client who is manifesting an extradural or subdural hemorrhage usually presents a deteriorating level of consciousness. Cerebral hemorrhage usually results in coma in a few minutes after its onset. However, this downward progression in level of consciousness may involve fluctuation of worsening and improving over a period of days and even from hour to hour. It is imperative, therefore, that the nurse make frequent and complete assessments of the level of consciousness to ensure diagnostic validation and to engage in appropriate intervention. It should be recalled that alcohol ingestion, certain drugs, and other coexistent brain pathological conditions may complicate the client's presentation, especially after trauma.

Respiratory pattern. The respiratory pattern depends on (1) the degree of cerebral anoxia imposed by circulatory impairment or dysfunctions of gaseous exchange and on (2) the degree of neuroanatomical damage in the brain's vital centers. It is essential for the nurse to evaluate and record all qualitative characteristics of respirations, not just the quantity. Because many different brain levels influence the act of breathing, certain conditions causing brain dysfunction induce respiratory abnormalities as well as make respiratory signs useful in diagnosis, and, finally, may suggest an urgent need for intervention. Increased and decreased respiratory efforts must be ascertained as truly reflecting hyperventilation or hypoventilation. For example, increased chest efforts are not really reflecting hyperventilation if they exist merely to overcome pneumonitis or respiratory obstruction. Conversely, shallow breathing may not be, in actuality, hypoventilation, because metabolic demands are greatly reduced in deep coma. Bedside observations should be tempered by CSF and arterial blood gas determinations at regular intervals to ensure that oxygenation is adequate and that the metabolic environment of the brain tissue is compatible with functional physiology. Shock increases cerebral ischemia by virtue of its hypotensive and hypoxic effects.

There may be accompanying injuries that interfere with breathing. Tracheal obstruction sometimes occurs as a result of neck and cervical cord trauma. The latter may also cause a neurological as well as mechanical interference with breathing. Chest trauma may also impair respiratory effort.

461

Nursing process for common health problems

The airway must be maintained at all times. It is the first priority in nursing care. Comatose clients are usually positioned supine and are susceptible to respiratory obstruction resulting from the tongue falling back and obstructing the posterior pharynx. Pulling the angle of the lower jaw forward will relieve the obstruction. Turning the client slightly so that the head will naturally lie on the side will help immensely in preventing the tongue from falling back.

Respiratory insufficiency may require mechanical ventilation with the aid of an endotracheal tube or a tracheostomy, especially for clients in coma or with cervical injuries.

Suctioning is an important adjunct in maintaining a natural or an artificial airway. It is frequently noted that clearing the airway may result in immediate improvement in the level of consciousness, a decrease in blood pressure, and a change from stertorous to normal respirations. Muscular twitchings, even seizures, may cease after correcting airway obstruction. It is recommended that sterile technique be employed to minimize the development of infections.

At the first signs of vomiting, immediate steps must be taken to prevent aspiration of vomitus. Turn the head forcibly to the side and lower the head below the level of the abdomen (even though the general rule in head trauma is to maintain elevation). If necessary, pull the client half out of bed and hold the thorax and head in an almost vertical head-down position. Suction the posterior pharynx until clear, and then return the individual to his precrisis position.

Pupil size and reaction. The size and reaction of the pupils are valuable guides in locating brain dysfunction and in monitoring its progression, because brainstem areas for controlling consciousness lie anatomically adjacent to those controlling pupils. Furthermore, because pupillary pathways are relatively resistant to metabolic insult, the presence or absence of the light reflex is the classical physical sign that can distinguish structural from metabolic causes.[17] In the overwhelming majority of brain hemorrhages the pupil is widely dilated on the ipsilateral side. (Pressure of the clot against cranial nerve III at the superior orbital fissure is thought to be responsible for this entity. Uncal herniation may also destroy cranial nerve III at the incisural gap.) It is important to note that after initial ipsilateral pupillary responses there may be contralateral dilatation as well. Retinal hemorrhages and engorged veins, additionally, are seen in most children.

Eye movements and oculovestibular responses. Eye movements and oculovestibular responses are valuable indicators for evaluating clients with altered levels of consciousness, because their anatomical pathways, again, are adjacent to brainstem areas necessary for consciousness. The extraocular movements in awake, cooperative clients can be examined for both voluntary and reflex activity. In stupor and coma, reflexes must suffice. The nurse should note the position of the eyes and the eyelids at rest and should watch for spontaneous eye movements. In coma the eyes are closed by tonic muscular contractions so that if the lid is lifted and released, it will close gradually. (Clients with psychogenic hysteria cannot duplicate this phenomenon.) Absence of tone or failure of the lid on either side to close may point to facial nerve dysfunction. Observe if blinking is present and under what circumstances. Is there a corneal reflex? There are several other neurological tests that are useful in evaluating eye movements and oculovestibular responses, including head-turning reflexes and caloric stimulation.

Motor responses from skeletal muscle. Motor function is often highly correlated with the depth of the coma, but this is misleading because pathways that regulate movement are far removed from those that mediate consciousness, either content or arousal. Motor decerebration can exist with full retention of consciousness, for example. The important aspect of motor assessment in brain hemorrhage is that it provides valuable information about the geographical distribution of dysfunction. Movements, reflex behavior, grasping responses, the presence of characteristic decorticate and decerebrate posturing, and responses to noxious stimuli are useful modes to assess motor functioning. Motor responses fluctuate with levels of consciousness, primarily because of physiological alterations in tissue circulation and metabolism.

Other assessments. Vital signs in hemorrhage and hematoma are variable. The pulse may be slow or full and bounding, or tachycardia may occur immediately after injury and in conjunction with a grave prognosis. Temperature is usually elevated to 101.1° to 103.2° F (38.4° to 39.6° C). Although the blood pressure may increase in elevated intracranial pressure, it is of little diagnostic value in assessing hemorrhage and hematoma.

The scalp should be examined at frequent intervals after trauma. Extradural lesions are often present as puffy areas, especially over the temporoparietal region. Palpable skull fractures may traverse the middle meningeal artery groove. (It has been noted that the incidence in children under 10 is less than adults because of greater adherence of dura to bone and lack of vascular depressions in bone.)

CSF may be bloody and under increased pressure. However, since the CSF circulation is characteristically slow, it may take up to 6 hours for blood to reach the lumbar region. Spinal taps therefore are seldom considered routine in the diagnosis of extradural and subdural hemorrhages.

Weighing the client and carefully assessing the fluid balance are essential. The nurse should remember to evaluate nebulized intake, since it may contribute up to 500 ml per day. A client with little or no caloric intake should lose about 400 g per day, and failure to lose this amount means that there is water retention.[2]

Extradural and subdural hemorrhages are surgically managed via burr holes, which permit clot aspiration. Children improve more rapidly than adults, but recovery is favorable for most clients. It is felt that children have reduced risks of transtentorial herniation because of its wider aperture and pliability. Nursing care related to such surgical procedures is discussed in relation to tumors (see discussions later in this chapter).

Planning and implementation. Frequently individuals may have reportedly incurred trauma to the head that is essentially asymptomatic at the time of injury. The question is often raised regarding under what circumstances seemingly minor bumps, blows, or scalp injuries can be safely managed without specific observation, x-ray films, or other medical intervention. It is virtually impossible to present a rule of thumb that is applicable in every circumstance. However, it is generally agreed that the following presenting signs or symptoms require prompt attention:

1. Deteriorating level of consciousness
2. Inequality of pupils
3. Otorrhea or rhinorrhea

4. Signs of increasing intracranial pressure, such as nausea, headache, vomiting, irritability, lethargy, or seizures
5. Depressed or open fracture
6. Unilateral or bilateral loss of sensory or motor functioning
7. Signs of meningeal irritation, such as nuchal rigidity, fever, or behavioral changes

Parents, babysitters, school nurses, teachers, and other individuals who are frequently responsible for children's postaccident observations should be aware of the "danger signs" of head injury, which could point to serious underlying pathological conditions. They should also understand that several days may elapse before some signs and symptoms become apparent; therefore historical perspective is always essential to communicate so that if any untoward manifestations are encountered, they can be interpreted appropriately in view of the injuries sustained.

Cerebral complication of trauma: fat embolism. Trauma may invite the serious complication of fat embolism, especially if there is a fracture of long bones. It is found in one fourth of all cases of death that occurs after the trauma. Clinicians believe that fat deposits of bone cannulae are released into circulation as fracture occurs. These lipid particles and possibly fibrin clots occlude small vessels, especially in the lung and brain tissue. Another point of view is that emboli originate from plasma proteins and that the fibrin plugging vessels is a by-product of disseminating intravascular coagulation.

Signs and symptoms of fat embolism may occur several hours after injury or within a 2- to 3-day time span. The temperature is elevated to 101.1° to 103.2° F (38.4° to 39.6° C), and there is marked tachycardia. Arterial blood gases reveal a decline in Po_2 and Pco_2. Serum lipase is elevated. Petechial rash appears on the neck, shoulders, anterior thorax, and eyegrounds. Biopsies of petechiae reveal lipid deposits. Two syndromes may appear clinically as fat embolism: respiratory and cerebral.

Respiratory fat emboli are marked by cough, chest pain, cyanosis, dyspnea, and rales. Fat in sputum or urine and chest x-ray films confirm the diagnosis. Complications from respiratory emboli often are responsible for deaths related to fat emboli.

Cerebral fat emboli may present insidiously with confusion, lethargy, stupor or coma, seizures, apahsia, and hemiplegia. Symptoms are thus easily mistaken for intracranial bleeding. One important diagnostic clue is that symptoms become most profound on the second day after trauma. Fat appearing in sputum or in the urine or papilledema may be the only cues to establishment of a diagnosis until the classic petechial rash appears after 48 to 72 hours.

With judicious medical and nursing management, most clients recover from fat embolism *if* the condition is promptly diagnosed and supportive therapy is begun. Nursing observations related to pulmonary functioning, behavior, neurological status, and skin eruptions are extremely important in helping the medical team confirm the existence of a fat embolism.

 Evaluation. Evaluation of the client with head injury is an ongoing component of the nursing process as care is planned and implemented.

EXPECTED OUTCOMES

The client and/or family can:
1. State limits of activity.

10 Neurological system

2. State plans for health maintenance.
3. State problems requiring emergency health care services.
4. Indicate plans for follow-up care and knowledge of community resources for health care.

SPINAL CORD INJURY

Although the spinal cord is protected by a bony encasement and the shock-absorbing cerebrospinal fluid, it is subject to injury from both internal and external sources.

The spinal cord does not move axially in the spinal canal but adapts to variations of canal length by shortening or elongating through plastic change of its substance. In flexion, it lengthens. In extension, it shortens by developing folds on its surface.

In youth the spinal cord is well protected mechanically and hydraulically. However, in aging, supportive tissues are altered, the spinal canal narrows, osteoporosis sets in, and there is general loss of elasticity of the intervertebral disks.

Besides gross trauma and penetrating wounds, such as stabbing, there are four basic types of spinal cord injuries. The usual mechanism of vertebral injury is a flexion-rotation force, with rotation being dominant in producing displacement (Fig. 10-33).

Types of spinal cord injuries

Flexion injury. In most instances flexion injury results from trauma and is likely to be a cervical wedge compression fracture with accompanying dislocation. The upper spine moves forward in relation to the lower spine, thus creating malalignment, which narrows the spinal canal and pinches or crushes the cord

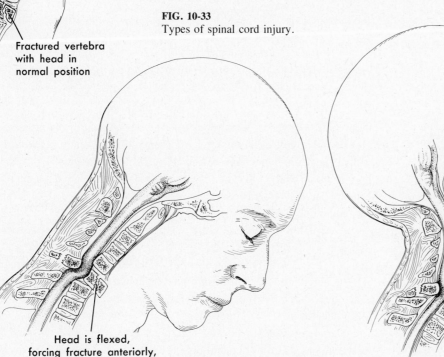

Base of spinal cord

Fractured vertebra with head in normal position

Head is flexed, forcing fracture anteriorly, pinching spinal cord

FIG. 10-33
Types of spinal cord injury.

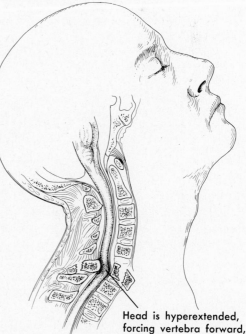

Head is hyperextended, forcing vertebra forward, pinching spinal cord

465

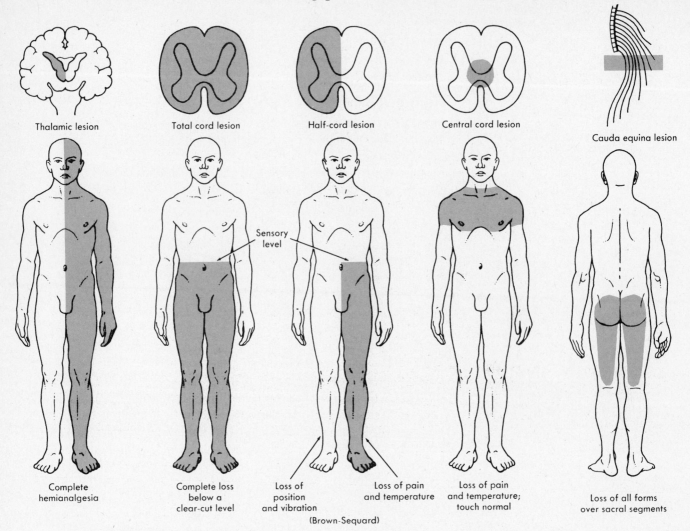

Thalamic lesion   Total cord lesion   Half-cord lesion   Central cord lesion   Cauda equina lesion

Sensory level

Complete
hemianalgesia

Complete loss
below a
clear-cut level

Loss of
position
and vibration

Loss of pain
and temperature
(Brown-Sequard)

Loss of pain
and temperature;
touch normal

Loss of all forms
over sacral segments

FIG. 10-34
Common patterns of sensory abnormality. Upper diagrams show site of lesion; lower diagrams show distribution of corresponding sensory loss. (From Budassi, Susan A., and Barber, Janet M.: Emergency nursing, principles and practice, St. Louis, 1981, The C.V. Mosby Co.)

between the lower vertebral body and the neural arch of the vertebra above. A flexion force will ordinarily create a compression fracture before rupturing the spinal ligaments, which are extremely resistant to flexion.

Rotation injury. Rotation is frequently combined with a flexion injury and is usually cervical. It involves trapping the cord between two separated portions of the spine that have been displaced by rotational force.

Compression injury. Compression cord damage is most typically lumbar but may be cervical. Force exerted to the whole spinal column is absorbed in lumbar region with resultant bursting of vertebral bodies. Bone fragments and disk material are forced backward into the spinal canal, thus damaging the cord. The vertebral bodies (not the articular facets) are affected because the latter are deep and strong.

Extension injury. An extension injury refers to hyperextension of the vertebral column caused by sudden force, such as striking the head on the windshield during an automobile accident. Hyperextension injuries of the cervical region with anterior and posterior cord compression may result in greater weakness of the upper limbs (rather than lower limbs), bladder dysfunction, and various degrees of sensory impairment. It is worthy to note that extension injuries can occur with seemingly minor trauma.

Brown-Sequard syndrome. A lateral lesion (Brown-Sequard) affects one half of the cord, producing ipsilateral paralysis and contralateral loss of pain and temperature. Penetrating trauma is the usual cause. Root syndrome often occurs, resulting from vertebral subluxation of acute herniated disks. Lost functions (sensory and motor) can return, because spinal roots and nerves are part of the peripheral nervous system, thus capable of regeneration if anatomical continuity has not been lost (Fig. 10-34).

• • •

In each of the preceding types of injury there is insult to meninges, blood vessels, and nerves with consequent edema formation, hemorrhage, and eventually degenerative fibrosis. Unfortunately spinal cord regeneration can occur only if axons have myelin derived from the Schwann cell sheath. Unmyelinated fibers are not capable of regeneration.

Assessment. An injury to the spinal cord should be suspected whenever any of the following conditions are present: (1) inability to move arms or legs, (2) unusual sensations in the extremities, (3) unexplained shock, (4) wounds of the face, head, neck, or shoulders, (5) unconsciousness after the injury, or (6) pain, tenderness, deformities, or muscle spasms adjacent to the vertebral column. *Whenever there is doubt regarding the presence of a spinal cord injury, manage the victim as if one were present.*

Always assess breathing first. If airway obstruction or inadequate ventilation exists, these problems must be managed *without extending the neck*. To open the airway, either place two fingers under the victim's jaw and lift it forward, or hook one thumb inside the victim's lower jaw and lift the chin forward. Determine if respirations are diaphragmatic. Since chest wall muscles may be paralyzed in neck injuries, all respiratory effort may be dependent on the diaphragm. If breathing assistance is necessary, it must be done without manipulating the neck. Suction may be required in some instances.

Neurogenic shock from vasomotor collapse may occur. Vessels, especially of the lower extremities, dilate rapidly and insufficient blood is returned to the heart. Elevation of the legs while keeping knees straight permits circulatory enhancement by gravitational return of blood to the heart.

The head and neck should be immobilized with a cervical collar or sandbags before transfer. A splinting board is used to ensure that the entire body is moved as a rigid unit, with firm support of all body parts and maintenance of alignment. Manual traction of the mandible, with the hands against the occiput, can be employed by a skilled person, or a prone position may be employed to hyperextend the spinal column, thus preventing further compression injury.

It is important that sudden jarring motions be avoided because they may result in (1) cord hemorrhage or edema, or (2) injury to the cord by tearing, compressing, or even severing.

Injudicious management of clients with cord injuries can result in permanent damage. It is advisable (even for nurses) to await the arrival of a qualified emergency medical technician or paramedic who is skilled and possesses essential equipment to properly manage and safely transfer such individuals from the accident scene to the hospital.

 Planning and implementation. The primary objective of the initial medical, surgical, and nursing management of the client with a spinal cord injury is to relieve compression and prevent further impairment.

Lifting and moving should always be accomplished by several individuals to ensure that the body is moved as a rigid unit to reduce pain, discomfort, and the possibility of additional injury. Traction, casts, braces, hyperextension techniques, and orthopedic frames may be employed to ensure achievement of this objective. When, however, it is determined that paralysis and loss of function below the level of damage is irreversible, the nurse needs to plan care for the long-term management of the client. See Table 10-8 for functional goals appropriate to various levels of spinal cord lesions.

General care should be appropriate for the immobilized client in relation to skin care, exercise, nutrition, hygiene, and socialization.

TABLE 10-8
Functional goals in spinal cord lesions

Spinal cord level	Key muscle control	Functional goals
C5	Neck Upper trapezius	Manipulate electric wheelchair with mouth stick Maintain limited self-care (feeding, make-up) using arm supports and externally powered hand splints
C6	Shoulder muscles Elbow flexors	Turn self in bed with overhead arm slings Transfer to and from bed with assistance Propel wheelchair with hand-rim projections Feed self with externally powered hand splints or clip-on equipment Maintain light hygiene (make-up, brushing teeth) Dress upper trunk
C7	Wrist extensors Supinators	Transfer to and from bed and car without assistance Transfer to commode chair with assistance Propel chair with hand-rim projections Feed self and maintain hygiene (shaving and grooming hair), dressing, writing, and skin inspection, using wrist-driven flexor-hinge hand splints where required Drive car with hand controls
C8	Elbow extensors Weak hand	Transfer independently to and from bed, car, and toilet Propel wheelchair without hand-rim projections Get wheelchair in and out of car Be independent in all self-care without hand splints or adapted equipment except catheter Do household activities from wheelchair
T1 to T8	Hand muscles	Get wheelchair up and down curb Transfer to and from tub Get wheelchair to floor and return Stand therapeutically with posterior leg splints Take care of catheter
T9 to T12	Trunk stability	Have wheelchair independence Ambulate physiologically with bilateral long leg braces and crutches Maintain complete self-care
L1 to L5	Pelvic stability	Ambulate with bilateral long leg braces and crutches
S1 to S2	Knee extension Hip flexion	Ambulate with short leg braces, crutches, or cane

Adapted from Feiring, Emanuel H., editor: Brock's injuries of the brain and spinal cord and their coverings, ed. 5. Copyright © 1974, New York, Springer Publishing Co., Inc.

Ultimately, the goal of rehabilitation of the cord-injured client is to return to his home, family, and a useful, productive pattern of living. Before this is possible, many weeks of painful processes must be endured, through varying levels of motivation, to accomplish (1) independence in activities of daily living (such as eating, toileting, and personal hygiene), (2) the learning of transfer techniques, and (3) vocational rehabilitation. Many agencies may be used in helping the client and his family toward the goal of returning to a meaningful life pattern.

Major problems of the client with spinal cord injury. The trauma that is felt by the client who learns that his cord injury has resulted in permanent damage is bound to evoke extreme depression and anger. It is thought that most persons encounter stages of grief similar to those related to death. After all, to the victim of paraplegia or quadriplegia, a very real loss of life has occurred. Considerable support from families, friends, and especially a spouse is essential for adjustment to a new mode of life. Since many spinal cord injuries involve young adults, especially those responsible for a family, the problems are compounded psychologically, socially, emotionally, and physically.

Spinal shock. Spinal shock is a transient condition effected by transection of the spinal cord. Two phenomena are at once present: (1) all voluntary motion in body parts innervated by the isolated spinal segments is permanently lost; (2) all sensation from those parts, which depends on the integrity of ascending spinal pathways, is abolished. Accompanying these two is a spinal areflexia or shock.[16] In addition to all reflexes and autonomic functions being absent, there is bilateral, flaccid paralysis below the transection (Fig. 10-35).

Reflexes may return as early as within the first 24 hours after the transection, but more commonly not for several weeks, especially if infection or toxic states exist. Rarely, reflexes do not return at all, probably because of actual destruction of cord tissue or related blood supply.

The acute period of spinal shock is followed by a period of minimal reflex activity. Then tone increases, flexor spasms develop, and Babinski's reflex becomes evident. Eventually, extensor activity appears and usually constitutes the dominant reflex pattern. The view that paraplegia in flexion is indicative of complete cord transection, whereas paraplegia in extension indicates an incomplete lesion, has been proved erroneous. Spinal shock may occur with partial cord lesions, also, but recovery is usually apparent in a period of hours or days.

Visceral reflexes associated with the bladder, bowel, vasomotor mechanisms, and sexual functioning are considered in depth, because they are intricately related to nursing care responsibilities.

Bladder. Immediately after cord transection, there is complete atony of the smooth muscle of the bladder wall. Concurrently there is an increase in constrictor tone of the sphincter because of loss of inhibitory influences. Consequently urine collects until the intravesical pressure overcomes sphincter resistance. Only small amounts of urine are allowed to escape (overflow incontinence). With return of somatic reflexes, reflex bladder emptying occurs, but residual urine remains in the incompletely evacuated bladder. More complete emptying can be encouraged if catheterization is employed to remove residual urine. Additionally, cutaneous stimuli delivered to the abdomen, perineum, or lower extremities can also facilitate this process. Reflex bladder action usually is established in 25 to 30 days after transection.[16]

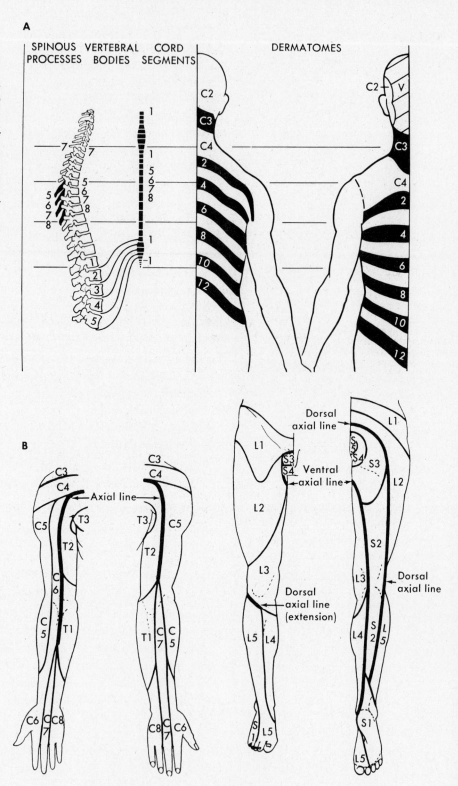

FIG. 10-35
Dermatomes indicate areas of body innervated by specific spinal cord segments. Note that spinal cord segments do not correspond with vertebral bodies and that spinous processes correspond with neither. **A,** Segmental innervation of trunk. **B,** Segmental innervation of upper and lower extremities. (**A** from Jennett, W. Bryan: Scientific foundations of surgery, London, William Heinemann Medical Books, Ltd.; **B** from Medical Research Council: War memorandum no. 7. Aids to the investigation of peripheral nerve injuries, London, H.M. Stationery Office.)

470

Some clients will require an indwelling catheter on a permanent basis. Because renal complications are the most common cause of death among clients with spinal cord injury, complications from long-term catheterization must be minimized by employing scrupulous catheter care practices.

Bowel. Processes of digestion and absorption seem to proceed normally following cord transection, but some difficulty is encountered in evacuating feces. Ordinarily the mere presence of fecal matter in intestines passively stretching the walls produces peristalsis and defecation. In spinal shock, however, the anal sphincter relaxes only slightly, despite distension of bowel walls, and elimination is impeded. Essentially a paralytic ileus occurs. With return of reflex excitability (as in the bladder), reflex emptying occurs. Again, this process can be facilitated by tactile stimulation of the skin area of the sacral segments or by manual dilation of the anal sphincter.

Oral intake is usually limited until bowel sounds return, and then a progressive regimen of bowel training is begun.

Because there is a complete sympathetic block from interruption of the descending and ascending visceral nerve pathways, vagal action and gastric acid production are thus unopposed. Stress ulcers are frequently discovered within a week or two after the transection. It is essential that the nurse observe for signs and symptoms of gastrointestinal bleeding, including progressive anemia.

Vasomotor mechanisms. In spinal shock there is a loss of vasoconstrictor tone, which creates hypotension that persists for several days (or up to 6 to 8 weeks). Eventually a tonic state returns, and blood pressure returns to a normal level. In addition, large muscles are no longer active in circulatory stimulation, and blood may pool in capillaries, thus shrinking circulating volume. Tachycardia, signs of fatigue, and orthostatic hypotension may occur. Thrombus formation may be a threat during prolonged periods of hemostasis. Elastic hose, for example, may augment position changes and range-of-motion exercises as measures to stimulate stagnant circulation.

Sweating does not occur below the level of injury, and thus the client has difficulty in maintenance of body temperature. Because of vasomotor interferences, the heart rate does not increase as body temperature elevations occur, and thus it is not unusual to have clients experience fever without the vital signs indices that usually accompany it.

Sexual function. The client with cord transection must undergo dramatic revisions of self-concept. Not only are there limitations of locomotion and elimination, but adjustments must be made regarding sexual role functioning.

Most victims of accidents that cause cord transection (automobile, motorcycle, skiing, and diving) are young adults. The special tragedy of sexual rehabilitation in youthful victims who have major tasks of life ahead is indeed a challenge for the nurse.

To understand the injured cord and its effect on sexual functioning, the nurse must consider the anatomical and physiological components of sexual intercourse.

PHYSIOLOGY. During the excitement phase of sexual activity, the descending corticomotor pathway or ascending sensory pathways transmit stimuli. The glans penis of the man and the clitoris of the woman are the focal receptive points for sensual stimuli, especially tactile, because they are well supplied with peripheral nerves. The afferent fibers of the pelvic and pudendal nerves convey im-

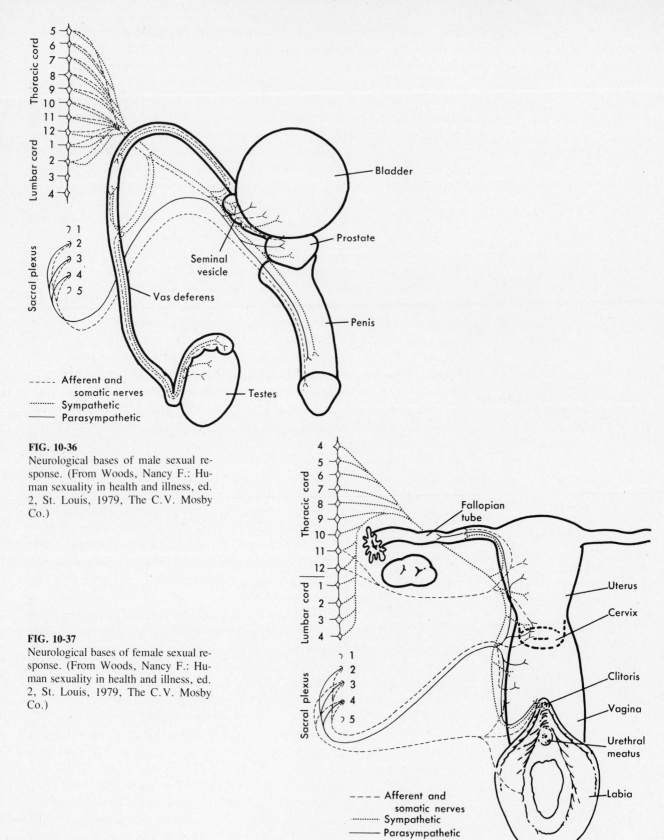

FIG. 10-36
Neurological bases of male sexual response. (From Woods, Nancy F.: Human sexuality in health and illness, ed. 2, St. Louis, 1979, The C.V. Mosby Co.)

FIG. 10-37
Neurological bases of female sexual response. (From Woods, Nancy F.: Human sexuality in health and illness, ed. 2, St. Louis, 1979, The C.V. Mosby Co.)

pulses to the sacral cord, where synapses with parasympathetic efferent nerves to the pelvis evoke reflex erectile responses in the penis or clitoris.

Male erection is influenced by parasympathetic impulses from the sacral cord transmitted through pelvic splanchnic nerves to the penis. Arteries of the penis dilate, veins constrict, and the cavernous sinuses become engorged, creating a larger, rigid organ for copulation.

Associated reflex centers may be activated in the brain, producing psychogenic erection. (In sacral cord dysfunction, thoracolumbar cord segments are believed to be responsible for reflex erection.) A similar phenomenon, which creates erection and vaginal lubrication, occurs in the clitoral region.

Parasympathetic impulses, active in excitement, cause mucus production in the glans of the man and just inside the vaginal opening in the woman. As intensity of the act increases, reflex centers of the thoracolumbar region transmit rhythmic impulses, and sympathetic nerves evoke the conveyance of sperm to the bladder neck region (emission). Emission stimulates afferent impulses that flow to the sacral cord and synapse with somatic efferent fibers of the pudendal nerve. This complex phenomenon ultimately yields the clonic contractions and pelvic floor motion responsible for ejaculation. Pelvic contractions in the woman occur essentially by the same mechanisms (Figs. 10-36 and 10-37).

Psychic stimuli seem to originate in the temporal lobe, in limbic system parts, and in the hypothalamus. Sensory stimulation creates impulses that are carried to the spinal cord via somatic and visceral efferent fibers.

PATHOPHYSIOLOGY. In transection of the spinal cord, sexual activity cannot be normally maintained, because important neurological mechanisms are inoperable.

The type of spinal cord injury (or transection) and whether it is complete or incomplete determine whether the client can achieve erection, ejaculation, and orgasm. However, the majority of injured persons can have erection and may be fertile unless there is extensive destruction at the sacral cord, cauda equina transection, or cord damage between the T6 and L3 segments sufficient to completely block sympathetic outflow. Reflex erections are possible for selected clients by either local or psychic stimulation. (Reflex erection should not be confused with *priapism,* an abnormal, painful, and continuous erection caused by cord lesions above the lumbar region, by peripheral sensory nerve irritants, or by organic disease that affects the associated nerve centers.) It is imperative that the paraplegic is not considered impotent because most are at least capable of erection. Orgasm may occur or orgasmic sensations may be experienced in the groin, on the inner thighs, or on the back and abdominal skin above the lesion's level. Intercourse is possible if erection can be attained and maintained, but gratification may be limited to satisfying the partner.

Paraplegic women, because their role can be passive, may enjoy intercourse and be perfectly capable of satisfying their mate. Little is known about their capacity for orgasm, however, because the majority of clients with paraplegia are men, victims of sporting or military combat accidents.

Sterility is not necessarily a consequence of paraplegia, although there is often testicular atrophy, and sperm viability may be adversely affected by loss of temperature regulatory control in the scrotum because of autonomic nerve loss. Fertility may be more influenced by the loss of the man's power of forceful ejaculatory projection, however.

TABLE 10-9

Type of spinal cord lesion and associated components of sexual function

Type of lesion	Erections	Ejaculation	Orgasm
Upper motor neuron			
Complete	Frequent (93%) Reflexogenic only	Rare	Absent
Incomplete	Most frequent (99%) Reflexogenic (80%) Reflexogenic and psychogenic (19%)	Less infrequent (32%) After reflexogenic erection (74%) After psychogenic erection (26%)	Present if ejaculation occurs
Lower motor neuron			
Complete	Infrequent (26%) Psychogenic only	Infrequent (18%)	Present if emission occurs
Incomplete	Frequent (90%) Psychogenic and reflexogenic	Frequent (70%) After psychogenic and reflexogenic erections	Present if ejaculation occurs

From Woods, Nancy Fugate: Human sexuality in health and illness, ed. 2, St. Louis, 1979, The C.V. Mosby Co. Based on the findings of Bors, E., and Comarr, A.E.: Neurological disturbances of sexual function, with special reference to 529 patients with spinal cord injury, Urological Survey **10:**191-222, 1960.

Women continue normal menstrual activity and seem to maintain fertility and the ability to bear children (Table 10-9).

 PLANNING AND IMPLEMENTATION. Usually within 6 months, a neurological evaluation will reveal the capacity for sexual activity, because most neurological processes will be stabilized. Special attention is given to assessment of sacral cord segments. Muscles essential to positioning for intercourse may be tested. Of course, the presence of incontinence may also influence sexual potential, but the presence of an indwelling catheter is not necessarily a deterrent. The attitude of the client and his partner is also important to determine, because success or failure at sexual role satisfaction is a joint responsibility of two individuals.

Some specific techniques have been found useful in enabling paraplegics to engage in intercourse.

Usually the paraplegic assumes a supine or sidelying position for intercourse because he is often unable to support his weight in the dominant position. The unaffected partner assumes the responsibility for pelvic thrusting in most instances.

A penis prosthesis (dildo) may be employed if the man is unable to achieve erection. Indwelling catheters left in place may help men to retain some penile rigidity. (The tubing is removed and the catheter merely folded back on itself and secured.) Women also may leave catheters in place. However, the bladder should be emptied before intercourse to avoid spasm-induced accidental voiding.

Both partners should cleanse genitalia before sexual activity, because chronic genitourinary infections may be transmitted or aggravated.

Sexual gratification must be achieved in other ways for some clients. Mechanical vibrators, oral-genital contact, and other modified stimulation of the partner may be tried.

Complications

Autonomic hyperreflexia. Autonomic hyperreflexia (or dysreflexia) is a crisis complication of spinal cord injury. Sensory excitement created by a phenomenon such as a distended bladder, fecal impaction, or decubitus ulcer triggers an exaggerated sympathetic discharge, uncontrolled by higher centers. There is a release of norepinephrine at the ganglia of the sympathetic nervous system, no longer under the influence of the spinal cord. This release creates a reflex vasoconstriction involving skin vessels and the splanchnic bed below the transection, and an immediate elevation of arterial pressure ensues. Such vasoconstriction and hypertension distend receptors in the aortic arch and carotid sinus and transmit impulses to the medulla oblongata. There, vasodilator and bradycardiac impulses are evoked. *Bradycardia* may be an early manifestation of hyperreflexia. If descending pathways are not intact, permitting the impulses to reach the effector organs, the hypertension creates a pounding headache instead.

Vasodilation can also occur above the level of the lesion if sympathetic pathways are intact, producing visible flushing, vein engorgement, and nasopharyngeal congestion. Sweating that occurs when the bladder is distended in clients with high cord lesions also typifies this classic autonomic response. The hyperreflexia syndrome may result in myocardial infarction or intracranial hemorrhage. It is interesting to note that strokes are the second most common cause of death in clients with long-term spinal cord lesions.

Autonomic hyperreflexia is heralded by hypertension, headache, diaphoresis, pilomotor erection (goose pimples), flushing of the skin above the lesion, nasal stuffiness, and bradycardia.

PLANNING AND IMPLEMENTATION. Emergency intervention is aimed at reducing hypertension. Assisting the client to a sitting position seems particularly beneficial in lowering blood pressure. The blood pressure should be constantly monitored and recorded, as often as every 3 to 5 minutes.

It is imperative to look for clues, such as a plugged catheter or a kink in urinary drainage tubing, that might have precipitated the crisis. Anesthetic agents are sometimes employed to reduce stimuli from distension until the bladder or bowel can be emptied safely.

Antihypertensive drugs or spinal anesthetics may be required if nursing measures are unsuccessful. Antidotes for antihypertensives should be at the bedside if undue pressure decreases are elicited.

Almost a year is required to evaluate if the hyperreflexia will continue when neurological stabilization is reached. If it does, surgical procedures such as posterior rhizotomy or nerve blocks may be performed to afford permanent relief.

Clients and their families should understand the likelihood of experiencing autonomic hyperreflexia and must be instructed regarding specific measures of intervention.[22]

Respiratory complications. Respiratory complications may accompany the cord injury. Tracheostomy or ventilatory support may be essential if there is paralysis of the respiratory mechanisms or the diaphragm. Diaphragm activity should be assessed by instructing the client to sniff. Breathing should be monitored regularly and frequently, especially during the first 48 hours when edema is developing at the injured site.

Skin complications. Skin complications are not unlike those associated with any immobility; however, there is added risk because of sensory and motor deficits in regions below the injured area. Because circulation in subtransection levels is impaired, injections in those sites should be avoided, and oral medications should be substituted, when possible, to minimize tissue trauma.

For a summary of selected nursing care for the client with a spinal cord injury, see Table 10-10.

TABLE 10-10

Client with spinal cord injury: model nursing care plan of selected problems

Problem	Planning and implementation	
	Strategies	**Instruction**
Anesthesia and analgesia	Protect from injury: check temperature of water with bath thermometer; no hot water bottles or heating pads; no razor blades; watch while smoking; file nails, do not cut	Teach client or family to examine body daily; take special care in buying shoes or braces that could cause skin trauma
Bladder atony and urinary stasis	Offer fluids on schedule; prepare for incontinence (exdwelling catheters, waterproof pants, and so forth; an indwelling catheter may be used to prevent distention and retention for some clients); maintain special protective care for skin	Teach reflex-trigger pattern or use Credé method as appropriate; teach catheter control if pertinent; monitor character and amount of urine; stress adequate hydration
Bowel atony and loss of motility Fecal impactions	Obtain elimination history (evacuation pattern, stimulant foods, time of evacuation, and so forth); establish elimination time; give prune juice in evening; administer suppository before breakfast and hot drink with meal; have client sit on toilet after breakfast at prescribed hour; use stool softeners and laxatives as necessary; maintain special protective care for skin	Teach bowel training program to family; instruct them in increasing dietary fiber and fluids; emphasize importance of relaxed, quiet, and private surrounding for elimination
Spastic paralysis	Do range of motion exercises at least q 6 h; plan physical therapy program including use of heat and cold; cooperate with occupational therapy for independent living activity program; prevent spasticity by reducing physical stimuli; use foot cradle; use slings and supports for affected extremities; elevate limbs and protect from pressure areas; use "thromboembolitic-prevention" elastic stockings; turn every 2 hours; support affected extremities in functional position	Teach client and family exercises and therapy programs; prepare client to use braces
Flaccid paralysis	Turn frequently; inspect skin regularly; do range-of-motion exercises	Teach client turning and skin protection regimens as well as exercises
Vascular tone decreased Blood pools in capillaries	Bathe daily and massage skin to stimulate circulation; employ range of motion exercises; use elastic supports on legs and abdomen; give injections above level of injury	Teach family associates skin condition assessments and care routines
Reflex automatism	Relieve any bowel or bladder obstructions at once; elevate head of bed	Explain automatic hyperreflexia to family associates
Respiratory distress	Anticipate cord edema and diaphragm paralysis in first 48 hours; have tracheostomy tray at hand; be prepared to provide ventilatory support; observe rate, rhythm, and quality of respirations; ask client to sniff to assess diaphragmatic functioning	Explain any respiratory assessments or mechanical aids; if respirator or tracheostomy is required, provide specific instruction
Excessive vagal influence on upper gastrointestinal tract and gastric acidity	Observe for stress ulcer development, especially during second week after injury; test stools for presence of occult blood; monitor hemoglobin levels to detect anemia; give antacids only as prescribed	Provide information regarding signs and symptoms of gastrointestinal bleeding; advise client to use antacids only with specific medical supervision

Abdominal injury masking. Abdominal injuries cannot be readily assessed in the presence of cord injury because usual clues, such as nausea, referred pain of diaphragmatic origin in the supraclavicular area, abdominal tenderness or rigidity, or ileus, may be obscured. (Ileus may be thought to be secondary to spinal cord trauma.) Fever may be attributed to a urinary tract infection rather than be linked to abdominal injury. If any client exhibits hypotension with tachycardia and lowered hematocrit, the nurse should suspect hemorrhage from an abdominal or chest source.

Stools and gastric contents should be tested for the presence of occult blood. Abdominal taps (paracentesis) may be indicated for detection of hemorrhage or peritonitis, especially in the presence of abdominal rigidity. Rigidity, however, may be solely caused by cord trauma.

Evaluation. Evaluation of the care plan for the client with spinal injury is an ongoing component of the nursing process.

EXPECTED OUTCOMES

The client and/or family can:

1. Demonstrate satisfactory adjustments of life-style imposed by the spinal cord injury.
2. Maintain a maximum level of activity within limitations imposed by the injury.
3. Explain the consequences of immobility and display behaviors to minimize such complications.
4. Exhibit caution in activity to facilitate personal safety, which is threatened by the spinal cord injury.
5. State plans for health maintenance.
6. State plans for follow-up care and problems requiring health care services.

Vertebral fractures. Vertebral fractures are caused by trauma incurred through automobile accidents, diving accidents, firearms, or severe blows. Persons who assist an injured individual should always be alert to the possibility of spinal cord injury. Injudicious but well-meaning bystanders who move or lift persons with spinal cord injuries can cause permanent damage to an already compressed cord. If the victim cannot move his arms or legs or has unusual sensations in the extremities, he should not be transferred until qualified personnel arrive.

Fracture symptoms of tenderness, deformity, and swelling may be present, but the most striking ones will undoubtedly relate to cord trauma caused by vertebral displacement. There may be loss of sensation and flaccid paralysis of all related muscles at the level of damage and below. Later such paralysis may become spastic and be accompanied by rigid spasms of muscles in the affected extremities.

Cervical vertebral fractures caused by hyperflexion of the neck may be managed by head halters (Fig. 10-38) and cervical (Crutchfield or Venke) tongs (Fig. 10-39), which hyperextend it. After 6 to 8 weeks a leather- or plastic-covered steel collar may be substituted. A *laminectomy* (removal of the dorsal

FIG. 10-38
Two methods of head-halter application. **A,** With client in bed. **B,** With client in chair, using over-door traction unit.

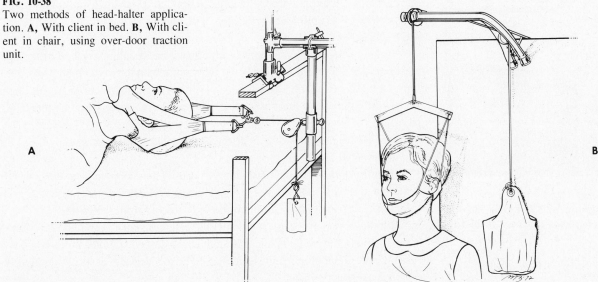

A

B

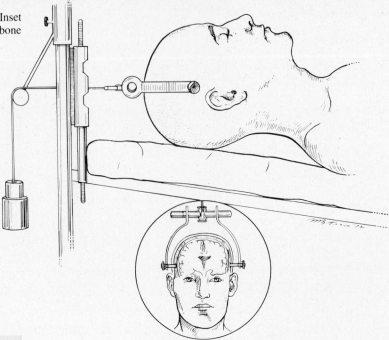

FIG. 10-39
Cervical traction with tongs. Inset shows position of tongs on skull bone structure.

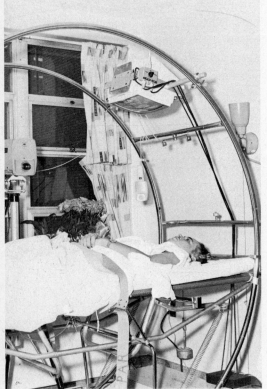

FIG. 10-40
A thoughtful staff has made viewing activity in room (via closed-circuit television) possible for this young client confined to CircOlectric bed. (Courtesy Methodist Hospital of Indiana, Inc., Indianapolis.)

478

arches of vertebrae to permit access to the cord) may be performed to relieve pressure on the cord. Intravenous muscle relaxants may be given to reduce spasms.

In addition to cervical tongs, a turning frame or CircOlectric bed (Fig. 10-40) may facilitate care of the client with a cervical fracture. Depending on their location and extent, other vertebral fractures may be managed by the use of (1) a prone, hyperextended position, (2) body casts, and (3) traction apparatus. Halo traction may be used to stabilize a vertebral fracture. This device permits easier turning, can be used with a regular bed, and reduces the period of immobility as much as 50%. After its removal, a brace is applied for about 4 weeks before the final phases of rehabilitation are begun. For nursing care of a client with casts and traction see Chapter 11.

For any person with a possible cord injury, the logrolling method of turning must be used to prevent any flexion, extension, or torsion of the spinal column. This is perhaps the cardinal skill necessary for the management of clients with spinal cord injuries. At least two nurses are required to accomplish the feat (Fig. 10-41).

Fig. 10-42 illustrates one method of positioning a client in a sidelying position after spinal cord surgery.

Whiplash injury. A whiplash injury is caused by violent hyperextension and flexion of the neck, usually as a result of a rear-end automobile accident. It is a common, recurring entity and often the only trauma from the crash.

Whiplash produces damage to muscles, disks, ligaments, and nervous tissue in the region of the cervical spine. If the injury is linked with head rotation, concussion and intracranial hemorrhage may be associated and deserve attention in the diagnostic assessment.

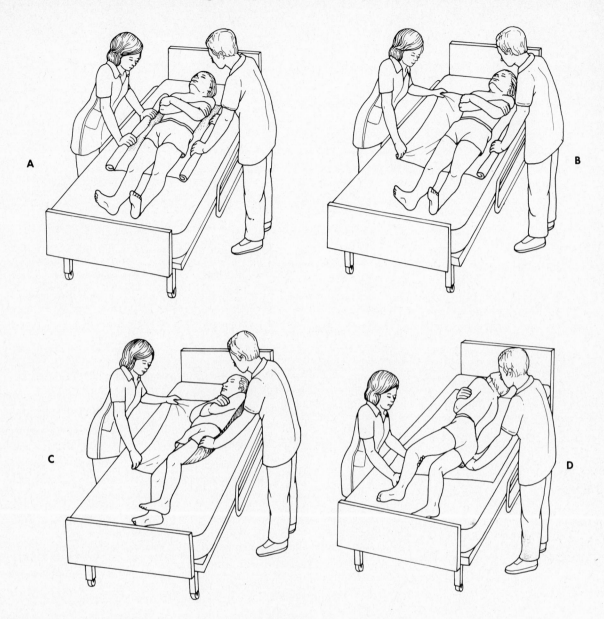

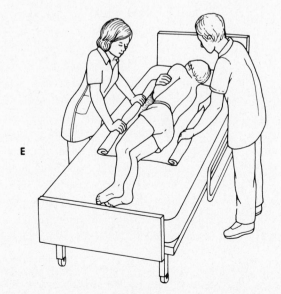

FIG. 10-41
Procedure for turning client (logrolling). **A,** Position preliminary to turning. **B,** Client has been moved to side of bed. **C,** Client is being turned onto right side. **D,** Buttocks are pulled out to maintain alignment of client's back. **E,** Client's back is supported while he is being turned to supine position.

FIG. 10-42
Client positioned on side with bed flat, as recommended, following surgery on spine. **A,** Anterior view. **B,** Posterior view.

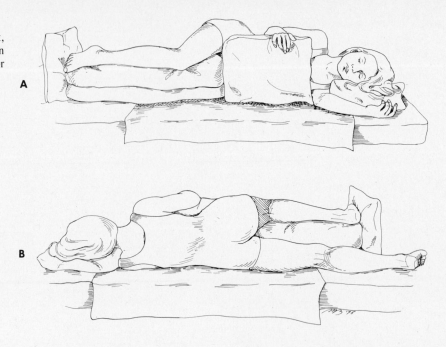

The client seen after the accident appears pale and dazed but rarely loses consciousness. He may exhibit weakness, gait disturbances, dizziness, and vomiting. Occipital headache may be severe and spread to temporal regions; it may be accompanied by nuchal rigidity and pain that radiates down the arms.

Younger clients usually recover with bed rest. Analgesics and hot packs to the neck are helpful in relieving symptoms. A plastic collar should be worn for several weeks to prevent aggravation of inflamed or bruised neck structures. Elderly clients may be slow to respond to treatment because of spondylosis (degeneration of vertebral structures) and vascular disease that interferes with the healing process.

All health team members should make frequent recordings of the behavioral responses of clients with whiplash injuries, since these frequently are a source of long litigations in insurance claims.

Compression injuries: ruptured disk. There are 23 intervertebral fibro-cartilages or disks. They (1) provide amphiarthrodial (slightly movable) articulations for vertebral bodies and (2) serve as shock absorbers for the spine. Disks comprise approximately one fourth of the length of the vertebral column if the first two vertebrae are excluded. The size, shape, and placement of individual disks determine, at least in part, the convexities characteristic of the cervical and lumbar regions, and the relative space they occupy accounts for the range of movement potential at various levels.

Each disk is made up of two parts: the circumferential portion (called the *anulus fibrosus*) and the center portion (called the *nucleus pulposus*). The latter semifluid substance is maintained under pressure by surrounding fibers, muscle tone, and the weight of the body on the spine. The nucleus pulposus obeys basic fluid laws. It is noncompressible, and it flattens, shortens, broadens, and distends as any applied force is equally transmitted over all opposing surfaces of the adjacent vertebrae. In children and young adults this nucleus pulposus has a high water content. However, in the processes of aging, this liquid is considerably reduced by the action of mucopolysaccharides, which also affect the maturation of collagen. Hence, structural degeneration occurs, which predisposes the disk to rupture.

Adult disks have no blood vessels. They are nourished from marrow by diffusion. However, in children, there is an identifiable blood supply arising from marrow spaces.

Lumbosacral disks are most subject to degeneration (especially L4 and L5, which act during flexion, the most extensive vertebral movement). If an individual lifts 100 pounds, it is estimated that the pressure exerted on these particular disks is up to 1600 pounds.[2]

The anulus fibrosus is prone to rupture, especially on the posterior portion, because of its considerably reduced thickness in that area. In flexion, the posterior aspect widens, with the anulus fibrosus stretched and the nucleus pulposus displaced posteriorly. Ninety-six percent of herniated disks involve the lumbar region, most (90%) affecting L4. Thoracic herniations are rare, but cervical herniations are fairly common.

The ruptured nucleus pulposus loses water, and fissures appear on the surface. Protrusion is followed by granulation and, ultimately, fusion.

A ruptured disk, or *herniated nucleus pulposus,* is usually caused by lifting a heavy object or a fall on the back. The disk capsule tears, allowing the softer fibrocartilaginous material to squeeze out and compress adjacent nerve roots against the vertebrae. Lumbar injury is most commonly caused by improper body mechanics (Fig. 10-43).

Assessment. Signs and symptoms associated with a herniated disk include back pain with radiation down the back of a leg, difficulty in walking, muscle spasm, and disorders of sensation. If the disk injury occurs near the thoracic or cervical region, there may be nuchal rigidity and pain radiating down the arm to the fingers.

Planning and implementation. If a single disk is involved, it may be surgically removed without disturbing any of the bony surroundings. However, spinal fusion (uniting two vertebrae) is usually performed if several disks are involved or if pain continues after the disk material has been removed. After fusion, a brace may be worn for about 6 weeks, or a body cast is applied. The client rests in a flat position with no elevation of the head. All turning is done by logrolling to reduce pain, discomfort, and the possibility of damaging the operative area. If x-ray films indicate that bone fusion is satisfactorily progressing after this 6 weeks, the client may be allowed gradual activity and increasing freedom from the regimen of immobilization therapy.

Conservative medical treatment with braces, casts, traction, prolonged bed rest, and physiotherapy has been successful in alleviating pain and annoying symptoms related to a herniated disk for some clients.

Sciatica

Sciatica is a syndrome that is characteristic of lumbosacral disk abnormality, and it derives its name from the sciatic nerve that it affects. The pain of sciatica usually begins in the buttocks and radiates down the back of the thigh to the ankle. It may be sharp or dull, intermittent or constant. The characteristic pain is precipitated by posture changes, prolonged standing or sitting in one position, or by acts that raise intracranial pressure, such as coughing, sneezing, or straining at the stool. Improper placement of intramuscular injections is yet another cause of sciatica.

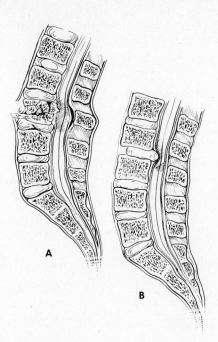

FIG. 10-43
Two causes of spinal cord compression. **A,** Compression fracture of vertebrae. **B,** Herniated nucleus pulposus.

Nursing process for common health problems

Sciatica is caused by nerve injury from compression or other trauma or to nerve irritation in association with toxic or metabolic disturbances or inflammations. Pregnancy may create mechanical compression of sciatic nerve roots in some instances.

The management depends on the cause. Physical therapy, heat, traction, immobilization, and muscle relaxants are among common modes of management.

Brain tumors

Tumors within the skull are managed in much the same way as hematomas, because the problems are essentially the same. Tumors also occupy space, extend, and create compressions and displacement of brain tissue (Fig. 10-44).

Intracranial tumors can arise from any structure present in the cranial vault—nerve tissue, blood vessels, neuroglia, or the pituitary gland. The greatest number (60%) begin in the neuroglia, the nonnerve support tissue of the brain. These tumors are called *gliomas*. They are not encapsulated and spread by direct extension. *Meningiomas* are benign tumors that arise from the meninges and account for about 15% of all brain tumors. Others involve acoustic neurons, pituitary tissue, or metastatic processes.

 Assessment. The presenting symptoms of brain tumors depend on the area and the extent of involvement. Early signs may include both motor and sensory phenomena. Visual disturbances, speech disorders, muscle weakness, headache, pain, paresthesia, and seizures are common presenting symptoms. Headache, seizures, and projectile vomiting are indicative of a tumor having grown to the size that it is creating intracranial pressure. *Papilledema* is the most important early sign of brain tumor and is often apparent long before any other specific signs or symptoms occur. Pituitary tumors present symptoms dependent on the type of structural cell involved and the age of the client when signs of pathological conditions first appear. If an eosinophilic tumor develops before the bones have ossified, overactivity of these cells responsible for growth may create gigantism, for example. Other endocrine-related symptoms such as Cushing's syndrome, acromegaly, and demasculinizing features may occur.

Diagnosis and localization involve isotope brain scans, x-ray films, echoencephalography, angiography, pneumoencephalography, and biopsy. Treatment may consist of chemotherapy, radiation, and surgery.

FIG. 10-44
Complications of intracranial tumor.

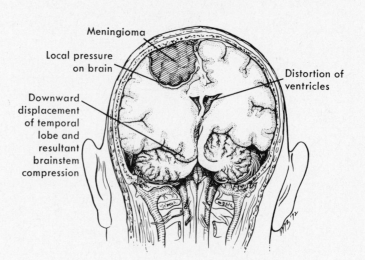

> **Data analysis**
> *Data analysis may reveal nursing diagnoses of self-care deficit, sensory perception alterations, alteration in thought processes, fear, and ineffective coping.*

Planning and implementation. The nursing care depends on the emotional needs of the client as well as the physical manifestations of the tumor. The prognosis depends on the nature and location of the tumor and its response to medical and surgical management.

The nursing assessments for the client with a brain tumor are similar to those made for other individuals with brain lesions. The factors of level of consciousness, ocular signs, cranial nerve checks, reflex and motor function, and vital signs make up the primary routine observations that determine the effect of the tumor on brain activity and detect the development of increased intracranial pressure.

The client with a brain tumor should remain as active as possible. If bed rest is necessary, the head should be elevated to minimize intracranial pressure and relieve headache. Frequent position changes are essential to prevent pulmonary complications and skin breakdown. Recommendations for these and other specific care measures regarding nutrition, exercise, hygiene, and elimination parallel those relevant to cerebrovascular accident.

Pain management is usually limited to headache relief. Codeine or aspirin is considered effective for most clients. Morphine is contraindicated because of its depressing action on the central nervous system and its tendency to obscure clinical neurological signs.

After the tumor is localized and evaluated, a biopsy may be performed to ascertain whether it is malignant or benign. A craniotomy or craniectomy is performed for biopsy, tumor removal, and relief of pressure.

Conditions that interfere with the integration of the cerebral hemispheres and the upper brainstem mechanisms and that therefore underlie stupor and coma fall into three categories: (1) supratentorial lesions, which secondarily encroach on deep diencephalic structures and damage physiological ascending reticular activating systems; (2) infratentorial lesions, which damage the central core of the brainstem, and (3) metabolic disorders, which widely interrupt brain function.

Clinicians caring for individuals with neurological dysfunction must ask: Where does the lesion lie? In what direction is the process evolving? While this determination is being made, the brain must be receiving adequate amounts of oxygen and glucose via the circulatory network.

Nurses who are observing individuals with neurological dysfunctioning are responsible for describing the level of consciousness. The detailed data that nurses regularly collect and record are extremely valuable to the physician in establishing a diagnosis and planning specific intervention. Rather than merely recording a single numerical level or related term, the nurse will find it is more useful to describe the behavior in regard to content and state of arousal. As is the case with many human phenomena, definitive classifications are not well circumscribed, and behavior may change readily during pathophysiological adjust-

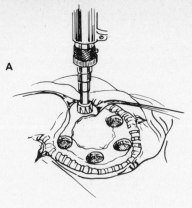

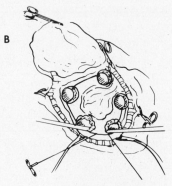

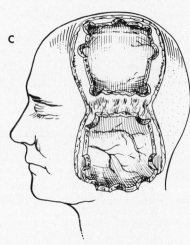

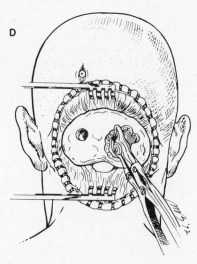

Nursing process for common health problems

ments. Objective records with hourly entries should be maintained for persons who have acute neurological problems or who have had recent surgical intervention or trauma.

Surgery. Cranial surgery demands that the nurse understand the factors of preoperative and postoperative care as well as how the brain responds to the trauma of the procedures. Because much of the postoperative care relates to monitoring intracranial pressure, it is imperative that this be understood thoroughly.

Cranial surgery may be performed to relieve intracranial pressure, to identify and remove space-occupying lesions (that is, tumors, hematomas), or to repair mechanical defects in vascular or bony tissue.

A *craniotomy* involves exposing the brain by creating a doorlike opening in the skull. A series of burr holes are drilled, and then the bone remaining between them is cut with a wirelike saw. One edge of the bony doorlike opening is usually left attached to muscle, creating a hinge. This is believed to benefit the reestablishment of blood supply to the area (Fig. 10-45).

A *craniectomy* involves the removal of bone to expose the brain and may be as simple as a single burr hole.

The choice of surgical exposure is determined by (1) location and (2) the nature and extent of the subject lesion.

Preoperative nursing care. Preoperative care for either procedure is similar. The client should be instructed about the surgical plan if his condition permits. He should be also informed about postsurgical routines such as range-of-motion and deep breathing exercises.

One of the most traumatic parts of preoperative care involves shaving of the head. The hair is placed in a receptacle for safekeeping, not destroyed. (It can be used to make a wig, for example.) The scalp is shampooed and covered with sterile towels or a turban dressing, for both aseptic and cosmetic considerations. (In some institutions, all such scalp preparation is done in the surgical suite immediately before the operative procedure.)

If ambulation is feasible, the client should be out of bed to stimulate circulation before the preoperative sedative is administered. Some clinicians routinely apply antiembolus hose before surgery to prevent venous stasis.

Dentures, if present, should be extracted and stored, and oral hygienic care administered. Rings are removed or secured with tape, and other jewelry is placed in safekeeping.

Enemas are usually omitted unless there are specific elimination problems, because they are fatiguing and tend to increase intracranial pressure.

It is essential to record immediate preoperative baseline vital and neurological signs for comparative purposes during and after surgery.

Other details for the nurse to attend to in this preoperative period include offering the bedpan and urinal, completing a check of preoperative laboratory values required by the institution (such as urinalysis, blood count, chest film, ECG), and permitting family and clergy to visit before administering the preoperative medications.

FIG. 10-45
Techniques of cranial surgery. **A,** Drilling burr holes. **B,** Using Gigli saw. **C,** Bone flap turned down. **D,** Modification for cerebellar craniotomy.

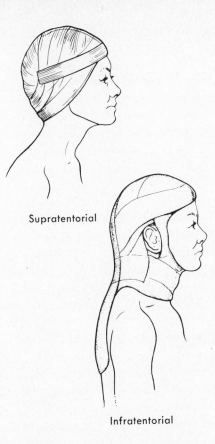

Supratentorial

Infratentorial

FIG. 10-46
Characteristic dressings after craniotomy. Supratentorial dressing is soft gauze wrapped turban style and secured with adhesive. Infratentorial dressing is more extensive and prevents flexion of neck or lateral movements of head. Usually it is protected with covering made of plaster of paris and requires same consideration as any cast.

The visitors should be informed that cranial procedures may last from 3 to 6 hours and that the client will remain in an intensive care setting until physiological stabilization is ensured. It is helpful to orient visitors to the waiting rooms, lounges, cafeterias, chapel, and other comfort facilities. They should also be instructed regarding the protocol for information exchanges with the surgery team postoperatively. Such routines, so familiar to hospital staff, are complex and foreign to many clients' visitors.

Postoperative nursing care. The client who has had cranial surgery usually receives his early postoperative care in a specialized intensive care unit. Postsurgical care is determined by the site and extent of the operative procedure. If the procedure was confined to the cerebrum or anterior of the brain, the supratentorial regimen is followed. If it involved the lower third of the brain, the infratentorial regimen is followed (Fig. 10-46). An outline of the two regimens may be found in Table 10-11.

When dressings are finally removed, the scalp is likely to be covered with crusts and scales. These may be softened with a petrolatum-based preparation and removed by shampooing. A cosmetic head covering or wig should be provided as soon as the wound is closed. Nurses must always remember that the

TABLE 10-11
Postoperative care for neurosurgical clients having supratentorial and infratentorial procedures

	Supratentorial	Commonalities	Infratentorial
Positioning	Semi-Fowler's position, because lowering head can cause venous congestion and bleeding; position *flat only in shock;* no Trendelenburg position, which would increase intracranial pressure.	Keep off operative site; turn every 2 hours; head on small pillow; mouth in dependent position to drain secretions.	Position flat on either side; keep off back because of impaired swallowing and gag reflexes; head may be gradually elevated on the third postoperative day.
Vital signs		Monitor vital signs; monitor neurological signs; observe for shock and increased intracranial pressure.	Be observant for respiratory difficulty.
Food and fluids	Limit to 1500 ml during first 24 hours to control edema; feed diet as tolerated after return of swallowing and gag reflexes.	Record intake and output.	No oral fluids or solids for 24 hours; begin oral fluids and diet on second postoperative day after ascertaining presence of swallowing and gag reflexes.
Other measures	1. Check dressing for clear drainage and excessive bleeding and reinforce as necessary. Restrain client if necessary to prevent disturbance of dressings. 2. Suction as necessary to clear mouth or airway, being careful not to stimulate the cough reflex, since this facilitates increasing intracranial pressure. 3. Encourage deep breathing; coughing should be discouraged. 4. Apply ice bag to head as necessary for headache. 5. Monitor bowel and bladder elimination. Catheterize if necessary. Avoid enemas, since they may increase the intracranial pressure. 6. Give analgesics, anticonvulsants, stimulants, or steroids as ordered. 7. Follow eye-care regimen if corneal reflex is absent. 8. Facilitate activity advances as indicated.		

Nursing process for common health problems

client is likely to be sensitive about his or her temporary baldness; therefore all scalp procedures should be done in privacy.

Complications following cranial surgery include hypovolemic shock, increased intracranial pressure, parotitis, meningitis, and pulmonary or wound infections. A few other potential complications deserve special attention.

Hyperthermia is a problem that may result from urinary or respiratory infection, meningeal irritation, thrombophlebitis, dehydration, or excessive metabolic activity related to the healing process. It may also partially result from hypothalamus dysfunction. Because temperature elevations ultimately contribute to further brain damage, several measures may be instituted to control fever. Some neurosurgical care units have specially controlled room temperatures of 68° F (20° C) to lessen environmental contributions to hyperthermia. Antipyretics, alcohol sponge baths, and hypothermia blankets may be useful in reducing fever. Adequate hydration is also an important adjunct in controlling hyperthermia.

Swallowing difficulties may be noted if there is cranial nerve injury. Evidence of such injury may be that the client cannot swallow without choking or regurgitating, has apparently no swallowing or gag reflexes, or experiences excessive salivation and drooling.

Fluid and food should be withheld until there is sure evidence that gagging and swallowing reflexes are present. Initial feedings are often given with the client elevated in a sidelying position. They should be, of course, carefully supervised with suction at hand. Nasogastric feedings may be required if oral ones are poorly tolerated.

Periocular edema is a frequent sequela to cranial surgery. Eye irrigations and alternating ice and heat applications may assist in its reduction. It usually subsides in 3 or 4 days.

Behavioral changes ranging from euphoria to irritability and aggression may occur. It is felt that these manifestations are the result of frontal lobe disturbances or diffuse brain dysfunction. Nurses should help family and significant others understand the cause of such behavioral changes and appreciate that they are most likely transient. Operant conditioning, tranquilizing medications, and sedatives may be useful, particularly for individuals who are resistive or assaultive. Since many clients are discharged to their homes without fully recovering independence, it is essential that considerable support, as well as instruction, be directed toward persons assuming such caring responsibility. Referrals to community agencies that can assist in rehabilitation should be initiated by the nurse.

Increased intracranial pressure (intracranial hypertension)

Increased intracranial pressure is a manifestation of brain compression. Any phenomena (edema, hemorrhage, or tumor) that occupies space within the skull does so at the expense of displacing brain tissue. Elevations of intracranial pressure are life-threatening, in that if pressure is not controlled, brain circulation is impaired, and, ultimately, vital centers controlling the heart and breathing mechanisms are destroyed by anoxia.

The signs and symptoms of intracranial pressure elevations depend on the type and amount of brain tissue affected by compression. A specific lesion such as a tumor or localized hemorrhage may disturb only a confined segment, but diffuse head trauma may cause widespread trauma. Tumors, hemorrhage, and other specific lesions are considered later in detail, but a general understanding of cerebral edema and increased intracranial pressure is pertinent to basic neurological assessment skills.

Growth and developmental considerations. As previously mentioned, the cranial vault of the young infant is not a totally confined space. The fontanels and suture lines allow for expansion; however, in the adult the skull is fused, and the bony structure completely covers the delicate brain. Intracranial volume is essentially unchanged beyond the second decade of life; nervous tissue volume, however, diminishes with aging. Older adults (55 to 75 years old) have up to 65 ml more space than does a 20-year-old.[2] Therefore older adults can tolerate more edema (or larger lesions) than younger persons without incurring compression damage to the brain.

Pathophysiology of cerebral edema. Cerebral edema results from increased permeability of the blood-brain barrier, which is induced by one of several mechanisms that alter ionic or vascular hemodynamics. Any insult to the blood vessels that permits plasma to escape into tissue can be responsible for edema formation. Hypothalamic injury that evokes loss or paralysis of vasomotor tone causes an increase in the volume of the cerebrovascular bed, and thus congestion and edema. However, these two causes are closely linked to a third mechanism, cerebral hypoxia, which must be understood to appreciate the potential consequences of cerebral edema.

Oxygen and glucose are essential factors in the maintenance of brain activity. The normal brain consumes oxygen at a constant rate (approximately 3.3 ml/100 g of brain tissue per minute) in both wakefulness and sleep. This represents about 20% of the total oxygen consumption of the body, although the brain comprises only about 2% of the body's weight.[17] Unlike glucose, which can be stored, the brain has only a 10-second reserve supply of oxygen, so that metabolic failure is almost instant in anoxia.

Cerebral blood flow is variable, depending on levels of activity and rest and on certain physiological stimuli. At rest, the blood flow rate is about 55 ml/100 g of brain tissue per minute; this represents 20% of the cardiac output. When the cerebral blood flow is initially reduced, the body compensates by extracting more oxygen per unit volume. If the arterial oxygen supply is normal, brain metabolism can continue temporarily with half the ordinary blood flow. However, as oxygen tension falls in tissue that is remote from capillaries, metabolism is impaired and anoxic neurons cause the individual to lose consciousness from a metabolic crisis.

Hypoxia and carbon dioxide retention precipitate cerebral edema from vascular dilatation and congestion. When vascular dilatation and congestion occur, medullary vasopressor mechanisms are activated to augment intracranial blood flow. This elevation in blood pressure further aggravates intracranial pressure and may even create arterial hemorrhage. This vicious cycle, especially when compounded by respiratory embarrassment, can produce rapid deteriorations in levels of consciousness. Coma, for example, may be caused solely by cellular anoxia and edema of vital brain tissue.

Assessment. Cerebral compression interferes with normal CSF production and flow, as well as with blood circulation and the normal functioning of the brain area involved. Table 10-12 outlines signs and symptoms of increased intracranial pressure, the underlying cause of signs and symptoms, and appropriate interventions. In addition to such clinical indices of intracranial hypertension, which are often vague and subject to considerable interpretation, there are specific devices that can measure intracranial pressure on a continuous or intermittent basis.

TABLE 10-12

Manifestations of increased intracranial pressure and related nursing care

Assessment	Underlying cause	Nursing implementation
Headache	Tension on intracranial vessels	Keep head elevated at least 30 degrees; post sign on bed—"No Trendelenburg"; give analgesics for headache as ordered (aspirin and narcotics are avoided, since they mask symptoms such as fever and pupillary signs, respectively).
Vomiting—unrelated to meals or nausea; is projectile	Pressure stimulation of medulla oblongata	Record nature and incidence of episodes; record intake and output; withhold oral fluids during persistent vomiting; have suction at hand; use nasogastric tube as indicated.
Slowing respiration	Pressure and anoxia of medulla	Monitor vital signs at least hourly; count respirations for 1 full minute; record observations; ventilatory support with a low level of oxygen.
Papilledema, visual impairment, and irregularity in size and response of pupils	Venous engorgement of central retinal area and lymphatic stases	Check pupils for equality and reaction to light (client may also report loss of visual acuity).
Loss of motor function	Pressure on motor centers	Record hemiparesis, bilateral paresis, or changes in cranial nerve signs; assess grasp reflexes bilaterally.
Seizures	Intracranial stimulation to brain by pressure	Carry out seizure precautions.
Loss of sphincter control	Cerebral pressure interferes with sphincter inhibitory control	Record intake and output; check for distension or incontinence; catheterize as required.
Temperature variations	Damage to hypothalamus or changes in metabolic environment of brain; may indicate development of meningitis	Give antipyretics, apply ice bags, give alcohol sponge baths; remove excessive covers for elevations; for hypothermia, prevent chilling by providing extra blankets; use temperature-control blanket for hyperthermia or hypothermia if available.
Changes in level of consciousness; derangements of behavior or sensorium	Pressure on cerebral cortex and reticular activating system	Note restlessness; rule out bladder distension; describe responses relating to level of consciousness; record behavior such as negativism, disorientation, hallucinations, irritability.
Elevation or displacement of bone flaps; bulging fontanels	Mechanical pressure	Report leakage of cerebrospinal fluid; reinforce dressings.

General measures:

Avoid straining at stool.*
Prevent coughing.*
Reduce environmental stimuli.
Restrain client as necessary.
Always assume that client can hear.
Intake and output.
Restrict sodium intake.

*Raises intracranial pressure.

Intracranial pressure monitoring. The direct measurement of intracranial pressure (ICP) is an important adjunct in the nursing care of clients with head injury or the possibility of cerebral edema from any cause. There are three basic methods in popular use at this time: (1) intraventricular, (2) epidural, and (3) subarachnoid.

The intraventricular method, as the name implies, involves the placement of a cannula within the ventricles, which is attached to a standard blood pressure transducer. This setup converts fluid pressure into an electrical signal that is visualized on a graph similar to an ECG or EEG. Although this method permits direct access to ventricles for the purposes of withdrawing CSF samples or removing fluid to control ICP, it can serve as a portal of entry for infections. Furthermore, frequent flushing is required to ensure patency of the system.

The epidural method relies on a sensing probe that is inserted between the skull and the dura. It is a superficial procedure and is less likely to introduce infections.

The subarachnoid monitoring device involves a sensor into the subarachnoid space. This approach, like the intraventricular cannula, requires attachment to a transducer using a stopcock and/or pressure tubing apparatus (Fig. 10-47).

Nursing responsibilities related to ICP monitoring vary considerably, depending on the type of equipment, and are not considered in detail in this text. However, it is crucial for a nurse to appreciate the factors that elevate pressure readings. Phenomena such as gagging, coughing, suctioning, vomiting, and defecation can cause dramatic rises in ICP on a temporary basis. Readings, therefore, should not be taken at these times.

The normal ICP is 4 to 14 mm Hg (50 to 200 mm H_2O). Rapid rises (in less than a half hour) to levels of 50 mm Hg or more signal a life-threatening emergency.

Planning and implementation. There are several methods currently in use to manage intracranial hypertension without surgical intervention: (1) de-

FIG. 10-47
Intracranial monitoring. **A,** Placement of epidural sensor between skull and dura to monitor intracranial pressure. **B,** External view of epidural sensor. **C,** Subarachnoid (left) and intraventricular (right) devices for measuring intracranial pressure; both require attachment to transducer using stopcock and/or pressure tubing. (From Budassi, Susan A., and Barber, Janet M.: Emergency nursing: principles and practice, St. Louis, 1981, The C.V. Mosby Co.)

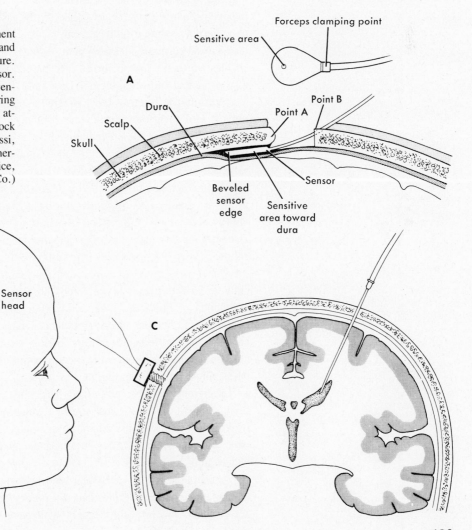

hydration, (2) steroids, (3) hypothermia, (4) barbiturate coma, and (5) controlled positive-negative pressure ventilation.

Dehydration. Although dehydration of the brain can be accomplished by several means, the use of osmolar agents, such as mannitol, or diuretics, such as furosemide (Lasix), are most popular. Urea is also used on a limited basis by some physicians.

Clients who are receiving these agents must be closely monitored for systemic dehydration and fluid and electrolyte imbalances. Intake and output, fluid restriction, sodium restriction, and frequent laboratory assessments of blood and urine usually accompany dehydration therapy.

Steroids. Steroids are controversial agents in the management of ICP, but research has indicated that they may prevent certain devastating consequences of cerebral edema. Dexamethasone (Decadron) is preferred by most clinicians because it has less sodium-retention properties than other steroids. It is thought that steroids stabilize the permeability of the blood-brain barrier, thus arresting progressive edema.

Hypothermia. Hypothermia is beneficial in combating cerebral edema because it decreases the metabolic demands of the cerebral tissue. Hypothermia may be achieved by (1) external surface cooling (by ice-water immersions, hypothermia blankets, or ice packs), (2) vascular cooling (by introducing a hypothermic solution into a ventricle or by removing and cooling venous blood and returning it to the body), or (3) internal surface cooling (by cold enemas, lavages, and so forth). The procedure is indicated for reducing fever as well as for controlling cerebral edema.

Various mechanical devices are available to achieve hypothermia, but nursing care measures during the procedure are essentially the same. If the client is conscious, the procedure should be carefully explained because it is an uncomfortable experience and because cooperation is more easily achieved if the rationale is understood. Record vital signs every 15 to 30 minutes, even after the desired temperature has been attained. (An electronic rectal thermometer probe is usually left in place during hypothermia.) Continue neurological checks and assess indices of impaired circulation, such as cyanosis, skin discoloration, or edema. Special attention should be given to avoiding complications, especially myocardial irritability evidenced by dysrhythmias. Because the client may have impaired reflexes, suctioning should be done periodically to maintain the airway, and the gag reflex should be elicited before oral foods or fluids are given. Shivering is normal for the client undergoing hypothermia, but the nurse should be aware that shivering exhausts the client, elevates the temperature, and offsets the effect of cooling. Drugs such as chlorpromazine hydrochloride, succinylcholine chloride, and phenobarbital may be used to control shivering.

If hypothermia is prolonged, the nurse should recognize that lowered body temperature may mask signs of inflammation and may alter the body's response to medications. Medications should be given intravenously, if possible, since absorption from intramuscular and subcutaneous routes is limited and unpredictable because of decreased peripheral perfusion.

Usually the client being managed by hypothermia is in an intensive care unit or in the surgical suite, and emergency equipment, drugs, and personnel are prepared to cope immediately with adverse responses, including cardiac arrest (Table 10-13).

TABLE 10-13

Guidelines for the client having hypothermia via hypothermia blanket or pad

Nursing considerations	Rationale
A. Preinductive period	
1. Take baseline vital signs and neurological signs, and begin ECG monitoring.	1. The cardiovascular and central nervous systems are profoundly affected by cold. Basal signs will be used for later comparisons (see B, 3).
2. Insert Foley catheter, weigh client, initiate intake and output record.	2. Urinary function is hypoactive during hypothermia. Overhydration is a potential problem.
3. Initiate parenteral fluid route if not already established.	3. Peripheral veins collapse later in the hypothermia, thus necessitating a venesection. Nutrition is supplied by parenteral route, because gag and swallowing reflexes are depressed and gastric absorption and utilization are hypoactive.
4. Begin seizure precautions (see p. 496).	4. Seizure threshold is reduced in hypothermia.
5. Review all medication orders with physician.	5. Drugs are slowly detoxified and excreted during hypothermia. Effects may be more profound and prolonged.
6. Review manufacturer's instruction for use of hypothermia equipment.	6. Maximum therapy safety requires thorough understanding of equipment and potential mechanical hazards.
B. Induction and maintenance period	
1. Set hypothermia equipment for desired temperature. Place bed in flat position. Cover pad with sheet for protection. Place client's back on hypothermia pad. Upper portion of pad should extend only to shoulders.	1. Desired temperature range can best be achieved when coolant can circulate freely in pad coils and with maximum surface exposed to client. *Head should never rest on pad.*
2. Insert rectal thermometer probe. Monitor vital signs and neurological signs at least every 15 to 30 minutes during induction when metabolic adjustments are being made. Watch for complications and untoward effects (respiratory distress, cyanosis, and heart failure). Pulse is taken apically.	2. Monitoring of temperatures is constant to prevent insidious skin and vital organ damage. Electronic temperature readings taken constantly indicate when the degree of hypothermia as ordered is reached. During induction vital signs rise as a result of vasoconstriction. As body metabolism is reduced, they fall (see also A, 1). Palpable pulses may be absent.
3. Specific problems	3.
a. Ventricular fibrillation and cardiac arrest.	a. Hypothermia creates changes in blood pH. Arrest may be caused by elevated serum potassium or a decrease in temperature to approximately 15° C.
b. Shivering. Administer medications (such as chlorpromazine hydrochloride, succinylcholine chloride, phenobarbital) prophylactically to inhibit response. Massage injection site to aid absorption.	b. Shivering is most likely during initial changes in temperature. It causes metabolic activity to increase 100%. Liver glycogen reserve can be depleted, causing hypoglycemia and elevation of serum potassium. Shivering also is responsible for rise in intracranial pressure, hyperventilation, and alkalosis.
c. Frostbite, burns, fat necrosis. Do not mummy client. Protect head, fingers, and toes from direct contact with pad. Turn every 2 hours from side to back to side. (All supports for positioning must be placed under the pad.) Observe security of rectal probe when turning to prevent dislodgement. *Observe for skin discoloration.* Give skin care using cool water *only.* Frequent deep massage of the limbs and trunk is recommended. Lotions may be applied.	c. Cold skin is hypersensitive to slight changes in temperature. Devices that retain heat are contraindicated. Client has reduced level of awareness, including sensation.
d. Protect eyes from trauma. Use artificial tears if indicated.	d. Hypothermia causes decrease in corneal reflexes and reduces secretions.
C. Rewarming period	
1. When equipment is discontinued, cover the client with blankets, allowing rewarming at his own rate.	1. Do not use hot water bottles or heating pads (see Rationale B, 3, c). Observe induction phase guidelines for complications as rewarming occurs.
2. Continue to monitor vital signs, ECG, and neurological signs.	2. As metabolism adjusts, complications similar to those during induction and maintenance can occur.

Nursing process for common health problems

Barbiturate coma. A barbiturate-induced coma is a new technique for lowering ICP and reducing brain metabolism. As the brain's requirements for oxygen are reduced, a "protecting" effect is achieved, permitting the damaged brain tissue to rest in a dormant state. A controlled coma is induced by an agent such as pentobarbital (Nembutal) and maintained for 2 weeks or more by continuous administration of the barbiturate. Intensive monitoring is essential, including CVP, ICP, urinary output, temperature, electrolytes, CBC, coagulation studies, and brainstem-evoked responses.

Controlled positive-negative pressure ventilation. There is an important association between adequate oxygenation of the brain tissue and the progression of cerebral edema. When the brain is insulted, there is increased blood flow to the area via activation of the medullary vasopressor mechanisms. As plasma escapes into tissue and vasopressor tone is eventually diminished, there is additional swelling. Finally, cerebral blood flow is further retarded, and the vicious cycle of hypertension is perpetuated.

Early attention to airway management, including intubation, if necessary, and the use of controlled mechanical ventilatory assistance can reduce cerebral hypertension. Therapy is designed to maintain the Po_2 above 100 and the Pco_2 below 25 to 30. Positive-end expiratory pressure (PEEP) may be used for some clients along with serial arterial blood gas sampling to guide the therapy. Conscious clients may be given high-flow humidified oxygen by mask at 10 to 12 L/min to control edema.

Other interventions. Clients with cerebral edema are often given intravenous fluid therapy for management of concurrent clinical problems and to ensure optimum caloric, fluid, and electrolyte status. This fluid must be judiciously calculated and monitored to prevent aggravation of the edematous state.

Analgesics may be required to help relieve headache that accompanies elevations in intracranial pressure; however, they are seldom used during initial evaluation because they may mask important changes in levels of consciousness. Because seizures are always a potential problem, standard precautions should be followed. Coughing, straining at stool, and emotional upsets also tend to aggravate the condition, and hence these problems require prompt attention by the clinical team.

The Trendelenburg position should not be used for clients with elevated intracranial pressure, even in the presence of shock, because it promotes venous stasis, increases intracranial tension, and permits abdominal contents to be pushed up against the diaphragm, impairing respiratory effort. A semi-Fowler's position (30- to 45-degree head elevation) is recommended because it reduces cerebral edema and promotes venous drainage from the brain.

Occasionally surgery must be employed to relieve elevated intracranial pressure when medical measures fail. Brain tissue and bony skull parts may be removed to prevent insult to vital centers by allowing room for brain expansion and/or by reducing compression.

Spinal cord tumors

Spinal cord tumors are space-occupying lesions that eventually cause compression of the cord as they grow.

Assessment. The symptoms are similar to those of a fracture but are slower in developing. They include disturbances in sensory and motor functioning, depending on the level of the mass. There may be sharp pain in

492

spinal roots arising from the cord in the affected area. A laminectomy is often performed for excision of the tumor and relief of pressure.

   Planning and implementation. Postsurgical management should include consideration of the open wound into the central nervous system, the threat of cerebrospinal fluid leakage, and meningitis. The dressing should be observed frequently and reinforced if necessary.

All tumors of the spinal cord cannot be managed successfully by surgery, and the client may progress to a state of paraplegia or quadriplegia if the tumor continues to create pressure.

Syncope (fainting)   Syncope is a transient loss of consciousness resulting from inadequate perfusion of the brain. It may be evoked by emotions, pain, or a sudden reduction in cardiac output or venous return from any cause.

   Assessment. Usually syncopal attacks occur while the client is standing or sitting. Peripheral vessels dilate; subsequently, heart rate is slowed and blood pressure fails (orthostatic hypotension).

Data analysis

Data analysis may reveal nursing diagnoses of alteration in cardiac output and potential for injury.

Planning and implementation. Nurses can prevent injuries related to syncope by permitting gradual posture changes of clients who are weak or under emotional stress or who have been on prolonged bed rest. It is wise for clients to dangle their feet for 30 seconds before standing and to stand for 30 seconds before walking. This is especially true for someone who has not been ambulatory for an extended period of time or who has cardiovascular dysfunctioning. If a client feels faint, he should be helped to his chair, the bed, or the floor, and his head should be positioned at the level of the heart or below. This measure is useful in averting syncope. For a fainting victim, aromatic spirits of ammonia, "smelling salts," or other noxious stimuli may be useful in bringing about recovery.

Seizures   Seizures are sudden changes in sensation, behaviors, muscular activity, or level of consciousness. They are beyond voluntary control and are caused by overactivity of the brain cells. The exact cause of seizures has been poorly understood, but they occur clinically as a result of inflammatory conditions, metabolic acidosis, alcoholism, tumors, intracranial vascular disturbances, pyrexia (fever), and trauma. All these conditions either affect the brain's structural cells or alter chemical and metabolic substances that bathe the tissue. The theory has been advanced that the glia cells of the brain may be more than support tissue for the neurons and have a vital role in the ion exchange process necessary for normal nervous impulses. It is thought that glia cells may be reservoirs for potassium ions and may not possess this capacity in damaged brains or unusual conditions of metabolism. As neurons discharge potassium during normal electrical impulse activity, the potassium may have no place to go and thus accumulate on the neuron walls, causing an electrical crisis. The result, therefore, is rapid and uncontrolled cellular activity, or a seizure.

Nursing process for common health problems

Growth and developmental considerations. Seizures in the neonate *(neonatal seizures)* are symptoms of central nervous system disease. Congenital anomalies, metabolic derangements, infection, and anoxia may be possible causes.

Infantile seizures are often missed by clinicians because they may be manifest in ways other than the tonic-clonic classic pattern. Transient abnormal posturing or rigidity, or even apneic episodes, may indicate that a seizure is occurring. Other clinical manifestations include repetitive flexion movements of the trunk, opisthotonic posturing, tremors, sudden loss of muscle tone, spasmodic crying, facial twitching or chewing movements, paroxysmal blinking or nystagmus, and hyperactivity unusual for the gestational age.

Nurses caring for infants should observe and carefully note signs of seizures. Data regarding the obstetrical history (such as infections, maternal diabetes, birth trauma, and anoxia) should be considered in regard to evaluation of etiology. In-depth physical examination, x-ray films, neurological tests, and laboratory procedures are usually important adjuncts to determining causation.

Therapy is directed to the cause of the seizures, if known. Undetermined, the seizure may need to be controlled by intravenous medications (such as diazepam [Valium] or phenobarbital) if symptoms are severe. Glucose, calcium, and magnesium are sometimes administered to correct metabolic disturbances.

Mortality from neonatal seizures in relatively high, and considerable neurological deficits have been observed in survivors. Prompt recognition and management are imperative to reducing neurological sequelae.

Infants with a history of seizures require long-term follow-up, and parents should be instructed accordingly.

Febrile seizures. Febrile seizures are induced by fever and usually occur in children from the ages of 6 months to 5 years. They result from the immature brain's response to a sudden increase in temperature.

Pathophysiology. During fever, cerebral blood flow accelerates and metabolic activity creates alterations of fluid and electrolyte balance in cerebral tissue. Thus the seizure threshold is reduced because of changes of membrane potential and excitability of neurons. The rapidity at which fever occurs seems to be a major factor, supposedly because the brain is not permitted to adjust gradually to the new chemical environment.

Assessment. Febrile convulsions are usually grand mal and of short duration. Recovery usually takes place in 15 minutes. They commonly occur in relation to upper respiratory tract infections with no previous client history of convulsions. Neurological examinations and electroencephalograms are normal.

Planning and implementation. Parents should be reassured that the child does not have epilepsy, although there is an increased risk of seizure disorder with an increase in number of seizures. The primary mode of prevention is to control fever.

Nurses who care for infants and young children should be well aware of the signs and symptoms of fever other than an elevated temperature. A flushed face, increased restlessness, tachycardia, and diaphoresis are common indices. Occasionally delirium will precede the febrile convulsion.

Forced fluids, tepid sponging, and the use of antipyretics are methods to control fever and may be instrumental in preventing complications such as seizure activity.

Seizures may be classified according to whether there is *generalized* or *localized* brain involvement. Generalized seizures include grand mal and petit mal seizures, and localized (focal seizures) include jacksonian and psychomotor seizures. Seizures frequently involve three phases: an aura, an ictus (seizure movement or sensation), and a postictal state.[24]

Grand mal seizures. The most dramatic type of seizure is grand mal. This seizure is generalized and sometimes referred to as a *convulsion*.

Assessment. It consists of sudden unconsciousness (from brain hypoxia) and alternating tonic (contractions) and clonic (successive contractions and relaxations) movements of extremities, which are involuntary. Respirations cease as intercostal muscles and the diaphragm become temporarily paralyzed; cyanosis may be marked. Muscles of the head and face jerk. There may be frothing from the mouth and dyspnea when breathing is finally resumed. Bladder control may be lost during the attack. Although the entire episode of a grand mal seizure may last only a few minutes, the nursing responsibilities are complex.

As tonic and clonic movements cease when the seizures terminate, there may be a remaining loss of consciousness for a few more minutes, and some clients appear exhausted, weak, and confused. A long sleep usually follows. Although they will not recall the seizure, clients often complain of severe muscle pain from the violent tonic and clonic movements and desire to sleep more than usual for several days.

Status epilepticus is a series of successive grand mal seizures occurring without an interim of regaining consciousness. This condition is extremely grave because of the effect of hypoxia on vital brain tissue. Prolonged seizures may result in respiratory arrest, hypertension, increased intracranial pressure, papilledema, and hyperthermia.

Data analysis
Data analysis may reveal nursing diagnoses of ineffective airway clearance, ineffective breathing, potential for injury, fear, and ineffective coping.

Planning and implementation. Nursing care is planned to maintain adequate ventilation, protect the client from injury, monitor the client's behavior, properly administer prescribed therapy, and educate the family about the problem.

Maintaining adequate ventilation. The nurse should ensure an adequate airway by positioning the head and placing the client in a sidelying position to facilitate drainage of secretions and to prevent the tongue from being bitten or falling backward to obstruct the nasopharynx. A padded tongue depressor or plastic airway may be used for this purpose. However, never attempt to pry open the mouth to insert it after a seizure begins, since damage to jaw muscles could result. A wad of linen, wash cloth, or other available safe object can be used in an emergency if a tongue depressor is not available. Never put fingers into the mouth of a convulsing client because a serious bite could result from this injudicious act. Nor should objects such as pens and pencils be used because of the potential damage to the client's mouth.

Ventilating can also be enhanced by loosening tight clothing about the client's neck, for example, loosening a collar, brassiere, or belt. Other tight clothing should be loosened or removed if possible.

Protecting from injury. Clients with clinical conditions known to produce seizures should be placed on *seizure precautions* and necessary equipment for managing the episode should be at hand. Such precautions include padded tongue blades, side rails, and headboards. A padded tongue depressor should be taped to the client's chair, bed, or transportation cart for immediate use when necessary. Other precautions include keeping side rails up and secure at all times and maintaining the bed in a low position.

Some clients have an aura (a highly individualized sensory experience, including auditory and visual hallucinations or gustatory or olfactory phenomena), which forewarns them of an impending crisis in sufficient time to call for help. Although the attack cannot be thwarted, efforts can be made to prevent injury, a major nursing responsibility.

If the client is not already lying down when a seizure occurs, the nurse should help him to the floor. No attempt should be made to use restraints. Torn soft tissues and fractures could result from such actions. Remove him from a place of danger, if possible. If the client's body hits surrounding objects, use any available soft objects to prevent him from striking his head or extremities against hard surfaces. Towels or blankets, pillows, or articles of clothing can be employed for padding.

Monitoring and reporting the client's behavior. Assessing the client's behavior is an important aspect of care. The time of onset and duration of the episode is to be noted. If an aura was present, it should be reported. Each phase of the seizure should be described, the kinds (for example, clonic or tonic) and anatomical location of movements. Were they general, or did they begin in one area and spread to others? Were there unusual eye movements? Incontinence? Was there a complete lack of consciousness at any point in the seizure or alterations in level of consciousness after the conclusion? The pupils should be checked during the seizure, if possible. If not, they should be checked as soon as possible after the seizure. (Pupils tend to dilate and are nonreactive during a true generalized seizure.) The respiratory rate and pattern, as well as the amount of perspiration, should be assessed. The cardiovascular status must also be monitored. Any paralysis or weakness after the attack or difficulty in speaking should be reported. It is also helpful to mention any injury or potential injury that occurred. If the client lapsed into sleep after the seizure, how long did he sleep? Any medications administered should be charted along with notations about their effect. Sedatives and anticonvulsant therapy may be prescribed after an attack.

Administering prescribed therapy. Several drugs are prescribed to decrease excitation of the neurons, for example, phenytoin (Dilantin), trimethadione (Tridione), and ethosuximide (Zarontin). The nurse must be familiar with these drugs and have them readily available for emergency use. Because of the value of these drugs in controlling seizures, the importance of these clients following prescribed drug therapy should be stressed. These drugs are taken for a lifetime if seizure control is to be established. Maintenance dosage must be followed. The nurse must instruct the client about the effect and side effects of these drugs.

Usually, attempts are made to establish well-defined blood levels until a therapeutic dose has been established. Clients should be encouraged to obtain blood level determinations as prescribed.

Informing family members. Another aspect of therapy is informing family members about seizures and the family's role in the care of the client. They should be informed of a potential seizure and instructed exactly what they should and should not do when a seizure occurs. They should also be instructed to obtain some type of emergency identification tag.

 Evaluation. Evaluation of the nursing plans for the client with seizures is an ongoing process.

EXPECTED OUTCOMES

The client and/or family can:
1. Describe seizures including factors that may precipitate them.
2. State plans for health maintenance.
3. State plans for follow-up care.
4. State use, dose, time, route, and side effects of any prescribed medications.
5. State indications requiring immediate health care services.
6. State intent to carry or wear some type of identification tag.
7. Demonstrate plan for emergency management during seizure attacks.

Petit mal seizures. These seizures are characterized by momentary episodes of loss of consciousness. The client may have a blank stare for a few seconds or may stop talking in the middle of a sentence. After the seizure the client is often unaware that he momentarily lost consciousness. There is no violent movement or loss of bladder control. Petit mal seizures are more common in children and may affect progress in school if not managed properly with medications.

Jacksonian seizures. Jacksonian seizures are focal, and only certain muscle groups are affected. There is generally no loss of consciousness. They may begin in one area, spreading to adjacent muscles on one side of the body, and can ultimately become generalized or grand mal.

Psychomotor seizures. Psychic phenomena are experienced with no recollection. Motor behavior may involve such things as wringing the hands, picking at objects, or undressing. The acts seem to be related to emotions such as frustration, fear, or rage. Speech may be affected, and the thought process seems rambling and perhaps nonsensical.

Headache (cephalgia)

Headache is a deep somatic pain in the head that indicates some unusual stress is affecting the body or its processes. Although the brain tissue itself is almost insensitive to pain, damage to the cranium, its blood supply, or the portion of the body it represents evokes a headache. Headaches are classified according to etiology; vascular or migraine, cluster, muscle contraction, nasomotor reactions, and a miscellaneous category are discussed.

Vascular, or migraine, headaches. Vascular or migraine headaches are headaches primarily occurring because of the painful dilation and distension of the extracranial and intracranial branches of the external carotid artery. These may be experienced by both adults and children, but they are most typical among women from menarche to menopause. There is a strong familial tendency toward development of migraine.

The painful migraine headache is theoretically linked to frustration and tension experiences by insecure, inflexible, meticulous, and conscientious individuals. It is thought that when such persons do not permit themselves to express emotions of anger and rage, these hostile and aggressive impulses are repressed and suppressed.

Considerable research has been done to discover the agents that play a part in the development of a migraine headache. Serotonin (5-hydroxytryptamine) has been investigated as a causative agent because the presence of its metabolites seem to be increased during headaches in 85% of the individuals studied.[20] Serotonin can act as a constricting or dilating stimulus, depending on the vascular bed, its resting tone, and the concentration of serotonin. (Ordinarily serotonin constricts large arteries and dilates smaller arterioles and capillaries.) Tyramine and phenylethyamine are also agents under study as causative factors in migraine because they liberate norepinephrine, a vasoconstrictor, from tissues. Since tyramine is contained in certain foods, dietary restrictions have been useful in some instances. Finally, the role of vasodilator polypeptides similar to bradykinin and prostaglandins seems to warrant additional research as they relate to migraine.

Pathophysiology. Theories of cranial arterial distension and dilation explain this type of headache. Exact pathophysiological mechanisms are unknown, but in the case of the classic migraine, it is presumed that tension caused by emotions creates a vasospasm that, in turn, produces local ischemia of the brain. After the intense spasm, the affected vessels presumably relax and become congested with blood for an extended period of time, even up to 48 hours. As the dilation progresses, there are excessive pulsations, especially of the temporal arteries. As the attack continues, edema fluid containing proteolytic enzymes and pain-provoking polypeptides collects in the extracranial perivascular tissue. The pain mechanisms of dilation and pulsations are thus augmented by chemical substances produced as by-products to vascular phenomena.[16] EEG changes may occur with migraine but are generally nonspecific.

Assessment. The client with classic migraine often experiences unusual disturbances (such as seeing stars) and a specific aura before the onset of the headache. Children are usually quiet. Some have visual disturbances, but listlessness is most common. Certain clients reportedly are pale and feel chilly at the onset of the migraine. These phenomena are thought to relate to the local cerebral ischemia from vasospasm.

Individuals with migraine headaches usually retreat to bed in a darkened, quiet room. They describe their distress vividly. The pain is usually unilateral at first, eventually extending throughout the cranium. Irritability, nausea, photophobia, and face pain may accompany the head pain. Vomiting, if it occurs, usually results in considerable relief for the victim. Sufferers of migraine seem to profit from the deep sleep that usually follows the acute episode.

Data analysis
Data analysis may reveal nursing diagnoses of alterations in comfort: pain.

Planning and implementation. Vasoconstricting drugs are useful in the prevention and control of migraine. Ergotamine tartrate (Gynergen) and ergotamine tartrate plus caffeine (Cafergot) are two preparations frequently employed.

These agents, especially ergotamine tartrate, cause nausea and vomiting. Intramuscular administration is therefore preferred. If relief is not obtained within 30 minutes, the dosage may be repeated. A few clients are maintained routinely on phenytoin (Dilantin) for symptomatic relief. Prophylactic agents for such vascular headaches include methysergide, cyproheptadine, diazepam (Valium), propranolol (Inderal), antihistamines, antiserotonin compounds, antiinflammatory drugs, and steroids.

Dietary restrictions aimed at avoidance of tyramine-containing foods are being tried by some clinicians to thwart migraines. Red wine, champagne, aged strong cheese, monosodium glutamate, cured meats (for example, ham, bacon, salami, hot dogs), chocolate, fatty and fried foods, chicken livers, pickled herring, bean pods, and selected fish contain tyramines and are therefore ill advised for clients with migraine headaches.

Psychotherapy aimed at treating anxiety and depression may be indicated. Warm baths and massage are helpful for some individuals in promoting relaxation. Scalp pressure over the superficial temporal arteries and carotid compression provide relief for others. Ice bags applied to the head and inhalation of 100% oxygen are additional measures occasionally useful in promoting reflex vasoconstriction. Biofeedback is also advantageous in controlling some clients' pain.

Cluster headache. A cluster headache is a vascular headache with periodic, closely occurring attacks separated by long remissions. They are usually brief in duration, often nocturnal, and marked by unilateral lacrimation and rhinorrhea. Flushing and sweating are not uncommonly associated. The management of cluster headaches is similar to that of migraine.

Muscle contraction headache. A muscle contraction headache is associated with sustained contraction of skeletal muscles of the face, head, and neck, usually bilateral, suboccipital, and stress related. Analgesics and physical therapy are usual modes of treatment.

Nasomotor reaction headaches. Nasomotor reaction headaches result from congestion and edema of nasal and paranasal mucous membranes. They may be related to allergens, infectious agents, or anatomical defects, although this has not been validated by controlled clinical research. Clients may refer to this pain as ''sinus headache.'' This complaint may be supported by x-ray evidence of sinusitis in some instances, and often there is local edema and tenderness. Treatment is aimed at the underlying cause and the relief of pain.

Other headaches. There are many other classifications of headache, including *traction headaches* (resulting from the stretching of intracranial structures by space-occupying lesions or loss of cerebrospinal fluid), *inflammatory headaches,* and those related to eye, ear, dental, and other cranial or neck structures. Some psychiatric phenomena have characteristic headache patterns that can be defined as *delusional, hypochondriacal,* or *conversional.*

Assessment. Signs of headache in children are vague and may be expressed by fretfulness, ear pulling, head rolling, and grimaces. Older children and adults are usually able to describe the nature of the pain and offer data regarding its onset, progression, duration, and location. They may, in addition, offer information about relationships of the headache to stress, changes in position, sleeping patterns, allergens, or injury. The nurse should record the client's descriptive terms of the experienced headache, such as ''sharp,'' ''dull,''

Nursing process for common health problems

"throbbing," "bandlike," "splitting." Associated phenomena such as nausea, vomiting, sleep disturbances, vertigo, visual or auditory disturbances, or light-headedness are noted. Neck and shoulder muscles should be palpated and the presence or absence of tension assessed. It is useful to determine what helps or worsens the nature of the headache, including postural changes, sleep, medications, air conditioning, or certain activity. For example, if the headache is caused by increased intracranial pressure, it becomes worse, as a rule, when the individual stoops or exercises, or when he arises in the morning. If it is caused by a deficient oxygen supply to the brain, it lessens with rest. Tension-related headaches improve with regular, sound patterns of sleep.

 Planning and implementation. The client who experiences an occasional headache usually resorts to over-the-counter remedies for pain relief such as aspirin, acetaminophen (Tylenol), or one of several other readily available analgesics. These preparations are basically safe, taken as directed, for episodic management of headache. However, their continued use over a long period of time may lead to serious complications. For example, gastritis and bleeding tendencies may be exacerbated by aspirin when taken frequently or in large quantities.

Clients should be instructed to seek medical attention for recurring or localized headaches accompanied by other somatic disturbances. They should also be cautioned in regard to side effects and hazards of regular or excessive use of common, over-the-counter drugs. The nurse must point out that many analgesics are combined with other preparations (caffeine, phenacetin, or buffers) and that they may interact adversely in combination with prescribed medications that the client may be taking to manage other health problems.

Headache is an important symptom, and it is often a valuable clue to a serious somatic disturbance. It is also the most frequent minor, or incidental complaint of clients. The nurse must be skilled in assessments related to headache. Unfortunately, data gathering is realistically confined to subjective reporting by the client, and little validation is possible for the majority of headaches, even with sophisticated diagnostic tests.

Infections   **Meningitis.** Meningitis is an infection of the meninges caused by bacteria or virus. Depending on the causative agent, meningitis may be divided into meningococcal, tuberculous, influenzal, pneumococcal, and staphylococcal types. The type, characteristics, and communicability as well as the drugs of choice are outlined in Table 10-14.

 Assessment

1. *Headache.* The primary symptom of most inflammations of the central nervous system is headache from an increase in cerebrospinal fluid pressure and stretching of the edematous nerve tissue. The headache is often localized frontally or occipitally, or it may extend down the back of the neck. It increases in severity with sudden movements of any type, especially forceful coughing.

2. *Nuchal rigidity.* The neck becomes rigid and resistant to flexion because of inflammation at the base of the brain. As the disease progresses, the rigidity becomes more intense.

3. *Brudzinski's sign.* A positive index of meningeal irritation, Brudzinski's sign, consists of flexion of the lower limbs on passive flexion of the head on the chest and is often present in meningitis.

4. *Kernig's sign.* Kernig's sign consists of pain and resistance on extend-

TABLE 10-14

Meningitis

Type and causative organisms	Characteristics	Communicability	Drugs of choice and prophylaxis
Meningococcal *Neisseria meningitidis*	Epidemic in winter or spring, especially in densely populated areas such as military camps, dormitories, and so on; "spotted fever" rash present in severe cases; purulent meningitis of most critical type; death often results; can be precursor to hydrocephalus if recovery is accomplished.	By droplet spray of nose and mouth of healthy carriers as well as victims; persons exposed should have prophylactic treatment.	Oral administration of sulfadiazine or penicillin Isolation precautions
Tuberculous *Mycobacterium tuberculosis*	Second most common type of meningitis; usually follows tuberculosis infection elsewhere in the body but may be only indication of tuberculous infection; primarily affects children from 1 to 5 years of age, especially those in crowded living conditions; stormy and unpredictable course; prognosis poor.		Streptomycin and isoniazid
Influenzal *Haemophilus influenzae*	Common in infants and young children; confused with respiratory infection in early stages; commonly associated or preceded by such infections; complications include paralysis, retardation, deafness, and hydrocephalus; prognosis good.		Chloramphenicol and sulfisoxazole
Pneumococcal *Pneumococcus*	Common in infants and young children; follows sinusitis, otitis, and pneumococcal pneumonia; good survival rate with prompt intervention.		Penicillin and sulfadiazine
Staphylococcal *Staphylococcus*	Common in newborns as a result of cutaneous lesions; frequently results in death caused by resistant organisms.		Penicillin, chloramphenicol, and erythromycin
Miscellaneous causative organisms *Escherichia coli, Streptococcus, Treponema pallidum, Pseudomonas aeruginosa,* and *Salmonella*	May be sequela to primary infections elsewhere in the body.		Varies with causative organism

ing the leg at the knee after flexing the thigh on the body. It indicates meningeal irritation of the lumbosacral roots and may be bilateral, unilateral, or completely absent in clinical cases of meningitis.

5. *Fever.* Fever is almost always present to some extent in cases of central nervous system inflammation. The severity varies widely in nature and extent and may be accompanied by chills, rapid pulse and respirations, and mental disturbances including seizures, especially in children.

Other signs and symptoms may include *opisthotonus* (an arched body position caused by tetanic spasm, with the feet and head on a surface), exaggerated deep reflexes, cranial nerve dysfunction, rash or petechiae in epidemic forms, hyperesthesia of the skin, photophobia, delirium, confusion, muscular twitching, spasms, cramps, choreic or athetoid movements, and signs of increased intracranial pressure.

The diagnostic assessment must include a history and physical and specific laboratory tests. In addition to the noting of the presenting features of the client, it is important to ascertain the history of trauma, recent infections, and possible contacts with diseased individuals. Causative organisms of meningitis can enter through the spinal cord pathway and by way of the bloodstream as well as by open lesions of the brain or cord sustained in trauma. The entity may be traced to an accident, diseases of the sinuses, mastoids, lungs, skin, or a relatively insignificant upper respiratory tract infection. A lumbar puncture, with subsequent smears and culture of cerebrospinal fluid and blood, confirms the diagnosis and identifies the causative factor in most cases. The spinal fluid is cloudy, high in protein, and low in glucose.

 Planning and implementation. The management of meningitis is aimed at combating the invading organisms or eliminating the original foci of infection or irritation.

Drugs are given parenterally in large doses, and if a demonstrable site of infection is present, it is specifically treated if possible.

Supportive management. The care of the client with meningitis is the same as for clients with other infectious diseases. Since fever and vomiting are often present, *fluid balance* is an important clinical consideration. If oral food is not tolerated well, gavage feedings may be necessary. *Rest* is of extreme importance. Barbiturates are often administered to ensure adequate rest. *Pain* can usually be controlled with aspirin and codeine, but occasionally even morphine may be indicated. *Elimination* is likely to be a nursing problem. Enemas, cathartics, and catheterizations are not uncommon in the care of a client with meningitis.

Because lumbar punctures may be performed more than once in the course of the illness, the nurse should explain to the client the importance of the procedure in the management of the disease and assist the physician in the performance of the puncture whenever necessary. Proper positioning is essential. The young child may need to be restrained. If available, an additional person can be instrumental in the restraining process.

It is essential, especially when meningococcal meningitis is diagnosed, to ascertain all recent contacts of the client so that prophylactic therapy can be administered to them. This preventive care is especially important during epidemics. Both sulfa drugs and penicillin may be used to reduce the risk of developing meningitis or becoming a carrier.

Persons with meningitis are usually admitted with an undifferentiated diagnosis, and respiratory isolation within a private room, employing masks, is carried out. When a specific organism or cause is identified, isolation precautions may be relaxed, giving consideration only to special handling of excreta.

Complications. Hydrocephalus, increased intracranial pressure, otitis media, arthritis, endocarditis, and pneumonia are among possible complications. Throughout the course of the illness and during the convalescent period the nurse should be observing for signs and symptoms of brain damage or further infection. Death occurs in approximately 10% of clients with meningococcal meningitis, considered to be the most severe type.

Encephalitis. Encephalitis is an inflammatory disease of the brain and spinal cord characterized by degeneration. It encompasses a broad spectrum of conditions, including rabies, poliomyelitis, and herpes, and should be considered a generic classification as opposed to a specific entity.

Because encephalitis occurs in both epidemic and nonepidemic form, it is difficult to make definite statements regarding the disease. However, some delineations are essential for descriptive management considerations.

Epidemic encephalitides important in North American include equine varieties and the St. Louis B virus. Equine encephalitis is transmitted from horses

502

to man by vectors, particularly mosquitoes and ticks. Certain birds harbor the virus. St. Louis encephalitis is also carried by vectors, and the chief reservoir of this virus seems to be domestic fowl. Transmission of the latter type is suspected to be as follows: (1) the virus is present in the chicken mite, which (2) transmits it to a host bird, which does not develop illness but which (3) serves as a source of infection for other mites and mosquito vectors, which (4) carry the virus to humans.

Nonepidemic forms that are prevalent in North American include rabies and hemorrhagic, toxic (especially from lead), and postinfection encephalitis. These last-named forms often follow diseases such as measles, scarlet fever, pertussis, chicken pox, vaccinations, pneumonia, mumps, and influenza.

Miscellaneous viral conditions that may lead to encephalitis include herpes, lymphogranuloma venereum, ECHO virus infections, poliomyelitis, and Guillain-Barré syndrome (Coxsackie virus infection). Guillain-Barré syndrome is characterized by pain in nerves and muscles, a loss of deep reflexes and sensation, and the preservation of superficial reflexes. The victim may recover, develop a chronic form of the disease, or die from respiratory failure caused by bulbar involvement.

Assessment. The onset of encephalitis is often sudden and characterized by a slight fever. Signs of disseminated meningeal irritation and brain disturbances are present in many clients. Vision and mobility may be impaired. Some persons call certain types of encephalitis "sleeping sickness" because of the profound drowsiness, which may progress to coma.

Encephalitis should be suspected when headache, fever, drowsiness, and focal or diffuse involvement of the brain are observed. An examination of cerebrospinal fluid as well as a history of recent infection assist in the establishment of a diagnosis.

Planning and implementation. Vaccines exist for active immunization against equine and St. Louis encephalitis, but they are not generally available, and their protective value has not been clearly established.

No therapeutic regimen is definitive, but supportive and symptomatic care principles are followed. Steroids and hypertonic solutions may be used in an attempt to control cerebral edema.

Mechanically assisted respirations should be considered as part of anticipatory management, since the respiratory center may be impaired.

Isolation is not necessary for equine or St. Louis encephalitis but is required for certain nonepidemic forms.

Because some encephalitic conditions result in demyelination and myelitis, those who survive the acute episode of the disease may have residual effects, including frequent seizures, spasticity, and mental deterioration. The prognosis and recovery depend considerably on the victim's age and the virus type.

Evaluation. Evaluation of the care plan of the client with encephalitis is an ongoing component of the nursing process.

EXPECTED OUTCOMES

The client and/or family can:
1. Describe encephalitis, including the basis for the problem.
2. State the importance of compliance to prescribed therapy.
3. State plans for health maintenance.
4. State plans for follow-up care and problems requiring health care services.

Nursing process for common health problems

Subacute sclerosing panencephalitis (Dawson's encephalitis). A particular type of postinfection encephalitis that is receiving considerable attention is subacute sclerosing panencephalitis (SSPE). The predominant diagnostic feature is the presence of measles antibodies in blood serum and cerebrospinal fluid. The typical client with SSPE is a 4- to 12-year-old boy who has had measles (rubeola) 2 to 10 years before the characteristic signs and symptoms of SSPE develop. (The incidence in boys is five times greater than that in girls.) The disease progresses through four distinct stages: (1) behavioral manifestations such as irritability, lethargy, speech problems, mental regression, drooling, and withdrawal; (2) myoclonic seizures, choreoathetoid movements, and tremor; (3) opisthotonus, decerebrate rigidity, and coma; and (4) loss of higher cerebral functions, mutism, myoclonus, and hypertonia.

The entire course of SSPE may be a few months or several years, but the outcome is always fatal because of degeneration of the central nervous system. Although no specific therapeutic regimen is currently considered successful, research efforts continue in an attempt to understand the pathology and course of the disease.

Rabies. Rabies is a form of encephalitis induced by the bite of a rabid animal. Dogs, cats, skunks, bats, and foxes are common carriers of the virus. The primary pathological involvement occurs in the brainstem, but extensive cord involvement also is present.

The incubation period of rabies varies from 2 weeks to 3 months or longer. Fever, restlessness, and apprehension are often the first indications of the disease. Next the victim experiences difficulty in breathing and swallowing. Spasms occur with increasing frequency and severity, at which time the client may find it impossible to swallow even saliva. This accounts for the characteristic frothing of the mouth. Seizures, delirium, intense excitability, and eventually coma ensue. Death occurs on about the seventh day of the disease. The chief cause of death is respiratory failure. If rabies is diagnosed, the client is placed on a strict isolation regimen.

The diagnosis of rabies depends on knowledge that the ill client has been bitten by a rabid animal. This can only be ascertained by killing the suspected animal and having its brain examined for Negri bodies (eosinophilic intracytoplasmic inclusions formed in ganglion cells in rabid animals). This extremely important clue to diagnosis is available only when one can determine the animal responsible for the bite and locate it for study. If it is determined that the animal is asymptomatic or has been protected by rabies vaccine, the victim will be spared the regimen of the vaccine series. However, if the animal is not recovered, it is likely that antirabies vaccine will be administered.

Bites from a suspected rabid animal should be thoroughly cleansed at once with soap or detergent and water or alcohol and treated with a strong mineral acid, a cationic detergent, or iodides. Some authorities believe that it may be beneficial to infiltrate antirabies vaccine around and in the wound. Immediate closure of the wound is not recommended, because it tends to contribute to spread of the virus.

Prophylaxis. The most frequent purveyors of rabies to humans are domestic pets, particularly dogs and cats. It is imperative that communities take rigorous measures to ensure that pets are immunized. Some have provided neighborhood clinics where free vaccine is given or sold for a minor charge. Programs to impound stray dogs are also considered useful.

Prophylaxis in humans is begun immediately in the following cases: (1) when the animal is known to be rabid; (2) if the animals cannot be found for observation and examination; and (3) if the person was bitten by a wild animal. The daily vaccine program usually lasts 21 days and is followed by booster doses.

Nurses who work in the community, particularly in schools, should be alert to animals, especially dogs, that are seemingly ownerless. If they exhibit unusual behavior such as agitation, viciousness, paralysis, or excessive foaming salivation, authorities should be notified to impound the animal.

Since the causative organism for rabies enters only through broken skin, every animal bite or scratch should be scrutinized. Even if the skin does not appear to have been penetrated at the point of contact, the nurse should be alert to other open lesions adjacent to the area where the organism might enter.

The nurse should give clients who have pets or live in areas where wild animals habitate information about preventing rabies, reporting suspect animals, tagging properly vaccinated animals for easy identification, and steps to be taken if someone is bitten. The fact should be stressed that once the symptoms of rabies appear in either animal or human, death is almost certain. It is therefore imperative to understand points of prevention and prophylaxis related to rabies.

Tetanus. Tetanus, like polio, was at one time a dreaded disease of humans, especially in wartime. Tetanus is an acute infectious disease of the central nervous system caused by *Clostridium tetani,* which is commonly found in the soil and in animal excreta. Tetanus is characterized by rather persistent tonic spasms of voluntary muscles and tonic seizures. Because the masseters are in characteristic spasm in acute cases, many lay persons refer to the illness as ''lockjaw.''

Clostridium tetani enters the body through open wounds. Since it is an anaerobic organism, it is most likely to be a threat in a deep penetration wound, especially a puncture. The incubation period is short (5 to 8 or 10 days) and symptoms progress rapidly; therefore a successful prophylaxis program must be pursued.

A program of immunization in childhood includes tetanus toxoid, and throughout childhood and adulthood, booster doses ought to be given periodically and when open wounds are encountered, especially if they have been incurred outdoors, in a barn, or by way of a puncture. Since the organism survives poorly in well-nourished and oxygenated tissue, wound cleansing and debridement are important. Antibiotic therapy is often coupled with the booster of toxoid.

If an individual has never been immunized or if a satisfactory history of immunization cannot be obtained, a tetanus-immune human globulin may be given. (Formerly, an antitoxin made from horse serum was used to provide passive immunization, but because of the risk of serum sickness, it is seldom used. If it is employed, it should always be preceded by careful skin testing.) The tetanus-immune human globulin can be safely given intramuscularly without skin tests. Although a local redness may occur after the injection, this should not be interpreted as an allergic reaction and thus cause the risk of withholding the preparation.

Tetanus can be avoided through a rigorous prophylaxis program as described, which begins in infancy and continues throughout life.

Abscesses. An abscess or collection of exudate may occur anywhere in the central nervous system, particularly the brain, as a result of a local infection or an infection elsewhere within the body. Infections of the bones, lungs, sinuses, or ears seem to predispose to brain abscess.

The signs and symptoms depend on the location and extent of the pus accumulation and may be similar to those associated with meningitis or increased intracranial pressure because of a brain tumor.

Antibiotics and surgical damage to relieve pressure are the major components of abscess management.

Poliomyelitis

Poliomyelitis is a viral disease of the spinomuscular level of the nervous system that chiefly involves the spinal portion. The anterior horn cells are affected by an acute inflammatory process that creates a flaccid paralysis of involved muscles or muscle groups. Atrophy follows, with loss of tendon reflexes and, ultimately, muscle and joint deterioration. It is particularly found in children. Although poliomyelitis was once a dreaded disease, it has been virtually eliminated by the regular use of immunization. In 1950, 33,300 cases of poliomyelitis were reported, but in recent years the numbers have been drastically reduced. The success of the Salk and Sabin vaccines in a worldwide distribution program have all but eliminated poliomyelitis as a threat to children and adults.

The Salk vaccine, which was introduced in 1955, employs a formalin-inactivated poliovirus and is injected parenterally. The Sabin vaccine contains a live, attenuated organism and is administered orally. The Sabin vaccine was licensed in the United States in 1961 and has several advantages over the Salk vaccine. It actually induces a poliovirus infection, which not only prompts a rise in antibodies but also induces a resistance to reinfection. Every person who has taken Sabin vaccine breaks a link in the natural chain of transmission, and thus if a high proportion of the population are immunized, the community is protected, as well as the individual client. The rapidly induced immunity that is associated with the oral vaccine is highly effective in arresting epidemics, and oral vaccines are easily administered in community-wide programs.

Many pediatricians advocate the use of both Salk and Sabin vaccines and administer them to every child. All preschoolers, school-age children, and adults should be immunized with at least one of the agents, preferably the oral Sabin vaccine that can be given easily by spoon or on a lump of sugar. Booster doses are required periodically with the Salk vaccine but are considered unnecessary when immunization has been completed with the Sabin live, attenuated poliovirus.

Evaluation

Evaluation, the final stage of the nursing process, encourages the nurse and client to make judgments about goal achievement relative to plans for health promotion maintenance and restoration for common problems of the neurological system. Nursing problems often include alteration in thought process, potential impairment of skin integrity, alterations in sensory perception, self-care deficit (for example, in feeding, bathing hygiene, dressing/grooming, toileting), disturbance in self-concept, impaired physical mobility, potential for injury, impaired home maintenance management, fear, grieving, diversional activity deficit, ineffective coping, alteration in bowel elimination, impaired verbal communication, and sexual dysfunction.

10 Neurological system

EXPECTED OUTCOMES

The client and/or family can:
1. Describe the basis for his neurological deficit and potential for recovery.
2. State plans for compliance to prescribed therapy, including medications, diet, and activity.
3. State plans for follow-up care.
4. Demonstrate satisfactory adjustments of life-style imposed by neurological deficits or dysfunctions.
5. Use appropriate agencies and resources to facilitate rehabilitation.
6. Strive to maintain a maximum level of activity within limitations imposed by the neurological deficit.
7. Explain the consequences of immobility and display behaviors to minimize such complications.
8. Exhibit caution in activity to facilitate personal safety, which is threatened by various neurological deficits.
9. Involve significant others in care planning.
10. Report signs and symptoms, which indicate a progression or regression in neurological status.

Summary   Caring for clients with nervous system disorders can be a challenging role for nurses. It involves keen assessment skills and a thorough knowledge of pathophysiology of conditions affecting the brain and spinal cord.

Special assessment modes include cranial nerve testing, reflex testing, and determining motor strength and power. Because developmental factors are closely related to nervous system functioning, the nurse must consider the client's history, growth pattern, and life-style when making assessments.

Although there are a number of diagnostic tests relevant to the brain and spinal cord, the lumbar puncture, with examination of CSF, is among the most revealing studies. Radiological procedures, isotope scanning, and electrical impulse response testing are also widely used. The most valid assessment tool, however, is the client's level of consciousness. The Glasgow Coma Scale is one method of quantitatively evaluating this factor.

The nurse must incorporate a knowledge of intracranial hypertension in a care plan of any client with central nervous system dysfunction. Intracranial pressure can be recognized by characteristic signs and symptoms, but can be accurately measured by intracranial monitoring devices. Increases in intracranial pressure must be promptly managed to prevent destruction of vital brain cells. Dehydration, steroids, hypothermia, barbiturate coma, and controlled positive-negative pressure ventilation are current methods.

Seizures reflect structural and metabolic aberrations of brain tissue and must be considered as a symptom, not a disease entity. Nursing care of a client with seizures involves physical protection measures and special attention to airway management, especially after a seizure.

The care of an individual who is unconscious is indeed challenging and incorporates airway management, maintenance of fluid and nutritional status, assessment of sensory functioning and elimination, and prevention of complications such as decubiti and deformities.

The client with a head injury must be carefully monitored in regard to

Nursing process for common health problems

metabolic, respiratory, cardiovascular, and gastrointestinal responses. Many specific nursing interventions will be based on a working knowledge of the physiological responses to head injury. The care of a client having cranial surgery is based on these tenets.

Common health problems of the neonate and infant largely result from congenital defects of the central nervous system. Hydrocephalus, spina bifida occulta, and myelomeningocele are examples.

Recurring health problems in children may include central nervous system dysfunction. Cerebral palsy, although often present at birth, is usually prevalent with its sensorimotor disturbances during childhood as independent activities are required. Management includes the specialized services of a multidisciplinary health care team. Minimal brain dysfunction, retardation, and muscular dystrophy are among other childhood nervous system problems that affect growth and development.

Epilepsy, a form of idiopathic seizures, may be manifest during childhood and adolescence as the body adjusts to the changing physiological demands. Most epilepsy is controlled by anticonvulsant drugs, avoidance of fatigue and stress, and the prevention of febrile illness.

Multiple sclerosis and myasthenia gravis are devastating degenerative diseases that affect young adults. Signs, symptoms, and prognosis are highly variable, but usually demand considerable life-style adaptations of the client.

The cerebrovascular accident (stroke) is one of the most dread conditions that may be experienced by the adult. Atherosclerosis, transient ischemia attacks, cerebral embolism, and cerebral infarction are among the causative factors. Nursing management after the acute period involves maintaining psychosocial function, coping with aphasia and perceptual defects, and promoting independence in the activities of daily living.

Common problems of the older adult include presenile dementia (normal pressure hydrocephalus, Huntington's chorea, and Alzheimer's and Pick's diseases). Management incorporates caring for the client in a protective environment with attention to social and behavioral responses.

Trauma is the most common problem of the central nervous system across the life span. Caring for the individual who has a head or spinal cord injury is complex and entails careful monitoring of brain activity. Assessments relating to levels of consciousness, respiratory pattern, pupil size and reaction, eye movements and oculovestibular responses, and motor responses from skeletal muscle are routine responsibilities of the nurse. For clients with permanent spinal cord injury, an extensive plan for long-term rehabilitation is required, with attention to bowel and bladder function, skin care, and psychosocial adjustments.

Other problems such as tumors of the brain or spinal cord and a variety of central nervous system infections can occur at any time during the life span. The nurse must be aware of surgical and other medical modes of management to plan nursing care.

References

1. Beland, Irene: Clinical nursing: pathophysiological and psychosocial approaches, New York, 1980, Macmillan Publishing Co., Inc.
2. Brock, Samuel: Injuries of brain and spinal cord and their coverings, ed. 5, New York, 1974, Springer Publishing Co.
3. Clipper, Margaret J.: Nursing care of the stroke patient. In Licht, Sidney, editor: Stroke and its rehabilitation, Baltimore, 1979, Waverly Press, Inc.
4. Conway-Rutkowski, Barbara Lang: Carini and Owens' neurological and neurosurgical nursing, ed. 8, St. Louis, 1982, The C.V. Mosby Co.
5. Davis, Joan E., and Mason, Celestine B.: Neurologic critical care, New York, 1979, Van Nostrand Reinhold Co.
6. DeJong, Russell N.: The neurological examination, ed. 4, Hagerstown, Md., 1979, Harper & Row.
7. Fisher, C. Miller, Mohr, Jay P., and Adams, Raymond D.: Cerebrovascular diseases. In Harrison's principles of internal medicine, ed. 9, New York, 1980, McGraw-Hill Book Co.
8. Gilroy, John, and Meyer, John Stirling: Cerebrovascular disease, Medical neurology, New York, 1969, Macmillan Publishing Co., Inc.
9. Guttman, L.: Problems of treatment of pressure sores in spinal paraplegia, Br. J. Plast. Surg. **8:**196-213, 1956.
10. Hayter, Jean: Patients who have Alzheimer's disease, Am. J. Nurs. **74:**1460-1463, August 1974.
11. Husain, Taffazzul: An experimental study of some pressure effects on tissue with reference to the bed sore problem, J. Pathol. Bacteriol. **66:**347-358, 1953.
12. Isselbacher, Kurt J., and LaMont, Thomas J.: Infiltrative and metabolic diseases affecting the liver. In Isselbacher, Kurt J., and others: Harrison's principles of internal medicine, ed. 9, New York, 1980, McGraw-Hill Book Co.
13. Kaplan, Gerald: The psychogenic etiology of headache post–lumbar puncture, Psychosom. Med. **29:**376-379, 1967.
14. Loetterle, Bridget C., and others: Cerebellar stimulation: pacing the brain, Am. J. Nurs. **75:**958-960, June 1975.
15. Meyer, John Stirling: New concepts of cerebrovascular disease, Med. Clin. North Am. **54:**349-360, March 1970.
16. Mountcastle, Vernon B., editor: Medical physiology, vol. 1, St. Louis, 1974, The C.V. Mosby Co.
17. Plum, Fred, and Posner, Jerome B.: Diagnosis of stupor and coma, ed. 2, Contemporary Neurology Series, Philadelphia, 1972, F.A. Davis Co.
18. Posner, Charles M.: The presenile dementias, J.A.M.A. **223:**81-84, July 1975.
19. Price, Sylvia Anderson, and Wilson, Lorraine McCarty: Pathophysiology and clinical concepts of disease processes, New York, 1978, McGraw-Hill Book Co.
20. Raskin, Neil H., and Appenzelle, Otto: Headache. In Smith, Lloyd H. Jr., editors: Series of major problems in internal medicine, vol. 19, Philadelphia, 1980, W.B. Saunders Co.
21. Salcman, Michael, editor: Neurologic emergencies: recognition and management, New York, 1980, Raven Press.
22. Taylor, Ann Gill: Autonomic dysreflexia in spinal cord injury, Nurs. Clin. North Am. **9:**717-725, December 1974.
23. Toole, James F., and Patel, Aneel N.: Cerebrovascular disorders, New York, 1967, McGraw-Hill Book Co.
24. Wilson, Susan Fickertt: Neuro-nursing, New York, 1979, Springer Publishing Co.
25. Wolf, John K.: Practical clinical neurology, New York, 1980, Medical Examination Publishing Co., Inc.
26. Wylie, Charles M.: Measuring and results of rehabilitation of patients with strokes, United States Public Health Service, Public Health Reports, Oct. 1967, pp. 893-898.

Suggested readings

Barber, Janet M., and Budassi, Susan A.: Mosby's manual of emergency care practices and procedures, St. Louis, 1979, The C.V. Mosby Co.

Budassi, Susan A., and Barber, Janet M.: Emergency nursing: principles and practice, St. Louis, 1981, The C.V. Mosby Co.

Burt, Margaret M.: Perceptual deficits in hemiplegia, Am. J. Nurs. **70:**1026-1029, May 1970.

Chippa, Keith H.: Evoked responses. Pt I. Pattern shift visual, Weekly update, Neurol. Neurosurg., vol. 2, Princeton, N.J., Bromedia, Inc.

Chippa, Keith H.: Evoked responses. Pt II. Brainstem auditory, Weekly update, Neurol. Neurosurg., vol. 2, no. 14, Princeton, N.J., Bromedia, Inc.

Dalessis, Donald J., editor: Wolff's headache and other head pain, ed. 4, Cambridge, England, 1980, Oxford University Press.

Frohlick, Edward: Pathophysiology, Philadelphia, 1972, J.B. Lippincott Co.

Harrington, Robert: Communication for the aphasic stroke patient: assessment and therapy, J. Am. Geriatr. Soc. **23:**254-257, June 1975.

Jackson, Pat Ludder: Ventriculaperitoneal shunts, Am. J. Nurs. **80:**1109, June 1980.

Kunkel, Joyce, and Wiley, John K.: Acute head injury: what to do when . . . and why, Nurs. 79, **9:**23-33, March 1979.

Liechty, Richard D., and Soper, Robert T.: Synopsis of surgery, ed. 3, St. Louis, 1976, The C.V. Mosby Co.

Meyer, John Stirling: New concepts of cerebrovascular disease, Med. Clin. North Am. **54**(2):349-360, March 1970.

Mooney, Thomas O., Cole, Thomas M., and Childgren, Richard A.: Sexual options for paraplegics and quadriplegics, Boston, 1975, Little Brown and Co.

McCormick, William F.: The pathology of stroke. In Licht, Sidney, editor: Stroke and its rehabilitation, Baltimore, 1979, Waverly Press.

Pierog, Sophie, and Ferrara, Angelo: Medical care of the sick newborn, ed. 2, St. Louis, 1976, The C.V. Mosby Co.

Plum, Fred, and Posner, Jerome B.: Diagnosis of stupor and coma, ed. 2, Contemporary Neurology Series, Philadelphia, 1972, F.A. Davis Co.

Sister Kenny Institute Staff: About stroke, Minneapolis, 1978, Sister Kenny Institute.

Tilbury, Mary: The intracranial pressure screw: a new assessment tool, Nurs. Clin. North Am. **9:**641-645, December 1974.

Woods, Nancy Fugate: Human sexuality in health and illness, ed. 2, St. Louis, 1979, The C.V. Mosby Co.

for clients with common health problems of the

11 Musculoskeletal system

Assessment

Data analysis

Planning

Implementation

Evaluation

Common health problems of the musculoskeletal system interfere with mobility throughout the life span and are often related to growth and development at specific ages. Birth injuries and congenital defects, for example, may inhibit neonates' and infants' range of motion. Children and young adults and older adults exhibit a high incidence rate for accidents, whereas adolescents are prone to structural defects often related to growth at this time. Rheumatoid arthritis is a major cause of disability that affects mostly women in middle adulthood. Osteoarthritis and osteoporosis are common to the aging process and produce changes in balance, posture, and mobility in older adults. The purpose of this chapter is to provide information for assessing the client's musculoskeletal system, maintaining health, planning care for the immobilized client, and implementing and evaluating a nursing care plan for clients with common health problems of the musculoskeletal system.

Overview of the musculoskeletal system

The musculoskeletal system provides structure and shape for the body and permits coordination of movement and activity. The system is composed of cartilage, bones, ligaments, tendons, and muscles.

Cartilage is a form of connective tissue that cushions bony prominences and offers protection where resiliency is required. The earlobes and nose are examples.

Bones provide rigid support and help maintain posture. The bones are protected by a lining of synovial cells and consist of an *epiphysis,* or cartilaginous growing end, and a *diaphysis,* or shaft. Epiphyseal cells are subject to hormonal regulation by the growth hormone from the anterior pituitary, causing chondrogenesis, calcification, and widening of epiphyseal plates. Skeletal growth ends during adolescence but growth hormone is present throughout the life span. A balance between deposition of new bone cells by osteoblasts and resorption is regulated by thyrocalcitonin, a thyroid hormone that regulates calcium metabolism and prevents resorption of bone minerals. Parathormone (a hormone from the parathyroid gland), thyroid hormone, and vitamin D regulate calcium and phosphorous deposition in the bones.

Articulation of bones occurs at the *joint*. The joint may be described as immovable, partially movable, or freely movable. *Synovial bursae* are located between movable joints as well as between tendons and muscles and bones. The membranes of these sacs secrete synovial fluid, which serves to reduce friction during movement.

Ligaments and *tendons* are primarily collagen and connect the bone to contiguous structures. Ligaments attach bone to bone, whereas tendons attach muscle to bone.

Skeletal *muscles,* comprising up to 50% of body weight, provide shape to the body, protect the bones, maintain posture, and by contracting, cause movement of various body parts. The muscles are attached to the skeleton at the point of origin and to the bones at the point of insertion. Skeletal muscles have properties of contraction and extension as well as elasticity that permit *isotonic* (shortening and thickening) or *isometric* (increased muscle tension) movement. Muscle contraction is initiated by nerve stimulation (see Chapter 10), and coordination of these systems is necessary for voluntary and involuntary movements.

Assessment
NURSING HISTORY

The nurse uses the health history and physical assessment to obtain data about individuals' usual patterns of mobility. The data are coordinated with a developmental history and information about the client's social and psychological background.

Health history

The health history should be obtained at the first contact with the client to establish baseline information and formulate nursing diagnoses. The health history should include information about the client's usual patterns of activity and exercise. The nurse inquires about the client's activities of daily living and records any limitations. The nurse also assesses the client's ambulation patterns and notes if the client requires ambulatory assist devices such as a wheelchair, cane, walker, or prosthesis. The nurse should ascertain if the client has stiffness, swelling, or pain in any joint and, if so, determine location, duration, and precipitating factors. Muscle pain, cramping, or weakness should likewise be noted.

The history should also be used to elicit information about previous musculoskeletal disorders. The nurse can inquire about presence of congenital defects, previous trauma, inflammations, or fractures.

The data collected from the history should be related to information from examination of other systems. A nutritional history, for example, may reveal dietary deficiencies or excess weight that could add stress to the skeleton.

When evaluating the client's potential or actual risk factors for musculoskeletal injury, the nurse should ask about the presence of congenital defects, family history of rheumatoid arthritis, poor nutrition, accident proneness, and use of safety devices when riding in a car. Individuals who play contact sports or who are employed in occupations that require lifting are at risk and should be so identified.

Developmental history

The needs for activity vary between individuals and are different during each developmental stage. The nurse should be aware of these differences when assessing the development of each client and when planning and implementing nursing care.

Neonate. The skeleton of the neonate is composed primarily of cartilage, and there is a considerable amount of fat surrounding the muscles and bones. For the first few days of life the posture of the neonate remains similar to that assumed in utero. The muscles are normally flexed, and muscle tone, the degree of flexion, and resistance to straightening can be rated by the Apgar scoring system (see Chapter 2). Muscles that are limp are rated 0, flexed muscles are rated 1, and muscles that are well flexed are given the highest rating of 2. Muscle tone is usually poor in hypoxic babies. Well, full-term neonates have full range of motion and a high degree of muscle tone. Upon initial appraisal, a slight incurvation of the ankles may be noted. This may be the result of fetal position. If the incurvation does not straighten during spontaneous movement or passive manipulation, further assessments for skeletal problems should be made.

Muscular activity is primarily involuntary; most movements are reflex responses to stimuli. These responses of sucking, swallowing, breathing, and grasping protect the newborn and help him cope with his new environment. Exploratory movements of the arms and legs help the newborn gain an awareness of himself in relation to his environment, achieve muscle control, and provide stress for bone ossification.

Infant. Activity becomes less a matter of survival and more a matter of musculoskeletal development and environmental exploration for the infant. The infant 1 to 3 months can turn his head when prone, raise his head and chest, and stretch his arms. The 3- to 6-month-old gains more control of his upper torso. He can support his head when sitting, sit with support, and roll over. He can shake objects with two hands and carry objects from his hand to his mouth. Erect body posture is assumed by 6 to 9 months, and the infant can sit up, hold a bottle or a cup, feed himself with his fingers, and grasp with one hand. Locomotive ability facilitates environmental exploration, and at 6 to 8 months the infant begins to crawl. The period from 9 to 18 months evidences more lower body control, and the infant pulls himself up, stands, and begins to walk.

Toddler and preschooler. The child from 15 months to 5 years begins to have more control over his own body and directs his activities to cope with the environment and his relationships to it. Pronation of the feet is normal in the toddler who has a wide-based gait, and no arch is observed in the foot until he starts to walk. There is fine muscle coordination, and basic walking skills improve. At about 15 months the toddler can climb, at about 18 months he can run, and at 30 months he can jump. When the child is around 2 years old, he walks up stairs; a few months later he can walk down stairs. At 4 he can walk forward and backward, hop, and skip. Self-care skills also develop during this period, and by 4 to 5 years of age the child can dress himself and, with direction, take care of his basic hygiene.

School-age child. From age 6 to age 13, muscular growth slows while the bones become elongated to give height to the youngster. Motor skills are more refined, and games of athletic skill are popular. Much of the child's time is spent in school and related activities.

Adolescent. Development of secondary sex characteristics changes the muscular shape and motor abilities of the adolescent. There is a spurt of growth in the long bones until late adolescence, when the epiphyses close and maximum height is attained. Increases in serum alkaline phosphatase are associated with increased velocity in growth in height. Many health problems of adolescence are related to this growth spurt. Ossification of bones generally occurs earlier in girls than boys because of the presence of estrogen. Paraspinal ligaments do not achieve full strength until adulthood; consequently, the adolescent may have the appearance of rounded shoulders. Adjustments to a new body image and use of newly developed muscles often make the adolescent appear awkward. The adolescent is usually active in school, and group activities often take precedence over individual activities.

Adult. Changes of the musculoskeletal system in middle adulthood are disconcerting to those who value the body image and musculoskeletal strength of early adulthood. In women osteoporotic changes are marked after menopause, and the skeleton becomes shorter and kyphotic. Subcutaneous fat deposits in both sexes increase in proportion to body mass, and there may be evidence of muscle disuse, depending on the activity of the individual.

Older adult. Physiological changes in the musculoskeletal system alter the physical appearance and well-being of the older adult. Calcification of ligaments and degeneration of cartilage and synovium as well as atrophy of the fibrocartilaginous disks of the vertebrae give a hunched and shortened stature to the older individual. There is an increase in the distribution of fatty tissue, a doubling between ages 25 to 75. Subcutaneous tissue diminishes, causing bony prominences to be apparent. Muscle mass shrinks, and there is less muscle strength. Active individuals, however, are slower to exhibit these changes.

The increased porosity of the bone causes the most serious consequences of aging. The degeneration of bone tissue that begins in middle adulthood is more evident in the later life span. Vertebral fractures caused by osteoporosis are not uncommon; even a sneeze may precipitate them. Changes in the angle of the neck of the femur cause lowered resistance to stress, and in fact a fracture here may cause a fall, rather than the accidental fall's causing the fracture of the femur.

Motor activity often diminishes as metabolism slows in older persons. Many older persons may have limited activity as a result of crippling diseases or bone degeneration or may have restrictions placed on their activity by illness. Physical activity is still important in older persons and should be encouraged within the limits of their ability and health.

11 Musculoskeletal system

Social history

The nurse should determine the educational, financial, religious, ethnic, and occupational factors that are significant to the history. The client's occupation, for example, is relevant if it puts the client at risk for musculoskeletal injury or requires physical strength and activity. Financial resources may be important if long-term hospitalization or disability is anticipated. The nurse should also determine the client's exercise pattern and if the exercise is obtained on a regular basis.

Psychological history

The nurse should determine the client's relationship with significant others and identify his usual coping styles. Interferences with mobility may require long-term hospitalization and adjustment to activity limitations, and the client's coping resources may be significant to the care plan.

Physical assessment

The physical examination of the musculoskeletal system involves *inspection* of the client's body build, posture, and gait and *palpation* of muscle function and joint range of motion. Assessment tools such as the Apgar score (Chapter 2) for neonatal muscle strength and the Denver Developmental Test (Appendix B) for activities related to growth and development in children may be used as guides for part of the physical appraisal in these age groups.

Inspection. Inspection of the client's body build, posture, and gait should be made at the onset of the examination. It is important for the nurse to relate normal changes in musculoskeletal development that occur during the life span and look for deviations that are associated with specific age groups.

The nurse should observe the client as he walks. Great differences in gait can be attributed to developmental stages, but generally the gait should be smooth, the body erect, the gaze forward, and the arms at the side.

FIG. 11-1
Posture changes across the life span: **A,** infant; **B,** toddler; **C,** child; **D,** adolescent; **E,** adult; **F,** older adult.

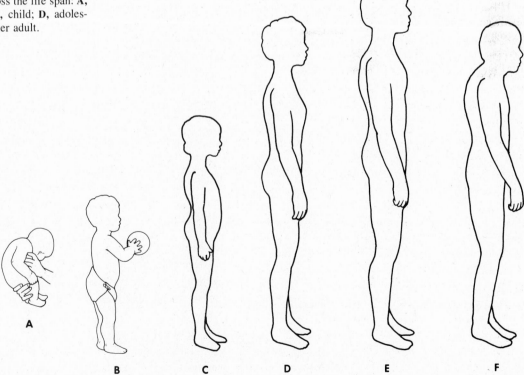

A   B   C   D   E   F

Nursing process for common health problems

The nurse should note the client's height and weight and observe the body build and proportion of body parts. The nurse should observe the client's posture from several angles. Posture refers to proportion, symmetry, and alignment and varies greatly across the life span (Fig. 11-1). The spine should be inspected for erectness. Lateral deviations (see discussion of scoliosis later in this chapter) and flexion (kyphosis) or extension (lordosis) deviations may contribute to impairment of mobility and should be identified in incipient states. The legs of children should be observed for bowing and the feet for eversion or inversion (see discussion of clubfoot later in this chapter). The hips of neonates and infants should be put through range of motion when the client is supine to detect congenital hip dislocation (discussed later in this chapter).

The muscles can be observed for obvious changes such as hypertrophy or atrophy. The muscle mass can be measured with a tape measure to document differences in symmetry.

Palpation. The musculoskeletal system can be palpated to detect changes in temperature of the skin and shape or function of the muscles. Muscle function and strength can be assessed by asking the client to flex and extend the muscle mass as well as to move the muscle against resistance. Muscle strength can be described as paralysis, severe weakness, moderate weakness, minimal weakness, and normal.

The joints are assessed as they perform active range of motion of abduction, adduction, flexion, extension, internal rotation, external rotation, and circumduction. If there is limitation, passive range of motion can be done by the nurse to detect true limitations. A goniometer can be used to measure more precisely the range of motion limits.

DIAGNOSTIC ASSESSMENT

Radiological studies

Roentgenograms. Roentgenograms (x-ray films) are used to determine injury to, or tumors of, bone and soft tissue. Clients suspected of having musculoskeletal injuries should be moved carefully when being transported and transferred.

Bone scans. Bone tumors can be detected early by bone scanning techniques. Several radionuclides are used, but ^{99}Tc-diphosphonate is favored because scanning can take place within 1 to 3 hours after injection. Others prefer gallium 72 (^{72}Ga); scintillation scanning can be done at 3 to 24 hours.

The client may be given pain medication before scanning to make him more comfortable. The radionuclide is administered intravenously, and the scan is done several hours later. Immediately before the scan the client should void to eliminate the radioactive material from the kidneys and bladder.

Arthrography. The structures of a joint can be viewed more specifically by injection of a dye or air into the joint for x-ray study. No special preparation of the client is needed.

Blood studies

Blood studies can be done to determine the presence of antibodies found in the blood of persons with rheumatoid arthritis. The rheumatoid factor, however, may also be present with aging, systemic lupus erythematosus, scleroderma, and other diseases. Normal values are absence of the factor; 80% is positive for rheumatoid arthritis in adults.

Other studies

Arthroscopy. The joint cavity can be visualized by insertion of a special endoscope (arthroscope) into the joint. This procedure is done to visualize, perform a biopsy of, or remove loose bodies. The client receives a local anesthetic before the procedure, which is usually done in a surgical area, where asepsis can be maintained. After the procedure a pressure dressing is applied, and the joint should remain immobilized for several hours, depending on the extent of the procedure.

Electromyography. The electrical activity of the muscles can be measured and recorded on an electromyogram (EMG). A needle electrode is inserted into the muscle to determine variations in muscle voltage. The electrical activity can be heard by an amplifier, viewed on an oscilloscope, or recorded on graph paper. Special preparations for this test are not necessary, but the nurse should explain to the client what to expect and reassure him that there is no undue pain or danger of electrical shock.

Data analysis

After obtaining information about the client's nursing history and physical examination, the nurse and client can identify actual and potential nursing problems or diagnoses. Potential or real nursing diagnoses may include impairment of mobility, alterations in comfort, knowledge deficit, self-care deficit, potential for injury, and disturbances in self-concept. The diagnoses should then be put in priority order and plans developed for each one.

Planning

PLANNING FOR HEALTH PROMOTION

Exercise

The nurse has a significant role in helping the client plan for health activities that preserve the integrity of the musculoskeletal system. Instruction may include information about exercise, body mechanics, diet, and risk management. The nurse must adapt instruction to the age of the client and his specific needs.

It is important that the client use his muscles, and the nurse should be aware of activities that will meet this need. The random movements of the newborn, for instance, should be encouraged. He should not be confined in a tiny bed, except for periods of rest, or wrapped so securely that he cannot move his limbs. Because the newborn cannot turn himself over, he should be repositioned occasionally so that he can flex and extend all muscle groups.

The infant needs ever-increasing opportunities to develop his motor abilities. He should not be confined to an area such as a playpen that inhibits crawling and walking. A safe area on the floor with a blanket spread out is helpful in promoting locomotor skills for the infant.

Young children and adolescents need opportunities to use their musculoskeletal system. They should have a safe play area in which they can run, jump, and play games. These activities are important in contributing to the growth of the body as well as in developing social skills.

Physical fitness is important to the adult. Even though the skeletal system is not growing, the adult must use muscles to retain tone. It is easy for adults to avoid exercise, because many conveniences in a technological society have removed the need to walk or exert energy. Exercise becomes increasingly important when metabolism slows. Moderate exercise is helpful in preventing obesity and stimulating organs to function at their peak capacity. The adult should have a daily exercise program based on his needs, abilities, and limitations. Rhythmic exercise such as walking, swimming, or bicycling and noncompetitive activity are advised for adults.

During later maturity, activity is necessary to maintain range of motion in the joints. Often, the older person has chronic illnesses that prevent him from enjoying unlimited activity, but he should be encouraged to be out of bed and participating in self-care activities. Those who are confined to bed or wheelchair can do limited rhythmic activities such as arm swinging that not only provide exercise but increase morale and well-being.

The nurse should be cognizant of the need for promoting musculoskeletal activity in bedridden persons. Active and passive range-of-motion exercises (see Chapter 10) should be performed several times a day. The client should turn in bed or, if unconscious, should be turned every 1 to 2 hours. Persons who are confined to bed for long periods of time can do exercises with uninvolved muscles.

Isometric exercises are exercises in which the individual exerts force without changing the length of the muscle, such as muscle-setting exercises (alternating tightening and relaxing the muscles). Such exercises help maintain muscle tone. *Gluteal muscle-setting exercises* can be done by contracting and relaxing the buttocks. *Quadriceps-setting exercises,* performed by pressing the popliteal space against the mattress, should also be done frequently. Isometric exercises raise the blood pressure, and the client should be cautioned against straining to do these exercises. In *isotonic exercises* the muscle contracts. Lifting is an example of an isotonic exercise. For the bedfast client, lifting weights is a useful isotonic exercise to promote musculoskeletal strength. In some settings the physical therapist may assist the client with these exercises.

Safe use of the musculoskeletal system: body mechanics

Musculoskeletal integrity is also promoted by the safe use of muscles. Body mechanics is the safe use of muscles of the body to accomplish mechanical tasks. Nurses should teach these principles to persons who must lift or use strenuous motion as well as incorporate them when giving nursing care. Long muscles should be used to lift heavy objects. The long muscles of the arms and legs are more effective than those of the back, and the person should bend his knees to lift objects from the floor. A wide base of support should be used when moving objects. This is done by placing the feet 12 to 18 inches apart. Tightening the abdominal muscles gives further support to the trunk when the person is lifting or carrying. Pulling is easier than pushing, and using wheels lessens the pulling force; hydraulic lifts are useful in lifting heavy persons out of bed (Fig. 11-2). Work is best accomplished at the center of gravity. Working at the waist level is most efficient, and holding objects near the body or working near the center of gravity conserves energy. Using these principles in daily work prevents undue stress on the musculoskeletal system.

Diet

A balanced diet is also important in maintaining the bones and muscles for optimum activity. The diet should meet nutritional needs, but overeating and obesity can put a strain on the musculoskeletal system and impair activity. The diet should contain adequate sources of calcium, phosphorus, and vitamin D for bone growth.

Risk management

The greatest threat to the musculoskeletal system is injury to muscle, soft tissue, or bones from traumatic injury. Accidental injury is the fourth cause of death for the total population and the leading cause of death in children and adolescents. Injuries are likely to occur from vehicle accidents including cars, motorcycles, and bicycles, job-related accidents, or sports injuries. Those at risk are

FIG. 11-2

Hydraulic lift. **A,** Roll patient on side away from attendant. Place sling folded half-way under patient so lower edge of seat is slightly below the knees—like placing a draw sheet. **B,** Roll patient back toward attendant. Pull sling through. If patient is in hospital bed, it will help to roll up the head of the bed. Hooks of the shortest straps of the web straps are hooked into the hole of the back part. **C,** Hook the center strap into top hole of seat, and the last strap into the last hole of the seat. Move Lifter so open end of horseshoe base is under the side of bed. Hook the D/rings of the web straps into end of swivel bar. Check to see that seat is close to knees for safety. **D,** Pump hydraulic handle. Steering handle may be held to steady the pumping. Make any needed adjustments for the patient's comfort. Attendant may assist by holding up patient's head as he is being lifted. **E,** When patient has been lifted just clear of bed, swing feet off bed. Grasp the steering handles and move patient away from bed. Wheel chair may be positioned under patient with brakes locked—or the U-base of the Lifter may be rolled to fit around the legs of a wheel chair or commode. **F,** Lower the patient by pressing handle toward jack. Guide his descent. Push gently on his knees as he is being lowered so correct sitting posture can be attained. **G,** After reaching seat, hold handle depressed and press down on boom. Detach web straps; move Lifter away. Patient may remain seated on sling. (Courtesy Ted Hoyer & Co., Inc., Oshkosh, Wis.)

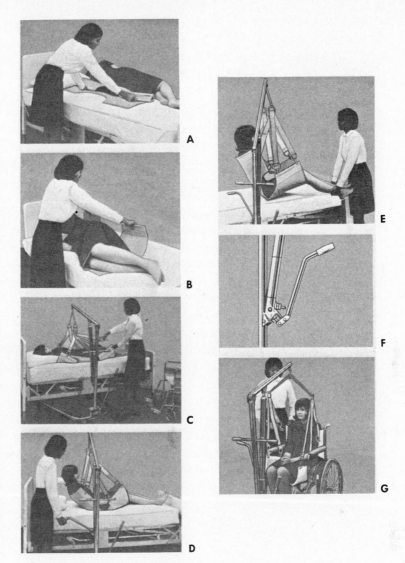

individuals who drive a lot, drive while drinking, do not wear seat belts, or ride motorcycles or bicycles without helmets; also at risk are those who have occupations that require heavy lifting or increased liability for injury and people who engage in contact sports or who participate in sports without being properly conditioned, as well as the elderly who, because of problems of balance or decreased hearing or sight, are prone to falls.

The nurse has a significant role in instructing clients about risk reduction. Information includes the use of seat belts, helmets, and other safety devices, and the avoidance of driving if drinking. Persons who are in high-risk occupations should use good body mechanics and protect themselves from the risk of injury. Persons who engage in contact sports should have a warm-up period before the activity and wear protective padding if possible. Safety in the home is especially important to older persons who are likely to trip or fall. Rugs should be secure and stairways lit and clear of debris.

Nursing process for common health problems

PLANNING FOR HEALTH MAINTENANCE AND RESTORATION

Clients with health problems of the musculoskeletal system may require immobilization of an extremity or the entire body to reduce pain and muscle spasm and facilitate healing. Casts, traction, cast-braces, and external fixation devices may be used to assure immobility. During this time the nursing care plan is developed with the client and his family to plan for immobilization during healing and for rehabilitation and return to the usual state of mobility. The nurse may plan with the physician, physical therapist, occupational therapist, or dietitian to meet these goals.

Casts

Casts are used to maintain external fixation, immobilize the bone, and permit active weight bearing. Casts applied to maintain fixation or shape of a body part are usually applied without surgical intervention, whereas those applied to immobilize the bone, after a compound fracture, for example, may be applied after surgery for internal reduction of the fracture. Casts are usually applied to include the joints distal and proximal to the involved part.

A cast can be described by the part that it contains (Fig. 11-3). A *cylinder* cast is used on a limb. A cylinder cast for the leg may have a heel plate put on so that the client can walk with the cast. A *spica* cast is used to immobilize the hips, shoulders, or thumb. The hip or shoulder spica cast covers part or all of the trunk and one or more of the extremities, whereas the thumb spica cast encloses the distal arm, wrist, and thumb. A *body cast* is used to immobilize the spine.

Nursing care of client in cast. Nursing care for the client in a cast is planned with the client and family and includes instructing the client about the application of the cast, care of the cast, and cast removal. Immobility depends on the type of cast and the reason for its use. The nurse and client plan for increasing independence as cast use and healing permit.

Cast application. Before the cast is applied, the nurse should explain the procedure to the client. The client may be in pain and upset if he has had a recent injury, and explanations may ease his fears. The nurse should be careful when moving the affected part in order not to cause additional pain. A child may be especially fearful of having a body part casted, and explanations should be pro-

FIG. 11-3
Types of casts: **A**, cylinder; **B**, hip spica; **C**, body cast.

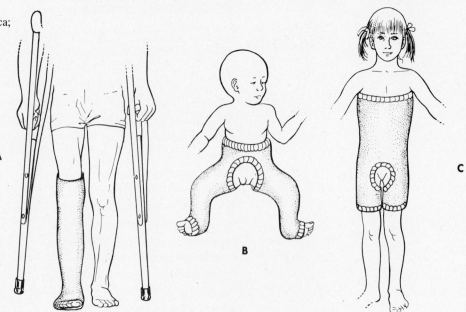

vided at his level of understanding. Often it is helpful to have a doll on which a small cast can be applied to demonstrate what is to occur. Older children may alleviate anxieties by applying the cast to the doll themselves.

Most casts are made of plaster, which comes in dry rolls. When these rolls are added to water, they form plaster of paris, which is molded to the limb or body to maintain the correct position. Before the plaster is put on, the limb is covered with stockinet, and the bony prominences are padded with sheet wadding, felt, or sponge rubber. The wet plaster rolls are then molded to the body, which is supported in proper alignment. Heat is generated when the chemical reaction occurs between the rolled plaster and water. Ice bags can be used on the client's head to keep him cool, but ice cannot be applied directly to the wet cast. When the cast is applied, the physician usually pulls the stockinet over the edge of the cast and secures it with a strip of tape or wet plaster so that the edges will not be rough against the skin. When casting is completed, the nurse can wipe off excess wet plaster from the skin before it dries and becomes difficult to remove.

Other casting materials, such as plastic, that are lighter weight and waterproof may be used. These plastic casts are one-third to one-fourth the weight of plaster and permit greater mobility and comfort.

The cast should be supported in a physiological position while drying. If the client is going home, the cast is supported in a sling or on pillows. The client who returns to the hospital room is put in a bed that has a firm board under the mattress and plastic-covered pillows. He should be positioned to support the cast, and extra pillows can be used in body bends to prevent cracking. Pillows should not be used under the head of a client in a body cast, to avoid pressure from the chest while the cast dries.

Cast care. The client should be turned every 2 to 4 hours to permit even drying of the cast. When individuals in a body or hip spica cast are turned for the first time, it is necessary to have three people turn them (Fig. 11-4). The palms of the hands should be used to lift the wet cast so that indentations are not made with the fingers. The three persons stand at the side of the *involved leg* and gently move the client to the side of the bed. Two people then go to the opposite side and arrange dry pillows to receive the client as he is turned on his *uninvolved leg*. The pillow from under the client's head is removed, and one person supports the shoulder and hip and the other the thigh and foot as the client is turned toward them.

When the client has been turned, the nurse should observe that he is in good alignment. The toes should be supported off the bed when he is on his stomach, and a foot rest may be used when he is on his back. When the cast is dry, the client can be more helpful in turning, and the procedure may be done with fewer helpers.

The plaster cast may take from 12 to 48 hours to dry, depending on its size. Cylinder casts may dry in 12 to 24 hours, but body casts usually take up to 48 hours to dry. Plastic casts usually dry in 8 to 10 hours. Air drying is the most efficient way for drying, and the air should be low in humidity to hasten evaporation of moisture from the cast. Some physicians may order a heat lamp or a heated fan dryer to facilitate drying. If these devices are used, the nurse should observe the client for burns or too rapid drying of the cast. The cast is dry when the plaster is white, shiny, hard, and resonant. Weight bearing should not be permitted until the cast has dried.

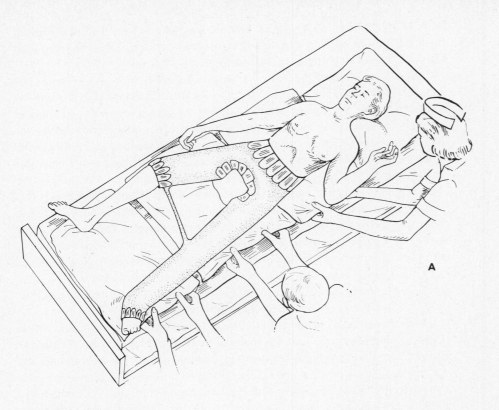

FIG. 11-4
Turning client in new cast. **A,** Three persons lift involved side of client. **B,** Two persons walk to the other side of bed to receive client as he turns on his uninvolved leg. **C,** Client is positioned in proper body alignment.

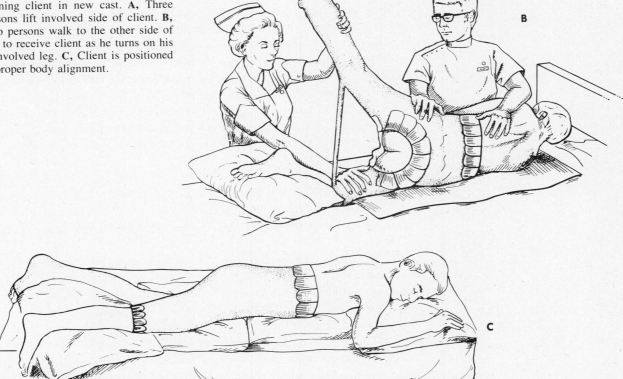

While the cast is drying and regularly thereafter, the nurse must evaluate the effect of the cast on the client. Swelling of the affected part or of the tissue distal to the cast may cause circulatory impairment or pressure on nerves. Unless these symptoms are detected immediately, permanent damage can result.

Circulatory status is evaluated by making sure that there is adequate circulation to points distal to the cast. The fingers or toes are pressed to see if they blanch, followed by capillary filling. Digits with adequate circulation are warm and have a healthy color when compared with the uninvolved digits. The cast should not be so tight that the nurse cannot insert one or two fingers between the body and the cast.

The nurse can assess pressure on nerves by asking the client to wiggle his digits, separate them, and flex them in a dorsal and plantar direction. Any numbness or tingling is indicative of abnormal pressure on the nerves.

Positioning the involved part on pillows or elevating the foot of the bed may prevent some edema. Slings may also be used to maintain the involved part in elevation.

Swelling that cannot be relieved by positioning should be reported to the physician. If the limb is casted, it may be necessary to bivalve the cast, that is, cut it from top to bottom and separate the plaster or plastic to increase the width of the cast. If the cast covers a large area, a "window" may be cut in the cast to relieve pressure. When swelling has subsided, the window is reinserted and secured.

If the cast has been applied after a surgical procedure, the nurse must assess the client for bleeding. The vital signs can be obtained frequently to detect incipient blood loss and shock. There may be some bleeding evident on the cast, and that area should be circled to detect further bleeding. Restlessness may be a sign of impending shock.

The client with a fracture may have pain for several days after surgery. Pain medication can be given as needed, and the client should be positioned to relieve any discomfort. Unusual pain that could be attributed to a tight cast should be reported to the physician.

FIG. 11-5
Petaling cast. **A,** Petals cut from tape with round or pointed edges. **B,** Petals placed inside of cast and secured to outside of cast. Overlapping petals ensure smooth edge to cast.

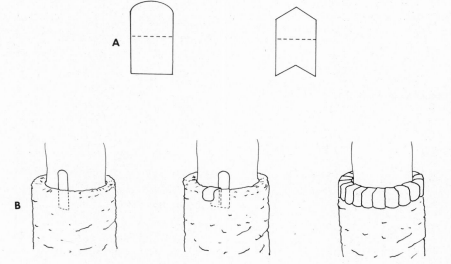

Nursing process for common health problems

Infection can occur under the cast, particularly if there have been lacerations, incisions, or pressure areas, which contribute to entry of microorganisms. The nurse should instruct the client to report any feelings of pressure, and the skin under the cast should be inspected with the eyes as far as possible. A flashlight may facilitate inspection. Odors that are indicative of infection may be perceived by smelling the cast. Elevated temperature is another cue of an infectious process. The nurse should be aware that children are not always reliable in reporting changes and should, therefore, make frequent assessments.

If there are sharp edges after the plaster has completely dried, the nurse may wish to make adhesive petals to protect the skin from flaking plaster and rough edges. The rough edges are trimmed, and excess plaster is removed. Strips of adhesive are cut in the shape of petals, either rounded or pointed (Fig. 11-5) to prevent curling after application. The petals are then placed from inside to outside of the cast in an overlapping fashion. A plaster-of-paris strip can be moistened and secured over the outside of the petals for additional support.

The cast should be maintained clean and dry. To this end the cast may be wiped with a damp cloth and powdered cleanser. The use of water and sponging should be avoided so that the plaster is not softened. When the cast has dried, shellac may be applied to keep it protected and clean.

If the client is in a body cast, it is necessary to keep the perineal area of the cast dry. This area may be lined with plastic wrap. No protective covering, however, should be put on until the cast is dried, to avoid mildew. Clients may find it easier to use a small bedpan and have the head of the bed slightly elevated so that urine does not run down the cast. Plastic-wrap linings can be applied to make a funnel to place in the bedpan if the client cannot use the bedpan easily. The nurse should anticipate when the client needs to void so that the wrap can be placed easily. A Bradford frame may be used to position incontinent children off the bed so that toileting can be accomplished without wetting the cast. Similar devices can be improvised for home use.

The skin under the cast often becomes dry and itches. When the nurse bathes the client, it is important to wash under the cast and massage the skin with rubbing alcohol, because 70% isopropyl alcohol (rubbing alcohol) strengthens the skin and prevents skin breakdown. Cotton swabs may be dipped in the alcohol and rubbed under the cast. The cotton swabs may also be used to clean between the toes. Some physicians may insert a strip of gauze under the cast. This gauze scratcher may be used to gently massage the skin. It may be changed by tying a clean strip of gauze to one end and bringing it through the other end. A vacuum or Asepto syringe may be used to blow air through the cast to provide relief from itching. However, sharp objects such as knitting needles, which could injure the skin, are not suitable scratchers. Children must be prevented from putting crumbs, food, toys, or paper down the cast.

The nurse must continuously evaluate the client with a cast to assure that objectives of the plan are met (see evaluation guide at left). Client expected outcomes include preservation of immobility of the casted part and prevention of complications.

Cast removal. The cast is removed when healing has occurred. The nurse should tell the client how the cast will be removed so that he is not frightened when the cast cutters are used. An electric cast saw is usually used to remove a cast. This saw vibrates against the plaster to separate it, but will not vibrate when in contact with the skin. The cast cutter is noisy, and the size of the equipment may overwhelm small children. It may be helpful to demonstrate the procedure on a doll to assure the client of its safety. Usually a long cylinder cast will be cut on two sides to bivalve the cast for easy removal. Nurses should know how to use the cast removal equipment in order to remove casts in emergency situations such as cardiac or respiratory arrest.

The skin beneath the cast is frequently dry with flakes of dead skin when the cast is removed. The nurse can wash the area with mild soap, taking care not to irritate the tender skin. Several washings are more effective than one vigorous bath. Lanolin can be used to soften the skin.

Muscles may be weak without the support from the cast, and initially the client may have aches and pains. Some physicians may bivalve the cast several days before cast removal so that the client can begin active and passive range-of-motion exercises. There may be some swelling as circulation is reestablished; elastic bandages may be used to minimize swelling. The limb can be elevated when the client rests to encourage adequate venous return.

Weight bearing is permitted gradually, and assistive walking devices such as crutches, canes, and walkers may be used to support weight bearing. The client who has had his arm in a cast should be advised not to lift heavy objects until muscle strength is restored.

After the cast is removed, the nurse can help the client learn about care of the involved part, muscle strengthening exericses, and weight bearing. Written instructions may particularly help the client or family who is immediately discharged after cast removal.

Cast-brace

The cast-brace (Fig. 11-6) is designed to allow increased mobility and early ambulation and weight bearing, particularly with femoral shaft fractures. The

FIG. 11-6
A, The three components of cast-brace. **B,** Comparative lengths of lever arms distal to fracture site with long-leg cast and with cast-brace. (From Larson, Carroll B., and Gould, Marjorie: Orthopedic nursing, ed. 9, St. Louis, 1978, The C.V. Mosby Co.)

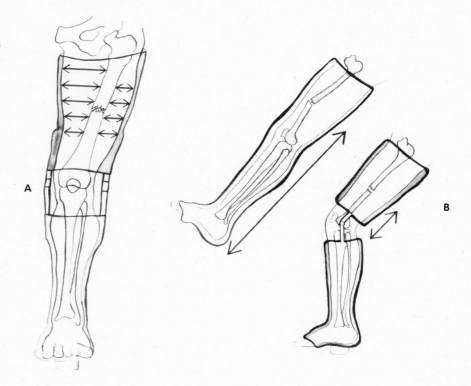

exercise increases circulation and blood supply to the bone and thereby hastens bone healing. The cast-brace, which has a thigh cuff, hinges at the knee, and a short leg walking cast, can be used in 2 to 6 weeks after immobilization in skeletal traction and replaces the hip spica cast, which limits mobility.[3]

External fixation devices   Complicated fractures of the arms, legs, or pelvis may be immobilized with an external fixation device used to maintain reduction of the fracture.[4] Pins or wires are passed through the involved bones and attached to the metal frame of the fixation device for stabilization. The use of this device facilitates mobility and ambulation and, therefore, is advantageous in preventing hazards of immobility and delayed healing.

Immediately after surgery the involved limb is elevated to reduce edema. Active range-of-motion exercise begins in 2 days to 2 to 3 weeks as healing begins. Ultimately weight bearing is permitted.

The nurse must observe the insertion sites of the pins or wires and report any indications of infection, such as drainage or odor. The insertion site should be cleansed daily with hydrogen peroxide and rinsed with sterile normal saline. Antibacterial ointment can then be applied to the site.

Traction   Traction is another way in which a fracture can be maintained in reduction and immobilized for healing. Traction is a pulling force exerted on bones when an overriding of a broken bone or muscle spasm interferes with the alignment of the fracture. Traction can also be used to maintain correct body alignment and to prevent deformities.

Traction may be achieved by a manual pull or by application of weights to the skin or skeleton. *Manual traction,* applied by the hands of a rescuer, is exerted by an even pull to separate bone ends. This is usually a temporary traction until other forms can be applied. *Skin traction* is produced by exerting a pulling force on the bone by weights that are attached to the skin by means of harnesses, adhesive strips, moleskin, or chin straps. Since the traction is applied to the skin, great care must be used to prevent excoriation. Skin traction that is not applied with adhesive may generally be removed to inspect the underlying skin. The nurse should validate with the physician, however, if there is any doubt. *Skeletal traction* is applied directly to the bone with wires or pins that are inserted during surgery. The wires or pins exit through the skin, and ropes with weights or bows or tongs with weights are added to create traction. The exit site provides a port of entry for microbes, and the nurse must inspect the site frequently for drainage, erythema, odor, or swelling, which might indicate infection. Some surgeons may order antibiotic ointments to prevent infection. These are applied daily as the dressing is changed. Others prefer that the sites not be disturbed because exposure increases opportunity for contamination. The nurse should observe that the exposed wires or pins are intact. Unequal lengths or bent pins can distort the traction and should be reported to the surgeon. Corks or tape can be used to cover the pins to prevent injury.

Traction may be continuous or intermittent. *Continuous traction* is usually used to stabilize a fracture and is not removed until the fracture has healed. The client is relatively immobile and confined to the bed. *Intermittent traction* is used to relieve muscle spasms or to correct or prevent deformities. The traction may be used for certain periods during the day and may be removed for eating and bathing.

Traction is further described by the line of its pull. *Running traction* is pulled in one direction against the long axis of the body or bone. The body acts as the countertraction. With this type of traction, the body must be aligned with the pulling force to be effective. *Balanced traction* is a combination of running traction plus a countertraction source other than the body. Usually a hammock or ring splint and a series of weights are used to achieve balanced traction. The client is permitted to raise himself up and turn slightly without disturbing the line of the traction.

Nursing care of client in traction. The nursing care plan for the client in traction is developed with the client and family. Before application of the traction, the nurse can explain the purpose of the traction and demonstrate the use of the equipment. As the traction devices are applied, the nurse can instruct the client about limits of activity and what actions the client can take to prevent hazards of immobility.

Cervical skin traction. Cervical skin traction can be used to alleviate painful muscle spasms of the neck, to create alignment, or to prevent deformities. The traction is applied with a cervical head halter, which may be used with weights suspended over the head of the bed when the client is lying on his back. The head of the bed may be elevated to provide countertraction. Cervical skin traction can also be applied by suspending the weights over the door with the client sitting in a chair. This type of traction is usually intermittent, and the client can remove it for daily activities.

The nurse should observe the client when he is in cervical skin traction to be sure that the halter is not putting pressure on the ears or chin. The ropes should not be frayed, and the weights should be suspended safely, out of the way of the client.

Pelvic skin traction. Pelvic skin traction is a running traction that is used to reduce muscle spasms of the lower back, relieve sciatica, immobilize a frac-

FIG. 11-7
Pelvic traction. Pelvic girdle is attached to spreader bar, and weights are added to create traction. Iliac crests are protected with padding, and foot of bed is raised for counter-traction.

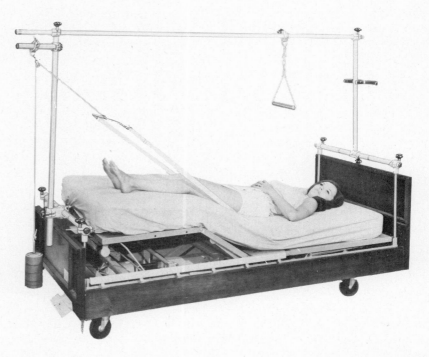

Nursing process for common health problems

tured pelvis, or correct lateral deviations of the spine. The traction may be continuous or intermittent, depending on the reason for its use. A pelvic girdle with extension straps is worn by the client.

In one method, ropes are tied to the extension straps and run through a pulley, and weights are applied for traction. The weights, 5 to 10 pounds (2.2 to 4.5 kg) for each leg, are suspended over the foot of the bed and should be attached to the extension straps simultaneously. The weights may also be applied by using a spreader bar to attach the extension straps (Fig. 11-7). In this case only one source of weights is needed. Because the client must lie on his back, it may be necessary to use foot supports to prevent foot drop.

The pelvic girdle is applied over the client's garments and exerts pressure on the iliac crest. These pressure areas should be padded to prevent skin breakdown. The client is positioned in semi-Fowler's position, with the knee of the bed gatched. Because the client is immobilized on his back, he should be encouraged to take several deep breaths every hour to prevent atelectasis.

Buck's traction. Buck's traction is a running skin traction that can be used temporarily to immobilize a fracture of the hip or femur until it is possible to do surgery. Buck's traction can also be used to relieve muscle spasms in the lower back, to prevent contractures after amputation, or to realign the vertebrae in a client with scoliosis. This traction can be continuous or intermittent.

The traction may be applied in several ways, all of which accomplish the same purpose. In one method a strip of moleskin or sponge rubber is placed on each side of one or both legs, with a loop left at the foot for the spreader bar. The strip is secured to the leg with elastic bandages, and the spreader bar is inserted in the loop and then attached to a rope that is run through a pulley, with prescribed weights (6 to 10 pounds, or 2.7 to 4.5 kg) added to create traction (Fig. 11-8).

FIG. 11-8
Buck's traction secured with elastic bandages. Notice alignment and use of foot support.

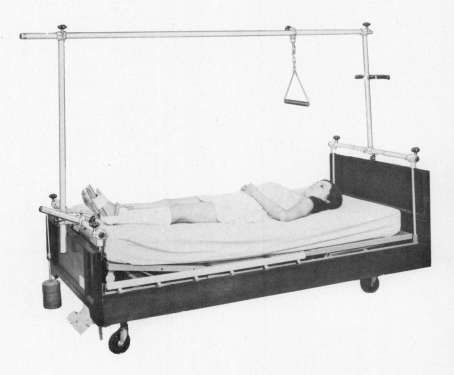

Another method is to use a polyurethane traction splint (Fig. 11-9), which is held in place with self-adhering tab fasteners. The weights are attached to the traction bar. The physician may leave an order for the foot of the bed to be elevated for countertraction.

Buck's traction should be used carefully with persons who have interference with the delivery of oxygen to the cells, such as in arteriosclerosis, varicose veins, or diabetes. The nurse should assess the skin for areas of irritation and observe that the spreader bar is not in contact with the sole of the foot. The heel should not rest on the mattress. The elastic bandages should be evaluated periodically to be sure that the traction is secure. Some physicians may request that the bandages be removed several times a day so that the skin can be inspected and the bandages rewrapped evenly.

The nurse should evaluate the client's position in bed. The client should be in the middle of the bed in a straight line with the traction. A foot plate or sandbag can be used to prevent foot drop. The uninvolved leg can be exercised frequently to prevent circulatory stasis. Since the client is lying on his back, he should have back rubs at least every 4 hours and the linens should be tight, to prevent skin irritation. A sheepskin pad or alternating–air pressure mattress can be used for clients who will have continuous Buck's traction for prolonged periods of time.

Bryant's traction. Bryant's traction is used to immobilize a fracture of the femur in children who weigh less than 40 pounds (18.2 kg). This skin traction is a simple running traction in which the legs are raised at a 90-degree angle to the body (Fig. 11-10). This position must be used because the weight of the child is insufficient to maintain countertraction. Both legs are held in traction for comfort and balance even though only one leg is affected. When the child is put in Bryant's traction, the legs are wrapped with padding at the heels that is secured with elastic bandages. The peroneal nerve should be checked frequently for signs indicative of undue pressure. A foot plate may be added to prevent foot drop. The weights should be suspended at the foot of the bed so that they do not hang over the child. When the traction is properly applied, the buttocks are suspended slightly off the mattress.

Nursing care for the child in Bryant's traction is directed at preventing com-

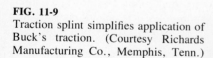

FIG. 11-9
Traction splint simplifies application of Buck's traction. (Courtesy Richards Manufacturing Co., Memphis, Tenn.)

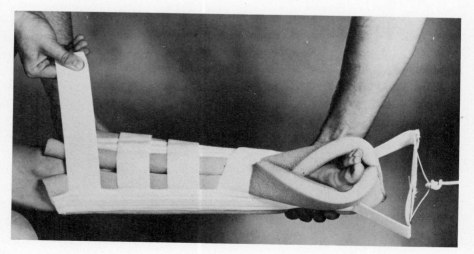

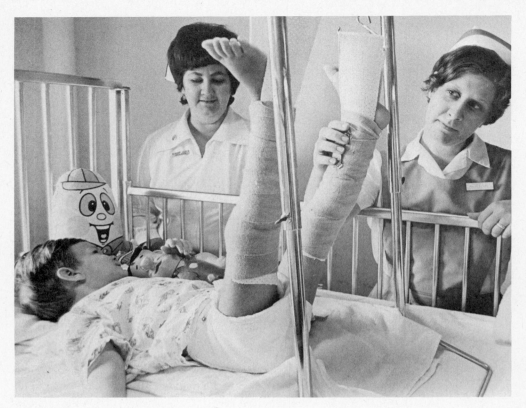

FIG. 11-10
Bryant's traction. Hips are slightly elevated to maintain traction, and weights are suspended safely at front of bed. Nursing student and her instructor provide sensorimotor experiences for this immobilized client. (Courtesy St. Francis Hospital Center, Beech Grove, Ind.)

plications of immobilization. The child is encouraged to cough and take deep breaths often. Blowing cotton balls or balloons can be made into a game to encourage the child to take deep breaths. Safety should be assured, and it may be necessary to restrain the very young child so that he will maintain the proper position.

The child may be in traction for 3 to 4 weeks until bone healing is accomplished. The parents should be encouraged to visit the child and participate in his care. Absence from the family for this period of time may be frightening to the child, and if possible, the parents can stay in the room with the child. The parents should convey affection to the child by their interest and attention. The child can participate in quiet playing if the bed is moved to the playroom. Activities that can be done in bed, such as being read to, listening to music, and playing with soft toys should be offered to provide sensory and social stimulation.

Russell's traction. Russell's traction is a balanced skin traction that is usually used to immobilize a fracture of the femur or hip. There is a continuous pull from the knee to an overhead pulley, with weights attached at the foot of the bed (Fig. 11-11, *A*). The foot of the bed may be elevated for countertraction. The client in Russell's traction may also have a cast to ensure immobilization, and a hammock sling or Thomas splint with a Pearson attachment (Fig. 11-11, *B*) may support the calf. The hip of the immobilized leg should be flexed at a 20-degree angle and may be supported with a pillow underneath the thigh. A foot plate is usually added to prevent foot drop, and the heel should be suspended off the mattress so that there is no source of irritation.

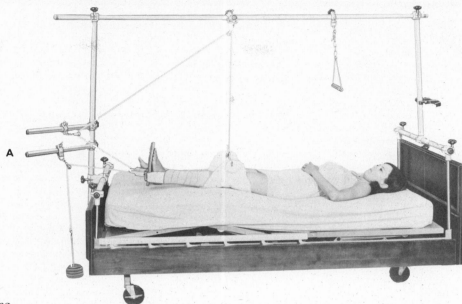

FIG. 11-11
A, Russell's traction. Hammock sling supports calf. Involved leg is positioned at a 20-degree angle, and foot support is used to prevent foot drop. **B,** Balanced traction using Thomas leg splint with Pearson attachment.

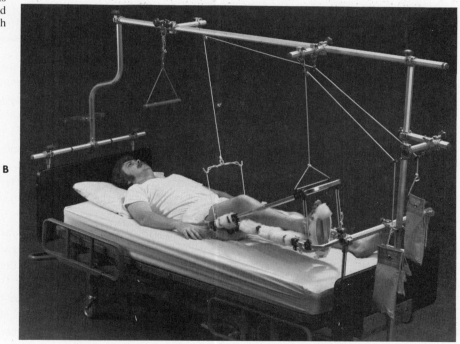

The client who is in balanced traction is permitted some movement and can assist with nursing care by lifting himself with an overhead trapeze when he uses the bedpan or when bed linens are changed.

It is important to assess the pressure points in clients who are in balanced traction. The circulation at the popliteal area should be verified, because the hammock can cause circulatory constriction there. The groin area should be inspected if a Thomas ring is being used.

EVALUATION GUIDE FOR CLIENTS IN TRACTION

1. General evaluations
   a. Are the ropes aligned? Not frayed? Free of knots or kinks?
   b. Are the weights hanging free? By the prescribed amount? Out of danger to the client?
   c. Is the bed in proper position? Should the head or foot be elevated?
   d. Is the groove of the pulley free moving and supporting the rope? Has it been lubricated with mineral oil?
   e. Is the line of the traction with the long axis of the bone?
   f. Is circulation impaired? Is there undue pressure on bony prominences or the peroneal nerve?
   g. Has there been a physician's order to change or remove the weights?
   h. Have the exit sites on skeletal traction been inspected for odor? Erythema? Drainage?
   i. Has the skin been inspected for pressure? Redness? Breakdown?
2. Cervical skin traction
   a. Is the chin strap causing undue pressure on the ears or under the chin?
   b. Are the weights suspended out of the way of the client?
3. Pelvic traction
   a. Are the weights applied to both legs at the same time?
   b. Is the client positioned in the center of the bed?
   c. Is the client taking deep breaths hourly?
   d. Are foot supports needed to prevent foot drop?
4. Bryant's traction
   a. Are the weights suspended at the foot of the bed?
   b. Are the client's buttocks slightly elevated off the bed?
   c. Is the environment safe? Free of unsafe toys? Should the child be restrained?
   d. Is the traction causing skin breakdown or restricting circulation? Is there pressure on the peroneal nerve?
5. Buck's traction
   a. Is the traction applied smoothly and securely?
   b. Has the skin been inspected for evidences of breakdown?
   c. Has the circulation in the foot been assessed by taking pedal pulses?
   d. Is the client in alignment with the traction?
   e. Is a foot plate or sandbag needed to prevent foot drop?
6. Russell's traction
   a. Is hip flexion 20 degrees?
   b. Is a foot plate being used to prevent foot drop?
   c. Has the skin under the popliteal and groin area been inspected for irritation?
   d. Have the femoral and popliteal pulses been assessed?

The uninvolved leg should be put through active and passive range-of-motion exercises several times a day. The client may tend to use this leg to push himself up in bed, and the nurse should inspect the heel for breakdown. When the client is resting, the uninvolved leg should be in proper alignment. A sandbag or trochanter roll can be used for support.

Cervical traction with tongs. Cervical traction with tongs (Crutchfield or Venke) is an example of skeletal traction that may be used for a fracture of the spine, a herniated disk, or muscle strain. The client is positioned on his back, and weights are attached to pins that have been inserted into the skull and suspended at the head of the bed (see Fig. 10-39).

Braces. Traction may also be maintained by braces that separate bone ends to reduce muscle spasms. A neck collar hyperextension brace for muscle spasms of the neck and the Milwaukee brace (see Fig. 11-23) for vertebrae alignment are examples of braces used for traction.

The nurse must continuously evaluate the client in traction (see evaluation guide above). Evaluation is specific for objectives of the nursing care plan. Expected outcomes of care include maintenance of traction and prevention of hazards of immobility.

Splints   Splints may be used to immobilize body parts, correct deformities, or protect joint or muscles from injury. The splint is made specifically for the client and must be observed frequently as the client grows or the deformity is corrected. Splints are discussed in detail where appropriate in the text.

Assisted locomotion   Assistance with locomotion may be needed for clients who have difficulty maintaining balance—those not permitted active weight bearing or who have an amputation of a leg, muscular weakness, or paralysis. Assistance in being mobile can be obtained from canes, walkers, crutches, or wheelchairs. The physician specifies the type of assistance that may be used, and the nurse or physical therapist helps the client learn how to use it.

Before beginning assisted locomotion, the client should do exercises that strengthen weight-bearing muscles of uninvolved limbs. Active and passive range-of-motion exercises can be done initially to maintain muscle strength. Later, other exercises are performed to develop muscles that will be used for ambulation. Push-ups and pull-ups with the overhead trapeze help develop triceps and biceps. The quadriceps can be strengthened with straight leg raises and quadriceps-setting exercises. These exercises should be done for 5 minutes every hour.

Immediately before walking with assistance, the client should dangle his legs and then stand at the bedside in supportive shoes to achieve a sense of balance. The client in a cast or with an amputation must adjust to a new balance of his weight. The client who has been in bed for several days must adjust to being in an upright position and must overcome orthostatic hypotension. In some instances adjustment to a vertical position can be achieved by the use of a tilt table, whereby the client is raised to a standing position slowly while being supported on the table. When standing, he should maintain correct posture. He may have a tendency to round his shoulders and look down to watch his steps. This can disrupt the balanced posture, and he should be encouraged to look straight ahead. A long mirror in front of him may be helpful to focus the eyes forward and permit him to observe himself as he walks.

FIG. 11-12
Using a walker to go up steps.

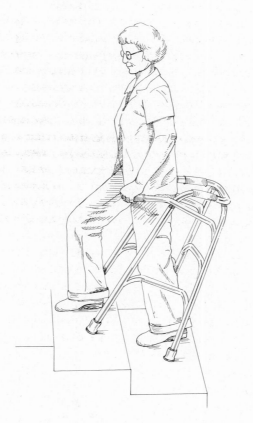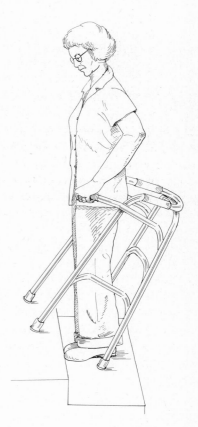

Nursing process for common health problems

As the client begins assisted locomotion, the nurse or physical therapist should stand nearby and steady him if necessary. Small, slow steps should be taken until he has mastered the new gaits.

Canes. Canes are used to provide a wide base of support and additional balance. When one cane is used for balance, it should be held in the hand opposite the involved leg. The cane should be measured from the floor to the client's waist, and the tip covered with a rubber cap to prevent slipping on the floor.

Walkers. Walkers are used primarily to provide balance for clients who can bear weight, although they may be used when only partial or limited weight bearing is permitted with the involved leg. The walker should be adjusted to the client's waist level and held in front of him with his hands on the sides of it. The client lifts the walker a few inches forward, places it firmly, and moves his body slowly toward it. Walkers can also be used to provide balance while ascending or descending steps. A special stair-climbing model with extended handles can be used. To negotiate up stairs, the client should hold the walker behind him (Fig. 11-12). Walkers are useful supports when showering, weighing, or when standing in other instances.

Crutches. Crutches are used to provide balance when there is partial or limited weight bearing. Crutches may be made of wood or aluminum and are measured to fit the individual client. There are several ways to measure crutches for a client. Most commonly the crutches are measured while the client is in the supine position with arms to the side, wearing his walking shoes. The measurement is taken from 2 inches (5 cm) below the axilla to 6 inches (13.2 cm) out from the heel. The armrest should be adjusted so that the arm is flexed at a 30-degree angle when holding the crutch.

If the client is able to stand, the crutches can be measured with the client standing next to a wall with his feet slightly apart and slightly away from the wall. A mark is placed on the floor 2 inches from the outside shoe at the toe and a second mark 6 inches from this. Another measurement is taken 2 inches below the axilla to the second mark on the floor. This measurement determines the length of the crutches.

FIG. 11-13
Three-point gait. (From Dison, Norma Greenler: Clinical nursing techniques, ed. 4, St. Louis, 1979, The C.V. Mosby Co.)

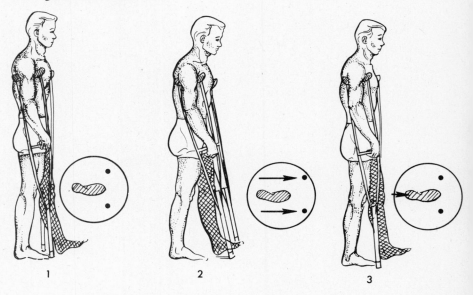

1   2   3

Crutchwalking gaits. After the client has stood with the crutches and maintained his balance, he is ready to walk with crutches. In the starting position the crutches are held 4 inches (10 cm) to the side of each foot and 4 inches (10 cm) in front of the toes. The weight is carried on the hands, and the armpits should not touch the armrest. Nerve damage can occur if the client persistently rests his arms on the top of the crutch.

Three-point gait. A three-point gait is used when there is to be little or no weight bearing on the affected extremity. Both crutches and the involved leg are advanced, followed by the uninvolved leg, which is brought to the crutches (Fig. 11-13). The client should take small steps and keep his head up to maintain proper balance.

Four-point gait. The four-point gait is used when there is partial weight bearing on each limb and additional support is needed for balance. One crutch is advanced and followed by the opposite leg; then the second crutch is advanced

FIG. 11-14
Four-point gait. (From Dison, Norma Greenler: Clinical nursing techniques, ed. 4, St. Louis, 1979, The C.V. Mosby Co.)

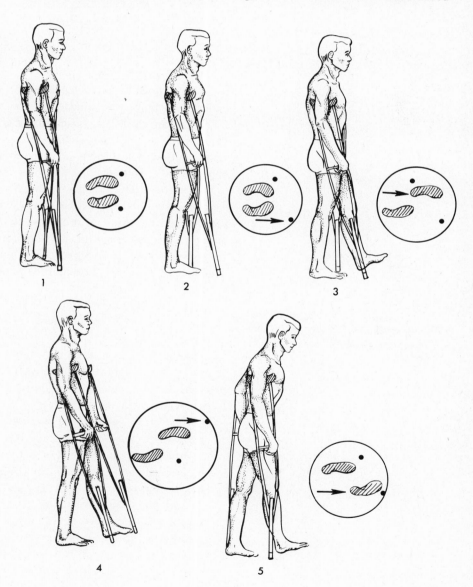

FIG. 11-15
Going up stairs, **A,** and down stairs, **B,** with crutches.

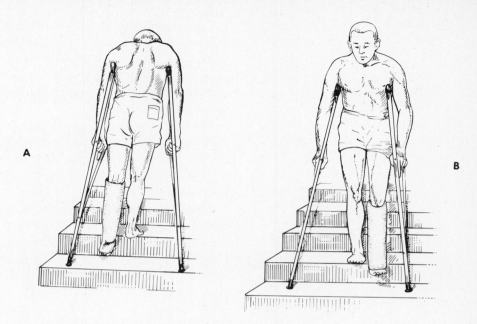

FIG. 11-15
Going up stairs, **A,** and down stairs, **B,** with crutches.

and followed by the second leg (Fig. 11-14). It is helpful to keep the steps small until the rhythm is established.

Two-point gait. The two-point gait is a faster version of the four-point gait. It is used after proficiency with the four-point gait has been established. The crutch and opposite leg are advanced together, and then the second crutch and opposite leg are advanced.

Swing-through gait. The swing-through gait is used when there may be weight bearing on both feet but there is need for support. Both crutches are advanced, and the legs are swung out past the crutches. The crutches are then brought to the legs, and the gait is repeated.

Swing-to gait. A swing-to gait is similar to the swing-through gait except that the legs are only brought to the crutches. This gait is useful in persons whose balance is not steady.

Going up and down stairs with crutches. To go *up* stairs, the client places the uninvolved leg on the step above and follows with the crutches and then the involved leg (Fig. 11-15, *A*). To go *down* stairs the process is reversed, so that weight bearing is balanced on the uninvolved leg. The crutches and involved leg are advanced and followed by the uninvolved leg (Fig. 11-15, *B*). Children may be more secure in going up and down steps by sitting on the step and scooting from one step to the next.

Transferring from sitting to standing with crutches. When transferring from a sitting to a standing position, the client should hold both crutches in one hand while pushing off the bed or chair to a standing position. To sit down, the client places the crutches in one hand, while the other hand balances on the bed or chair to receive body weight (Fig. 11-16).

Wheelchairs. Wheelchairs may be used by clients who are unable to use other measures of locomotion. The use of a wheelchair can give independence to one who might otherwise be confined to a bed or chair. Motor-driven wheelchairs may be obtained, as well as collapsible chairs that can be transferred to a car. The wheelchair should be selected for the size and needs of the client. Many

FIG. 11-16
Transferring from sitting to standing with crutches.

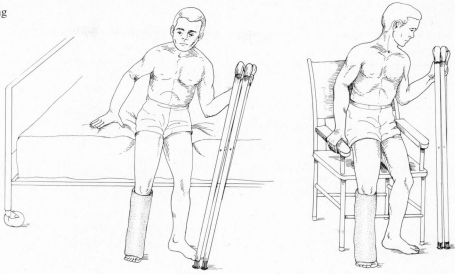

public places have ramps, lavatories, water fountains, and telephone booths that are designed to be used by persons who must depend on a wheelchair for locomotion. When assisting an individual in a wheelchair to go down a curb or ramp, the nurse should reverse the wheelchair and be in position to control the chair down the curb by standing between the chair and the curb.

Evaluation. The nurse should evaluate the client as he uses assisted locomotion and should help him incorporate these skills in activities of daily living. The nurse can help the client anticipate the use of assisted locomotion in his home or at his place of employment. It is helpful to anticipate obstacles to locomotion so that the client can adjust to his new mobility. The community health nurse or occupational health nurse should be aware of the client's need, and nursing care plans that reflect continuity of care should be developed.

The immobilized client

Immobility imposed by therapeutic interventions (such as casts, traction, or braces) or by other instances of bedfastness alters total biopsychosocial responses. The limits placed on activity interfere with physiological and psychological needs and with normal development. The nurse should use the nursing process to identify actual or potential problems and plan to prevent the hazardous consequences of immobility that can occur throughout the life span (Table 11-1).

Hazards of immobility

Sensory alterations. Persons who are immobilized are likely to have pressure on nerves because of the required maintenance of unfavorable positions. The client must therefore turn or be repositioned frequently. *Foot drop* is a particularly hazardous outcome of immobility. Foot drop is caused from peroneal nerve damage and also from shortening of the Achilles tendon. If possible the client should exercise against a foot board and change positions frequently. Bed rest further restricts sensory input and proprioception; monotony and boredom give rise to states of *sensory deprivation.* For more information see Chapter 8. It is imperative for the nurse and client to plan opportunities for social contact, orientation as to time and place, and varieties of sensory stimulation.

Skin integrity impairment. Clients restricted to bed are often unaware that

537

TABLE 11-1

Nursing process for immobilized clients

Nursing diagnosis (actual or potential)	Assessment	Planning and implementation	Evaluation: client outcomes
Sensory alterations			
Nerve impingement	Touch, numbness, and tingling; separate and extend digits, plantarflex and dorsiflex hands and feet; pin prick for sensation; foot drop	Turn; prevent pressure from casts, traction, and position; use footboard and footplate.	Able to freely move all extremities; sense of touch intact
Sensory deprivation	Boredom, monotony, restlessness, apathy, disorientation, and depression	Touch; offer visual and auditory stimulation; encourage visitors; change environment if possible; use orientation strategies such as clocks, television, newspaper, and calendar; encourage diversion, crafts, use of glasses, hearing aid.	Oriented, relaxed
Skin integrity impairment			
Skin breakdown (decubitus ulcer)	Inspection of bony prominences, pressure areas, redness, and open skin areas	Turn; avoid pressure; protect bony prominences with foam or sheepskin; use alternating air pressure mattress, flotation pad, or sheepskin; cleanse skin; lubricate or strengthen with skin preparations as needed; encourage fluid intake.	Skin intact; no redness or evidence of pressure
Impaired mobility			
Ankylosis	Limitation of range of motion	Turn; do range-of-motion exercises; encourage self-care activities.	Full range of motion
Decreased muscle mass	Weakness	Do range-of-motion exercises	Usual muscle mass
Decreased muscle strength	Weakness	Do muscle-setting and active-resistive exercises.	Usual muscle strength
Contractures of muscles	Limitation of range of motion	Position to prevent contractures; do range-of-motion exercises.	No contractures, usual range of motion
Osteoporosis	Demineralization of bone (calcium loss); pain on weight bearing; pathological fractures	Provide stress on bone; tilt table; do active-resistive exercises; use parallel bars; position carefully to avoid sudden stress on bones.	Calcium levels normal; no fractures, no osteoporosis on x-ray studies
Alterations in patterns of sexuality			
Role changes	Expression of feelings about role changes	Encourage ventilation of feelings; assist with planning for economic resources; assist with planning for home management resources.	Adapts to role changes, verbalizes feelings
Sexual deprivation	Masturbation; flirtatious behavior; acting out and testing behaviors	Provide privacy; encourage visits from significant family and friends; encourage use of own clothing, make-up, grooming habits.	Sexuality needs met; relationships maintained with significant others
Nutritional alteration			
Decreased metabolic rate	Increased catabolism; decreased anabolism; decreased production of adrenocortical hormones; weight gain	Increase protein in diet; decrease calories; turn; exercise muscles.	Weight maintained; appropriate diet
Negative nitrogen balance	Muscle wasting; anorexia	Increase protein; use favorite foods; perform mouth care before meals.	Adequate diet for protein needs; muscle mass normal

TABLE 11-1

Nursing process for immobilized clients—cont'd

Nursing diagnosis (actual or potential)	Assessment	Planning and implementation	Evaluation: client outcomes
Alterations of urinary elimination			
Renal calculi	Flank pain; calculi in urine	Force fluids; give acid residue diet (meats, fish, nuts, and cereals).	No calculi
Urinary stasis	Urinary output increase caused by increased perfusion of kidneys; intake and output, color, odor, concentration of urine	Turn if possible to avoid stasis; encourage voiding in natural positions; force fluids.	No stasis; normal volume output
Urinary retention	Bladder distension; intake and output	Position to void; encourage voiding with running water, and so forth; force fluids; if necessary to catheterize, use strict asepsis; clamp and drain catheter to prevent loss of bladder tone.	No retention; voids freely
Alterations in bowel elimination			
Constipation	Previous bowel habits; color, amount, consistency of stool; headache, anorexia, decreased abdominal tone, sacral pain, decreased defecation reflex	Maintain established bowel habits, time and frequency; defecate when reflex cues are present; force fluids; add bulk to diet; do abdominal muscle-setting exercises; position in anatomical position; provide privacy; give stool softeners, laxatives, enemas.	Usual bowel habits maintained
Impaction	Cramping pain, diarrhea stool; abdominal distension; elevated temperature	Prevent by above interventions; give enemas; perform digital stimulation of anal sphincter; perform digital removal of impaction.	No impaction
Ineffective airway clearance			
Atelectasis	Increased respirations, pulse; change in chest sounds: rales, ronchi; color and consistency of mucus, sputum; cyanosis, dyspnea	Position to facilitate chest expansion; turn; cough, deep breathing, chest physiotherapy; use blow bottles, blow gloves; limit use of sedatives and narcotics.	No atelectasis; lungs clear to auscultation
Decreased tidal volume	Blood gas changes; hypercapnia, hypoxia	Encourage oxygen exchange with deep breathing.	Tidal volume normal for client
Decreased chest excursions	Shallow breaths	Encourage deep breathing.	Chest expansion normal
Pneumonia	Increased temperature; microbes in sputum	Force fluids; give antibiotics as ordered.	No evidence of microbial growth in sputum
Alterations in cardiac output			
Increased cardiac output	Increased pulse	Sit up and rest in chair if possible.	Normal heart rate, blood pressure
Increased blood volume	Increased blood pressure	Exhale when straining such as when turning, using trapeze, or when defecating; exhalation prevents Valsalva's maneuver.	Normal heart rate, blood pressure
Increased workload of heart	Increased pulse and blood pressure	Change positions as possible.	Normal heart rate, blood pressure
Postural hypotension	Decreased blood pressure, dizziness	Turn; force fluids; use elastic stockings; tilt table; CirOlectric bed.	Normal blood pressure
Venous stasis	Edema	Force fluids.	No stasis
Thrombophlebitis	Pain, redness, warmth, positive Homan's sign	Do active and passive range-of-motion exercises.	No inflammation of veins
Embolism	Pain, hypotension	Turn; give anticoagulants as ordered; report any calf pain or sudden pain in chest; encourage fluid intake; exercise uninvolved extremities	No evidence of embolism

pressure is exerted on the skin surfaces and that breakdown can occur in a matter of hours. The nurse should be aware of the many nursing actions that prevent skin breakdown (Chapter 10) and should use them appropriately. Skin breakdown should be observed carefully in individuals with casts or traction where friction may irritate the skin.

Mobility. Mobility is impaired when the client is immobile. Disuse of joints produces stiffening and ankylosis, whereas muscle disuse reduces strength by as much as 5% per day. Disuse also decreases muscle mass and reduces endurance for physical activity, and contractures may ultimately result. Bones not subject to stress tend to become osteoporotic because of decalcification and imbalance in favor of osteoclastic activity. These effects can be prevented by rigorous attention to range-of-motion exercises, muscle-setting exercises, and active-resistive exercises (see Chapter 10) as well as stress on bone through exercising, turning, and use of tilt tables. These exercises can be incorporated into games for children and into meaningful recreational activities for adults.

Sexuality. Sexuality may not pose imminent threats to the immobilized individual, but the nurse should be cognizant of the effects on body image and role perception resulting from this unnatural state. Masturbation and seductive behavior may increase. The client should be offered privacy, particularly during visits from a spouse or friends.

Alterations in bowel elimination, body fluids, digestion, or nutrition. Nutrition and elimination patterns are altered by prolonged periods of rest. The metabolic rate decreases, resulting in fewer caloric requirements for basal needs. *Negative nitrogen balances* can occur when tissue catabolism prevails. High-protein foods should therefore be encouraged. A negative calcium balance may also arise as a result of osteoporotic processes. The calcium withdrawn from the bone is excreted by the kidneys, which in addition to *urinary stasis* from bed rest may cause urinary calculi, also known as *stones of recumbency* (see Chapter 18). Because calcium is more easily excreted in diluted urine and favorable urinary pH, it is imperative to force fluids. Some physicians also suggest a special acid residue diet, including foods such as cereals, meats, and fish. *Urinary retention* may occur if the individual must be positioned in a manner that makes voiding difficult. If at all possible, the client should be permitted to void naturally, using such strategies to stimulate voiding as running water, pouring warm water over the perineum, and so forth. Constipation, a common consequence of immobility, can be prevented by forcing fluids, by including bulk in the diet, and by exercising abdominal muscles. Laxatives and enemas may be necessary to prevent fecal impactions.

Alterations in cardiac output and ineffective respirations. Changes in the lungs, cardiac output, and circulation, which result during periods of immobility, affect oxygen transport. When persons are resting in bed, the tidal volume in the lungs is reduced, and the effort to expand the lungs increases. For this reason it is important for the client to turn, cough, and breathe deeply frequently. Incentive spirometry may be used to encourage deep inspirations. If at all possible, the client should rest in semi-Fowler's position to facilitate lung expansion and turn from side to side and from front to back to prevent atelectasis.

Bed rest increases the work of the heart, creates postural hypotension (decreased vasoconstriction), and slows circulation. To prevent the dangers of cardiac stress, the client should turn frequently, if possible. Tilt tables or

CircOlectric beds are often used to prevent postural hypotension. Elastic stockings can be used to promote venous return and casted parts elevated to prevent swelling or edema. Thromboembolic diseases are serious hazards of immobility, often causing pulmonary emboli (see Chapter 21); turning, active and passive range-of-motion exercise, and antiembolic stockings assist in prevention. Clients with known cardiac problems must be cautioned not to hold their breath against a closed glottis when exercising, turning, defecating, or using the overbed frame, because Valsalva's maneuver can cause cardiac dysrhythmias or release of an embolus.

Developmental considerations

Infant and preschooler. The infant or preschooler who is immobilized is limited in activity at a time when weaning, toilet training, and motor and vocabulary development are important tasks. The nurse should plan with the parents, physician, and client to promote growth and development within the limits of activity. Young children adapt easily and can learn to feed themselves in spite of limitations from casts or traction. Eating is encouraged by the parents' visiting the child during mealtime or by the child's being taken to the dining room with other children. Toilet training can be continued when the nurse helps the child use his own words to indicate the need to void or defecate. The uninvolved limbs should be used so that motor development is not retarded. The child in a body cast can be put on a low cart and can use crawling movements of the arms. Sensory development can be implemented with soft toys and mobiles and by moving the crib into the playroom for contact with others. Reading and talking with the child develop his vocabulary skills.

School-age child. It is important for the school-age child to have motor and intellectual stimulation while activity is limited. Uninvolved parts of the body should be used in a normal way, and the child should be permitted to participate in group activities with other children. The child should keep up with his schoolwork, and if hospitalization is to be prolonged, the family may wish to explore resources for a classroom telephone hook-up. There may be classrooms at rehabilitation centers or special schools where children with limited movement can participate in the teaching/learning process.

Adolescent. Adolescence is a time of developing self-confidence, and the need for peer approval is paramount. Being immobilized interferes with these normal needs. The nurse can help the adolescent meet these needs by providing opportunities for self-development. If the client is out of bed, the nurse can suggest clothing that will focus attention away from a cast or brace. Activities that the client enjoys should be permitted within his limits. There are also special nutritional needs during adolescence, and the diet should contain sufficient calories and protein to support growth as well as healing. Favorite snack foods can be permitted to ensure caloric intake. Puberty brings bodily changes, and the nurse should encourage appropriate hygiene. Perspiration may be increased, and the skin under the cast or brace should be inspected and washed frequently. The adolescent requires more time for sleep, and the understanding nurse does not chide the client for wanting to sleep late in the morning. If the adolescent is in a section of the hospital where the other clients are primarily children, he should be permitted independence in determining his sleep needs.

Adult. Immobilization for adults may represent an economic loss and disruption of career and family responsibilities. The breadwinner who is confined to bed may have his ego shattered and may not have adequate income for household expenses. The parent who is hospitalized may be concerned over the management of the household and family. The nurse understands these feelings and may suggest appropriate resources. Unemployment compensation and Social Security benefits may be explored as financial resources. Family service agencies may be able to provide a temporary homemaker to meet the family needs during this crisis. The hospitalized parent can also be encouraged to keep in contact with the family by telephone and Visit Vision. Psychological security of the adult may be threatened if rehabilitation is lengthy or involves changes of employment. Diversional activities may absorb anxiety and release the frustrations of being immobile. The occupational therapist can provide diversion as well as a sense of accomplishment.

Older adult. The older adult has additional difficulties coping with prolonged immobilization, because healing is slower and body processes may be impaired by other illnesses. There are often circulatory problems. The client should be turned every 2 to 4 hours, if possible, to promote circulation and prevent skin breakdown. Unaffected limbs should be put through range-of-motion exercises to prevent ankylosis of the joints. Sensory deprivation is inherent in the elderly, and confinement makes it more acute. If the client wears glasses or uses a hearing aid, the nurse can stimulate the senses by encouraging him to wear them. Providing an access to the outside world by a wheelchair, television set, newspaper, radio, or visitors may prevent disorientation. A clock and a calendar can be used to keep the client in contact with time. The nurse should be aware of the change in the cycle of rest and activity in older persons and plan to assure a proper balance. Constipation, normally caused by the sluggish gastrointestinal tract in older persons, is compounded by immobilization. The nurse should encourage a diet with adequate fluids and bulk to prevent constipation. The diet should also be reduced in calories, because metabolic processes are slower in older persons.

Implementation

COMMON HEALTH PROBLEMS OF THE NEONATE AND INFANT

Congenital hip dysplasia

Congenital hip dysplasia is an inclusive term referring to various malformations of the hip. The most common is *hip dislocation,* which may occur in one or both hips.

Pathophysiology. Congenital dislocation of the hip occurs when the acetabulum is unable to hold the head of the femur. The dislocation may be partial, subluxated, or complete. In *partial dislocation* there is a shallowness of the acetabulum but the femoral head remains in the acetabulum. *Subluxation* is an incomplete dislocation in which the head of the femur remains in contact with the acetabulum but rides up and out of the acetabulum. *Complete dislocation* is the total disarticulation of the joint.

The cause of congenital hip dysplasia is unknown. Prenatal factors such as intrauterine position (breech) or hormonal factors may be implicated. Cultural factors may also be responsible, because there is an increased incidence in cultures where the infant is strapped to a cradle board as opposed to those in which the infant is carried on the parents' hips with the infant's legs abducted.

Congenital hip dislocation occurs in 1 in 500 to 1000 births. There is an increased incidence with breech delivery, and more girls are affected.

Assessment. The nurse can observe the presence of a dislocated hip during neonatal appraisals or subsequent well-child examinations. The symptoms are related to the dislocation and are observed as differences in the shape of the lower extremity and, when the child can walk, unevenness of gait.

Inspection reveals uneven gluteal folds on the involved side and a prominent trochanter (Fig. 11-17). There may be pain on abduction or the infant may not be able to fully abduct the involved leg. If the infant is placed on his back with his legs flexed, it is possible to elicit a click in the involved hip as the hip is carried to abduction *(Ortolani's click)* (Fig. 11-18). The thigh level appears uneven, and the limb is shorter on the affected side *(Allis's sign)*.

When the child is old enough to stand and walk, the signs become more evident. *Trendelenburg's test* is used when the child stands on the involved leg with the stable leg elevated. There is pelvic dropping if the hip is dislocated. The child is late in walking at 12 to 18 months and when he does, the gait is uneven and the child appears to limp.

The dislocation may be unilateral or bilateral. A *unilateral* dislocation is noticed by the uneven gluteal folds and limping gait. A *bilateral* dislocation is noticed by a wide perineum and prominence of the hip. When walking, the child has a waddling gait. Diagnosis is based on the signs and confirmed by x-ray studies.

FIG. 11-17
Extra gluteal folds and prominent trochanter are indications of congenital hip dislocation. (From Larson, Carroll B., and Gould, Marjorie: Orthopedic nursing, ed. 9, St. Louis, 1978, The C.V. Mosby Co.)

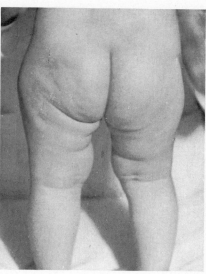

FIG. 11-18
Ortolani's click. Flexed legs are carried to abduction to note characteristic click.

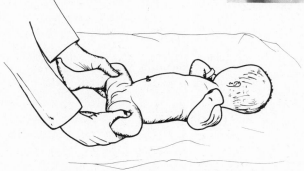

Nursing process for common health problems

Planning and implementation. The nurse develops a plan with the client and his family to reestablish mobility and self-care activities. The objective of medical treatment is to reduce the dislocation with the hip in abduction while the acetabulum develops. The type of treatment depends on the extent of dislocation and the age of the client, but may include splinting or closed reduction, and the nursing care plan is developed accordingly.

Splinting. If there is only partial dislocation, the femur is held in abduction while the acetabulum develops. In early infancy this may be accomplished with the use of three diapers to abduct the legs. Later, special pillow splints that maintain the hip in abduction can be used. Several splints such as the Craig adjustable hip splint are made commercially (Fig. 11-19). A splint may also be improvised with soft pillows placed between the legs. The splint is worn over the diaper and should be protected with plastic so that it does not become soiled. The parents should learn how to apply the splint because it must be removed and reapplied with each change of the diaper.

While the infant is wearing the splint, the parents should encourage normal growth and development. Feeding patterns should promote finger feeding and weaning. The splint limits movement, but the infant should be given opportunities to reach, grasp, hold objects, and play with soft toys. The parents can move the child from room to room so that he has a change of environment. They should also touch and hold the child to express affection and reinforce security.

The splint is worn for several months before correction is obtained, and x-ray films are taken periodically to determine the development of the acetabulum. When the splint is removed, the parents should observe the child's growth. X-ray examinations may be made later to be sure that reduction is maintained during periods of growth.

Closed reduction. Infants and children with subluxation and complete dislocation usually require closed reduction (correction without a surgical incision) of the dislocation. The hip is immobilized in abduction while the infant is

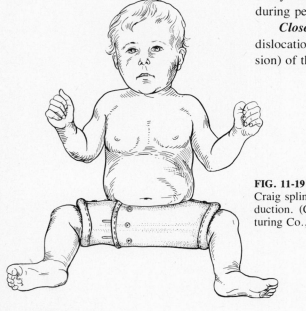

FIG. 11-19
Craig splint is used to maintain hip abduction. (Courtesy Richards Manufacturing Co., Memphis, Tenn.)

under anesthesia. A hip spica cast, which extends from above the waist to below the knee of the affected leg is applied to maintain abduction during healing.

When the infant returns from surgery, the nurse must evaluate the cast to be sure that there is no circulatory or nerve impairment. This is done by taking the pulse and checking color and movement of the extremities. The infant in the wet cast should be turned frequently to assure drying and prevent unnatural molding of the cast.

The infant in a hip spica cast should be positioned so that he does not soil the cast. A Bradford frame, which is suspended from the crib, may be used. There is an opening for a bedpan under the frame, so that the infant has less chance of lying in wet or soiled diapers. Pillows can also be placed in the bed to support the infant and allow for toileting. Plastic wrap can be used around the cast so that it does not become wet. Double folds of diaper may prevent soiling, if changed often. One diaper is folded and used as a perineal pad, and the other diaper is secured to hold the folded diaper in place.

The child in the hip spica cast has limited activity, and the nurse should therefore plan activities that will promote muscle development. The crib may be wheeled into the playroom so that the child may play with others. Hanging mobiles and soft toys develop sensorimotor learning. Some hospitals have a special cart in which the child can sit; it has a wide base and a high back to support the cast, and the legs are on casters so that it can move easily.

If the child is cared for at home, the parents should be shown how to adapt hospital procedures to home use. A mobile crib, wagon, or cart can be devised to make lifting and transporting the child easier. The parents should continue to observe the skin for breakdown or circulatory impairment; they should also notice how the child is growing and if the cast is becoming too small. A tight cast can cause circulatory impairment and should be changed if the child outgrows it.

When x-ray films show that the acetabulum will hold the head of the femur, the cast is removed. The child's legs are exercised gradually before weight bearing is permitted. Physical therapy administered by a therapist, nurse, or parent is used to strengthen the muscles of inward rotation so that they will give sufficient support for walking.

The prognosis for congenital hip dislocation is good if treated early. Normal activity progresses naturally, but the parents are encouraged to have follow-up appointments with the physician so that the child can be observed during later periods of growth. If reduction is not maintained, it may be necessary to employ operative procedures (*open reduction*) at a later time.

 Evaluation. Evaluation of the nursing plans for the young client with congenital hip dysplasia is an ongoing component of the nursing process as the congenital defect is corrected and mobility increases.

EXPECTED OUTCOMES

The client and/or family can:
1. Describe congenital hip dysplasia.
2. Demonstrate plans for care of the infant in a cast or splint.
3. State limits of activity.
4. Describe patterns of growth and development of the infant and child and plans to foster these.
5. State problems requiring health care services.
6. Indicate plans for follow-up care, and state knowledge of community resources for health care.

545

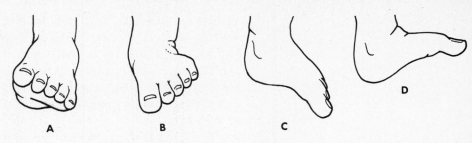

FIG. 11-20
Types of clubfoot deformities: **A,** varus; **B,** valgus; **C,** equinus; **D,** calcaneus.

Clubfoot

Clubfoot is a rarely occurring malposition of the foot. The foot may be out of position in several directions, and Latin terms are used to describe the defect (Fig. 11-20). *Talipes* refers to the foot and is used with *varus* for inversion, *valgus* for eversion, *equinus* for plantar flexion, and *calcaneus* for dorsiflexion. Talipes equinovarus is the most common type of clubfoot. The malposition may occur in one or both feet, with varying degrees of severity. The cause is not known, but is attributed to genetic defects or fetal malposition in utero. Clubfoot occurs in 1 in 700 to 1000 live births.

 Assessment. Clubfoot is noticed by the malformation of the foot. Although slight eversion of the foot is normal in neonates, the foot can be rotated. In neonates with clubfoot, however, the foot cannot be repositioned. The diagnosis is made by the appearance of the foot and the inability to rotate the foot.

 Planning and implementation. Treatment for clubfoot depends on the degree of version and flexion. Manipulation, splinting, or casting are used to reposition the foot. A slight malposition may respond to a routine of regularly manipulating the foot into the correct position. The physician or nurse instructs the parent how to massage the foot, and the exercise is done every 4 hours until correction is obtained. The exercises should not be done near mealtime, so that the infant will not associate the discomfort of exercising with eating.

Splints or casts may be used to effect continuous alignment of the foot. A Denis Browne splint (Fig. 11-21) is taped to the infant's feet and gradually adjusted to bring the feet into proper alignment. As the child moves his legs, the spreader bar of the splint directs the affected foot into alignment. Movement of the legs is limited when the child wears this splint, and the parents should pick the child up, hold him, and turn him frequently.

Casts may also be used to obtain alignment of malpositioned feet. In one procedure the casts are used initially and changed every few weeks; then when the casts are removed, a modified Denis Browne splint is worn at night to maintain correction. There is considerable pressure on the tendons and blood vessels when casts are used to correct clubfoot, and the parents must observe the toes for adequate circulation. Many visits to the physician are necessary while the casts are changed and refitted, and the family must follow through with this therapy.

Brachial nerve palsy

Brachial nerve palsy is a rare complication of vaginal delivery. Paralysis of the muscles of the arm occurs because of stretching, pressure, or laceration of the nerves from the neck to the shoulder and the arms during difficult delivery.

 Assessment. The nurse caring for the neonate must be alert to this possible problem and assess reflexes as well as noting any abnormalities in arm positioning or movements. The absence of bilateral symmetry of the upper extremities in the Moro reflex is often indicative of damage to the brachial nerve plexus.

FIG. 11-21
Denis Browne splint is used to realign clubfoot. The feet are taped to foot plate, and spreader bar and foot plate are adjusted periodically. (Courtesy Arthur Steindler, M.D., Iowa City, Iowa.)

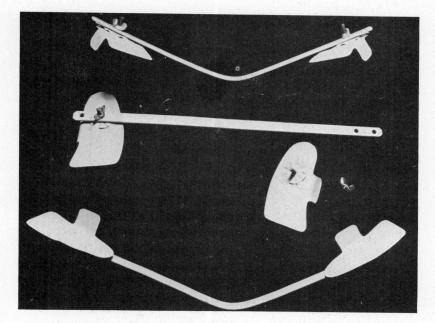

☞   **Planning and implementation.** Treatment is directed toward recovery of function in the involved muscles and maintenance of optimum function in uninvolved ones. Positioning techniques, exercise, and massage are employed. The outcome of the injury depends on the type and extent of trauma. If nerves are not actually lacerated, recovery may be accomplished within a few months.

Torticollis   Torticollis (wryneck) is caused by overstretching the sternocleidomastoid muscle during birth. The stretching causes hemorrhage, scar formation, and contracture of the muscle. This seems to happen most frequently in girls, but it is a rare congenital defect.

☞   **Assessment.** The nurse can observe torticollis when the infant holds the head to the affected side and the shoulder on the affected side is raised. There may be a palpable hematoma at the muscle site.

☞   **Planning and implementation.** If the symptoms are noted early, heat and massage can be used to stretch the muscle. Correction can also be achieved by turning the neck 25 times, three times a day, to stretch the muscle and prevent contractures. If torticollis is not treated early, the tendon must be resected, and the infant must be put in a cast for 6 weeks while the muscle heals. The cast is not applied until the day after surgery so that the infant can expand the chest normally to prevent atelectasis and to prevent aspiration from postoperative vomiting.

COMMON HEALTH PROBLEMS OF THE CHILD

Osteomyelitis

Osteomyelitis is an infection of the bone marrow of long bones caused by microorganisms such as *Staphylococcus aureus,* and less frequently, *Haemophilus influenzae.* The organisms can enter the bone through open wounds, fractures, or surgical incisions, or by way of the blood stream from other foci such as upper respiratory tract infections, tonsilitis, tooth abscess, skin lesions, or pyelonephritis. The microorganisms migrate through the blood stream to the bone metaphysis where infection ensues, and if not treated, results in abscess formation and bone destruction. As the abscess enlarges, it ruptures into subperiosteal space and causes necrosis.

547

Osteomyelitis is primarily a disease of children and adolescents, although debilitated individuals of all ages may be at risk. Boys are affected twice as often as girls.

 Assessment. The infection causes tenderness and swelling at the site. Additionally there are systemic effects of the infection such as increased temperature, tachycardia, restlessness, leukocytosis, and dehydration.

 Planning and implementation. Objectives of therapy are to reduce the inflammation and relieve the pain. Antibiotics such as penicillin or ampicillin are given in large doses. The bone may be irrigated and drained to relieve the abscess. Two catheters may be inserted into the area, one for continuous irrigation with an antibiotic and the other to drain the fluid. Wound precautions should be instituted and strict asepsis observed while irrigating catheters are used.

The involved extremity is immobilized, and the client is placed on bed rest. Analgesics and narcotics are offered to relieve the pain.

Fluids and nutrition should be planned to prevent dehydration and promote healing. Antipyretics may be used while the temperature is elevated.

If the infection becomes chronic, it may be necessary to remove the affected part of the bone. Necrotic tissue that appears after an infection of the bone is called *sequestrum;* when it is removed, the surgery is called *sequestrectomy.* Amputation is a final consideration if the infection in the involved area is not resolved or the area of necrosis is large.

Juvenile rheumatoid arthritis

Juvenile rheumatoid arthritis (JRA, Still's disease) is a form of rheumatoid arthritis observed in children. The disease occurs at two peaks, ages 2 to 5 and 9 to 12. Manifestations of clinical evidence are usually more overt than in adults and may involve one or more joints. Growth may be disrupted depending on the age of the child at onset.

 Assessment. In children, diagnostic indicators of JRA, unlike those for adults, include high fever, rheumatoid rash, generalized lymphadenopathy, splenomegaly, and leukocytosis. Streptococcal infections may be inciting factors, because the ASO titer is increased in one third of clients diagnosed with JRA. The rheumatoid factor used for diagnosis in adults is not diagnostic for JRA.

There are several types of onset, and the clinical course differs for each. In the *systemic* onset, fever, rash, and lymphadenopathy are predominant. In a *pauciarticular* onset, there are fewer systemic effects, but one joint, usually the knee, is involved. With *polyarticular* onset there is synovitis of more than four joints.

 Planning and implementation. JRA is managed to reduce inflammation and prevent deformities. Remission occurs in one half of affected individuals. Surgery to restore function may be performed for late stages of the disease. A complete discussion of the nursing care for a client with rheumatoid arthritis is presented later in this chapter.

Legg-Calvé-Perthes disease

Legg-Calvé-Perthes disease (coxa plana, osteochodritis deformans juvenilis) is an aseptic necrosis of the head of the femur. The cause of the necrosis is unknown, but it is assumed to be associated with decreased circulation to the femoral capital epiphysis, which results in ischemia and necrosis. The disease is self-limiting in 18 months to 3 years. In the initial (avascular) stage there is aseptic necrosis and flattening of the head of the femur. Later there is revascularization and resorption of the epiphysis. Finally, new bone regenerates (regenerative stage).

This is a disease of young children, usually 3 to 12. Boys 4 to 8 are more affected and it is seen more often in whites.

 Assessment. The nurse has a significant role in identifying clients with Legg-Calvé-Perthes disease during well-child appraisals. The problem is noticed by pain and a limp. There may be joint dysfunction and limited movement. The diagnosis is confirmed by x-ray films. The disease may involve one or both legs.

 Planning and implementation. The goal of therapy is to keep the head of the femur in the acetabulum until bone regeneration occurs. This can be accomplished by a brace or cast, which may be used for several years. Surgical correction is an alternative, and recovery is considerably shorter: 3 to 4 months. The prognosis for return to normal mobility is favorable if treated early.

Rickets

Rickets occurs in children 3 months to 3 years of age who do not have an adequate dietary source of vitamin D, the vitamin necessary for absorption of calcium and phosphorus. The intake may be poor because of inadequate vitamin D in the formula or in breast milk. Lack of sunshine can diminish the supply of vitamin D, and rickets occasionally occurs in areas of air pollution where sunlight is poor. Heredity and prematurity may also cause rickets.

Assessment. When vitamin D is insufficient, calcium deposits in the long bones are decreased. There may be pain, muscle weakness, kyphosis, or scoliosis. If the disease is not treated, the child will have misshapen limbs, usually bowed legs. A rachitic rosary (beading on the costochondral junctions) is another sign of rickets. The diagnosis is based on clinical symptoms and hypocalcemia.

Planning and implementation. The bone regeneration is reversed when the intake of vitamin D is improved. Vitamin D may be given orally to supplement dietary sources. Sunlight is a good source of vitamin D, and the child should be encouraged to play outside.

Nursing care for the child with rickets should be supportive of the musculoskeletal system. The nurse can position the client carefully to avoid deformities. When the child is turned, great care should be taken not to put stress on the bones. As the diet improves, the bones regenerate, and the prognosis is favorable when nutrition is adequate.

COMMON HEALTH PROBLEMS OF THE ADOLESCENT

Scoliosis

Scoliosis is the lateral deviation of one or more vertebrae of the spine, usually accompanied by a rotary deformity. There are two types of scoliosis: functional (nonstructural) and structural. *Functional scoliosis,* which accounts for 10% to 20% of cases of scoliosis, is a flexible deviation that corrects by bending. It is caused by poor posture. *Structural (idiopathic) scoliosis* is inherited as an autosomal dominant characteristic, although there may be neurogenic or myopathic causes. There is an apparent involvement of the epiphysis, and changes occur at the spinal curve.[8] The scoliosis may be described as thoracic, lumbar, or thoracolumbar, depending on the segment involved.

Scoliosis is a disease of early adolescence but can be diagnosed earlier. Girls are affected 10 times more frequently than boys. The incidence is 140 in 100,000.

Assessment. Scoliosis is noted during periods of growth, particularly in early puberty. Because changes in the spine can be easily detected, the nurse has a significant role in assessing young girls during health appraisals and instructing

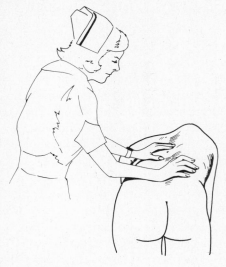

FIG. 11-22
Assessing spine. Palpation reveals rib hump and unevenness of spine.

others who are in contact with young girls, such as schoolteachers, to also assess the deviations of the spine.

The curvature of the vertebrae can be noticed by poor posture and unevenness of the hips. The posture improves in a recumbent position if the scoliosis is functional.

Structural scoliosis, however, is manifested by loss of flexibility and inability to correct the spinal deviation. Unevenness of the scapulae or flank may be noticed, particularly when the child bends forward at the waist (Fig. 11-22). Palpation in this position further reveals enlarged paravertebral masses and an alteration of the iliac crest. The shoulder may be uneven or one breast more prominent. Often the clothing or hemlines may appear uneven. Thoracic involvement causes decrease in pulmonary function; if not treated, reduced lung capacity and increased dead space can ensue.

The diagnosis is made by inspection and confirmed by x-ray examination. At the time of diagnosis, baseline measurements are taken to determine the upper and lower end vertebrae of the curve so that progress from therapy can be evaluated.

Data analysis
Data analysis may include nursing diagnoses of alterations in comfort, impaired mobility, self-care deficit, and disturbances in self-concept.

Planning and implementation. The goal of therapy is to prevent progression of mild scoliosis and to correct more severe deformities. Therapy may include exercises, electrostimulation, braces, traction, casts, or surgery, depending on the curvature of the spine. The nurse plans with the client and family to provide knowledge necessary to comply with the therapy or to cope with altered mobility, self-care, and disturbances in self-concept if traction, casts, or surgery is required.

Exercises. Exercises can be used to treat functional scoliosis or as an adjunct to the use of the Milwaukee brace. Exercises include the pelvic tilt (lying supine with the knees flexed, the buttocks are tightened, and the small of the back pushed to the floor with the abdominal muscles); sit-up with pelvic tilt, and push-ups with the pelvic tilt.[8] The nurse can help the client learn these exercises and encourage compliance.

Electrostimulation. Another nonsurgical approach to correction of the deviation is muscle electrostimulation. A stimulator is implanted or attached to the skin that delivers a small electric current to stimulate muscles attached to the vertebral column. The muscle contraction pulls the vertebral column toward alignment and thereby prevents further deformity.

Braces. The Milwaukee brace (Fig. 11-23) is the most common brace used to treat scoliosis. It is used to prevent further deviation when the girl is still growing and the degree of curvature is less than 30% to 50%.[5] The brace extends from the back of the head to the hips and includes a throat mold to prevent forward flexion of the neck and side pads that encourage active correction as the girl moves the spine to avoid the pads. The brace is worn 23 hours a day. A bra and a soft shirt can be worn under the brace, but underpants should be worn over

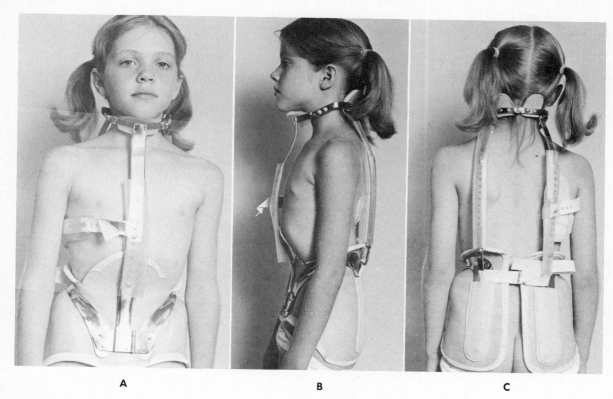

A   B   C

FIG. 11-23
Milwaukee brace: **A,** front view, **B,** side view; **C,** rear view. (Courtesy Walter P. Blount, MD, Minneapolis, personal research.)

the brace to prevent skin irritation from rubbing. The brace is worn until the client is grown as evidenced by closure of the thoracic vertebral apophyses. This may take as long as 5 years. Exercises as described above may be prescribed as adjuncts to the brace.

The use of a brace may impose limits on the adolescent's mobility and create body image changes at a crucial point in the life span. The nurse should plan with the client and family ways to provide activities that are consistent with the therapeutic plan yet allow peer relations and a positive development of self-concept.

The nurse can also help the client and family comply with the therapy. Often the use of the brace is long-term, and motivation to do exercises and wear restrictive braces decreases. The nurse can be a source of encouragement and support at this time.

Casts. Casts are used to provide forcible correction of the curvature. The Risser turnbuckle cast (Fig. 11-24) is applied over stockinet from the chin to the knee. Wedges of the cast are cut out at the curvature, and turnbuckles are added at the concavity. The turnbuckles are adjusted periodically to achieve correction.

Traction. Traction may be used to straighten the spine, particularly before surgical approaches. *Cotrel traction* may be used for curvatures less than 40 degrees. This traction includes a cervical halter to pull proximally and a pelvic girdle to pull longitudinally. Weights are increased gradually. (See discussion earlier in this chapter for nursing care of clients in traction.) Spinal *skeletal traction* is used if the curvature is 60 to 90 degrees. *Halo-femoral traction* or *halo-pelvic traction* (Fig. 11-25) are examples. These devices are attached to the

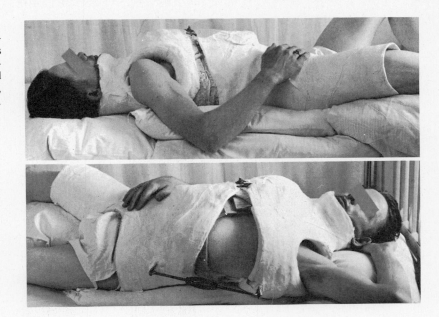

FIG. 11-24
Turnbuckle cast is applied to force correction of deviated spine. Adjustments in turnbuckle gradually create alignment. (From Larson, Carroll B., and Gould, Marjorie: Orthopedic nursing, ed. 7, St. Louis, 1970, The C.V. Mosby Co.)

skull and femur (or pelvis) and weights gradually increased to 50 pounds (110 kg).

Surgery. Surgical correction with a spinal fusion is used for severe deformities and is usually preceded or followed (or both) by the use of casts, braces, or traction. The surgery is usually not done until the child is about 14 years old and bone growth is complete. The surgery may include a spinal fusion; in addition to fusion, some use a distraction rod *(Harrington rod),* which is attached to the posterior aspects of the spinal column on the concave curve (Fig. 11-26). A compression rod is placed on the convex side to force the spine into alignment. These rods are removed when straightening is complete.

After fusion, the client is put in a body cast for 6 to 12 months until the spine heals. The client is confined to bed for several months and then permitted increasing mobility. Most often the client can be cared for at home after the immediate postoperative recovery period. Nursing care for the client in a cast is discussed earlier in this chapter.

 Evaluation. The adolescent with scoliosis plans with the nurse to restore mobility and maintain self-care activities. Evaluation of the plans are ongoing.

EXPECTED OUTCOMES

The client and/or family can:
1. Describe scoliosis.
2. Demonstrate plans for implementing therapeutic intervention (cast, brace, exercises).
3. Demonstrate sensitivity to changes in self-concept.
4. State limits of activity and alternative plans for exercise.
5. State plans for health maintenance:
   a. Rest and activity
   b. Diet, and weight control
   c. Hygiene and skin care
   d. Adequate urinary and bowel elimination
6. State use, dosage, time, route, and side effects of any medications prescribed.
7. State plans for follow-up care and problems requiring health care services.

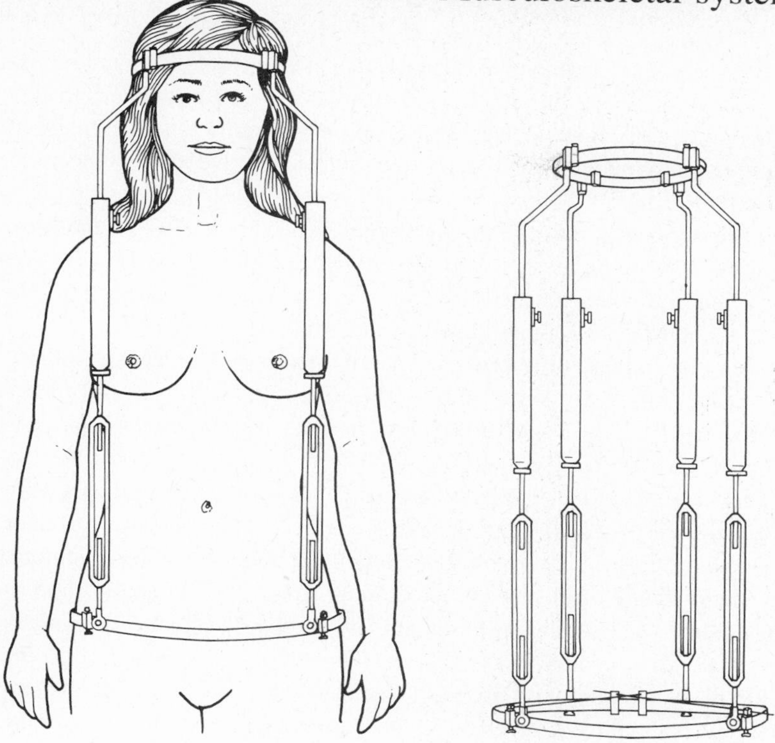

FIG. 11-25
Halo pelvic traction.

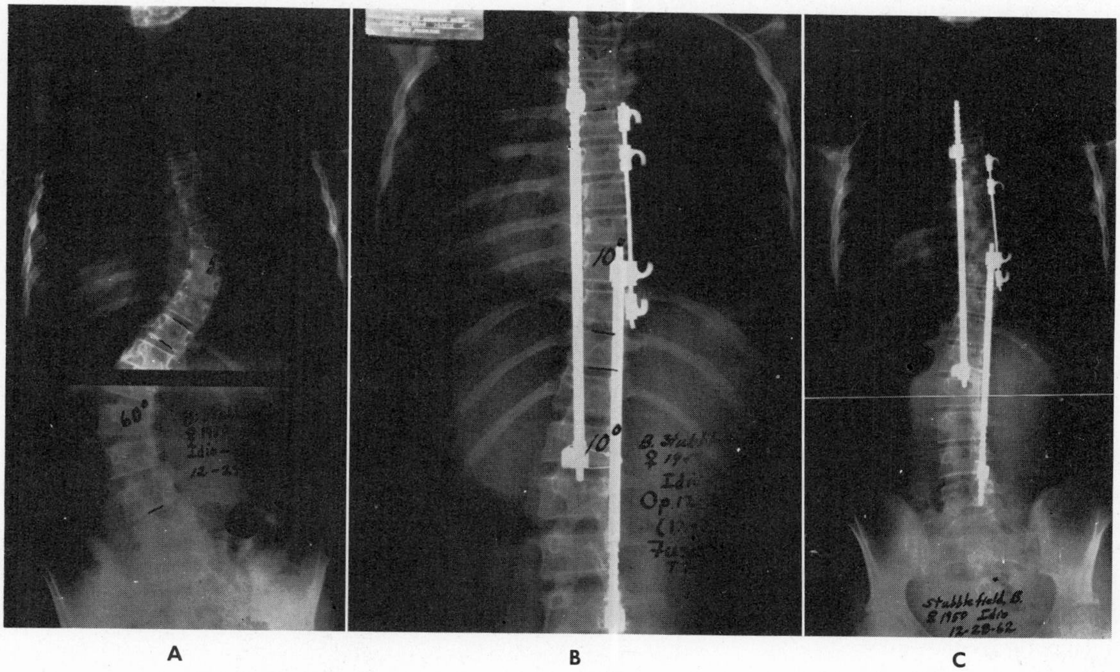

A   B   C

FIG. 11-26
Harrington treatment by instrumentation and fusion. **A,** Spine of 11-year-old girl with idiopathic scoliosis with right dorsal primary curve of 55 degrees and left lumbar one of 60 degrees. **B,** Spine after curves have been corrected to 10 degrees each by instrumentation; spine has been fused by Moe technique. **C,** Spine 2 years after fusion. Note that ossification of iliac epiphyses is complete. About 5 degrees of correction have been lost, but spine is stable and patient is free of discomfort. Removing instruments 5 years after surgery is planned. (Courtesy Paul R. Harrington, M.D.)

553

Nursing process for common health problems

Epiphysitis of the tibial tubercle

Epiphysitis of the tibial tubercle (Osgood-Schlatter disease) is an inflammation of the epiphysis of the tibia, believed to be caused by a circulatory disturbance of the epiphyseal centers. The disease occurs primarily in adolescents, in boys more frequently than girls. Boys and girls who are active in sports seem to be at greater risk.

Assessment. Pain is the primary symptom. It occurs just below the knee joint and occurs with activity. There is a prominence of the tibial tubercle that is extremely painful when touched. The diagnosis is based on inspection and palpation and confirmed by x-ray studies of the tibial tubercle.

Planning and implementation. The goal of therapy is to reduce the inflammation by immobilizing the knee. Frequently, immobility is self-enforced because the pain is too great to permit activity. In other instances splints or casts may be used to immobilize the knee.

Slipped femoral capital epiphysis

A slipped capital femoral epiphysis (coxa vara) is a downward and backward displacement of the epiphysis. The femoral epiphysis becomes weakened or stressed and slides upward. There is rarefaction of the bone on the lower femoral epiphysis and widening of the growth plate. With stress, the femoral portion of the epiphysis slides up, causing posterior and inferior displacement. The cause is unknown, although it occurs more frequently in obese children and it occurs during puberty. Adolescent boys are most frequently affected. The contralateral femoral epiphysis should also be assessed, because subsequent involvement may occur.

Assessment. The slipped epiphysis is noticed by the pain in the lower one third of the thigh and may be referred to the groin or knee. There is external rotation of the lower extremity, and the client has difficulty in abduction and internal rotation of the hip, which is noticed as a limp.

Planning and implementation. Internal fixation is necessary to repair the slipped epiphysis. Pins are used to align the femoral head until healing takes place. A cast may be used to maintain immobility during healing.

COMMON HEALTH PROBLEMS OF THE YOUNG ADULT

Osteogenic sarcoma

Osteogenic sarcoma is a primary tumor of the diaphysis of long bones, particularly the femur, tibia, ileum, and humerus. The cause of the tumor is not known, although the cancer cells originate in the bone-forming mesenchyme and produce malignant osteoid tissue. The tumor generally occurs in young adults (peak incidence 10 to 25 years) and in men more frequently than women.

Assessment. The growth of the tumor is evidenced by pain and swelling that is not attributed to injury or infection. If the tumor is in the tibia or femur, the client may limp. There may be fever and fatigue associated with tumor growth. The diagnosis is based on the symptoms, biopsy, elevated alkaline phosphatase, and x-ray studies.

Planning and implementation. Therapeutic intervention involves radical surgery to remove the tumor and surrounding tissue. Amputation may include an extremity, hemipelvectomy, or forequarter amputation (arm, scapula, and clavicle). Radiation therapy or chemotherapy may be used singly or as adjuncts to surgical amputation.

In specialized clinical settings, *femur replacement* is being used as an alternative to amputation. The client is treated with high doses of methotrexate, which causes tumor cell death and ultimately necrosis of bone cells. When methotrexate is used, intravenous fluids with sodium bicarbonate are administered before and after each treatment to increase the alkalinity of the urine and prevent renal damage. Citrovorum factor (folinic acid or Leucovorin) is used to minimize toxic effects of methotrexate on normal cells (citrovorum rescue). The necrotic bone tissue can then be removed and replaced by a metallic prosthesis. Although healing requires long periods of immobilization, this intervention preserves body function and maintains self-image in adolescents for whom these concerns are significant.

The nursing care plan should be developed with the client and family to emphasize the client's individual needs. An honest approach facilitates communications and the client should be informed about his therapeutic plan.

When amputation is necessary, the nurse plans for perioperative care that is based on the client's individual needs. Time should be allowed for grieving and acceptance of change in body image. After surgery many clients can use a prosthesis, and the nurse and health team members can help the client adapt to this change in locomotion. Nutritional requirements may increase, and fluids and foods should be planned accordingly. The prognosis for long-term survival is not favorable and psychological support for the client and family must be provided throughout.

COMMON HEALTH PROBLEMS OF THE ADULT

Adult rheumatoid arthritis

Rheumatoid arthritis (RA, atrophic arthritis deformans) is a chronic systemic inflammation of the synovial membrane of diarthroidal joints, particularly the knees, ankles, wrists, fingers, hips, shoulders, elbows, spine, and occasionally the temporomandibular or intervertebral facetal joints. The onset may be *episodic* or *sustained,* and if the disease is sustained it follows a course of remissions and exacerbations. In a small number of individuals with RA, the disease may progress rapidly, with joint destruction and other systemic effects and is known as *malignant rheumatic disease.*

The cause of RA is unknown, but several factors are believed to incite the inflammation.[1] The most widely held theory is that an autoimmune response precipitates inflammation. Others favor environmental factors, because the symptoms of RA increase in the spring and when the humidity is high. The inflammation may be caused by a viral or streptococcal infection. Others believe that "personality types" are prone to RA or that there are strong correlations with psychological or physiological stress. Another possibility is a genetic basis for RA, because familial tendencies have been noted. A multifactoral causation theory suggests that an individual with a genetic predisposition to RA is susceptible to an infectious agent that produces the inflammation of the synovial membrane. RA is frequently classified as a collagen disease, but because the manifestations of the disease affect mobility, it is discussed in this chapter.

Nearly 4 million individuals are affected by some form of RA. The disease characteristically involves middle-aged women. The peak incidence is between 20 to 60 years, and women are three times more affected than men. Three fourths of those with episodic onset may only have active symptoms for less than a year and may have complete remission.

Pathophysiology. Inflammation of the joints begin at the synovial membrane, which is infiltrated by leukocytes causing congestion and *edema.* The involved joints become *stiff* (particularly early in the morning and lasting longer than 1 hour), *red, swollen,* and *painful* on motion and at rest. *Pain* is attributed to the pressure on sensory nerve endings, and there may be paresthesias of the first three fingers of the involved hand.

555

FIG. 11-27
Arthritic deformities: **A,** boutonnière; **B,** swan neck; **C,** ulnar deviation.

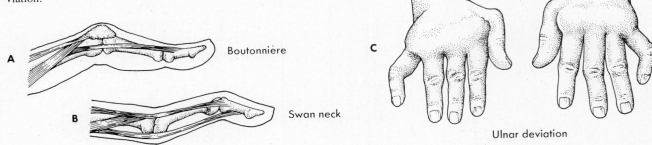

As the disease progresses with cellular infiltration, the tendon sheath becomes inflamed. The client experiences more pain and increasing immobility as flexion and extension of the joint are limited. There may be tendon contraction, causing characteristic ulnar deviation and other deformities such as the "swan neck" and "boutonnière" deformities (Fig. 11-27).

As the inflammatory exudate accumulates, it spills into joint capsules and produces joint effusion. The client notices boggy, swollen joints (Fig. 11-28). The joint capsule becomes thickened with connective tissue. Granulation tissue or proliferating fibroblasts and blood vessels (pannus) forms at the site and eventually erodes the articular cartilage and subchondral bone.

Ultimately, surrounding connective tissue is inflamed, producing weakness of tendons and ligaments. Muscles may atrophy from disuse *(disuse atrophy)*. Destructive changes of the joint cause subluxation of the involved joint, deformities, pain, and immobility.

RA is invariably accompanied by systemic or extraarticular manifestations. These are caused by the generalized inflammation and may include (1) systemic complications, (2) organ involvement, (3) rheumatoid granulomas, and (4) vasculitis.

Systemic effects can be noted in individuals with RA. There may be decreases in hemoglobin, which result in anemia, weakness, and fatigue. *Felty's syndrome* (leukopenia and splenomegaly) and *Sjögren's syndrome* (decreased secretions of lacrimal and salivary glands) are other systemic manifestations.

Major organs can be affected by RA. There may be *cardiomyopathy,* which is usually asymptomatic, and *pulmonary nodules*. Clumping of cells in the anterior chamber of the eye causes *iridocyclitis,* which predisposes the client to glaucoma or cataracts. *Nephropathy* and *neuropathy* may also be evident.

Rheumatoid granulomas are subcutaneous nodules that appear over tendon sheaths. They are particularly evident over pressure areas such as the elbow. Twenty percent of individuals with RA have nodules.

Vascular manifestations include changes in venules, arterioles, and arteries. *Raynaud's phenomenon* occurs in about 10% of clients.

Assessment. The nurse can gather information about the course of the disease and its effect on the client's mobility. The nurse should inspect all joints and ascertain range of motion and presence of deformities. The ability to perform activities of daily living should also be noted. Pain is characteristic of RA, and

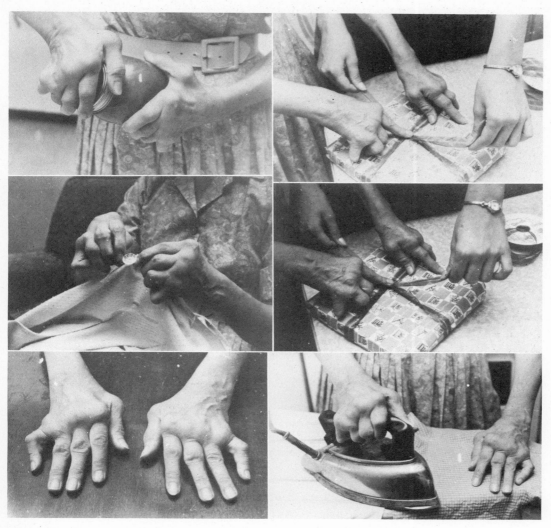

FIG. 11-28
Arthritic joints make simple tasks diffi-cult. Note atrophy and contractures. (Courtesy Indiana Chapter, The Arthri-tis Foundation, Indianapolis.)

the nurse can determine the degree of pain, when it occurs, where it occurs, and what affords the client relief from pain.

The diagnosis is based on the clinical changes as well as on x-ray studies, and blood studies. The x-ray films may show joint effusions. An elevated sedimentation rate, leukocytosis, anemia, and the presence of the rheumatoid factor and C-reactive protein may be evident, but because they are present in other diseases, they are not specifically diagnostic for RA. Synovial fluid analy-sis and synovial tissue biopsy may also be used in diagnosis.

RA has been described in clinical stages and by functional classification to facilitate diagnosis and planning for care (see material, p. 558).

> **Data analysis**
> *Data analysis may reveal nursing diagnoses of pain, impaired mobility, self-care deficit, and disturbance in self-concept.*

Nursing process for common health problems

RHEUMATOID ARTHRITIS

Clinical stages

Stage I, early
1. X-ray films show no evidence of destructive changes.
2. X-ray films may show evidence of osteoporosis.

Stage II, moderate
1. X-ray films show evidence of osteoporosis, possibly with slight destruction of cartilage or subchondral bone.
2. Joints are not deformed, but mobility may be limited.
3. Adjacent muscles are atrophied.
4. Extraarticular soft-tissue lesions (such as nodules and tenovaginitis) may be present.

Stage III, severe
1. X-ray films show cartilage and bone destruction, as well as osteoporosis.
2. Joint deformity (such as subluxation, ulnar deviation, or hyperextension) exists but not fibrous or bony ankylosis.
3. Muscle atrophy is extensive.
4. Extraarticular soft-tissue lesions (such as nodules and tenovaginitis) are often present.

Stage IV, terminal
1. Fibrous or bony ankylosis exists in addition to all criteria listed for stage III.

Functional classification

Class I
No loss of functional capacity.

Class II
Functional capacity impaired but sufficient for normal activities despite joint pain or limited mobility.

Class III
Functional capacity adequate to perform few if any occupational or self-care tasks.

Class IV
Client confined to bed or wheelchair and capable of little or no self-care.

Planning and implementation. In the early stages of the disease the foundations of medical management are salicylates, simple exercises, localized heat, as well as physical and emotional rest and a well-balanced diet. As the disease progresses, antiinflammatory agents, steroids, potent analgesics, and splints may be necessary. In later stages gold therapy, synovectomy, and reconstructive surgery may be employed. The nursing care plan for a client with RA depends on the stage of the disease and the client's problems with pain, self-care activities, and mobility. At times the nurse may be more involved with care, but as the client is able, the nurse assumes a supportive and instructive role. General goals are to reduce inflammation, relieve pain, provide rest, maintain mobility, restore function, and help the client manage the therapeutic plan for health maintenance with a chronic illness.

Reducing inflammation. At the onset of RA, the inflammation is controlled with acetylsalicylic acid *(aspirin);* 5 to 6 g are given in divided doses four times a day. It is imperative for the client to take the drug regularly to maintain effective blood levels at 20% to 30%. Because aspirin is irritating to the gastric mucosa, it should be taken after meals or with antacids. Buffered or enteric coated forms of aspirin are available but more expensive. Side effects, in addition to gastritis, are tinnitus and prolonged bleeding time. The client may adjust his dose to minimize tinnitus by gradually reducing the dosage by 1 or 2 tablets a day until the tinnitus stops. The client should also observe bleeding precautions and avoid cuts and bruises.

If the high doses of aspirin are not tolerated or if aspirin is ineffective in reducing inflammation and pain, nonsteroid antiinflammatory agents may be used. These are: indomethacin (Indocin), phenylbutazone (Butazolidin), oxyphenbutazone (Tandearil), fenoprofen (Nalfon), ibuprofen (Motrin), sulindac (Clinoril), and naprosyn (Naproxen). Indomethacin has analgesic, antipyretic, and antiinflammatory effects. Side effects include anorexia, nausea and vomiting, peptic ulcer, depression, confusion, and psychosis. Because of the side effects, indomethacin is not recommended for long-term use. Phenylbutazone and oxyphenbutazone are antiinflammatory analgesics. These drugs also have many toxic effects such as peptic ulcer, dermatitis, sodium retention, anemia, leukopenia and thrombocytopenia; long-term use is not advised. Frequent blood studies should be performed if the drugs are used for long periods of time. Ibuprofen, fenoprofen, and sulindac have antiinflammatory and analgesic properties and because the side effects are fewer, these drugs can be used for longer periods of time. Side effects are rash, nausea and vomiting, dizziness, and decreased prothrombin time. The nurse should instruct the client about these effects and urge frequent blood tests for prothrombin time. Antimalarial drugs such as hydroxychloroquine (Plaquenil) offer antiinflammatory effects for some clients. Beneficial effects of these drugs often do not occur for 3 to 6 months. Side effects include neuromyopathy, leukopenia, and retinal changes. Clients who are on this therapy should have a regular eye examination.

Corticosteroids offer the best antiinflammatory response and are used when previous therapy with aspirin and nonsteroid antiinflammatory agents is not effective. The purpose of the corticosteroids is to relieve the symptoms, particularly during acute exacerbations, and because they do not prevent joint destruction they must be given in addition to aspirin therapy. The side effects of electrolyte imbalance, edema, and pathological fractures make long-term use prohibitive. The client who is receiving steroids should be closely monitored. Doses are increased and decreased gradually and given at specific time intervals to enhance metabolism of the drug. The client must be instructed about the use of the drug so he can comply with the therapy. If the client undergoes surgery he will require additional steroids to prevent adrenal insufficiency after surgery. Steroids are administered orally, intramuscularly, or intraarticularly to specific joints. The dose of the drug is individual to the client's needs.

Gold therapy is another therapeutic modality that is used when inflammation is not relieved by previously discussed drugs. Aurothioglucose (Solganal) and gold sodium thiomalate (Myochrysine) are the most common preparations. It is not known how this drug acts, but the ultimate effect is reduction of the synovitis.[7] The drug is given intramuscularly, with a 10-mg test dose given initially. If no vasomotor effects such as flushing or fainting occur, the dose is followed a week later with a 25-mg dose. If tolerated, the dose is increased to 50 mg weekly to a total dose of 1 g. Drug levels are then maintained by tapering the dose of 50 mg every other week to every third or fourth week, depending on the recurrence of symptoms. Side effects include dermatitis, stomatitis, skin rash with pruritus, and gold deposits on the cornea. Kidney damage and nephritis are not uncommon, and the client's urine should be tested for proteinuria when receiving gold therapy. If any symptoms of the side effects occur, the drug is discontinued.

Nursing process for common health problems

Penicillamine is another drug that may be used to reduce the inflammation and subsequent pain and morning stiffness of RA. The action is unknown, but it is presumed to act on the immune system and reduce immune complexes in the serum and synovial fluid. The drug is given in initial doses of 250 mg daily and increased over 6 to 12 weeks to 500 to 750 mg daily. Side effects include pruritus, rash, anorexia, nausea, and vomiting. Bone marrow depression and nephropathy are toxic effects of use, and the nurse should encourage the client to be monitored for blood count and urinalysis.

As a final approach for clients who are unresponsive to other therapies, *immunosuppressive agents* such as azathioprine (Imuran) or cyclophosphamide (Cytoxan) may be used.

Relieving pain. Pain compounds immobility by causing discomfort as the client moves. Often simple activities of raising an arm or turning to the side are unbearable. Unless the pain is relieved, the dangerous cycle of pain, immobility, and contractures may result.

The need for pain relief should be anticipated by the nurse and client. Periods of immobility, particularly during sleeping, make the client more susceptible to stiffness and pain. Pain is relieved by analgesics and applications of heat or cold, as well as by supporting the joints with splints.

Pain relief from analgesics may be obtained from the analgesic properties of the drugs used to reduce inflammation. Analgesics such as acetaminophen (Tylenol) or dextropropoxyphene (Darvon) may also be used. The client should be instructed that these drugs are for pain relief and he should continue to take the other antiinflammatory drugs as prescribed. Narcotic analgesics are generally avoided, because pain relief therapy may be of a long duration. The pain medication should be taken on a schedule that offers the most relief and is suited to the client's life style. Because pain and stiffness are greater after periods of immobility, the client may plan to take analgesics 30 minutes before rising or before exercise or planned activities.

Applications of dry or moist heat may be used over the entire body to manage generalized pain or locally for involved joints. Heat relaxes muscles, reduces edema, and stimulates circulation. A hot tub or shower is the most convenient way to apply heat. A hot bath in the morning followed by 20 minutes of rest may help the client be more comfortable in carrying out daily activities. Warm soaks may be applied to aching joints. A towel that has been soaked in warm water and wrung out may be applied to the limbs. A plastic sheet can be wrapped around the towel to hold in the heat and prevent wetness. The heat usually lasts about 20 to 30 minutes and must be reapplied.

Penetrating heat can be obtained from dipping the affected joints in hot paraffin. The client is instructed to heat 4 pounds (1.8 kg) of paraffin with 2 to 4 ounces of mineral oil in a double boiler. The mixture is heated over low heat until it melts and then is cooled until a white film appears. The affected part should be shaved before it is dipped into the paraffin. It is immersed eight or ten times and covered with a towel and plastic to hold the heat. A paintbrush may be used to apply the paraffin to larger, inaccessible areas. The paraffin may be left on the involved part for 30 to 90 minutes and then peeled off and saved for reuse.

Heat may also be given by diathermy or ultrasound treatments or by the heat from an electric light bulb. Heat from an electric bulb is given at a distance of 12 to 18 inches with caution for safety.

The Hubbard tank may be used to relieve pain. The buoyant water reduces weight bearing, and warmth relaxes tense muscles. Hubbard tank therapy is particularly helpful in relieving pain so that range of motion can be improved.

Cold applications are used occasionally on the premise that the cold decreases the joint pain during acute exacerbations. The applications can be made from ice wrapped in a plastic bag and applied to the involved joint or by rubbing an ice cube over the involved area. Cold applications should be used for only 20 minutes at a time.

Providing for rest. Systemic effects of the disease such as fatigue, as well as the pain and inflammation, increase the client's needs for rest. Rest includes the physical and emotional rest, as well as localized rest of the involved joints. During the acute stage the client may be on bed rest to permit inflamed joints to rest and to relieve musculoskeletal stress.

When the client is in bed, he should be positioned to prevent contractures. A firm mattress with a board under it supports the body. Bedboards can be improvised for the bed at home with large plywood panels. It is most important to prevent flexion deformities. When the client is positioned on his back, there should be no pillows under his knees and only a small pillow under his head. A footboard can be used to prevent foot drop, and a trochanter roll used to prevent external rotation. The supine position prevents flexion contractures of the knees and spine. When the client is prone or sidelying, he should be in equally good alignment.

Localized rest of the involved joints may be obtained from splints, braces, or traction. These devices may be particularly useful during sleep when flexion is dominant to protect the joint. The nurse can explain the use of the equipment to the client and teach a family member how to apply the brace, splint, or traction.

Later, as the client improves, he should plan periods of activity alternated with rest to prevent fatigue. A time for a nap should be a specific part of each day's activities.

Maintaining mobility. It is imperative that the client with RA maintain mobility and range of joint motion. The extent of mobility varies with the course of the disease, but exercises and activities of daily living should be planned to maintain and increase mobility.

The client is encouraged to do as much for himself as possible. It is often easy for the nurse to do things for the client because the pain, discomfort, and dependency can elicit sympathy. The nurse should understand these problems but should gently encourage the client to be independent. The client should be permitted to move at his own pace when performing his activities. The nurse should not convey a feeling of hurry or impatience. There is a psychological benefit from mobility. The client who can get up, dress, and groom himself ultimately feels better. Simple chores or diversional activity may add to a feeling of usefulness.

If the client is on bed rest during a period of exacerbation, he should do active and passive range-of-motion exercises to prevent contractures that limit mobility. Later, a specific exercise program may be developed to promote muscle strengthening and to teach the client appropriate methods of using the muscles to maintain mobility. Exercises are done slowly, increased gradually, and not carried past the point of being painful. Different types of exercises are used, and the nurse works with the physical therapist, client, and family to develop an exercise program compatible with the client's needs.

Passive exercises are done by the nurse, physical therapist or client's family while the client relaxes his muscles. These exercises maintain and improve range of motion, particularly in acute exacerbations when joints are severely inflamed.

Isometric exercises are accomplished by muscle setting and do not involve joint motion. They are done to preserve muscle strength. The client is instructed to contract the particular muscle group for 6 to 10 seconds and relax for an equal time. These should be done several times a day.

Resistive exercises are those done actively by the client with manual or mechanical resistance. The purpose of these exercises is to develop muscle strength. To do these exercises, the client pushes against a resistance such as the hand of the nurse, therapist, or family member or against a fixed object such as a foot board.

Activity should be planned to conserve energy and prevent stress on the joints, as well as preserve range of motion. Many aids can be devised to save motion. A trapeze, for instance, can help the client get out of bed.

When the client is out of bed, he should use proper body mechanics. He should wear shoes that give support. The chair should be firm, fit the height of the client, and have arm rests. Low, soft chairs are not suitable for the client with arthritis. If necessary, the toilet seat can be adapted with a special elevated seat so that the client does not have to bend to sit on the toilet. After sitting, he may find that his joints have become stiff. Flexing the legs several times before rising prepares the muscles to support the body.

Clothing may be difficult to put on, and the nurse can suggest ways to dress. Dresses that zip in the front, for instance, are easiest to wear. There are special long-handled devices that can be used to pull up zippers and put on shoes and stockings. Zippers are easier to use than buttons; often clothing can be redesigned. The range of motion used in dressing provides exercise and gives the client a sense of independence and accomplishment without undue frustration.

Restoring function. Surgery is indicated when medical therapy fails to reduce inflammation and pain is to the point that the client is unable to perform his daily activities. There are several types of surgery that can be used, and the decision to perform surgery is based on the progress of the disease, attitude of the client toward surgery, and the expected outcome.

A *synovectomy* is a palliative procedure done to remove excess synovial fluid and tissue in order to prevent recurrence of inflammation. It can produce a drastic improvement in range of motion, particularly of the knee, elbow, and wrist joints. After a synovectomy, a compression dressing is applied. Activity is resumed gradually, and muscle-setting exercises are done before weight bearing to prepare for full range of motion.

An *arthrotomy* is an opening in the joint that in this instance is created to remove damaged tissue or calcium deposits. A compression dressing is applied after surgery and the joint protected until healing takes place. Activity is increased gradually and strength restored with active exercise.

An *arthrodesis* is the fusion of the joint to give stability, correct deformity, and reduce pain. A cast is applied after surgery until healing and fixation have occurred. Because fusion is permanent and limits motion, this surgery is done only when other approaches are not useful.

Arthroplasty is the plastic reconstruction of a joint to permit mobility and weight bearing and alleviate pain. The shoulders, elbows, wrists, hands, fingers, hips, knees, ankles, and feet can be reconstructed with rearrangement of the existing joint or insertion of a prosthesis. The most common surgeries, however, are those of the hip, knee, and hand.

Hip arthroplasty. Total hip arthroplasty involves reconstruction of one or both hips so the client can walk without pain. Usually the acetabulum is reamed out and a polyethylene cup is affixed with special cement. The head of the femur is replaced with a prosthesis and fitted into the cup (Fig. 11-29).

PREOPERATIVE NURSING CARE. Before surgery the client should receive instructions about the surgery and postoperative course. He should practice coughing and deep breathing exercises, using the overbed frame with a trapeze, and toileting in a recumbent position. Muscle-setting exercises that will be used after surgery can be practiced at this time.

POSTOPERATIVE NURSING CARE. The care plan after surgery includes the following goals: to maintain immobility during the immediate postoperative period, prevent cardiopulmonary complications, prevent infection, manage pain, and prepare for weight bearing.

1. *Maintaining immobility.* Nursing care after a total hip replacement is directed toward maintaining the leg in abduction for healing and later toward helping the client resume normal activity. Immediately after the operation, the hip is maintained in abduction and internal rotation with splints or with sandbags and traction. Russell's traction may be used to reduce muscle spasm and maintain abduction.

FIG. 11-29
Austin Moore prosthesis. (From Edmonson, A., and Crenshaw, A.H., editors: Campbell's operative orthopedics, ed. 6, St. Louis, 1980, The C.V. Mosby Co.)

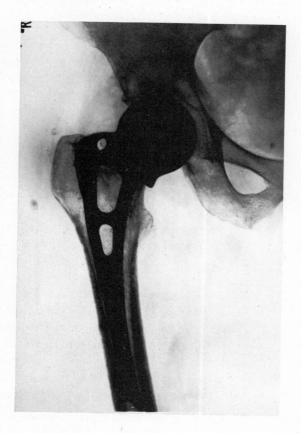

Nursing process for common health problems

Because the client must maintain this position for several days after surgery, his bed should be made with an air pressure mattress or similar device. The client can raise himself up with a trapeze to assist the nurses when back care is given or when he is using the bedpan. When the bed is changed, several personnel should support the client off the bed while the linens are changed quickly. Because the client is immobilized, the nurse must also plan to prevent hazards of immobility.

2. *Preventing cardiopulmonary complications.* After surgery the nurse should assess the surgery site for bleeding. A Hemovac drain may be inserted and should be emptied as needed. The client is encouraged to cough and take deep breaths. Intermittent positive pressure breathing (IPPB) treatments may also be ordered and thigh-high elastic hose worn to prevent circulatory stasis and thromboembolism. The nurse should promote adequate circulation and observe the alignment of splints, sandbags, or traction. The uninvolved limbs should be put through full range-of-motion exercises. Both limbs should be assessed for circulation and neurological status.

3. *Preventing infection.* The infection rate after surgery has been observed to be as great as 2% to 11% and may occur during the immediate postoperative period or be delayed. The nurse should maintain asepsis with dressing changes and report fever, pain, or drainage from the operative site. Antibiotics and wound irrigations may be used to treat the infection; occasionally the prosthesis must be removed and the insertion of a new prosthesis or hip pinning attempted.

4. *Managing pain.* For the first few days after surgery the client may experience pain from the incision and muscle spasms. Narcotic analgesics and muscle relaxants may be used regularly to provide pain relief. The nurse should consider the client's age, respiratory status and the client's pain threshold when administering narcotics, but the drugs should not be withheld to the point of discomfort for the client. Other pain relief strategies such as positioning and relaxation exercises can also be used.

5. *Preparing for weight bearing.* After surgery the client begins to prepare for weight bearing. On the first postoperative day he can begin active foot and ankle extension and flexion exercises as well as knee flexion exercises. On the fourth or fifth postoperative day, the client may be instructed to do gluteal and quadriceps muscle-setting exercises. As strength improves, the client progressively stands at the bedside and walks and learns transfer activities to the toilet and chair. A cane or walker may be used for the first few days to provide balance.

DISCHARGE INSTRUCTIONS. When the client returns home, he should be aware of maintaining alignment of the involved hip and be instructed about preventing stress of adduction until his examination by the surgeon in 4 to 6 weeks. The client should not cross his legs for 3 months. He should sit in chairs with high supportive seats and a straight back and should not bend his hip more than 90 degrees. An elevated toilet seat may be more comfortable to use. Riding in a car for more than an hour is not advisable. When sleeping, the client should place a pillow between his knees if in a sidelying position, or otherwise sleep on his back. Later, exercises may be added to increase strength and mobility, and eventually the client can resume most previously enjoyed activities.

Arthroplasty of the knee. Total knee arthroplasty can be performed to reduce pain and to increase stability. Knees are generally not as easily replaced as hips; consequently clients are selected judiciously for this procedure.

The procedure involves removing synovial tissue and inserting a tibial plateau prosthesis. A compression dressing or cast is applied following insertion of the prosthesis to maintain immobility during healing. A Hemovac drainage apparatus may be used to collect drainage. The nurse should make careful assessments about the amount and location of any bleeding.

An exercise regimen is initiated on the first or second day after surgery. The cast may be bivalved to permit quadricep and hamstring muscle-setting exercises. Ankle flexion and extension are also permitted at this time. Active-assistive range-of-motion exercises are started on the second to fifth day. Partial weight bearing with the use of crutches or walkers is usually permitted on the fourth or fifth day, but full weight bearing is not allowed for 3 months until the cement used with the prosthesis is set up. Rocking chair and bicycling exercises are helpful for increasing strength during recovery.

Arthroplasty of the hands and elbows. Mobility in arthritic joints of the hands and elbows can be achieved by the removal of synovial tissue and the insertion of Silastic prostheses that serve as joints. As healing begins, the client performs range-of-motion exercises to achieve maximum use of the affected joints.

Following the therapeutic plan for health maintenance. Rheumatoid arthritis occurs at the age of greatest productivity and may interrupt the client's home and career plans. Injury to body organs can produce changes in body image, and the client may feel depressed. Chronic illnesses and pain are wearing on the individual, and it becomes increasingly difficult to maintain a normal lifestyle. The nurse can help the client set practical goals and maintain optimum health.

The client should plan to follow health maintenance activities that include a well-balanced diet, rest, and prevention of the systemic effects of RA.

The diet should be planned for the client's calorie needs, and if he is overweight may include calorie reduction. If the client is anemic, additional iron and protein should be included in the diet. It should be emphasized that fad diets are not cures for RA and the client's sensible diet is for his best health.

A community health nurse may visit the client in the home to make suggestions on adapting home activities to the client's abilities. Often, the nurse and client can develop a daily activity schedule for the client to assume realistic responsibilities while coping with arthritis. The Arthritis Foundation also has many helpful suggestions for modifying home activities to make life more comfortable.

Sexual activities may be disrupted by painful crippling, fatigue, or depression. The person with arthritis may find that sexual activities may be enjoyed if initiated at the time of day he feels best, perhaps after use of analgesia and heat therapy. Modification of position may also make sexual intercourse more comfortable. Steroids released during intercourse have a beneficial effect on the inflammatory nature of the disease.

Some individuals with rheumatoid arthritis are prone to iridocyclitis, which can cause glaucoma or cataracts. The client should, therefore, be advised to have a slit-lamp examination every 3 to 6 months. Mydriatics and steroids are used to manage the iridocyclitis.

It may be necessary to change career objectives, and the client can be referred to several community agencies. Vocational rehabilitation, sheltered workshops, and rehabilitation centers offer employment retraining for persons with arthritis. If the client is unemployed, he should be directed to sources of financial aid, such as Social Security benefits or unemployment compensation.

Persons with chronic illnesses are often willing to try anything to find a cure. Clients with rheumatoid arthritis should be counseled to avoid quick cure remedies and patent medicines. Therapeutic intervention directed by health professionals is the best means for coping with arthritis.

 Evaluation. Evaluation of the nursing care plan for the client with rheumatoid arthritis is continuous and provides information for modification of plans as the client's status changes with increasing or decreasing mobility.

EXPECTED OUTCOMES

The client and/or family can:
1. Describe arthritis.
2. Describe plans for preventing or managing joint inflammation (rest, splints, anti-inflammatory agents).
3. Describe plans for preventing or managing pain (analgesics, rest, applications of heat or cold).
4. Describe plans for maintaining mobility (exercises, splints, self-care activities).
5. State limits of activity.
6. State use, dosage, time, route, and side effects of prescribed medications.
7. Describe plans for health maintenance (rest, adequate diet, weight control, adequate urinary and bowel elimination).
8. Describe plans for follow-up care and use of community resources.

Gout

Gout is an inflammatory disease of the joints. The onset is abrupt and usually involves the big toe. Gout is a genetic defect of purine metabolism in which there is an elevated blood level of uric acid and crystallate deposits *(tophi)* in the joints. Gout affects men 20 to 60, primarily those over 40. The predisposition for gout is inherited.

 Assessment. The symptoms of gout are caused by the deposition of uric acid crystals in the joint. The joint becomes reddened and painful, and tophi may appear. The disease is characterized by remissions and exacerbations, although some individuals have only several attacks whereas others have progressive disease.

Planning and intervention. Objectives of treatment are to reduce the serum purine levels and relieve the pain. Purine metabolism can be reduced by certain drugs and by eliminating purine from the diet. Uricosuric drugs such as probenecid (Benemid) and salicylates increase the output of uric acid and hence lower serum uric acid levels. Allopurinol (Zyloprim) inhibits production of the enzyme that causes the formation of the uric acid crystals. This drug may be taken to prevent exacerbations of gout and should be taken daily even if the client is not experiencing pain.

Foods that are high in purine should be eliminated from the diet. These include shellfish, sardines, anchovies, liver, kidneys, and mushrooms. Fats and alcohol may precipitate an attack of gout and should be avoided.

When the pain is severe, the client may be instructed to rest. The nurse can suggest the use of a bed cradle to keep the covers off painful joints. Analgesics can be used to overcome the pain. Colchicine is particularly useful during an attack of gout. Colchicine may be given intravenously, followed by oral doses, until pain relief is obtained. The drug may cause severe nausea, vomiting, or diarrhea and should be discontinued when these symptoms appear. Indomethacin and phenylbutazone may also be used for pain relief.

Surgery may be done to remove tophi or improve joint mobility. The surgery is done when the acute exacerbation has subsided.

Bursitis

Bursitis is a painful inflammation of the connective tissue sac between the muscles, tendons, and bones, particularly of the shoulder, elbow, and knee. It occurs primarily in middle-aged persons, usually the result of repeated stress and pressure at the joint. "Tennis elbow" or "housemaid's knee" are common examples of acute bursitis. Toxins or infectious agents can also cause bursitis.

Planning and implementation. The inflammation may be treated by resting the affected part, splinting, applying dry heat, draining the bursa, aspirating calcium deposits, or injecting cortisone into the bursa. Analgesics may be given to relieve the pain, and physical therapy may be instituted to reestablish mobility of the affected joint.

Tenosynovitis

Tenosynovitis is an inflammation of the synovial sheath surrounding the tendon, which results from overstretching. The pain and swelling are relieved by moist heat and analgesics.

Carpal tunnel syndrome

The carpal tunnel is an area of the wrist bounded on three sides by bone and on the fourth by the transverse carpal ligament. Nine tendons and the median nerve pass through this tunnel. Compression of the nerve at this point is called the carpal tunnel syndrome (CTS).

Carpal tunnel syndrome is caused by the compression of the median nerve at the wrist. The compression can be precipitated by trauma, rheumatoid arthritis, a fracture, tumors, or simply by the chronic thickening of the synovial sheath of tendons. The syndrome occurs more frequently in women near menopause, raising the possibility of a hormonal relationship.

Assessment. The compression of the median nerve causes burning pain in the thumb, index, and middle fingers. In the morning the fingers may be swollen and stiff. Numbness and tingling may be present and are aggravated by repeated movement such as typing. Atrophy of the thumb can occur if not treated. The syndrome is diagnosed by the symptoms, electromyogram, and decreased nerve conduction time. The symptoms can be elicited by tapping the median nerve at the wrist (Tinel's sign).

Planning and implementation. The nerve compression can be relieved medically or surgically. In conservative therapy cortisone can be injected into the tunnel and the joint splinted. In the surgical approach the client receives a local, regional, or general anesthetic, and the transverse carpal ligament is resected to relieve pressure on the median nerve. After surgery a compression dressing is applied and a splint used to support the wrist and ulnar aspect of the hand. The client should be encouraged to exercise the fingers by making a fist and releasing it several times each hour. Pain relief is provided with analgesics, and the sutures are removed in 10 to 14 days.

Osteomalacia

Osteomalacia is a decalcification of the bone from a poor dietary intake of vitamin D, absence of exposure to sunlight, or from intestinal malabsorption. This disease occurs in adults, particularly those with intestinal malabsorption syndromes (see Chapter 18). The bones become soft, and there may be pathological fractures. The degenerative process is reversed with adequate nutrition, sunshine, and vitamin D supplements.

Nursing process for common health problems

Multiple myeloma

Multiple myeloma is a malignant growth of the plasma cells of the bone marrow. The cause of the growth is unknown, but it involves protein synthesis, particularly in flat bones such as the skull, ribs, vertebrae, and pelvis.

Multiple myeloma is the most frequently occurring bone tumor. Men are affected two to three times more often than women, and the age of peak incidence is 50 to 60.

 Assessment. The symptoms of the tumor have slow onset and are often vague. There may be weight loss, weakness, anemia, back pain, or pathological fractures of the ribs or vertebrae. The diagnosis is based on x-ray studies and a biopsy specimen of the bone, increased serum calcium levels, and the presence of the *Bence-Jones protein* in the urine. Because the Bence-Jones protein only occurs in multiple myeloma, the test confirms the diagnosis.

 Planning and implementation. The disease is treated with radiation or various combinations of chemotherapy, or both. The nurse should be familiar with the specific therapy and plan care accordingly. (See Chapter 6 for discussion of the client receiving radiation therapy and for the client receiving chemotherapy.) Additional attention should be given to the client's nutritional status. Safety measures must be employed with turning, ambulation, and transfer because the client is susceptible to pathological fractures. Psychological support is necessary as the client adapts to terminal illness.

Osteoporosis

Osteoporosis is a degeneration of bone tissue because of an imbalance between the normal deposition of bone tissue and its withdrawal. The imbalance can be caused by endocrine diseases such as hyperparathyroidism, Cushing's disease, and diabetes mellitus. Women who are past menopause often have osteoporosis caused by estrogen withdrawal. Osteoporosis can also result from inactivity when the stress placed on the bones is insufficient for deposition of bone tissue. This type of osteoporosis is noted in aging persons and those persons who have had prolonged bed rest.

 Assessment. Persons with osteoporosis may complain of low back pain or musculoskeletal aching. The bone mass may decrease as a result of absorption of protein and minerals. There may also be pathological fractures caused by the increased porosity of the bones. The degenerative process is also reflected in diminution of stature. Furthermore, there may be an increase in urinary calcium, especially at night as calcium withdrawal increases.

Planning and implementation. Treatment is directed toward preserving skeletal strength and correcting hormonal imbalances. Corsets or braces may be used to support the body or limbs. Weight-bearing activity, such as walking, or active exercises in bed or using a tilt table help promote bone tissue regeneration. The nurse should encourage clients who can be out of bed to do so, and those who are in bed should engage in active or passive range-of-motion exercises.

Estrogens may be given to postmenopausal women to combat the degenerative process. The diet should be adequate in vitamin D and calcium to promote bone strength. Osteoporosis is reversed when endocrine imbalances are corrected.

Degenerative joint disease

Degenerative joint disease (osteoarthritis) is a noninflammatory degeneration and atrophy of the cartilage. Degeneration of the joints is a normal process of aging that begins around age 20. The weight-bearing joints of the lower extremities are involved initially. There is a proliferation of fibroblasts and deposition of bone at the joint capsule and a thickening of the synovium. The joint destruction is usually not severe and only one or two joints are affected. There is no systemic involvement.

Because osteoarthritis is a normal process of aging, the incidence is widespread. The disease is not usually manifested until after age 40 and is aggravated by poor posture, trauma, stress on the involved joints, and obesity.

Osteoarthritis is recognized by muscle spasms that produce pain. The pain increases as the day progresses. There is stiffness, particularly after rest. Ultimately there may be contractures.

The symptoms of osteoarthritis are alleviated by rest and mild analgesics, such as aspirin or antiinflammatory analgesics such as ibuprofen (Motrin). Clients usually adapt to the degenerative changes as a part of aging and can maintain most normal activity. The nurse should encourage the usual activities of daily living that involve the use of all joints. If the client can lose weight, less stress will be put on the muscles and weight-bearing joints and range of motion will be more easily maintained. A balance of rest and activity is necessary for optimum health for these individuals.

COMMON HEALTH PROBLEMS THAT OCCUR ACROSS THE LIFE SPAN
Musculoskeletal trauma

The musculoskeletal system has elastic limits, and the stress placed on the muscles, tendons, ligaments, cartilage, and bones is proportional to the force exerted. When stress is placed on these tissues at rest, they change to accommodate the stress. Stress injuries to musculoskeletal tissue can result from a striking force, unequal pressure, or tissue weakness; the muscles and tendons may be stretched or torn, and the bones fractured. Specific musculoskeletal trauma such as fracture, injury to soft tissue (strain, sprain, contusion), dislocation, multiple trauma, and battering involve individuals of all ages and are significant causes of death or disability for specific age groups.

Fracture. A fracture is a break in any bone of the body and can be described by the type, the extent of injury, and the line of the fracture.

There are two types of fractures: complete and incomplete. A *complete* fracture involves separation of bone ends. In an *incomplete* fracture, the bone ends do not separate. Children whose bones are more flexible often have an incomplete fracture, known as a greenstick fracture.

A fracture may be identified by the extent of injury to surrounding tissue. A *simple* fracture does not break the skin or damage other tissue. A *compound* fracture produces an opening in the skin, and the bone protrudes. There is more pain and chance for infection with a compound fracture. A *complicated* fracture produces injury to organs as the bone ends pierce other structures. Injuries to the bladder or lungs are common examples of a complicated fracture.

The *line* of the fracture describes the injury to the bone. A directional description is given by the terms *spiral, transverse,* and *oblique* fractures. In a *comminuted* fracture the bone is broken into several chips. An *impacted* fracture occurs when the bone ends are telescoped by the force of the injury (Fig. 11-30).

Fractures are caused by trauma or stress on weakened bones. The type of force causing the injury determines the type and extent of the fracture. The force can be *tensile,* in which case the bones are pulled apart, or *compressive,* in which the bones are impacted. A *shearing* force causes the bones to break at a point distal to the force.

Fractures can also be caused by inadequate bone mineralization. These are

FIG. 11-30
Types and line of fractures. (From Ingalls, A. Joy, and Salerno, M. Constance: Maternal and child health nursing, ed. 4, St. Louis, 1979, The C.V. Mosby Co.)

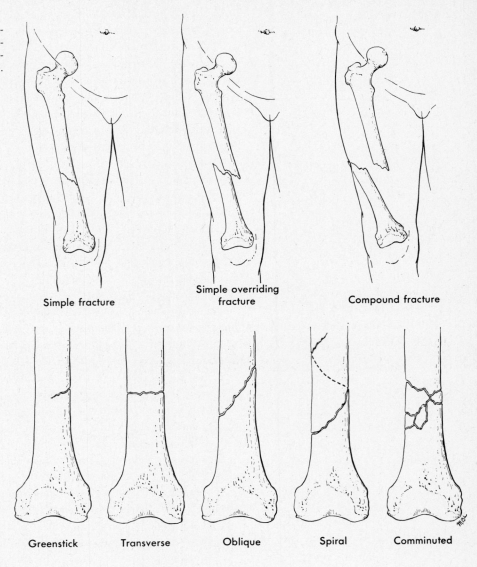

Simple fracture

Simple overriding
fracture

Compound fracture

Greenstick

Transverse

Oblique

Spiral

Comminuted

referred to as *pathological fractures* and can occur from long-term steroid therapy, estrogen withdrawal, osteoporosis, prolonged inactivity, or bone cancer.

Fractures are common throughout the life span. Interestingly, the type of fracture is frequently specific to an age group. Fractures in neonates may be caused by birth injuries. Young children are prone to fractures of the humerus, clavicle, femur, and tibia, which usually result from falls. Adolescents and young adults may have a Colles' fracture of the wrist, which occurs when the hands are outstretched to prevent a fall. The most common fracture in adults is a fracture of the pelvis and ribs from automobile accidents. Older persons are most susceptible to fractures caused by normal demineralization of bone and diminished sensory acuity. The most common fractures in older adults are fractures of the hip or femur, and women are more likely to suffer these fractures.

Persons at risk for fractures are those who are involved in sports activities. Others are those who do not wear seat belts in cars or helmets when cycle riding or who drive while drinking. Also at risk are those clients with bone cancer, the elderly, or individuals receiving steroid therapy. Care plans should reflect safety measures for these clients.

 Assessment. When obtaining a nursing history from a client with a fracture, the nurse should ascertain a brief account of the events preceding the fracture and inspect and palpate the involved area as well as surrounding tissue. The initial indication of a fracture is *pain,* which occurs at the site of the fracture. Pain may be more intense if the fracture is compound or complicated and there is damage to surrounding tissue or organs. There is *swelling* and *ecchymosis* at the site. *Muscle spasm* may produce shortening of the involved limb, and range of joint motion is painful or impossible. *Crepitus,* a grating sound of tissue, may be evident if the fracture is compound.

When assessing the client who has had a fracture, the nurse must also determine the extent of injury to other tissues and organs and identify other problems associated with the accident. Bleeding may be apparent, as well as evidence of lung injury, skull fracture, contusion, confusion, paresthesia, numbness, tingling, or spinal cord injury. (See discussion of the multiply injured client later in this chapter.)

There is increased likelihood of *fat embolism* with compound fractures because minute globules of fat may be dislodged as the fractured bone protrudes through tissue. The nurse should therefore assess the client for petechiae in buccal membranes and conjunctival sacs, chest pain, increased temperature, dyspnea, cough, or confusion that might indicate the presence of fat embolism. See Chapters 20 and 21 for further discussion of embolism. The diagnosis of a fracture is based on the history of the injury and the clinical symptoms and confirmed by x-ray studies.

> **Data analysis**
> Data analysis may reveal nursing diagnoses of pain, fear, impaired mobility, and self-care deficits.

Planning and implementation. The nursing care plan begins at the time of the accident, continues through definitive care that follows reduction and immobilization for healing, and concludes during the rehabilitation stage as the client prepares for return to his usual state of mobility. The roles of the nurse and the client throughout the care plan change as the nurse assumes more responsibility for self-care activities at the time of the injury and immobilization to the point that the client assumes responsibility for his care during rehabilitation.

Immediate care. Initial treatment for any type of fracture is to immobilize the joints above and below the fractured bone. Items from the scene of the accident may be improvised to splint the fracture. Boards, rolled newspaper, or cardboard may be used to support the limb and maintain alignment. Emergency vehicles are often equipped with plastic inflatable casts that can be used to support the involved limb while the client is transported. Utmost care must be used to prevent further injury. No attempt should be made to reduce the fracture or realign the bone. If there is a break in the skin, it should be covered with a clean (or sterile, if available) dressing. Bleeding can be controlled by direct pressure. Cold compresses can be applied to reduce swelling and pain. To prevent shock, the client should be kept quiet, lying down, and warm. Medication for pain relief and muscle relaxants to prevent muscle spasm should be obtained as soon as possible.

Transportation of the client with a fracture should be planned before he is moved. The fracture must be supported and immobilized while the client is moved to a car or ambulance. If there is suspicion of a back injury, the client should be transported on a firm surface and logrolled to prevent twisting the spine (see Fig. 10-41). General principles of splinting before transportation apply in most instances. Victims of accidents should be splinted where they are with minimal movement to change position. A continuous pull should be exerted while splinting. Special devices such as the half-ring splint may be used by qualified emergency personnel. Wounds should be covered before splinting. Finally, assessments should be made to ensure that the splint is not interfering with circulation or putting pressure on any area. The splint can be padded if needed.

If other injuries are present, these should be managed before transportation. Priorities include airway maintenance, control of hemorrhage, and treatment of shock. Airway management and insertion of an intravenous catheter for intravenous infusions may be done at this time.

Reduction and healing. Fractures in which there is bone discontinuity must be reduced, aligned, and maintained in approximation for healing. Reduction of the fracture can be accomplished manually by exerting a pull to realign the bones. This is referred to as *closed reduction,* because surgical intervention is not required, although anesthesia may be used to induce muscle relaxation. *Open reduction* is a surgical approach that involves an incision of the involved area to manipulate the bones to alignment.

Reduction is maintained by external or internal fixation. *External fixation* can be achieved with the use of casts and/or traction for immobilization. *Internal fixation* is accomplished by the insertion of plates, pins or wires at the time of surgery. Common examples are the Jewett nail, Steinmann pin, and the Kirschner wire. With fixation, the client has more mobility while healing takes place and may be out of bed and have limited weight bearing on the fracture.

Bone healing begins several hours after the fracture. A *hematoma* forms around the broken bone ends to secure them. This hematoma is unique because it is not absorbed. Instead it forms a base for granulation tissue that provides support during healing. Within one day after the injury *cellular growth* is evident as capillaries extend into the hematoma and fibroblasts proliferate. By the sixth to tenth day the tissue contains calcium, cartilage, and osteoblasts and is referred to as a *provisional callus,* which secures the bones but does not support weight bearing. Within 3 weeks osteoblasts form an osteoid matrix, and *true callus* continues to support the fracture. Blood vessels develop within 2 to 3 months in adults (earlier in children). Stress on the bone increases osteoblastic activity to produce tissue resembling the parent bone, a process known as *modeling.* In children the process of healing a fracture before the age of epiphyseal closure is known as *remodeling.* The irregularities of the bone caused by the fracture are filled in and the angles rounded off, giving a straighter appearance to the bone; the callus provides structure despite malalignment. The younger the child and the closer the fracture to the growth plate the greater the extent of remodeling, even to spontaneously correcting the deformity. The final stage of healing occurs as the callus is absorbed and union, or *ossification,* is achieved.

The rate and result of bone healing depend on the age of the client and the type of bone injured. Children, whose bones normally have more stress and are more elastic, heal rapidly. In addition callus formation and absorption are increased in children, whereas in adults the callus may be present for 2 to 3 months. Older persons usually have less stress on the bones and may have osteoporosis or arteriosclerosis, which further delays healing.

Healing is facilitated by increased blood supply and stress on the involved bone. For this reason exercises that increase circulation and mobility as well as early ambulation are advised. Devices such as casts, cast-braces, or external fixation devices permit immobilization of the fracture while allowing mobility. In some instances when bone healing is slow, an electrical stimulator may be implanted in the bone to induce osteogenesis.

If the fracture occurs in flat bones or bones with a good blood supply, healing time is shorter. If the fracture is at the epiphysis, premature fusion and the curtailment of bone growth are matters of concern in children and adolescents.

Union of the fracture depends on the regenerative abilities of the bone. There may be *delayed union,* in which healing time is longer than anticipated. This may be caused by an infection or by stress on the bone before healing is completed. *Nonunion* is the inability of the fracture to heal. In cases of nonunion, it may be necessary to reset the bone or to devise other means for establishing bone continuity.

Complications of healing include infection, nerve damage, circulatory impairment, contractures, and posttraumatic arthritis.

Evaluation. The nurse should continually evaluate the client during the healing process and report any untoward signs.

EXPECTED OUTCOMES

The client and/or family can:
1. Describe fracture.
2. Maintain reduction of fracture with external or internal fixation.
3. Describe care of cast if discharged with applied cast.
4. Return to usual state of mobility and self-care.
5. State indication for need for health care services and knowledge of community resources.

Injury to soft tissue

Sprain. A sprain is an injury of a ligament. Sprains result from complete tear injuries or stretching of the ligament, as occurs during a fall that causes hyperextension of a joint and stretching of the ligament. Sprains are frequently caused by sports injuries and may occur secondary to a dislocation.

Sprains are more likely to occur at the knee, wrist, or ankle where twisting motion accompanies a force. Those who are active in sports are at a greater risk for sprains.

Assessment. The symptoms of a sprain result from the tearing or stretching of the ligament. The client experiences *pain* and *swelling*. An x-ray film may be taken to rule out a fracture.

Planning and implementation. The objective of care for a client with a sprain is to decrease swelling and relieve the pain. The painful swelling that follows a sprain can be minimized by *initial* applications of cold for 30 minutes to constrict blood vessels and prevent edema. If the injury has occurred several hours before treatment, applications of cold are not advisable. Rather, applications of

Nursing process for common health problems

heat to dilate the blood vessels and decrease edema of the involved area are used. The involved part should be elevated, and a splint or supportive bandage may be applied to provide support and decrease pain.

Internal derangement of the knee. A special sprain common to adolescents and young adults is an internal derangement of the knee.

ASSESSMENT. The internal and external lateral ligaments, posterior and anterior cruciate ligaments, and the internal and external semilunar cartilage provide stability for the knee. These are apt to be torn when stress is placed on the knee, as often occurs when the knee is rotated and the foot remains on the ground.

PLANNING AND IMPLEMENTATION. Torn ligaments may heal spontaneously with immobilization and rest or may be replaced with strips of fascia or tendons. The client is usually in a cast for 3 to 4 weeks and uses a knee support for several weeks after cast removal.

Torn cartilage is usually managed by immobilization or, if the symptoms are not relieved, by removal of the cartilage. A compression dressing is used after surgery, and the client may be permitted partial weight bearing in 24 to 36 hours. Quadriceps setting, patella setting, and straight leg raises improve strength. Full recovery can be expected in 3 months.

Strain. A strain is an injury to muscle caused by trauma or excessive stretching. There is pain and muscle spasm, which can be relieved by initial applications of cold, followed by applications of heat. Traction and muscle relaxants are used to prevent or manage muscle spasm.

Contusion. A contusion is an injury to soft tissue by a blunt force. The affected part is painful, swollen, and discolored. There may be bleeding, bruising, or hematoma formation. The contusion is treated symptomatically by reducing swelling and relieving pain. To reduce initial swelling, cold applications are used in order to constrict the blood vessels. Later, applications of heat may be used to promote absorption of fluid in edematous tissues. Elevating the affected part prevents swelling by promoting venous return. Pain can be managed with analgesics and limiting the movement of the affected part.

Dislocation. A dislocation is the disjoining of bones from their sockets. A dislocation can be caused by genetic defects of the socket (congenital hip dislocation is discussed earlier in this chapter) or from trauma to the joint. The force that causes the trauma is greater than that which produces a strain or sprain, and the joint becomes dislocated. Individuals who play contact sports are at particular risk for this injury.

Assessment. A dislocated joint is assessed by the history of the injury and observation on the involved joint. The joint is painful, and there is a change in the shape of the joint, loss of mobility, and a shortening in the length of the affected extremity. There may be hemorrhage, soft tissue injury, and tearing of surrounding ligaments. The nurse should assess the client for nerve and blood vessel damage distal to the dislocation by checking the pulse and evaluating movement and absence of numbness and tingling.

Planning and implementation. The initial objective of treatment is to immobilize the joint to prevent further tearing. A dislocated shoulder can be temporarily immobilized by putting the involved arm in a sling and securing the arm across the chest with a bandage (Fig. 11-31). A dislocated hip may be immobilized by placing a firm surface at the lateral side of the affected hip and leg and securing it to the body or the uninvolved leg. Applications of ice may be used to reduce swelling, and muscle relaxants are given as soon as feasible to prevent muscle spasm and further injury.

Reduction of the dislocated joint is accomplished by manipulating the joint back into the socket. This is done under general anesthesia when muscles are relaxed. After reduction of the dislocation has been achieved, the involved part is put into a cast to immobilize the joint until it heals.

Multiple trauma. Multiple trauma (multiple injuries) is a term used to describe a client who has several injuries from one incident. The trauma usually involves the musculoskeletal system as contusions, sprains, strains, fractures, and dislocations and may include other injuries such as head injuries (concussion), chest injuries (flail chest, wounds, tension pneumothorax), abdominal injuries, hemorrhage, and shock.

The multiple trauma is usually caused by an accident. Industrial accidents, automobile accidents, and motorcycle and bicycle accidents are common causes.

Assessment. The evidence of multiple trauma is varied, depending on the extent and location of the injury. Because more than one system may be involved, the nurse must set priorities for assessment that are inclusive as well as relevant to the injury. Priorities for assessment include the airway, breathing, circulation, bleeding, shock, chest injuries, spinal injuries, and level of consciousness. Other injuries such as fractures, sprains, and minor lacerations are assessed last because they do not present immediate threat to life.

The multiply injured young child requires special assessments. The child's head is large, and the liver and spleen are proportionately large for the child's small body. More injuries occur here, and the nurse should make special observation for cranial and abdominal injuries. The airway is also small and is easily obstructed with blood or mucus, requiring immediate intervention.

Planning and implementation. Intervention is initiated at the scene of the accident and is planned to deal with the most life-threatening aspects of the injury. Priorities for assessment and management are presented on p. 576. The client is usually transported to a critical care unit for further treatment of the injury and continuous monitoring.

Battering. Battering (child beating, battered child syndrome; battered wife syndrome, wife abuse, abused woman; elderly battering) is a part of a larger problem of abuse that includes neglect and emotional, sexual, or intellectual abuse. Battering is more appropriately considered a symptom of an interpersonal or family problem in which the dynamics of interpersonal relationships are in disequilibrium. Attention can be focused on the battered individual or the person doing the battering, but in essence the root of the problem is in the relationship in which there is (1) a potential for an individual to become abusive, (2) the unique situation of the powerlessness of the abused, and (3) a crisis that precipitates the physical abuse.[6]

Factors that have been identified that predispose to battering are unhealthy self-concept, family history of abuse models, fear of leaving the situation, or in the case of children, the inability to leave the situation.

The incidence of battering is difficult to ascertain, because many instances of battering are not reported. It is estimated that 4 million individuals are battered yearly.[2] Of these as many as 29% are adolescents.[6] Many states have laws that protect professionals from legal involvement when they report battering or

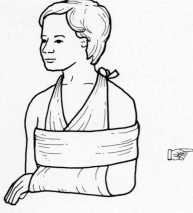

FIG. 11-31
Immobilizing dislocated shoulder with sling and bandage.

Nursing process for common health problems

PRIORITIES FOR ASSESSMENT AND MANAGEMENT OF MULTIPLE TRAUMA

A 60-second evaluation to assess for life-threatening conditions should be conducted and should include:

1. Airway
   a. Use head tilt, jaw thrust, airway adjuncts (including the esophageal obturator airway, endotracheal tube, and cricothyrotomy) as indicated.
   b. Prevent aspiration; have suction ready.
   c. Clear airway of debris.
2. Breathing
   a. Assure adequate oxygenation; do not withhold oxygen from a chronic obstructive lung disease patient.
   b. Assess lung sounds.
   c. Obtain arterial blood gas determinations if possible.
3. Circulation
   a. Assess pulses (carotid and femoral).
   b. Perform external cardiac massage if necessary.
4. Assess the vital signs for a baseline.
5. Correct hypovolemia.
   a. Initiate two or three IV infusions of Ringer's lactate solution with 14-gauge intracatheters into antecubital veins, a basilic cutdown, a saphenous cutdown, or a subclavian stick.
   b. Place antishock trousers under the patient.
   c. Inflate the antishock trousers if the systolic pressure drops below 100 mm Hg.
6. Protect the cervical spine.
   a. Apply a cervical collar and immobilize with sandbags.
   b. Place the patient on a backboard.
7. Control external bleeding.
   a. Direct pressure.
   b. Pressure points.
   c. Apply a tourniquet if it is a life-threatening situation.
   d. Estimate blood loss.
8. Evaluate the chest (quickly).
   a. Tension pneumothorax.
   b. Open chest wounds.
   c. Cardiac tamponade.
   d. Other major chest injuries.
9. Evaluate the neurological condition (quickly).
   a. Level of consciousness.
   b. Pupil size and reaction to light.
10. Splint fractures.
    a. Evaluate neurovascular status distal to the fracture site.
    b. Cover open wounds.
11. Transport.
12. Obtain and interpret a cross-table lateral cervical spine film.
13. Undress the patient completely.
14. Rapidly reevaluate airway, breathing, and circulation and vital signs.
15. Make a rapid systemic evaluation.
    a. Head, for lacerations and fractures.
    b. Ears, nose, and throat, for cerebrospinal fluid leak.
    c. Eyes, for trauma and pupil reactivity.
    d. Neck, for wounds.
    e. Chest, for wounds, heart sounds, and lung sounds.
    f. Abdomen for rigidity, pain, tenderness, and wounds.
    g. Spine, for trauma.
    h. Extremities, for movement, fractures, and neurovascular status.
    i. Hips, for fractures of hips and/or pelvis.
    j. Perineum, for blood or urine extravasation.
    k. Buttocks, for wounds.
    l. Back, for wounds.
16. Tetanus prophylaxis
17. Type and cross-match for six units of whole blood cells.
18. Obtain blood for testing: for hematocrit, hemoglobin, complete blood count, serum amylase level, prothrombin time, and partial thromboplastin time.
19. Place a Foley catheter; perform an IVP if indicated.
20. Insert a nasogastric tube.
21. Perform peritoneal lavage if indicated.
22. Antibiotics.
23. Steroids.
24. Consultation with surgical and medical specialties.

Immediate intervention is indicated for the following life-threatening emergencies:
Upper airway obstruction
Lower airway obstruction
Fractured larynx
Flail chest
Bilateral pneumothorax
Severe tension pneumothorax
Severe neurological trauma
Ruptured great vessel
Rapidly deteriorating vital signs
Cardiac arrest, pulmonary arrest, or both

From Barber, Janet, and Budassi, Susan: Mosby's manual of emergency care, St. Louis, 1979, The C.V. Mosby Co.

abuse and make the reporting of suspected abuse mandatory. Nurses should be familiar with the laws in the state in which they practice because they are often the first professionals to detect or suspect abuse.

☞ *Assessment.* The nurse is often the health care professional who observes the battered individual and obtains a family history presumptive of battering. The appearance and behavior of the battered individual are generally characteristic and include the results of burns, beatings, twisting of extremities, or battering against walls or furnishings. Poor hygiene and nutrition are also likely to be noted. Body bruises, unusual marks on the trunk or limbs, fractures or dislocations of extremities, cuts, burned areas, intracranial trauma, hematomas, abrasions, lacerations, and soft tissue swelling invite concern, especially when coupled with accounts of the accident.

Parents who batter their children often go from one hospital to another to avoid suspicion of willful infliction of trauma. They are poor history-givers, often providing conflicting data and creating unexplained discrepancies in their relating of an incident leading to the "accident." X-ray films or detailed physical findings are not congruent with the history. Abused adults often demonstrate the same pattern of visits to several health care facilities and incongruent histories.

The behavior of the battered child is often marked with helplessness and hopelessness. Retardation, mental dullness, or failure to thrive may also be apparent. The battered adult may also demonstrate depression or fear.

Planning and implementation. The victim of a battering incident is often seen in an emergency department or community clinic where the results of the battering force the victim or relatives to request assistance. The goal of intervention at this time is to treat the physical effects of battering and help the client initiate changes in the relationship in which the violence exists.

Family service agencies and other community services are prepared to deal with families facing such crises. In some communities, parents who have abused children have formed self-help groups to cope with episodic stresses, thus preventing recurrences. In rare instances, law enforcement is required to remove the child to protective custody until home problems are resolved. Similar services may be available for battered adults. Therapy groups, women's shelters, and counseling services are several resources that might be available.

Amputation. Amputation of a limb may be accidental or operative. Accidents involving motorcycles, automobiles, military combat, and industry account for many *accidental amputations*. The limb is severed, and the tissues, nerves, and blood supply are inadequate to support cell life. *Operative amputations* may be necessary to preserve life and function in a limb that has an inadequate oxygen supply to the cells. Inadequate oxygen supply may be caused by obstructive processes such as arteriosclerosis, tumors, or by anaerobic infections such as gangrene. These illnesses occur primarily in older persons, and operative amputation may be complicated by other disorders.

Planning and implementation. The approaches to management of an amputation depend on whether the amputation is traumatic or operative. Traumatic amputation necessitates emergency actions and offers no opportunity for presurgical preparation. Operative amputation, on the other hand, can be anticipated and the client prepared for surgery.

Immediate care for an accidental amputation is to control bleeding and prevent shock. Direct pressure is applied to stop bleeding, and the client should be kept warm and lying down. The body part should be saved and wrapped in a sterile or clean cloth. If there is only partial amputation, the limb should be supported in a functional position.

Many trauma centers and hospitals with emergency department facilities are achieving increasing success with limb preservation and reattachment. Nursing care in these instances is directed toward preserving function and mobility.

Operative amputation is considered carefully, and the life-saving necessity to amputate outweighs the loss of function. Amputations are described by the joint that is amputated. Common amputations are below the knee (BK), above the knee (AK), below the elbow (BE), and above the elbow (AE). A Syme amputation removes the foot at the ankle joint.

Several surgical approaches may be used to amputate a limb. In a *guillotine* operation the limb is amputated by cutting the skin, tissue, and bone. Healing takes longer, and there may be drainage for several weeks. Another approach is to create a flap of skin from the excised limb to cover the stump. This is not always possible, however, if there is inadequate oxygen to the tissues. Attempts are made to create a stump that has smooth, healthy skin and is free of nerve endings. If a prosthesis will be used, the scar should not be over the weight-bearing portion of the bone.

After the amputation, the stump may be dressed in several ways. A soft dressing may be applied and secured with elastic bandages. This dressing permits easy inspection of the stump's healing but delays prosthesis fitting because of edema and because the bandages need to be rewrapped frequently to contour and shrink the stump.

FIG. 11-32
Wrapping a stump.

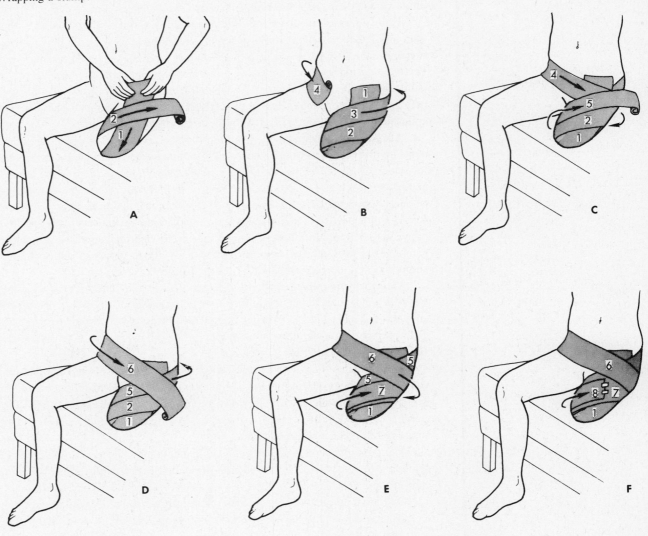

The elastic bandage should be rewrapped daily or as needed to assure compression (Fig. 11-32). The client may be instructed to do this himself, particularly if he will need to wrap the stump at home.

Plaster dressings are used in other instances. With this dressing there is less edema and contractures. The prosthesis may be fitted in 1 to 2 weeks.

Many physicians use an immediate postoperative prosthesis. Applying the prosthesis during, or several days after, surgery minimizes bleeding and edema and gives the client immediate mobility. Physical and psychological recovery are hastened, and pain is diminished by the use of the immediate post-

FIG. 11-33
Immediate postoperative prosthesis is applied during surgery or within a week of amputation. **A,** Stump is being readied for cast. **B,** Cast is applied. **C,** Cast with attachment for pylon. **D,** Pylon is attached. **E,** Client walks on his temporary prosthesis.

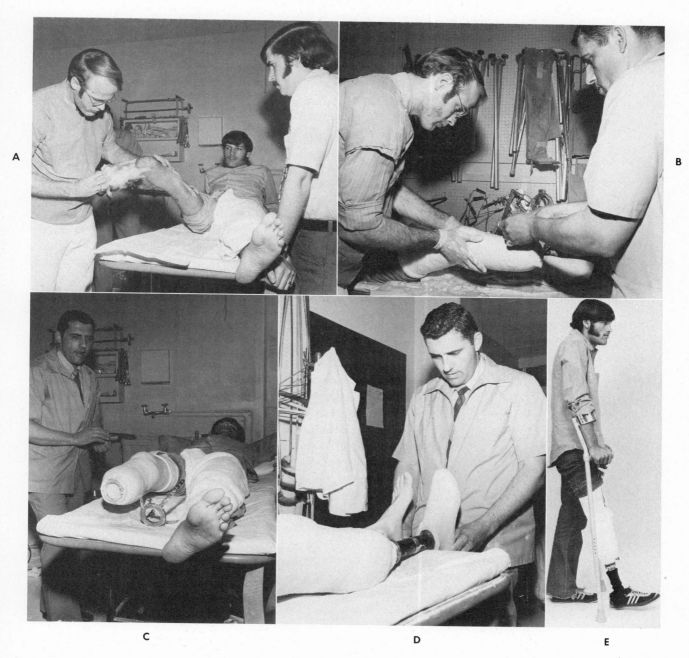

A   B   C   D   E

operative prosthesis. When this prosthesis is used, a plaster cast is put on the stump after surgery. After the plaster has dried, a pylon (temporary prosthesis consisting of the foot and attachment) is secured to the plaster (Fig. 11-33). The limb is elevated for the first day, and then the client may be up walking. When healing is complete, a permanent prosthesis is fitted.

Preoperative nursing care. Rehabilitation of the client who is to have an operative amputation begins before surgery. The physician discusses the surgery with the client and plans with him for the use of a prosthesis. Not all clients can wear a prosthesis, but for those who can, it is important to develop accessory muscles and learn balance.

Exercises are done before surgery to strengthen muscles that will be used to support the prosthesis and promote mobility. Push-ups can be done to develop arm muscles for turning in bed and transferring out of bed. If the leg is to be amputated, the cient should do exercises such as leg raises to strengthen abdominal muscles for walking with a prosthesis. The client can simulate daily activities without the limb to practice getting out of bed, walking, or dressing.

Clients who face operative amputation have some time to prepare psychologically for the loss of the limb. Dismemberment is an overwhelming thought to the client, and his body image as well as his physical health is at stake. To help the grieving process, the nurse should be an active listener when the client expresses his feelings about his amputation.

Postoperative nursing care. Postoperative nursing care should be planned to control bleeding, prevent edema, relieve psychological and physical pain, assure body alignment, and prepare the client for mobility. The nursing care depends on the type of amputation and the use of a postoperative prosthesis.

CONTROLLING BLEEDING. After surgery, the compression bandage or plaster cast is applied to control bleeding. Slight bleeding may be noted on the dressing, and the nurse should circle the area with a pen and observe any increase. Hemorrhage can be an immediate threat to life, and a tourniquet may be left at the bedside so that it can be applied immediately if bleeding becomes severe.

PREVENTING EDEMA. A certain amount of edema is usually present after surgical amputation. The use of a heavy compression dressing, cast, or immediate postoperative prosthesis minimizes some swelling. For the first 24 hours the involved limb is elevated to promote circulatory return and decrease swelling. Later, as the client exercises, swelling decreases. Compression bandages may be rewrapped at the physician's direction for several weeks after surgery to give the stump proper contour. If the client has an immediate postoperative prosthesis, the nurse should verify the security of the cast. Should the cast come off, the nurse must notify the physician and rewrap the affected limb with elastic bandages as indicated.

RELIEVING PAIN. Postoperative pain is normal. The nurse assures the client of comfort by giving medication that will alleviate pain. The client may be better able to move in bed and get up if he is free of pain.

After surgery the client may experience phantom limb sensations or phantom limb pain. The *phantom limb sensations* are sensations of the presence of the limb. The client reports itching or throbbing and often responds as if the limb were present. These sensations, however, provide useful proprioceptive stimuli for prosthesis use.

Phantom limb pain occurs several weeks after the surgery and may persist for months or years. It is believed that this pain is caused by the disruption of the neural reflex pathways. The pain tends to be more evident in persons who had a painful limb before surgery. About one third of amputees experience phantom limb pain at some time. This pain is occasionally treated with hypnosis, biofeedback, or distraction as methods of obtaining pain relief (see Chapter 8 for further discussion of pain). Occasionally reamputation is done in an attempt to restructure nerve endings.

Loss of a body part is psychologically painful, and adjustment to a new body image is not easy. Clients may grieve over the missing part and should be permitted to work through the grief process. A stable preoperative personality contributes to postoperative adjustment, and the nurse draws on these strengths to support the client at this time. Psychological counseling may be an adjunct to promoting recovery.

ASSURING BODY ALIGNMENT. Proper body alignment is essential for healing and rehabilitation. The client should be on a firm mattress, and all body parts in proper alignment. After the first 24 hours the involved limb should not be elevated. If the amputation is above or below the knee, the leg should rest flat on the bed, and no pillows are used at the hip, knee, or back. The client should be instructed not to bend his knee or put pillows between his thighs. When the client is sitting up in bed or in a wheelchair, the stump should be supported in a straight line. The stump should not hang over the bed or wheelchair. Flexion is normal for muscles, and flexion contractures must be avoided. To prevent flexion contractures, the client is turned frequently and should lie prone for 30 minutes at least twice a day.

PREPARING FOR LOCOMOTION. The stump should be prepared for the use of the prosthesis. When the stump has healed, it is washed daily with soap and water and dried carefully. No harsh soaps or antiseptics should be used on the stump. The client should be instructed to inspect the stump daily for signs of irritation, infection, or skin breakdown.

Exercises can be done in preparation for walking. Quadriceps-setting exercises develop strength for supporting the prosthesis. When the client is prone, he can bring the stump to the uninvolved leg and raise it off the bed. Squeezing a pillow between the legs also strengthens the involved limb. Later the client may walk with parallel bars, crutches, or a walker to establish a sense of balance.

Prosthesis fitting may be done 2 to 3 months after healing, and the client may be referred to a prosthetist who will fit the appropriate prosthesis. The client should be encouraged to follow through with wearing the prosthesis so that he will be mobile and will establish a healthy body image.

The older person who has had an amputation presents several unique problems. Often this individual has peripheral vascular disease, which impairs stump healing or may present complications that delay prosthesis fitting. Considerations must be given to the physical and psychological adaptations that will be required by the older person using the prosthesis. Some older individuals have decreased strength, and the energy expenditure required to use the prosthesis may be too great, particularly for those with compromised cardiac status. Unsteady gait and poor eyesight may also contribute to difficulties in prosthesis use.

The success of rehabilitation depends on the motivation of the client. Generally the client resumes his former life-style. It is reasonable to expect that the person who has led an active life will continue to do so and equally likely to expect that a person who has been confined to a wheelchair may not be enthusiastic about becoming ambulatory. Community resources may be available to those who need continuing rehabilitation or job training, and the nurse should help the client seek these resources.

Evaluation

Evaluation, the final stage of the nursing process, encourages the nurse and client to make judgments about goal achievement relative to plans for health promotion, maintenance, and restoration for common problems of the musculoskeletal system, Nursing problems often include impaired mobility, self-care deficit, alterations in comfort, knowledge deficit, potential for injury, and disturbances in self-concept.

EXPECTED OUTCOMES

The client and/or family can:
1. State plans for safety and protection of the musculoskeletal system, including use of body mechanics and protective devices such as seat belts and safety helmets.
2. Describe patterns of growth and development of the musculoskeletal system throughout the life span.
3. State plans for health maintenance, including balance of activity and rest, range-of-motion exercises, weight control.
4. Manage self-care activities during immobility imposed by immobilization devices, pain, or surgery.
5. Manage pain by using analgesics, immobilization and protection of involved part, applications of heat or cold.
6. State plans for health restoration, including use of medication, diet, activity restriction, or immobilization devices.
7. State indications for health care and/or plans for follow-up care and use of community resources.

The nurse and client may determine that the problem has been resolved and terminate the nurse-client relationship. In other instances the problem is not resolved and nursing care continues with appropriate modification of the diagnosis, plans, or implementation, so that the client can attain his optimum level of wellness.

Summary

The nursing process provides a framework for planning nursing care for clients with common health problems of the musculoskeletal system. The relationship of the nurse and the client changes because the client is dependent on the nurse when mobility is impaired and less dependent as he is increasingly able to perform his own self-care activities.

During the assessment stage of the nursing process, the nurse collects and analyzes data relative to the client's musculoskeletal system. The health history, developmental, social, and psychological histories, and physical assessment are tools for collecting data, which are then used to formulate a list of nursing problems or diagnoses. These may include alteration in comfort, self-care deficit, impaired mobility, altered self-concept, knowledge deficit, and potential for injury.

During the planning stage the nurse and client establish goals and objectives for health promotion, maintenance, and restoration. Health promotion may include instruction about exercise, body mechanics, diet, and risk management. Casts, cast-braces, braces, traction, and external fixation devices may be used to maintain or restore mobility; and the nurse and client plan for care when these devices are used.

Health problems of the musculoskeletal system occur throughout the life span. Problems of the neonate and infant may include congenital defects such as hip dysplasia or clubfoot. Trauma and inflammatory diseases are common in childhood, whereas structural defects such as scoliosis or epiphysitis may occur during adolescence. Adulthood is noted by inflammatory and degenerative processes such as rheumatoid arthritis, gout, bursitis, and degenerative joint disease. Trauma and battering occur across the life span and contribute to significant mortality from accidental injury, particularly in older adult, adolescent, and young adult age groups. Plans are implemented for these problems to restore the client to his highest level of wellness.

The nurse and client evaluate objectives formulated during the planning stage. Client expected outcomes are specific for each client and reflect his needs and stage of growth and development. Ultimate outcomes are that the client is able to maintain health of the musculoskeletal system for maximum mobility and independence in self-care activities.

References

1. Groer, Maureen, and Shekleton, Maureen: Basic pathophysiology, a conceptual approach, St. Louis, 1979, The C.V. Mosby Co.
2. Iyer, Patricia: The battered wife, Nurs. 80, **10**(7):53, 1980.
3. Farrell, Jane: Nursing care of the patient in a cast-brace, Nurs. Clin. North Am. **11**(4):717-724, 1976.
4. Kryschyshen, Patt, and Fischer, David: External fixation for complicated fractures, Am. J. Nurs. **80**(2):256, 1980.
5. Love-Mignogna, Susan: Scoliosis, Nurs. 77, **7**(5):51-55, 1977.
6. McKeel, Nancy: Child abuse can be prevented, Am. J. Nurs. **78**(9):1478, 1978.
7. Spruck, Marie: Gold therapy for rheumatoid arthritis, Am. J. Nurs. **79**(7):1246, 1979.
8. Tibbits, Carole: Adolescent idiopathic scoliosis, Nurse Practitioner, **5**(2):11, 1980.

Additional readings

Alexander, Mary, and Brown, Marie Scott: Physical examination: the musculoskeletal system, Nurs. 76, **6**(4):51-56, 1976.

Anderson, Beverly, and D'Ambra, Phyllis: The adolescent patient with scoliosis, Nurs. Clin. North Am. **11**(4):699-708, 1976.

Berger, M.R.: Dupuytren's contracture, Am. J. Nurs. **78**(2):244-245, 1978.

Berger, M.R., and Froimson, Avrum: Hands that hurt: carpal tunnel syndrome, Am. J. Nurs. **79**(2):264-266, 1979.

Borgman, Mary Frances: Carpal tunnel syndrome, Nurse Practitioner, **5**(3):21, 1980.

Bosanko, Lydia: Immediate post-operative prosthesis, Am. J. Nurs. **71**(2):281-283, 1971.

Bowden, Susan: New surgery for arthritic hands, Nurs. 76, **6**(8):46-48, 1976.

Brower, Eleanor, and Nash, Clyde: Evaluating growth and posture in school-age children, Nurs. 79, **9**(4):58-63, 1979.

Buck, Barbara, and Lee, Allen: Amputation: two views, Nurs. Clin. North Am. **11**(4):641-657, 1976.

Clark, Helen: Osteoarthritis: an interesting case? Nurs. Clin. North Am. **11**:199-206, 1976.

Deyerle, William, and Crossland, Sharon: Broken legs are to be walked on, Am. J. Nurs. **77**(12):1927-1930, 1977.

Dickinson, Glenda: A home care program for patients with rheumatoid arthritis, Nurs. Clin. North Am. **15**(2):403, 1980.

Nursing process for common health problems

Drury, Lawrence: Evacuation and early care of the trauma patient, Heart Lung **7**(2):249, 1978.

Engstrand, Janet: Rehabilitation of the patient with a lower extremity amputation, Nurs. Clin. North Am. **11**(4):659-669, 1976.

Farrell, Jane: Casts, your patients and you, part 2: a review of arm and leg cast procedures, Nurs. 78, **8**(11):57-64, 1978.

Farrell, Jane: Casts, your patients and you, part 3: a review of hip-spica procedures, Nurs. 78, **8**(12):53-57, 1978.

Gilroy, Ann, and Caldwell, Elaine: Initial assessment of the multiply injured patient, Nurs. Clin. North Am. **13**(2):177, 1978.

Hilt, Nancy, and Schmitt, E. William: Pediatric orthopedic nursing, St. Louis, 1975, The C.V. Mosby Co.

Jennings, Kate R.: The cheerful operation: total hip replacement, Nurs. 76, **6**(7):32-37, 1976.

Larson, Carroll B., and Gould, Marjorie: Orthopedic nursing, ed. 9, St. Louis, 1978, The C.V. Mosby Co.

Leaman, Karen: Recognizing and helping the abused child, Nurs. 79, **9**(2):64-67, 1979.

McClinton, Virginia: Nursing of the upper extremity amputee and preparation for prosthetic training, Nurs. Clin. North Am. **11**(4):671-677, 1976.

Meyers, Marin, and others: Total hip replacement—a team effort, Am. J. Nurs. **78**(9):1485-1488, 1968.

Miller, Barbara: How to spot and treat carpal tunnel syndrome early, Nurs. 80, **10**(3):50, 1980.

Nirenberg, Anita: High-dose methotrexate for the patient with osteogenic sarcoma, Am. J. Nurs. **76**(11):1776-1780, 1976.

Pasnau, Robert, and Pfefferbaum, Betty: Psychologic aspects of post-amputation pain, Nurs. Clin. North Am. **11**(4):679-685, 1976.

Pfefferbaum, Betty, and Pasnau, Robert: Post-amputation grief, Nurs. Clin. North Am. **11**(4): 687-690, 1976.

Rickel, Linda: Emotional support for the multiple myeloma patient, Nurs. 76, **6**(4):76-80, 1976.

Rodgers, Bradley: Trauma and the child, Heart Lung **6**(6):1052, 1977.

Rutecki, Barbara, and Seligson, David: Caring for the patient in a halo apparatus, Nurs. 80, **10**(10): 73-77, 1980.

Schwaid, Madeline: Advice to arthritics: keep moving, Am. J. Nurs. **78**(10):1708, 1978.

Sculco, Cynthia, and Sculco, Thomas: Management of the patient with an infected total hip arthroplasty, Am. J. Nurs. **76**(4):584-587, 1976.

Segil, Clive: Current concepts in the management of scoliosis, Nurs. Clin. North Am. **11**(4):691-698, 1976.

Stright, Patricia: How to help the patient with a dislocated shoulder, Am. J. Nurs. **79**(4):666-669, 1969.

Townley, Charles, and Hill, Leslie: Total knee replacement, Am. J. Nurs. **74**(9):1612-1617, 1974.

Witte, Natalie: Why the elderly fall, Am. J. Nurs. **79**(11):1950-1952, 1979.

NURSING PROCESS

for clients with common health problems of the

12 Reproductive system

Assessment

Data analysis

Planning

Implementation

Evaluation

Sexuality is the totality of being an individual. It includes the foundation the reproductive system provides for gender identification as well as biological, psychological, sociological, and cultural variables associated with being male or female. An individual's sexuality is subject to dynamic changes as a variety of forces contribute to reproductive and sexual growth throughout the life span.

Health problems may interfere with the reproductive system and sexuality. Congenital defects of neonates and infants, for example, may confuse gender identification and early sexual development. Sexually transmitted diseases, prevalent among adolescents and young adults, may interfere with reproductive health. In adulthood, tumors of the reproductive organs are a significant health problem and may disrupt childbearing and sexual functioning.

The purpose of this chapter is to provide information about the reproductive system that will help the nurse assess the client's health and sexuality; maintain health; and plan, implement, and evaluate nursing care for clients with common health problems of the reproductive system.

Overview of the reproductive system

The reproductive system includes the breasts and genitalia of the male and female as well as the accessory organs. The endocrine system influences sexual and reproductive development, whereas the nervous system mediates human sexual response; they are considered here in relationship to sexual development and sexuality.

Nursing process for common health problems

FEMALE SYSTEM

The female reproductive organs are differentiated by location and are referred to as external or internal organs.

The external genitalia, known as the *vulva,* includes the *mons pubis,* fatty tissue in front of the symphysis pubis, the *labia majora* and *labia minora,* and the vaginal outlet. The *clitoris* is located near the anterior folds of the labia minora. During sexual stimulation it enlarges and is a site of female orgasm. The *vagina* is an organ of sexual pleasure, and outlet for menstrual flow, and the birth canal during delivery. The vagina is lubricated by secretions from *Bartholin's* and *Skene's glands* and from its own cells. Estrogen and the presence of Doderlein bacilli regulate the pH of the vagina. Normal pH after puberty is 4.0 to 5.0. The vagina is protected by a thin membrane, the *hymen,* which may become separated during exercise, trauma, digital examination, or coitus.

The internal reproductive organs (*uterus, fallopian tubes,* and *ovaries*) are contained in the pelvic cavity. The uterus, a muscular organ, is composed of three layers: the inner *endometrial* layer (which, in response to cyclical hormonal changes, is shed during menstruation), the middle layer, or *myometrium,* and the outer layer, or *perimetrium.* The muscle layers are necessary for the birth process and have properties of contractibility and retractability. The uterus is suspended in the pelvic cavity by the *round, broad,* and *uterosacral ligaments.* Frequent or difficult deliveries may stretch these ligaments, causing prolapse of the uterus.

The fallopian tubes and ovaries are essential for reproduction and hormonal regulation. In the mature woman the ovaries each month release an ovum, which is transported by the fallopian tube where it is either fertilized and propelled to the uterus for implantation or shed with the endometrial lining of the uterus in the menstrual fluid.

The female breasts are considered a part of the reproductive system because of their response to hormonal and physical changes during puberty, menstruation, pregnancy, and sexual excitement. The female breast is composed of *acini* (milk-producing glands), *lactiferous ducts,* and the *nipple.* The breast is given form by subcutaneous tissue and retromammary fat supported by the pectoralis major and minor muscles. The center of the breast is known as the *areola* and has darker pigmentation than the surrounding breast tissue. The pigment deepens during pregnancy and with the use of oral contraceptives. The nipple, an erectile tissue, is located in the center of the areola and in most women is everted. Elevations on the areola surrounding the nipple are known as *Montgomery's glands,* which secrete a lubricating substance that protects the nipple during lactation. *Striae,* or stretch marks, may appear on the breast during periods of rapid growth such as during pregnancy.

The female breast is rich in lymphatic drainage systems. Lymph drains from the cutaneous, areolar, and deep mammary tissue. The cutaneous lymphatic system drains from the skin surface areas into the ipsilateral axillary nodes (mammary, scapular, brachial, and intermediate nodes). The lymph from the areola and nipple flows into anterior axillary nodes (mammary nodes), and lymph from the deep mammary tissue drains into the anterior axillary nodes as well as apical, subclavian, infraclavicular, and supraclavicular nodes.

MALE SYSTEM

The reproductive organs of the male include the penis, testes, vas deferens, seminal vesicle, prostate gland, and breast. The *penis* is the primary organ of sexual pleasure and also contains the *urethra,* which serves as an outlet for urine from the bladder. The urethra is surrounded by the *prostate gland,* which secretes an alkaline fluid transported by ejaculatory ducts that pass through the prostate.

The *testes,* which produce sperm and testosterone, are enclosed in the *scrotum* and suspended outside the body to maintain the sperm at a temperature lower than the rest of the body. As sperm are produced in the mature male, they collect in the *epididymis* and are transported through the *vas deferens* to the *seminal vesicle.* Here is added seminal fluid from the seminal vesicle and prostate. During coitus, the seminal fluid and sperm are deposited from the penis into the vagina.

The breasts of the male do not contain the glandular or subcutaneous tissue of the female breast. The breast does, however, enlarge in response to hormonal changes during puberty or in disease states such as cirrhosis. Abnormal enlargement of the male breast is referred to as *gynecomastia.*

PUBERTY, MENARCHE, CLIMACTERIC: RELATIONSHIPS WITH THE ENDOCRINE SYSTEM

Puberty

The pituitary gland regulates ovarian and testicular function for two significant events in the life span of both sexes: puberty and climacteric.

Preparation for reproductive ability is called puberty and occurs at about age 10 for girls and age 12 for boys. There is increased growth in body size, and the reproductive organs are stimulated by neural regulatory mechanisms toward maturity.

Puberty in girls. In girls the reproductive organs increase in size, and the uterus becomes anteflexed in preparation for childbearing. The breasts enlarge, and the nipples protrude. Axillary and pubic hair increases in density and darkness, and the girl takes on a female appearance as fat distribution increases around the thighs.

Menarche, the onset of menstruation, occurs at about age 12 or 13. The onset of menarche is species specific and, in humans, maturation is signalled by body weight sufficient to support pregnancy (about 35 pounds of stored fat).[11,16] Follicle-stimulating hormone from the anterior pituitary stimulates the ovary to produce estrogen and an ovarian follicle containing the ovum. When the ovum is released (every 26 to 30 days), the luteinizing hormone stimulates the corpus luteum to produce estrogen and progesterone. These hormones prepare the endometrial lining of the uterus to receive the fertilized egg. If conception does not occur, the endometrial lining is shed as menstrual fluid, and the menstrual cycle begins again.

Menstrual fluid appears as dark red drainage and may contain small clots. A characteristic odor may be identified with the menstrual fluid. Generally no more than 60 to 150 ml of menstrual fluid is shed during menstruation, and if dietary intake contains sufficient iron, nutritional losses from this bleeding are negligible. The menstrual period usually lasts 4 to 5 days but varies greatly for each woman.

Early menstrual flow is spotty, irregular, and anovulatory. Within 2 years, however, a normal cycle is established, and the girl will ovulate every 26 to 30 days. The menstrual cycle may be altered by emotional and physical stress, illness, or climate changes. Absence of a menstrual cycle, *amenorrhea,* may be occasional during the early establishment of the cycle. The cycles become more regular and during early adulthood average every 28 days. As the woman approaches age 40, the cycles may change; cycles of 18 to 45 days may be normal and vary from month to month. (Amenorrhea may also indicate pregnancy or hormonal imbalances and should be evaluated by a physician if the condition persists or occurs after the establishment of a regular cycle.)

Puberty in boys. Male characteristics appear in boys 2 to 3 years later than female characteristics in girls. The sexual organs increase in size, and follicle-stimulating hormone stimulates continuous production of sperm in the testes. There are nocturnal seminal emissions around age 14 as the reproductive apparatus becomes functional. The voice deepens because of enlargement of the larynx, and facial, axillary, and pubic hair appears. The muscles become larger, particularly in the shoulders, and the boy takes on a male appearance.

Climacteric

Middle adulthood is noted by a change in reproductive ability. This "change of life" is known as the climacteric and signals the onset of declining reproductive ability in men and women.

Climacteric in women. Climacteric in women is also referred to as *menopause*. Follicle-stimulating hormone begins to decrease when the woman is between ages 45 and 50, causing irregular menstrual periods. As the menstrual flow decreases, the cycle gradually shortens, and within 1 to 2 years becomes absent altogether. Menopause is not considered to have occurred, however, until the menses have stopped for 1 year. Until that time there exists the possibility of ovulation and pregnancy, and the woman should use conception control measures if she does not wish to become pregnant.

Climacteric in men. Climacteric is usually less pronounced in men and may not even be apparent in many men. Frequently reproductive ability does not cease in men; in fact, sperm production may never diminish. There may be certain physiological and psychological changes, however, such as flushing and chills. The man may be at the peak of his career and may view future retirement as a loss of sexual power. He, too, is adjusting to the change in family structure and coping with changes in life-style at this time in his life.

HUMAN SEXUAL RESPONSE: RELATIONSHIPS WITH THE NERVOUS SYSTEM

Human sexual response is a complex interaction of psychological and physiological forces that culminate in orgasmic release. Sexual response depends on intact cortical pathways, peripheral nerves, autonomic pathways, afferent nerves, pathways to and from the spinal cord, reflex centers, and, of course, intact genitalia responsive to sexual stimulation. Basically, sexual response in both sexes follows similar nerve pathways from tactile or psychogenic stimulation of the clitoris or glans penis through peripheral nerves, to afferent fibers of pudendal and pelvic nerves, to the sacral area of the spinal cord, and return through parasympathetic efferent nerves, resulting in vasocongestion of the penis or clitoris.

Several researchers have provided theoretical frameworks for describing human sexual response. One prominent theory is that of Masters and Johnson, who describe human sexual response in four phases.[12] (The nurse should be aware that there are variations in intensity and duration of responses and that any framework is only a basis for understanding this phenomenon.)

According to Masters and Johnson, human sexual response begins with the *excitement phase,* in which a variety of somatogenic and psychogenic stimuli trigger central nervous system and musculoskeletal responses. The penis becomes erect, and lubrication of the vagina begins. In the *plateau phase,* sexual tensions heighten. The blood pressure and pulse increase. There is vasocongestion in the genital areas and increasing muscle tension. Preejaculatory emissions and mucoid emissions from Bartholin's glands occur during this phase. During the *orgasmic phase* sexual tensions are released. The male ejaculates, and the female experiences uterine and vaginal contractions. Muscles relax and vasoconcentration decreases. Subjective pleasurable feelings are associated with the vagina, clitoris, uterus, penis, prostate, and seminal vesicles. The *resolution phase* describes the resolve from the height of orgasmic response. The resolution phase is longer in women, and many can be restimulated to orgasm during this period. In the male there is a refractory period, during which he returns to the early excitement phase level and cannot be restimulated until the resolution phase has been completed.

Assessment

NURSING HISTORY

The nursing history is used to obtain data about the client's reproductive system and perceptions of sexuality that are used in identifying nursing problems and formulating nursing diagnoses. Gathering data about an individual's reproductive health and sexuality may be a sensitive issue for both the nurse and the client. Factors that influence the interview and examination are the comfort of the nurse in assessing reproductive health and sexuality, the comfort of the client, the age and developmental stage of both the client and nurse, the sex of both the nurse and the client, the openness of the client during the interview, the purpose of the interview, and the type of information being discussed.

FIG. 12-1
Sexual health model. (From Sexuality, a nursing perspective by Fern Mims and Melinda Swenson. © 1980 McGraw-Hill Book Co. Used with the permission of McGraw-Hill Book Co.)

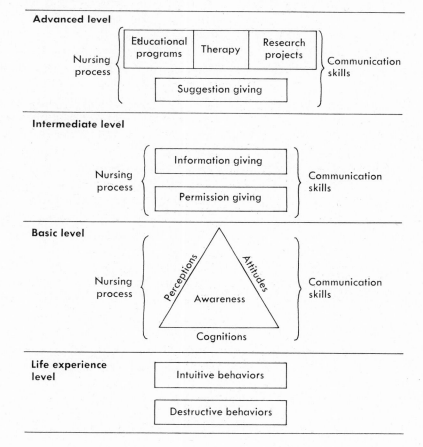

Nursing process for common health problems

Mims and Swenson offer a sexual health model (Fig. 12-1) for self-assessment and client assessment and intervention.[14] Their model presents four levels of knowledge and interventions at which nurses and clients can discuss sexual health and sexuality. At the first level the nurse and client operate with intuitive knowledge about sexual anatomy, physiology, and psychosexual development. Some attitudes and knowledge may be erroneous or include destructive behaviors that inhibit communication and must be clarified. At the basic level it is imperative for nurses to become aware of their own sexuality, values, and knowledge, and be nonjudgmental about the values of others. The intermediate level includes communication skills used in the nursing process for giving permission to discuss topics related to sexuality and giving information. At the advanced level the nurse and client may be involved in suggestion giving, therapy, educational programs, or research. This level requires advanced knowledge and skills in human sexuality. Nurses can use this model when obtaining a nursing history and performing physical assessment, because the model can be adapted to the needs of the nurse and client throughout the life span.

Health history Information about the client's reproductive health and sexuality can be obtained from a health history. The history format must be adapted to the age and sex of the client to obtain information relevant to the client's developmental stage.

Female client. The history for *infants* and *children* includes information about psychosexual development and general health. The history may be obtained from the parent and may provide an opportunity to clarify misconceptions about sexual behavior of the child or offer information about sexual development.

The history for *adolescent* and *adult* women focuses on the menstrual history, gynecological history, and obstetrical history. The nurse should note the age of menarche (and climacteric, if appropriate), the date of the last menstrual period, the usual amount of flow, presence of dysmenorrhea, menorrhagia (heavy flow), or metrorrhagia (spotting between periods). The gynecological history includes presence of vaginal discharge, odor, color, frequency and duration of discharge, and presence of pruritis. The type of birth control method, if any used, should be noted, as well as the date of the last Pap smear. The nurse should ask the client if she has noticed breast masses; nipple discharge; soreness, tenderness, or pain in the breasts; and if she performs monthly breast self-examination. If the woman has conceived, the nurse should note the client's parity (number of pregnancies, abortions, and living children).

Information relevant to the woman's sexuality may be obtained at this time. The woman's attitudes or willingness to discuss sexuality are often ascertained during the reproductive health history. Other questions may include the ability to perform and enjoy sex and how health problems, if present, will affect sexuality.

Male client. The health history for the infant or child is designed to obtain information about the boy's psychosexual development and presence of health problems. The nurse should particularly inquire if the boy has difficulty voiding.

Data to be obtained from adolescent and adult males include a urological history and information about reproductive health. The nurse should inquire whether the client has difficulty voiding, a history of prostate problems, testicular changes, lesions on the penis, or discharge from the urethra.

Information about the client's sexuality can be obtained by asking about his ability to perform and enjoy sex. The nurse can also ask the client what changes he anticipates if a reproductive health problem is evident.

Risk factors. The health history should also include information about risk factors related to reproductive health problems for both sexes. Sexually transmitted diseases and cancer of the reproductive organs are two significant health problems that affect sexuality. Individuals' risk should be identified, and those at risk should be encouraged to have frequent physical examinations.

Developmental history

Information about the developmental stages that are manifested by physical as well as psychosexual development contributes to client assessment. This information is particularly useful in determining the client's need and readiness for explanations and information about sexual health.

Neonate. The newborn has sexual anatomy that is proportionate in size to the rest of his body. Newborn girls often have an engorged clitoris and labia because of maternal estrogen stimulation. The labia minora are often larger than the labia majora, particularly in preterm neonates. There may be a white, mucoid vaginal discharge for the first few weeks of life. The vaginal discharge may also be blood tinged and should be considered normal during the first few weeks.

Newborn boys often have slight swelling of the scrotum that disappears in a few weeks. During the neonatal appraisal the nurse should verify the presence of the testes in the scrotal sac. The testes of the premature neonate may not be fully descended and are often found in the inguinal canal. Foreskin covers the penis of the newborn and should be retracted on initial health appraisal to verify an outlet for urine. Several days later the parents may wish to have the foreskin removed (circumcised) for health or religious reasons. Although not necessary for health reasons, removal of the foreskin makes cleaning the penis easier.[7] Jewish boys are usually circumcised in a special ceremony called *Berith,* which takes place 8 days after birth.

Sexual pleasure is recognized by the neonate by the warmth, holding, and cuddling from adults. The nurse and parents provide an important beginning for developing human sexuality by providing this pleasurable stimulation.

Infant. The infant has a beginning awareness of sensations in the genital organs. Sexual satisfaction for the infant comes from expressions of love by parents or parent substitutes as they meet his basic needs. Changing wet diapers, holding, rocking, and cuddling of infants stimulate pleasurable sexual feelings.

Toddler and preschooler. The young child is learning to cope with his environment. He is curious about himself and his relationships with others. His curiosity also includes his sexual role. The child observes his own body and the differences in the opposite sex. He wants to know the name of his body parts and their function. Parents help the child accept his body and its sexual functioning as they teach appropriate names for all body parts. To ignore the penis or vagina or call them by incorrect names may draw attention to their special nature. Children of 3 and 4 years of age begin to ask parents how babies are conceived and born. Parents are encouraged to give simple and honest answers that are appropriate to the child's understanding. These answers serve to satisfy curiosity and clarify fantasies.

The preschooler observes aspects of behavior that differentiate sexual roles and then imitates them. Sexual role satisfaction is also learned as the toddler observes the interactions of his parents. Loving relationships between adults who feel comfortable in their sexual roles form the basis for later sexual identity.

The preschooler becomes more aware of the pleasure from stimulation of the genital organs. Bathing or pulling on the penis may produce an erection in boys. Rocking or rubbing the labia to stimulate the clitoris is satisfying to girls. This self-stimulation, or *masturbation,* is a normal outlet for sexual tensions in young children. Parents help the child by not drawing attention to the behavior with scolding or punishment. If masturbation is excessive, the parents can redirect the child's activity to seek additional satisfying experiences.

The most important task in the later preschool years is to establish a sexual identity. By age 5 the child is acutely aware of sex-typing behaviors, and it is important for parents to be supportive of appropriate sexual behavior while encouraging individual development without sex stereotypes. Parenting techniques that are not seductive or overwhelming but that clearly respond to the child's sexuality are most helpful in helping the child develop gender identity.

School-age child. Sexual role identification intensifies during the school years. Cultural pressures of peer groups, television, and magazines further separate sex roles. The child learns that his parents are not the only examples of sexual roles, and he may try a variety of behaviors in his continuing search for sexual identity. Curiosity about sexual differences may stimulate children to explore each other's bodies. Explorative play and group activities with the same sex are common at this time and do not need parental interference unless persistent or unusual.

Adolescent. Physiological and psychological changes are characteristic of adolescent sexual development. Puberty is often the hallmark for increased sexual awareness. Sexual activity gradually changes from the autoerotic interest of childhood to adult sexuality. Adolescence is a period of finding one's identity, and finding sexual identity is an important maturational task. Other tasks of the adolescent include adopting a code of sexual behavior and establishing moral and social responsibilities involved in a sexual relationship. Social activities such as parties, dating, and courtship prepare the adolescent for selecting a sex partner.

In the United States there is a cultural lag between adolescence and adulthood that must be overcome by sublimation of emerging sexual feelings. The need to release sexual tension is usually met by an increase in masturbatory activity. Many adolescents will engage in foreplay. Others may have intercourse to satisfy these intense sexual feelings. Adolescent pregnancy is a significant problem in the United States. It is estimated that one in four adolescent women has been pregnant by age 19.[9]

Adult. Many sexual role adjustments take place during adulthood. In early adulthood most adults select a mate and prepare to be married or cohabitate. Early in the family cycle the individual adjusts to being a spouse and a parent. There are responsibilities for providing economic security and planning for family size. Parents then act as role models and help their own children achieve sexual identity. Later, as reproductive and child-rearing responsibilities end, there is a reshaping of sexual roles.

Middle adulthood is a significant period of readjustment. Goals for career and family planning may have been reached, and life may appear to offer fewer challenges. Many persons feel discouraged because they perceive aging as causing them to be unable to do the things they did when they were younger.

Men and women cope with physiological and psychological changes of climacteric, and sexual needs may vary during this adjustment.

Sexual relationships need not terminate when reproductive activity ends. Some couples feel relieved of the fear of an unwanted pregnancy and are better able to enjoy intercourse. This feeling of shared intimacy may help the couple adjust to the changes in sexual role satisfaction in the middle adult years. Women report increased enjoyment in intercourse, and although full erection is slower for men, it is also sustained longer, increasing sexual satisfaction for both partners.

Older adult. As with all needs, the aging process is evident in the need for continued satisfying sexual relationships. Unfortunately, myths continue to prevail about sexuality in older individuals and tend to inhibit continuing enjoyment of sexual relationships.

The effects of aging in women are primarily related to estrogen withdrawal. The labia become pendulous as subcutaneous fat is lost, the vagina shortens and is less elastic, and the thin mucosa may cause *dyspareunia* (painful intercourse) and increased susceptibility to infection. Furthermore, the pH of the vagina becomes more alkaline, providing a medium for bacterial growth. Pelvic support structures weaken, and there may be dysuria and frequency of urination. The breasts lose elasticity and become smaller and pendulous. The hair becomes coarser, and the woman may become hirsute.

The man is subject to loss of skin tone and change in distribution of body hair. Hypertrophy of the prostate may cause dysuria, frequency of urination, and incontinence.

In spite of physical changes, the need for satisfying relationships between the sexes continues. It has been found that interest in sexual activities does not diminish with age but is a continuation of previously enjoyed relationships. Masters and Johnson report that human sexual response occurs in the same phases in the older adult but with less intensity.[12] Others have described slower sexual arousal, erections to be longer to achieve (but can be sustained longer), and less elasticity of the vagina. Contrary to prevalent beliefs, older adults can and do enjoy sexual relationships.

Determinants of sexual behavior in older individuals are past enjoyment, current health, and availability of a partner. Frequency of intercourse also determines enjoyment because regular stimulation facilitates sexual response.

Later maturity also brings adjustment to roles as parents become grandparents and once again enjoy the perpetuation of the life cycle. Many couples must also adjust to the death of the spouse and the possibility of remarriage or to changes in economic or health status.

Social history

Attitudes about reproductive and sexual health are rooted in an individual's social environment. It is useful for the nurse and client to be aware of these values and how they relate to the client's current health status.

The client's religious and ethical views may be significant to attitudes about reproduction, birth control, sexual roles, and homosexual and heterosexual relationships. The nurse should determine the meaning these values hold for the client.

Culture and ethnicity contribute significantly to the client's sexuality. Styles of dress, subtleties of stance and body behavior, as well as sex-descriptive employment roles are examples of cultural influences on sexuality. Dress styles, although tending to be less differentiating, are often encouraged by parents and peers as outward reflections of gender identity.

Less obvious sex discriminations are in societal descriptions of masculine or feminine behavior. Body stance, ways of crossing arms or legs, and the manner of expressing joy or sorrow are learned behaviors reinforced by the larger social group. The nurse should be aware of various cultural and ethnic implications of sexual behavior to interpret and promote gender role assumption.

Societal tasks may also be sex related and culturally influenced. In some cultures, women were traditionally involved in housekeeping and childrearing whereas men were assigned tasks of food gathering and other aspects of family welfare. Currently, in the United States great emphasis is focused on equality in work-related roles, and there is increasing comfort with these role-sharing approaches.

Gender roles may also be related to socioeconomic class. Roles in the lower economic groups may be more rigid.[10] Sexual behavior may also vary among ethnic groups, and the nurse should be aware of the client's perception and values related to sexuality.

Social attitudes about sexuality, social roles, and reproductive health are promoted by a variety of interest groups such as the women's movement, gay liberation movement, "right-to-life" groups, and others. These groups have increased society's awareness of issues pertaining to sexuality and in many instances have lobbied for local, state, and federal laws that are continuing to influence social values.

Psychological history

In addition to the nursing history, developmental, and social histories, the nurse obtains information about the client's psychological strengths and limitations. The nurse should determine how the client's coping behaviors relate to his sexuality and use this information to predict how interferences with reproductive health might impinge on the client's sexuality. The nurse should identify individuals significant to the client and their relationship to him. Spouse, parents, children, and friends are a part of the client's sexual role system and must be included in the care plan.

PHYSICAL ASSESSMENT

The physical examination of the reproductive system includes *inspection* and *palpation* of the female and male genitalia and breasts for lesions, changes in shape, and presence of discharge. The nurse must consider the age and developmental stage of the client and be respectful of the need for privacy. The examination should be performed in a warm room with provision for draping the client to avoid unnecessary exposure.

Female client

Inspection of the female genitalia involves examination of the labia majora for lesions, parasites, leukoplakia, swelling, and abnormal pigment changes. The labia are palpated for size, shape, and tenderness. Normal labia are soft and of a consistent texture. The labia of young girls are flat in appearance, whereas the labia of older women may be atrophic. If the woman has had several pregnancies, the labia may be gaping. If discharge is present, a culture or smear may be obtained for diagnosis.

The breasts should be inspected and palpated for growths, because breast cancer is the major cause of cancer death in women.[8] The procedure is similar to that described for breast self-examination, and the nurse should inspect and palpate the breasts for changes in color, shape, discharge, and consistency.

12 Reproductive system

Male client   Physical examination of the male includes inspection and palpation of the external genitals. The penis should be inspected for the presence and position of the meatus. In neonates and uncircumcised children or adults the prepuce (foreskin) must be retracted to make this observation. If the prepuce does not retract easily, *phimosis* may be suspected. The meatus should be positioned centrally on the glans. Deviations include epispadias or hypospadias. The penis should also be observed for swelling, lesions, and discharges. If a discharge is present, a culture or smear may be obtained. The scrotum should be observed for size, symmetry, and presence of both testicles. The normal scrotum may be asymmetrical, because the left testis is often lower than the right. The size of the scrotum may depend on the cremesteric muscle, which contracts when cold. The testes should be palpated and both testes identified. The testes should be palpated simultaneously to detect masses, swelling, differences in size, or movability.

The prostate gland can be palpated through the rectum. A gloved and lubricated finger can be inserted into the rectum to palpate the prostate for size, contour, and consistency.

The male breasts should be inspected and palpated for lesions, discharge, or masses. Although the incidence of cancer of the male breast is less than 1%, men should also be encouraged to report changes in size, shape, color, or presence of discharge.

DIAGNOSTIC ASSESSMENT

Direct visualization procedures

Pelvic examination. A pelvic examination involves visual inspection and palpation of the external genitalia, vagina, and internal reproductive organs and should be a part of a physical examination of all adult women. Some advise performing the examination after the onset of menstruation, at which time the hymen may be excised or dilated.

The nurse has the role of explaining the examination to the woman, instructing her to relax by taking deep breaths, and observing the examination. In some settings, nurses with advanced physical assessment skills may perform the examination themselves. Young women may be modest or fearful, particularly if this is the first examination. Older women may need additional help in being positioned for safety and comfort.

Before the examination the woman should remove all underclothing and constricting garments. The woman also should void so that the bladder is empty and does not interfere with digital examination of the pelvic structures. If a cytopathological smear is to be taken during the pelvic examination, the woman should be instructed not to have intercourse, take a tub bath, or douche 24 hours before the examination to prevent lavage of loosened cells. The woman should also not have a curettage or catheterization 2 weeks before cytopathological examination, because abnormal tissues may have been dislodged.

The pelvic examination is usually performed on an examining table with foot supports or stirrups, but it can be performed on a bed or with a regular examination table (Fig. 12-2). Several positions may be used for the examination. The most common is the *lithotomy* position. The woman is placed on her back, and her feet are placed in stirrups or foot supports or are positioned next to her body. The legs should be placed in the stirrups and lowered at the same time to avoid straining the leg muscles. If stirrups are used, they should be padded to prevent pressure on the popliteal area. In *Sims'* position the woman lies on her left side, with her left arm behind her back, and the right thigh and

Nursing process for common health problems

FIG. 12-2
A, Lithotomy position for a pelvic examination. **B,** Bivalve speculum in position for visualization of cervix.

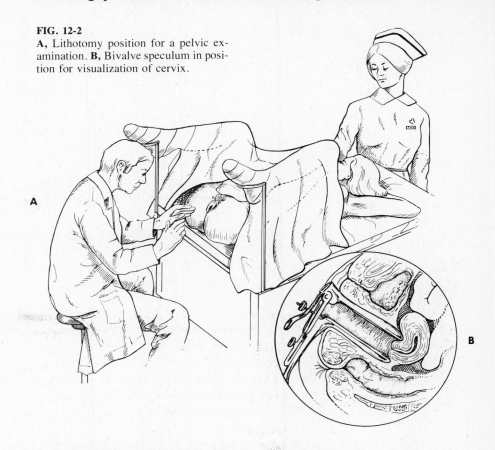

knee flexed. The *knee-chest* position is an alternative position. In this position the woman kneels on the bed or examining table with her feet over the side. The chest is positioned on the pillow and the head turned to one side, resting on the pillow. After the woman has been positioned comfortably, she is draped to preserve modesty.

The physician begins the examination by inspecting the vulva for abnormalities, irritation, swelling, or discharge. A gooseneck lamp facilitates observation. The labia majora and minora are spread, and the vestibule is examined. Digital examination of the vagina precedes visual examination. The visual examination is accomplished with the use of a bivalve speculum that supports the vagina. The speculum comes in several sizes, and the nurse should select the appropriate one for the age, size, and parity of the client. The speculum may be warmed under a lightbulb or with warm water. A lubricant is not used if cultures or Pap smears are to be obtained.

After obtaining the Pap smear, the physician bimanually examines the internal organs for growths on the ovaries, fallopian tubes, or uterus. Normal position and mobility of the uterus can also be detected. A rectal examination is also done to palpate the pelvic floor, and lubricant is used liberally as the physician palpates the rectum and vaginal wall.

When the examination is completed, the nurse should help the woman into a more comfortable position. Tissue paper is used to remove lubricant and secretions from the perianal area, and the client should be allowed to sit on the examining table for a few minutes to regain her balance before standing.

FIG. 12-3
Culdoscope is used to visualize internal reproductive organs in women.

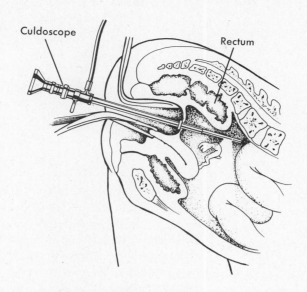

Culdoscopy. The internal organs of the female can be observed directly by inserting a lighted tube, the culdoscope, through the vagina to the posterior fornix and cul de sac (Fig. 12-3). The ovaries, fallopian tubes, uterus, and small intestines can be examined for endometriosis, cysts, or tumors. The procedure is usually done with a local anesthetic, rarely with a general anesthetic. The woman should be positioned in the knee-chest position before the culdoscope is inserted.

After the procedure the woman is positioned on her abdomen, with a pillow beneath her so that the air that has entered the abdominal cavity will be expelled. The nurse should assess the vital signs and observe the client for vaginal bleeding. Analgesia and backrubs can be used to relieve temporary discomforts. The woman should not have intercourse or douche until advised by the physician that the entry site has healed.

Colposcopy. Colposcopy involves visualization of the cervix with a colposcope, an instrument that magnifies tissue, thereby facilitating inspection of cervical cells and obtaining specimens for biopsy.

The client is prepared as for a pelvic examination. The colposcope is inserted in the vagina through the speculum. Tissues are then observed for color, shape, vasculature, and presence of lesions. In some settings nurses are prepared to perform colposcopic examinations.

Laparoscopy. Structures in the pelvic cavity may be viewed with a lighted laparoscope that is inserted through a stab wound beneath the umbilicus (Fig. 12-4). While the cervix is grasped with tenaculum forceps, the laparoscope is inserted through the abdomen. At this time, carbon dioxide may be introduced to distend the abdomen for easier visualization. A second incision may be made in the lower quadrant of the abdomen for insertion of biopsy instruments or manipulation of the organs. Masses on the ovaries or fallopian tubes, pelvic inflammatory disease, adhesions, or an ectopic pregnancy can be visualized by laparoscopy, and tubal ligations can be performed. When the procedure is completed, the carbon dioxide is released, and the incision is covered with a dressing.

This procedure is usually done with a general anesthetic. Preparation includes inserting a Foley catheter to maintain bladder decompression. After the

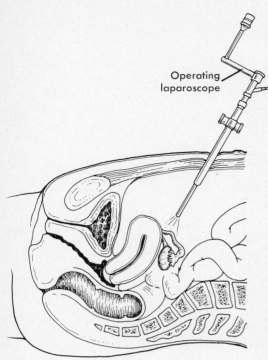

Operating
laparoscope

FIG. 12-4
Laparoscope is used to visualize organs in abdominal cavity.

Cytopathological examinations

procedure the client may be out of bed and have a regular diet. The woman is usually dismissed in 24 hours with instructions to report any bleeding from the incision.

Cystoscopy. The prostate and bladder of the male can be examined by passing a lighted cystoscope through the urethra to the bladder. Enlargement of the prostate is noted as the cystoscope is passed through the urethra. The man should have had nothing to eat or drink since midnight and is given a sedative before the procedure. The examination is usually done without anesthesia, but a local anesthetic may be instilled into the bladder. After cystoscopy the nurse should evaluate vital signs, note that the man has voided, and report any bleeding to the physician. Hot packs to the lower abdomen may be ordered to relieve minor discomfort. Cystoscopic examinations may also be done to detect bladder infections or tumors for both men and women, and the procedure may be modified.

Cells from the vagina, cervix, uterus, and breast can be obtained and examined for abnormal cells. These specimens provide cells for early diagnosis, often before clinical symptoms are evident, and are useful adjuncts to yearly physical examinations and health hazard appraisals.

Cervical Pap smear. The Pap (Papanicolaou) smear for cytology is taken from cells that have become loosened from the vagina, cervix, posterior fornix, and occasionally from the endocervix. It is recommended that this test be performed every 3 years for asymptomatic women over age 20 after two negative tests performed a year apart. Sexually active women under age 20 should also follow this practice. A pelvic examination should be done along with a physical examination every 3 years for women ages 20 to 40 and annually thereafter. Women at high risk for cervical cancer should be examined more frequently.[8] A wooden spatula, pipette, or applicator stick may be used to obtain the specimens. After the specimens have been obtained, they are spread on glass slides with a paper clip separating them. The labeled slides are placed in a container with a preservative and sent to the laboratory where they are examined for atypical cells. The nurse should mark the identification slip with the date, time of last menstrual period, and a notation whether the woman is taking estrogens or birth control pills.

Pap smears can be taken by women in their own homes with a pipette and bulb syringe to aspirate cells from the cervix and vagina. These smears, which are sent to a central laboratory for evaluation, are helpful in women who have had suspicious findings or who live great distances from medical supervision. Even though the kits are readily available, they are not intended to be used for self-diagnosis.

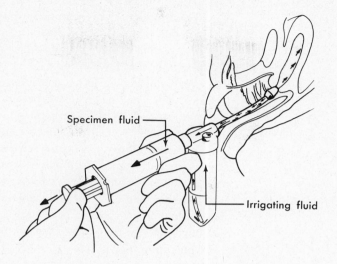

Specimen fluid

Irrigating fluid

Endometrial lavage. Cells from the endometrial lining of the uterus may be obtained by the use of the Gravlee Jet Washer (Fig. 12-5), which is used to lavage the uterus with sterile normal saline under negative pressure to obtain loosened cells for examination.

A pelvic examination is done first, and after the depth of the uterus is determined, the washer is inserted and the endometrial cavity is lavaged. The washings are then used for cytopathological examination.

Biopsies

Biopsies are samples of tissue taken for cytopathological evaluation, which are used to confirm or locate a malignant lesion. Biopsies may be obtained by aspirating tissue cells with special needles or by making an incision and removing selected tissue.

Cervical biopsy. A cervical biopsy is done to detect cancer of the cervix. The biopsy is usually obtained without anesthesia, because the cervix has no pain receptors. The cervix is dilated and scraped with a curette to obtain specimens of cervical and endometrial tissue, and gauze packing is inserted to provide hemostasis. After the procedure the woman should be observed for bleeding, and she is advised not to douche or have intercourse for several weeks after the biopsy.

Dilation and curettage. Dilation and curettage (D and C) are done to obtain tissue for biopsy or to treat excessive bleeding. The client is prepared for general surgery and given an enema to empty the rectum. A catheter is usually inserted during surgery to maintain bladder decompression. The cervix is then dilated and scraped to obtain tissue for biopsy or to aspirate bleeding tissue. A packing may be inserted after surgery for hemostasis, and a sterile perineal pad is worn for protection from drainage. The nurse should observe and record the amount of drainage on the perineal pad. The woman may be out of bed when she has recovered from anesthesia, and the nurse should encourage the client to void as soon as possible to prevent urinary retention. Analgesics may be given for cramping. The woman is usually dismissed from the hospital in a few hours and should be reminded not to douche or have intercourse until advised by her physician (about 2 to 4 weeks). Bleeding may occur for several days, but is excessive if it saturates more than one pad (changed hourly) in 8 hours and should be reported to the surgeon.

Breast biopsy. Breast biopsies may be obtained by incision or aspiration and are done with a local or general anesthetic, depending on the size of the tumor. A section of the tissue may be frozen and stained for rapid diagnosis. This *frozen section* provides rapid diagnosis but may not be as accurate as more extensive cytopathological examinations. Many surgeons also do a "mirror biopsy" on the contralateral breast because there is a 10% incidence of cancer in the opposite breast. A pressure dressing is usually used after a breast biopsy, and the nurse should observe the client for any bleeding on the dressing.

Testicular biopsy. Testicular biopsies can be done to detect abnormal cells and presence of sperm. The biopsies can be incisional or aspirational, and the anesthesia varies with the type of biopsy. A scrotal support may be worn to prevent bleeding, and ice bags and analgesic drugs can relieve minor discomfort. A heat lamp or sitz bath can be used if there is swelling. Any unusual bleeding should be reported to the physician.

Conization. See p. 641.

Cultures and smears

Cultures and smears are done to identify infectious processes, presence of abnormal cells, and hormonal changes in reproductive tissue. The specimens that are taken from an exudate or suspected infection should be obtained with aseptic technique. The nurse should be cautious when handling these specimens and observe good handwashing procedures to prevent the spread of microorganisms.

Cultures. Cultures may be taken from exudates of the vagina, breast, penis, and foreskin. Syphilis, gonorrhea, mastitis, and balanitis (inflammation of the glans penis) are diagnosed by isolating the causative organism.

Prostatic smear. A prostatic smear is obtained to detect microorganisms or tumor cells in the prostate. After the physician massages the prostate through the rectum, the client voids into a sterile specimen container to which a preservative has been added. The specimen is then examined for microorganisms and tumor cells.

Schiller's test. Schiller's test may be done to detect cervical cancer by applying an iodine preparation to the cervix. Normal vaginal cells will be stained brown by the iodine, whereas immature or abnormal cells will not absorb the dye. The client is prepared in the same manner as for a pelvic examination, and the dye is painted on the cervix. After the procedure the nurse can suggest that the woman wear a perineal pad for several hours to prevent iodine stain on the clothing.

Radiographic examinations

Radiographic examinations are done to detect abnormal tissue, to indicate the presence and position of structures, and to discover the patency of ducts.

Hysterogram and hysterosalpingogram. A hysterogram and hysterosalpingogram are done to outline abnormal structures of the uterus or of the uterus, tubes, and ovaries. The client is placed in the lithotomy position, and the dye is inserted through the vagina to the uterus and fallopian tubes. After the procedure the woman may be fatigued and may wish to rest. A perineal pad can be used as dye drains, and analgesics offered as necessary for cramping or discomfort.

Pelvic pneumoperitoneum. A pelvic pneumoperitoneum (nitrous oxide gynecogram) involves the introduction of gas into the pelvic cavity through the abdomen to outline the uterus, tubes, and ovaries. After the procedure the client is placed in the Trendelenburg position for 2 hours so that the gas will rise and be expelled. The woman may experience some pain when the phrenic nerve is stimulated by the excess gas in the pelvic cavity. Backrubs and analgesia usually relieve any discomfort.

Mammography. Mammograms or xeromammograms are used to detect tumors of the breast. X-ray films of the breast are taken from various angles to identify tumors before the appearance of clinical symptoms. The average breast tumor is believed to be present for 8 years before being palpable, thus making mammography a useful screening procedure for those at risk for breast cancer.

The woman undresses to the waist and, when seated, a cone-shaped x-ray beam is focused on the breast from a caudal exposure and, in the supine position, from a medial-lateral angle. The x-rays provide views of the breast as negative images on film (mammogram) or as positive images on paper (xeromammogram).

The use of mammography in routine screening and diagnosis is a controversial issue. Many believe that the risk of cancer induced by repeated x-rays does not justify its use. It is recommended, therefore, that mammography as a diagnostic procedure be reserved for women over age 50; for women ages 40 to 49 with a history of relatives with breast cancer or a personal history of breast cancer; or women ages 35 to 39 only with a personal history of breast cancer.[2,8]

Thermography. Thermography is used to detect changes in circulation in breast tissue by infrared photography. There is increased heat in areas of increased blood supply, indicating a tumor process. For this test the woman sits undressed to the waist for 10 minutes in a room maintained at 69° F (19° C) so that the breast tissue is at basal levels. The temperature recording is then made.

The advantage of this diagnostic test is the absence of exposure to ionizing radiation. The test is used infrequently, however, because accuracy of the results varies widely.

Data analysis

After gathering data about the client's reproductive health and sexuality, the nurse compares the data with norms and, along with the client and/or family, formulates a list of actual or potential nursing diagnoses. Although the nursing diagnoses are unique to the client and derived from specific data, possible priority diagnoses related to reproductive health and sexuality might include ineffective coping, fear, grieving, disturbance in self-concept, sexual dysfunction, alterations in patterns of urinary elimination, self-care deficit, alteration in comfort, and rape-trauma syndrome.

Planning

PLANNING FOR HEALTH PROMOTION

The nurse has an important role in helping clients promote reproductive and sexual health. The nurse may have an opportunity to instruct or counsel clients about personal hygiene, sex education, menstrual health, menopause, conception, infertility, and birth control. Information should be provided with consideration for the client's age, sex, and stage of psychosexual development.

Personal hygiene

Hygiene involves keeping the reproductive organs clean and observing changes in the size and shape of the organs, which could interfere with normal sexual development or signal the onset of disease. Personal cleanliness is a health habit that should be promoted for all clients and implemented in each care plan.

Female client. Cleansing of the female external genitalia should be done with a clean washcloth or cotton balls and soap and water. The labia are separated and cleansed from the pubis to the rectum to avoid contamination. The external labia should be cleansed first, followed by cleansing of the internal labia and finally the urinary meatus and vaginal orifice. A clean part of the cloth should be used for each area. The external genitalia should also be cleansed in this manner after defecation to avoid transfer of microorganisms from the rectum to the vagina or urinary meatus. If the woman is unable to cleanse herself, the nurse should do it for her.

Hygiene is particularly important during adolescence when sweat glands are hyperactive. Taking a daily bath or shower cleanses the skin and reduces body odors, and a deodorant can be used to prevent undesirable body odors. The hair should be washed as often as necessary to keep it clean.

In older women who are prone to senile vulvitis, keeping the vulva clean and dry is an important aspect of feminine hygiene. After the area is thoroughly cleansed, it should be dried with an absorbent towel. An electric hair dryer can be used when pendulous skin folds make drying difficult. Cornstarch, applied after washing, may be used to absorb additional body perspiration. To maintain dryness, cotton underwear is preferred. Nylon pantyhose and tight-fitting slacks cause retention of moisture and should not be used for long periods of time.

Daily cleansing with soap and water is sufficient to control odors, but many women feel the need to use feminine hygiene products such as vaginal sprays and suppositories. Although these products contribute to a feeling of cleanliness, they are not necessary. Some women may be allergic to the chemicals in these products and should inspect the perineal area for rash or signs of inflammation such as rash, burning, or urethritis.

Douching. Douching is generally not a part of feminine hygiene. In fact, repeated douching changes the protective bacterial flora of the vagina and predisposes the woman to infection.

If, however, douching is done occasionally for cleanliness, to remove purulent discharge, or to instill medication, the woman should be taught how to douche. A douche bag with a blunt-ended nozzle to spray all parts of the vagina is preferred. Bulb syringes that force solution and air into the vagina should not be used, because irritation and air emboli may result. The douche is given most safely in the bathtub in the recumbent position. Some women may consider sitting on the toilet seat more comfortable, but this position does not allow the douching solution to adequately contact the vaginal mucosa. If the douche must be given when the woman is in bed, she should be positioned on the bedpan in a semirecumbent position.

The solution should be warmed to 105° F (40.5° C) and administered slowly from a height of 12 to 18 inches (30 to 45 cm) above the vagina. The woman should be instructed to alternately open and close the labia every 15 seconds so that the irrigating solution can contact the mucosa. A continuous douching shield can be attached to the douche bag tubing to control outflow of the solution. If this attachment is used, it is not necessary to hold the labia. During the procedure the nozzle should be rotated to ensure adequate penetration of the vagina. After the procedure the woman should rest in the tub until the solution is expelled. The bathtub should be cleaned, and the douche tip boiled for 15 minutes and stored in a clean container.

Breast self-examination. Examination of the breasts should be a monthly health habit for all adult women. Cancer of the breast is the most frequent cause of death in young women, and tumor growths can be detected when the woman regularly examines her own breasts.

The best time to perform the examination is a week after the onset of the menstrual period so that the normal breast engorgement of menstruation is not confused with abnormal growths. Additionally, this set time serves as a reminder to do the examination. Women who are pregnant or not menstruating should examine their breasts regularly. A specific day each month should be designated for this purpose.

The first step of the examination involves inspecting the breasts in a mirror (Fig. 12-6, *A*). Initial examination is done with the arms at the side. Next, the woman should raise her arms above her head to observe the lifted breasts (Fig. 12-6, *B*). Finally, the woman should place her hands on her hips, lean forward slightly and press her hands against the hips (Fig. 12-6, *C*). Muscle contraction caused by this maneuver aids visualization of dimpling or retraction. During each

FIG. 12-6
Breast self-examination. **A,** Inspection. **B,** Inspection with arms raised. **C,** Inspection with muscles contracted. **D,** Circular pattern of palpation. **E,** Palpation of inner aspect of breast with arms raised. **F,** Palpation of outer aspect with arm lowered.

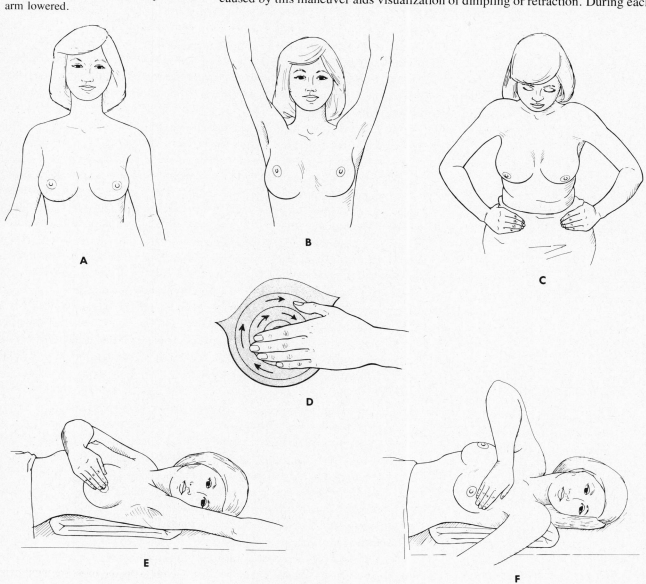

inspection phase the woman should note changes in size of breasts, symmetry, dimpling, changes in color or outline, sores, discharge, puckering of the skin, change of nipple position, or nipple discharge.

The next step of the examination is to palpate each breast to detect unusual growths. Palpation should first be performed in the shower or tub when the skin is wet and easy to palpate. The flat part of the fingers of the right hand is used to palpate the left breast, using a small circular motion to palpate each area. One of two patterns are suggested to ensure careful examination. The woman can palpate the breast in a circular manner starting from the outer aspect of the breast (Fig. 12-6, *D*) to the nipple, or the woman can imagine the breast as a wheel with spokes and follow the spokes to the hub as she palpates. Special attention should be given to the upper outer quadrant and the axillary tail where most tumors are found. The same procedure is then followed for the other breast.

A more complete examination of the breast is done next, with the woman lying on her bed. A small pillow or folded towel should be placed under the shoulder of the breast to be palpated to support the breast tissue and make palpation easier, (Fig. 12-6, *E*). The arm is raised above the head and the inner aspect of the breast carefully examined as described above. The arm is then lowered (Fig. 12-6, *F*), and the outer aspect of the breast is palpated. Others suggest a final examination in the sitting position with one arm above the head, using the opposite hand for palpation.

Finally, the nipple should be held and gently pressed. Secretions or discharge should not be present unless the woman is lactating.

In doing breast self-examination, the woman soon learns what her breasts feel like and what is normal for her. The woman should not be alarmed by certain normal anatomical structures. There may be ridges or cysts in normal breast tissue, and it is not unusual for the breasts to enlarge and feel painful before the menstrual period.

Lumps, pain unrelated to the menstrual cycle, or bleeding from the nipple are the most notable changes indicating abnormalities. These should be reported to the physician at once.

Many women find it difficult to examine their breasts regularly. Some may fear cancer and bodily disfigurement, or some may be embarrassed to inspect or touch their breasts. In a survey of women's attitudes regarding breast cancer, it was learned that lack of knowledge about the proper technique for breast examination was a major factor in infrequency of breast examinations.[23] When breast examination is taught personally by a health professional, the chances of the woman doing the examination herself are increased. The role of the nurse in teaching breast self-examination, therefore, cannot be emphasized too strongly.

Examination of the vulva. In addition to a monthly examination of the breast, women should be encouraged to inspect and palpate the vulva (labia majora, labia minora, clitoris, vaginal orifice) for changes in color, size, or shape. The nurse can instruct the woman to use a mirror to identify normal structures and be familiar with what is normal for her. Ulcerations, rashes, nodules, or other lesions should be reported to a physician.

Male client. Cleansing of the male genitalia is done with a washcloth and soap and water. If the man is not circumcised, it is necessary to retract the foreskin to cleanse the penis. The foreskin should not remain retracted, however, because constriction may cause edema, pain, dysuria, reduced blood supply, and necrosis. If the nurse or mother is cleansing the boy, it may be easier to wash the scrotum first to prevent penile erection.

During puberty and adolescence the boy should be encouraged to bathe daily. Hyperactive sweat glands produce a body odor that can be controlled by bathing and using a deodorant. The adolescent usually begins to be more aware of his appearance and more willing to bathe, shave, and groom himself than he was as a school-age boy.

Testicular self-examination. The nurse can instruct the man to inspect and palpate the testes for changes in color or shape. The testes are best palpated in the bath or shower when the cremesteric muscles relax and the testes are pendulous. The man supports the testes in the palm of one hand and gently palpates with the testes between the thumb and forefinger. Growths, lesions, or nodules should be reported to the physician.

Promotion of health during menstruation

Menstruation is a normal aspect of a woman's health. The nurse has the responsibility to foster positive attitudes toward menstruation and provide information as needed or requested by the client. Menstruation should not be considered an illness, and phrases such as "the curse" should be avoided in favor of "menstruating" or "the period."

When counseling a girl or woman about menstruation, the nurse must assess the client's knowledge of menstruation. From this point the nurse can clarify misconceptions and supply appropriate knowledge. Knowledge should, furthermore, be provided at times suitable to the client's development and before the need for its use.

Instruction generally centers around the understanding of the process of menstruation, use of sanitary protection, and management of minor discomforts. Additionally, the client should be aware of her normal menstrual cycle and what problems she should report to a health professional.

Before a girl begins to menstruate, she should receive instruction about the process of menstruation. Instruction may come from parents, friends, organized instruction programs, or health personnel, and the nurse may assist any of these by offering information.

The nurse can also instruct the girl about the use of sanitary napkins and tampons. Although there may be individual preferences as to the use of a method of sanitary protection, it is recommended that if the client uses tampons, they should be alternated in a 24-hour time period with sanitary napkins to prevent menstrual back flow and toxic shock syndrome.[17] Napkins should be attached and removed from front to back to prevent contamination. The napkin may be self-adhering or used with an elastic belt. Unless there is difficulty or contraindication to insertion, many girls prefer the use of tampons. Tampons may be lubricated with water soluble gel to make insertion easier. Napkins and tampons should be changed every 3 to 4 hours to prevent irritation and odor.

Premenstrual syndrome. As many as 30% of women experience irritability, anxiety, depression, dizziness, sensations of being bloated, and other discomforts 1 to 12 days before the onset of menstruation. Additionally, migraine headaches, asthma, and glaucoma may be aggravated at this time. It is believed that the physiological basis for these discomforts is an alteration of the renin-angiotensin-aldosterone cycle. Rest and fluid restriction alleviate some of the discomforts. Progesterone may be used to correct ovarian hormone imbalances.

Immediately before the onset of menstruation, many women experience

605

weight gain and enlargement of the breasts. This is caused by progesterone production that causes sodium and water retention. Sodium restriction in the diet and diuretics may be prescribed to alleviate these symptoms.

Before or during menstruation, some women experience mild muscle cramps in the lower abdomen and across the back. Exercise, heat, and mild analgesics usually relieve cramping. Cramping can also be prevented or minimized by maintaining good posture to alleviate strain on sacral muscles and ligaments and by observing health habits of diet, rest, and exercise. Exercise is important to the sense of well-being and to prevent discomfort from menstrual cramps (dysmenorrhea) by breaking up clot formations. Walking and bicycling are relaxing to the pelvic muscles. All sports activities, including swimming, may be done during menstruation, but some women may find that they need extra rest at this time.

Promotion of health during menopause

Menopause is a normal event in the woman's life span. The nurse may have an opportunity to clarify myths and facilitate health instruction at this time.

Physical and psychological changes accompany menopause. Women may experience vasomotor effects of estrogen withdrawal such as hot flushes, palpitations, sweating, chills, headaches, numbness, or tingling. Estrogen withdrawal produces other changes. Osteoporosis resulting from estrogen depletion causes a shortening in stature. The woman may experience abdominal pain and backaches. There may be decreased elasticity of the skin and increases in fat deposits. Furthermore, coronary atherosclerosis is thought by some to be caused by estrogen withdrawal because the incidence of coronary artery disease increases after menopause.

The physical changes may be accompanied by psychological periods of depression and withdrawal. The woman may feel nervous, anxious, or fatigued. Often the woman feels that she is useless when her reproductive ability ceases.

The effects of menopause may be minimized by hormonal supplements. Estrogens may be given to decrease the flushes, sweating, or vaginitis. Few advise that these supplements be continued on an indefinite basis, and it is recommended that they be given in a cyclic manner such as 5 days on the pill and 2 days off. Estrogens are generally not advised for women with a history of cancer, hypertension, diabetes, or thromboembolism. The woman is furthermore assisted by the understanding of her husband, family, and friends. Finding satisfying outlets in a job or volunteer activity often detracts from depression and feelings of uselessness.

Sex education

Individuals' information about reproduction and sexuality come from many sources, including friends, literature, parents, siblings, school or religious education programs, or health professionals. The nurse may have an opportunity to be a part of a sex education curriculum or may be active in counseling parents and children and should offer information within the framework of the family's values and the objectives of the sex education curriculum.

Education regarding sexual activities should be given to individuals before they need to use the information. It is unfortunate for a girl to begin to menstruate or a boy to have seminal emissions without understanding the purpose. Health education information should be correct and discussed at the individual's level of understanding. The preschooler does not need an explanation of the process of conception, delivery, and postpartum care when he asks how are babies born, but the adolescent does.

Sex education should include appropriate information about conception, birth, venereal disease, conception control, and family living. The information may be given in the home, church, school, or community organizations. Many pamphlets, films, and educational curricula are available to students, families, parents, teachers, and group leaders. The nurse may help community agencies locate and use these resources.

Attitudes that develop in the formative years establish the basis for adult sexuality. Marital problems may be related to misunderstandings and misconceptions, and persons with these problems can be referred to their physician or family counseling agencies. Much research has been done on sexual compatibility and happiness in sex relations, and there are several books and articles that may be helpful to married couples and health team members.

Birth control planning

Advances in drug therapy and family planning technology have made available a range of options for individuals wishing to prevent or plan conception. Birth control planning involves moral, religious, cultural, and personal values, and the nurse should be sensitive to these factors when discussing birth control with clients.

There are several types of birth control procedures or devices that can be employed. The selection of the particular method should be based on the health of the individual, effectiveness, cost, ease of use, age, and parity of the client, willingness of the client to comply with use, and preference of the individual and sex partner. The nurse can help the client obtain information about each method and the relationship to the individual's needs so that the client can make an informed choice.

Sterilization. Sterilization is a permanent, effective method of birth control, which can be performed for men or women. Many states have laws regulating who can use this method of birth control, and the husband and wife must both sign a permit for the operative procedure. Sterilization is generally not done for persons who have not had children.

Sterilization of the man. A *vasectomy* is the operation performed on a man to terminate the passage of sperm through the vas deferens. There are several ways to perform this procedure, and it can generally be done in a physician's office or in an ambulatory care clinic. In one approach the client is given a local anesthetic, and an incision is made in the scrotum to clip, clamp, or crush the vas deferens or to remove ¼ to ½ inch of the vas deferens (0.6 to 1.2 cm). This operation is permanent, and chances of reanastomosis are minimal. After surgery there is slight swelling of the scrotum, and the client should wear a scrotal support for several days; hot baths may be used to reduce the swelling. The client can have intercourse when the pain subsides, but he must have several successive negative sperm counts from seminal emissions before he can be assured that conception will not occur, because residual sperm are present in the vas deferens. This usually takes from 1 to 3 months, and other methods of birth control should be used in the meantime.

Although the procedure is intended to be permanent, the client may wish to reverse the procedure because of remarriage or death of a child. In some instances the vas deferens may be reanastomosed in a surgical procedure known as a *vasovasotomy*. Research is also being conducted to develop a device that permits a reversible vasectomy. These devices, now in trial use, are inserted in the vas deferens and have a valve that can be turned off or on to allow passage of sperm.

607

Sterilization of the woman. Sterilization for women can be accomplished by *tubal ligation.* The fallopian tubes are tied or cauterized during an operation that is done through an abdominal incision. In this type of surgery the woman is exposed to routine operative risks and must be hospitalized for several days.

In another approach to tubal ligation, a *laparoscope* is passed through a puncture wound near the umbilicus. A small incision is made 2 inches (5 cm) from the insertion of the laparoscope, and when the fallopian tubes are visualized, they are cauterized, ligated, crushed, clipped, or resected by means of instruments inserted in the incision. A bandage is placed over the incision, hence the term "Band-Aid surgery." This method of tubal ligation can be performed with a local or short-acting general anesthetic and may be done in a clinic. Recovery is rapid, and there is no unsightly scar from an abdominal incision.

In the culdoscopic approach to tubal ligation, a culdoscope is inserted through the vagina to the cul de sac and the tubes coagulated with an electric cautery. Shorter hospitalization time is required with this method.

When the woman has recovered from the surgery, ova will not pass through the fallopian tubes. The menstrual cycle, however, will remain normal because the ovaries continue to produce estrogen. Reconstruction of the tubes is possible, and success rates of reconstruction approach 50%.

Hysterectomy (removal of the uterus) and oophorectomy (removal of the ovaries) are other surgical procedures that will cause the woman to be sterile.

Oral contraceptives. Oral contraceptives (birth control pills) are a popular and easy form of contraception that is close to 100% effective. The pill, which is taken by the woman, inhibits release of follicle-stimulating hormone, and subsequently the menstrual cycles are anovulatory. Some pills contain estrogen only; others combine a progestogen in the last five or six pills of the cycle. Others are dispensed in 28-day cycles, with the last seven pills containing inert substances. The birth control pills are taken in a cyclical fashion beginning on the fifth day of the cycle. (Day 1 of the cycle begins with the onset of menstruation.) The pills are continued at the same time daily for 20 to 21 days. Several days later the woman menstruates, and the cycle is repeated.

Birth control pills have the advantages of being easy to take, not requiring use of a contraceptive device before intercourse, and being highly effective. They are prescribed by a physician, and the woman should have a yearly physical examination while taking birth control pills. The woman must remember to take the pill daily. If she forgets to take one, she is usually advised to take two the next day. If she misses more than two pills she should stop taking the pills for that cycle for 7 days and then restart the cycle. It is advisable to use another form of contraception for that cycle.

The pills should be stored carefully. They are affected by high humidity and should be kept in a dry place; extreme heat should be avoided because heat can decrease potency of the pills.

Some women experience various side effects when using the pills, particularly during the first few months. The symptoms are usually similar to those of the first trimester of pregnancy: nausea and vomiting, weight gain, and swelling of the breasts. The pills can be taken after a meal to lessen the nausea. It is also helpful to take the pills at the same time each day.

Birth control pills tend to increase the alkalinity of the vagina and thereby cause the woman to be more susceptible to vaginal infections. Monilial infections *(Candida albicans)* are particularly common.

Oral contraceptives have been demonstrated to have a relationship to certain cardiovascular disorders, and consequently women with hypertension, thromboembolic diseases, or a history of circulatory disease, varicosities, or diabetes mellitus should be discouraged from using birth control pills. Smoking increases the risk of cardiovascular complications in women taking birth control pills.

Other side effects are often related to birth control use. As research findings are published, more information is available to use in considering birth control pills as a method for contraception. The nurse should help the client interpret the information for her individual needs.

Intrauterine devices. Intrauterine devices (IUDs) are also nearly 100% effective. These devices are inserted into the uterus by a physician. It is not known exactly how these devices prevent pregnancy, presumably by causing degeneration of the fertilized egg or by rendering the uterine wall impervious to implantation. The Lippes loop, Birnberg bow, Copper T, and Margulies coil (Fig. 12-7, *A*) are examples of commonly used IUDs. The device should be inserted during menstruation when the cervix is dilated and it is assured that the woman is not pregnant. The devices do not interrupt the menstrual cycle, and the

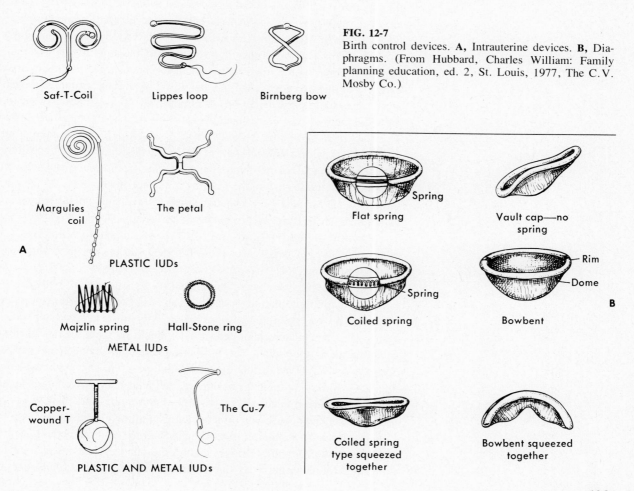

FIG. 12-7
Birth control devices. **A,** Intrauterine devices. **B,** Diaphragms. (From Hubbard, Charles William: Family planning education, ed. 2, St. Louis, 1977, The C.V. Mosby Co.)

Saf-T-Coil   Lippes loop   Birnberg bow

Margulies coil   The petal

A

PLASTIC IUDs

Majzlin spring   Hall-Stone ring

METAL IUDs

Copper-wound T   The Cu-7

PLASTIC AND METAL IUDs

Flat spring   Vault cap—no spring

Coiled spring   Bowbent · Rim · Dome

B

Coiled spring type squeezed together   Bowbent squeezed together side effects are minimal, although the woman may have cramping or excessive menstrual flow for 2 to 3 months. These devices are usually used for women who have had at least one pregnancy.

The most common side effect of IUD use is infection. Because the infection rate is high, it is advisable that this form of birth control not be used for young or nulliparous women. Pelvic inflammatory disease, intermenstrual bleeding, and uterine perforations are complications of IUD use.

The woman should check every few weeks for the presence of the IUD in the uterus by feeling the string or plastic bead that is suspended in the vagina. The woman should also check after each voiding or change of perineal pad or tampon to be sure that the device has not become dislodged. The device is usually replaced every 2 to 3 years.

Condom. The condom offers a simple, effective method of birth control. Condoms have the additional benefit of preventing venereal disease. The latex rubber sheath fits over the penis and prevents ejaculate and sperm from entering the vagina. Condoms are easy to use, easily obtained, and relatively inexpensive, but some tactile pleasure may be lost with their use. Good-quality condoms should be purchased, then discarded after each use.

Diaphragm. The diaphragm is a highly effective (97%) method of birth control if used correctly. A flexible rubber ring with a latex cup is inserted into the vagina and released to cover the cervix (Fig. 12-7, *B*). When in position, the diaphragm prevents sperm from entering the cervix. Spermicidal gel should be used with the diaphragm to increase its effectiveness. The diaphragm is fitted by a physician, and the woman is given instruction about its use. The diaphragm may be inserted before intercourse but must remain in place 6 hours after intercourse. Additional spermicidal gel should be used if the couple has intercourse again, and the diaphragm can be left in place for up to 24 hours. After each use, the diaphragm should be washed, observed for tears, and stored in a dry place. The diaphragm should be refitted every 2 years as well as after each pregnancy.

Vaginal spermicides. Spermicidal foams, jellies, and suppositories are almost as effective as the diaphragm. They are inserted into the vagina before intercourse to interfere with the viability of the sperm and prevent their entry into the cervix. These methods of contraception are available without medical supervision and can be purchased without a prescription.

Rhythm method. The rhythm method of birth control is not as effective as other methods, but it is acceptable to religious groups who do not support the methods of birth control previously described. This method is based on the regularity of ovulation, which can be detected by the lowering of body temperature before ovulation and the slight rise during ovulation. The temperature must be taken rectally each morning before rising and recorded to note temperature variations. A thermometer calibrated in 0.1° should be used for this purpose. Because sperm may be viable for 48 hours, the couple should abstain from intercourse for several days before and after ovulation. The menstrual cycle is easily altered by illness, hormonal imbalances, and physical or psychological stresses, so that this method is not always reliable. Furthermore, the method is even less reliable near menopause when menstrual cycles become irregular.

In the *ovulation method,* a modification of the rhythm method of birth control, the woman identifies changes that occur in the cervical mucus during ovulation and abstains for the 3 days surrounding ovulation. The cervical mucus thickens and may be yellow or cloudy during ovulation. The ovulation method of birth control has been 98% effective in women instructed in this method and offers an inexpensive, natural alternative for contraception. Problems exist, however, if there are changes in the cycle because of illness or stress.

Coitus interruptus. Coitus interruptus is a primitive form of contraception of questionable effectiveness. The man withdraws his penis before ejaculation to avoid depositing sperm into the vagina. Sperm may be present, however, in seminal fluid, which is emitted before ejaculation, and this can cause an unwanted pregnancy. Coitus interruptus is usually not psychologically satisfying to either partner.

Other methods. Other forms of birth control are in experimental stages. Attempts are being made to develop an effective progestational drug that may be administered monthly. Research is also being done to explore chemotherapeutic birth control for men. Other research efforts are directed toward a "morning-after" pill, potent synthetic estrogens to be used after intercourse.

Improvised, noncommercial products are not contraceptive devices and will not prevent pregnancy. Douches do not provide contraceptive protection and, in fact, may force the sperm into the cervix. The nurse can assist clients by explaining which contraceptive measures are successful in preventing pregnancy.

Implementation

COMMON HEALTH PROBLEMS OF THE NEONATE AND INFANT

Phimosis

Phimosis is the narrowing of the foreskin of the penis. When the foreskin is completely constricted, urine flow is obstructed, and the client is predisposed to urinary tract infection. Phimosis usually appears as a congenital defect but can be acquired if smegma accumulates under the foreskin and infection develops, causing the foreskin to adhere.

The tightened foreskin can be removed easily in a simple procedure known as *circumcision*. In this operation a special instrument is placed over the tip of the penis to excise the foreskin. No anesthesia is used when the procedure is performed on neonates. Gauze saturated with petrolatum is placed over the penis to prevent irritation. After the circumcision, the nurse should record the first voiding to indicate urinary tract patency. The petrolatum-smeared gauze should be changed after each voiding. The client usually goes home the day after the circumcision, and the nurse should instruct that the gauze be changed and the area kept dry until the skin has healed. Unusual bleeding should be reported to the physician.

Hypospadias

Hypospadias is an opening of the urinary meatus on the ventral surface of the penis (Fig. 12-8). Ventral bowing (chordee) usually accompanies hypospadias. Hypospadias is a congenital defect that may occur along with other defects such as undescended testicles. If the meatal opening is large, it is possible to confuse the gender identity of the neonate, and further tests such as chromosome analysis may be necessary.

This defect is surgically corrected when the boy is 1 to 3 years old. If the meatal defect is small, it may only be necessary to correct the ventral bowing because spontaneous closure of the meatus may occur. If the defect is large, the surgery is done in two stages, first to correct the ventral bowing and later to correct the hypospadias. When the hypospadias is corrected, a suprapubic cystostomy catheter is inserted into the bladder for urinary drainage. The catheter is

611

FIG. 12-8
Hypospadias. Note opening of meatus on ventral surface of penis. (Courtesy Dr. Matthew C. Gleason, San Diego, Calif.)

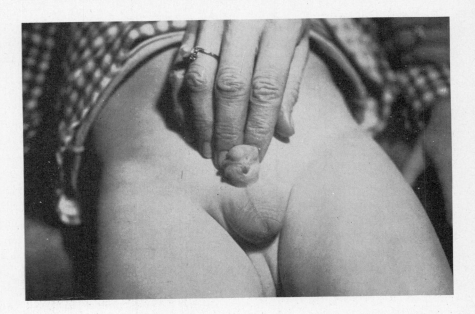

removed after healing, and the nurse should observe the first voiding through the newly positioned meatus. The parents are encouraged to observe the child's voiding for several years after surgery because scar tissue may cause urethral stricture and impair urination. The parents should help the child maintain cleanliness to avoid infection.

During hospitalization and subsequent recovery, the child should be reassured that the problem is congenital and not caused by masturbation or sex fantasies. The child should be approached with respect for his modesty and given straightforward answers to questions about the surgery.

Epispadias

Epispadias is a malposition of the urinary meatus on the dorsal surface of the penis. The defect can be small or large and include extrophy of the bladder.

This defect is corrected by surgical repair as soon as the child can tolerate surgery. The surgery may be performed in one or two stages, depending on the size of the defect. Nursing care is similar to that of the child with hypospadias repair.

Cryptorchidism

Cryptorchidism (undescended testicle) occurs when one or both testicles do not descend into the scrotum. In *true cryptorchidism* the testicles remain in the abdominal cavity, whereas in *ectopic cryptorchidism* they remain in the inguinal canal. There is an increased incidence of cryptorchidism in premature births because the testicles do not descend until the seventh to ninth months of gestation. The nurse should palpate the scrotum of neonates to verify the presence of the testicles, because diagnosis of the defect can be made during this initial health appraisal.

If the undescended testicle remains in the abdominal cavity or the inguinal canal, it is susceptible to crushing abdominal injury. There are also increased chances for neoplastic growth and damage to sperm production from body heat if the testicles remain undescended after the fifth year. It is important, therefore, to correct the defect within the first few years of life.

If true cryptorchidism exists, conservative therapy may be used. Chorionic gonadotropic hormone is given to stimulate the testicles to descend spontaneously.

If there is ectopic cryptorchidism or if there is no response to conservative therapy, the testicles may be repositioned surgically in a procedure known as *orchidopexy*. This procedure is usually done before the child enters school. An incision is made in the inguinal canal, and the testis is brought down into the scrotum. Traction may be applied from the scrotum to the thigh with a suture, to ensure that the testis will remain in proper position until healing occurs.

After surgery the nurse should ensure that traction is maintained and prevent contamination of the suture line. Antibiotics may be used to prevent infection. The nurse should plan care appropriate to the boy's age and social development and be sensitive to his needs for privacy.

COMMON HEALTH PROBLEMS OF THE ADOLESCENT AND YOUNG ADULT

Sexually transmitted diseases (venereal diseases)

Sexually transmitted diseases (STD) include those infections of the reproductive system that are transmitted by any form of sexual contact. The most common are gonorrhea, herpes genitalis II, syphilis, trichomoniasis, and moniliasis. Less common are lymphogranuloma venereum, granuloma inguinale, chancroid, condylomata acuminatum, and cytomegalovirus (Table 12-1).

Transmission of venereal diseases usually occurs during intercourse, but noncoital contact of mucous membranes with involved individuals can also spread these diseases. Examples are gonorrheal ophthalmia acquired by the newborn during delivery and gonorrhea contracted by youngsters sleeping in the same bed with infected adults.

Sexually transmitted diseases are a significant health problem in the United States. Although the true incidence is difficult to estimate because many cases go unreported, STDs exist in epidemic proportions and are considered to be the number one cause of communicable disease in individuals 15 to 30 years of age.[9] This fact is more astounding when one considers that methods or prevention and treatment are readily available. Many reasons are offered for this persistent prevalence of venereal diseases; some are improved birth control methods, changes in moral standards, and mobility of populations.

The nurse has an important role in working with other health team members in preventing the spread of venereal disease. Education is the primary tool of prevention. Information can be offered about the consequences of sexual contact and how to recognize indications of infection. The information should be given in a nonthreatening manner with respect for the client's sexual mores. Some methods of prevention are using condoms and washing involved parts before and after sexual contact.

Once venereal disease is suspected, the client should be encouraged to seek medical attention immediately. Some states do not require parental consent for minors to be treated. Health care workers will also need to ascertain contacts of the involved individuals so that they can be discreetly approached and advised to seek medical intervention. Venereal diseases should be reported to the local board of health for epidemiological study and contact investigation. Finally, once the client is being treated, he should be given instruction and support. He should be encouraged to follow the medical therapy and abstain from intercourse until he is no longer infectious.

Gonorrhea. Gonorrhea (clap, whites, the dose, the drips) is caused by the gonococcus *Neisseria gonorrhoeae*. There are four types of gonococci, types 1

TABLE 12-1
Sexually transmitted diseases

	Causative organism	Incubation period	Period of communicability	Diagnostic test	Clinical manifestations	Medical therapy (males and females [nonpregnant women])
Gonorrhea	Neisseria gonorrhoeae	3 to 5 days	When infected	Culture, gram stain	Urethritis; purulent, yellow-green discharge	Aqueous penicillin, 4.8 million U IM with 1 g probenecid
Herpes genitalis II	Herpesvirus hominis type 2	3 to 6 days	When lesion present	Virology of lesion cytology	Vesicles or ulcers on vulva, perineum, vagina, penis	Symptomatic treatment of pain and secondary infection; miconazole nitrate topically and intravaginally
Syphilis	Treponema pallidum	3 weeks	Primary stage: exudate or lesions; Secondary stage: blood contains microorganism; Latent: 2 years	Culture, serological tests	Primary stage: chancre on mucous membranes; Secondary stage: vague symptoms, headache, anorexia; Late stage: gummas on organs, paresis, somnolence	Benzathine penicillin, 4.8 million U IM; procaine penicillin, 600,000 U orally, up to 12 days
Trichomoniasis	Trichomonas vaginalis	4 to 28 days	When infected	Culture, cytology	Pruritus; thin, frothy, white, green, yellow, or yellow-green discharge; dysuria	Metronidazole (Flagyl), 2 g orally or 250 mg orally three times daily for 7 days
Moniliasis	Candida albicans	Variable	When infected	Culture, gram stains	Pruritus; thick, curdlike discharge	Nystatin (Monistat) vaginal suppositories, 100,000 U twice daily for 14 days; nystatin ointment to penis twice a day for 14 days
Chancroid	Haemophilus ducreyi	4 to 5 days		Gram stain	Macule proceeding to pustules and ulcerated lesions	Sulfonamide, 1 g orally every 6 hr for 14 days
Lymphogranuloma venereum	Chlamydia organisms	7 to 12 days		Complement-fixation tests	Papule or vesicle	Tetracycline, 500 mg four times daily for 3 weeks
Condyloma acuminatum	Papilloma viruses			Biopsy	Verrucous growth on genitourinary organs	25% Podophyllin in tincture of benzoin one or two times a week; electrocautery
Granuloma inguinale	Calymmatobacterium granulomatis	8 to 12 weeks		Tissue stain for Donovan bodies	Lesions on genitals	Tetracycline, 500 mg four times daily for 14 days

and 2 have hairlike projections that attach to mucous membranes. These types are pathogenic, whereas types 3 and 4 are not.

Gonorrhea is the most common of the sexually transmitted diseases. It is the most common in the 20- to 24-year age group followed by the 15- to 19-year age group.[9] Those at risk are all sexually active individuals and those women who use birth control pills or are otherwise susceptible to infection. Three times as many men are affected as women, and the symptoms are more pronounced in men.

☞ *Assessment.* The indications of an infection in the man include urethritis, burning on urination, frequency, and dysuria. These are followed by a yellowish-green discharge from the urethra. The presence of these symptoms may motivate the client to seek health care assistance.

Eighty percent of women who have gonorrhea are asymptomatic, and because of this many are not treated until complications such as pelvic inflammatory disease are evident. Early signs include labial tenderness, low back pain, and a slightly purulent discharge. If the bladder is involved, there may be symptoms of cystitis such as frequency and burning on urination.

The diagnosis of gonorrhea is made by direct smear or culture of the organism. Smears are difficult to obtain from women, and cultures should be obtained from the cervix, urethra, and anus to confirm the diagnosis. A presumptive diagnosis may be made on the clinical evidence so that therapy can begin immediately.

☞ *Planning and implementation.* Gonorrhea is treated with antibiotics and symptomatically. Penicillin, 4.8 million U aqueous penicillin IM in divided doses, is given with 1 g probenecid orally. The probenecid competes with the penicillin for excretion by the kidneys and thereby delays excretion of the penicillin. Tetracyclines may be used if the client is allergic to penicillin.

The client is encouraged to drink fluids to promote urination. Sitz baths may be used to relieve local discomfort. The nurse should emphasize the importance of good handwashing techniques after urinating. The man may wear an athletic support if drainage is severe. Women should wear a perineal pad if there is a vaginal discharge.

If gonorrhea is not treated, the gonococcus invades the prostate and epididymis or the fallopian tubes. If these infections are untreated, sterility may result from adhesions.

Gonorrhea can be transmitted to the mucous membranes of the eyes of newborns if the mother has a gonococcal infection. Silver nitrate or antibiotics are used prophylactically in the eyes of all newborns to prevent *ophthalmia neonatorum,* which produces blindness. Gonorrhea can also be transmitted to young girls as a vulvovaginitis if they are sleeping next to women with gonococcal infections, and for this reason it is advisable that children sleep in separate beds.

Herpes genitalis II. Herpes genitalis is a venereal disease caused by a virus, herpesvirus hominis type 2 (HVH-2), which produces vesicles on the genitalia. Herpes genitalis has become the second most common sexually transmitted disease.[9] Those at risk are sexually active individuals and persons with low resistance to infection. It is believed that lesions are associated with cancer of the cervix. Additionally, if the woman is in the first trimester of pregnancy, there is an increased incidence of abortion; congenital anomalies are rare. If the lesions are present at the time of delivery, a cesarean section may be used to prevent transmission to the neonate.

615

Assessment. In women the virus appears as tender vesicles on the vulva, vagina, or perineum. There is pain and tenderness of the vulva, vaginal discharge, and pruritus. In men the vesicle appears on the penis, and there is urethral discharge, pain, pruritus, and dysuria.

The disease is characterized by recurrent infection. The infection may be exacerbated by stress, fever, overexposure to heat or sun, and emotional upset. The client may experience parasthesias at the site before eruption of the lesion, a premonitory sign that the disease is once again active. The disease is diagnosed by virological or cytological examination of aspirate of the lesions.

Planning and implementation. To date, no treatment has been proved effective for cure of herpes genitalis. Some approaches to treatment have included the use of photodynamic dye therapy or topical application of ether. A new drug, miconazole nitrate (2-deoxy-D glucose) is being used with success.[1] The drug is applied as a gel topically or intravaginally four times a day.

Other treatment is directed to preventing infection and treating the symptoms. Antibiotics may be used as well as analgesic ointments, steroid creams, and Burow's solution.

The nurse helps the client learn to manage the treatment plan. Because the lesion appears at times of physical or emotional stress, the client should plan to use stress management strategies and maintain health habits of adequate rest, nutrition, and hygiene. The nurse should also counsel the client that the disease is communicable when lesions reappear.

Syphilis. Syphilis is an infection caused by the spirochete *Treponema pallidum*. This organism thrives in warm parts of the body but is killed by soap and exposure to sunlight. The organism is spread by direct contact through openings in the mucous membranes of genital organs, the anus, or mouth, or it may be transmitted across the placenta to the fetus. The spirochete can also be transmitted by blood transfusion, although it is killed within 3 hours if the blood is stored at a cool temperature.

Syphilis is estimated to be the third most common sexually transmitted disease. The ease of treatment at one time reduced the incidence, but changes in sexual mores and decreased use of condoms as a contraceptive device have been attributed to an increased incidence of syphilis.

Assessment. The symptoms of the infection follow a pattern that has been defined in stages: primary, secondary, latent, and late.

Primary. The incubation of syphilis (the time from when the spirochetes enter the body until symptoms occur) is about 3 weeks. At this time a lesion, the *chancre,* appears at the site of exposure—the labia, penis, mouth, anus, or nipple. The chancre is a painless, reddened macule that becomes ulcerated. It often goes unnoticed. If no treatment is instituted, the chancre heals within 3 to 8 weeks. During this period the client is highly contagious.

Secondary. Secondary symptoms of the disease occur within 2 to 4 weeks to 6 months of exposure, and even as late as 2 years, because the spirochetes invade the bloodstream. These symptoms include a rash on the palms and soles or elsewhere on the body, papules called *mucous patches* in the mouth, sore throat, or loss of hair. There may even be anorexia, fever, headache, anemia, or weight loss. The person is able to transmit the disease if he is not treated.

Latent stage. The *early latent stage* of syphilis occurs from 2 to 4 years after infection. The serological tests are positive, and the disease is transmissible. If the body defenses are not adequate, the symptoms may be exacerbated. During the *late latent stage,* reappearance of the infection is unlikely. It is rare that the disease could be transmitted at this time. Eighty percent of clients remain asymptomatic. The other 20% develop systemic symptoms.

Late (tertiary stage). The spirochetes in the body form gummas (cellular deposits) on various organs of the body, which can impair their function. The heart, aorta, and blood vessels are common sites. The gummas often cause valvular disease and aneurysms of the arteries. The central nervous system may be affected, and blindness, crippling, lack of coordination, paralysis, and slurred speech may result.

A presumptive diagnosis can be made by history, but the diagnosis is confirmed by culture or serological tests. The spirochetes can be detected by the culture of the open lesion (chancre). The client should not wash the chancre or apply topical medication because this will destroy the spirochete for culture.

Serological tests for syphilis are determined by the antigen-antibody reaction that occurs between the antigen *(T pallidum)* and the host antibody. Two types of antibodies are produced, specific and nonspecific reagins, and the tests are based on these antibodies.

The nontreponemal (reagin) test is the Venereal Disease Research Laboratory (VDRL) test. The VDRL test is a flocculation test in which any reagin of the spirochete present forms a precipitate. The Wasserman and Kolmer tests are complement-fixation tests. These rapid plasma reagin (RPR) tests can give false-positive results if the person has a collagen disease. These tests are not positive until 1 to 4 weeks after the appearance of the chancre.

Treponemal tests are more specific. Two are the *Treponema pallidum* immobilization (TPI) test and the fluorescent treponemal antibody absorption (FTA-ABS) test. These tests remain positive even after treatment.

Planning and implementation. Syphilis is treated with massive doses of penicillin. A dosage of 600,000 U of procaine penicillin G may be given every day for 10 to 12 days. Benzathine penicillin G (Bicillin) may also be used as a one-time dose of 2.4 million U in both buttocks. If the client is allergic to penicillin, tetracyclines are prescribed.

Congenital syphilis. Congenital syphilis is passed to the fetus through the placenta of a mother who has syphilis. The neonate with congenital syphilis is observed to have rhinitis, skin rashes, cutaneous lesions, osteochondritis, or fissures on the lips, nares, or anus. Later signs may include saddlenose, saw-teeth, saber shin, and other congenital deformities. If the mother is treated before the eighteenth week of the pregnancy, the chances of congenital syphilis are reduced because penicillin crosses the placental barrier.

Trichomoniasis. Trichomoniasis is a venereal disease caused by the protozoan *Trichomonas vaginalis.* Those at risk for this infection are sexually active women and women who have changes in vaginal pH from taking antibiotics.

Assessment. In women, trichomoniasis produces a characteristic frothy-discharge that may be white, yellow, yellowish-green, or green. Pruritus and subsequent excoriation of the vulva and vagina are common. Dysuria, frequency, and dyspareunia may also occur. In men, although usually asymptomatic, the infection is evidenced by pruritus, burning, urethritis, and purulent discharge.

Planning and implementation. Metronidazole (Flagyl), 250 mg orally for 7 to 10 days, or one dose of 2 g orally, is used to treat trichomoniasis. The sex

Nursing process for common health problems

partner must also be treated to prevent cross-infection. Metronidazole may have effects similar to disulfiram (Antabuse), and the client should be instructed not to drink alcoholic beverages while using the drug to prevent the unpleasant symptoms. Side effects include gastrointestinal upset, headache, metallic taste in the mouth, and stomatitis.

Moniliasis. Monilial infections are caused by fungus, *Candida albicans*. There is controversy if, in fact, moniliasis is a sexually transmitted disease, but because it can be spread by sexual contact, it is often so classified. Monilial infections are common, particularly in women. The incidence of infection is increased in women with diabetes mellitus because the fungus thrives on the glucose spilled in the urine. The fungus also thrives in a vaginal flora that has been changed by the use of systemic antibiotic therapy or birth control pills.

 Assessment. In women a monilial infection is characterized by thick, white, cheesy vaginal discharge. There is intense pruritus, and the vulva may become inflamed. In men there may be symptoms of balanitis. The diagnosis is confirmed by the symptoms and microscopic examination of the discharge.

Planning and implementation. Moniliasis is treated with sulfonamide vaginal suppositories or ointment, or oral tetracyclines. Gentian violet painted in the vagina is rarely used. Nystatin (Mycostatin) vaginal suppositories, 100,000 U and miconazole (Monistat) cream are commonly used. These drugs must be used regularly twice a day for 2 weeks, including during menstruation when the pH of the vagina is more conducive to the growth of *Candida albicans*. When vaginal suppositories are used, they should be inserted high in the vagina and the woman should remain recumbent for 30 minutes to increase absorption. Tampons should not be used during treatment because they absorb the medication. A perineal pad can be used to prevent staining clothing during treatment. Men are treated with nystatin ointment to the penis twice a day for 2 weeks.

Chancroid. Chancroid, caused by *Haemophilus ducreyi,* is a rare venereal disease more prevalent in men. The symptoms of chancroid include inflamed macules that proceed to a vesicle, pustule, and ulcerated lesions. Diagnosis is based on identification of the organism by Gram stain. The disease is treated with oral sulfonamides, 1 g every 6 hours for 10 to 14 days.

Lymphogranuloma venereum. Lymphogranuloma venereum (LGV), caused by a virus, produces lesions on involved parts. There may be pustule formation, vulvar edema, ulcer formation, and scarring. Sulfonamides and tetracyclines are used in treatment (Table 12-1). Tetracycline, 500 mg orally twice a day for 3 weeks is recommended treatment.

Condyloma acuminatum. Condyloma acuminatum, another viral inflammation, produces verrucae (warts) on the genitalia. The warts can be cauterized or treated with applications of podophyllin (Table 12-1).

Granuloma inguinale. Granuloma inguinale (donovanosis) is a bacterial infection that produces ulcers on involved parts. Chloramphenicol or tetracyclines are used in treatment (Table 12-1).

 Evaluation. Evaluation of the nursing care plan for the client with a sexually transmitted disease is ongoing as the client learns to manage his health problem.

EXPECTED OUTCOMES

The client and/or family can:
1. Describe the sexually transmitted disease.
2. State use, time, dose, route, and side effect of prescribed medications (penicillin, tetracyclines, metronidazole, nystatin).

618

3. Describe plans for prevention of transmission of the disease (abstinence from sexual contact until no longer infective).
4. Describe plans for health maintenance.
   a. Adequate intake of nutrition and fluids.
   b. Body hygiene practices.
5. State plans for follow-up care and identify available community resources.

**COMMON HEALTH
PROBLEMS OF THE ADULT**

Infertility

Childbearing for many individuals is a natural outcome of sexual maturity. For some, childbearing solidifies the sexual role; for others, it gives additional meaning to the marriage. For these reasons, involuntary childlessness may be a source of great concern to the couple who wish to have their own family.

Fertility may be influenced by age, frequency of intercourse, and length of time during which conception has been desired. Peak fertility ages are slightly different in men and women, with the man's most fertile years usually between 25 to 40 years, whereas fertile years for women are ages 24 to 30. Those not in these age ranges may be considered at risk for fertility problems. The frequency with which the couple has intercourse also affects chances of conception. Because it is believed that frequent ejaculation increases motility of sperm, intercourse three to four times a week is recommended for those desiring conception. In 25% of couples wishing a family, pregnancy will occur within 1 month, and in 18 months 90% will be pregnant.

Childlessness is not unusual; one out of every six to ten couples may have difficulty in conceiving. Men and women contribute equally to the childless marriage and may either be infertile or sterile. *Infertility* arises when the person is unable to conceive because of organic difficulties, many of which can be remedied. *Sterility* occurs when sperm or ova are absent.

If conception does not occur within a year of attempting to have a family, the couple may wish to consult their physician or a specialist in fertility counseling.

 Assessment. Initial evaluation for couples who have difficulty in conceiving includes a history and physical examination of each partner and an evaluation of their attempts at conception. The physician may suggest that the couple improve chances for conception by having intercourse during the woman's fertile period, the time of ovulation, which may be detected by the 1° F drop in body temperature and subsequent 1° to 2° F elevation above normal. The woman should take a rectal temperature every morning before rising and record the temperature on a graph, so that ovulation can be detected.

Further examinations may be necessary if repeated attempts at pregnancy are not successful. The man should be examined first because his tests are simpler and less expensive. *Sperm counts* are the most basic examination and are taken from a sample of seminal fluid, which is collected in a specimen container by masturbation or by withdrawal before ejaculation. A condom is not a suitable receptacle for sperm analysis, because it contains a spermicidal powder. Testicular biopsy gives more accurate information about the sperm count and indicates if the problem is a blockage in the ducts instead of a low sperm count. If no sperm are produced *(azoospermia),* the man is considered sterile.

The examination for the infertile woman includes a physical examination, pelvic examination, laparoscopy, and x-ray examination to indicate the position and patency of the reproductive organs. X-ray films of the uterus and tubes, *hysterogram* and *hysterosalpingogram,* are taken to outline the uterus and fallopian tubes. There may be tumors or malpositions of these organs, which interfere

619

with conception. The *Rubin* test is done to detect the patency of the fallopian tubes. Compressed air or carbon dioxide is inserted in the fallopian tubes through the uterus, and the physician listens with a stethoscope for gas in the abdominal cavity. The client may feel subscapular pain as the patent tube permits the gas to pass and irritate the phrenic nerve. The insertion of this gas may be sufficient to force a stricture to dilate and is referred to as *tubal insufflation*. After the procedure the woman is placed on her abdomen with a pillow under her hips to help expel the gas.

Further examinations may be necessary to evaluate hormonal function and chemical compatibility of the sperm in the vagina. Endocrine studies are done to detect anovulatory cycles or hypothyroid or hyperthyroid diseases that could interfere with conception. An *endometrial biopsy* may be performed to evaluate cyclical changes in the endometrium. The *pH* of the vagina is often assessed to detect compatibility with sperm. Seminal fluid is alkaline, the pH of the vagina is slightly acid, and the pH of the cervix is alkaline. If the environment is incompatible, the sperm are killed. The *Huhner* test is used to examine the viability of the sperm in the cervical mucus. The woman goes to the physician within 1 hour after intercourse. She should be instructed not to void or douche and to wear a perineal pad to prevent loss of fluid. The physician then aspirates the secretions from the vagina and cervix and examines the sperm for number and motility. The presence of immotile sperm usually indicates a chemical incompatibility. A *maturation index* is a simple test in which a smear from the vaginal mucosa can be obtained to determine estrogen levels, an indicator of hormonal imbalances.

Planning and implementation. Because the ability to conceive is an important aspect of sexuality, infertility may be disappointing to the couple. Fortunately, various attempts can be made to overcome the cause of infertility, and many couples are able to have their own children.

Therapeutic intervention for any infertile woman depends on the cause of infertility. Cervical and uterine problems account for approximately 20% of all infertility problems, and correction of an incompetent cervix or repair of anatomical defects of the uterine position may be sufficient to make conception possible. In instances of tubal factors causing infertility, the tubes may be repaired or opened by tubal insufflation.

When the cause of infertility is hormonal, clomiphene citrate (Clomid) may be used if absence of menstrual cycles is caused by lack of pituitary function. This drug induces ovulation. Side effects include those similar to pregnancy, gastrointestinal disturbances, and weight gain. Incidences of multiple pregnancies have been reported.

Human menopausal gonadotropins (HMG) may be used if treatment with clomiphene is not successful. The drug (Pergonal) is extracted from the urine of postmenopausal women and is used to promote follicular growth and maturation. The woman therefore must have adequate ovarian function. The drug is given intramuscularly, and the woman should have intercourse on the day of injection as well as for 2 days afterward.

Therapeutic intervention for men with inadequate sperm count varies according to the cause. If there is a stricture in the ducts, plastic surgery can be attempted to anastomose the ducts. If the sperm count is low *(oligospermia)*, testosterone and a diet high in vitamins A and E may be prescribed. Abstinence from sexual relations for several days before intercourse at the time of ovulation may increase the sperm count, though others feel that abstinence reduces motility even though sperm become more concentrated. Sperm may also be concentrated from ejaculate and deposited in the cervix by the physician to assure maximum chances of conception (artificial insemination).

Artificial insemination to promote fertility can be accomplished by using sperm from the partner or a donor and depositing the seminal sample in the cervix of the woman. Artificial insemination with the partner's sperm (AIH) can be done when the sperm and the vaginal or cervical mucus are chemically incompatible, the cervix is obstructed, the partner's sperm count is low, or he has a spinal cord injury. If the man is to undergo surgery that will render him sterile, he may collect a seminal specimen that can be frozen and stored for future use.

If the man is sterile, the couple may wish to consider artificial insemination with donor sperm, or AID. When donor sperm are used, there is great respect for anonymity of the donor. Married men, over 21, who have children are usually used as donors. Their genetic background is screened and matched with the characteristics of the male partner. The sperm are obtained by masturbation and may be used immediately or frozen and stored for future use. Sperm banks are located in several large cities, and the sperm are categorized genetically and can be stored until there is a request for a donor.

The seminal sample is introduced into the female during her most fertile period, which is determined by careful basal body temperature readings. The woman visits the physician at the appropriate time, and the sperm are injected into the cervix. A cup with additional semen is placed over the cervix for 6 to 8 hours to enhance the chances of conception. The woman goes home and is instructed not to douche, swim, or have vaginal entry and then removes the cup in 6 to 8 hours. Rarely, if there is an incompatible cervical mucus, the sperm are introduced into the uterus. Several injections of sperm may be needed before conception occurs.

There are many legal and moral questions raised when a couple uses donor sperm to promote fertility. Generally the child is considered to be the male partner's and does not need to be adopted. Most churches accept artificial insemination as a method of promoting fertility. Nurses should be familiar, however, with statutes of the state in which they practice.

If the couple do not wish to use artificial insemination and are otherwise sterile, they may wish to consider adoption. They can be referred to community adoption agencies where they may request a child of a certain age or sex.

Genetic engineering: embryo transplants and cloning. Other options for facilitating conception are currently available because of rapid advances in reproductive technology. It is possible to unite sperm and ova for implantation in the uterus. The concept of the *test-tube baby* gives hope to many childless couples who may consider this option. Cloning, the reproduction of an individual from a single cell producing an individual genetically identical to the donor, is a scientific possibility, although at this time morally, ethically, and legally unfeasible. The nurse must be aware of advances in science as well as social values about futuristic conception technology.

Infections of reproductive organs

Vaginal infections. Vaginal infections are a common health problem of women. The infections are caused by an imbalance in the flora of the vagina produced by microorganisms such as *Staphylococcus aureus* and *S albus, E coli, Aerobacter* organisms, *Pseudomonas, Micrococcus,* and *Streptococcus.* Vaginal infections also include those considered to be sexually transmitted diseases (gonorrhea, trichomoniasis, and moniliasis). Other types are simple vaginitis, nonspecific vaginitis, senile (atrophic) vaginitis, and toxic shock syndrome.

The vagina is lubricated by flora containing Döderlein's bacillus, an acid pH, and secretions from the vaginal and cervical cells, which produce a gray-white, nonbloody discharge, *leukorrhea*. The discharge varies in color, odor, and amount. The discharge increases at ovulation and before menstruation. When the flora and the acidity of the vagina are changed by medications such as antibiotics or birth control pills, stress, malnutrition, aging, douching, or disease, the opportunities for infection increase.

The concept of a "normal" vaginal flora has changed recently as a variety of pathogens have been found in asymptomatic women. Vaginitis is now considered more than a cause-and-effect relationship between pathogens and decreased resistance to infection.[11] Rather, a variety of variables contribute to causation. These factors may include genetic conditions favorable to infection, physiological changes, and social factors. Malnutrition appears to have a significant relationship to vaginitis, not only because malnourished individuals are susceptible to infection, but also because there is decreased leukocytosis and reduced bactericidal and glycolytic activity of the leukocytes.

Simple vaginitis. Simple vaginitis is the most common vaginal infection. It is usually caused by *E coli,* a microorganism found in the stools and rectum, but it may be caused by staphylococcal and streptococcal infections. A yellow discharge and vaginal itching are present. There may be burning and edema. Simple vaginitis is treated with douches or antibiotics. A vinegar douche of 1 tablespoon of vinegar to 1 quart of water is used to change the bacterial flora. The physician may also order antibiotic creams. These are applied after douching, with an applicator that is inserted deep into the vagina. The applicator should be cleansed after each use. Additionally, sitz baths may be used to reduce inflammation and promote healing.

Nonspecific vaginitis. Nonspecific vaginitis refers to vaginal infections that are difficult to diagnose but are presumed to be of a bacterial origin. Pathogens may include *E coli, Proteus* organisms, *Staphylococcus* organisms, or *Streptococcus* organisms. A sulfa vaginal cream is used for treatment.

Senile vaginitis. Senile vaginitis (atrophic vaginitis) occurs in women after menopause. The mucosa of the vulva and vagina become atrophied because of estrogen withdrawal and are easily invaded by bacteria. Estrogen and antibiotic vaginal suppositories and ointments may be applied to the vagina and vulva. The nurse can suggest that the woman keep her fingernails cut so that further infection does not come from scratching the area. Soothing perineal care and sitz baths promote healing and comfort.

Toxic shock syndrome. Toxic shock syndrome (TSS) is a rarely occurring (3 per 100,000 women) infection, primarily affecting young women during or immediately subsequent to their menstrual periods.[21] Although the pathogenesis is not understood, the disease is associated with the identification of *Staphylococcus aureus* and the use of tampons. The syndrome, however, may also occur in nonmenstruating women and even men.

The syndrome is recognized by a sudden onset of a high fever with vomiting, diarrhea, drop in systolic blood pressure below 90 mm Hg, and an erythematous rash of the palms and soles that desquamates in 7 to 14 days.[15] There is also potential involvement of the kidneys, central nervous system, gastrointestinal system, hematological system, or the cardiopulmonary system, and involvement in at least four of these systems constitutes criteria for diagnosis.[17] Laboratory studies reveal an elevated BUN, serum creatinine, CPK, SGOT, bilirubin, and leukocytosis.

Early diagnosis and teratment are imperative because fatality may be as high as 10%. Fluid and electrolyte replacement and beta-lactamase-resistant anti-staphylococcal antibiotics are instituted immediately. The client may be in an intensive care setting to ensure frequent monitoring of fluid status and vital signs.[17]

After recovery the woman should observe appropriate menstrual hygiene habits and should not use tampons for several cycles. Recurrence may be as high as 30%.[21]

Cervicitis. Cervicitis is an infection of the cervix that can occur from vaginal infections but most commonly follows a laceration incurred during childbirth or abortion. There is a leukorrheal discharge, backache, and menstrual irregularities. The treatment consists of antibiotic suppositories, douches, and, if necessary, cauterization to remove the infected tissue. If the infected tissue is cauterized, the woman may notice vaginal discharge 4 to 5 days after surgery as necrotic tissue is sloughed. Frequent bathing and hygienic measures minimize the odor and discomfort. If the infection is not treated, it may invade other pelvic organs.

Bartholinitis. Bartholinitis is an infection of Bartholin's gland. It is usually caused by the gonococcus and occasionally by *E coli, Staphylococcus* organisms, and *Streptococcus* organisms. The infection is treated with systemic antibiotics. If an abscess forms, incision and drainage may be necessary.

Pelvic inflammatory disease. A local infection that is not treated can ascend to infect the fallopian tubes, ovaries, and other organs and is termed pelvic inflammatory disease (PID). *Neisseria gonorrhoeae* and *Streptococcus* and *Staphylococcus* organisms and tubercule bacilli are the common causative organisms. There is a generalized infection, with malaise, fever, abdominal pain, leukocytosis, and a vaginal discharge. The infection is serious because it can cause adhesions that may produce sterility.

The client is usually hospitalized to isolate the organism and plan treatment. The nurse should assess the communicability of the organism and institute precautions or isolation as needed. Perineal pads are worn if there is a vaginal drainage. The nurse observes the amount, color, and odor of any drainage. The pads should be disposed of in a sanitary manner. Tampons should not be used when there is a vaginal infection, because they block drainage. The nurse should also instruct the client about perineal care. If the nurse assists the client, gloves should be worn to prevent spread of the infection. The nurse also stresses handwashing to the client and other personnel so that the infection is not spread.

Systemic antibiotics, which may be given intramuscularly or intravenously, are used to treat the infection. Fluids can be forced to reduce dehydration from the fever. Warm douches may also be ordered to increase circulation and promote drainage. The client should be positioned in semi-Fowler's position to promote drainage.

The nurse should help the client plan for rest and assure comfort measures. Pain medication can be offered as needed.

Nursing process for common health problems

Before discharge the nurse can instruct the woman about hygiene practices and indications of infection to report such as unusual drainage, fever, or pain.

Puerperal infections. *Staphylococcus, Streptococcus,* and other microorganisms can invade the uterus after childbirth or abortion. Antibiotics may be given to control the infection, or it may be necessary to perform a D and C to remove placental fragments or other infected tissue.

Mastitis. Mastitis is an infection of the breast that usually occurs during lactation. The infection may result from inadequate cleanliness of the breasts or an infection in the infant, or the infection may be blood-borne. The breasts become reddened, inflamed, and tender. There may be an exudate from the nipples, fever, fatigue, and leukocytosis. Pain may arise from stagnation of the milk in the lobules. The woman must stop breast-feeding temporarily and is given systemic antibiotics. Warm packs may be used to promote drainage, and progesterone may be given to inhibit lactation and reduce the pain. A tight brassiere can be worn to give support to the breasts.

Chronic cystic mastitis. Chronic cystic mastitis occurs in women between ages 30 and 50 when there is increased fibrosis of the tissue surrounding the mammary ducts. The fibrosis forms small cysts that are palpable on breast examination. Biopsies of the cysts are done at intervals to detect malignancy.

Urethritis. Urethritis is an infection of the urethra caused by the gonococcus or *Streptococcus* organisms. It occurs most frequently in men because of the presence of microorganisms as they ascend the urethra. Systemic antibiotics and sulfonamides are used, and the client is encouraged to force fluids to prevent dehydration and to flush organisms out of the urethra during voiding.

Prostatitis. Prostatitis is frequently a sequela of urethritis. It may also be caused by pressure from an enlarged prostate gland. Treatment is with systemic antibiotics. Rectal irrigations of warm saline give relief from internal congestion, promote drainage, and reduce pain. The enema tip is introduced just inside of the rectum, and the fluid is allowed to run in slowly and return.

Epididymitis. Epididymitis is a serious infection of the epididymis, commonly caused by gonococcal or tubercle infections. There is severe pain, difficulty in walking, and dysuria. If not treated, the infection can cause sterility. Antibiotics or antituberculosis drugs are used, and the client is placed on bed rest with the scrotum elevated on a towel. The client is encouraged to force fluids to flush out the microorganisms, and ice packs may be used to reduce pain.

Orchitis. Orchitis is an infection of the testes that can be caused by the virus of mumps or occur as a complication of gonorrhea or syphilis. This infection is painful and can cause sterility if contracted after puberty. If the client is exposed to the mumps virus, gamma globulin can be given prophylactically to prevent serious inflammation. Specific drugs are used for other causative organisms. Ice can be applied to the scrotum to reduce swelling, and the man rests in bed until the infection is controlled.

Cancer of the breast

Cancer of the breast is a rapidly growing tumor. The cause of the tumor is not known. Genetic influences are implicated because of an increased incidence of breast cancer in certain families. Other research indicates hormonal influences. The incidence of breast cancer is lower in women who have had several pregnancies and a late menarche and early menopause, supporting a theory of a relationship of frequent ovulation and breast cancer.

Cancer of the breast is the most common cancer in women and the leading

624

cause of death for women ages 40 to 44.[2] Currently about 1 in 11 women will develop breast cancer.[8] The incidence of breast cancer in males is rare, less than 1%. Women at risk are those who experienced early menarche and/or late menopause, have had one breast removed for malignancy, have a family history of breast cancer, have had hormonal therapy, or have used oral contraceptives, those women over age 35 who had their first baby after age 35, women who have had fewer than two pregnancies, and those who have never had children. Increased consumption of animal fat and protein may also be a risk factor because the incidence is lower in Asia and Africa where diets are lower in these nutrients.[2]

Pathophysiology. Most tumors of the breast are adenocarcinomas originating in the lactiferous ducts (intraductal carcinoma). The primary cancer exists in multiple foci in one half of the clients with breast cancer.[19] The spread of the tumor may occur through lymphatic channels, but may also enter the bloodstream directly. Metastasis occurs commonly to the axillary nodes and ultimately to the brain, bones, lungs, and liver.

Assessment. The nurse has an opportunity to assess breast disease in women in a variety of settings and should emphasize the need for monthly assessment, particularly in high-risk women.

Fifty percent of the tumors are located in the upper outer quadrant of the breast, 20% in the medial half, 20% around the nipple, and 10% in the lower outer quadrant. Ninety-five percent of tumors are found by women themselves during breast self-examination. Breast tumors are usually noticed as small, movable, painless lumps with distinct edges in the breast. There may be a rash, change in color of the skin, pain, tenderness, puckering, dimpling (described as orange-peel skin), nipple retraction, axillary adenopathy, or nipple discharge.

The tumor is diagnosed by mammography and confirmed by biopsy. Because incisional biopsy is a surgical procedure, the client may be scheduled for surgical removal of the breast if the frozen section of the tissue demonstrates the malignant tumor. This reduces the risk of performing surgery twice. Others, however, prefer to schedule the surgery after the biopsy report has been discussed with the woman and her family and the treatment options fully considered. In addition to the biopsy, radiographic studies of the brain, chest, liver, and bones may be obtained to detect metastasis. Arm lymphangiography may be done to identify axillary and supraclavicular nodes. The tumor is staged to plan therapy (see staging of cancer of the breast, p. 626).

> **Data analysis**
> *Data analysis helps the nurse and client identify actual and potential nursing diagnoses. These may include sexual dysfunction, disturbances in self-concept, alteration in comfort, self-care deficit, and grieving.*

Planning and implementation. The nursing care plan is developed for the unique needs of the client. Women may experience several stages of behavior as they learn of the diagnosis and plan for treatment.[22] The first is the prediagnostic stage when the woman suspects or learns from health care personnel that she has a breast tumor. Shock, confusion, conflict, withdrawal, fear, and perhaps avoidance of health care services are a part of this stage. In the diagnostic stage

Nursing process for common health problems

STAGING OF CANCER OF THE BREAST

TNM CLASSIFICATION
Primary tumor (T)

Clinical-diagnostic classification

TX Tumor cannot be assessed
T0 No evidence of primary tumor
TIS Paget's disease of the nipple with no demonstrable tumor
  NOTE: *Paget's disease with a demonstrable tumor is classified according to size of the tumor.*
T1* Tumor 2 cm or less in greatest dimension
  T1a No fixation to underlying pectoral fascia or muscle
  T1b Fixation to underlying pectoral fascia and/or muscle
T2* Tumor more than 2 cm but not more than 5 cm in its greatest dimension
  T2a No fixation to underlying pectoral fascia and/or muscle
  T2b Fixation to underlying pectoral fascia and/or muscle
T3* Tumor more than 5 cm in its greatest dimension
  T3a No fixation to underlying pectoral fascia and/or muscle
  T3b Fixation to underlying pectoral fascia and/or muscle
T4 Tumor of any size with direct extension to chest wall or skin
  NOTE: *Chest wall includes ribs, intercostal muscles, and serratus anterior muscle, but not pectoral muscle.*
  T4a Fixation to chest wall
  T4b Edema (including peau d'orange), ulceration of the skin of the breast, or satellite skin nodules confined to the same breast
  T4c Both of above
  T4d Inflammatory carcinoma

Postsurgical treatment-pathologic classification

TX Tumor cannot be assessed
T0 No evidence of primary tumor
TIS Preinvasive carcinoma (carcinoma in situ), noninfiltrating intraductal carcinoma, or Paget's disease of nipple
T1 **T1a** Same as clinical-diagnostic classification
  T1b i: tumor < 0.5 cm
    ii: tumor 0.5-0.9 cm
    iii: tumor 0.1-1.9 cm
T2 **T2a** **T2b** Same as clinical-diagnostic classification
T3 **T3a** **T3b** Same as clinical-diagnostic classification
T4 **T4a** **T4b** **T4c** **T4d** Same as clinical-diagnostic classification

Nodal involvement (N)

Clinical-diagnostic classification

NX Regional lymph nodes cannot be assessed clinically
N0 No palpable homolateral axillary nodes
N1 Movable homolateral axillary nodes
  N1a Nodes not considered to contain growth
  N1b Nodes considered to contain growth
N2 **Ho** Homolateral axillary nodes considered to contain growth and fixed to one another or to other structures
N3 Homolateral supraclavicular or infraclavicular nodes considered to contain growth or edema of the arm

From Rubin, Philip, editor: Clinical oncology for medical students and physicians, a multidisciplinary approach, ed. 5, Rochester, N.Y., 1979, American Cancer Society. Dimpling of the skin, nipple retraction, or any other skin changes except those in T4b may occur in T1, T2, or T3 without the classification.

the woman marshals resources for coping, seeks health care services, and the diagnosis is confirmed. The next stages relate to intervention and involve the preoperative phase, postoperative phase, adjuvant treatment (if needed), and the recovery or terminal illness period. The nursing care plan is developed for special needs during these stages and the nurse-client relationship may vary from dependence to independence during the course of care.

The type of therapeutic intervention for tumors of the breast depends on the stage of the tumor and the age and health of the client. Surgery, radiation, and chemotherapy are the usual modes of treatment. Radiation therapy (external beam radiation or radium implant) may be used with stages I or II tumors or used as an adjunct to surgery. Chemotherapy is often used to treat advanced breast cancer.

Surgery, however, is the primary intervention for cancer of the breast. Several surgical approaches are used, and the nurse should be familiar with these in order to help the woman make an informed decision and consent for surgery. Types of surgery include the following:

1. A *partial mastectomy* (lumpectomy) is the removal of involved breast tissue (about one third of the breast), thus preserving contour and muscle

function. This surgery is usually done when the lesion is small and peripheral.

2. A *subcutaneous mastectomy* (adenomastectomy) may be performed for premalignant lesions. In this surgery, breast tissue is removed, and the skin and nipple remain intact. In some instances a prosthesis can be implanted at the time of surgery.
3. A *simple mastectomy* involves the removal of the entire breast, and a skin flap is used to cover the area.
4. A *radical mastectomy* is usually performed when tumor cells can be demonstrated. The major and minor pectoral muscles, all lymph nodes, fat, and fascia are removed. A skin graft may be used to cover the area.
5. In a *modified radical mastectomy* the breast, axillary nodes, and pectoral or superior apical nodes are removed. The major and minor pectoral muscles are preserved, although occasionally resection of the minor pectoral muscle may be required.
6. In an *extended radical mastectomy* the chest wall is resected.
7. In a *superradical mastectomy* the sternum is split and lymph nodes dissected from the mediastinum. Some surgeons also consider it safe practice to do a biopsy of the contralateral breast and, if necessary, consider prophylactic removal.

Nursing care plan for a client having breast surgery. The nurse plans with the client and her family or significant others to develop a plan that reflects continuity of care from diagnosis to discharge. Data gathered from the nursing history and information about the client's psychological and social status help the nurse and client formulate nursing diagnoses and develop a care plan for the client.

Preoperative nursing care. Facing the loss of a breast is a traumatic event for a woman and her family. The nurse and client should plan before surgery for psychological preparation for the loss of the breast as well as for providing specific preoperative instructions and preparation for the surgery.

PSYCHOLOGICAL PREPARATION. Women will react to breast surgery in many ways, and the nurse should accept each woman as an individual and permit her to express her feelings. Losing a breast may interfere with roles of being a wife and mother; the woman may fear rejection from her husband or may be disappointed at not being able to breast-feed. It is helpful if the husband and family visit the woman and give her support at this time. When the family can indicate that loss of a breast will not alter their feelings for her, the woman may be less apprehensive about her surgery.

Many women can be reassured about the outcome of a mastectomy by talking with someone who has had the same operation. "Reach to Recovery" is a program of the American Cancer Society, Inc. in which women who have had a mastectomy visit the client in the hospital to offer reassurance. If the physician approves, the visit should be arranged before surgery. Many women will be less apprehensive about surgery when they know that ultimately no one will be able to tell that they have had a breast removed.

PREOPERATIVE INSTRUCTION. The nurse should discuss the postoperative course with the client to gain cooperation for recovery. The nurse can demonstrate and observe the client as she practices turning, coughing, and deep breath-

627

ing. The nurse should explain that a pressure dressing will be on the mastectomy site and that a drain may be inserted to remove excess fluid.

Most women will do exercises after surgery to prevent shoulder contractures and increase range of motion. If the physician permits and if the woman is interested, some of these exercises can be demonstrated and practiced before surgery. The nurse should also reassure the client that pain medication will be available if she needs it.

Postoperative nursing care. The postoperative nursing care plan is directed toward (1) preventing complications, (2) preventing edema, (3) preventing muscle contractures, and (4) helping the client adjust to the change in body image.

PREVENTING COMPLICATIONS. After surgery the nurse should assess the client's vital signs and inspect the dressing for bleeding. A pressure dressing is usually applied to the surgical site to prevent bleeding and accumulation of fluids, and the nurse should make a point of looking under the client where the drainage may be seeping during recumbency.

Many surgeons use a Hemovac (a closed-wound suction drain, Fig. 12-9) or a Penrose drain to provide an outlet for fluid that would otherwise accumulate and be a medium for infection or cause pressure on the surgical site. Suction is created in the Hemovac by the negative pressure in the collection apparatus, and the Hemovac should be emptied before it becomes full. The Penrose drain may be attached to a wall or portable suction. Regardless of the type of suction, the nurse should observe and record the amount of drainage. The drain is usually removed in 3 to 5 days when the drainage is less than 100 ml in 24 hrs.

Healing is individual and depends on the extent of surgery and cosmetic repair. The dressing should be changed frequently to minimize odor. The surrounding area can be washed with mild soap and water. Deodorant should not be used, however, until the incision is healed and the sutures are removed.

The woman may experience incisional pain for several days and for sometime thereafter when exercising. Some women may experience referred pain or numbness in the involved arm and behind the shoulders after a radical mastectomy because of severing of peripheral nerves. In most instances nerve regenera-

FIG. 12-9
A, Hemovac closed drainage suction is used to remove fluids after mastectomy. **B,** Compression of Hemovac creates suction.

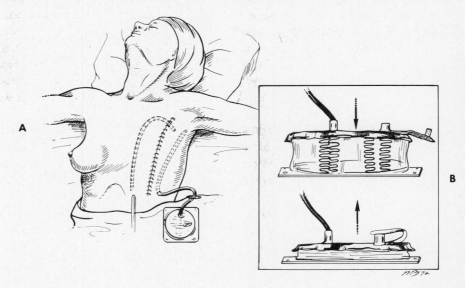

tion will occur, but occasionally the woman will have residual numbness in the arm or chest wall. The woman should be instructed to differentiate this numbness from incisional pain.

The client is usually permitted to be out of bed after surgery and can be encouraged to exercise the uninvolved limbs and to cough and breathe deeply to prevent cardiopulmonary complications. The woman may feel more like moving if she is given pain medication as she needs it. When the client ambulates for the first time, the nurse should accompany her, because she may be slightly unbalanced from the removal of the breast, and the dressing may be bulky and constricting.

If a radical mastectomy has been performed, the defense against infection is lessened because of the removal of the lymph nodes. The involved arm should be kept clean and dry and should not be used for intramuscular injections, venipunctures, or skin tests that could cause entry of microorganisms.

PREVENTING LYMPHEDEMA. When the lymph glands are removed, there is a tendency for the lymph circulation to pool in the involved arm. Lymphedema may occur within a week because of operative trauma or several weeks later because of wound infection, delayed healing, or damage to lymphatic channels by radiation therapy. Obesity also aggravates lymphedema, and the woman should be encouraged to lose weight. It is estimated that about 50% of women have lymphedema after radical surgery, but in most instances the edema will subside. Edema that occurs months after the surgery tends to be persistent.

The amount of lymphedema can be determined by daily measurement of the involved arm. A tape measure should be used at a point 5 inches (12.7 cm) above the elbow and 5 inches (12.7 cm) below the shoulder.[6] The measurement should be taken daily and compared with the uninvolved arm to assess incipient lymphedema and monitor changes. Several nursing actions can be used to prevent lymphedema. The arm on the involved side should be positioned on a pillow, with each joint higher than the proximal joint. Furthermore the woman should be advised not to sleep on the involved arm. Elevating the arm in this manner uses gravity to promote return of fluid to the lymphatic circulation.

Exercising the involved arm increases circulation and the development of collateral lymphatics. To this end the woman is encouraged to use the involved arm in daily care activities. Even though it may be uncomfortable, the woman should use her arm to eat, brush her hair, and bathe herself.

Isometric exercises can also be instituted, with the physician's approval, immediately after surgery. These simple exercises promote lymphatic drainage by muscle contractions. Squeezing a rubber ball or a rolled bandage or opening and closing the fingers in a fist will accomplish the necessary isometric movements.

The woman can be encouraged to wear loose clothing so that there is no constriction of circulation in the involved arm. Nightgowns with elastic sleeves and tight sweaters are not advisable, and the woman should wear her watch on the uninvolved arm. Blood pressure determinations should be obtained using the uninvolved arm to avoid constriction.

If lymphedema is severe, the physician may order a lymphedema sleeve (an elastic sleeve that extends from the wrist to the shoulder, Fig. 12-10) or intermittent compression therapy (a mechanical compression of the arm by automatic inflation and deflation of a pneumomassage sleeve applied to the arm). These

FIG 12-10
Lymphedema sleeve. (Courtesy Camp
International, Inc.)

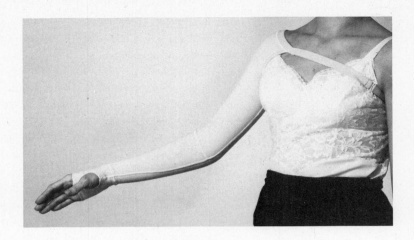

appliances improve circulation by pressure on the muscles, which enhances venous return. Digital massage, which serves to break up lymphatic pools, may be done by the physical therapist, or it may later be taught to a family member. Diuretics and low sodium diets may also be used to treat persistent or continued lymphedema.

The woman who experiences lymphedema persisting after surgery may be instructed by the physician, physical therapist, or nurse to continue isometric and range-of-motion exercises. The exercises may be taught by the physician, nurse, physical therapist, or Reach to Recovery volunteer. In some settings the exercises may be done in groups where women derive support from each other, though emphasis is placed on individualization of exercising.

Gravitational exercises may also be taught to help reduce edema. These include holding the involved arm above the head for 1 minute followed by 1 minute of rest. Next the woman holds her arm above her head and bends and straightens her arm at the elbow. This exercise is also done for 1 minute. The third exercise involves holding the raised arm above her head while alternately squeezing and releasing her fist. Finally the arm is held overhead, making a large circle. All four exercises should be done several times each day while the lymphedema persists.

When the woman begins to do the exercises, she should do them slowly, in sequence, and should gradually increase the number until each exercise is done three to four times, five times each day. All exercises (see below) with the exception of the pendulum may be done from a sitting position. If the woman prefers to stand, she should use good posture and a wide base of support. Both arms are used in most exercises to promote balance and symmetrical movements. When the woman experiences discomfort, she can be instructed to take a deep breath (exercise 4) and continue the exercises, until the point of pain or incisional pull.

PREVENTING MUSCLE CONTRACTURES AND LIMITING SHOULDER MOVEMENT. Flexion contractures and limitation of movement in the involved shoulder are likely to occur if the involved arm is not exercised. Initially a small pillow placed between the trunk and arm may be used, even when the woman ambulates, to maintain abduction, and to prevent dangling of the arm and gravitational pull. Activities of daily living such as combing the hair, eating, or putting on clothing are natural movements that encourage range of motion. Pain medication used judiciously will help maintain comfort and promote freedom of movement.

Specific exercises may be ordered by the physician. The aim of the exercises is to restore muscle strength and full range of motion, though each depends on the type of surgery performed and individual variances between women. An added benefit of the exercises is the pain relief that results when the muscles are relaxed. The exercises are usually instituted on the second or third postoperative day but may be postponed if there is an elevated temperature, excessive drainage, or problems with wound healing.

Suggested exercises follow:

1. *Ball squeezing* is a simple exercise to strengthen the use of the hand and arm and promote circulation. A rubber ball or a crumpled newspaper is squeezed in the hand of the involved side. This exercise should be done periodically throughout the day.

2. *Wall climbing* promotes extension of the involved arm (Fig. 12-11, *A*). The woman sits or stands facing the wall, with her toes next to the wall. Both hands are placed on the wall, with the uninvolved arm followed by the involved arm. When the client reaches the point of pain, she works her hand down to the starting position. A mark is made on the wall, and when the exercises are done the next time, she tries to go beyond that point.

3. *Pendulum* or *arm swinging* loosens the shoulder and develops accessory muscles (Fig. 12-11, *B*). The woman bends at the waist and swings her arms from side to side without bending her elbows. The nurse should stand beside the woman the first time to be sure that she does not become dizzy. This exercise should not be done excessively, because gravitational pull and the dependent position can increase lymphedema.

4. *Deep breathing* can be done not only to prevent atelectasis, but also to relax muscles, decrease tautness on the side of the surgery, and improve posture. The woman, sitting in a chair, places her hand over the involved portion of her chest and takes a deep breath through the nose, feeling her chest expand as the breath is inhaled. As the breath is exhaled, her chest and shoulders sag and relax (Fig. 12-11, *C*). An added benefit of this exercise is encouraging the woman to touch the incisional area.

5. *Lifting clasped hands* increases range of motion. In this exercise the woman clasps her hands and lifts them slowly over her head, keeping the elbows straight. When the point of pain is reached, she should take a deep breath and try to raise the arms higher (Fig. 12-11, *D*).

6. *Pulley* or *rope pulling* is done to encourage shoulder movement (Fig. 12-11, *E*). A rope or string is placed over a shower curtain rod, closet rod, or IV pole. The woman pulls the string down, and the opposite arm is raised. The process is then reversed, increasing the height each time the exercise is done.

When the woman returns home, she should continue to do these exercises until full range of motion is attained and stiffness is relieved. Full range of motion is determined by being able to fully extend both arms above the head, elbows next to the head (Fig. 12-11, *F*). Many exercises can be incorporated into activities of daily living and housekeeping tasks such as sweeping and putting dishes in the cupboard. The woman should be instructed to maintain activity and full use of the involved arm for the rest of her life.

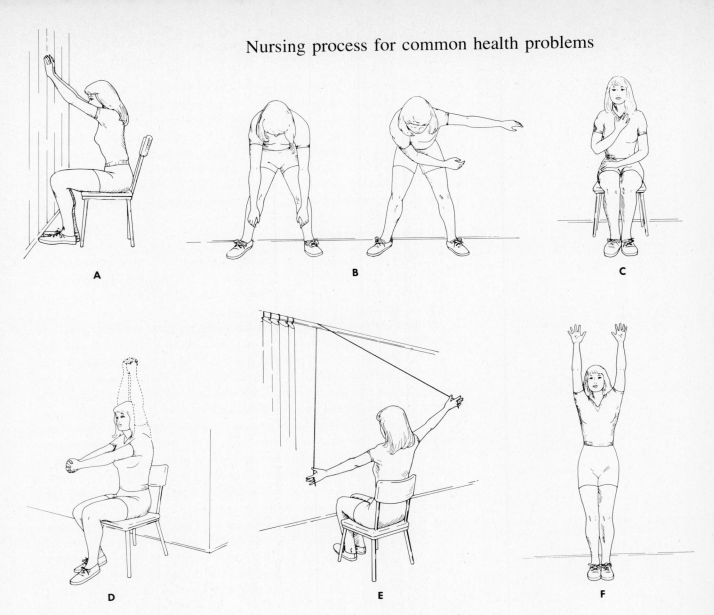

FIG. 12-11
Postmastectomy exercises. **A,** Wall climbing. **B,** Pendulum. **C,** Deep breathing. **D,** Lifting clasped hands. **E,** Pulley. **F,** Full extension.

PROMOTING ACCEPTANCE OF SELF-CONCEPT. Depression and grieving for a lost body part are normal after breast surgery. The woman can be assisted to work through these feelings with support from her family and the nursing personnel.

The woman's husband or a significant other should be encouraged to visit frequently and observe the surgical area before the woman goes home. Acceptance will do much to encourage the woman and alleviate fears of rejection. Sexual role adjustments depend on the woman's preoperative role security and the value placed on the breasts for sexual esteem and pleasure, and the nurse should help the client and family anticipate these feelings that usually occur.

The woman will be more relaxed by a comfortable feeling that she has about her appearance. The nurse can encourage the woman to feel attractive by daily bathing and application of makeup. The client may feel more feminine if she wears her own nightgown or bedjacket.

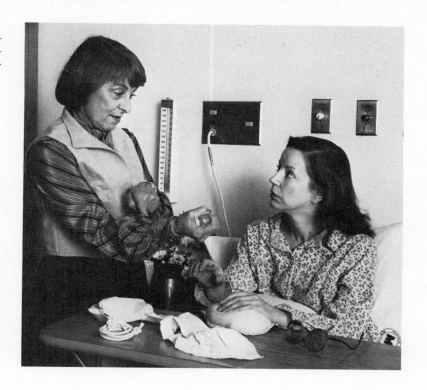

The incision may initially appear red and swollen but will gradually become less discolored and uncomfortable. The woman may be instructed to gently massage the incision with cocoa butter, cold cream, or petroleum jelly to make the incision softer. Powder or cornstarch may be used to absorb perspiration and relieve itching.

Some women may experience phantom breast sensations similar to an individual who has had a body part amputated. These sensations tend to be more evident in women who attach emotional significance to the breasts. Encouraging expression of feeling and reassurance as to positive sexuality are helpful interventions.

Before the woman goes home, she will want to pad her brassiere to give shape to her clothing. Permanent breast forms cannot be worn until healing has completely occurred (in about 6 weeks), but in the meantime it is possible to make a temporary padding from tissues, a perineal pad, or cotton put in the brassiere cup. A soft, Dacron-filled form insert is provided in the Reach to Recovery kit (Fig. 12-12). The padding should be secured with elastic to the panties, girdle, or garter belt so that it will not ride up, and the woman may lengthen the shoulder strap of her slip and add elastic for comfort. The woman can wear her own bra if it is not constricting and she has sufficient range of motion to fasten it. Bra extenders can be purchased to enlarge her own bras, particularly if the bra is being worn over a bulky dressing. The nurse can suggest that the woman wear loose-fitting clothing such as blouses and shift dresses, and above all the woman should stand straight. Much confidence is obtained when the woman sees that no one will be able to detect that she has had a breast removed.

When healing has occurred and the physician has given approval, the woman may invest in a breast form (prosthesis). There are many types of breast forms available, and the prosthesis is selected to match contour and weight of the breast. The complexion of the prosthesis can be changed to match skin tones by soaking the prosthesis in tea or coffee to stain it or by dying the prosthesis. Most department stores, lingerie shops, or surgical supply houses have employees who are qualified to fit them. The husband is encouraged to shop with his wife to give her support and approval. Foam rubber inserts are the least expensive and fit in the cup of the brassiere. A backing can be made for the brassiere to hold the insert in place. Foam forms are rigid and do not give with body movement. Fluid-filled prostheses have contour and are flexible when the woman bends; these must be returned to the manufacturer periodically for replacement. Silicone prostheses are most lifelike and even "heal" if accidentally punctured. These forms, which are more expensive, are more lasting. They can be cleaned with soap and water and are easily worn. There are also special breast forms available that can be worn with bathing suits and nightgowns. The woman should select the form that suits her budget and taste. Most important, she should feel confident when wearing it.

BREAST RECONSTRUCTION. Insertion of a prosthesis after mastectomy is possible in some instances. The surgery may be done if the client is uncomfortable from uneven chest weight, has difficulty wearing a breast form, or has a difficult emotional adjustment to the use of a breast form. Women with small tumors (less than 2 cm and fewer than three positive nodes) who are young and in good health are better candidates for reconstructive surgery. The procedure is contraindicated if there is a likelihood of metastasis or if there is not sufficient tissue for implantation and healing.

Two types of implants may be used: the inflatable implant filled with saline or the silicone gel implant. The implants are inserted underneath breast skin or occasionally under the pectoralis major muscle.

After implantation the client should wear a bra continuously to maintain alignment of the prosthesis. This may be necessary for as long as 2 to 3 months. Range-of-motion exercises are initiated several days after surgery and should be increased gradually. The elbow should be kept close to the side for several weeks and total range of motion obtained in 1 month.

Discharge instructions. Before the woman goes home, the nurse should instruct her to continue hygiene practices that will prevent infection of the involved arm (see hand and arm care, opposite). Breaks in the skin provide an entry for microorganisms, and the woman should wear gloves when she is washing or gardening. She should also take care when she shaves her underarms and may wish to use an electric razor. Wearing a thimble when sewing prevents accidental skin puncture. Use of gloves for dishwashing and laundry are advisable. Insect repellent should be worn if one is in infested areas. Heavy purses and packages may pull on the arm and should be carried with the uninvolved arm. The client should also protect her involved arm from sunburn and blistering by wearing a beach jacket or shirt. Any signs indicative of infection such as redness, pain, or swelling should be reported to the physician.

Many women begin to think of preparing to resume sexual relations at this time, and the nurse can help the client anticipate questions or anxieties that might occur. The husband, family, or close friends also will require time for adjustment to the changed body image. The incisional area will be sensitive for some time after surgery, and changes in positions for coitus may be modified to prevent

---

**HAND AND ARM CARE
AFTER BREAST SURGERY**

1. Prevention of infection:
   a. Wear gloves when cleaning with harsh detergent.
   b. Wear gloves when gardening.
   c. Avoid injections, vaccinations, venipuncture in involved arm.
   d. Use cuticle remover in preference to cutting cuticles.
   e. Sew with thimble.
   f. Avoid chapping of hands; use lanolin cream daily.
   g. Take care when using equipment that might cut, scrape, or be abrasive.
   h. Shave underarms with electric razor.
   i. Avoid insect bites; use insect repellent.
2. Prevention of constricting circulation:
   a. Do not take blood pressure in involved arm.
   b. Wear loose clothing; avoid tight bra straps or tight sleeves.
   c. Wear watch or jewelry on uninvolved arm.
   d. Carry purse on uninvolved arm or shoulder.
3. Prevention of burns:
   a. Wear padded mitts to reach in oven; use potholders.
   b. Hold cigarette in uninvolved hand.
   c. Prevent sunburn; use tanning creams or sunscreens; cover arms during prolonged exposure.
4. Prevention of drag or pull:
   a. Carry heavy packages in uninvolved arm.
   b. Avoid motions that increase centrifugal force.
   c. Carry purse on uninvolved arm or shoulder.

Report any signs of redness, swelling, warmth, or pain.

pressure on the area. Openness in discussion may make resumption of sexual relations easier for the client.

Various community resources are available to mastectomees, and the nurse may wish to refer the client to these services. The local chapter of the American Cancer Society, in addition to the Reach to Recovery Program, may provide dressings to women who may need them.

Some communities have nurses who are specially trained in oncology nursing and offer services to clients and the health team. The community health nurse or visiting nurse may also be referred to the client who may wish follow-up nursing care in the home. Community clinics are becoming more involved in the early detection and treatment of cancer of the breast in an attempt to maintain the woman in her role in the family and community.

Advanced breast cancer. Breast cancer in advanced stages may be evident as primary tumors too invasive to resect, or there may be dissemination to other parts of the body, particularly bone, lungs, liver, and brain with concomitant organ involvement. Indications of metastasis may be noticed in the bone by pathological fractures, pain, and limitations of range of motion; in the lungs by hemoptysis, dyspnea, and shortness of breath; in the liver by jaundice, ascites, and coma; and in the brain by confusion, personality changes, ataxia, and seizures. In these instances therapy is directed toward controlling metastasis and maintaining quality of life in terminal stages of breast cancer.

Several approaches may be used to induce remission or prevent tumor spread. Radiation therapy, alteration of hormonal environment, chemotherapy, and immunotherapy are most commonly used. The nurse has a significant role in offering psychological support to clients receiving these therapies as well as implementing nursing intervention to provide comfort for physiological changes resulting from therapy.

Radiation therapy may be an adjunctive or the primary treatment mode in advanced breast cancer. Depending on the site radiated, many systemic reactions to therapy may be evident, and the nurse should employ interventions to minimize these discomforts. Esophagitis, pneumonitis, or difficulties in digestion may result from radiation therapy of the breast. The nurse should be alert for dysphagia, dyspnea, nausea, or vomiting and help the client maintain optimal respiratory and nutritional status.

Alterations of hormonal environment is another approach and, depending on the woman's menopausal state, may be additive or ablative.

A hormone receptor assay that determines the presence of estrogen receptor sites is used to identify those women who can benefit from antiestrogen therapy. About one third of the tumors are hormone dependent.[20] Nolvadex (tamoxifen citrate) is an antiestrogen used as palliative therapy in advanced breast cancer. This drug inhibits estrogen from binding with the tumor and thereby decreases cell division. The side effects of the drug are few; nausea and vomiting are the most common.

The hormonal environment may also be altered by adding hormones, primarily estrogens and androgens. Estrogens are usually used if the woman is past menopause. Varied side effects, especially hypercalcemia (indicated by nausea, vomiting, constipation, and confusion), should be anticipated and corrected. Androgens may be used for women before menopause. These hormones produce masculinizing effects, and the nurse should help the client cope with these changes.

635

Nursing process for common health problems

The hormonal environment can be additionally modified by removing hormone-producing glands: the ovaries (oophorectomy), adrenal glands (adrenalectomy), and the pituitary gland (hypophysectomy). Removal of these glands is based on the theory that estrogens stimulate tumor growth and spread. These surgeries produce significant changes in metabolism, and careful monitoring is imperative. Often supplemental hormones may be used to maintain homeostasis.

Chemotherapy is another option for management and palliation of advanced breast cancer. Antineoplastic drugs may be used singly or in combination. One such therapy program uses methotrexate (Amethopterin), 5-fluorouracil (Fluorouracil), and prednisone. Others use cytotoxic drugs such as cytarabine (Cytosar), cyclophosphamide (Cytoxan), melphalan (Alkeran), or doxorubicin hydrochloride (Adriamycin). The nurse should be familiar with the untoward effects of these drugs and help the client maintain maximum comfort.

Nursing care in terminal breast cancer. Although survival rates are improving with early diagnosis and treatment, not all clients respond to therapeutic intervention; they face imminent death. During this time the nurse should be sensitive to the predictable stages of dying and the client's and family's coping mechanisms. The nurse can help the client and family face death and maintain quality of life during this time. Special attention can be given to pain relief, comfort measures, nutritional status, and psychological and spiritual support. Hospices and community-based programs that facilitate care for the dying client and her family may be appropriate resources for the woman dying from breast cancer.

 Evaluation. Evaluation of the nursing care plan for the client with cancer of the breast occurs throughout the course of hospitalization, particularly before surgery, after surgery, and during rehabilitation as nursing problems of pain, alteration in self-concept, and sexuality are resolved.

EXPECTED OUTCOMES

The client and/or her family can:
1. Describe cancer of the breast.
2. Use appropriate coping resources for adjustment to a life-threatening health problem.
3. State plans for care of incision.
4. State plans for preventing and/or managing lymphedema (isometric and gravitational exercises).
5. State plans for attaining and maintaining full range of motion (exercises, positioning).
6. State plans for prevention of infection in involved arm.
7. State use, dosage, time, route, and side effects of prescribed medication.
8. Describe plans for health maintenance, including rest, exercise, nutrition, and elimination.
9. Anticipate changes in body image and establish positive relationships with family and sexual partner. State plans for use of a prosthesis.
10. State plans for follow-up care and knowledge of community resources for clients with cancer of the breast.

Fibrocystic disease of the breast

Benign cysts of the breast are common in women over age 30 and those near menopause. The cysts are affected by the hormones of the menstrual cycle and subside during pregnancy, lactation, or after menopause. They are soft, tender, and freely movable and become enlarged during menstruation. They are not usually removed but may be aspirated to reduce discomfort. Any unusual change in shape or size should be reported to the physician at once because cystic disease may predispose to malignancy.

Fibroadenoma of the breast

Fibroadenoma of the breast occurs in women under age 25. The fibroadenomas are encapsulated, round, freely movable, nontender growths. Biopsies of the tumors are done to rule out malignancy, and the tumors may be removed if necessary.

Hypoplasia and hyperplasia of the breast

Breast size may be an important component of sexuality to some women. Breasts that are too small may not fit the woman's concept of beauty; breasts that are too large are pendulous and painful and may cause the woman to be off-balance. Cosmetic surgery procedures have been developed, which women may elect to undergo to obtain desired breast size.

An *augmentation mammoplasty* is performed to enlarge the size and symmetry of the breasts. Silicone inserts are placed under breast tissue to provide safe cosmetic improvement of the breast contour. After surgery, pressure dressings are applied, and the woman wears a tight brassiere for support. There may be initial swelling and discoloration, but the woman is usually pleased with her new figure. Arm movement may be restricted for several days, and the nurse may need to help with the bath.

The woman should understand that augmentation mammoplasty will not change her personality or solve existing problems. The nurse can give the client support as she adjusts to her new figure and should avoid judgmental comments about the need for the surgery.

When the breast tissue is excessive, a *reduction mammoplasty* may be performed. In this operation the excessive tissue is removed and the nipple relocated. Lactation is possible if the mammary ducts are anastomosed to the nipple. A pressure dressing is used for several days to prevent bleeding, and a drain may be used to prevent swelling.

Adjustment to a new body image and posture is as important for the woman who has a reduction mammoplasty as it is for the woman who has an augmentation mammoplasty. The nurse should indicate support and interest as the woman adjusts to her new figure.

Cancer of the uterus

Malignant tumor cells may invade the uterus at two distinct sites: the fundus and the cervix. The type of tumor, client at risk, and clinical manifestations, however, are different for each.

Pathophysiology. Cancer of the *cervix* arises from squamous cells. The tumor is invasive and, unless treated in early stages, ultimately invades the vagina, pelvic wall, bladder, rectum, and regional lymph nodes (see staging of cancer of the cervix, p. 638). Cancer of the *uterine fundus* (endometrial cancer) is usually an adenocarcinoma. The tumor is more likely to be localized, but may spread to the cervix, bladder, rectum, and surrounding lymph nodes (see staging of cancer of the endometrium, p. 638).

Cancer of the *uterus* is the fourth most common site of cancer in women.[24] Cancer of the *cervix* accounts for 4% of cancer in women and occurs in women ages 30 to 50.[8] Those at risk are women with cervical infections, frequent type II herpesvirus, venereal disease, multiple pregnancies, an active sex life, and those women who are malnourished or have vitamin A deficiencies. Furthermore, the incidence is higher in lower socioeconomic groups, perhaps owing to malnutrition from lack of economic resources.

Cancer of the *uterine fundus* as a primary site is more than twice as common

STAGING OF CANCER OF THE CERVIX

Stage 0	**(TIS)**	Carcinoma in situ
Stage I	**(T1)**	Carcinoma confined to cervix
IA	**(T1a)**	Microinvasive carcinoma
IB	**(T1b)**	All other cases of stage I
Stage II	**(T2)**	Carcinoma extends beyond cervix but not to pelvic wall or lower vagina
IIA	**(T2a)**	No obvious parametrial involvement
IIB	**(T2b)**	Obvious parametrial involvement
Stage III	**(T3)**	Carcinoma to pelvic wall or lower vagina, or ureteral obstruction
IIIA	**(T3a)**	No extension of pelvic wall
IIIB	**(T3b)**	Extension to one or both pelvic walls, or ureteral obstruction
Stage IV	**(T4)**	Carcinoma beyond true pelvis or invading bladder or rectum
IVA	**(T4a)**	Spread to adjacent organs
IVB	**(T4b)**	Spread to distant organs

Uniform TNM classification

Nodes

NX	Not possible to assess regional nodes
N0	No evidence of regional node involvement
N1	Evidence of regional node involvement
N3	Fixed or ulcerated regional nodes
N4	Juxtaregional node involvement

Distant metastasis (M)

MX	Not assessed
M0	No (known) distant metastasis
M1	Distant metastasis present
	Specify _____

Specify sites according to the following notations:

Pulmonary—PUL	Bone marrow—MAR
Osseous—OSS	Pleura—PLE
Hepatic—HEP	Skin—SKI
Brain—BRA	Eye—EYE
Lymph nodes—LYM	Other—OTH

From Rubin, Philip, editor: Clinical oncology for medical students and physicians, and a multidisciplinary approach, ed. 5, Rochester, N.Y., 1979, American Cancer Society.

STAGING OF CANCER OF THE ENDOMETRIUM

Stage 0	**(TIS)**	Carcinoma in situ
Stage I	**(T1)**	Carcinoma confined to the corpus
IA	**(T1a)**	Uterine cavity 8 cm or less in length
IB	**(T1b)**	Uterine cavity greater than 8 cm in length
		Stage 1 should be subgrouped by histology as follows:
		G1—highly differentiated, G2—moderately differentiated, G3—undifferentiated

Stage II	**(T2)**	Extension to cervix only
Stage III	**(T3)**	Extension outside the uterus but confined to true pelvis
Stage IV	**(T4)**	Extension beyond true pelvis or invading bladder or rectum

See Cervix for uniform TNM classification

From Rubin, Philip, editor: Clinical oncology for medical students and physicians, a multidisciplinary approach, ed. 5, Rochester, N.Y., 1979, American Cancer Society.

as cancer of the cervix.[24] Those at risk are women with a past history of irregular menstruation, difficulties during menopause, use of continuous estrogens without progesterone to treat postmenopausal symptoms, and chronic disease such as diabetes mellitus or hypertension. The tumor generally occurs in women past menopause (age 50 to 64) and is slow growing.

 Assessment. Because cancer of the uterus is a significant health problem, the nurse helps the client report and identify changes in reproductive or sexual health. Assessment is accomplished by use of the health history and physical assessment and is directed toward noting early symptoms of cancer of the cervix and/or fundus. Early symptoms of cancer of the *cervix* are a watery discharge, irregular menstrual bleeding, and *metrorrhagia* (excessive menstrual bleeding). Later, the discharge becomes dark from sloughing necrotic tissue. The discharge increases with douching, intercourse, or defecation. As the cancer of the cervix becomes more invasive, the pelvic nodes enlarge and spread to the fundus, vagina, bladder, rectum, and sacrum. At this point the client experiences pain, weight loss, anemia, fever, and malaise.

Early diagnosis can be made by a Pap smear, and survival is 100% if detected in situ. Additional diagnostic studies such as an intravenous pyelogram, cystoscopy, sigmoidoscopy, or liver function studies are often done to determine the extent of invasion.

Women with cancer of the *fundus* present with vaginal bleeding. Pelvic pain or lower back pain is a late sign. A boggy uterus is an ominous sign indicative of advanced disease. Diagnosis is based on clinical evidence, radiography, and tissue biopsy.

Data analysis
Data analysis may reveal nursing diagnoses of sexual dysfunction, alteration in comfort: pain, or disturbances in self-concept. Plans are developed for each diagnosis.

Planning and implementation. The type of treatment for cancer of the uterus and female reproductive organs depends on the site involved, the stage of the cancer, age and parity of the client, and the woman's general health. Radiation therapy, chemotherapy, and surgery are the most common management modalities and may be used singly or in combination.

Radiation therapy. Radiation therapy may be used to deter tumor growth and metastatic invasion of the pelvic cavity when the primary tumor is located in the cervix or uterus. Radiation therapy may include the use of external beam radiation, particularly as an adjunct to surgery for cancer of the uterine fundus or as an intracavitary implant for cancer of the cervix.

Nursing care for the client with an intravaginal radium implant. Tumors of the cervix are amenable to treatment with radiation because they are confined and easily accessible for therapy. Cobalt, cesium, or radium is commonly used as an intracavitary implant. A colpostat or Ernst applicator, which holds the radioactive material, is inserted through the vagina and dilated cervix to the uterus (Fig. 12-13). The radiation source is directed at the cervix from the uterus and vaginal vault.

Before the radiation therapy begins, the client is readied for the therapy. The physician explains the type, amount, and length of time of the therapy. Two or three days is an average treatment time for cancer of the cervix. A Foley catheter is inserted to decompress the bladder to avoid irradiation, and an enema may be given before insertion to empty the rectum. A low-residue diet is usually given during the course of therapy to prevent gastrointestinal distension, bowel movements, and flatus. An irrigating catheter may be inserted into the vagina so that a solution can be instilled to soothe irritated mucosa and remove necrotic tissue.

While the client is receiving radiation to the cervix, the nurse should help her be comfortable, lessen the discomforts of prolonged bed rest, and assure safety of the radiation source. The woman must lie on her back to maintain the proper position of the implant. She may, however, turn slightly from side to side and raise her hips to use the bedpan and have her back washed. A fracture pan is

FIG. 12-13
Radium implant for cancer of cervix. Note catheter in bladder to maintain decompression.

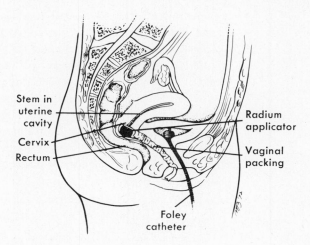

Stem in
uterine
cavity

Cervix

Rectum

Radium
applicator

Vaginal
packing

Foley
catheter

used more comfortably if the woman has a bowel movement. The nurse should assist the woman with her daily bath and rub her back frequently to relieve minor aches and prevent skin breakdown. Analgesics may be used to reduce pain from cramping that results when the cervix is dilated. Antiemetics may be used for nausea. A perineal pad is used to collect drainage of sloughing tissue, and it should be changed frequently for comfort and to prevent odors from accumulating. If there is a disturbing odor, a room deodorizer may be used.

Complications of bed rest are limited by the short time the woman must maintain this position. To prevent respiratory and circulatory complications, however, the woman should take deep breaths to aerate the lungs and should flex and extend the legs. Because the client cannot be turned to different positions, the nurse should encourage activity within the bed.

The nurse must plan care to ensure maximum safety for the client, visitors, and personnel; the principles of *time, distance,* and *shielding* should be incorporated in the care plan. When nursing care is given, it is given in enough time to complete the care and at a safe distance; the client should not feel hurried or isolated when receiving radiation therapy, and several nurses can plan to participate in nursing care. Pregnant nurses and those in childbearing years are usually not assigned to clients with radiation implants, however. Visitors are usually not permitted unless there is a need, and their time with the client is limited and shields used as necessary. A sign indicating that the client is receiving radiation should be put on the chart and door of the room to alert personnel of the necessity for safety. If the implant is accidentally dislodged, the radiation officer should be called, and only long-handled forceps used to retrieve the implant.

After removal of the implant the woman is assisted to be comfortable. An enema may be ordered to empty the rectum. The catheter is removed, and the nurse notes the time and amount of the first voiding to be sure urinary output is not impaired. A douche may be ordered to soothe irritated mucosa and remove necrotic tissue.

The client may experience some systemic and local reactions to the radiation. Nausea, vomiting, and diarrhea are common and are treated symptomatically. Local reactions may include cystitis and proctitis. The woman should increase fluid intake to prevent cystitis. Soothing ointments may be used to relieve proc-

640

titis or pruritus. Fistulas or hemorrhage are serious complications and require additional therapy.

The woman is encouraged to keep follow-up appointments and to report any unusual problems to the physician. Slight vaginal bleeding is not unusual for 1 to 3 months. Sexual relations can be resumed in 7 to 10 days.

Conization. Conization is the removal of a cone-shaped section of the cervix for diagnosis, or conization may be used to remove eroded or infected tissue. This small section of tissue also may be removed when the tumor is in stage 0 (confined to the epithelial tissue). This operation is particularly useful to preserve childbearing function.

After surgery, packing is inserted into the cervix to control hemorrhage. The client is observed for bleeding, given frequent perineal cleanses, and may be discharged from the hospital on the same day. The client is encouraged to have frequent follow-up visits to the physician and avoid vaginal entry until advised by her physician.

Hysterectomy. Hysterectomy is the surgical removal of the uterus. This operation may be necessary for benign or malignant tumors of the uterus or when the uterus is prolapsed from weakened pelvic muscles. Various terms are used to describe the removal of the uterus, and the nurse should be familiar with the surgical approach and what alterations are caused by a hysterectomy.

In a *subtotal hysterectomy,* only the fundus is removed; the distal portion of the uterus and cervix remain intact, and the woman will menstruate. A *total hysterectomy* is the removal of the entire uterus. The vagina remains intact, and intercourse is possible even though childbearing is not. Estrogens are still released, and menopause will occur naturally. A *panhysterosalpingo-oophorectomy* is the removal of the uterus, fallopian tubes, and ovaries; a *radical hysterectomy* also includes the removal of the lymph nodes. In these operations there is a surgically induced menopause, but sexual relations may be maintained.

A hysterectomy can be performed from two surgical approaches. An *abdominal hysterectomy* is done if the fallopian tubes and ovaries are to be removed. The abdominal approach is also used if it is necessary to explore the pelvic cavity. A midline incision is usually made above the symphysis pubis, and postoperative nursing care is similar to that for a client who has had abdominal surgery. A *vaginal hysterectomy* can be done when the uterus has prolapsed or when the client is unable to tolerate abdominal surgery. The uterus is removed through the vagina, and there is no abdominal incision.

Nursing care of a client having a hysterectomy. Before surgery the nurse and client plan to prepare for the impending surgery. Clients who are psychologically and physically prepared for surgery have shorter recovery and fewer complications after surgery.

PREOPERATIVE NURSING CARE. The preoperative nursing care plan should include goals for psychological preparation, instructions about surgery, and preparation for surgery.

1. Psychological preparation. Removal of the uterus may be a traumatic experience for the client. Young women who are in the childbearing years may be upset over the loss of reproductive abilities. For other women the uterus may be a symbol of femininity, and they may fear the consequences of a change in their body image. Some women may be embarrassed about a scar on the abdomen or fear the rejection of their husband.

Nursing process for common health problems

The nurse should understand that the woman's age, marital status, parity, and socioeconomic, ethnic, and religious background may influence the ability to cope with the sexual role changes that occur when the client has a hysterectomy. The nurse should encourage the woman to express her feelings and fears and should offer understanding as she prepares for this surgery.

2. Preoperative instructions. The physician should explain what type of surgery will be done and what approach will be used. The physician should also anticipate the woman's questions about her sexual function and indicate when she will be able to resume sexual relations, whether she will have a surgical menopause, and whether she will be able to have children. Many women are unfamiliar with the reproductive anatomy and may wonder just what is going to happen to them. When the physician has explained the surgery, the nurse can reinforce the explanation and answer questions that the woman might have.

Additional preoperative instruction is given to help the woman prepare for recovery after surgery. The nurse should instruct the woman how to turn, cough, and breathe deeply and should practice with her. The nurse should also teach the woman how to do perineal cleanses and show her the procedure that she will use after surgery. If there will be any special equipment such as an intravenous infusion, nasogastric tube, or Foley catheter, the nurse should tell the woman they will be used and offer explanations of their use.

3. Preparation for surgery. Before vaginal or abdominal removal of the uterus, the rectum is emptied to prevent pressure on the surgical area. The woman may be on a low-residue diet for several days before surgery, and enemas may be given before surgery.

The bladder must also be decompressed to prevent pressure on the site and to protect it from accidental trauma during surgery. An indwelling catheter is inserted in the bladder before surgery and will usually remain in place for several days after surgery.

Occasionally an antiseptic vaginal douche may be ordered to decrease microbial invasion of the surgical site. The douche may be given in the bathtub or when the woman is comfortably supported on the bedpan. If the woman is able, she may prefer to douche herself.

If the surgeon anticipates excessive manipulation of the intestines, a nasogastric tube may be inserted before surgery to prevent abdominal distension. The nurse should explain the use of this tube to the woman and tell her that it will be kept in place for a few days after surgery.

POSTOPERATIVE NURSING CARE. In planning postoperative nursing care, the nurse should know which surgical approach was used and whether there were any complications. The nursing care at this time should be directed toward (1) preventing complications, (2) promoting urinary drainage, (3) promoting feminine hygiene, (4) facilitating nutrition and elimination, and (5) helping the woman adjust to body image changes.

1. Preventing complications. After surgery the nurse should assess the vital signs and dressings to detect bleeding. The woman who has had an abdominal hysterectomy will have an abdominal dressing and a perineal dressing, whereas the woman who has had a vaginal hysterectomy will have only the perineal dressing. The vaginal (and abdominal) dressing should be inspected frequently for bleeding or foul-smelling drainage. After an abdominal hysterectomy a binder may be used to support the abdominal structures, particularly if a large

tumor has been removed, and the nurse should observe the dressing under the binder for bleeding.

To maintain circulation and prevent circulatory and respiratory complications, the woman is encouraged to turn, cough, and deep breathe. The client is usually permitted to be out of bed on the second postoperative day, but the nurse should encourage the client to dangle her legs and sit on the side of the bed before standing and walking to prevent the effects of postural hypotension. Antiembolic stockings may be used to prevent thrombus or embolus formation, and the legs should be exercised frequently when the woman is in bed to prevent pooling of venous blood. The woman should also avoid bending her knees and gatching the bed, activities that could cause pooling of blood in the pelvic cavity and constrict popliteal circulation with resultant dependent blood pooling. Women at risk for thromboembolic disease (elderly women and those with cardiovascular disease) may receive low-dose heparin to prevent thrombus formation.

If both ovaries have been removed at the time of the hysterectomy, a surgical menopause will be created. Some recommended use of estrogen replacement in the immediate postoperative stage. Estradiol valerate (Delestrogen) is one commonly used estrogen, administered intramuscularly for sustained estrogenic effects for 3 weeks. Estrogens should be used with extreme caution in women with cancer of the breast or uterus because of the hormonal relationship believed to exist with these malignancies.

The use of estrogens for replacement therapy after bilateral oophorectomy in premenopausal women is controversial. Some believe the incidence of cardiovascular disease and osteoporosis increases without estrogen replacement and prescribe low-dose estrogen (1.5 mg daily). The estrogen is given in a cyclic fashion 5 days on and 2 days off; therapy may be continued until the client is about age 50. The incidence of breast cancer may be increased with estrogen use, and these women are closely monitored.

Pain medication may be given as needed. It is particularly helpful to give the medication before the woman gets out of bed or has visitors. When an abdominal approach to the surgery has been used, the client may have more pain and need medication more frequently.

2. Promoting urinary drainage. A Foley or suprapubic cystostomy catheter is used after surgery if there is bladder atony; the decompressed bladder also allows pelvic healing. The nurse should observe the catheter for patency and record the urinary output. The catheter is usually removed on the third or fourth postoperative day, and the nurse should note the time and amount of the first voiding. Some physicians may order a catheterized specimen for residual urine after the first voiding. If over 100 to 200 ml of residual urine is obtained at this time, the catheter may be reinserted. When the catheter is removed, the woman is encouraged to drink fluids to promote urinary drainage and encourage spontaneous voiding so that she will not need to be catheterized again.

3. Promoting feminine hygiene. Vaginal drainage is present from both abdominal and vaginal surgery, and a perineal pad is worn until the drainage ceases. Some physicians prefer using a sterile perineal pad for the first few days after surgery; the pads should be counted, and the amount, color, and odor of drainage should be recorded. The perineal area should be cleansed with each change of the perineal pad. Antiseptic wipes or cotton balls with an antiseptic solution are used to give perineal care, and the client is instructed to wipe from

front to back and use only one wipe for each cleansing. Perineal care is given not only for comfort and cleanliness but also to prevent accumulation of microorganisms around the indwelling catheter. Some hospital procedures require the use of an antibiotic ointment around the urinary meatus after each perineal cleanse.

The nurse should help the woman with her bath as needed. Frequent backrubs and position changes help with promoting comfort. The woman should be encouraged to put on makeup and make herself attractive for her family and visitors.

4. Facilitating nutrition and elimination. Unless there has been gastrointestinal interference, the woman receives a liquid diet after surgery and is advanced to a regular diet as tolerated.

A rectal tube may be ordered to relieve pressure caused by flatus. Carminatives such as simethicone (Mylicon) may be used to decrease discomfort caused by flatulence. The woman is encouraged to force fluids and exercise to prevent constipation and straining to defecate. A stool softener or laxative can be ordered to prevent constipation and pressure in the pelvic cavity.

5. Promoting acceptance of self-concept. A hysterectomy may be depressing surgery for a woman. She may feel threatened by not being able to have children, and since femininity may be associated with the uterus, its removal may precipitate strong feelings. The woman may cry and work through a grieving process for several days after surgery. The family is encouraged to understand the woman's feelings and be patient as she adjusts to the change in body image.

DISCHARGE INSTRUCTIONS. Before the woman's discharge, the physician should explain to the woman and her partner that there should be no vaginal entry, douching, or intercourse for 4 to 6 weeks after the surgery. If there has been an abdominal incision, there may be further restrictions on heavy lifting, walking up and down stairs, and riding in the car because sitting may cause pelvic pooling. The family should understand these restrictions and help plan for assistance in doing housework. The woman can be reminded to return to her physician for a follow-up visit in 4 to 6 weeks.

Evaluation. The woman who has had a hysterectomy experiences physical and psychological changes, and the nursing care plan is developed to help the client cope with problems of pain and alterations in sexuality and self-concept. Evaluation of the plan provides information about achievement of client objectives.

EXPECTED OUTCOMES

The client and/or family can:
1. Describe the health problem, type of surgery, and reason for surgery.
2. Use appropriate coping resources.
3. Describe limits on activity during immediate recovery period (no lifting or driving for 2 to 6 weeks).
4. State use, dosage, time, route, and side effects of prescribed medications (analgesics, estrogens).
5. State plans for health maintenance, including rest and exercise, adequate nutrition, and hygiene (no vaginal entry for 4 to 6 weeks).
6. Anticipate changes in self-concept and plans for coping.
7. State plans for follow-up care and identify community resources.

Pelvic exenteration. Pelvic exenteration is the more complex therapeutic intervention for metastasis in which all the reproductive organs, including the vagina, pelvic lymph nodes, peritoneum, and other pelvic structures are removed. An *anterior exenteration* involves the additional removal of the bladder and ureters and the creation of an ileal bladder (conduit) from a loop of ileum. In a *posterior exenteration* the colon and rectum are removed, and a colostomy (an opening in the colon) is created to provide for fecal elimination. A *total exenteration* is radical surgery used to remove tumors that involve all the pelvic organs. The client has an ileal bladder and a colostomy in addition to the removal of the reproductive organs.

The client who has a pelvic exenteration not only copes with changes in sexuality but also with alternative methods of urinary and fecal elimination, and the nurse should plan to assist in adjustment to these changes. Recovery is often slow, and the client may be referred to a continuing care facility until she can be independent in her care.

Uterine fibroids

Uterine fibroids (myomas) are benign tumors of the uterus. They can occur outside the uterus, in the uterus, or on the endometrial lining. The cause of the fibroids is unknown, but there may be a relationship with the endocrine system, because the fibroids disappear after menopause. Fibroids are believed to predispose to cancer of the uterus and are therefore evaluated frequently.

Fibroid tumors occur in about 20% of women between ages 25 and 50. Fibroids are more common in black women and women who have not conceived.

The tumors produce backache, constipation, menorrhagia, and pain. If the tumor is large, there is subsequent ureteral obstruction. Fibroids are diagnosed by the clinical symptoms and radiographic evidence.

A hysterectomy is usually done to relieve the symptoms caused by the fibroids and remove a possible source of malignant tumor formation. If the woman is in the childbearing years, a partial resection of the uterus, a *myomectomy* can be done. Nursing care for a client having a hysterectomy is discussed in the preceding section.

Endometriosis

Endometriosis is the proliferation of aberrant endometrial tissue outside the uterus. The tissue can be found on the ovaries, fallopian tubes, uterus, and within the abdominal cavity and vagina.

It is not known how the tissue spreads, but it may be by lymphatic circulation or menstrual backflow to the fallopian tubes and pelvic cavity. Another theory is that there is congenital displacement of endometrial cells. The endometrial tissue responds to the normal cyclical stimulation of the ovaries and bleeds each month. If the bleeding occurs in tissue on the ovaries, there is no outlet for the blood, and an *endometrial cyst* may form. These cysts may then rupture and cause further spread of the endometrial tissue.

Endometriosis occurs in about one fourth of women over age 30. Women who have not conceived or lactated are at greater risk. Endometriosis appears to be a disease of American upper socioeconomic classes and may reflect the nutritional and delayed childbearing practices of this group.

Early symptoms of endometriosis include backaches from strain on the ureterosacral muscles, menstrual irregularities such as menorrhagia or metrorrhagia, increasing dysmenorrhea, and dyspareunia. The proliferated endometrial tissue can also produce adhesions, which cause sterility. The uterus is not freely movable when examined, and the aberrant tissue can be observed on culdoscopy.

The treatment of endometriosis depends on the severity of the symptoms, size of the tumors, and the age and parity of the client. Conservative treatment is aimed at preventing ovulation, which is the stimulus for the proliferation of endometrial tissue. Antiovulatory drugs in doses higher than normal are used to inhibit ovulation, but the dose is increased gradually to minimize side effects of nausea. Danazol, an antigonadotropin, may be used to decrease pituitary-ovarian stimulation and thereby reduce endometrial stimulation. Side effects are minimal: weight gain and breakthrough bleeding. The woman is encouraged to have her family early because pregnancy causes abatement of symptoms, and, later, sterility may be caused by adhesions. Endometriosis subsides after menopause when there is no longer ovulatory stimulation.

Surgery is indicated if the endometrial tissue obstructs other reproductive organs. Generally the surgical approach is avoided if the woman is in her childbearing years, but eventually a hysterectomy or panhysterosalpingo-oophorectomy may be performed.

Cancer of the ovary or fallopian tube

Cancer of the ovary may be a primary tumor or represent metastasis from cancer of the uterus. The cause of the tumor is unknown, although it is believed that primary tumors may arise from ovarian cysts.[19]

The ovaries are the sixth most common site of cancer in women.[24] The tumor occurs in women ages 40 to 60, and women with increased risk are those who have family histories of ovarian cancer, are nulliparous, have endometriosis, and have ovarian cysts.

The onset of symptoms of ovarian cancer is insidious. There may be menstrual irregularities or a palpable tumor accompanied by abdominal pain. Ascites is a late sign because the tumor metastasizes to the omentum. The tumor may be diagnosed during a pelvic examination and is confirmed by x-ray studies, ultrasound, and biopsy.

Cancer of the fallopian tube is rare, accounting for less than 0.5% of cancers of the female reproductive system. Middle-aged women are at greatest risk. The onset of the tumor is insidious and may only be noted by unusual vaginal bleeding. Diagnosis is made by laparotomy.

Tumors of the ovary or fallopian tube are removed surgically. Follow-up therapy may include radiation or chemotherapy. Palliative chemotherapy may be used in advanced disease. Surgical removal of an ovary is called *oophorectomy;* removal of a fallopian tube, *salpingectomy;* removal of both organs is called *salpingo-oophorectomy.* Bilateral salpingo-oophorectomy renders the woman sterile and produces a surgically induced menopause.

Nursing care for a woman having removal of ovary(ies) and/or tube(s) is similar to that of a client having abdominal surgery and abdominal hysterectomy.

Ovarian cysts

Ovarian cysts are benign tumors that arise from dermoid cells of the ovary or from a cystic corpus luteum or graafian follicle. They enlarge and are palpable on examination. The cysts are usually removed before they become malignant or obstruct blood supply to the ovaries. Nursing care is similar to that for the client having an abdominal hysterectomy, and the nurse should make special observations for abdominal distension and shifting of internal organs when a large mass is removed from the abdominal cavity.

Cancer of the vulva

Cancer of the vulva is a rarely occurring tumor of squamous cell origin. The cancer occurs primarily in women in the fifth or sixth decade of life and accounts for less than 1% of tumors of the female reproductive tract. This tumor is often associated with women who have diabetes mellitus or syphilis, and consequently these women may be at risk for cancer of the vulva.

Tumors of the vulva are slow growing and may be first recognized as nodules on the vulva. There may be pruritus or leukoplakia. Occasionally there is an ulcerated area that does not heal and is painful and may become infected or produce a bloody discharge. Later there may be burning on urination. Women often delay seeking medical consultation because of embarrassment and hope that the ulceration will disappear. If treatment is not instituted promptly, the tumor cells metastasize to the lymph glands. Early diagnosis is confirmed by biopsy. Later there is radiographic evidence of lymph gland involvement.

Surgery is indicated to excise the tumor. If the tumor is diagnosed early, a simple vulvectomy may be performed to remove the tissue. If metastasis has occurred, it is necessary to do a radical vulvectomy, which involves the removal of the vulva and surrounding lymph nodes.

Nursing care of a client having a vulvectomy. The nurse and the client plan to prepare for surgical intervention. The care plan includes preoperative preparation as well as postoperative care during the potentially debilitating recovery.

Preoperative nursing care. Preoperative nursing care is planned to help the client prepare for physical and psychological changes incurred by surgery. Client outcomes during this time include adequate nutrition and hydration and an understanding of the surgery and postoperative course.

Postoperative nursing care. Postoperative nursing care is directed at preventing wound infection and promoting healing. A Foley catheter is inserted during surgery to prevent bladder distension and infection from urinary drainage. Perineal cleanses are given with dilute hydrogen peroxide, 0.5% silver nitrate, or saline to prevent contamination from the rectum. The cleanses should be given with aseptic technique to avoid contamination.

A Penrose drain or Hemovac may be used to provide an outlet for drainage, as much as 300 to 500 ml per day for the first 3 to 4 days. If a Penrose drain is used, dressings should be changed frequently to avoid excoriation and media for bacterial growth and to prevent odor accumulation.

Healing is slow in these clients not only because of age factors but also because the fascia is removed and only a thin layer of skin, which has minimal blood supply, remains. Nursing care is directed toward increasing the circulation in the perineal area to promote wound healing. Sitz baths may be preferred by some physicians to promote circulation; others feel they are a source of contamination and only deter wound healing. Heat lamps are also used to increase circulation, and the nurse should place them at a safe distance and observe for untoward reactions such as burns or a rash. The client should be turned from side to side frequently to prevent circulatory stasis and pressure sores, and a pillow may be placed between the legs to make turning more comfortable. The physician usually permits the woman to be out of bed in 3 to 4 days after surgery. Although this may be uncomfortable for the client, it is important in stimulating circulation.

When lymph nodes are removed from the groin, there is tendency for fluid accumulation. Thigh-high elastic hose should be used immediately after surgery to promote circulation and prevent embolism. Ambulation also increases circulation, and as previously mentioned, the woman should be encouraged to walk as much as she can tolerate. Elevation of the legs while in bed aids venous return. When the woman returns home, she should continue to wear the elastic hose because chronic leg edema occurs in as many as one third of clients with radical vulvectomies.

The woman may be depressed about the time required for healing and amount of disfiguration. The nurse should understand these feelings and help her and her husband cope with them. Because healing is slow, the woman may be transferred to a continuing care facility, and the nurse should initiate an intra-agency care plan to ensure continuity of care.

Discharge instructions. When the woman returns home, she may be concerned about resumption of sexual relations. She should understand that only her external organs, the labia and subcutaneous tissue, have been removed; the vagina is still intact. Lubricants may be used if the vaginal wall is atrophied or uncomfortable. Less deep intromission of the penis may also reduce discomfort. Discussing and anticipating these questions will make sexual role adjustments easier for this client.

Dysmenorrhea

Dysmenorrhea is a severe discomfort before the onset of or during menstruation. It differs from the premenstrual syndrome with respect to cause and severity of discomfort.

Dysmenorrhea is described as primary or secondary. *Primary dysmenorrhea* is not attributed to organic pathological conditions. The discomfort comes with vascular changes of the blood vessels in the endometrial lining. Although psychological factors such as stress, the woman's attitude toward herself, or cultural or ethnic attitudes toward menstruation and pain may influence the course of dysmenorrhea, recent evidence links dysmenorrhea to increased prostaglandin levels in the blood.[18] It has been noted that there is a correlation between the increased prostaglandins and the pelvic pain of dysmenorrhea. The theory is further supported by the fact that dysmenorrhea does not occur during anovulatory cycles of early menarche or in women who use birth control pills and endometrial prostaglandins are not elevated. *Secondary dysmenorrhea,* on the other hand, is attributed to pelvic pathological conditions such as endometriosis, pelvic inflammatory disease, or adhesions.

 Assessment. The nurse can gather health information about the client's menstrual history and help her identify the extent of discomfort. The woman may report spasmodic, cramping pain unrelieved by nonnarcotic analgesics. There may be backache, headache, nausea, vomiting, and chills. Secondary dysmenorrhea tends to occur before the period and radiates to the abdomen and legs and may be associated with pelvic congestion. The medical diagnosis is based on the clinical symptoms and gynecological examination that is done to determine possible causes of the dysmenorrhea.

> **Data analysis**
> *Data analysis may reveal nursing diagnoses of alterations in comfort and sexual dysfunction.*

 Planning and implementation. The nurse helps the client plan to manage the pain and discomfort. Antiprostaglandin drugs such as ibuprofen (Motrin), or indomethacin (Indocin) may be used to relieve the pain. These drugs inhibit prostaglandin synthesis and relieve uterine pressure. The drugs should be given several days before the onset of menstruation for maximum pain relief. Symptomatic relief can be obtained by the application of heat to the abdomen and the use of analgesics, narcotics, or antispasmodics. Exercises such as pelvic rocking and waist bending or relaxation exercises may also be useful to prevent or manage pain. The nurse should instruct the client in health measures of good nutrition, adequate exercise, sufficient fluid intake, and stress management that contribute to health and well-being. The nurse should also urge the client to seek health care services to rule out or treat secondary dysmenorrhea.

☞ **Evaluation.** The nurse and client evaluate the plans for prevention and management of pain and discomfort associated with dysmenorrhea.

EXPECTED OUTCOMES

The client and/or family can:
1. Describe dysmenorrhea.
2. State plans to manage pain (exercise, application of heat, analgesics).
3. State plans for health maintenance, including rest and exercise, nutrition, fluids, and elimination.
4. State use, dosage, time, route, and side effects of prescribed medications (antiprostaglandin drugs, analgesics, antispasmodics).
5. State indications for health care follow-up.

Abortion

An abortion (miscarriage) is the interruption of fetal growth before viability. The fetus is usually considered viable after twenty-eight weeks of fetal life or when it weighs 1000 g. Interruption of pregnancy after that time is called *premature labor*. With improved prenatal health care practices, many fetuses weighing 1000 g survive. Consequently the definition of abortion in some areas is considered to be a fetus weighing 500 g, and the fetus weighing 500 to 1000 g is termed *immature*.

There are several types of abortions. A *spontaneous abortion* occurs when there is no outside interference to disrupt fetal life. An *induced abortion* results from outside interference and may be planned by the physician (*therapeutic abortion*) or done outside the confines of the law (*criminal abortion*). When the abortion occurs three successive times in one woman, it is known as a *habitual abortion*. In a *missed abortion,* the fetus dies but is not delivered for several months.

Spontaneous abortion. A spontaneous abortion is the termination of pregnancy that occurs without external intervention. The cause of the abortion is not known, although many embryos aborted within the first trimester are not normal.

A spontaneous abortion may be either complete or incomplete, depending on the degree to which fetal products are expelled. In a *complete abortion,* the products of conception are observed intact. In an *incomplete abortion,* there may be copious bleeding with part of the products of conception expelled, usually the secundines (placental fragments). Any tissue that is expelled is saved for pathological analysis.

It is estimated that one in five pregnancies is terminated by spontaneous abortion. Maternal risk factors such as malnutrition, incompetent cervix, anomalies of the reproductive tract, and chronic disease may contribute to spontaneous abortion.

A spontaneous abortion may be threatened, inevitable, or imminent, and the clinical signs and intervention differ slightly for each.

Threatened abortion. A threatened abortion is marked by the onset of cramping and vaginal bleeding, but the cervix does not dilate. The woman may be put on strict bed rest at home or in the hospital to maintain the pregnancy, and she may be given a tranquilizer or a sedative to facilitate rest. Progesterones may be used to supplement the endometrium in maintaining the pregnancy. The woman should avoid straining at stool, lifting, and coughing, which could cause abortion of the fetus. The number of perineal pads used are counted so that the physician will have an indication of the amount of vaginal bleeding.

Inevitable abortion. An inevitable abortion occurs when the cervix begins to dilate and there is cramping and bleeding. The woman is often hospitalized and placed on bed rest. The nurse should observe the perineal pads and the bedpan for the lost products of conception, which appear as tissue fragments or fetal tissue within the placenta.

Imminent abortion. An imminent abortion occurs when there is copious vaginal bleeding, cervical dilation, and rupture of the amniotic sac. The woman may be placed on bed rest and given progesterones in an attempt to save the pregnancy. The nurse should observe the woman for signs of shock caused by blood loss. A transfusion may be necessary if there has been hemorrhage. To assure that the products of conception have been expelled and that bleeding has stopped, it is usually necessary to use oxytocic drugs and dilate and curette the uterus. The surgery is referred to as *evacuation of retained secundines* (ERS). The woman is prepared for vaginal surgery, and the uterus is evacuated under anesthesia. Packing may be inserted to assure hemostasis.

The nurse should consider the woman's age, marital status, parity, and sexual role development when planning nursing care for a client who has had a spontaneous abortion. The woman may feel depressed or guilty, and her sexuality disrupted. The nurse should be sensitive to the needs of the client and avoid moral and critical judgments.

After surgery the woman should be assessed for vaginal bleeding, cramping, and shock. The nurse should note the time of the first voiding, because a distended bladder can be painful and predispose to infection. Difficulty in voiding is not uncommon as a result of the manipulation of the bladder during surgery, and if the woman does not void within 8 hours after surgery, the physician may leave an order for her to be catheterized. Pain medication is used to promote comfort.

The woman is usually discharged from the hospital in several days. The physician advises her not to douche or have intercourse until her follow-up visit in several weeks.

Induced abortion. An induced abortion is one in which plans are made to terminate the pregnancy by one of several different methods. The abortion may be done for the health of the mother or the fetus, or to terminate the pregnancy for reasons of family planning. It is estimated that one third of teenage pregnancies are terminated by abortion.[9]

Induced abortions are influenced by federal and state laws as well as religious and moral tenets about terminating life. Changes in legal, moral, and ethical values have produced conflict as to the advisability of therapeutic abortions. The issue is polarized by the feminist and "right-to-life" groups. Feminists argue that a woman should have control of her body and reproductive decisions. This group resists interferences from laws that perpetuate female dependency, male superiority, and sex-oriented social roles. They believe abortion is a right and an option for conception control. The "right-to-life" or "pronatalists," on the other hand, believe that voluntary abortion is a criminal act. They affirm life at conception, and the right to life for that newly conceived individual should be protected. Their position is that abortion should be performed only if the life of the mother is in jeopardy.

Several procedures may be used to induce abortion. The type used depends primarily on fetal gestation. The nurse may have an opportunity to counsel women about abortion and the types and availability of health care services. Because the type of abortion and risks are more complicated after the first trimester, decisions must be made as soon as possible. The counseling and nursing care plan should be developed for the individual client with respect for her social, ethical, and religious views as well as health care needs. Follow-up counseling or referral following the abortion may be included in the care plan.

Menstrual induction (menstrual extraction, endometrial aspiration, mini abortion). This procedure can be done on an outpatient basis 5 to 7 weeks after the missed menstrual period. The endometrium is aspirated with low-pressure suction applied to a plastic cannula. The woman is premedicated with diazepam (Valium) and given a local anesthetic as a paracervical block. This procedure can be done early in the pregnancy with minimal side effects for the woman.

Curettage. Abortions that are performed early in the first trimester of pregnancy, up to 12 weeks, can be done by suction curettage (vacuum aspiration, dilation, and evacuation), a procedure in which a suction source is applied to a curette and the uterine contents are evacuated. This procedure is usually done with a local anesthetic and premedication with diazepam (Valium). The procedure takes about 2 minutes. The recovery period is short, and there is minimal bleeding. Antibiotics may be given for several days after the abortion, and the woman should be instructed to report any vaginal bleeding. Vaginal entry is usually prohibited for 4 to 6 weeks.

Saline abortion. A therapeutic abortion can also be induced by instilling hypertonic saline into the amniotic cavity to cause fetal dehydration and death. Saline abortions are best done after the fourteenth week of gestation when the fundus has enlarged. Before the procedure is started, a test dose of saline is inserted to locate the amniotic cavity, and then 200 ml of the hypertonic saline is instilled as amniotic fluid is withdrawn. Fetal death occurs within an hour. Oxytocic drugs are then given intravenously to produce cervical dilation. Labor usually begins in 12 to 72 hours, and the fetus is expelled. This procedure can be done without anesthesia, and minimal hospitalization is required.

Drug-induced abortion. Second-trimester pregnancies can also be terminated by the use of a prostaglandin abortifacient drug, dinoprost tromethamine (Prostin F2 Alpha). Prostaglandins are also oxytocic drugs, but their effect on stimulation of abortion is not known; perhaps they cause a disruption of the implanted ovum.[11] Side effects are vomiting, diarrhea, shaking, and fever. The drug is injected into the amniotic fluid in a manner similar to the saline abortion. The drug causes contractions similar to labor, and the fetus is expelled. The drug is easier to use than saline and reduces the chances of disseminated intravascular coagulation.

Prostaglandins can also be administered intramuscularly between the twelfth and sixteenth week of gestation. The drug is administered every 2 hours until abortion occurs, up to 24 hours of therapy. The side effects of the drug, nausea, vomiting, and fever should be monitored and supportive care provided. The procedure is done in a hospital setting.

Hysterotomy. An abortion can also be performed by way of an incision in the uterus through which the products of conception are removed. This approach is used if the pregnancy is greater than 16 weeks or if tubal ligation is also being performed. Nursing care is similar to that of a woman having an abdominal hysterectomy.

Parturitional trauma

Prolonged labor or difficult delivery may cause lacerations of the cervix, vagina, or perineum. These lacerations are usually detected during postpartum examinations and can be sutured if they do not heal spontaneously. All women should have a pelvic examination 4 to 6 weeks after delivery to be sure there are no injuries to the reproductive organs.

Vaginal fistulas

A fistula is an abnormal connection through openings in two organs. Fistulas of the female reproductive tract occur between the vagina and rectum, vagina and bladder, or vagina and ureter. Fistulas of the female reproductive organs may be caused by radiation therapy, surgical intervention, or weakness caused by pregnancies. They are named for the parts that are connected (Fig. 12-14). A *rectovaginal fistula* drains fecal material from the rectum through the vagina. In a *urethrovaginal fistula*, urine escapes into the vagina and produces an irritation. A *ureterovaginal fistula* is usually caused by a damaged ureter. There may be urine drainage through the vagina. A *vesicovaginal fistula* occurs between the bladder and the vagina, and there is usually a bladder infection.

Fistulas are recognized by the vaginal drainage, which contains feces or urine. There is odor and vaginal irritation. Fistulas are diagnosed by pelvic examination and radiography. If the fistula is small, it may heal spontaneously. Often a Foley catheter can be inserted for several months to prevent irritation and promote healing of a ureterovaginal fistula. The drainage of fecal material from a rectovaginal fistula can be controlled by giving high enemas to force expulsion of the feces before it enters the vagina. The woman should wear protective undergarments and a perineal pad to protect herself from embarrassing drainage.

FIG. 12-14
Vaginal fistulas.

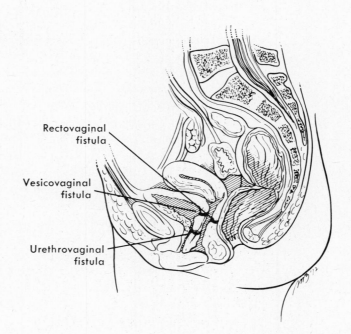

If the fistula does not heal, surgery is necessary to close the openings. The surgical approach is similar to an anterior or posterior colporrhaphy. Nursing care is directed at preventing pressure on the surgical area by using liquid diets, preventing constipation, and promoting bladder drainage by forcing fluids. Healing is promoted by heat lamps, sitz baths, and scrupulous perineal cleansings. Rarely, it may be necessary to create an ileal bladder to prevent continuous urine drainage through a large vesicovaginal fistula.

Fistulas are annoying to the woman, and the healing process may be prolonged. Hygiene is important; deodorants and frequent changes of underclothing will help control odors produced from urine or fecal drainage. The partner and family offer their support by understanding the woman's feelings at this time. Intercourse can be resumed when the fistula is healed.

Uterine displacements

Uterine displacements are usually caused by the weakening of pelvic muscles. The displacements may be retrograde (*retroversion* or *retroflexion*), causing the woman symptoms of backache, fatigue, muscle strain, or leukorrhea; forward displacements of the uterus are *anteflexion* or *anteversion* (Fig. 12-15). Uterine displacements are uncomfortable and may cause dysmenorrhea and infertility. The displacements are diagnosed by x-ray films and pelvic examination.

The displacements may be corrected by muscle-strengthening exercises, support of the uterus by a pessary, or surgical shortening of the muscles. The nurse should help the woman understand and follow the therapeutic approach.

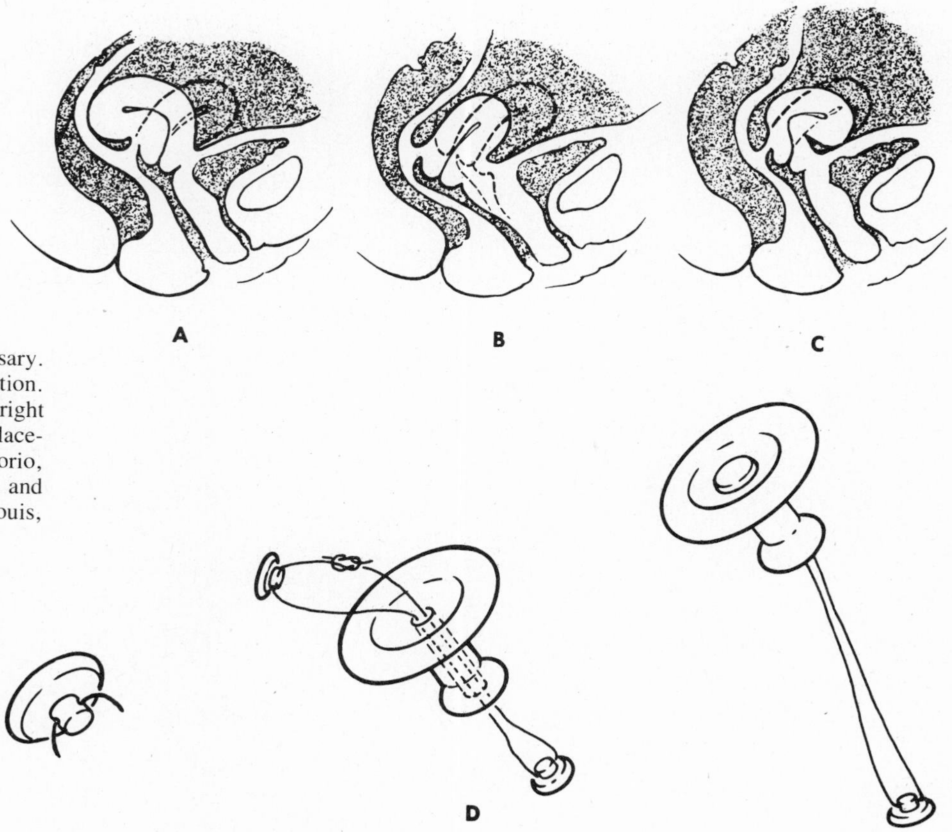

FIG. 12-15
Uterine displacements and pessary. Dotted lines represent normal position. **A,** Forward displacement. **B,** Upright displacement. **C,** Retrograde displacement. **D,** Gelhorn pessary. (From Iorio, Josephine: Principles of obstetrics and gynecology for nurses, ed. 2, St. Louis, 1971, The C.V. Mosby Co.)

Uterine prolapse, cystocele, and rectocele

The internal reproductive organs of the woman are supported by pelvic muscles. When these muscles atrophy with age or become weakened by childbearing, they are no longer able to provide support. The uterus may prolapse and impinge on other structures, or the bladder or rectum may prolapse through the vaginal wall.

Uterine prolapse. A uterine prolapse is the collapse of the uterus into the vagina (Fig. 12-16). The woman notices urinary incontinence, retention, constipation, backache, and vaginal discharge, from the increased pressure exerted by the prolapsed uterus. The symptoms increase with coughing or prolonged standing. The diagnosis is confirmed during a pelvic examination.

The prolapse can be treated by supporting the uterus with a pessary or by removing the uterus. If the woman is unable to withstand surgery or is in her childbearing years, a pessary may be used. The pessary, a firm rubber form that supports the uterus (see Fig. 12-15, *D*), is inserted through the vagina by the physician. The woman must check frequently to be sure that it is in place. A hysterectomy is the preferred corrective therapeutic intervention.

Cystocele. A cystocele is the protrusion of the bladder through the vaginal wall because of weakening of the pelvic musculature (Fig. 12-17). The woman experiences interference with voiding, such as frequency, urgency, and stress incontinence. The cystocele can be diagnosed by the presence of these symptoms and by visual inspection during a pelvic examination.

The cystocele is corrected by tightening the pelvic muscles so that the bladder is supported. Mild prolapses may be treated by exercising the pelvic muscles, but permanent correction is achieved by surgically shortening the muscles that support the bladder. A vaginal approach is used, and the surgery is known as an *anterior colporrhaphy,* or anterior repair. Nursing care is similar to that for a client who has had a vaginal hysterectomy.

Rectocele. A rectocele is the protrusion of the rectum through the vaginal wall (Fig. 12-17). There are symptoms of rectal pressure such as constipation, heaviness, and hemorrhoids. The rectocele is diagnosed by pelvic examination and gastrointestinal x-ray films.

Surgery is indicated to strengthen the weakened muscles. The operation is called a *posterior colporrhaphy,* and if it is done at the same time that a cystocele

FIG. 12-16
Uterine prolapse. (From Iorio, Josephine: Principles of obstetrics and gynecology for nurses, ed. 2, St. Louis, 1971, The C.V. Mosby Co.)

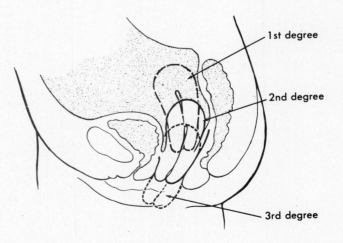

1st degree

2nd degree

3rd degree

is repaired, it is referred to as an *anterior-posterior colporrhaphy* (anterior-posterior repair). Before surgery the woman is given a cathartic to empty the bowel. A low-residue diet may also be used. Postoperative care is similar to that for a client with rectal surgery. The client should avoid any increased rectal pressure from straining at stool, and a high-residue diet and stool softeners are given to prevent constipation until the area has healed.

Benign prostatic hypertrophy

Benign prostatic hypertrophy (BPH) is an enlargement of the glandular and cellular tissue of the prostate. The prostate surrounds the urethra and, as it enlarges, causes pressure and obstruction of urinary flow. The cause of BPH is unknown.

BPH is a common health problem of middle-aged men. More than one half of men over age 50 have BPH, and the incidence increases with age.

 Assessment. The symptoms of BPH are related to the pressure of the enlarged gland on the urethra. There is dysuria, frequency of urination, urgency, hesitancy, and nocturia. Incomplete bladder emptying with residual urine causes collection of urine, which then provides a medium for infection. Later there may be cystitis, hydroureter, hydronephrosis, or urinary calculi. The diagnosis is made by rectal examination, cystoscopy, and radiography of the kidneys, ureter, and bladder. Laboratory studies such as BUN and creatine may be done to assess renal function.

Data analysis

Data analysis may reveal nursing diagnoses of alterations in urinary elimination, alteration in comfort, sexual dysfunction, and disturbances in self-concept.

Planning and implementation. The nursing care plan is developed to relieve the immediate problems of urinary elimination. The nurse plans with the client and in the context of medical management to comply with therapeutic interventions.

Medical management of the enlarged prostate may include conservative measures to reduce prostatic congestion or surgery to relieve the obstruction. If the prostate is not too enlarged or if the client is a poor surgery risk, the prostate

FIG. 12-17
Cystocele and rectocele. (From Iorio, Josephine: Principles of obstetrics and gynecology for nurses, ed. 2, St. Louis, 1971, The C.V. Mosby Co.)

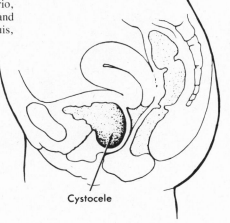

Cystocele

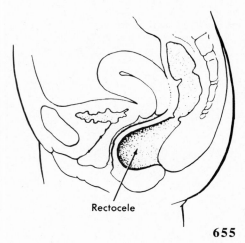

Rectocele

655

Nursing process for common health problems

gland can be massaged to reduce prostatic congestion. Warm sitz baths may also be used to stimulate the gland to release fluid and thereby relieve edema of the gland and urethral obstruction.

Most often, however, surgical intervention is indicated to relieve obstruction. Four basic surgical approaches can be used to remove the prostate. The approach depends on the size and position of the tumor.

1. A *suprapubic prostatectomy* is performed from an abdominal incision through the bladder to the anterior aspect of the prostate. After this surgery a Foley catheter and a suprapubic cystostomy catheter are inserted to maintain bladder decompression until edema subsides. Hemostasis may be accomplished with packing.

2. A *retropubic* incision can be made in the lower abdomen to approach the prostate. This approach is useful when the prostate is large. The client will have a Foley catheter to facilitate urinary drainage and a Penrose drain to remove the drainage from the incisional area.

3. The *perineal approach* involves an incision through the scrotum and rectum. The client is prepared for rectal surgery with enemas, antibiotics, and a low-residue diet. After surgery, sitz baths may be used to promote healing.

4. A *transurethral resection* (TUR) is the most common approach to remove the hypertrophied prostate. A resectoscope is passed through the urethra to excise and cauterize the excessive prostatic tissue (Fig. 12-18). A large, three-way Foley catheter is inserted to provide hemostasis and facilitate urinary drainage. A vasectomy may also be done at this time to prevent infection of the epididymis.

5. A *radical prostatectomy* may be done to resect cancer of the prostate. In this procedure the prostate gland, seminal vesicles, and the cuff of the bladder neck are removed by a retropubic or transpubic route. After this surgery the client will be impotent and possibly incontinent.

Nursing care plan for a client having prostate surgery

Preoperative nursing care. Before surgery the nurse plans with the client to prepare for surgery and recovery. Objectives before any approach to prostatic surgery are to (1) promote urinary drainage, (2) assure nutritional status, and (3) give the client preoperative instructions. The nurse should be aware that the

FIG. 12-18
Resectoscope is used to remove hypertrophied prostatic tissue. (From Liechty, Richard D., and Soper, Robert T.: Synopsis of surgery, ed. 4, St. Louis, 1980, The C.V. Mosby Co.)

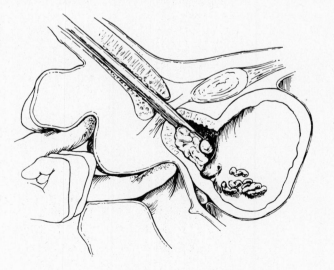

client may feel that his sexuality is threatened and should approach him with respect for his privacy and masculinity.

PROMOTING URINARY DRAINAGE. If the client is unable to void or has urinary retention from prostatic obstruction, a catheter is inserted to provide urinary drainage. A filiform catheter, which has more rigidity, may be required to pass through the obstructed urethra. Occasionally it may be necessary to use decompression drainage so that the bladder tone will not be lost by sudden emptying of the bladder. If urine flow has been obstructed for some time, kidney damage may have occurred, and kidney function studies may be done before surgery.

ASSURING NUTRITION. The nutritional status influences recovery, and for this reason the client should obtain a well-balanced diet for several days before surgery. There may be a fluid and electrolyte imbalance if the client has had urinary retention, and this must be corrected before surgery.

PROVIDING INSTRUCTION. The client may be apprehensive about what will be done to his prostate and how it will affect his sexual functioning. The physician should explain the surgical approach and reassure the man about his sexual capabilities.

The nurse can further relieve the client's anxiety by explaining that he will have one or two catheters to drain urine from his bladder. The nurse should instruct the man that he may feel like voiding, but he should not strain to void around the catheter. Preoperative instruction should also be given about the client's responsibilities in turning, coughing, and deep breathing.

Postoperative nursing care. Objectives of postoperative nursing care are to (1) prevent complications, (2) provide urinary drainage, (3) promote healing, and (4) adjust to changes in sexual function or self-concept. The care plan should be based on the surgical approach used to remove the prostate and the client's response to surgery.

PREVENTING COMPLICATIONS. Immediately after surgery and routinely thereafter the nurse should assess the vital signs and observe for shock. The most common complication of prostate surgery is *hemorrhage,* which is noted by copious, bright red blood in the urine.

Arterial bleeding should be distinguished from venous bleeding. Arterial bleeding, which is indicative of hemorrhage, is noticed by red, viscous blood and passing of clots. The bleeding is accompanied by a drop in blood pressure and other signs of shock such as increased pulse, cold clammy skin, and pallor. The surgeon should be notified immediately of the presence of hemorrhage. Venous bleeding, on the other hand, is darker red and contains fewer clots. This bleeding is not unusual for the first 48 hours after surgery and again at 6 to 10 days as necrotic tissue is passed or after straining at stool or prolonged sitting.

Thrombus and *embolism* are prevented by turning in bed and exercising the legs. The client is usually permitted to be out of bed the day after surgery and should be encouraged to ambulate.

Bladder spasms are not uncommon after removal of the prostate, and antispasmodics may be ordered prophylactically. Ambulation reduces bladder spasms, and the client should be encouraged to take short, frequent walks. If the client does complain of pain or bladder spasm, the nurse should determine the patency of the catheter and irrigate it as ordered by the surgeon.

Bladder spasms may be aggravated by trying to void around the catheter. The nurse should tell the client the purpose of the catheter and remind him not to attempt to void. The frequency of the spasms should decrease in 24 to 48 hours. Continual bladder spasms may indicate injury to the urinary sphincter and should be reported to the physician.

The client should avoid becoming constipated or straining to have a bowel movement because rectal pressure can precipitate bleeding from the surgery site. Stool softeners and increased bulk in the diet are usually given after surgery to prevent constipation. Enemas, however, should not be used for several weeks after surgery. Rectal temperatures should not be taken.

URINARY DRAINAGE. Urinary drainage is promoted by a catheter in the bladder. After a transurethral resection or retropubic resection, a large (no. 18 to 22) three-way Foley catheter is used to provide hemostasis and an outlet for urine; in the suprapubic approach, the client will have a suprapubic cystostomy catheter and a Foley catheter.

The catheters must remain unobstructed. This is accomplished by continuous or manual irrigation. The nurse should explain the irrigation procedure and approach the client tactfully. If a Foley catheter and suprapubic catheter are irrigated, two separate irrigating sets should be used, and care taken to assure aseptic technique with each catheter.

The nurse should offer fluids frequently to keep the urine dilute and to minimize infection and obstruction of the catheter. An intake and output record should be kept. The nurse should also monitor the irrigating solution to prevent *water intoxication* from absorption of irrigating solution through the venous sinusoids.

When the catheter is removed, about 3 to 7 days after surgery, the client should void within 5 or 6 hours. It is normal for the client to experience some urgency, frequency, dysuria, and occasional dribbling when the catheter is removed, but incontinence is not normal and may be caused by bladder spasms. The time and amount of the first voiding should be recorded on the intake and output record. The client should continue to drink 12 to 14 glasses of water a day to irrigate the urinary tract and reestablish normal urination habits.

Exercises can be done to strengthen perineal muscles to achieve urinary control. These exercises are done by pressing the buttocks together, followed by relaxing the muscles. The exercises should be done 10 to 20 times each hour. Urinary control may not be achieved for several weeks, and the client should be given understanding during this frustrating period.

HEALING. Health habits of adequate nutrition, and rest help promote healing, particularly in older, debilitated clients. The nurse should help the client obtain a balance of activity and rest.

If a perineal approach was used to remove the prostate, the physician may order a sitz bath or warm compresses to be applied to the perineum. These treatments are usually given several times a day to increase circulation and promote healing.

ADJUSTING TO CHANGES IN SELF-CONCEPT. The nurse can help the client discuss problems of sexuality and body image changes by indications of interest and acceptance. The man may be depressed and withdrawn, or he may react to his surgery by being aggressive and exerting his independence. The nurse should understand that this behavior is a possible reaction to sexual role interference. The client's wife and family are encouraged to visit and demonstrate their continuing interest.

Clients who have had prostatic surgery may have permanent or temporary interference with sexual functioning. Those surgeries, such as radical perineal prostatectomy, which affect nerves, blood supply, or tissues that are necessary to achieve or maintain an erection, will cause impotence. This may be treated by penile implants. Sterility will be a consequence of severing the vas deferens in attempts to prevent secondary infection. Both these outcomes should be discussed with the client before surgery. In some instances there may be a temporary retrograde ejaculation because of damage to the internal sphincter. The semen is discharged into the bladder, and the client may notice a cloudy urine because of the semen voided in the urine.

Discharge instructions. The client is ready to go home in 7 to 8 days, when he is able to empty his bladder spontaneously. The physician usually advises him not to do any heavy lifting or have intercourse for 6 weeks after surgery. Hematuria may continue as tissue continues to slough, but the client should report bright red bleeding or inability to void.

 Evaluation. The evaluation component of the nursing process for a client having prostate surgery is ongoing and evaluates plans made for preoperative and postoperative nursing care.

EXPECTED OUTCOMES

The client and/or family can:
1. Describe the health problem, surgical intervention, and reasons for surgery.
2. Use appropriate coping resources.
3. Maintain adequate urinary flow.
4. State plans for limitations of activity during recovery.
5. State use, dosage, time, route, and side effects of prescribed medications (antispasmodics, analgesics, antibiotics).
6. State plans for follow-up health care.

Cancer of the prostate

Cancer of the prostate is a proliferation of cells originating in the posterior lobe of the prostate. There is no known cause, although theories of hormonal imbalances have been postulated. Most tumors are adenocarcinomas and frequently invade the entire prostate as well as the seminal vesicles, urethra, bladder, and rectum. Distant metastasis may occur to lymph glands, bones, lungs, and liver.

Cancer of the prostate usually occurs in middle-aged men. It is the second most common site for cancer of male reproductive organs and accounts for 17% of cancer in men.[24] Men over age 50 and with a family history of cancer of the prostate are at risk. There is a possible association of BPH and cancer of the prostate because they occur together frequently.

Symptoms of cancer of the prostate are related to the pressure of the prostate on the urethra. There is urgency, frequency, and urinary retention. Back pain or pain radiating down the leg is often the only warning symptom. The diagnosis is confirmed by biopsy. The tumor can be staged to facilitate diagnosis and treatment (see staging of cancer of the prostate, p. 660).

Treatment may be curative or palliative. The tumor may be removed surgically, with radiation therapy and chemotherapy used as adjuncts. Surgical intervention involves removal of the prostate gland and if there is metastasis, the seminal vesicles and part of the urethra may also be excised. A perineal or retropubic approach is used, and if the urethra is removed, an anastomosis is done to provide urinary drainage.

STAGING OF CANCER OF THE PROSTATE

TNM CLASSIFICATION
Primary tumor (T)

TX   Minimum requirements cannot be met

T0   No tumor palpable; includes incidental findings of cancer in a biopsy or operative specimen. Assign all such cases a G, N, or M category

T1   Tumor intracapsular surrounded by normal gland

T2   Tumor confined to gland, deforming contour, and invading capsule, but lateral sulci and seminal vesicles are not involved

T3   Tumor extends beyond capsule with or without involvement of lateral sulci and/or seminal vesicles

T4   Tumor fixed or involving neighboring structures. Add suffix (m) after "T" to indicate multiple tumors (for example, T2m)

Nodal involvement (N)

NX   Minimum requirements cannot be met

N0   No involvement of regional lymph nodes

N1   Involvement of a single regional lymph node

N2   Involvement of multiple regional lymph nodes

N3   Free space between tumor and fixed pelvic wall mass

N4   Involvement of juxtaregional nodes

NOTE: *If N category is determined by lymphangiography or isotope scans, insert "1" or "i" between "N" and appropriate number (for example, N12 or Ni2). If nodes are histologically positive after surgery, add " + "; if negative, add " −."*

Distant metastasis (M)

MX   Not assessed

M0   No (known) distant metastasis

M1   Distant metastasis present

Specify _____

Specify sites according to the following notations:

Pulmonary—PUL	Bone marrow—MAR
Osseous—OSS	Pleura—PLE
Hepatic—HEP	Skin—SKI
Brain—BRA	Eye—EYE
Lymph nodes—LYM	Other—OTH

NOTE: *Add " + " to the abbreviated notation to indicate that the pathology (p) is proved.*

STAGE GROUPING

No stage grouping is recommended at this time.

From Rubin, Philip, editor: Clinical oncology for medical students and physicians, a multidisciplinary approach, ed. 5, Rochester, N.Y., 1979, American Cancer Society.

Hormonal and chemotherapy with estrogen such as diethylstilbestrol may be given as a palliative measure to relieve pain and retard metastasis. Feminizing side effects of a higher-pitched voice, redistribution of body hair, or breast enlargement may be disturbing to the client who already is coping with an adjustment in sexuality. The physician should explain these side effects before instituting therapy, and the nurse should support the client as he adjusts to these changes.

Alterations in the hormonal environment can also be achieved by orchiectomy (removal of the testes), adrenalectomy, and hypophysectomy.

Radiation therapy may be used before surgery to reduce the size of the tumor or as palliation in advanced cancers. Radiation may be administered externally or interstitially.

Cancer of the penis   The penis as a site for cancer is rare and usually occurs in men over age 50. Those men who have not been circumcised, maintain poor hygiene, or have had frequent venereal infections are at risk.

The tumor is noticed as a lesion on the glans. Metastasis to the inguinal nodes and adjacent organs is common. The diagnosis is confirmed by biopsy.

Therapeutic intervention requires excision of the tumor while leaving as much tissue as possible. Often there is metastasis, and it is necessary to do more radical surgery. Pelvic exenteration (hemipelvectomy) involves the removal of the bladder and rectum as well as the penis. Outlets for urinary and fecal elimination are provided by creating an ileal bladder and a colostomy.

Cancer of the testis

Cancer of the testis is a rarely occurring cancer of the male reproductive organs that affects adults ages 20 to 35. The tumor is usually germ cell in origin and metastasizes rapidly to the brain and lungs. Forty percent of the tumors are seminomas, and 25% are teratomas. Those at risk are men with undescended testes, although this cancer accounts for only 1% to 3% of cancer in males.[19]

The symptoms of testicular cancer are painless swelling of the testicle, which may follow an injury. There may be backaches, heaviness of the scrotum, weight loss, and weakness. The diagnosis of malignancy is confirmed by biopsy.

Testicular cancer is treated by removing the testis (orchiectomy) or chemotherapy or radiation therapy. The prognosis is not favorable, and death occurs within months or years.

Surgical removal of the testis and radical node dissection, if there is metastasis, is done to remove the tumor. Following surgery the nursing care plan should be developed with the client to prevent postoperative complications and manage pain.

Radiation therapy may be used after surgery to retard metastasis. The nurse should be alert to systemic and external reactions to the therapy and develop a plan to minimize these adverse effects. Chemotherapy may be used if the tumor is a seminoma. Vinblastine (Velban), bleomycin, or platinum (Cisplatin) may be used.

COMMON HEALTH PROBLEMS THAT OCCUR ACROSS THE LIFE SPAN

Sexual trauma

Sexual trauma (sexual abuse and sexual assault) is a traumatic event that can happen to victims of all ages. The situation occurs when an individual is pressured into sexual activity by another who has power, physical or psychological, over him. Children, women, and the elderly are often the victims of sexual trauma.

The two most common forms of sexual trauma are molestation and rape. The former occurs primarily in children, whereas rape victims are more likely to be adolescents and adults.

Molestation. Sexual molestation is defined as noncoital contact without consent. Children are usually the victims of molestation and are enticed by offerings of candy or money or by adult permission and sanction to be molested. The child is pressured into not reporting the act, and that the child has been molested is therefore not known for long periods of time. The child may eventually describe the situation, or the parent may observe a change in behavior such as withdrawal, refusal to go outside or to school, crying, regression, or physical complaints.

When the evidence of sexual trauma is known, the parents or health professional should encourage the child to talk about the incident and his perceptions of it. The parents should be encouraged to offer support to the child and avoid display of anger or shame. The child should resume his normal activities, and the parents should provide opportunities to discuss the event as long as necessary. If the child continues to be distressed, family and/or child counseling may be considered.

Rape. Rape is defined as coitus without consent, although forcible insertion of the penis between the labia without penetration of the vagina and ejaculation is also considered rape. *Statutory rape* involves coitus with a victim below the age of consent.

The incidence of rape is difficult to determine because many instances are not reported. Rape can occur in either sex across the life span, but in most instances a woman is the victim. Over one half of reported rape victims are adolescents.

Data have now been gathered about the offender and his motivation for rape. Rapists are usually young and under 25 years of age.[10] Most rapists do not commit rape with intent to kill, although many are motivated by aggression, violence, and impulse of the moment as well as sexual pleasure. The offender in adult rapes is generally unknown to the victim, and the rape frequently represents an act of violence. The offender in rapes of adolescents and young children, however, is often known to the victim and may be a friend or relative. The sexual abuse may continue for months and, if it involves immediate family members, may be an aspect of child abuse.

Prevention of rape. Individuals should be instructed from an early age to avoid situations that make them vulnerable to sexual assault.[5] The child should be made aware of the possible dangers of contacts with strangers. This information should be given explicitly but without alarm or inhibiting the child's natural friendliness. During adolescence and adulthood the information can be more specific. Some examples are:

1. Do not hitchhike or pick up hitchhikers.
2. Maintain security in the dwelling; lock doors, keep windows closed.
3. Hang up and report obscene telephone calls.
4. Do not walk alone at night.
5. Do not wear enticing clothing.
6. Be discreet when unescorted; do not encourage encounters with unknown individuals.
7. Lock car doors; park in well-lighted areas.
8. Avoid deserted places.
9. Do not admit strangers to the home; verify identification of service personnel.
10. Do not enter elevators with strangers.

If the individual is assaulted, the perpetrator should be considered dangerous. Most rapes are committed for the thrill of violence, not for sexual pleasure. If possible, the victim should remain calm and talk the perpetrator out of the act; screams and protests may excite the rapist. Using elements of surprise or self-defense skills such as karate, however, may enable the victim to become free, and some stress the need for women to be able to protect themselves. If these measures are not successful, some suggest screaming "fire" as the most dramatic way to arouse help.

Crisis intervention. If the rape does occur, the victim may be overwhelmed with feelings of fear, anger, or guilt. It is at this time that the individual most needs supportive assistance from a friend, trained volunteer, or health professional.[3,13] Many communities have crisis intervention centers in which personnel are available to assist the victim with physical and psychological recovery from the sexual trauma.

After the rape the victim must consider seeking medical intervention. Many prefer to maintain secrecy about the event, carrying a silent burden for many years. Communities in which crisis centers, emergency units, and women's activist groups provide supportive services for the rape victim encourage reporting and obtaining medical assistance for the rape victim.

If clients do seek medical intervention, they should be instructed to come to the medical facility immediately, to save clothing, not to bathe, and if the victim is a woman, not to douche. The medical examination that follows is performed to evaluate bodily injury and extent of trauma and to obtain evidence of sexual assault. Because evidence for prosecution of the offender may be obtained at this time, strict protocols of examination may be necessary. Adolescent victims, if mature or if the parents are unavailable, may usually be examined without parental consent. This may be a humiliating experience for the client. Women may feel more at ease with a female nurse or volunteer offering support during the examination.

The nurse may assist with obtaining a history of the event. The information should be obtained with consideration for the client's anxiety and include date, time, location, description of the rape, as well as a description of the events subsequent to the rape, such as urination, defecation, douching, or clothing change. Reproductive history data is also relevant, and the date of the last menstrual period and use of contraceptives should be recorded.

The physical examination of the woman involves inspection of the external genitalia and examination of the vagina and cervix. Specimens may be obtained from the vagina to determine presence of sperm or evidence of blood and to obtain cultures for venereal disease.

Treatment for venereal disease or suspected pregnancy is given at this time. Antibiotics such as penicillin may be used prophylactically to prevent venereal disease. If the rape occurred during or near ovulation, high doses of estrogen such as diethylstilbestrol, 25 mg twice daily for 5 days, may be given to prevent implantation of a fertilized ovum. This drug may cause nausea, vomiting, breast engorgement, anorexia, or temporary disruption of the menstrual cycle. The woman should be instructed to anticipate some of these effects. A dilation and curettage and menstrual extraction are other approaches that may be used to prevent pregnancy.

Questioning by the police may precede or follow the medical examination. Many police departments are becoming aware of the psychological trauma involved and in some areas have trained investigators, many of whom are women, to obtain needed information in a supportive manner. If the victim wishes to prosecute, there may be further questions involving hearings, court appearances, and trials. This repeated reliving of the experience may be overwhelming, and for this reason many choose not to follow through the legal process of prosecution. Changes in local laws and support from interested women's groups are two factors that are influencing expedition of trial and conviction of sex offenders.

The trauma of rape does not end with the physical examination and police questioning but involves a long-term process of psychological reorganization. Nurses who have interviewed rape victims have noted a variety of responses.[4] Initially there may be expressed anger, fear, disbelief, or shock; others react in silence. Behavioral manifestations may include crying, edginess, and nervousness. Several weeks after the rape, clients may react by changing their address or telephone number, or by experiencing nightmares or a multitude of phobias. A later period of outward readjustment may be followed by depression. It is only much later that total reintegration of the experience occurs, and victims return to former life-styles.

It is during the immediate and long-term crisis that the nurse plays a vital role in supporting the victim during reintegration. Crisis counseling should be available in the medical facility with provisions for follow-up support during the long-term psychological rebuilding that these clients encounter.

Evaluation

Clients with health problems of the reproductive system may have nursing problems of sexual dysfunction, disturbance in self-concept, ineffective coping, fear, grieving, alterations in patterns of urinary elimination, self-care deficit, alterations in comfort, and rape-trauma syndrome. The nurse and client evaluate plans made for these problems.

EXPECTED OUTCOMES

The client and/or family can:
1. Recognize own sexuality.
2. Describe psychosexual development throughout the life span.
3. State plans for health promotion for the reproductive system, including identification of risk for health problems, personal hygiene, self-examination of external genitalia and breast, and birth control planning.
4. State plans for health maintenance, including adequate diet, rest, and urinary and bowel elimination.
5. Recognize impact of health problem of the reproductive system on sexuality and self-concept and use appropriate coping resources.
6. State plans for health restoration, including use of medications, radiation therapy, chemotherapy, and immunotherapy.
7. State indications for health care and/or plans for follow-up care and use of community resources.

Evaluation of nursing care is ongoing as the nurse and client meet goals for health care of the reproductive system. The nurse-client relationship may continue as evaluation indicates the need for modification or continuity of the nursing diagnosis, plans, or implementation; or terminate as problems are resolved and the client demonstrates his optimal level of health.

Summary

The nursing process provides a framework for assessing, planning, implementing, and evaluating nursing care for clients with common health problems of the reproductive system. The nurse and client collaborate for health promotion, maintenance, and restoration.

During the assessment stage of the nursing process the nurse gathers information about the client's reproductive system and perceptions of sexuality. The health history, developmental, social, and psychological histories, and physical assessment tools facilitate systematic data collection. Data analysis may discover nursing problems or nursing diagnoses of sexual dysfunction, disturbance in self-concept, alterations in comfort, alterations in patterns of urinary elimination, ineffective coping, fear, grieving, self-care deficit, and rape-trauma syndrome.

Planning includes establishing goals for health promotion, maintenance, and restoration. Health promotion may include instruction about personal hygiene, promotion of health during menstruation and menopause, and information about birth control options.

Health problems of the reproductive system occur throughout the life span and often impinge on psychosexual growth and development. Congenital defects are detected during the neonatal period or in infancy and may include phimosis, hypospadias, epispadias, or cryptorchidism. Sexually transmitted diseases have their highest incidence in the adolescent and young adult populations and continue to be significant health problems in the United States. Cancer of the reproductive organs is a major health problem of adults. Other health problems include infections and benign tumors. Sexual trauma is a risk for all age groups, notably young children and women. Plans are implemented for these problems to restore the client to his highest level of health.

Evaluation is an ongoing component of the nursing process, and the nurse and client measure client outcomes against criteria established in the nursing care plan. Ultimate outcomes are that the client can obtain optimal health of the reproductive system to enhance sexuality and self-concept.

References

1. Blough, Herbert, and Giuntoli, Robert: Successful treatment of human genital herpes infections with 2 deoxy-D-glucose, J.A.M.A. **241**:2798, 1979.
2. The breast cancer digest, a guide to medical care, emotional support, educational programs, and resources, Washington, D.C., 1979, U.S. Dept. of Health, Education, and Welfare.
3. Burgess, Ann Wolbert, and Holmstrom, Lynda Lytle: The rape victim in the emergency ward, Am. J. Nurs. **73**(10):1741-1745, 1973.
4. Burgess, Ann Wolbert, and Holmstrom, Lynda Lytle: Rape: victims of crises, Bowie, Md., 1974, Robert J. Brady Co.
5. Csida, June Bundy, and Csida, Joseph: Rape—how to avoid it and what to do about it if you can't, Chatsworth, Calif., 1974, Books for Better Living.
6. Foss, Georgia: Post-mastectomy exercises: how to make them painless, more effective, Nurs. 74 **4**(6):23-27, 1974.
7. Grimes, David: Routine circumcision reconsidered, Am. J. Nurs. **80**(1):108-109, 1980.
8. Guidelines for the cancer-related checkup, Cancer J. Clin. **30**(4):194-240, 1980.
9. Healthy people, The Surgeon General's report on health promotion and disease prevention, Washington, D.C., 1979, U.S. Dept. of Health, Education, and Welfare.
10. Hyde, Janet: Understanding human sexuality, New York, 1979, McGraw-Hill Book Co.
11. Martin, Leonide: Health care of women, New York, 1978, J.B. Lippincott Co.
12. Masters, W. H., and Johnson, V.E.: Human sexual response, Boston, 1966, Little, Brown and Co.
13. Medea, Andra, and Thompson, Kathleen: Against rape, New York, 1974, Farrar, Straus and Giroux.
14. Mims, Fern, and Swenson, Melinda: Sexuality: a nursing perspective, New York, 1980, McGraw-Hill Book Co.
15. Morbidity and Mortality Weekly Reports, Sept. 19, 1980, vol. 29, no. 37, U.S. Dept. of Health and Human Services.
16. Overfield, Theresa: Obesity: prevention is easier than cure, Nurse Pract. **5**(5):25, 1980.
17. Richmond, Julius: Advisory on toxic shock syndrome, FDA Bull. **10**(2):10-11, 1980.
18. Roberts, Susan: Dysmenorrhea, Nurse Pract. **5**(4):9-10, 1980.
19. Rubin, Philip, editor: Clinical oncology for medical students and physicians, a multidisciplinary approach, ed. 5, Rochester, N.Y., 1979, American Cancer Society.
20. Schwartz, Morton: Breast cancer, alternative therapy: hormone receptor assay, Am. J. Nurs. **77**(9):1445-1446, 1977.
21. The sexism of toxic shock, Emerg. Med. **12**(17):63, 1980.
22. Thomas, S.G.: Breast cancer, the psychosocial issues, Cancer Nurs. **1**(1):53-60, 1978.
23. Women's attitudes regarding breast cancer (summary), Princeton, 1974, The Gallup Organization, Inc., from American Cancer Society.
24. 1981 Cancer facts and figures, New York, 1980, American Cancer Society, Inc.

Additional readings

Barglow, Peter: Abortion in 1975: the psychiatric perspective, J. Obstet. Gynecol. Neonatal Nurs. **5**:41-47, 1976.

Boston Women's Health Book Collective: Our bodies, our selves, New York, 1971, Simon & Schuster.

Britt, Sylvia: Fertility awareness: four methods of natural family planning, J. Obstet. Gynecol. Neonatal Nurs. **6**(2):9-18, 1977.

Brown, Marie Scott, and Alexander, Mary: Physical examination: female genitalia, Nurs. 76 **3**(3): 39-41, 1976.

Burger, Doris: Breast self-examination, Am. J. Nurs. **79**(6):1088-1089, 1979.

Burgess, Ann Wolbert, and Holmstrom, Lynda Lytle: Sexual trauma of children and adolescents, Nurs. Clin. North Am. **10**(3):551-563, 1975.

Campbell, Charles, and Herten, Jeffrey: VD to STD: redefining venereal disease, Am. J. Nurs. **81**(9):1629-1635, 1981.

Cosper, Bonnie, and others: Characteristics of posthospitalization recovery following hysterectomy, J. Obstet. Gynecol. Neonatal Nurs. **7**(3):7-11, 1978.

Cowart, Marie, and Newton, David: Oral contraceptives, Nurs. 76 **76**(6):44-48, 1976.

Edwards, Martha: Venereal herpes: a nursing overview, J. Obstet. Gynecol. Neonatal Nurs. **7**(5): 7-15, 1978.

Field, Peggy, and Funke, Jeannette: The premenstrual syndrome: current findings, treatment, and implications for nurses, J. Obstet. Gynecol. Neonatal Nurs. **5**(5):23-26, 1976.

Fogel, C.I., and Woods, N.F.: Health care of women, a nursing perspective, St. Louis, 1981, The C.V. Mosby Co.

Galloway, Karen: The change of life, Am. J. Nurs. **75**(6):1006-1011, 1975.

Gault, Patricia: The prostate: coping with dangerous and disturbing complications, Nurs. 77 **7**(4): 34-38, 1977.

Gorline, Lynne: Teaching successful use of the diaphragm, Am. J. Nurs. **79**(10):1732-1735, 1979.

Gorringe, Ray, and others: The mammography controversy, a case for breast self-examination, J. Obstet. Gynecol. Neonatal Nurs. **7**(4):7-12, 1978.

Hebert, Patricia, and others: Colposcopy—what is it? J. Obstet. Gynecol. Neonatal Nurs. **5**(3):29-32, 1976.

Hildebrand, Barbara: Nursing process and chemotherapy for the woman with cancer of the reproductive system, Nurs. Clin. North Am. **13**(2):351-368, 1978.

Holmstrom, Lynda, and Burgess, Ann: Assessing trauma in the rape victim, Am. J. Nurs. **75**(8): 1288-1291, 1975.

Hubbard, Charles: Family planning education, ed. 2, St. Louis, 1977, The C.V. Mosby Co.

Houde, Charlotte: Adolescent contraceptive counseling, J. Obstet. Gynecol. Neonatal Nurs. **5**:52-54, 1976.

Katzman, Elaine: Common disorders of female genitalia from birth to older years: implications for nursing intervention, J. Obstet. Gynecol. Neonatal Nurs. **6**(3):19-21, 1977.

Kilroy, Patricia: Feminine hygiene products—issues and answers, J. Obstet. Gynecol. Neonatal Nurs. **6**(1):37-41, 1977.

Kjervik, Diane, and Martism, Ida, editors: Women in stress: a nursing perspective, New York, 1979, Appleton-Century-Crofts.

Koch, Sharon: Augmentation mammoplasty, Am. J. Nurs. **80**(8):1480-1484, 1980.

Kyndely, Katie: The sexuality of women in pregnancy and postpartum: a review, J. Obstet. Gynecol. Neonatal Nurs. **7**(1):28-32, 1978.

Laatsch, Nancy: Nursing the woman receiving adjuvant chemotherapy for breast cancer, Nurs. Clin. North Am. **13**(2):337-349, 1978.

Leaman, Karen: The sexually abused child, Nurs. 77 **7**(5):68-72, 1977.

Levene, Martin: Breast cancer: alternative therapy, a new role for radiation therapy, Am. J. Nurs. **77**(7):1443-1444, 1977.

Liston, Joneen, and Liston, Edward: The mirror pelvic examination: assessment in a clinic setting, J. Obstet. Gynecol. Neonatal Nurs. **7**(2):47-49, 1978.

McGuire, Linda: Chronic vaginitis masking serious affective disorder: an illustrative case, J. Obstet. Gynecol. Neonatal Nurs. **7**(2):13-16, 1978.

Murray, Barbara, and Wilcox, Linda: Testicular self-examination, Am. J. Nurs. **78**(12):2074-2075, 1978.

Palmore, Erdman, editor: Normal aging II, Durham, N.C., 1974, Duke University Press.

Robbie, Marilyn: Contraceptive counseling for the younger adolescent woman, a suggested solution to the problem, J. Obstet. Gynecol. Neonatal Nurs. **7**(4):29-33, 1978.

Roznoy, Melinda: Taking a sexual history, Am. J. Nurs. **76**(8):1279-1282, 1976.

Stanford, Dennyse: All about sex after middle age, Am. J. Nurs. **77**(4):608-611, 1977.

Thomas, Sally, and Yates, Marilyn: Breast reconstruction after mastectomy, Am. J. Nurs. **77**(9): 1438-1442, 1977.

Timby, Barbara: Ovulation method of birth control, Am. J. Nurs. **76:**928-929, 1976.

Tobiason, Sarah Jane: Benign prostatic hypertrophy, Am. J. Nurs. **79**(2):286-290, 1979.

Tucker, Sherry Jill: The menopause: how much soma and how much psyche? J. Obstet. Gynecol. Neonatal Nurs. **6**(5):40-48, 1977.

Tully, Joanne, and Wagner, Beatrice: Breast cancer: helping the mastectomy patient live life fully, Nurs. 78 **8**(1):18-25, 1978.

Wahl, Theresa, and Blythe, James: Chemotherapy in gynecological malignancies and its nursing aspects, J. Obstet. Gynecol. Neonatal Nurs. **5:**9-14, 1976.

Wiehe, Vernon: Psychological reactions to infertility: implications for nursing in resolving feelings of disappointment and inadequacy, J. Obstet. Gynecol. Neonatal Nurs. **5**(4):28-32, 1976.

Winkler, Win Ann: Breast cancer, confronting one's changed image: choosing the prosthesis and clothing, Am. J. Nurs. **77**(9):1433-1436, 1977.

Wood, Robin, and Rose, Karla: Penile implants for impotence, Am. J. Nurs. **78**(2):234-238, 1978.

Woods, Nancy Fugate: Human sexuality in health and illness, ed. 2, St. Louis, 1979, The C.V. Mosby Co.

Woods, Nancy Fugate: Influences on sexual adaptation to mastectomy, J. Obstet. Gynecol. Neonatal Nurs. **4**(3):33-37, 1975.

Wroblewski, Sandra: Toxic shock syndrome, Am. J. Nurs. **81**(1):82-85, 1981.

NURSING PROCESS

for clients with common health problems of the

13 Visual system

Assessment

Data analysis

Planning

Implementation

Evaluation

Common health problems affecting the visual system may occur across the life span. These problems may occur either from trauma or infections. The visual system is essential to feelings of security. Therefore, alterations in visual acuity that occur as a result of a health problem are likely to have both physical and psychosocial implications. The individual's mobility and participation in varied activities will be altered. Subsequently alternate modes of self-care must be established. This chapter discusses the nursing process as it relates to common health problems affecting the eye. A complete discussion of the assessment skills necessary for examining the visual system is presented as well as essential strategies of care that deal with health promotion, maintenance, and restoration.

Overview of the eye

The eye is the organ of vision. It is through vision that we are able to get a detailed report of the outside world, view the size, shape, color, form, and position of objects, carry out daily activities, and enjoy the beauty of nature and activities within the environment.

The eye is equipped with various structures. Some of these structures function primarily in relation to vision, whereas others serve to protect the eye from dangers. For example, the *iris,* a circular muscle, determines the size of the pupil. The *pupil* controls the amount of light that enters the eye. The cornea, aqueous humor, lens, vitreous humor, and retina are passageways for light rays. More specifically, the *cornea* is a transparent avascular tissue that functions as a refractive and protective membrane through which light rays pass en route to the retina. The *aqueous humor* is a clear fluid. The *lens,* also avascular, focuses light rays on the retina, whereas the *vitreous humor,* another nonvascular structure, functions to maintain transparency and shape of the eye. Light rays pass from these optical structures and focus on the outer layer of the *retina* (the rods and cones). The retina, a multilayered sheet of neural tissue, receives the visual images, partially analyzes them, and transmits the information to the visual cortex in the brain. As a result, visual images are formed.

Movement of the eye is controlled by six muscles. Four cranial nerves innervate the eye: the *optic nerve* mediates vision; the *oculomotor nerve,* in addition to controlling anatomical function, controls four eye muscles; the *trochlear* and the *abducens nerves* innervate the other two eye muscles.

The appendages of the eyes, along with the orbits of the eye, protect the eyes from dangers. The *eyelids,* movable folds of tissue, fulfill their protective function by closing reflexly—blinking—at the sight of danger. When a particle enters the eye, the eyelids immediately close in an effort to relieve the eye of the offending agent. The average person blinks about 25 times per minute. In addition to protecting the eyes from injury, blinking helps regulate the amount of light that enters them and keeps the eyeballs clean, warm, and moist by conveying tears over them. This secretion also permits the eyes to open and close without discomfort or pain. *Tears,* constantly produced by the *lacrimal glands* and spread by blinking, drain across the eyes to prevent damage to the epithelial cells. Two small *lacrimal ducts* convey tears from the eye into the lacrimal sac, and then the nasolacrimal ducts drain into the nose and nasopharynx. An antibacterial enzyme, *lysozyme,* contained in tears is effective in inhibiting growth of microorganisms on the conjunctiva or cornea and thus helps maintain healthy eyes.

The *eyelashes* line the upper and lower lid margins and curve upward and outward to protect the eyes from particles that may enter them from either direction. The conjunctiva and cornea contain nerve cells. These structures are therefore very sensitive to even the smallest particle that might enter the eye.

Assessment
NURSING HISTORY

The taking of a nursing history is essential in developing a plan of care for clients. A complete history should include data about the client's health, development, and social and psychological status. Such information should be obtained during the initial contact, then analyzed and used as a basis for planning and implementing care.

Health history

The health history should include information about health status including specific diseases and any complaints of visual disturbance such as pain, discomfort, or drainage. In obtaining data about the *health status,* the nurse should elicit specific information about health problems such as diabetes, hypertension, and blood dyscrasias. The presence of these will necessitate a detailed ophthalmoscopic examination, because specific eye changes frequently occur with these problems. Because many diseases have a genetic pattern, it will also be useful to obtain information about the family history of eye problems.

When information is obtained about *visual acuity,* it is essential to inquire about the *onset* and *duration,* using questions such as: Is visual acuity the same as it has been throughout life? When was the problem first noticed? Has the change occurred gradually, or did the change occur suddenly? Is there any difference in the eyes? Has there always been a difference? A comparison should be made of both eyes.

Any complaint of *visual disturbance* should be assessed in terms of *onset, duration,* and *relationship to visual acuity.* Be alert for complaints such as diplopia, photophobia (sensitivity to light), and blurred vision. When these are experienced, it is helpful to assess whether the client has taken medications. If a medication has been taken, it is necessary to obtain information about the type. Inquire about spots before the eyes, which are often associated with vitreous opacities, and halos or rings seen around lights or bright objects. The latter commonly occur in glaucoma. Inquire about fogginess and ability to see straight ahead.

Information should also be obtained about *night blindness,* (nyctalopia). More specifically, assess for difficulty in seeing in the dark, distortion of normal shapes of objects (metamorphopsia), and color changes (chromatopsia). Be alert for complaints of yellow, white, or red vision. The presence of these warrant further assessments about health problems such as jaundice, or the use of medications such as cardiotonic glycosides. Yellow or white vision may be experienced in digitalis toxicity. *Amaurosis fugax* (momentary loss of vision) usually indicates impending cerebrovascular accident.

Pain and discomfort. When assessing for pain and discomfort, the nurse should consider the duration, onset, and relationship of the following symptoms to visual acuity: photophobia, burning, headache, eye ache, itching, and fatigue (which is often described as tired eyes or feeling of pressure). Eye ache often occurs during extreme fatigue. Burning and itching are often indicative of eye strain, inflammation, or allergy.

Discharge. In assessing information about *drainage,* nurses should note the type, amount, color, and whether or not crusting occurs. They should also assess whether or not the discharge is associated with symptoms such as redness, pain, or photophobia. In infectious conditions, the drainage may be purulent.

Developmental history

Neonate. The neonate's eyes, anatomically larger in comparison with body size than in later life and functionally immature, are hyperopic as determined by the short anteroposterior diameter. Because of the immature neuromuscular system, the pupils are constricted and may be unequal, but within the first weeks of life they attain equality. The cornea is larger and flatter than the adult cornea.[1] Often the eyelids are edematous for a couple of days, and the neonate may open his eyes infrequently. A few days after birth, he responds to a flash of light to the eyes by closing his lids. The pupils dilate, and eye movements are not coordinated because of the slow development of the reflexes. For this reason, the eyes may appear crossed. The lacrimal glands are absent for the first 2 weeks of life.

Infant. As development proceeds, changes are noted in the degree of functional and anatomical maturity (Table 13-1). For example, the pupils are smaller than they were at birth, and tears may flow from the eyes in response to emotions. Around 1 month of age the infant focuses on stationary objects within his line of vision. By 2 months of age, he is able to follow moving objects such as

TABLE 13-1

Development of visual acuity

Age	Visual acuity	
	Meters	Feet
2 months	6/120	20/400
6 months	6/60	20/200
1 year	6/30	20/100
2 years	6/18	20/60
3 years	6/9	20/30
4-5 years	6/6	20/20

Reproduced, with permission, from Vaughan, Daniel, and Asbury, Taylor: General ophthalmology, ed. 9. Copyright 1980 by Lange Medical Publications, Los Altos, California.

light and bright colors. At 3 months of age, the infant focuses on objects that are within easy reach with both eyes, which indicates increasing binocular coordination. He reflexively blinks at any object that threatens his eyes. Failure of tear development by 3 months warrants attention. By 4 to 6 months of age, central visual acuity improves to 20/200, the infant shows interest in stimuli more than 3 feet away, and he is able to recognize strangers. He can follow moving objects well, stares at objects placed in his hands, and takes them to his mouth. Such response indicates development of eye-hand coordination. Between 5 and 7 months of age, preference is shown to bright colors, particularly reds and yellows. By 9 months of age, visual acuity increases and hand preference begins, as evidenced by the infant's fascination with, and his ability to pick up, tiny objects. At 1 year of age, visual acuity is approximately 20/100, and eye muscles are mature. The cornea reaches its adult size about 2 years of age.

Child. During the first 3 years of life, the eyes become anatomically mature, and binocular vision fully develops. Central visual acuity approaches 20/60 by 2 years of age and 20/30 by age 3. The child's attention span increases to approximately 1 minute, as evidenced by fixation on small pictures and toys.

During the preschool period, visual acuity reaches 20/30, and the child may show a readiness for reading. Stereoscopic vision (depth sense) is present, and the lacrimal glands are fully developed. By age 5, color recognition is established, and the child knows at least two colors well.

By the school-age period, visual maturity develops. Visual acuity approaches 20/20. Physiological hyperopia (farsightedness) gradually decreases toward emmetropia (normal refraction). Characteristic changes are noted in the attention span. Gross attention span lengthens to about 20 minutes, but attention for details may last only 2 minutes. The school-age child can differentiate shades of color.

Adolescent. Emmetropia is well established, and the eyeball attains its adult size.

Adult. As age increases, the lens of the eyes becomes less elastic, and as a result, the ability to focus is lost. This process (presbyopia), or the gradual loss of the power of accommodation, occurs gradually, usually beginning between 42 and 45 years of age. A common complaint is not being able to see. It is not uncommon to observe persons with presbyopia reading a paper at arm's length. Having arms too short to read the paper is often expressed. In addition to this complaint, individuals may complain of not being able to thread a needle.

Social history

The social history should include data about the age, occupation, and leisure time activities.

Obtaining information about the *age* of the client provides a basis for the comparison of data against established norms for a given age period. For example, "normal" visual acuity usually does not develop until around the school-age period. Subsequently such information helps the nurse provide support to the client and family members about specific changes that occur throughout development. It is not uncommon for visual acuity not to be corrected in the very young child because the demand for distant vision is less than for the older school-age child.[5] Being aware that presbyopia develops during the middle adult period enables the nurse to provide information to clients when they express concern about problems or changes that occur.

Data about the *occupation* should include information about whether the

Nursing process for common health problems

client works with small objects or at close distance from objects. Such information may be useful in evaluating complaints such as "tired eyes" or "pressure in eyes." For *leisure time activities,* it is important to inquire if the client engages in hobbies that require close work.

Psychological history

It will be helpful for the nurse to elicit information about the client's behavior and reactions to the visual impairment (if present), coping behaviors, and the family's or significant others' reaction to the problem.

Physical assessment

The physical assessment skill used to obtain data about the eye is *inspection.* An orderly plan must be developed in doing an assessment of the eye. Ophthalmoscopic examination enables the clinician to examine the interior of the eye in more detail with the use of an ophthalmoscope. A small beam of light is reflected through the pupil as the examiner looks through a tiny opening in the mirror of the instrument. Abnormalities of the fundus, optic disk, and vessels of the eye can be detected. Because of the difficulty in viewing through the small pupil, mydriatics are instilled into the eye before examination. The lids may be everted (Fig. 13-1), or a retractor may be used to open the lids. If retractors are used, an ophthalmic anesthetic is instilled in the eye. The examination should be carried out in a dark room to facilitate pupillary dilation. Young children should be immobilized in a recumbent position, whereas older children and adults may be examined in a sitting position. When medications are instilled, diplopia and blurred vision may be experienced for a short time after the test. The client should therefore be forewarned so that preparation can be made for transportation to and from the health care facility.

Although the ophthalmoscopic examination is an essential part of the physical examination, a presentation of this aspect of the examination is beyond the scope of this chapter. A complete physical assessment of the external eye structures should include inspection of structures such as the lids, lashes, lacrimal apparatus, and conjunctiva. When applicable, the color, position, and presence of any growth, swelling, or secretions should be noted.

Assessing external structures

Lids. The lids are assessed for color and redness. Evaluation of the conjunctiva indicates discoloration and inflammation.

Position. The lids should completely cover the eyes. This should be an initial assessment. Assess whether the lid sags outward (ectropion), sags inward (entropion), or droops (ptosis). Ptosis may be indicative of paralysis, meningitis, tumor, or the maturational level of the client. Ptosis is sometimes present at birth but later disappears with maturation.

Growths. Any growth on the lid is abnormal. Growths that may appear on the lid include styes and chalazion.

Swelling. Assess whether one or both lids are swollen. Swollen lids may indicate hypothyroidism, kidney disease, and allergies.

Excessive blinking. Assess whether the excessive blinking is a habit, or whether it is the result of some other problem such as eyestrain.

Lacrimal apparatus. Assess the amount and character of lacrimation: increased, decreased, or excessive (epiphora). Sufficient lacrimal fluid may not be secreted to produce tearing during the first month of life. If the lacrimal duct is not patent, excessive tearing may be observed. Allergic conditions, inflammation, and a foreign body may also cause increased lacrimation. After this has been accomplished, assess the size or position of the eye as well as specific structures including the conjunctiva, cornea, sclera, iris, and pupils.

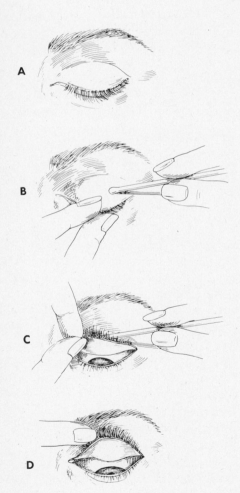

FIG. 13-1
Steps in everting the eyelid. **A,** Client looks downward. **B,** Examiner pulls lid down with fingers. **C,** Lid is pulled over rod by examiner. **D,** Lid is everted.

Size of the eye. Note whether the eye is small (microphthalmos), normal (enophthalmos), or prominent (exophthalmos). An exophthalmometer is used to measure the exact amount of exophthalmos.

Conjunctiva. The conjunctiva is assessed for color and growths.

Color. The conjunctiva is normally transparent. Redness is indicative of inflammation; pallor may be indicative of anemia; yellow discoloration may be a first sign of liver disease.

Growths. Growths on the conjunctiva are abnormal. A common growth found on the conjunctiva is a pterygium.

Cornea. The color is normally transparent. Assess for any evidence of abrasion, irritation, or opacities. Fluorescein, an indicator dye, is used to identify defects of the cornea.

Sclera. The normal color is clear and white. Variations in color may be apparent depending on the individual's age. For example, the sclera of the infant and young child may be bluish because of its thinness and because of the prominence of the *pigmented choroid*. In the adult it is white and opaqe. The sclera during later maturity may appear yellowish because of the presence of fat and because of degenerative changes. A blue discoloration is abnormal and is indicative of some pathological process, such as otogenesis imperfecta. A yellow discoloration of the sclera is associated with jaundice; whereas a dark discoloration is often indicative of long-standing use of silver compounds, or of sclera thinning or degeneration.[5]

Iris. The irides of both eyes are normally the same color. A difference in color indicates congenital abnormalities, tumors, or the presence of an intraocular foreign body.

Pupils. The pupils should be inspected for location, size, equality, color, shape, and reaction to the stimulation of light.

Location. The pupils are centrally located and round.

Size. The size of the pupil varies according to the age of the client. The pupils tend to be small during infancy, larger in the child, and progressively smaller during advancing age. The average diameter of the pupil is 3 to 4 mm. However, individuals with blue eyes are thought to have larger pupils.

REGULATION OF PUPILLARY SIZE. The sympathetic and parasympathetic divisions of the autonomic nervous system influence pupillary size. Parasympathetic stimulation causes pupillary constriction by contracting the sphincter muscle in response to light and accommodation, whereas sympathetic stimuli produce dilation by contracting the dilator muscles of the iris.

VARIABLES AFFECTING PUPILLARY SIZE. Certain conditions may alter the size of the pupils. These include rest, drugs, excitement, and health state. During rest, the pupils continuously fluctuate, minutely, from constriction to dilation. Certain drugs may also affect the size and ability of the eye to react to light. For example, cycloplegic drugs such as atropine may dilate and immobilize the pupil. As a result, the pupils may not constrict on light stimulation. Drugs such as amphetamines and cocaine may dilate the pupils through sympathetic activity. Drugs that may cause constriction of the pupils are medications such as pilocarpine used for treating glaucoma. Morphine causes pupillary constriction, and an overdose of the drug characteristically produces small pinpointed pupils. Dilation of the pupils may also be evident when an individual is anxious or afraid. Pain in the eye constricts the pupils, whereas other types of pain cause the

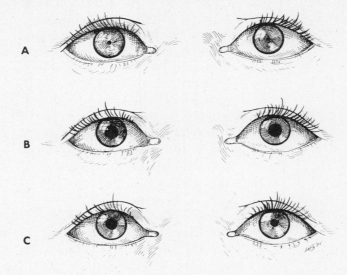

FIG. 13-2
Variations in pupil size. **A,** Constriction. **B,** Dilation. **C,** Unequal pupil (anisocoria).

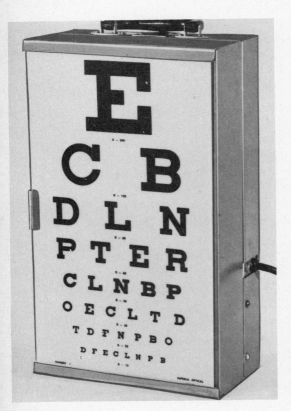

FIG. 13-3
Snellen visual acuity chart. (From Stein, Harold A., and Slatt, Bernard J.: The ophthalmic assistant, ed. 4, St. Louis, 1982, The C.V. Mosby Co.)

pupils to dilate. Health problems such as iritis and lesions of the cornea may cause unilateral constriction. Problems such as paralysis of cranial nerve III, intracranial damage, acute narrow-angle glaucoma, or those involving the retina and optic nerve cause dilation. Conditions involving the retina and optic nerve may also produce an immobile and unresponsive pupil.

EQUALITY OF SIZE. The pupils are normally equal in size. Anisocoria (difference in pupil size) occurs in a small percentage of the population (Fig. 13-2). Inequality in the size of the pupils may be evident in conditions characterized by a tonic pupil (such as in *Adie's Syndrome*), which is slow response of the pupil to light stimulation. *Argyll Robertson* pupils, characteristic of late syphilis, are small (less than 3 mm), irregular in shape, and do not react to light stimulation. They do, however, constrict with accommodation.[5]

Shape. Irregularities in shape of the pupil most likely result from congenital abnormalities, inflammatory and traumatic instabilities, and surgical interventions (such as iridectomy).

Reaction to light. The pupils' normal reaction to light is brisk, with prompt constriction. They normally react equally to light stimulation. Two methods of assessment may be employed: direct and consensual. With the *direct method,* a light is brought from the side and directed into the pupil. Assessment should be made of the pupil on the side being examined. For the *consensual method,* the light is shone into one eye and the assessment is made in the opposite (unilluminated) eye. The nurse should note the speed (rapid or slow) of the response. One condition essential for accuracy of this assessment is room illumination, because light affects the responses of the normal pupils. A dimly lighted room, with the light evenly distributed is recommended. An excessive amount of light causes the pupils, by action of the sphincter muscles of the iris, to constrict; whereas an opposite effect (such as poor illumination) causes the pupil to dilate. A small penlight is recommended for this assessment; however, a flashlight may be used. The client should be resting.

Following examination of the structures of the eye, attention should be directed toward assessing visual acuity, color vision, alignment, refractive errors, and intraocular pressure.

Assessing visual acuity. Assessments of visual acuity should be made across the life span. Some ophthalmologists recommend that an examination be performed as early as the first year of life. The National Society for the Prevention of Blindness recommends the following schedule: kindergarten or first grades (5 to 6 years), second grade (7 years), fifth grade (10 to 11 years), eighth grade (13 years), eleventh grade (16 years), and thereafter every 2 years.

Before the screening test is started, specific instructions should be given about the test. For example, if the illiterate E is used for testing, the child should be taught to point his finger in the direction that the legs of the E extend. If the child is not able to perform, he may benefit from brief instruction periods at home with the parents or with the nurse.

Visual acuity is most commonly tested with the use of the Snellen chart or one of its modifications. The Snellen test measures the difference in visual acuity between both eyes. It is composed of lines of letters of various sizes (Fig. 13-3). This test is performed with the client at a distance of 20 feet (6 meters) from the chart. At this distance rays of light from an object are practically parallel, and no effort of accommodation is necessary to focus on the object. One who is able to read the 20-foot line of letters at a distance of 20 feet has vision that is expressed by the fraction 20/20 (6/6). The numerator denotes the distance at which the test is conducted, and the denominator denotes the distance at which the smallest letter can be read. If an individual is not able to read all the letters on a given line (such as the 70 line), the acuity may be recorded as 20/70-1.

The test is done by having the individual cover one eye at a time. The acuity of the right eye is generally assessed first, then the left eye. If the client wears corrective glasses, the test is carried out with and without them and the results recorded as corrected or uncorrected. During the test, one eye should be covered with an occluder rather than with the client's hand. This practice prevents peeking through the fingers and irritating the eye.

Modifications of the Snellen Test are used for children who may not be familiar with the alphabet. Examples of the modifications are the illiterate E, pictures, numbers, symbols, non-Arabic letters (Fig. 13-4). The letter E is presented in any one of four directions—right, left, up, or down—and the person is asked to point in the direction of the legs of the E. The picture visual acuity chart,

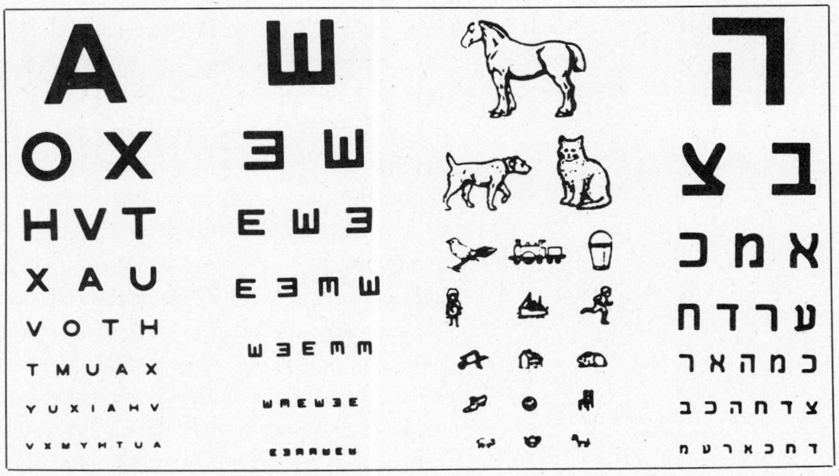

FIG. 13-4
Examples of Snellen Test Card with variations used for testing visual acuity in illiterates, young children, and patients of varying ethnic backgrounds. (From Rose, Clifford F., editor: Medical ophthalmology, St. Louis, 1976, The C.V. Mosby Co.)

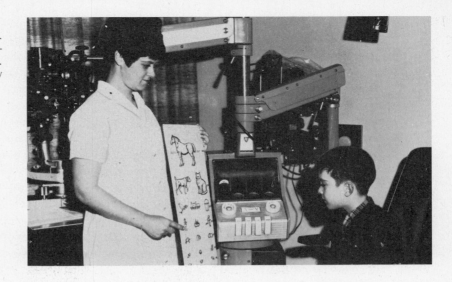

although less accurate, has proved to be a useful method for testing young children and the retarded. Pictures of familiar objects (horse, dog, cat, bird, train, and so on) are presented in various sizes at a distance of 1 foot as a picture game (Fig. 13-5). A distance of 1 foot is used because this is the natural distance for playing a game. The child is asked to identify the picture. If he cannot do so, the picture on the card is identified, and the child is retested. Flash cards, a modification of the picture chart, have also been developed.

Assessing color vision. It is generally recommended that an assessment of color perception be administered at least once during the school-age period, preferably during kindergarten. Thereafter this assessment is made during examination for the military and for occupations that require the best possible color perception.[5]

An assessment of color vision is made with the use of Ishihara polychromatic plates, Stilling, and Harvey-Rand-Rittler plates.[1] The Ishihara plates (commonly used to detect red/green defects) contain dots of primary colors printed in the background of similar dots in several colors. The dots are outlined in a pattern (for example, in numbers) that can easily be identified by individuals with normal color vision: the color-deficient individual cannot identify the pattern, as evidenced by interpreting the dots as forming completely different numbers. For clients who cannot read numbers, plates with colored winding lines, which can be traced, are used. The Harvey-Rand-Rittler (HRR) plates are similar to the Ishihara plates, but permit detection of red/green as well as blue/yellow defects. Good lighting, whether natural or artificial, is essential for this assessment.

Assessing alignment of the eye. The *cover-uncover test* is a method of evaluating the degree of *phoria* or *tropia* and is useful in differentiating various types of strabismus. The test may be performed as early as 3 months of age and periodically during the preschool period. It is accomplished by covering one eye with an opaque object. The uncovered eye is observed for movement (Fig. 13-6). In normal conditions, no movement is noted in the uncovered eye, whereas with an abnormality, the uncovered eye moves in an effort to focus on the designated point. It is essential that fixation be assured during the test. There-

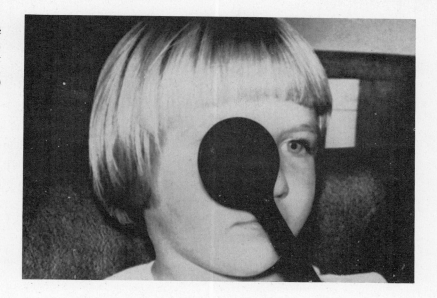

fore, the examiner uses an article such as a brightly colored or squeaky toy, that will attract a child's attention. Other than giving explanations about the test, no other preparation is necessary.

Assessing refractive errors. Retinoscopy is an objective method for determining the refractive error of an eye. When a retinoscopic examination is performed, the examiner directs a light through a pupil and observes the light rays as they reflect from the retina. Each corrective lens has a characteristic pattern, and therefore the error can readily be identified. Cycloplegics are often administered before retinoscopy to abolish accommodation. It is generally recommended to test children for refractive errors around 4 years of age.

Assessing intraocular pressure. *Tonometry* is the measure of intraocular pressure. This measurement is accomplished with the use of a tonometer. Two types of tonometers may be used to assess intraocular pressure: an applanation tonometer and an indentation tonometer.

The *indentation tonometer* (for example, a Schiøtz tonometer, Fig. 13-7, *A*) measures intraocular pressure by indentation of the cornea by a plunger. With the tonometer in the vertical position, the footplate is placed lightly on the center of the anesthetized cornea. A scale on the instrument enables the examiner to read the amount of indentation produced by weights on the plunger. The amount of indentation of the cornea depends on the intraocular pressure. The harder the eye, the less amount of indentation will occur, the lower the scale reading, and the higher the intraocular pressure. If the eye is soft, the more indentation occurs, the higher the scale readings, and the lower the pressure. Recordings are made in millimeters of mercury. The test is performed with the client in the recumbent position.

The *applanation tonometer* flattens a small area of the cornea (Fig. 13-7, *B*). Tension recordings may be made with a special hand device or with the use of a slit-lamp microscope. With use of the latter, the client must be in a sitting position, whereas, with the former, readings may be taken while the client assumes either a recumbent or sitting position. It is recommended that after 35 years of age, the assessment of intraocular pressure be made every 2 years.

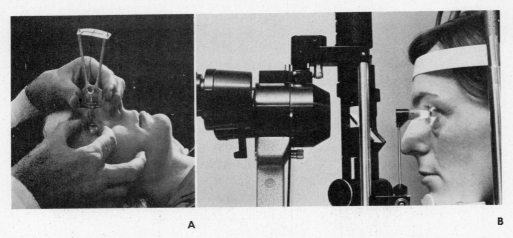

FIG. 13-7
A, Measurement of ocular tension with the Schiøtz tonometer. The examiner must be careful not to exert pressure on the globe through the eyelids. **B,** Measurement of the ocular tension with a Goldmann applanation tonometer. This method is more sensitive than Schiøtz tonometry, but it requires an expensive biomicroscope. (From Newell, Frank W.: Ophthalmology: principles and concepts, ed. 4, St. Louis, 1978, The C.V. Mosby Co.)

Preparation for measurement of intraocular pressure. To ensure accurate readings, the client should be adequately prepared for tonometry. The nurse should assess for the presence of contact lenses. If present, they should be removed. Explanations should be given about the nature of the examination. The client should be informed of behaviors that will affect pressure readings. For example, straining, squeezing of the lids, coughing, breath holding, and wandering eye movements will increase the tension and result in false readings. Instructions should be given to refrain from rubbing the eyes once the eye drops are instilled because of loss of pain sensation from the anesthetic. Consequently, the cornea could become abraded. Therefore, if tears are formed, they should be blotted with a tissue rather than rubbed. Before the test, one or two drops of a topical anesthetic, such as 1% tetracaine (Pontocaine) or 0.5% proparacaine (Ophthaine), are instilled into the conjunctival sac.

Relaxation should be encouraged during the test, and the client is instructed to look upward at some fixed object. Because intraocular pressure may vary over the course of the day, a notation should be made of the time of day. This information can be used in evaluation of the reading.

DIAGNOSTIC ASSESSMENT

A variety of diagnostic tests may be used to obtain information about the condition of the eye; some of these follow.

Electroretinography

Electroretinography (electroretinogram, ERG) is a measure of the changes in electrical potential that occur in the retina after exposure to light. Since electrical potential exists between the cornea and retina, changes in the intensity of light that enters the eye and the state of adaptation will alter it. Because some diseases of the retina and choroid alter the ERG, it is a useful diagnostic tool.

When the test is performed, a contact lens electrode is placed on the eye, and the client is instructed to look straight ahead. Blinking is discouraged.

678

13   Visual system

Echoophthalmography

Echoophthalmography (ultrasonography, ultrasound, echography) is useful in diagnosing ocular and orbital growths. It employs a sound probe that transforms high frequency electrical pulses into ultrasonic waves directed in the form of a beam.[1] The echoes from tissues are converted into electrical impulses and displayed on a screen. The echo signals may be displayed as vertical defections or as bright spots.

Fluorescein angiography

Fluorescein angiography, a dye (sodium fluorescein) is injected in the antecubital vein as rapidly as possible,[4] following which multiple photographs of the retina are taken at specified intervals with a retina camera. The film records the flow of the dye through the retina and choroid.

Shortly after the dye is injected, the client may experience transient nausea and vomiting. The urine will take on a yellowish appearance for about 2 days. Therefore, to decrease apprehension, the client should be informed of this.

Since, occasionally, individuals may be allergic to the dye, allergies to specific substances should be well established before the test. Drugs to combat allergic responses should be readily available.

Phosphorus 32 radioactive uptake

Phosphorus 32 radioactive uptake is a test to gain information about an ocular tumor. Radioactive phosphorus is injected intravenously. Forty-eight hours after the substance is injected, a count is made of the radioactivity by using a Geiger counter during surgery. Malignant tissue retains more radioactive phosphorus when compared with normal tissue.

Tonography

Tonography, commonly referred to as aqueous outflow study, measures the rate at which the intraocular pressure decreases when the eye is compressed by means of an indentation tonometer on the eye.[4] The reading is generally taken over a 4-minute period and recorded on a graph similar to an electrocardiogram.

Gonioscopy

Gonioscopy is a biomicroscopic examination that visualizes the anterior chamber angle, the area where aqueous humor leaves the eye. The examiner places a special gonioscopic contact lens over the cornea and examines the area with a microscope. This technique is useful in diagnosing congenital and secondary glaucoma, in evaluating angle closure preoperatively, and in evaluating the success of ocular surgery postoperatively.

Perimetry

Perimetry, measurement of the peripheral field, can detect a loss of peripheral vision, which commonly occurs in glaucoma.

Data analysis

After necessary data have been obtained about the client, the nurse should compare the data with norms appropriate to the client's age, sex, and developmental level. Social and psychological data should be considered as the data are analyzed in preparation for the formulation of nursing diagnoses. Data analysis may reveal nursing diagnoses of alterations in sensory perception, grieving, alteration in self-care activities, alterations in body image, alterations in comfort, fear, ineffective coping, and disturbance in self-concept.

Planning

As care is planned for the client, consideration must be given to aspects of health promotion as well as strategies and measures essential to maintenance and restoration of health.

PLANNING FOR HEALTH PROMOTION

The nurse's role in promotion of eye health cannot be overemphasized. The provision of information is one way in which the nurse can facilitate health promotion. Information may range from the answer to one question about the eyes to providing detailed facts about ocular and general health and about ways of protecting the visual system. The community health or visiting nurse, through home visits, or the occupational health nurse can be instrumental in teaching about eye safety.

Explanations may be given about the proper environment, nutrition, and relaxation. In addition, information about the stages of development is valuable. Explanations of the role of vision in intellectual development, reading, and study, and also of changes that occur with age and what should be done for the conservation of vision are often necessary. The information provided might be based on observations that are made, on expressed misconceptions, or on questions that are raised by the client. For example, information may be given regarding eye specialists and their roles and the care of the eyes, including the use of medication, prevention of eye fatigue and eye injuries, illumination, principles of first aid, danger signals of visual disorders, and proper use of dark glasses.

Eye specialists

Clients often are not aware of the differences between the various eye specialists and consequently do not understand the role of each. The nurse is one health care provider who can provide information about these specialists. Following are definitions of eye specialists.

Optometrist. An optometrist (OD) is a licensed nonmedical practitioner who is qualified to measure refractive errors and eye muscle disturbances. He does not treat or diagnose diseases of the eye.

Optician. An optician is a technician who prepares and grinds lenses, fits them into a proper frame, and adjusts the frames to the wearer.

Ophthalmologist. An ophthalmologist (oculist) is an MD who specializes in diagnosis and treatment of defects and diseases of the eyes, performs surgery when necessary, and prescribes other types of treatment including glasses and care for refractive problems.

Orthoptist. An orthoptist is a medical technician who assists the oculist in the examination and care of clients with disorders of ocular movements.

Care of the eyes

Use of medications. Many persons have a tendency to use over-the-counter eye drops for cleansing purposes. Because the eyes are equipped with an efficient cleansing mechanism, this practice should be discouraged. Tears are produced by the lacrimal glands and are therefore the best fluid for cleansing the eyes. Basically, tears are a saline solution with protein components that help reduce surface tension and efficiently wet the corneal surface. An element is present in tears that acts as a lubricant. They also contain a lysozyme, beta lysin, IgA, and IgG, all of which inhibit bacterial growth.[5] These properties make it unnecessary to wash healthy eyes. Frequent use of eye drops may only serve to introduce bacteria into the eye or destroy the normal protective mechanism of the eye. Clients therefore should not be instructed to use eye medications unless prescribed by a physician.

Eye fatigue. Eye fatigue (often described as pressure, tired eyes) commonly occurs when reading materials are placed too close to the eyes. Printed matter should therefore be held at least 14 inches from the eye. Eye muscles become tired after long periods of reading or close work; therefore frequent rest periods should be planned to relax the eye muscles. To reduce fatigue, for example, from watching television, individuals must be reminded to sit 10 to 12 feet away from the screen.

Prevention of eye injuries. Instructions regarding eye hazards should be directed to children as well as adults. Instructions about measures to protect the visual system in the home, school, automobile industry, and other environments are essential. For example, parents should be given information about safe toys and toys that promote visual and intellectual development. BB guns, bows and arrows, and other potentially dangerous toys should not be purchased. Children, particularly, should be advised against running with sharp objects or swinging belts and buckles. Those who wear glasses and engage in sports activities should be encouraged to use protective eyewear over glasses.

Individuals who work in factories with metal and strong chemicals should wear a protective face shield (goggles, glasses). Those who work in extremely bright light should wear eye shields to reduce the amount of light that enters the eye. A government regulation requires the lenses in glasses to be made of safety glass or plastic.

First aid principles. Instructions should also be provided about the proper first aid principles when a foreign body enters the eye. Application of these principles is important in preventing visual damage and blindness.

1. Wash chemical eye burns immediately with plain water for at least 15 minutes.
2. Refrain from touching the eye when an object penetrates the eye. Cover the eye with a shield to protect the eye from accidental pressure. Seek medical help immediately.
3. If bleeding is noted from the eye, let it bleed. Do not try to stop the bleeding, because pressure will cause more damage to the eye.
4. If a foreign body gets into the cornea, seek medical help immediately, so that the object can be removed under sterile conditions. Do not rub.
5. If a foreign body gets on the conjunctiva and can be readily seen, carefully pick the object out with a clean handkerchief, moistened wisp of cotton, or some other clean object.
6. When a black eye is sustained, seek medical help because more damage may have been suffered than is readily noted.

Danger signals of visual disorders. Clients should be informed of the seven danger symptoms that indicate the need to seek health care. These symptoms may occur at any age.

1. Persistent redness of the eye
2. Continued discomfort or pain about the eye, especially following an injury
3. Crossing of the eyes, especially in children
4. Visual disturbances such as blurred vision or spots before the eyes
5. Growth on the eye or eyelid or opacities visible in the normally transparent part of the eye
6. Continual discharge, crusting, or tearing of the eye
7. Pupil irregularities

Illumination. Proper light conserves vision and reduces eyestrain, whether the person is reading or engaging in other activities. Individuals ought to be encouraged to read in an environment illuminated by bulbs of 100 to 150 watts. The light should come from behind and not reflect a glare. Activities such as watching television should be done in a room that has adequate illumination.

Use of dark glasses. The pupil, by changing in size, normally helps regulate the amount of light that enters the eye. Therefore, under normal conditions dark glasses are not necessary. Occasionally the amount of light that enters the eye is excessive and may cause acute discomfort, for example, light reflected from snow or water. Most individuals work in factories, shops, offices, and stores where illumination is less than normal daylight; consequently, a change from the working environment to sunlight may be uncomfortable. Under these circumstances, tinted or dark glasses are necessary to promote eye comfort.

Phototropic lenses, commonly referred to as photograys, have gained wide attention. These lenses automatically change their light-absorbing power under lighting conditions. As a result, they protect the eyes of individuals who change environments by becoming lighter as the individual enters a dark environment and darker as he enters sunlight.

PLANNING FOR HEALTH MAINTENANCE AND RESTORATION

Instillation of eye drops

Measures that must be considered in planning for the care of clients with problems of the eye include proper instillation of medications and specific care of contact lens.

Before instilling any medications into the eye, the nurse should be aware of factors that are necessary for effects of the drug. Certain medications may cause systemic reactions if absorbed into the lacrimal duct. The nurse must therefore press the inner angle of the eye after instillation, to prevent systemic absorption. All equipment used for instillation should be sterile, and the medications should

FIG. 13-8
Method for instilling eye drops in eye. Client tilts head backward and looks upward. Nurse pulls lower lid downward and places drops in conjunctival sac. Note that nurse may rest finger on client's forehead to facilitate steadying the hand.

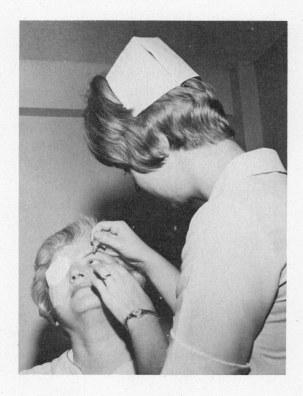

be instilled properly. The eye drop should be instilled in the lower conjunctival sac, and instructions should be given not to squeeze the eye or close the eyes tightly because this only serves to express the medications from the eye. If two drops are prescribed, the client should be permitted to blink before the second drop is instilled. To facilitate correct placement of the drops, the client should be instructed to look up at the ceiling or at some fixed object as the drop is placed into the pouch (Fig. 13-8) and then to look downward while the nurse slowly releases the skin of the eyelid. The procedure may be carried out with the client in a sitting or lying position. The nurse may steady the client's head to prevent the dropper from touching the eyelids or eye. If this happens, another sterile dropper must be obtained.

Instillation of ointments

Ointments are applied directly into the eye from the tube. A small amount of ointment is squeezed along the inside of the lower eyelid. The same principles discussed under eye drops apply for application of ointments. Warming the ointment tube in the hand a few minutes before application prevents the ointment from sliding along the lower lid.

The nurse must also direct efforts toward maintaining cleanliness. Handwashing before instilling medications or examining the eyes is an absolute necessity. Care must be maintained in using eye droppers. The dropper should not be touched with the hand or by the cornea or eyelashes. The eyelids should always be cleansed with a clean, damp cloth. The direction of cleansing should be from the inner canthus outward to prevent the spread of contaminants into the lacrimal duct.

COMMON OPHTHALMIC SYMBOLS

OD	Oculus dexter (right eye, RE)
OS	Oculus sinister (left eye, LE)
OU	Oculi uterque (both eyes)
EOM	Extraocular muscles
gtt(s)	Gutta, guttae (drop, drops)
IOP	Intraocular pressure

Often it is necessary for clients to continue ophthalmic medications at home; therefore, to facilitate continuity in care, ample instructions should be given regarding instillation techniques, the rationale for these, and the importance of maintaining asepsis. The nurse should be familiar with common ophthalmic symbols (see material on this page).

Glasses

Glasses may be worn almost at any age. Younger children, more so than older ones, tend to "like to wear glasses." Older children generally find it more difficult to accept them because of the belief that glasses change their appearance. If this is the case and if glasses are needed, the nurse, in addition to explaining the need, should suggest the use of attractive frames. Properly fitting glasses should be encouraged. Children should have glasses changed as recommended by the ophthalmologist to keep pace with growth changes and shifts in visual acuity.

Contact lenses

Two types of contact lenses are presently used: scleral and corneal.

Scleral contact lenses fit over the cornea and the conjunctiva covering the sclera. They are used in pathological conditions such as corneal ulcers or corneal burns and in cases where corneal lenses cannot be worn. These are less popular than corneal lenses.

Corneal contact lenses are tiny disks that are contoured to fit the anterior cornea. The lenses float freely on the tear film and are held to the cornea through capillary attraction. Because of the difficulty many people have in successfully adjusting to contact lenses and because of complications that can arise, they should be fitted only under the supervision of an ophthalmologist.

Contact lenses may be hard or soft, both of which have advantages and disadvantages. Soft, or hydrophilic, lenses are relatively new. They are malleable and easily conform to the shape of the cornea.

Nursing process for common health problems

When instructing clients about contact lenses, the nurse should stress the advantages as well as the disadvantages. The advantages include more than cosmetic effects. With hard or soft contact lenses there is no bother with dirty glasses or loose frames, and they can be worn during most athletic activities. Because of the softness of the edges of soft lenses, they are nonirritating to ocular tissue, more comfortable, and easy to adapt. As a result, even during the initial period, they can be tolerated for an extensive period of time. They are ideal for young children, older adults, and individuals who have had difficulty adjusting to hard lenses. Because soft lenses are hydrophilic, they tend to absorb chemicals; therefore, instructions are usually given for clients not to wear them while they swim unless goggles or a mask is used. Contact lenses can be better tolerated in occupations where misting of glasses makes vision difficult. Certain disorders (such as keratoconus, severe myopia, and hyperopia) can be treated with contact lenses. They also afford adequate vision after cataract surgery.

The disadvantages of contact lenses are many. They are expensive, and the wearer must receive considerable instruction in insertion and removal. With hard lenses, prolonged minor discomfort may be endured while the client is developing corneal tolerance. Occasionally corneal abrasions occur. Contact lenses are contraindicated in disease of the anterior segment, such as conjunctivitis, keratitis, iritis, and closed-angle glaucoma.

Individuals who wear contact lenses are carefully instructed in their insertion, removal, and care. Various methods have been recommended for insertion, removal, and storage. The client should be encouraged to follow the instruction given by the ophthalmologist. The importance of the client's remaining under the care of the ophthalmologist cannot be overemphasized.

The wetting solution used with contact lenses should be sterile. Some contact wearers have a tendency to use saliva as a wetting agent. Although effective, its use should be discouraged because saliva contains mineral salts and protein material that increases the risk of bacterial contamination.[10] Water, even distilled water, should not be used for cleaning because of the possible presence of chlorine, minerals, and bacterial contamination. In addition, water is hypotonic in relation to tear fluid; therefore, it may cause some discomfort.

Assessing for the presence of contact lenses. When individuals are admitted to health care facilities, particularly in emergency situations, the nurse should assess whether they are wearing contact lenses.

1. Ask the conscious individual if he wears contact lenses.
2. Check identification to determine whether or not mention is made of contact lenses.
3. Separate the eyelids and observe for their presence; shining a light over the eye may prove helpful.

If contact lenses are present:
1. Determine the type.
2. Assess the position of the lens.

Those individuals who are alert will likely be able to inform the nurse of the presence of contact lenses and may even remove them or help remove them. However, for those who are unconscious, it becomes the responsibility of the nurse to remove the lenses. Serious damage can occur if contact lenses remain on the eye for extended periods.

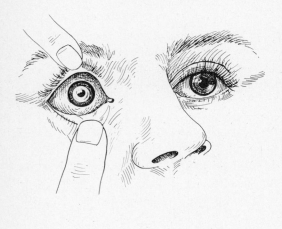

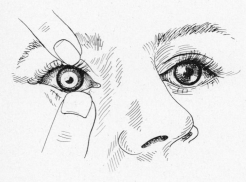

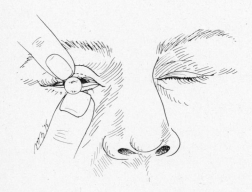

FIG. 13-9
Technique for removing contact lens from an individual's eye.

684

Methods for removal. Several methods have been suggested for removing contact lenses. One method involves the use of a suction tip. Once the lens position is determined, the tip should be placed over the lens and the lens lifted off the cornea. Another method involves the two-hand approach (Fig. 13-9). If the lens is not over the cornea, gently move the eyelid and slide the lens over the cornea. In using the two-hand method, the person removing the lens uses the thumbs of both hands.

1. The thumb of the right hand should be placed close to the edge of the upper lid, and the thumb of the left hand placed near the edge of the lower lid. (The thumb of the left hand and the forefinger of the right hand may also be used.) The lids should be held taut.
2. The lids are then gently but firmly pushed toward the contact lens. This maneuver breaks capillarity and facilitates removal of the lens. The lens should slide out between the lids. Once the lenses are removed, care should be taken to keep the right and left lens identified and appropriately marked when placed in a container.

Care of the client with variations in visual impairment

Normal visual acuity varies according to age. From established norms, varying degrees of impairment range from partial sight to blindness. The individual who is considered partially sighted may have a visual acuity ranging from 20/70 to 20/200. An individual with a visual acuity of 20/70 generally requires special services because of the impairment in vision. An individual whose vision is 20/200 or less in the better eye with corrective lenses is considered *legally blind*. Some individuals in this category can distinguish only light and darkness or varying shapes and patterns, and many of these people are eligible for tax deductions. An individual who has totally lost his ability to see is considered *blind*.

A partial loss of vision or total blindness may occur at any age. Some infants are born blind and thus have *congenital blindness*. Those individuals who lose their sight during infancy, childhood, adolescence, adulthood, or during the aging process are considered to have *acquired blindness*.

Improvements in preventive research and medical therapy have helped to decrease the incidence of blindness in the United States. Knowledge about the cause of *retrolental fibroplasia* has helped decrease the incidence of blindness in premature infants. Preventive measures taken at birth have decreased the incidence of *ophthalmia neonatorum*, which at one time was responsible for a large percentage of blindness in infancy. Accidents and trauma account for a large percentage of blindness in younger life, whereas the conditions of glaucoma or cataracts are responsible for increasing blindness in the older population.

Assessment of visual impairment. The nurse should be cognizant of normal visual development patterns so that comparative assessments can be made on any child whose development deviates from the normal pattern. A delay in certain developmental activities may elicit cues to visual impairment. For example, at *1 month* certain visual responses should have been acquired (see Chapter 2). Failure to acquire these should arouse concern, and the child should be referred to an ophthalmologist.

The nurse can observe the child's behavior and reactions to detect cues that indicate visual impairment. The *infant* or *young child* who tilts or twists the head while looking at or holding objects, frowns or squints when looking at distant objects, holds objects close to the eyes, rubs the eyes in an attempt to rub away a blur, stumbles over objects, is markedly sensitive to light, or is not aware of colors by age 4 should be referred to an ophthalmologist.

In addition to signs that are peculiar to young children, the *school-age child* may present cues that are related to schoolwork and games. He may hold a book at a peculiar distance from the face—either too far away or too close. He may not pay attention to reading or chalkboard activities, may show a general lack of interest, or may fail to participate in certain games and group activities. He may complain of dizziness or headache, itching, burning, or scratchy eyes after close work. Poor body alignment while doing written activities, shutting one eye when reading, or an unusual use of colors are cues that should alert the school nurse, teacher, or parents to the need for seeking health care.

Blindness

Reactions and adjustments to blindness. The age and onset at which an individual becomes blind may totally affect his adjustment. The person who is born blind cannot visualize or form visual concepts. Sighted language must be used if he is to form ideas about reality. All who deal with the congenitally blind should use descriptive, vivid terms to give a clear mental picture of objects. The person who acquires blindness after visual concepts have already been developed may not need the same type of mental picture painted.

Individuals who become blind during adolescence or early adulthood are faced with problems different from those of persons who acquire blindness during the aging process. The impairment may impose limitations in one's way of life. The adult may be the breadwinner for the family. Depending on his line of work, financial problems may arise. The family may be plagued with problems because the person so close to them can no longer see. They may have feelings of guilt and worry about the individual's welfare. Nurses must help the family understand blindness, the grief process, and how they can best work with him.

Suddenness of onset is another factor that may affect adjustment. An individual who loses his vision suddenly, as might result from a traumatic injury or accident, is faced with problems different from those of one whose vision is lost gradually. The latter individual has time to adjust to the loss and prepare for it. The family and close associates also have time to adjust to the loss.

Shortly after a person becomes blind, he and his family are likely to experience various reactions (such as shock or depression). These responses are healthy, natural, and necessary because they help the individual reorganize his body image and self-concept. Shock is the first stage experienced. This stage may last from a few days to weeks or months. It is characterized by an inability of the person to think or feel emotionally. The shorter the period, the sooner the individual adjusts to blindness. Following the stage of shock is the stage of depression. The individual may also go through a period of grieving in which he actually mourns for his eyes.

Health team members must help individuals, their families and their friends understand blindness and the importance of the grief process. They must be given ample time to work through their feelings. Opportunities should be provided for them to discuss their thoughts, fears, and inadequacies. Nurses must also understand their own feelings about blindness. This is essential for assisting the individual in rehabilitation.

Developmental considerations and the blind child. Physical maturation of the blind or partially sighted child differs very little from that of a sighted child. Motor development and neuromuscular coordination in the blind child will be noted at approximately the same age as in the sighted child. He will lift his head as if to view objects within the environment. Such behavior must be encouraged. Mothers should be encouraged to prop the child with pillows to facilitate this developmental pattern.

During the time when the child's quest for exploration dominates, he must be allowed to develop through exploring the environment. He should be permitted to crawl, wander, and climb at the same age at which he normally would crawl, wander, and climb. Some authorities contend it might even be beneficial to place fewer restrictions on the blind child, since he has to learn through the other sensory modalities of tasting, touching, smelling, and hearing. All children tend to explore the environment through "mouthing"; the blind child should be permitted to learn the same way.

Parents should be encouraged to play with the child. Playing games such as pat-a-cake encourages midline organization. When the child progresses to a walker, toys should be placed directly in front of him. In this way the child learns where to obtain a toy. As he moves about, more toys with different sounds and textures can be placed around him. This is one way of helping the child learn through hearing (differing sounds) and through touching (hard or soft objects).

The blind child has the same needs as the sighted child. He should be treated as normally as possible and helped to become as independent as possible. He has the need to feel independent at certain activities such as self-feeding. As the child learns to feed himself, frankfurters, crackers, and other finger foods should be offered to permit the child to become accustomed to self-feeding. When this is accomplished, the use of the spoon can be introduced with minimal assistance. Parents should be sensitive to indications of the child's readiness to carry out certain activities and allow him to do so, as they would the sighted child. Just as limits must be set for the sighted child, they must also be set for the blind child.

Education for individuals with visual impairment. Some form of education must be provided for persons with visual impairment. Various educational settings may be used. Children with subnormal vision may be educated in local public or private schools. In some communities public schools have special resource rooms within the educational facility. When this is the case, the child attends classes in which instruction is provided by a teacher with unique skills for educating the blind. Provisions are also made for special teaching aids. The child may also attend some classes with sighted children. Use of books with large print makes this approach possible. Group participation with children having normal vision affords an opportunity to prepare the children for future roles and responsibilities as citizens.

If such facilities are not available, the child may be educated in a residential school away from home. With this approach, the child lives and boards at school during the school year and spends vacations and the summer at home with the family. In some communities, the child is permitted to attend special schools for the blind during the day and spend the night at home. Fortunately, greater emphasis is being placed on educating the child within the community. The general feeling about this approach is that if the child is allowed to live at home and attend regular school, chances for isolation and dependency are reduced, which subsequently enhances the secure feeling of being a part of the family.

In instructing families about an educational setting, the nurse should encourage them to enroll the child in the kind of educational setting from which he can benefit most.

Once the child completes high school, he may attend college with the sighted. However, inasmuch as success in most colleges depends on the ability to see, the blind student may find it difficult to adjust. The federally supported Gallaudet College in Washington, D.C. is the only college for the blind in the United States. Students should be informed of this special resource.

The Pratt-Smoot Act authorizes the federal government to coordinate library services for the blind, both nationally and regionally. Resources such as Braille books, talking-book tapes, records of lectures, and other services are provided for the legally blind. Postal regulations enable Braille books to be sent free from the library for the blind.

The American Foundation for the Blind and The National Society for the Prevention of Blindness are the major national organizations that provide educational material on the problems of blindness and carry out research in the area.

Rehabilitation. Rehabilitation, which must be individualized, is an important element in education for persons with visual impairment. The goal must be to help each person lead as normal a life as possible. They must become independent in activities of daily living, employment, and community activities. Many special services are available.

Braille, a kind of code made up of raised pinpricks, is available for independent reading and writing (Fig. 13-10). It uses tactile sensitivity and at one time was the leading method for reading by the blind. However, recently a pen has been developed that enables blind clients to "see" words printed on a *flat* page. The pen emits a tiny laser beam that scans a fraction of a letter at a time. When the beam hits a white space, a reed on the side of the pen vibrates against the reader's finger. The vibrations stop when the beam hits black print. With the start-and-stop vibrations, the blind individual can trace each letter. One of the disadvantages is that only large print can be read. It is hoped that by the time these are commercially available, they will be refined and will be able to trace fine print and letters.

Aids for the blind. There are a number of aids on the market that enhance the client's ability to become independent.

Canes are useful instruments to assist the blind client in orientation and mobility. With a cane, the client can explore by touching objects within his immediate environment. Many types of canes are available commercially. The white cane has become a symbol for the blind.

The *seeing-eye dog,* or *guide dog,* permits the blind individual to travel and explore areas where he would otherwise be hesitant to venture by himself. The dog is a constant companion and is instrumental in enhancing the client's safety and security. With a dog, the client can become independent in travel and employment.

Other devices have been developed that enable the blind client to cope with everyday living. A Braille *watch* is available to help him keep abreast with time (Fig. 13-11). Available kitchen devices enable the homemaker to carry out household activities. Pressure cookers with Braille timers and controls, pie

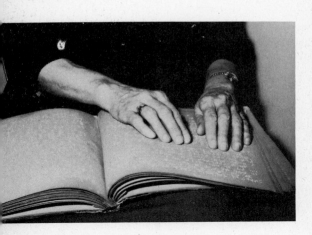

FIG. 13-10
Blind client reads Braille. (From Stein, Harold A., and Slatt, Bernard J.: The ophthalmic assistant, ed. 4, St. Louis, 1982, The C.V. Mosby Co.)

FIG. 13-11
Blind client can keep track of time with Braille watch. (From Stein, Harold A., and Slatt, Bernard J.: The ophthalmic assistant, ed. 4, St. Louis, 1982, The C.V. Mosby Co.)

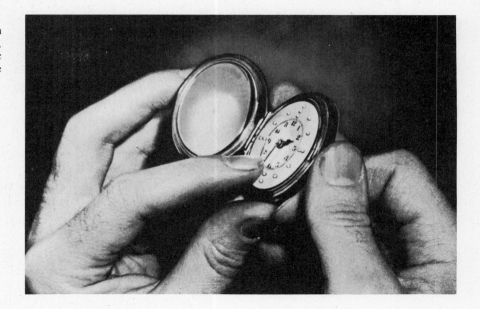

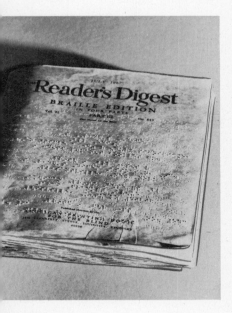

FIG. 13-12
Blind client can enjoy popular magazines in Braille. (From Stein, Harold A., and Slatt, Bernard J.: The ophthalmic assistant, ed. 4, St. Louis, 1982, The C.V. Mosby Co.)

cutters, automatic turners for pancakes, self-threading needles, and tape measures are available. The markings on the tape measure are elevated at the inch mark. Special telephones have been developed. Braille telephone directories, cookbooks, and special editions of magazines are also obtainable (Fig. 13-12).

Medical aids are also available to help the client maintain independence in the home. Braille thermometers with raised dots and insulin syringes with tactile markings that enable the client to draw up the desired amount of insulin are examples.

Recreation. Leisure time activities should also be a part of rehabilitation for the blind client. Special toys are available for children that enable them to engage in softball and other recreational activities. Special checkers and checkerboards, chess, Scrabble, and Braille cards can be purchased. They may also engage in arts and crafts. Films, plays, and lectures are great sources of stimulation. Fishing is an excellent outdoor sport. Young clients should be encouraged to engage in physical sports to relieve aggression and hostility. Engaging in sports with the sighted should also be encouraged.

Aids for the partially sighted. Books and newspapers are available in large print to enable the partially sighted client to cope with his condition as well as to continue contact with the outside world of pleasure and companionship. The type in these books is twice as large as the usual print, and the ink is much darker. These books are available in most libraries.

The hospitalized client with visual impairment. When the blind client is seen in the clinic, physician's office, or hospital, he should be oriented to his environment. He should be greeted warmly, introduced to the staff, addressed by name, and permitted to shake their hands. Such actions give the client information about the age, physical strength, and personality of the staff members. When orienting him, the nurse should encourage use of the tactile sense by allowing him to locate the call light, furniture, windows, bathrooms, nursing station, and other objects within the environment. He should be told the relationship of each object to his room. Efforts should be made to keep equipment

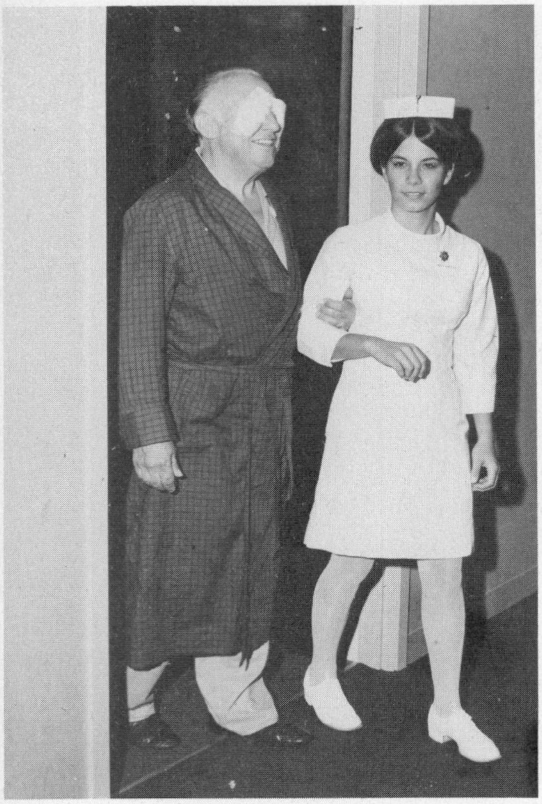

Nursing process for common health problems

FIG. 13-13
Client with bilateral eye patches should hold nurse's elbow as he ambulates.

in the same place. If furniture or personal belongings have to be moved, the client should be informed of the changes. He should also be oriented to the various sounds of the hospital environment.

When it is necessary to ambulate an older child or adult, the nurse should permit him to follow by resting his hand on the nurse's arm (Fig. 13-13). This approach places the client a step behind the person assisting him. As a result, it serves as a means of protection as each movement helps the client anticipate change in direction.

Another approach that has been suggested is the hand-shoulder method. The client stands behind the person and places the hands on the shoulder of the person who is guiding him. This approach affords an added sense of balance and security and is considered to be a safe method of maneuvering around objects.

The principles discussed in the following paragraphs are guidelines for all clients regardless of age.

As much as possible, the nurse should walk in a straight path. When deviations are necessary, the nurse must give a step-by-step account of the change. When the way leads up or down stairs, the nurse should pause for a brief period, inform the client, and then proceed. When guided properly, he can feel the movements as each step is made. If handrails are available, he ought to be encouraged to use them, because they provide added security. When helping him sit in a chair, the nurse should place his hand on the arm or back of the chair. Doors must never be left partially open. It is imperative that they always be completely opened or closed, to prevent the client from walking into the door's edge and injuring himself.

Nurses should address the client by name, always introduce themselves, and give the reason for being there when entering the room of a blind client. When the nurse leaves, the client should be informed. He might also be told the possible time when someone will return. It is necessary that all procedures be explained in advance. When they are actually performed, he should be given a step-by-step account of the procedure. Personnel should be encouraged to use terms that refer to sight (such as look or see) and should not hesitate to name a specific color when talking with these clients.

The blind client should be allowed to be as independent as possible in order to restore or maintain his sense of well-being and adequacy. The nurse must be helpful, but not too helpful. Assistance should be given when needed. It may be difficult to determine how much help to give, and when to stop. This must be decided on the basis of each client. It may be frustrating to watch the blind client eat—especially if he has problems picking food up with the fork—but health care personnel must not let the frustration overshadow the goal of helping him become independent.

When the nurse feeds the client, a clear description of the color, texture, and location of the food should be given. If he feeds himself, the nurse may find it very helpful to use the clock-hand position to help him determine where various foods are placed. "The meat is at 12 o'clock." He should specifically be told where hot foods are located. Consistency is very important. As much as possible specific foods should be in the same position at each meal. To prevent food from being scraped into the lap, divided plates or plates with ridges may be helpful, particularly for children. The continued use of the same kind of dinnerware may help eliminate confusion.

The nurse may find individually filled packets of sugar, salt, pepper, and other condiments useful in helping the client judge quantities. When helping the client fill a water glass, encourage him to place the tips of his fingers on the edge of the glass to prevent overrunning it. As much as possible, he should be allowed to explore and devise techniques for himself.

Ample time should be allowed for meals. The client should not have to rush through his meal. Soft music may help put him at ease. If the client is fed by the nurse or relative, he should not be fed too fast or too slowly. The entire time allotted for feeding should be devoted to the client, with conversation carried on as is normally done during mealtime. In this and all other activities, individuals caring for the blind must show patience, acceptance, and understanding.

As much as possible, hospitalized clients and clients at home should be encouraged to engage in recreational and leisure time activities. Items such as talking books (that is, book and magazine recordings) are available for all age groups in public libraries. A favorite radio program may also be an excellent source of diversion. They should be included in conversations and visited frequently to help decrease boredom and loneliness. Planned activities, whether at home or in the hospital, should take into consideration the client's likes, age, and abilities.

Implementation

COMMON HEALTH PROBLEMS OF THE NEONATE

Retrolental fibroplasia

Retrolental fibroplasia (RLF) is a bilateral retinal disease of premature infants. It occurs in infants who receive excessive concentrations of oxygen (greater than 40%) for even short periods of time.

Pathophysiology. In premature infants, retinal vascularization is incomplete, but under normal conditions, it develops by proliferation of the vessels. However, excessive oxygen concentrations cause the retinal vessels to constrict, and if the high oxygen concentration continues for 48 to 72 hours, the vessels become badly damaged and may undergo several changes, which may range from spasms to edema of the retina, dilation of the vessels, retinal hemorrhage, and proliferation to detachment of the retina. If the disease is arrested during an early stage, vision may be saved. Beyond this, severe visual impairment or blindness may result.

 Assessment. Retrolental fibroplasia usually occurs during the first few days of life and progresses to blindness over a period of weeks. Restoration of sight is impossible once blindness occurs. However, reports have been made of regression occuring in either one or both eyes.[5]

Data analysis
Data analysis may reveal family members who are disturbed about the established diagnosis. Nursing diagnoses of fear, grieving, and sensory perception alteration may be established.

 Planning and implementation. The incidence of RLF has decreased with improved methods and control in oxygen administration. Some recommendations that have been made in regard to oxygen administration include that (1) a prescription for oxygen be specific in regard to the duration and concentration,

(2) the prescribed concentration be the minimal amount needed to maintain adequate blood oxygen tension,[1] and (3) the oxygen administration be controlled by analysis of blood gases. Nurses who work in nurseries should therefore constantly observe infants who receive oxygen therapy for signs indicative of oxygen need and for signs that indicate improvement. When improvements are noted, the physician should be notified so that a decision can be made about the administration of oxygen.

 Evaluation. The nursing care plan for the infant with retrolental fibroplasia is developed around diagnoses such as fear, grieving, and sensory perception alteration.

EXPECTED OUTCOMES:

The family can:
1. Describe retrolental fibroplasia.
2. State plans for health maintenance.
3. Verbalize plans for follow-up health care and use of community resources.
4. Verbalize feelings about retrolental fibroplasia.

Conjunctivitis of the newborn   In the neonate conjunctivitis, an inflammation of the conjunctiva, may be caused by chemicals, bacteria or viruses.

Pathophysiology. The symptoms commonly associated with conjunctivitis are redness, swelling of the eyelids, and lacrimation. These symptoms can be directly related to the structure of the conjunctiva. For example, the conjunctiva is loose, contains numerous blood vessels, lymphoid tissue, and mucus-secreting glands. As a result, when the blood vessels become congested, the conjunctiva takes on a reddened appearance, hence the common name, pink-eye.

Chemical conjunctivitis is caused by the instillation of silver nitrate into the conjunctival sac of the newborn at birth. The eyes become inflamed shortly after the drops are instilled, and the inflammation becomes greatest during the first and second day, and clears up shortly thereafter without treatment.

Ophthalmia neonatorum (neonatal gonococcal conjunctivitis) is one type of bacterial conjunctivitis, which is contracted as the baby passes through the birth canal of the mother infected with the gonococcus organism *(Neisseria gonorrhoeae).*

 Assessment. Signs of inflammation (redness, edema of the eyelids, and exudation) usually occur within 24 to 48 hours after birth. The exudate is at first serous and then purulent. Bacterial cultures and smears of the secretions are obtained to confirm the diagnosis. Corneal damage may result.

> **Data analysis**
> *Data analysis may reveal nursing diagnoses of fear and sensory perception alteration.*

 Planning and implementation. Therapy is planned to control infection. Antibacterial agents such as bacitracin, tetracycline, and neomycin may be instilled into the eye, even before the results of the culture.

Planning for prevention. Prophylactic measures, required by law in all states, are carried out shortly after birth to prevent the occurrence of ophthalmia neonatorum. A commonly employed method is the Credé method. If this method is used, one drop of 1% silver nitrate is instilled in the conjunctiva of each eye immediately after delivery. Some institutions repeat this within 2 or 3 hours after the infant has been bathed and dressed. A more recent measure is to introduce an antibiotic such as penicillin into the eye of the infant. Some arguments against the use of antibiotics are that (1) they are not germicidal and must therefore be instilled several times a day for approximately a week and (2) many strains of gonococci are resistant to a number of antibiotics.

 Evaluation. The nursing care plan for the infant with ophthalmia neonatorum is developed around diagnoses such as sensory perception alteration and fear.

EXPECTED OUTCOMES
The family can:
1. Describe conjunctivitis.
2. State plans for health maintenance and care.
3. Demonstrate proper technique for administration of prescribed therapy and medications.
4. Verbalize plans for follow-up health care and use of community resources.

COMMON HEALTH PROBLEMS OF THE INFANT AND CHILD

Congenital cataracts

Congenital cataracts are genetically determined,[5] or they occur as a result of congenital malformation of the lens. The malformation may result from maternal rubella occurring during the first trimester of pregnancy. They may also result from injury or an inflammatory disease. They are generally bilateral. Infants and children with congenital cataracts usually have white pupils, and are usually observed not to see well during their early life. Surgery (lens extraction) is performed around 6 months of age to permit normal visual development.

Strabismus

Strabismus (squint, crossed eyes) refers to an imbalance of the extraocular muscles. As a result, the eyes deviate rather than function as a unit. Strabismus may occur as a result of eye disease or a central nervous system disease.

Pathophysiology. Two types of strabismus have been identified: *nonparalytic* (comitant) and *paralytic* (noncomitant). The term comitant refers to equal deviation on all directions of gaze; noncomitant means variation of the deviation in different directions of the gaze. In nonparalytic strabismus, there is no muscle weakness, whereas in paralytic strabismus, the misalignment of the visual axis is the result of weakness, paralysis, or restriction of one or more of the ocular muscles.[4]

 Assessment. Diplopia is a characteristic symptom. A deviation in the position of the eye can be readily observed. For example, the eyes may deviate in varied directions: inward deviation (toward the nose) is *esotropia,* or convergent strabismus; outward deviation is *exotropia,* or divergent strabismus; upward is *hypertropia;* and downward is *hypotropia.* Terms using the suffix *phoria* are also used to describe the deviation. *Esophoria* refers to medial deviation; *exophoria* to lateral deviation; and *hyperphoria* to upward deviation.

Data analysis
Data analysis may reveal nursing diagnoses of sensory perception alteration and fear.

Nursing process for common health problems

Planning and implementation. The nurse should instruct families about the importance of early detection. Instructions should specifically include information about possible behavior of a child with strabismus, as well as the potential harmful effect of strabismus. The child who tilts his head in order to focus or who has difficulty in coordination (peers at objects with one eye closed) should be suspected of having strabismus. Families sometimes take the "wait and see" attitude, thinking that the child will outgrow the defect. Because infections and central nervous system disturbances may be responsible for the strabismus and because psychological and physiological manifestations (such as monocular blindness) may result, parents should be encouraged to seek health care when the signs and symptoms are first noted. Constant *suppression* or nonuse of the deviating eye will also lead to a condition known as suppression amblyopia (lazy eye), which may result in monocular blindness. This is another reason that early medical attention should be encouraged.

Therapy for strabismus varies according to the degree of deviation. The *objectives of therapy* are to develop visual acuity in both eyes, to straighten the eyes, and to develop coordinate function of the eyes.[5] These objectives may be accomplished with the use of nonsurgical therapy, including occlusion, properly fitted glasses, orthoptic exercises, and surgery. Nonsurgical therapy is usually started by the age of 6.[1,4]

Improving visual acuity. The occlusion method involves covering the unaffected eye in an effort to improve visual acuity in the squinting eye. The child may wear the patch for weeks or even months. It should completely cover the eye and be kept on during waking hours, and the child should be instructed not to take the patch off.

Straightening the eyes. Corrective glasses may be worn at any age. They are prescribed to improve visual acuity, to straighten the eyes, and to help the eyes see as a unit. Glasses may also be combined with other forms of therapy.

Coordinating function. The use of orthoptic exercises as a form of treatment requires that the child be mature enough to understand; therefore exercises are generally started around school age. They consist of a series of muscle exercises that are designed to strengthen fusion so that the eyes will move together as a unit rather than deviate. These exercises are adjuncts to other forms of therapy.

When these measures fail, surgery may be performed to weaken or strengthen the recti muscles in order to improve alignment of the eyes. A number of surgical procedures may be performed. These include recession, resection, myotomy, and tenotomy. A *recession* involves removing a muscle from its insertion and placing it farther back on the sclera. *Resection* involves removing the muscle and reattaching it to its original position. This results in shortening of the muscle, whereas recession results in lengthening of the muscle. A *myotomy* involves making overlapping cuts on each side of the muscle to lengthen it. With a *tenotomy,* the muscle is severed and permitted to retract.

Preoperative care. Parents should be given instructions as to what to expect in the postoperative period. The eyes are covered for 24 hours after surgery. It will be helpful to consult the child or parents about some strategies for diversion during this period. They should also be given instructions as to expectations. For example the child's eye will appear red for a few days postoperatively, then the redness will gradually decrease. The parents and the child should be made aware that this is an expected phenomenon.

694

Postoperative care. Limitations placed on the child postoperatively will depend on the preference of the physician. Usually the eyes are covered for 24 hours, and the child can resume normal activities (such as school activities) within a couple of days. Contact sports are likely not to be permitted for a couple of weeks. Parents should be instructed about these guidelines and given instructions as to expectations.

Information should be provided about symptoms that should be reported to the physician (increased pain, drainage) and about community resources that may be useful.

 Evaluation. The child with strabismus may experience alterations in sensory function and fear; therefore the plan must be continually evaluated on *an ongoing basis* to facilitate maintenance of sensory function.

EXPECTED OUTCOMES

The child and/or family can:
1. Describe strabismus.
2. Describe plans for maintaining sensory function.
3. State indications of health problems requiring health care.
4. State plans for follow-up health care.
5. State resources for continuity of care.

Retinoblastoma

Retinoblastoma is a malignant intraocular tumor of the retina that commonly occurs during childhood. It occurs most commonly in the first 5 years of life, usually before the end of 3 years and rarely occurs during later stages of development. Retinoblastoma is hereditary, and results from mutation of an autosomal dominant gene.

Pathophysiology. The tumor originates in the retina, tends to grow rapidly, and is spread by way of the optic nerve choroidal blood vessels and orbital lymphatics.[4]

 Assessment. Signs of the tumor may appear as discoloration of the pupils (whitish glow, or cat's eye reflex), which is usually the first indication; strabismus, red, painful eye accompanied by glaucoma, and retinal detachment. The diagnosis is made by ophthalmoscopic examination. If the iris or anterior chamber is involved, aspiration and examination of the tumor cells may help confirm the diagnosis.

Data analysis

Data analysis may reveal nursing diagnoses of sensory perception alteration, fear, and alterations in comfort.

Planning and implementation. Therapy for retinoblastoma varies according to the extent of involvement. If both eyes are affected, the eye with the greater involvement is enucleated. The other is treated by means of radiation therapy combined with chemotherapy, but later the eye may be enucleated. Local irradiation (which has been most successful), diathermy, photocoagulation, and cryotherapy, are other forms of therapy.

Photocoagulation is a technique whereby a laser beam is directed through the transparent part of the eye onto the tumor. Because of the intensity of the light, the tumor is burned as a piece of paper would be by sunlight focused

695

through a magnifying glass. This is considered a useful form of therapy when less than one-third of the retina is involved.[9] Parents who have one child with the tumor should receive genetic counseling.

 Evaluation. Evaluation of the care plan for a child who has retinoblastoma must be ongoing.

EXPECTED OUTCOMES

The child (depending on age) and/or family can:
1. Describe plans for maintaining sensory function.
2. State indications of health problems requiring health care.
3. State plans for follow-up health care.
4. Describe community resources that may be used for continuity of care.

Blepharitis

Blepharitis is a bilateral inflammation of the lid margins. It generally starts in childhood, continues through life, and is characterized by remissions and exacerbations.

 Assessment. During exacerbations the lid margins are inflamed and covered with crusts and scales. During remission these symptoms disappear, except that the lids remain hyperemic. There are two main types: staphylococcal and seborrheic. In the staphylococcal type, the scales are dry, ulcerations appear along the lid margins, and the area is hyperemic. In the seborrheic type, the scales are greasy in appearance and the area is less red.

> **Data analysis**
> *Data analysis may reveal nursing diagnoses of sensory perception alterations and alterations in comfort.*

 Planning and implementation. The use of wet compresses three to four times a day softens the crust and scales and enables removal. For staphylococcal blepharitis, antibiotic ointments are applied to the lid margins to control infection. In the seborrheic type, therapy is directed toward controlling this condition, for example, maintaining cleanliness by washing the area with soap and water. In addition to compresses as mentioned above, applicators may be used to facilitate removal of the scales.

COMMON HEALTH PROBLEMS OF THE ADULT

Retinal detachment

Retinal detachment is a condition in which the retina (rods-and-cones layer) becomes separated from the choroid (pigmented layer). It commonly occurs in elderly individuals; however, it may occur at any age. Its occurrence in children is more likely to result from trauma. The client who has a family history of retinal detachment or other ocular diseases is also more prone than most individuals.

Pathophysiology. The retina is firmly attached only at the optic nerve and ora serrata. It is loosely attached at the choroid. Therefore, when a tear occurs, fluids can seep through the retina and elevate it away from the choroid. The separation may be precipitated by trauma or degenerative conditions of the retina.

 Assessment. The onset of retinal detachment may be sudden or gradual. The appearance of floating spots before the eyes is a characteristic symptom. These spots are caused by the accumulation of red blood cells in the vitreous at the time of the retinal tear. Blurred or smoky vision, often described as the sensation of a veil covering the eye, is another symptom. Diagnosis is usually made through visualization with an indirect ophthalmoscope. Vision is seriously compromised if therapy is delayed.

Data analysis
Data analysis may reveal nursing diagnoses of sensory perception alteration, fear, and alterations in comfort.

Planning and implementation. Therapy is directed toward reattaching the retina, which is accomplished by nonsurgical methods or surgery.

Nonsurgical methods. Photocoagulation and cryotherapy are nonsurgical methods employed to seal retinal breaks before the retina becomes detached. With *photocoagulation,* a small burn is made in the retina by shining a very bright light through the pupil. With *cryotherapy,* a cold probe is applied to the outer wall of the eye to "freeze" the retina. The former is used to treat breaks located in the front half of the eye, and the latter is useful in treated breaks at the posterior half of the eye.

Surgical methods. Surgical therapy for retinal detachment is aimed at sealing the retinal break, reattaching the retina, and preventing the retina from redetaching. One surgical approach commonly employed is *scleral buckling.* Fluid that has accumulated under the retina is released, and the wall of the eye is buckled (that is, indented) to facilitate contact with the detached retina. A small piece of silicone rubber is embedded in the sclera at points where the break occurs, and a high and permanent ridge is created to ensure sealing of the retinal break. A small silicone belt may be placed around the implanted silicone to permanently maintain the indentation and thus prevent traction that may be the result of stretched vitreous bands and membranes.

Advanced cases of retinal detachment are treated with *intravitreal surgery.* With this method the vitreous is replaced with saline, air, donor vitreous, spinal fluid, blood serum, or liquid silicone. As a result, the vitreous volume is increased, which facilitates the replacement of the separated retina into position. If liquid silicone is used, it occupies the vitreous cavity permanently.

Preoperative nursing care. Before surgery the client is placed on bed rest, and the eyes are covered to prevent ocular movement, thus facilitating transitory settling of the detached retina. The client may be positioned so that the area of the detachment is dependent. The rationale for this dependent position is that it permits the vitreous to act as a tamponade. With the area of the tear uppermost, the rationale is to permit the retina to settle against the choroid by force of gravity. Usually the pupils are dilated by a mydriatic such as phenylephrine (Neo-Synephrine). A cycloplegic such as cyclopentolate (Cyclogyl) is used to facilitate visualization of the retina and to decrease movement of the intraocular structures.

Although most retinal tears are tiny, occasionally the break may be extensive. With extensive tears, a specially designed table, which uses the force of gravity, is used to unfold the torn retina. When this table is used, the client is securely anchored, and the table is tilted in multiple positions as the physician determines the position that will most likely unfold the tear. Once the determination is made, surgery is performed to reattach the retina.

A consequence of large retinal tears is the formation of adhesions by scar

697

Nursing process for common health problems

tissue. In such instances, a small intraocular balloon is placed under the overlapping retina and is inflated to break through the adhesions and thus unfold the retina.

Postoperative nursing care. Nursing care in the postoperative period is directed toward minimizing movement in the eyes and head, thus preventing an increase in venous pressure about the head. Because of restrictions in activities, the client is dependent on the nurse to meet his hygienic needs. He must be logrolled (see Chapter 10) and his position changed frequently to prevent skin breakdown. Principles of care that apply to the care of a bedridden client also apply to these clients.

Discharge instructions. The client must be instructed to avoid strenuous exercise and activity for at least 6 months. Contact sports are restricted for the remainder of the client's life. The client should also avoid sudden jarring and motions of the head. Movements of the eyes do not precipitate recurrence, and therefore no restrictions are placed on the use of the eyes.

 Evaluation. Evaluation of the care plan for a client with retinal detachment must be ongoing.

EXPECTED OUTCOMES

The client and/or family can:
1. Describe retinal detachment, including signs indicative of further development of the problem.
2. State indications of problems requiring health care.
3. State plans for follow-up care.
4. Verbalize the limitations placed on activity.
5. Describe community resources that may be used for continuity of care.

FIG. 13-14
Comparison of the normal angle of the eye with closed-angle glaucoma.

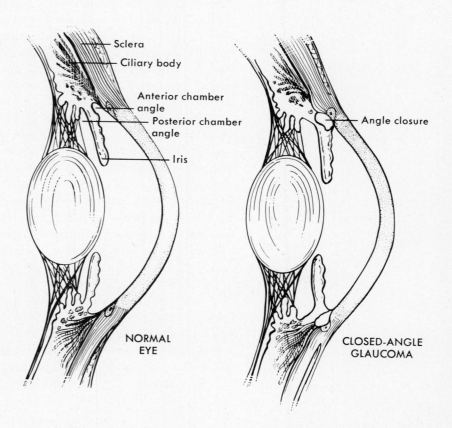

Glaucoma

Glaucoma is a disease characterized by an increase in intraocular pressure (it may increase as much as 4 to 5 times the normal pressure). The pressure increases because of a disturbance in the circulation of the aqueous fluid. Aqueous humor, a fluid secreted by the epithelium of the ciliary processes, passes into the posterior chamber through the pupil into the anterior chamber. As the fluid flows into the anterior chamber, it reaches the surface toward the trabecular meshwork and flows into Schlemm's canal, ultimately entering the venous system through the aqueous veins. Normally the amount of fluid that enters the eye is balanced by the amount that leaves, maintaining a normal level of 14 to 20 mm Hg. A disturbance in the circulation of aqueous fluid through Schlemm's canal results in an increase in intraocular pressure. Such a pressure increase characterizes glaucoma.

Two types of glaucoma that commonly occur are *open-angle glaucoma* and *closed-angle glaucoma* (Fig. 13-14). These angles, opened or closed, are used in reference to the angle of the anterior chamber where the cornea and iris meet.

Open-angle glaucoma. Open-angle glaucoma (also referred to as chronic, simple, or wide-angle glaucoma) is most common, occuring in 90% to 95% of those individuals with glaucoma. It is hereditary and affects the older age group. It is a major cause of blindness.

Pathophysiology. Degenerative changes occur in the aqueous drainage channels (trabeculum, Schlemm's canal, and surrounding structures). As a result of the degenerative changes, an obstruction occurs to the outflow of aqueous fluid.

 Assessment. Open-angle glaucoma is thought to be more dangerous than closed-angle glaucoma because of its gradual, painless onset. The increase in pressure occurs over a period of years. Peripheral vision is progressively lost without the client's being aware of it because central visual acuity is normal (Fig. 13-15). Because pain and headache are absent, the optic nerve may be seriously affected before glaucoma is detected.

> ***Data analysis***
> *Data analysis may reveal nursing diagnoses of sensory perception alteration, alterations in comfort, and fear.*

 Planning and implementation. Therapy for open-angle glaucoma is directed toward reducing the intraocular pressure. This may be accomplished by

FIG. 13-15
Glaucoma results in loss of peripheral vision.

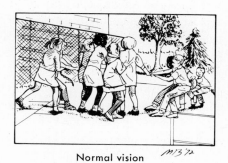
Normal vision

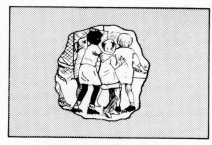
Advanced glaucoma

increasing the outflow or by decreasing the rate of aqueous secretion. Drugs used to reduce intraocular pressure include carbonic anhydrase inhibitors such as acetazolamide (Diamox), which act by blocking the secretion of sodium, thereby reducing the rate of formation of aqueous fluid by the ciliary processes. Other drugs used include *parasympathomimetics* (such as pilocarpine, usually in concentrations ranging from 1% to 4%), which facilitate aqueous outflow; *sympathomimetics* (such as epinephrine), which decrease secretions of aqueous and facilitate outflow; and recently beta-adrenergic blockers have been employed.

Many clients with glaucoma are at one time or another admitted to the hospital for problems other than glaucoma. If the client states that he uses eye drops, the nurse should determine the type and obtain the necessary order for the medication. Often clients are permitted to use their own drops rather than obtain a new prescription. The nurse should also permit the client to follow his home routine of administration rather than conform to the routine of the hospital.

Client instruction. The nurse has an important responsibility in educating the client about the nature of glaucoma and its therapy. Often if the client and family understand the disease, they will follow the prescribed therapeutic plan. The client and his family must understand the need for lifetime therapy. Certain limitations are not necessary, provided the client practices moderation. For example, he may drink a normal amount of coffee or tea (one or two cups) and alcoholic beverages, but not excessive quantities. The major problem caused by drinking excessive alcoholic beverages is that if the client becomes intoxicated, he will be unable to follow his prescribed therapy.

Since miotic therapy is an important means of intervention, the nurse should teach the client and family the correct way of instilling eye drops. Before discharge, the nurse must be sure that he understands when and how to instill eye drops. Intraocular pressure is usually higher on arising in the morning; therefore drops are usually prescribed for early morning. They are also prescribed for intervals during the day and at bedtime.

The use of miotics poses several problems. Side effects can occur from their use. The client should therefore be informed about possible side effects and encouraged to consult his physician if they occur. Since mydriasis (pupillary dilation) does not occur, the client may have difficulty in seeing in dark places. Providing extra lighting usually proves helpful. The client should be encouraged to be extremely cautious when driving at night and when climbing stairs. Leisure time activities such as reading and games should be done at intervals rather than for long periods of time, because accommodation is lost.

No restrictions should be placed on visitation to theaters or other darkened areas. However, some authorities suggest instilling drops into the eyes before such activity, particularly if the time for the medication comes while the client engages in leisure time activities. Some also encourage that drops be instilled if the client is awakened in the middle of the night when the light is out and if he has difficulty going to sleep.

When therapy with drugs fails, surgery may be performed to maintain the intraocular pressure within normal limits. Surgery is also recommended when there is progressive loss of the visual field because of optic nerve drainage.[5]

Several filtering procedures may be performed to improve aqueous outflow. These include the trephine procedure, sclerectomy, trabeculectomy, and the

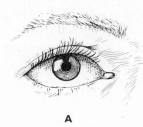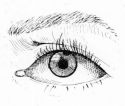

A   **B**

trephine operation in conjunction with an iridectomy. A small opening is made through the corneoscleral junction, thus facilitating drainage of aqueous fluid from the anterior chamber into the space between the conjunctiva and Tenon's capsule. A complete or peripheral iridectomy (Fig. 13-16) is usually performed by bringing the iris through the small opening. The conjunctival sac is sutured in place. Aqueous fluid thereafter leaks through the small opening into the subconjunctival space where some is absorbed into the lymphatic channels.

Iridencleisis, another filtering procedure, may also be performed. It involves making an incision at the corneoscleral junction into the anterior chamber. A segment of the iris is permitted to fall back in the eye, and the other segment is incarcerated into the incision to act as a wick, thus permitting a permanent drainage system into the subconjunctival space.

Other filtering procedures include sclerectomy and cyclodialysis. *Sclerectomy* is the removal of a small portion of the sclera at the superior junction of the cornea and sclera. This procedure also provides a permanent drainage channel for aqueous fluid from the anterior chamber to an area beneath the conjunctiva. *Cyclodialysis* is the creation of an opening between the anterior chamber and suprachoroidal space.

Microsurgical techniques that are frequently used are *trabeculectomy* and *trabeculotomy.*[1] A trabeculectomy involves the excision of a rectangle of the sclera that includes the trabeculum, Schlemm's canal, and scleral spur. In addition, a peripheral iridectomy is performed, a scleral flap is created, and the conjunctiva is sutured over it. A trabeculotomy involves the insertion of a small probe into the canal. This results in the exposure of Schlemm's canal directly to the anterior chamber.[5] The end result is that it relieves any block to the aqueous outflow.

A peripheral iridectomy, removal of a portion of the iris at the surface, may be performed to create an opening between the anterior and posterior chambers. Subsequently, it relieves pupillary block and permits the root of the iris to fall away from the filtration angle, thus establishing the outflow for aqueous fluid by normal channels.

A nonsurgical procedure sometimes employed is cyclocryosurgery. A cryoprobe is applied to the conjunctiva, thus destroying the ciliary body. The end result of this procedure is a reduction in aqueous production because of decreased functioning of the ciliary body.

Primary closed-angle glaucoma. Closed-angle glaucoma (narrow-angle or acute congestive glaucoma) occurs less frequently than open-angle glaucoma.

Pathophysiology. It is characterized by a sudden rise in intraocular pressure because of a blockage of the angle of the anterior chamber by the root of the iris, which blocks off aqueous outflow. (The aqueous drainage channels are normal.)

Nursing process for common health problems

Factors that may predispose to closed-angle glaucoma include (1) hypermetropia (because of a narrow anterior chamber), (2) pupillary block, and (3) mydriasis (which causes an increased thickness of the iris). With pupillary block, adhesions form between the lens and the iris, thus obstructing the normal pathway of aqueous humor from the posterior chamber to the anterior chamber. Emotional stress (anger and fright) may precipitate an attack of acute glaucoma, which may be related to mydriasis because in "fight or flight" the pupils dilate.

 Assessment. Pain, which is severe and occurs suddenly, is at first localized in the eye but later radiates to any part of the head, even down toward the teeth. Often such pain is confused with dental pain. The pain may also be accompanied by nausea and vomiting, which is thought to be caused by an oculovagal reflex.[5] Corneal edema may be present and may result in blurred vision. As the pressure builds, fluid is forced into the cornea and collects in tiny droplets, and the client experiences an impression of halos or rainbows around lights. The redness that is often observed is caused by passive venous congestion secondary to increased intraocular pressure.

Data analysis
Data analysis may reveal problems with vision and pain. Therefore nursing diagnoses of sensory perception alteration, pain, and fear may be established.

 Planning and implementation. Therapy is directed toward decreasing the intraocular pressure and relieving pain and nausea. When the client is seen in a health care facility, miotic therapy, and osmotic agents are started promptly. Pilocarpine (2% or 4%) may be instilled in the eyes at frequent intervals, such as a 5- to 10-minute intervals for a few hours. It decreases the intraocular pressure by pulling the iris away from the chamber angle, thus resulting in free drainage of fluid.

The commonly used osmotic agent, glycerin (Glyrol) is administered in a cold 50% solution mixed with chilled lemon juice. This hypertonic solution draws fluid from the eye, and subsequently reduces the pressure. There have also been reports of intravenous mannitol being used when glycerin is not successful.[3] Acetazolamide (Diamox) may be administered to lower intraocular pressure. Systemic analgesics such as meperidine (Demerol) or morphine produce miosis and decrease intraocular pressure and may therefore be administered to relieve pain. If the emergency treatment is successful, surgery may be delayed for a couple of days until the eye is less inflamed.

Once intraocular pressure is reduced, surgery (such as a peripheral iridectomy) may be performed. This may be performed surgically or with the use of ruby or argon laser. An iridectomy consists of removal of a portion of the iris. The opening that is created provides a channel through which aqueous fluid can escape from the posterior into the anterior chamber. The response to surgery is usually good. Postoperative care is the same as for other forms of intraocular surgery.

Planning for prevention. Because the end result of glaucoma could be blindness, the importance of early detection and early health intervention cannot be overemphasized. The National Society for the Prevention of Blindness has established the following six danger signals of glaucoma:

1. Frequent changes in glasses, none of which is satisfactory
2. Blurred or foggy vision that clears up for a while
3. Loss of peripheral vision
4. Rainbow-colored rings around lights
5. Difficulty in adjusting to dark rooms such as movie theaters
6. Difficulty in focusing on close work

Clients with any of these symptoms should be encouraged to consult a physician, and all persons over 35 years of age should have a complete eye examination every 2 years, including tonometry.

Evaluation. The nursing plan for a client with glaucoma is evaluated on an ongoing basis.

EXPECTED OUTCOMES

The client and/or family can:
1. Describe glaucoma.
2. Describe the anticipated effects of therapy, including medications and surgery.
3. Describe plans for health maintenance.
4. State the needs for lifetime use of ocular medications.
5. State use, dosage, time, route, frequency, and side effects of prescribed ocular medications.
6. Describe preventive strategies, including keeping extra bottle of eye drops and carrying some form of identification.
7. Verbalize fears and concerns.
8. State plans for follow-up health care and use of community resources.
9. State signs indicative of need for emergency care.

Cataracts   A cataract is opacification or clouding of the lens of the eye. Opacity may be the result of anything that causes physical or chemical changes in the lens protein and may vary from a few small spots to an area involving much of the lens. The protein content of the lens is higher than any other tissue. A normal balance between the soluble and insoluble (such as albuminoid) proteins is an important factor in determining lens transparency. The protein molecules of the lens are strategically arranged so that a transparent mass is formed. However, in the presence of an instability in the eye, a cataract may form. As fluid accumulates between the fibers, degeneration and disintegration of the fibers occur and subsequently block the passage of light rays to the retina, resulting in visual impairment (Fig. 13-17). *Senile cataracts* occur in the older age group as a result of the aging process.

FIG. 13-17
Light rays pass lens and focus on retina (left). Clouded lens from cataracts block light rays and prevents them from reaching retina (right). (Reproduced by permission of the National Society for the Prevention of Blindness, Inc., New York.)

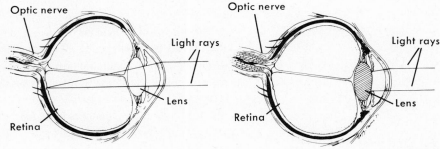

Pathophysiology. With age, fibers of the lens become more dense and change in color. The amount of insoluble protein increases relative to soluble protein, and a reduction is noted in the synthesizing proteins. As a result, opacification begins.

 Assessment. The most common symptoms of senile cataracts are diminished visual acuity, blurred vision, and diplopia. These clients may give a history of frequent changes in eyeglasses, or they may complain of having to hold objects or reading materials close to their eyes in order to see them. Other complaints may be seeing spots before the eyes and foggy vision. The course of the disease varies. Vision may be severely impaired, and blindness may eventually occur unless treatment is obtained.

> **Data analysis**
> *Data analysis may reveal nursing diagnoses of sensory perception alterations, potential for injury, and alteration in self-concept.*

 Planning and implementation. To date there is no known local or medical therapy that can stop the progress of senile cataracts. The only known effective treatment is surgery. The objective of surgery is to restore visual acuity. Surgery is indicated whenever the reduction of vision interferes with the client's normal activities.

Surgical procedures. The methods used to extract the lens are the intracapsular and extracapsular methods.

Intracapsular method. The intracapsular method makes it possible to remove the cataract before it becomes mature. This method involves removing the whole lens intact in its capsule. Before this method was developed, it was necessary to wait until the lens became completely opaque, or "ripe," for easy removal. Presently the intracapsular method is the operation of choice.

Enzymatic zonulolysis is a technique that involves injecting alpha chymotrypsin, a fibrinolytic and proteolytic enzyme, into the anterior chamber angle. This enzyme frees the attachment of the zonules to the lens capsule and thereby facilitates removal of the lens without tearing the lens in the process of removing it. The method is generally used for individuals between the second and fifth decades. It is not used for clients under 20 because, up to this age, the lens is attached to the vitreous; therefore use of this method, according to authorities, leads to loss of vitreous and could possibly destroy the eye.[5] The aspiration and irrigation technique is considered beneficial in clients under 30 because the cataracts are softer and subsequently more easily liquified. Before intracapsular surgery is performed, osmotic agents may be prescribed to reduce intraocular pressure.

Extracapsular method. The extracapsular extraction consists of cutting through the anterior capsule of the lens and expressing the opaque lens material. A newer extracapsular method for removing cataracts is *phacoemulsification*. This technique combines ultrasonic vibrations to emulsify the lens with the use of a tiny suction tip and irrigating fluid to aspirate and wash out the lens fragments through a small incision made at the corneal scleral junction. Convalescence and visual rehabilitation are considerably shortened. Usually the client can be ambulatory after he completely recovers from anesthesia, and contact lenses are generally prescribed 3 weeks after surgery.

Preoperative nursing care. Preoperative instruction should include the fact that vision will be poor in the early postoperative period. The client must also be informed about the adjustments that must be made in the use of glasses.[2] He must relearn to judge space in varied daily activities, such as walking, driving, climbing stairs, crossing the street, and performing even simpler tasks such as reaching for a glass of liquid.

Cataract glasses are thicker and heavier than conventional glasses. They magnify everything about one-third its original size. Instructions should be given about the magnification of the glasses and some of the problems that will ensue. Objects will appear closer. It will take time for the client to learn to judge distance; therefore, during the first few months, the client should be told to pour milk or other liquids in front of the glass rather than in it. He might be encouraged to use break-resistant dishes.

Images, as seen through the periphery of the glasses, are distorted. The distortions that occur cause objects to take on a curved appearance. As a result, peripheral vision is poor. Because he can generally see best through the center of the lens, he should be instructed to turn his head rather than his eyes in order to facilitate looking through the center of the lens.

There is a blind area between about 11 and 20 feet away in which the client cannot see at all. People and objects seem to come and go in this area so quickly that they can be said to "pop in and out." An explanation should be given to the client that this is expected and that with time he will become accustomed to it. He should be encouraged to keep his appointments with the oculist so that adjustments can be made in lenses as needed.

Contact lenses produce less magnification because the corrected lens is closer to the retina. They are also frequently prescribed to correct distortion defects. The client is therefore able to maintain binocular vision. Diplopia is often experienced because the unoperated eye has normal vision and vision of the operative eye is magnified. Except for difficulty that the client experiences in learning to insert and remove the lens, contact lenses have an advantage over glasses. Though still in the experimental stage, intraocular lenses have been tried to correct aphakia. With the intraocular lens, the magnification problem is nil. Also in the investigative stages, reports exist of *intraocular lenses* being inserted into the pupillary space at the time that the cataract is removed.[5] This procedure is thought to produce less distortion of vision and magnification.

Postoperative nursing care. Although postoperative vision is usually improved in the majority of clients, they must undergo a period of adjustment and depend on a pair of heavy "cataract glasses" or contact lenses. Glasses are ordinarily used if the client has a bilateral lens extraction.

However, permanent cataract glasses are not prescribed until about 3 months after the operation because curvature of the cornea continually changes during the early months of healing.

During the period of healing, temporary glasses or contact lenses are prescribed, especially if the vision in the unoperated eye is poor. Community health nurses and office nurses are in a particularly good position to give the client the needed support when new glasses are prescribed.

Discharge instructions. Clients who have had cataract operations are usually discharged from the hospital within 10 days. Both the client and his family must be well aware of his limitations before discharge. He should not exert himself to the point of raising venous pressure. He must not perform household duties or go back to work immediately. The eyes must be protected from bright light by the wearing of dark glasses. General activities are limited to those that will not increase intraocular pressure.

☞ **Evaluation.** The nursing plan for the client with cataracts is evaluated on an ongoing basis.

EXPECTED OUTCOMES

The client and/or family can:
1. Describe cataracts.
2. Describe the anticipated effects of surgery.
3. Describe limitations of activity.
4. Describe plans for health maintenance.
5. Demonstrate the correct method of changing eye dressing.
6. State needs for follow-up care by an ophthalmologist.

Other eye surgery

Types of eye surgery. Several surgeries may be performed for problems of the eye. These include enucleation, evisceration, exenteration, and blepharoplasty.

Enucleation is the removal of the eye. Severe eye injuries, malignant tumors, and sympathetic ophthalmia are common reasons for performing an enucleation. Clients who are blind may have an eye enucleated for cosmetic reasons. After removal, an implant of glass, fat, or bone may be put in the fascia of the eyeball to prevent a deep socket from forming and to maintain the normal shape of the lids. The rectus muscles are attached to the implant to provide movement of the prosthetic eye. After surgery, a conformer, which resembles the prosthesis, is worn for a few days or weeks. When edema subsides, the client is fitted for a permanent prosthesis.

Whenever the enucleation is performed, the client is likely to experience a change in body image. The nurse must provide psychological support during hospitalization. Explanations should be given to the family as to the reasons for reactions and behaviors of the client as he experiences the mourning period. This period is necessary if he is to reorganize his self-image.

An *evisceration* is the removal of the contents of the eye except the sclera. *Exenteration* is the removal of the eye plus the surrounding structure.

Blepharoplasty is the surgical removal of excess skin and fat pockets in the upper and lower eyelids.

Eye transplants. Certain structures of the eye can be used to restore sight in individuals whose vision has become severely impaired or destroyed by traumatic eye injuries or diseases. The structures usually used for transplants are the cornea, sclera, and vitreous.

Keratoplasty (corneal transplantation). A corneal transplant is the excision of corneal tissue and its replacement by a cornea from a human donor.[4] It is indicated when vision is severely impaired from conditions such as corneal scars, corneal inflammations, or keratoconus. Conditions that contraindicate a transplant include hepatitis, tumors of the eye structures, and leukemia.

Preoperative nursing care. The nurse must be familiar with the procedure, requirements, and laws regarding transplants to relay correct information to prospective donors.

The nurse should be aware that the eyes must be enucleated as soon as possible after the death of a donor. It is recommended that they be removed within 2 to 6 hours after death. If they cannot be used immediately, they are stored at a temperature of 4° C. When a possible donor dies, the eyelids should be closed, and a piece of gauze that has been moistened with saline placed over the eyes to prevent drying and subsequent damage to the cornea.

The nurse must reassure the family of a prospective donor, because they may worry about the appearance or features of the deceased without eyes. The nurse should reassure them that morticians are skillful and can make features appear unchanged and that usually prostheses are placed in the eye cavities to prevent deformities.

Often, the nurse is called on to interpret facts about corneal grafts to a client. Questions may be raised regarding "willing" eyes and making special requests. The nurse must be aware that eyes are donated, not willed. Because a time limit is imposed on the removal of eyes after death, the impracticality of donors' making special bequests to specific persons should be stressed. Specific information may be obtained from the Eye Bank Association of America. This association coordinates the donation of eyes in the United States, sets standards for each eye bank, solicits eye pledges, and coordinates supply and demand in the United States.

The fact that corneal grafts are not a cure-all should also be stressed. These grafts are useful only for treating disease of the cornea. All the other eye structures must be in good functioning condition.

FIG. 13-18
Corneal transplant. **A,** Lamellar, or partial-penetrating, corneal transplant. Clouded outer portion of cornea is removed and replaced with clear donor cornea. **B,** Penetrating, or full-thickness, corneal transplant. Entire central portion of clouded cornea is removed and replaced with clear donor cornea. (From Stein, Harold A., and Slatt, Bernard J.: The ophthalmic assistant, ed. 4, St. Louis, 1982, The C.V. Mosby Co.)

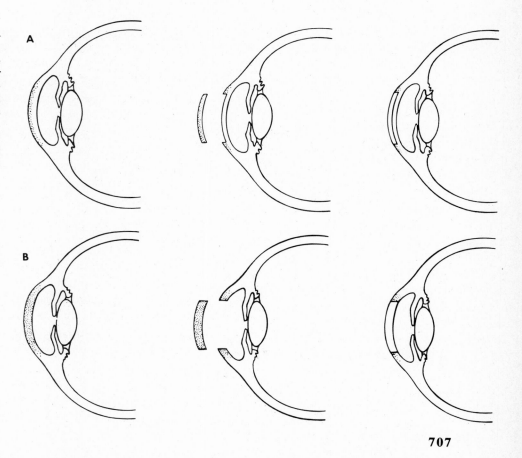

There are various types of grafts (Fig. 13-18). The type that is performed depends on the extent of the eye disease. A *penetrating,* or full-thickness, graft is one in which the entire thickness of the cornea is removed and replaced by transparent corneal tissue. *Lamellar,* or partial-penetrating grafts, or nonpenetrating grafts involve removal of the superficial layer and replacement by a graft without entry into the anterior chamber. The *mushroom* graft, a combination of the two, is used when a heavily vascularized scar is present. It is so named because it resembles a mushroom. The surgery may be performed in two stages. During the first stage a lamellar graft is done to improve the environmental condition, and a smaller graft is done later.

Postoperative nursing care. Nursing care after corneal grafts is similar to the care given to clients with other types of intraocular surgery. One exception is care after a penetrating graft. With this type of graft, the eye is opened, and therefore the integrity of the anterior chamber is lost. The client's activity is generally restricted for 48 hours. He must be kept flat in bed during this time. He usually is hospitalized for about 3 weeks.

Scleral and vitreous transplants. Scleral transplants are generally used in reconstruction surgery, whereas vitreous transplants are used in retinal detachment or in instabilities where vitreous has been lost from the eye. Once the cornea is removed, these structures are removed and may be stored. They may remain viable for up to 1 year.

Keratoprosthesis. A keratoprosthesis (corneal implant) may be performed in individuals in whom corneal transplantation was previously contraindicated because of excessive scarring.[4]

Planning and implementation

Preoperative nursing care. When a client is admitted for eye surgery, the nurse should obtain baseline data by assessing both the ability to see and the overall physical condition, and ascertaining the knowledge base of the client in regard to his condition and the possible surgical procedure. All the client's questions must be answered, all misconceptions about surgery must be cleared, and information must be provided about preoperative routines.

One such routine is preparation of the periorbital area. The eyebrow and eyelashes are shaved after cleaning the area with a germicidal soap (a clean cotton ball can be used for application) then rinsing with an irrigating solution.

When the eyebrow and eyelashes are shaved, measures should be taken to promote comfort and minimize injury. The following measures are useful:

1. To promote comfort:
   a. Shave the brow from the medial to the lateral aspects.
   b. Shave in the direction of the grain of the eyebrow.
2. To minimize injury in trimming the lashes:
   a. Use small scissors that have blunt ends. (Scissors with blunt ends conform to the shape of the eyelid.)
   b. Coat the blades of the scissors with a lubricant (such as petroleum jelly). This measure is instrumental in preventing lashes from falling into the client's eyes.
   c. Instruct the client to look in the direction opposite the lashes being trimmed. For example, the client should look upward when the lower lashes are being trimmed and vice versa.

Another important part of preoperative preparation is teaching the client about *postoperative restrictions*. As a general rule, improved methods of suturing and operative techniques have decreased the need for extensive restrictions in the postoperative period. However, certain restrictions may be placed on the client to prevent an increase in ocular pressure and consequently prevent pressure on the suture line.

To prevent increase in pressure, activity is restricted in the early postoperative period; for example, clients are instructed not to bend over the side of the bed until permission is granted. Sneezing, coughing, blowing the nose, nausea and vomiting, and restlessness may produce added pressure on the operative site; therefore, the client should be aware that specified medications for cough, nausea, and pain will be available. Restrictions may also be placed on activities of daily living. He may not be allowed to shave or comb his hair without permission. If certain activities are permitted (such as brushing the teeth and combing the hair), they should be done gently. He should be fed until he can feed himself.

A metal shield is worn in the postoperative period for protective purposes. The client should be encouraged not to squeeze the eye by tightly closing the lid, because injury might result.

Whether the client has one or both eyes bandaged, certain behavioral changes such as disorientation may be evident. Because vision depends on sensory input from the environment, a sudden loss of the ability to see (such as from bandages) makes one feel isolated from his environment. Therefore the nurse must use varied interventions to help the client remain oriented to reality. See Chapter 8 for a complete discussion of sensory deprivation.

Restrictions in movement should also be discussed. After surgery, movement may be permitted to the unoperated side. When the client is moved, he will be moved gently. Because of the restrictions that will be placed on head movement, it is desirable before surgery to carry out range-of-motion exercises to improve postoperative circulation and prevent postoperative fatigue. Deep breathing exercises to prevent pulmonary complications and limb movements to increase circulation should be encouraged.

In addition, it may be helpful to plan for the postoperative period by allowing the client to engage in routines that will be experienced postoperatively. For example, in the preoperative period the nurse might shield the client's eye and permit him to assist with feeding or similar activities.

Postoperative nursing care. In the immediate postoperative period, the client must be observed closely for complications such as hemorrhage or rupture of the suture line. In monitoring for these complications, the vital signs should be checked at frequent intervals, and any significant changes should be reported. The dressing should be checked for the presence of blood. The client may experience some discomfort in the eye, but sharp pain generally indicates rupture of the suture line and should be reported immediately. Any unusual restlessness, nausea, vomiting, and coughing should also be reported to the physician. Inasmuch as the client may not be permitted to sleep or lie on the operated side, belongings may be placed on the nonoperated side. The signal cord should be placed within easy reach by pinning it to the client's gown or pillow. For other pointers relating to management of a client with ocular surgery, review the section on the care of the blind client earlier in this chapter.

Nursing process for common health problems

If proper preoperative teaching has been done, efforts in the postoperative period should be directed toward seeing that measures taught in the preoperative period are carried out, and toward guiding the client to a successful recovery. The physician's orders should be followed regarding positioning and activity. The client should be kept quiet and protected from injury. For example, the side rails should be kept in the up position until the nurse is assured that it is safe for them to be left down.

Later, teaching should be directed toward preparation of the client and his family for discharge. Such instructions should include the proper way of instilling eye drops and the proper care of the eyes. Activities that must be avoided should be stressed. Light tasks such as drying dishes may be done from the start, but heavy household duties and activities that might increase venous pressure in the head should be delayed. Stooping and bending should be avoided for a month after surgery. To avoid stooping, the client should be encouraged to wear shoes that can be slipped into rather than tied. The client should be instructed to keep his head high and to use proper body mechanics when sitting and walking. Cathartics may be needed for bowel elimination to prevent straining and subsequent increased intraocular pressure. Soft foods and adequate bulk are recommended.

Artificial eyes. Prostheses are made of plastic or glass. Both types look the same and allow the same amount of movement; however, plastic eyes are nonbreakable and are therefore more serviceable. Glass may break or crack, particularly in hot weather as the gas within it expands.

The client should be encouraged to follow the instructions of the physician precisely. For the first few weeks after surgery, a moderate amount of secretion may occur. If the secretion increases in amount and duration, an infection may be present. If this happens, the client should be instructed to see his physician. To remove the drainage, the client should carry clean tissue with him at all times. The use of the fingers and handkerchiefs for cleansing must be totally discouraged. If he swims, he should not allow the socket to get wet. The client must be instructed to wash his hands thoroughly before touching the prosthesis or eye socket.

Although the client generally cares for his own artificial eye, the nurse must also be familiar with how to care for it, as well as how to remove and insert it. Scrupulous care must be given to the artificial eye and the socket. Warm soap and water may be used to cleanse the prosthesis. Extremely hot or cold water or alcohol should never be used for cleansing. A soft cloth or tissue is recommended for polishing the eye. When the eye is not worn, it should be stored in plain water and always be cleansed before storage. The eye socket should be washed daily or as prescribed. A normal saline solution is usually recommended to cleanse the socket.

The steps of inserting and removing an artificial eye follow:

1. Insertion. The upper lid should be raised, and the eye should be slipped beneath it. After the eye is in place, the lid should be released, and the lower lid should be supported and drawn over the lower edge of the eye.
2. Removal. The lower lid should be drawn downward, and the eye should be slipped forward over the lower lid and removed.

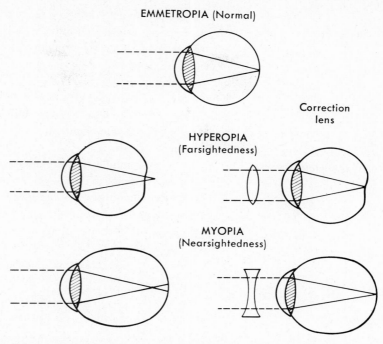

EMMETROPIA (Normal)

Correction lens

HYPEROPIA (Farsightedness)

MYOPIA (Nearsightedness)

COMMON HEALTH PROBLEMS THAT OCCUR ACROSS THE LIFE SPAN

Errors of refraction

Light rays pass to the retina through the refractive media: the cornea, aqueous, lens, and vitreous. Varied optical densities of these structures cause the light rays to change direction as they pass through these media (Fig. 13-19). Normal refraction is referred to as a *emmetropia*. The emmetropic eye is one in which parallel rays of light focus on the fovea without the use of accommodation.

When light rays do not focus directly on the retina, refractive areas occur, and are referred to as *ametropia*. Forms of ametropia include: hyperopia, hypermetropia (farsightedness), and myopia (nearsightedness). Heredity, various diseases, injuries, or degenerative changes may be responsible for causing the refractive error. The hyperopic eye fails to converge the light rays upon the fovea without the use of accommodation. Consequently, the rays of light entering the eye are focused behind the retina. It is the most common refractive error and occurs in about 80% of all infants because of the small size of the eye. As the child grows, the error gradually becomes lessened and may disappear. Individuals with hyperopia have better distance vision than near vision. Therefore they have a tendency to be less interested in near objects. Problems may be experienced in reading because of inability to sustain a sharp image for a long period of time, because the correction is obtained with the use of convex lens.

In myopia the light rays focus in front of the retina. The eyeballs are characteristically long, and therefore the distance between the lens and retina is increased. Individuals with myopic eyes have normal near vision but very poor distance vision. Myopia usually develops after the child starts school, gradually increases during the growing period, and stabilizes about age 25. Individuals with myopia may have problems when attempting to review objects from a distance such as a chalkboard in school or road signs. Frowning or squinting is not uncommon in these individuals. This is an attempt to make acuity sharper by eliminating peripheral rays of light entering the eye. Other symptoms that commonly are experienced are headaches and lid irritations.

Nursing process for common health problems

To correct myopia, concave lens are used. These cause the light rays to diverge and focus on the retina.

Astigmatism is a common optical condition in which the refractory power of an eye is not the same in all meridians. [6] It may occur with hyperopia or myopia, or it may occur alone. Children with astigmatism tend to hold reading material close, and have a tendency to frown, which consequently causes a headache. Lenses with a cylindrical correction are used to correct astigmatism.

Anisometropia is a condition characterized by a difference in the refractive error of the two eyes.

Foreign bodies in the eye

It is not uncommon for an individual to get a foreign body in the eye. In everyday life, particles of dust, cloth, sand, and eyelashes may enter the eye and lodge in the conjunctival sac or cornea.

 Assessment. When an object enters the eye, it generally causes some discomfort because of irritation to the conjunctiva. Pain, lacrimation, and congestion are also common symptoms of a foreign body on the conjunctiva or cornea.

Data analysis
Data analysis may reveal nursing diagnoses of sensory perception alteration and alterations in comfort.

Planning and implementation. Any foreign object that enters the conjunctiva can be removed by the client, the nurse, a family member, or friend. However, before attempts are made to remove it, adequate lighting must be provided in order to determine whether the foreign object is on the conjunctiva or cornea. If the object cannot be readily seen, it may be necessary to evert the lids to permit adequate inspection.

Adequate hygiene measures should be followed. The hands should be clean, and all equipment used should be sterile.

The client should be encouraged to hold his head perfectly still to prevent damaging the eye. It may be necessary to mummify the small child in a sheet. If this does not keep the child immobile—or if the client is extremely apprehensive—a general anesthetic may be administered.

Removing an object from the conjunctiva. To properly remove an object from the conjunctiva, a piece of twisted cotton or an applicator stick moistened with water or saline should be used. If dry cotton is used, a wisp of it may be left in the eye, thus causing as much irritation as the foreign body. An irrigating solution may also be used to remove a foreign body. When the latter is used, the same procedure as for instillation of eye drops can be followed.

Removing an object from the cornea. If the foreign body enters the cornea, no attempt should be made by the nurse or lay person to remove it, because considerable damage might be done to the delicate epithelium of the cornea. Also, the cornea is less resistant to infection, and corneal abrasions may easily occur and result in visual impairment. Therefore foreign bodies on the cornea should be removed only by the ophthalmologist.

Foreign bodies on the cornea are not easily detected. Therefore the cornea must be stained with a fluorescein strip to outline the object before removal is attempted. To facilitate examination of the tissue and to detect the extent of epithelial damage, a biomicroscope is used in order to detect the object. An x-ray film may be taken to confirm the location. Nonmetal objects may be removed with the use of a hypodermic needle. A magnet is used to remove metal foreign objects.

After removal of the foreign body, small amounts of antibiotic or sulfonamide eye ointment may be instilled into the eye to prevent infection. An eye patch may be prescribed to be worn until healing takes place, which usually takes 24 hours. There may be some discomfort after foreign body removal, and therefore the client may require sedation.

Eye injuries   Eye injuries are common. These injuries may be nonpenetrating or penetrating.

Nonpenetrating injuries. Nonpenetrating injuries are those that result from blunt objects as might occur when one is hit in the eye while engaging in sport or work activities. The effect of the blow may vary from a small corneal abrasion to rupture of the globe. Because it is difficult to determine the extent of the damage that might have resulted from the injury, the client should be seen by an ophthalmologist.

Abrasions, superficial scratches of the lids, cornea, or conjunctiva, usually occur after injuries caused by objects such as paper or fingernails. The client who has an abrasion of the cornea often complains of a foreign body sensation in the eye. Individuals who complain of this sensation should be encouraged to consult a physician. When the client is examined, the ophthalmologist stains the eye with fluorescein and carefully examines the eye with the use of magnifying glasses. The usual treatment is to tightly patch the eye for a period of approximately 24 hours. A patch lessens discomfort and promotes healing by preventing the lids from moving over the involved area. Local anesthetics are thought to delay epithelization, and are therefore contraindicated.

Contusion of the eyeballs and surrounding structures occurs as a result of an injury to the eye from a blunt object. After the injury, a large amount of blood escapes underneath the skin and is responsible for the discoloration about the eye (ecchymosis, commonly referred to as black eye). The appearance of the eye frequently causes the individual to become alarmed.

When the injury is experienced, immediate health assistance should be obtained. This is essential because once swelling occurs, examination becomes difficult. Another reason for immediate care is that damage may have been sustained to other structures of the eye.

Initial therapy includes application of cold compresses to reduce swelling and administration of analgesics for pain. Usually within a week the swelling subsides and the color returns to a more normal appearance.

Penetrating injuries. Penetrating injuries are caused by objects that actually pierce the eye, such as scissors, knives, or sticks. Children are prone to sustain eye injuries from mobile objects such as BB guns, arrows, and similar items that are part of childhood games. In industrial settings, pointed or sharp objects may cause injuries ranging from a small break in the tissue to collapse of the globe.

Penetrating injuries in which a foreign object is retained are more likely to occur in industrial settings where high-powered grinding and drilling machines are used. Steel that breaks off from a hammer and chisel is also a common source. The particles that enter the eye generally do so at a high speed. As a result, the individual may be unaware of its entrance. However, he usually is aware that something is wrong with the eye. When a penetrating injury is sustained or suspected, first-aid principles should be applied immediately. On impulse, the client will attempt to protect the eye by applying pressure. This practice should not be allowed. Therefore the most important first-aid principle to apply is to prevent any pressure on the eye because pressure may cause the object to be driven farther into the eye, subsequently causing more damage. The eye should be protected by a metal shield or a light patch, or no form of treatment should be attempted. Activities such as bending, lifting, and coughing have a tendency to raise intraocular pressure and may result in loss of intraocular contents. These activities should therefore be prohibited, and the client instructed to remain as quiet as possible.

After first-aid management, the client should be referred to an ophthalmologist for treatment. There is a direct relationship between promptness in treatment and conservation of sight. The earlier a penetrating injury is treated, the better the chance of saving vision. Some authorities contend that clients who receive competent care within the first 24 hours are about three times more likely to retain useful vision than those treated later. Therapy is likely to follow the same general principles as discussed under foreign bodies. Antibiotics are prescribed to prevent infection. Depending on the extent of the injury, surgery may be performed to repair the damage.

Complications of penetrating injuries. Sympathetic ophthalmia (sympathetic uveitis) is a bilateral inflammation of the uveal tract that usually occurs as a result of a penetrating injury to the eye. The exact cause is unknown; however, it is contended that it may be an autoimmune hypersensitivity reaction to uveal pigment.[6] The condition occurs gradually over a period of 3 weeks after the injury, when the injured eye does not respond to therapy.

Blindness may occur in both eyes unless the injured eye (exciting eye) is enucleated before the disease progresses to the fellow eye. When the sympathizing eye (noninjured or fellow eye) becomes affected, photophobia, lacrimation, pain, and dimness of vision are the major symptoms.

Planning and implementation. As much as possible, measures are planned to prevent sympathetic ophthalmia by enucleating the exciting eye before the fellow eye is involved. Once the sympathizing eye becomes involved, enucleation of the exciting eye is not recommended because it may eventually be the better of the two bad eyes.[1] Salicylates, antibiotics, or steroids may be prescribed to control pain and inflammation. If no treatment is instituted, bilateral blindness occurs.

Burns

Chemical burns. Of the burns of the eye, chemical burns are perhaps the most common and the most serious. They often result in corneal ulceration, opacities, or perforations. Burns from chemicals generally take place in laboratories, industrial plants, and the home. The offending agents are usually cleansers, insecticides, acids, or alkalis, all of which may cause considerable damage to the eye.

The extent of damage is determined by the nature of the chemical and the length of time the substance remains in the eye. Strong acids and alkalis are dangerous because they may cause opacification and destruction of the corneal tissue by breaking down the collagen structure and damaging the epithelium. Initially, acid burns appear more severe; however, alkali burns are more damaging because alkalis are proteolytic. Consequently, they destroy proteins and form

714

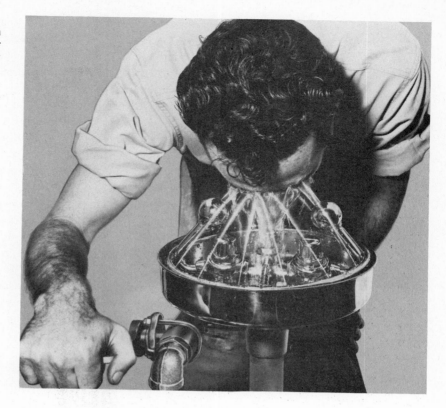

more toxic alkaline products. These products tend to penetrate the soft tissue. When acids enter the eye, they are quickly buffered by the tissue,[4] which generally prevents penetration of acid into the tissue. Acid burns are therefore self-limiting.

First aid. Regardless of the cause of the chemical burn or the setting of the accident, emergency treatment is the same. The importance of speed cannot be overemphasized. The eye(s) must be washed immediately with copious amounts of water. Time should not be wasted in trying to find a specific antidote if the cornea is to be saved. Irrigation should be performed continuously for 15 to 20 minutes to prevent permanent scarring of the eye. Water may be poured onto the eye from a large drinking glass or quart jar, or the eye may be held directly under the faucet (Fig. 13-20). Another effective method is to place the entire face into a container of water, and then open the eyes under water.[4] Spasms of the eyes sometimes prevent the eyes from opening. To facilitate opening the eye, it may be necessary to forcibly separate the lids while the eye is being irrigated.

Follow-up therapy. After first-aid therapy has been administered, the client should be taken to the nearest health care facility. Here the initial treatment is likely to be repeated, and saline, which has the advantage of not causing edema of the cornea, may be used. An IV flask of normal saline (attached to tubing) may be used to facilitate continuous irrigation. The eye may be further examined to determine the extent of damage. Sedatives or narcotics may be used to control pain. Anesthetics may be used for the initial examination; however, repeated use of anesthetics is discouraged because they tend to inhibit healing. Topical atropine may be used to dilate the pupils and to paralyze the ciliary muscle. Steroids may be used to lessen the inflammatory reaction, thus preventing scar formation, and topical and systemic antibiotics may be ordered to prevent infection.

Radiation burns. Radiation burns of the eye fall into two categories: ultraviolet burns and infrared burns.

Ultraviolet burns are least serious and usually occur as a result of exposing the naked eye to sun lamps. They also occur in welders, mountain climbers, and those exposed to snow fields. Snow blindness is caused by ultraviolet rays' being reflected into the eyes from the snow. Pain, the leading symptom, may not be produced until several hours after exposure. The client may be awakened from sleep with severe pain. Photophobia, blepharospasm, and lacrimation are usually present. Surface anesthesia in the form of an ointment is generally used to control the pain and cycloplegics to counteract ciliary spasm. Sedation may also be necessary. In order to keep the eye quiet, an eye patch is usually prescribed for 1 or 2 days. Ultraviolet burns are generally self-limiting.[4]

Infrared burns of the eyes are more serious because permanent visual damage may result. Common causes are exposure to lightning or the short exposure to a high tension electrical system. Eclipse blindness, which may occur while the person is watching an eclipse of the sun, is another common cause. Medical therapy is of no avail after injury occurs. Therefore instruction should be directed toward prevention.

Thermal burns. Thermal burns are common occupational hazards in adults. They are most likely caused by hot metals, flash burns, steam, and gasoline. Therapy consists of sedation, adequate cleansing, cycloplegics, sterile ointments, and patching of both eyes.

When facial burns are sustained, it is not unusual for the lids to be affected. Edema often makes it difficult for the client to open his eyes. An ophthalmologist is likely to examine the eyes to determine the extent of damage, if any. If the results from the examination are negative, the client should be reassured that ability to see will improve as the swelling subsides. When the client is not able to close his eyes completely, eye irrigations, usually with normal saline, and ophthalmic ointments are prescribed. Generally, ointments containing steroids are not used, because they retard the protective inflammatory process and an intraocular infection may result. During the period when the client is unable to see, the nurse should apply principles of care associated with blindness (see discussion earlier in this chapter).

Infections and inflammations

Bacterial conjunctivitis. Bacterial conjunctivitis usually results from gonococcal, staphylococcal, pneumococcal, *Hemophilus,* or *Pseudomonas* organisms. Conjunctivitis of bacterial origin usually occurs between the second and fifth day of life.[5] Because corneal damage may result, conjunctivitis caused by the gonococcal organism is thought to be most serious.

Viral conjunctivitis. Viral conjunctivitis may be caused by infection with one of the adenoviruses. It is characterized by edema and hyperemia, a watery discharge that usually clears up within 2 to 3 weeks without treatment. However, topical antibiotics are often employed to prevent secondary infection, as are warm moist compresses to remove crusts.

Allergic conjunctivitis. Allergic conjunctivitis may be iatrogenic or may occur in conjunction with a number of allergic manifestations. One common example of the latter is hay fever. Symptoms characteristic of allergic conjunctivitis include lacrimation, itching, redness, and a mucoid discharge. Hydrocortisone ophthalmic ointment is usually prescribed for acute forms. In chronic states, attempts are made to eliminate contact with offending allergens.

Hordeolum. Hordeolum (stye) is a suppurative inflammation of the hair follicle and accessory glands of the anterior lid margin. The usual cause is the staphylococcal organism. Tenderness, usually the initial symptom, and swelling, redness, and pain are characteristic. A small abscess forms. Application of warm compresses three to four times a day may be prescribed to hasten the pointing of the abscess. Antibiotic therapy may be prescribed to prevent involvement of the adjacent tissue. When the stye points, it is usually incised and drained. Clients should be instructed not to squeeze the area because of the danger of spreading the infection and causing lid cellulitis.

Chalazion. Chalazion is an inflammatory cyst of the meibomian glands (a sebaceous gland of the eyelids). It is caused by obstruction of the ducts. Painless swelling of the gland is characteristic. Complete excision or incision and drainage of the cyst are accepted forms of therapy; however, sometimes the mass disappears spontaneously.

Keratitis. Keratitis is an inflammation of the cornea. The two main types of keratitis are superficial keratitis and deep keratitis. Superficial keratitis is generally associated with either a viral infection of the conjunctiva or cornea or an upper respiratory tract infection. Herpes simplex is a common viral disease that causes superficial keratitis. Deep keratitis results from the spread of a systemic disease such as tuberculosis to the cornea. The major symptoms include photophobia, pain, redness, and lacrimation. Cultures are usually taken to determine the nature of the organism. Antibiotics and hot compresses are useful forms of therapy for both types. Steroids are prescribed, except in herpes simplex, to relieve the inflammatory reaction and prevent scarring.

Uveitis. Uveitis is an inflammation of the uveal tract (iris, ciliary body, choroid). Inflammation of a single structure seldom occurs and generally involves two structures simultaneously because of the proximity of the structures. For example, inflammation of the iris (iritis) and ciliary body (cyclitis) usually occurs at the same time and is referred to as iridocyclitis. Inflammation of the choroid (choroiditis) usually involves inflammation of the retina (retinitis), hence the inflammation is retinochoroiditis. Uveitis is usually unilateral and most often affects school-age children and middle-aged adults.

Uveitis may be caused by local or systemic infections. Rheumatoid arthritis and toxoplasmosis are common conditions that are thought to cause uveitis. In many cases the cause cannot be determined. Symptoms depend on the part of the uveal tract involved. If the iris is affected, lacrimation, pain, and photophobia are main symptoms. Visual blurring and the appearance of "floaters" are major symptoms when the ciliary body and choroid are involved. Decreased visual acuity is also present in choroiditis.

To prevent the formation of adhesions between the iris and the anterior lens capsule, mydriatics are used to dilate the pupil. Symptomatic relief may be obtained by using warm compresses and analgesics to control pain and dark glasses to relieve photophobia. Antibiotics may be prescribed to control infection, and steroids for their antiinflammatory effect.

Evaluation

Evaluation, the final stage of the nursing process, is ongoing. Clients with health problems of the visual system may have problems of sensory perception alteration, grieving, alteration in self-care activities, alterations in comfort, alterations in body image, and ineffective coping, fear, and disturbance in self-concept.

EXPECTED OUTCOMES

The client and/or family can:
1. State the specific health problem.
2. Explain plans for maintaining a safe environment (such as removal of potential dangerous objects in the environment and keeping doors opened or closed.)
3. State plans for maintaining independence in activities of daily living.
4. Demonstrate the correct use of special lenses (for example, contact lenses, eye glasses).
5. State symptoms indicative of follow-up health care.
6. State use, dosage, time, frequency and method of administration, and side effects of prescribed medications.
7. Demonstrate instillation of special medications for the eye in a safe manner.
8. State plans for follow-up care.
9. Identify appropriate community resources that can be used as the need arises.

Summary

The care of clients with problems of the visual system is based on a thorough knowledge of the pathophysiology of conditions affecting the eye. Such care involves using the nursing process. The nursing process commences with assessment through the acquisition of data through the taking of a nursing history. Components of this history include health, developmental, social, and psychological elements. The physical assessment skill essential to acquiring information about the visual system is inspection. Screening tests and diagnostic parameters are also used to provide information about the state of the client. Screening tests include those used to assess visual acuity, color vision, refractive errors, and intraocular pressure. Specific diagnostic tests include electroretinography, echo-ophthalmography, fluorescein angiography, phosphorus 32 radioactive uptake, tonography, gonioscopy, and perimetry. Information obtained from assessment of these components is analyzed and used as a basis for planning and implementing and evaluating care.

Nursing care is planned to promote visual health as well as to maintain and restore vision. The nurse plays an important role in each of these. Instructions and care center around providing the client with information about the visual specialist, the care of the eyes including the use of medications, frequency of care, illumination, prevention of injuries, principles of first aid, danger signals of visual problems, and use of glasses. The care of the client with varied aspects of visual impairment is challenging and at the same time rewarding as the nurse facilitates the client's enjoyment of the environment and things about him. The care provided is evaluated on an ongoing basis.

Common health problems of the neonate are conjunctivitis (chemical conjunctivitis and ophthalmia neonatorum), congenital cataracts, and strabismus. Retinoblastoma and blepharitis are common among infants and young children.

13 Visual system

Retina detachment, glaucoma, and cataracts are common during the adult years. A number of surgical procedures may be used to correct or maintain visual problems. Transplants are used to restore sight in individuals with severe visual disturbances. Accidents affecting the eye are not uncommon in the home and work environments. Infections may affect the visual system at varied times across the life span.

References

1. Cooke, Robert E., and Levin, Sidney, editors: The biologic basis of pediatric practice, New York, 1968, McGraw-Hill Book Co.
2. Emery, Jared, M.: Cataract treatment and rehabilitation, A.O.R.N. J. **20**:992-995, December 1974.
3. Fraunfelder, F.T.: Current ocular therapy, Philadelphia, 1980, W.B. Saunders Co.
4. Newell, Frank W.: Ophthalmology: principles and concepts, ed. 4, St. Louis, 1978, The C.V. Mosby Co.
5. Vaughan, Daniel, and Asbury, Taylor: General ophthalmology, ed. 9, Los Altos, Calif., 1980, Lange Medical Publications.
6. Vale, Janet, and Cox, B.: Drugs and the eye, Boston, 1978, Butterworths.

Additional readings

Alexander, Mary M., and Brown, Marie Scott: Pediatric physical diagnosis for nurses, New York, 1974, McGraw-Hill Book Co.

Feman, Stephen S., and Reinecke, Robert D.: Handbook of pediatric ophthalmology, New York, 1978, Grune & Stratton.

Fernsebner, Wilhelmina: Etiology and treatment of glaucoma, A.O.R.N. J. **20**:996-1001, December 1974.

Friedman, Ephrain, and Lessell, Simmons: Diseases of the eye and ocular manifestations of systemic diseases. In Keefer, Chester S., and Wilkins, Robert W., Essentials of clinical practice, Boston, 1970, Little Brown & Co.

Jaffe, Norman S., Cataract surgery and its complications, ed. 3, St. Louis, 1981, The C.V. Mosby Co.

Liebman, Summer D., and Gellis, Sydney S., editors: The pediatrician's ophthalmology, St. Louis, 1966, The C.V. Mosby Co.

Mayer, Walter: Cryopreserved corneal grafting, A.O.R.N. J. **20**:973-976, December 1974.

Ohno, Mary I.: The eye-patched patient, Am. J. Nurs. **71**:271-274, February 1971.

Pilgrim, Margaret, and Sigler, Barbara: Phaco-emulsification of cataracts, Am. J. Nurs. **75**:976-978, June 1975.

Portney, Gerald L., Glaucoma guidebook, Philadelphia, 1977, Lea and Febiger.

Rose, F. Clifford, editor: Medical ophthalmology, St. Louis, 1976, The C.V. Mosby Co.

Salmon, Donald L.: Low vision and public health, Can. J. Public Health **69**:35-38, November/December 1978.

Saunders, William H., and others: Nursing care in eye, ear, nose, and throat disorders, ed. 4, St. Louis, 1979, The C.V. Mosby Co.

Sharpe, Ann: Helping parents in the developmental rearing of a blind child, Clinical Nurse Specialist Symposium, Ann Arbor, 1972, Department of Nursing, University of Michigan.

Sloan, Louise L.: Recommended aids for the partially sighted, New York, 1971, National Society for the Prevention of Blindness, Inc.

Smith, Taylor R.: Malignant tumors of the eye, Cancer **19**(6):360-363, November-December 1969.

Stein, Harold A., and Slatt, Bernard J.: The ophthalmic assistant: fundamentals and clinical practice, ed. 4, St. Louis, 1982, The C.V. Mosby Co.

Victor, Maurice, and Adams, Raymond D.: Common disturbances of vision, ocular movement, and hearing. In Harrison's Principles of Internal Medicine, ed. 9, New York, 1980, McGraw-Hill Book Co.

Wov, Georgé: Age and its effect in vision, Can. J. Public Health **69**:29-31, November/December 1978.

for clients with common health problems of the

14 Auditory system and speech

Assessment

Data analysis

Planning

Implementation

Evaluation

The patterns in development of hearing are unique, as evidenced by the various responses to sound and other environmental stimulations. Common health problems affecting the auditory system occur across the life span and may result from infection, trauma, or degeneration.

Alteration in hearing ability has both physical and psychosocial implications. Varying degrees of hearing impairment may be produced; the exact extent depends on the degree of involvement. The assessment portion of the nursing process can be used to obtain sufficient information to begin an individualized plan of care. This chapter presents information about common health problems. Such information can help the nurse and the client promote, maintain, or restore health.

FIG. 14-1
Comparison of anatomy of the ear of adult and young child. Notice that ossicles, semicircular canals, and cochlea are almost fully grown in young child. (From Chinn, Peggy L.: Child health maintenance: concepts in family-centered care, ed. 2, St. Louis, 1979, The C.V. Mosby Co.)

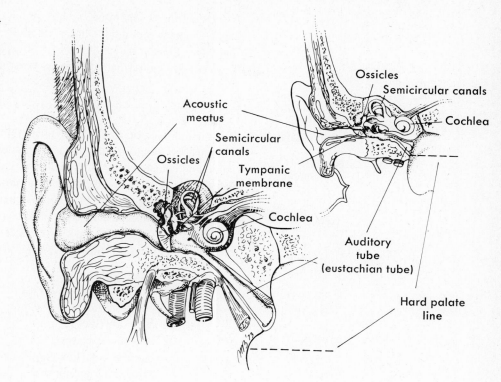

The auditory system

Overview of the ear

The ear, the organ of hearing and balance, anatomically is divided into the *external, middle,* and *inner* ear (Fig. 14-1). The *external ear* is composed of the auricle and external auricle canal and functions to transmit sound to the middle ear. The *middle ear* contains the tympanic cavity in which three ossicles (tiny bones) are found—the malleus (hammer), incus (anvil), and stapes (stirrup). These bones transmit sound vibrations to the cochlea. The eustachian tube, which connects the middle ear with the nasopharynx, is contiguous with air-filled cells, and is instrumental in regulating air pressure. The *inner ear* is the organ of equilibrium. It contains membranous and bony labyrinths and the distal terminations of the cochlear and vestibular branches of the acoustic nerve. The organ of corti, found within the cochlea, is the end organ of hearing. It contains tiny hair cells that are bent by sound waves and converts them from a mechanical force to an electrochemical impulse that travels to the brain by way of the acoustic nerve. It is at this point that one hears sound.

The sense of hearing is important in that it not only enables one to perceive the many sounds within the environment but it also facilitates oral communication. Subsequently, hearing affords us the opportunity to exchange ideas and opinions through speech. It enables us to be aware of environmental dangers. For example, with an intact auditory system we can hear the blast of the train that warns us it is approaching, the horn of an automobile that warns us to be careful in crossing the street, or a fire alarm that alerts us to fire. Hearing also enables us to enjoy certain pleasures of life. For example, we can enjoy the voice of a

721

Nursing process for common health problems

loved one, the beauty of music, and other pleasurable sounds within the environment. Inherent within this sense is its ability to provide both protective and social functions. Loss of the ability to hear affects one's personal safety, and the realization of this causes one to become more insecure and more hesitant in actions.

Assessment
NURSING HISTORY

Health history

The nursing history should be obtained during the initial contact with the client. This history should include assessments regarding the client's health, development, and social and psychological state. Such information should be evaluated and used as a basis for formulating a nursing diagnosis, and subsequently for developing a nursing care plan for the client.

The health history can be obtained as the physical assessment is performed. Questions the nurse might ask to facilitate understanding of the client and his problems include the following:

1. What is the problem?
   a. Do you have problems with ringing (tinnitus) or buzzing in the ears? Discomfort? Itching? If either is present, does it interfere with sleep or other activities?
   b. Have you experienced dizzy spells? Loss of balance? Over what period of time? How long does it last? When was it first noticed? For example, after an upper respiratory infection? After an airplane trip? After swimming? Do you experience any other symptoms during the attack? Nausea or vomiting? Lightheadedness? Headache?
   c. Do you experience pain in the ear? If so, describe it. When does it occur? And where is the pain located?
   d. Do you have earaches? How often?
   e. Have you noted any drainage or discharge from the ear? When did you first notice the drainage? What does the drainage look like? What color is it? Is it blood tinged? Serous? Mucoid? Purulent?
   f. Are you on any special medications? What are they?
   g. Do you have difficulty hearing? Do you have a hearing loss? If yes, did the problem occur suddenly? Gradually? Were other symptoms experienced when you first noted the hearing problem? Is the problem experienced in one ear? Both ears? Does the hearing problem interfere with normal conversation?
   h. Are you frequently exposed to loud noises? For example, rock music or machinery?
2. Questions related to hearing loss that may be specific if the client is a child include the following:
   a. When did you first suspect the child might have a hearing problem?
   b. Did the child have an infectious disease shortly after birth?
   c. At what age was the hearing impairment first noticed?
   d. Had the child started to talk? If yes, what changes were noticed in his speech pattern?
   e. Has the child had any childhood diseases? If yes, which ones? At what age?
   f. Has the child's hearing been tested?

3. Questions for the mother, and specifically related to the pregnancy, include the following:
   a. Assess whether the mother had a "childhood" disease during the pregnancy. If yes, which childhood disease? At what trimester of pregnancy?
   b. Did the mother take any medications during the pregnancy? What were they?
4. Assess past ear history.
   a. Have you had any type of ear surgery? If yes, when? What type was it? Why was it done?

Developmental history

Much has been written about the developmental stages of hearing. However, some stages have been more clearly defined than others. Characteristic changes may be noted in the hearing ability as the individual progresses through the developmental stages. The ability of the client to hear or not hear may be assessed on the basis of behaviors.

Neonate. Hearing in the neonate is thought to occur after the first cry. However, response to sound is reflexive and may not be noted until 3 or 4 days after birth. Responses to sound may be manifested by the Moro (startle) reflex and may be accompanied by grimacing or crying. The body's startle response is thought to be a protective reaction and is more likely to occur if the sound is loud and unexpected. Blinking, a form of autopalpebral response, and clenching the eyes may also be manifestations of responses to sound. The latter is more likely to occur when the neonate is asleep, whereas the former may be observed during the waking hours.[8]

Infant. The infant reacts to the voice of his mother and responds to his name by smiling. At about 3 to 4 months he begins to localize sound by turning his head toward the source. This will especially be observed if the sounds are pleasant—mother's voice, a rattle, a feeding utensil, or playing children. Similar stimuli will also elicit responses such as a smile or a coo. Unpleasant, loud sounds (a vacuum cleaner or a lawn mower) are more likely to elicit crying. By the end of the first year, the infant is thought to be able to localize sound just as well as an older child or adult.[6]

Child. The toddler period is characterized by an increase in listening skills. It is not uncommon to see the toddler moving in response to the rhythm of songs. He also attempts to imitate the sounds within his environment. However, by the end of this period, the child tends to be more selective in listening, as evidenced by the fact that he tends to ignore many commands that are given by persons in the environment.

As the child approaches school age, hearing development is characterized by a continued refinement in the skills that are developed during the first 3 years of life. During the preschool years, incantations are frequently expressed. At various times during the school-age period, "tuning out" may be noted.

Adult. Although *presbycusis* (a progressive hearing loss caused by degeneration of the sensory process in the elderly) generally develops later, a premature form may occur during the early adult years.

Older adult. Presbycusis generally develops during the sixth decade. It occurs in most adults as a result of deterioration of the structures of the cochlear duct. With age, the organ of Corti and surrounding structures atrophy. As a

Nursing process for common health problems

result, an impairment is noted in the individual's ability to hear high tones. Hearing for speech is vastly affected, especially in a crowd. The elderly person tends to depend on his sight as a means of coping with the impairment.

Social history

Data should be obtained about the client's education, background, life-style, and occupation. It will also be useful to determine whether anyone in the family has a problem with hearing. If a child is of school age, it will be useful to determine the type of school the child attends. For example, does the child attend school or classes with children who hear normally or only with those who are hard of hearing? Does he attend special classes? If the child is not in school, determine what the plans are for education.

Determine whether the client wears a hearing aid. If yes, determine what type. How long has he worn the aid? How much is it worn each day? Determine the client's feelings about the aid. Does he enjoy it? Resent wearing it?

If the client is employed, determine the type of occupation and whether he is employed in a noise-polluted environment.

This information will be useful in preparing an individualized plan of care.

Psychological history

As the nurse takes the psychological history, focus should be placed on information such as the client's feelings about the hearing impairment and his coping patterns. It will also be useful to observe the client's behavior during the history, because valuable information might be obtained. Inquire about the family's reaction and feelings about the problem. If aids are used (for example, hearing aid), obtaining information about adjustment to such devices will also be valid information as the care plan is developed.

Physical assessment

The physical assessment skill necessary for examination of the ear is *inspection*. Adequate illumination is essential for this examination. Examination of the infant and young child requires the assistance of a second person because young children tend to resist examination and frequently struggle during the process. The parent can be a helpful assistant. Depending on how much the child struggles, it may be necessary to use retraints. If these are required, they should be applied carefully.

The position the client assumes during the examination depends on his stage of development. For example, the infant or child can be placed in a supine position, whereas the older child and adult may be examined in a sitting position. The child's arms should be held in an extended position close to the side of the head, with the head turned in the opposite direction of the ear being examined. The client should be informed of his role during the examination.

A systematic examination should be made of the ear, including the position and configuration, size, location of auricle, symmetry, patency, and presence of deformities. For better visualization of the external auditory canal, pull the auricle down and back for the child and up and out for the adult (Fig. 14-2). On performing this part of the examination, pay close attention to the color, texture, and odor of cerumen.

An *otoscope,* which is used to inspect the structure of the external canal, tympanic membrane, middle ear, and eustachian tube, facilitates this portion of the examination. Such examination requires special skills. An ear speculum is used to dilate the canal to permit greater visibility. This examination rules out involvement in the conductive apparatus and is best carried out with the client in the sitting position. Observation should also be made of the amount and type of drainage.

FIG. 14-2
Comparison of maneuver required to alter contour of external canal for visualization of adult tympanic membrane and young child's tympanic membrane. (From Chinn, Peggy L.: Child health maintenance, ed. 2, St. Louis, 1979, The C.V. Mosby Co.)

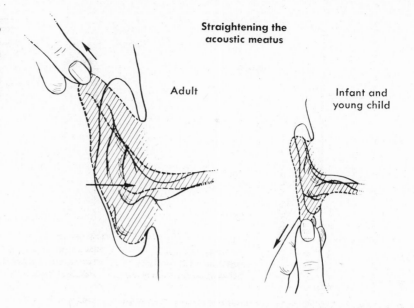

Straightening the acoustic meatus

Adult

Infant and young child

The ears normally join the scalp on or above an imaginary line drawn across the inner and outer canthus of the eye. Abnormally low-set auricles may be indicative of a congenital defect.

Assessment of hearing ability. Lack of development of expected behaviors or changes in the client's behavior often indicate some degree of hearing impairment. Because of the close relationship of hearing and speech, assessments should be made in both areas. Some of the cues that may suggest hearing impairment in various age groups are listed below.

In the *infant* the nurse should be alert to the following:
1. Failure of the infant to blink at sudden and often loud noises.
2. Failure of the infant to turn his head toward the source of sound.
3. A failure of the infant to imitate words.

In the *preschool child* the nurse should be alert to the following:
1. Absence of babbling in a baby. At the age of 9 months a baby should produce two- to three-syllable babbling (such as "ma-ma" or "da-da").
2. Develops speech slowly. A normal 2½-year-old child has a vocabulary of 300 to 400 words and considerable skill in communication.
3. Responds more to vibrations and touch than to airborne sound. One may note that to waken a child with a hearing impairment, it may be necessary to touch him.
4. Expresses wants by pointing, grunting, or placing the hand on the desired object.
5. Responds mainly to loud sounds. He may exhibit behavioral disorders because of frustrations with communication. The child is often described as being physically aggressive and unmanageable.

In the *school-age child* the nurse should be alert to the following[11]:
1. Gives irrelevant answers, may not follow directions, or may follow them incorrectly.

2. Requests to have words repeated frequently.
3. Is inattentive and daydreams.
4. Performs scholastically below the level of his apparent ability.
5. Hears much better when watching the speaker's face. May respond to changes in facial expressions more readily than to words.
6. Tends to withdraw from activities necessitating conversation. He often is not interested in casual conversation.
7. Deviates in speech-sound articulation.
8. Responds more to movement than to sound.
9. Is often described as shy, timid, and dreamy.

Other cues that should alert the nurse and family to a hearing impairment are the development of behavioral problems and failure to listen to the radio or watch television at normal volume. He may turn up the volume so high that discomfort is experienced among others in the environment. In the classroom the child may cup his hand behind his ear in an attempt to hear conversations.

Hearing impairment in the adult may be noted by an increasing difficulty in communication, which is more pronounced when he engages in group conversation or when he listens in a noisy environment. Other behaviors are similar to those that have been discussed previously, for example, lack of normal response to sound, inattentiveness, difficulty in following verbal directions, failure to respond when spoken to, frequent requests to repeat previous statements, tendency to turn one ear toward the speaker, monotonous or unusual voice quality, and unusually loud or soft speech.[2] These behaviors are also common among older adults.

DIAGNOSTIC ASSESSMENT

Auditory screening

Auditory screening, used to detect defective hearing, should be a part of the routine examination in the nursery (Fig. 14-3), during infancy, in the preschool, school age (Fig. 14-4), and adolescent period. This is especially indicated if the individual has borderline hearing acuity. The choice of screening test usually depends on the maturational level of the client.

Screening test during the preschool period. Since auditory behavior during the *first 3 months* of life is mainly reflexive, hearing tests for the very young infant are those that require him to perform some action in response to sound. One of the first tests that may be performed is one using a noisemaker. Horns, rattles, an alarm clock, or a bell may be sounded, and a notation made of the child's response. Generalized body activity indicates that the infant hears. Other expected responses are eye-blinking and eye-clenching, movement of the fingers or toes, alteration in the breathing pattern, and head-rolling or movement of the eyes.

The child between *3 and 12 months* will attempt to localize the sound by moving his head in the direction of the sound or rolling his eyes. The older child's responses may range from a smile to cessation of activity.

The child may also be placed in a room with a high-fidelity amplifying system with speakers in several locations. The child's responses to the sounds coming from various directions are noted.

Around *1 year* of age the child responds better to soft, quiet noises. Therefore a *voice test* may be performed on a child up to *18 to 24 months* of age to give an estimate of the child's hearing ability. This test is not considered ex-

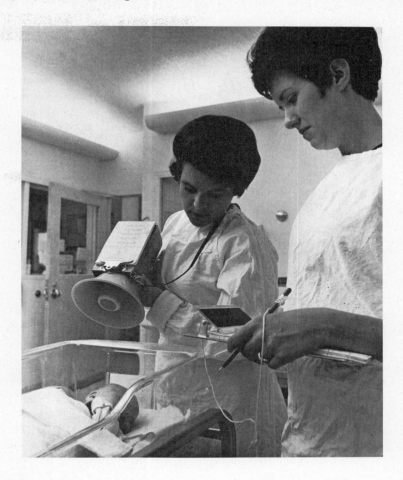

FIG. 14-3
Nurses performing auditory screening on newborn. One nurse uses infant audiometer to present sounds of selected intensities while other nurse records responses. (Courtesy Tracor, Inc., Austin, Tex.)

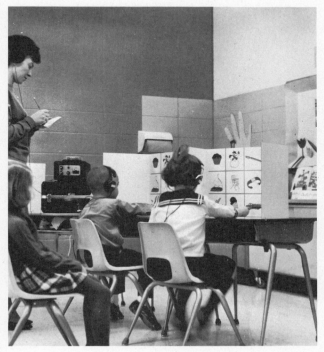

FIG. 14-4
Auditory screening being performed on school-age children. Recorded words identifying pictures are presented through earphones at predetermined intensity. If incorrect pictures are selected, child is given more detailed test on individual basis. Note one-to-one observation. (Courtesy Zenith Hearing Instrument Corporation, a subsidiary of Zenith Radio Corporation, Chicago.)

tremely accurate unless the pitch and voice are controlled electronically. The examiner may softly call the child's name or repeat soft syllables. The child around 2 *years* of age may be asked to respond to specific requests such as "show me your finger" or "point to your ear."

Audiometric screening tests. Audiometric screening may be performed for children 3 years of age and older.

Pure tone audiometry determines the client's ability to discriminate pure tones of different frequencies and intensities. The pure tones may be barely audible or extremely loud. Sounds are usually presented through earphones.

This method uses electronic equipment to evaluate the degree and type of hearing loss for pure tone and speech. The measurement of hearing is represented by the use of an audiogram, a graph on which an individual's hearing threshold at varied frequencies is recorded (Fig. 14-5). An audiometer is the instrument used to measure hearing, and the unit of measurement for determining hearing is the decibel. The decibel is represented on the horizontal lines of the audiogram. The N line (0 db) represents normal hearing thresholds for all frequencies. The lines above it are used to record better than average hearing scores. In contrast, the bottom line (100 db) represents the deafness level. The vertical lines represent the frequencies that are usually tested (measured in cycles per second, or hertz [Hz]): 125, 250, 500, 1,000, 2,000, 4,000, and 8,000 Hz.

The examiner's voice or the phonograph record of a voice are used in *speech audiometry*. The voice is presented through gradually decreasing volumes until the threshold level is determined. The voice is transmitted through earphones or a loud speaker. When the voice is presented through earphones, the test may be administered individually or in groups.

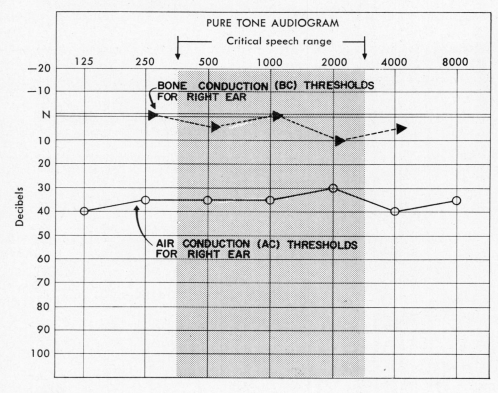

FIG. 14-5
Audiogram gives graphic outline of individual's hearing as measured by pure tones. (From Saunders, William H., and others: Nursing care in eye, ear, nose, and throat disorders, ed. 4, St. Louis, 1979, The C.V. Mosby Co.)

Cortical audiometry is a computerized form of brain-wave analysis similar to the electroencephalogram. Sounds are presented through an earphone, and the responses are recorded. Cortical audiometry is usually performed after previous tests indicate some degree of hearing loss. The client is sedated before the examination.

Speech discrimination determines how well speech is heard. The client is given a list of phonetically balanced words (such as deck and peck) about 30 db above the speech reception threshold. If the client is not able to discriminate, he may complain that the words seem to run together or he may complain of difficulty in understanding the spoken word.

The nurse should plan so that the chances of getting false-positive results are decreased. It may be helpful to allow the young child to practice the test step by step before the actual testing. Any measure that will help maintain confidence should be tried. For example, the child may be permitted to handle the equipment. The environment should be friendly. During the test, the infant or young child may be permitted to sit on the mother's lap. The nurse should also observe the client for the presence of aural drainage. If it is present, the physician should be notified, and the test should be rescheduled after the drainage ceases. The child should not be tired, fretful, or hungry, because all these feelings may result in false-positive results. The test should therefore be performed between feeding schedules.

It is best to perform the audiometric test in a soundproof room. If such a room is not available, the nurse should be sure that the testing room is free from distracting noises. Care must also be maintained not to distract the client, particularly the small infant, since any movement or shadow may cause him to turn toward the stimulus. This will give the impression that he hears when, in fact, he may not.

Tuning fork tests. A number of tests may be used to detect hearing loss. Included among these are tuning fork tests. The nurse, to facilitate preparation of a plan of care, must be familiar with these tests.

The Weber, Rinne, and Schwabach tests are tuning fork tests used to evaluate conductive and sensorineural hearing loss. An activated tuning fork is used for each of these. To test air conduction, the fork is held close to the external auditory meatus. Bone conduction is tested by pressing the base of the vibrating fork against the skull or mastoid.

The *Weber test* compares bone conduction of both ears. A tuning fork is placed against the client's forehead, and the client is asked to announce when he hears the sound. If the sound is heard better in the affected ear, the impairment is of the conductive type. If the vibration is heard better in the normal ear, the hearing loss in the affected ear is thought to be of the sensorineural type.

The *Rinne test* compares the client's acuity for air conduction with his acuity for bone conduction. The fork is placed against the mastoid bone of the ear being tested. When the vibrations cannot be heard by the client through the mastoid bone, the fork is transferred to the external auditory meatus, where it remains until sound is no longer heard. A comparison is made of the results of the two testing positions. Normally air conduction is about twice as long as bone conduction. If this is the case in the test, the individual has positive Rinne test results.

The *Schwabach test* compares the bone conduction of the individual being tested with normal hearing (usually the examiner's). The examiner places the fork on the mastoid of the client. The fork is left in place until the tone is no longer heard. At this time, the fork is transferred to the examiner's mastoid. If the tone is still heard, it indicates that the client may have a sensorineural hearing loss.

One of the major drawbacks of these tests is that they do not give quantitative information. Therefore, before therapeutic intervention is started, audiometric tests must be performed.

Tests of vestibular function. Certain tests are useful in evaluating labyrinth function. These include caloric and rotation tests.

Labyrinth function is stimulated when the temperature of the labyrinth fluid is raised or lowered. This is the basic principle used in the *caloric test*. The ear canal is filled with a determined amount of warm or cold water as the head is tilted backward. Nystagmus will be produced as the head is tilted in various positions. Cold water should produce a nystagmus that moves away from the stimulated ear, and the opposite effect should be produced when warm water is used.

For the *rotation test,* the client is placed in a rotating chair. Young children are thought to do best if they are allowed to sit in the mother's or nurse's lap during the test. The chair is rotated to the right and left for a specified length of time and a specified number of times. If the labyrinth is functioning normally, the nystagmus will be in the direction opposite of the rotation.

Tests to determine vestibular function may be administered in the nursery and periodically throughout life.

Data analysis

After necessary data have been obtained about the client, the nurse should compare the data with norms appropriate to the client's age, sex, and developmental level. Considerations should be given to the client's family, social background, and health status as the data are analyzed in preparation for the formulation of nursing diagnoses. Potential or actual diagnoses may include grief, disturbance in self-concept, sensory perception alteration, fear, alteration in comfort, impaired verbal communication, ineffective coping, and potential for injury.

Planning
PLANNING FOR HEALTH PROMOTION

An essential aspect of care is health promotion. Hearing plays such an important part in speech and language development that individuals should be aware of ways to preserve auditory function. Knowledge about the care of the ears is important and basic to preventing hearing problems. Instruction should start with the mother in the early antenatal period. The importance of antenatal care should be stressed. With adequate care and instructions, conditions that can lead to premature births are more likely to be detected and prevented. The expectant mother should be instructed to avoid infections that may affect the auditory development of the fetus, for example, childhood diseases. In the infancy period, proper immunization schedules should be followed so that childhood diseases, which may result in hearing impairment, can be prevented.

The nurse can further instruct individuals of precautionary measures against infections and injuries and the proper care of their ears. Some individuals have a tendency to irrigate their ears because of cerumen (wax) accumulation. This practice should be discouraged, because the wax affords some protection for the middle ear. When performed, it should be carried out by a physician under sterile conditions. Individuals should also be instructed on how to properly blow their noses. This should be done gently, with the nares and eyes open.

Because infections are common causes of hearing impairment, individuals should be informed about the signs of an ear infection. When these signs are experienced, instruction should be given to seek health care assistance so that proper therapy can be implemented. Frequent colds and other upper respiratory tract infections are conditions that commonly lead to ear infection; therefore proper rest and adequate nutrition should be encouraged to help the client maintain his resistance against infection.

Prevention of injuries such as tympanic rupture is important. Children and adults should be informed of the possible consequences of slapping another individual on the ear. Individuals who have a tendency to put sharp objects into the ear for cleaning purposes should be discouraged from doing so, because such practice may injure the tympanic membrane and thus affect hearing.

Following are several consequences that may result when hearing problems are not detected early:

1. The child may fail to develop normal language and speech. Hearing is essential if the child is to learn to talk. Distorted speech is likely to result when only partial sounds are heard.
2. The child becomes deprived of the give-and-take relationship with the family and surroundings, which is basic for speech and language development and for personal growth and satisfaction.
3. The educational process will be interfered with if language cannot be comprehended. If the child fails to achieve, he may be classed as being mentally retarded.
4. Adjustment problems may become manifested. Children may become overaggressive, disobedient, or withdrawn.
5. Family relationships may be affected because of anxiety, guilt feelings, or shame about the impairment.

Since speech development and emotional growth depend on the ability to hear, early detection of hearing impairment is essential. The nurse should encourage a periodic auditory examination, particularly in those with a family history of deafness and in children whose mother had a viral infection in early pregnancy. Adults who work in loud industrial noise should also have frequent auditory tests.

When a hearing impairment is suspected, the client should be referred to an otologist or an otolaryngologist.

PLANNING FOR HEALTH MAINTENANCE AND RESTORATION

Ear drops and irrigation

Ear drops and ear irrigations may be prescribed for clients who have conditions associated with the ear. Since the client or a family member may be the one to actually perform these irrigations, instructions should be given to the essential principles regarding *temperature, pressure,* and *position.*

The *temperature* of ear drops or solutions should be near body temperature (about 100° F or 37.7° C) because vertigo may occur if the temperature of the solution is too high or too low. Solutions can easily be warmed by holding the bottle in the palms of the hands.

Nursing process for common health problems

To ensure proper *placement* of ear drops, place drops so that they run in the wall of the canal and so that air does not become entrapped. The auricle should be moved gently down and back in the child to straighten the ear canal, thus permitting the medicine to be properly placed.

During irrigation the client (or family member) must be concerned about the *pressure* of the flow of solution. The pressure should be low to prevent damage to the eardrum. To control the pressure flow, the height of the container or the force applied to the bulb must be controlled.

Health effects of noise

Excessive noise has been documented to overstimulate the hair cells within the inner ear and subsequently result in degeneration of the organ of Corti. Hearing loss from noise is a slow, gradual process, and tends to be permanent. Health care personnel should therefore inform individuals about the effects that noise has on health, as well as means of prevention. (See also Chapter 4.)

Individuals who work in loud industrial or entertainment settings should be encouraged to wear some type of hearing protector. Some forms of earplugs have been demonstrated that reduce noise by 20 to 35 db. However, to be effective, the plugs must fit directly in the meatus. It may be necessary to consult a physician to ensure a proper fit. When plugs are worn, instructions should be given regarding the importance of keeping them clean so that chances of developing an ear infection are decreased. Earmuffs are also useful. They are worn over the ear and come in various shapes. Both earplugs and earmuffs are relatively inexpensive. Rubber, plastic, and wax-impregnated cotton are helpful and provide a similar form of protection. Ordinary cotton and swimming earplugs should not be used for noise protection because they do not provide the same degree of protection against loud noise.

Clients who work in noisy environments (industrial or entertainment settings) should be encouraged to have periodic examinations so that changes in hearing acuity can be detected early.

Caring for the client with hearing impairment

Often the client with a hearing impairment is able to manage at home, but when he is in the hospital or an unfamiliar environment, his hearing may seem to diminish. (This may occur even in the client with normal hearing.) Anxiety and lack of security provided by unfamiliar surroundings are often responsible for this reaction. Therefore health care personnel should be aware of ways of communicating with him. The following guide will prove helpful to the nurse and families of hard-of-hearing clients.

1. Avoid using gestures without speech. Gestures may be used in combination with speech. Facial expression and physical contact should be used to convey the warmth, understanding, or concern that is normally expressed verbally. On the other hand, for the *deaf* client, a warm smile and touch are more effective than the usual verbal greeting.
2. Face the client when talking to him. The person with a hearing impairment becomes an expert at lipreading; therefore by facing him movements can be readily seen. Light on the speaker's face should be adequate and without glare. Conversing with the hard-of-hearing client in a dim, shadowy room may result in the client's not understanding what is being said. The nurse might stand near a window to avoid confusing shadows across the face.
3. Speak in a natural tone of voice and keep your voice at about the same

volume. *Do not* shout. Raising the voice only confuses the client, because such practice causes the sounds to become distorted. Second, speaking loudly is a common way to express anger. Such clients may therefore misinterpret loud speech as an expression of anger.

4. Speak distinctly and as close to the client as possible.

5. Allow time for cues to reach the client and to be integrated at the cortical level.

6. Use short phrases and sentences. Subject-verb-object is the expected sequence and more easily understood than complicated dependent clauses.

7. Assess the client for signs that indicate lack of understanding: a puzzled expression or inappropriate response. When this happens, rephrase the sentence in simpler language.

8. Long drawn-out conversations should be avoided because they cause frustration and fatigue in the client, who must strain in order to hear.

9. Do not communicate with someone else in front of the hard-of-hearing or deaf client without cueing him in, because this may lead him to suspect that the conversation is about him and may result in hurt feelings and misunderstandings.

10. Provide paper and pencil when necessary.

11. If the client wears glasses, allow him to wear them as he desires. This is important because a hearing impairment, especially in the older client, is often accompanied by decreased visual acuity. Without glasses, he cannot make full use of visual cues, which help him to compensate for the hearing deficit.

Implementation

COMMON HEALTH PROBLEMS OF THE NEONATE

Congenital anomalies of the ear

Congenital anomalies of the ear are common and may involve the auricle, external, middle, or inner ear. The auricle may be partially or completely absent. The external ear canal may not be patent, and as a result the neonate will experience some hearing impairment.

Macrotia (excessively large auricles), *microtia* (small auricles of normal shape, *anotia* (complete absence of the auricle), and *polyotia* (the presence of a number of auricles on the same side) are congenital disorders. Except for the psychological impact, macrotia is the least serious. Microtia is more serious, especially when it occurs bilaterally, because it may be accompanied by atresia of the external auditory meatus and maldevelopment of the middle ear, eustachian tube, and mastoid process. Deafness may also accompany this disorder.

Parents of children with ear deformities may be alarmed when they find out about the deformity. This is a normal reaction, and the nurse must allow them to express their feelings. All their questions should be answered, and they should not be made to feel guilty. The nurse should be familiar with available resources so that necessary information can be given to the parents. If the child's ear is absent, a prosthesis may be purchased. This may be glued to the side of the head. Young individuals may be terribly upset about a deformed ear. They can be encouraged to wear their hair in a way that hides the deformity until reconstructive surgery can be performed. Reconstructive surgery should be performed as early as possible.

Congenital atresia, an absence of the auditory meatus, is usually associated with microtia. Usually it is unilateral and is accompanied by normal internal ear structures. When this is the case, therapy is delayed because hearing and speech development will not be impaired. At the age of 3 or 4, plastic reconstruction of the ear may be performed to restore the meatus. However, if the atresia is bilateral, surgery may be performed during infancy to prevent retardation of hearing and speech.

COMMON HEALTH PROBLEMS OF INFANTS AND CHILDREN

Otitis media

Otitis media, an infection of the lining of the middle ear, is usually caused by beta hemolytic streptococci, pneumococci, and *Haemophilus influenzae.* Since the lining of the middle ear is continuous with the tympanic membrane and mastoid cells, infection of one structure usually leads to infection of the others.

In infants and children, *acute otitis media* is usually secondary to an upper respiratory tract infection because of the shortness and position of the eustachian tube and its relationship to the nasopharynx. The short eustachian tube provides a ready path for the entrance of infection into the middle ear. The incidence of acute otitis media is also thought to be higher in bottle-fed babies because of the horizontal position of the eustachian tube and the position commonly used in feeding. Breast-fed babies are normally held more or less upright, whereas bottle-fed babies may be allowed to lie on their backs. As a result of the latter, milk may migrate into the nasopharynx and tympanic cavity by way of the eustachian tube, thereby becoming a source of inflammation. In older persons, excessive nose blowing and unwise syringing of the nasal passages may cause secretions to be forced into the middle ear and may set up an infection. In an adult the eustachian tube becomes less of a causative factor because it is elongated and narrower and assumes a 45-degree angle.

Assessment. Pain, which is caused by irritation of the nerve endings in the inflamed ear, is the main symptom. The infant or young child may indicate pain by crying, rolling the head, tugging at the ears, or tilting the head to one side. The older child and adult describe the pain as being sharp and lancinating. Restlessness and irritability are not uncommon. Pyrexia, chills, nausea, and vomiting may also be present. As the fluid pressure builds up within the ear, pain becomes more severe, and the membrane may rupture. The appearance of purulent or serosanguineous drainage from the ear canal is an indication of a ruptured membrane. Following the rupture, pain is relieved.

> **Data analysis**
> *Data analysis may reveal nursing diagnoses of alterations in comfort and sensory perception alterations.*

Planning and implementation. Therapy is planned to prevent further infection and promote comfort. Antibiotics are prescribed and are specific to the organism causing the infection. Antibiotics commonly used are ampicillin, amoxicillin, or penicillin with sulfa. In addition to antibiotic therapy, decongestants such as syrup of ephedrine or elixir of phenylephrine may be used. Decongestants are useful in that they tend to shrink mucous membranes. Such effects, in turn, facilitate drainage from the middle ear. Either of these is usually admin-

734

istered until the infection is eradicated. The ears should be cleansed with dry wipes, while employing aseptic principles.

A *myringotomy* may be performed if the tympanic membrane bulges and if the client is in considerable pain. This is a procedure in which an incision is made into the tympanic membrane to release purulent fluid, thereby relieving pain and facilitating healing of the drum. Healing usually takes place within 24 hours after the procedure. If repeated attacks of otitis media occur, the physician may implant a tympanic membrane button in the ear to facilitate drainage.

 Evaluation. The nursing care plan for the client with otitis media is developed around diagnoses related to alterations in comfort and sensory perception alteration. This component of the process is ongoing.

EXPECTED OUTCOMES
The child and/or family can:
1. Describe otitis media.
2. State plans for preventing further infection and promoting comfort.
3. State use, dosage, time, route, and side effects of prescribed medications.
4. State limitation of activity (for example, swimming).
5. State indications requiring follow-up health care.
6. State plans for follow-up health care.

Chronic otitis media Chronic otitis media is a middle ear infection that occurs as a result of bacterial infection of the tympanic membrane.[7]

Pathophysiology. Repeated infections may cause necrotic changes in the tympanic membrane or the formation of cholesteatoma. As a result, a purulent discharge drains from the ear. If the infection is allowed to progress, the hair cells and mastoid bone become involved.

Data analysis
Data analysis may reveal nursing diagnoses of alterations in comfort and sensory perception alterations.

 Planning and implementation. Aural hygiene and antibiotics are important therapeutic measures. All debris should be removed from the ear by cleansing or irrigation before instilling the medication (for example, antibiotics). Such measures promote healing. Hydrogen peroxide solution may be used to assist with cleansing. The solution may be instilled with the child on his side. The position should be maintained for several minutes. Instructions are usually given to clients to keep their ears dry to prevent the infection from becoming reactivated. Swimming is discouraged.

Evaluation. The nursing care plan for the client with chronic otitis media is developed around diagnoses related to alterations in comfort and sensory perception alteration. This component of the process is ongoing.

EXPECTED OUTCOMES
The child and/or family can:
1. Describe chronic otitis media.
2. State plans for preventing further infection and promoting comfort.
3. State use, dosage, time, route, and side effects of prescribed medications.
4. Demonstrate proper technique for cleansing the ear canal.
5. State limitation of activity (for example, swimming).
6. State indications requiring follow-up health care.
7. State plans for follow-up health care.

735

Nursing process for common health problems

Foreign bodies

Children are prone to place objects in their ears—beads, erasers, crayons, paper, peas, or seeds. This may be done out of boredom or curiosity or to relieve irritation. Live insects may find their way into the ears of persons sleeping in the open, such as on a camping trip. At any age, pieces of sand, gravel, and food particles may accidentally become lodged in the ear.

 Assessment. The presence of a foreign body may be detected immediately, or weeks may pass before it is detected. The nature of the object may determine whether it is noticed immediately or later. For example, insects move within the ear and cause loud noises, tickling, and discomfort. Seldom do they cause trauma. Sharp mineral objects may damage the middle ear. Vegetable foreign bodies have a tendency to swell and cause local inflammation. An impairment of hearing may be one of the first signs to indicate that a foreign object is within the ear. The development of a local cellulitis may cause pain.

> **Data analysis**
> *Data analysis may reveal nursing diagnoses of alterations in comfort, sensory perception alterations, and potential for injury.*

 Planning and implementation. No attempt should be made by an unskilled person to remove a foreign object from the ear because such action may result in damage to the eardrum or the object may be embedded deeper. Rather than run these risks, the client should be seen by a physician so that the object can be removed safely.

Preparation for removal. Before attempts are made to remove the foreign object, the client's cooperation must be obtained. Explanations should be given about the purpose and expectations of the procedure. It may be necessary to restrain the young child with mummy restraints. The nurse positions the client so that the involved ear is uppermost. Occasionally an anesthetic may have to be administered as a precautionary measure if the child struggles to resist treatment.

Removal of the foreign object. The procedure used for removing an object depends on its nature and position. Foreign bodies of vegetable composition may have swollen by absorbing moisture and thus may have become impacted. Therefore water or fluids are not used in removing these because fluids tend to create additional swelling and cause the object to become wedged in the bony canal in such a way as to cause severe pain and make removal more difficult. Foreign bodies of a nonvegetable nature, such as beads or rubber, are best removed by irrigation. Insects may be killed by instilling a few drops of an oily substance, or drowned with water and then removed by syringing or with forceps. Specially designed forceps may be used to remove foreign objects that have not penetrated beyond the isthmus. If the object cannot be removed by syringing or with forceps, the physician may extract it through a postauricular incision. This method, however, is seldom necessary. After removal, antibiotics may be instilled into the ear to prevent infection. Once the object is removed, the nurse should instruct the child about the hazards of such acts and encourage him not to do it again.

 Evaluation. The client who inserts a foreign object into the ear has problems of alterations in comfort, sensory perception alterations, and potential for injury. The nursing care plan should focus on measures for comfort, communication, and client instruction.

EXPECTED OUTCOMES

The client and/or family can:
1. Describe potential sources of foreign objects.
2. Describe signs indicative of a foreign object in the ear.
3. State plans for prevention of recurrences.
4. State indications requiring follow-up health care.

COMMON HEALTH PROBLEMS OF THE YOUNG ADULT

Otosclerosis

Otosclerosis is caused by the replacement of normal bone by a spongy bone, and the condition invades the labyrinth and fixes (ankyloses), the footplate of the stapes.[12] As a result, the vibration system of the middle ear is impaired. The client is therefore unable to hear sounds conducted by air vibration. The exact cause of otosclerosis is unknown. It is thought to be hereditary and is commonly found in females after puberty and during pregnancy, the puerperium, or menopause.

 Assessment. Otosclerosis usually begins with a gradual loss of hearing and tinnitus. Clients with otosclerosis often have difficulty in hearing a whisper or understanding a person speaking from a distance. Their own voice sounds seem unusually loud, and so, to compensate, they speak in such low voices that they can barely be understood. As bone conduction increases, even the sounds of chewing become intensified. They therefore hear poorly during meals. This is often a factor that intensifies problems related to family and social life. The client tends to withdraw from conversation because of the embarrassment experienced from constantly asking friends and relatives to repeat. At the same time, his family and friends may grow tired of constantly having to talk louder and therefore tend to leave the client out of conversations. Clients usually give a history of being able to hear better in noisy surroundings. This is related to the fact that people tend to raise their voices in noisy surroundings.

Audiometric and tuning fork tests usually make the diagnosis evident. In the tuning fork test, bone conduction is better than air conduction, which is the opposite of the normal condition.

Hearing loss may be corrected by the use of a hearing aid or surgery.

> **Data analysis**
> *Data analysis may reveal nursing diagnoses of alterations in comfort and sensory perception alterations.*

 Planning and implementation. Surgery is the primary form of therapy. When surgery is performed for otosclerosis, one of three operations may be performed: stapedectomy, fenestration, or stapes mobilization. At present, stapedectomy is the operation of choice because it affords a higher level of hearing than the other operations and hospitalization is shortened to 2 or 3 days. Surgery is performed with the client under local anesthesia and with the aid of a microscope. Vertigo and dizziness, which occur as a result of stimulation of the inner ear during surgery, are common complaints after each operation.

In a *stapedectomy* procedure the entire stapes is removed, and a bone, fat, or stainless steel prosthesis is inserted to replace the stapes. The prosthesis restores normal air-conduction hearing by providing a new movable pathway across the middle of the inner ear. In the *stapes mobilization* operation, the footplate of the stapes is loosened to permit the stapes to vibrate.

737

With the *fenestration operation* a new window is created, which redirects vibrations by allowing them to pass from the external auditory canal to the inner ear. The procedure is more extensive than the stapedectomy or stapes mobilization. The fenestration operative procedure requires the client to spend a week in the hospital, a couple of weeks convalescing, and a refrain from any strenuous activity during this time.

Care of the client having ear surgery

Preoperative nursing care. During the preoperative period the client should be adequately prepared for surgery. The physician instructs the client about the potential of hearing improvement and the hazards of the surgery. The nurse must be aware of what the client knows and should reinforce instructions by basing explanations on what he has been told by the physician. Instructions should also be given about preoperative and postoperative care. These explanations may be given by the office nurse before the client is admitted for surgery. Generally the preoperative routines do not differ significantly from routines for general surgery. However, some of the specifics that should be discussed include measures related to maintenance of safety and prevention of complications.

The client is instructed to shampoo the hair before the surgery. It is important to keep water out of the involved ear. The head movements required for shampooing will increase sensations of dizziness.

The client must be told that during surgery the head will be kept absolutely still. Because equilibrium is disturbed postoperatively, the client is cautioned not to attempt to get out of bed without assistance and to avoid nose blowing for at least a week after surgery. Blowing the nose might cause air to be forced into the eustachian tube, thus causing the eardrum to become loosened. Mucus is also forced into the eustachian tube, which may become a source of infection. To avoid complications, the client is instructed in the proper way to blow the nose: blowing gently, with the nostrils unrestricted and the eyes open.

Postoperative nursing care. In the postoperative period, therapy is planned to promote comfort and safety, promote psychological well-being, and prevent complications.

PROMOTING COMFORT AND SAFETY. Postoperatively, particularly after a stapedectomy, head movements should be kept at a minimum. Bed rest is usually prescribed for at least 24 hours, and the client is encouraged to remain flat, even for meals. This precaution lessens the chances of the prosthesis slipping out of position. The client should be discouraged from watching fast-moving objects, especially on television, because this increases the sensation of vertigo. Passive range-of-motion exercises should be performed to enhance relaxation of muscles, improve circulation, and prevent joint stiffness.

Medications for pain should be administered as often as necessary. Sedatives may also be prescribed for restlessness, and antibiotics to prevent infection and promote healing.

Because of disturbance of the semicircular canals during surgery, the client must be assisted when he ambulates. As he changes from a lying to a standing position, the nurse should use the same guidelines that would be used for a client who has been on bed rest for prolonged periods. The client should be allowed to sit up before assuming a standing position, and on standing, he should be encouraged to look straight ahead rather than look down. This helps him maintain his balance.

PROMOTING PSYCHOLOGICAL WELL-BEING. The client needs reassurance about diminished hearing acuity. This may be caused by swelling within the ear canal or the presence of a dressing. He may be concerned over hearing fluid "slushing" within the ear. The appearance of this symptom should be brought to the attention of the physician because it indicates that serous fluid is collecting within the middle ear.

OBSERVING FOR DEVELOPMENT OF COMPLICATIONS. The nurse should be aware of conditions that are likely to occur after surgery of the inner ear. Bleeding, meningitis, and facial nerve involvement are common complications. The appearance of these or related signs should be reported to the physician.

Frequent assessments should be made of the vital signs and visible bleeding on the dressing.

The facial nerve (a mixed nerve) passes within the bony canal through the middle ear. As a result, it may be affected during surgery. The motor branches go to the muscle of the cheek, lips, forehead, and eyelids. Signs indicative of facial nerve involvement include facial paralysis or facial weakness. To assess facial nerve damage, the nurse should instruct the client to show his teeth, wrinkle his forehead, raise his eyebrows, or close his eyes. Inability to perform these activities may indicate facial nerve involvement. Other indications include a pulling of the mouth toward the unaffected side, while the weakened or paralyzed side remains immobile. The unaffected eye closes tightly, but the paralyzed eyelid remains open. The mouth droops, and the client is unable to drink fluids without their dripping from the mouth. He may not be able to whistle.

The chorda tympani branch of the facial nerve carries sensory nerve fibers from the sweet and sour taste buds in the anterior two thirds of the tongue. It also carries secretion-stimulating fibers for the submaxillary and sublingual glands. Damage to the chorda tympani may result in symptoms of mouth dryness and a bitter, metallic taste. Awareness of the potential for these symptoms to develop will enable the nurse to allay the client's fears if they are experienced.

Signs of meningeal irritation may be caused by bacterial contamination by inner ear fluid. If this occurs, organisms could be transmitted to the cerebrospinal fluid because there is a communication between the inner ear and subarachnoid spaces. The nurse should report to the physician immediately such signs as persistent headache, temperature elevation, chills, nuchal rigidity, nausea, and vomiting.

Because of the proximity of some vagal fibers to the middle ear, symptoms of pallor, nausea, and vomiting may be experienced. A quiet and comfortable environment usually helps relieve these symptoms.

Discharge instructions. Instructions for home care should be given before the client leaves the hospital. Since the client is usually discharged with a dressing, instructions should include principles of sterile technique. The client and a family member should be instructed about changing the dressing properly. Directions should be given *not* to touch the inside of the cotton pad or dressing and to refrain from getting the dressing wet while showering. Some type of plastic material may be placed over the dressing to keep it dry. Sudden movements should be avoided. It may be necessary to advise the client against riding in elevators. Adequate rest should be encouraged, and he should avoid people who have upper respiratory tract infections.

Evaluation. The nursing care plan for the client with otosclerosis is developed around diagnoses related to comfort and sensory perception.

EXPECTED OUTCOMES

The client and/or family can:
1. Describe otosclerosis.
2. Verbalize limitations.
3. State plans for health maintenance and care.
4. Demonstrate proper technique for dressing change.
5. Verbalize plans for follow-up care.

Meniere's disease

Meniere's disease is a chronic inner ear disease caused by an increase in endolymphatic pressure. It affects both sexes and usually occurs between the third and sixth decades.

Assessment. Tinnitus, unilateral hearing loss, and vertigo are characteristic symptoms. During the early stages of the disease, tinnitus is intermittent and is associated with a vertigo attack. It may, however, occur in the absence of vertigo. As the disease progresses, the symptoms, which are often described as a hissing, roaring, or ringing sensation, increase in frequency and severity.

Attacks of vertigo usually occur suddenly without warning. The client becomes frightened and feels as though the environment is spinning. Even a slight movement of the head intensifies the sensation. Nausea and vomiting, sweating, pallor, and nystagmus may accompany the attack. These attacks may last for only a few minutes or persist for many hours or days. During attacks the client stays in bed but may carry on normal activities when the attack is over. An attack of vertigo may incapacitate a client for weeks. It may be necessary to delay household, employment, and social activities.

Because of the effect of the disease on equilibrium, the nurse should teach the client ways of preventing accidents within the environment.

Hearing loss associated with Meniere's disease is usually unilateral and may occur with the vertigo or occur months before the vertigo attack. Because the hearing loss occurs gradually, the client may not be aware of hearing impairment. Diagnosis is made on the basis of the presenting symptoms and results of the caloric test.

> **Data analysis**
> *Data analysis may reveal nursing diagnoses of alteration in comfort, sensory perception alterations, and potential for injury.*

Planning and implementation. Therapy is symptomatic and supportive. Bed rest is encouraged. A sedative (such as phenobarbital) may be prescribed. Antiemetics and antihistamines are prescribed to suppress motion sickness. Dimenhydrinate (Dramamine) is often prescribed for this purpose. The client should be reassured by providing support and answering questions.

Between attacks, preventive measures are often prescribed to prevent recurrences. A low-salt diet may be prescribed to reduce the disturbance in water metabolism that is thought to be responsible for causing the attacks. A vasodilator (nicotinic acid), diuretics, and antihistamines may also be prescribed.

Surgery may be delayed until the client's hearing is below the serviceable level as indicated by pure audiometry. The surgical procedures used are destruction of the labyrinth and cryosurgery of the labyrinth. Cryosurgery involves application of intense cold to the semicircular canal. The cryogenic probe is applied to the area for three 2-minute applications.

Evaluation. The nursing care plan for the client with Meniere's disease should be evaluated on an ongoing basis.

EXPECTED OUTCOMES

The client and/or family can:
1. Describe Meniere's disease.
2. State plans for health maintenance and care.
3. State use, dosage, time, route, and side effects of prescribed medications.
4. State plans for follow-up care.

COMMON HEALTH PROBLEMS THAT OCCUR ACROSS THE LIFE SPAN

Otitis externa

Otitis externa is an inflammation of the external ear caused by bacteria, fungi, virus, allergy, or chemicals. Although more common in children, it may occur at any age. Unlike other forms of otitis, it may occur as a result of small abrasions that come in contact with contaminated water while swimming, or careless use of soaps or shampoo. Otitis externa may be acute or chronic.

Assessment. In the acute stage, pain is severe, the ear is tender to the touch, and the glands in front of the tragus are enlarged. Pain is caused by edema of the skin overlying the bony ear canal, an area where there is little room to accommodate swelling.

> **Data analysis**
> *Data analysis may reveal nursing diagnoses of alterations in comfort and sensory perception alterations.*

Planning and implementation. Therapy for acute otitis externa is planned to promote cleanliness, control infection, and relieve pain. Hospitalization may be necessary. Some form of irrigation is ordered to keep the ear clean. Hot compresses may be applied for brief periods, every 2 to 3 hours, to mobilize the body defenses and for soothing purposes. A mixture of antibiotics and steroids may be applied topically to control infection and reduce inflammation. Polymyxin B sulfate, neomycin sulfate, and hydrocortisone are often prescribed for these purposes. An analgesic such as codeine may be prescribed to relieve pain, thereby facilitating sleep.

Chronic otitis externa

Chronic otitis externa is associated with a longstanding infection or with skin disorders such as psoriasis and dermatitis.

Assessment. Pain is generally not a problem, but itching and hearing loss are prominent symptoms.

Planning and implementation. For the chronic form of otitis, therapy is directed toward relieving itching and preventing consequent reinfection. Topical cream such as hydrocortisone may be prescribed. Instruction should be given to the clients to avoid irritating the ear. The client should be instructed to refrain from getting water, other contaminants, or any form of soap in the ear. Swimming should be discouraged until the symptoms have subsided. During bathing or swimming, a cotton plug may be placed into the ear. After bathing and swim-

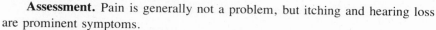

ming, the ears should be dried thoroughly with dry cotton. These practices lessen the chances of the ear's becoming reinfected.

 Evaluation. The care plan for the client with chronic otitis externa centers around alterations in comfort and sensory perception alterations.

EXPECTED OUTCOMES

The client and/or family can:
1. Describe chronic otitis externa.
2. State plans for health maintenance.
3. State use, dosage, route, frequency, and side effects of prescribed medications.
4. State plans for preventing further infection.
5. State indications for follow-up care.

Labyrinthitis

Labyrinthitis is an inflammation of the bony or membranous labyrinth that usually occurs as a result of infection of the middle ear. Two forms may occur: serous and purulent. Pain, hearing impairment, vertigo, vomiting, and loss of equilibrium are common symptoms. The infection is controlled with the use of antibiotics and sulfonamides.

Rupture of the tympanic membrane

Ruptured eardrums may be caused by varied types of trauma such as blows on the side of the head, as well as by the introduction of sharp objects, such as pencils and hairpins, into the ear. The latter is the most common cause, because many individuals deliberately introduce objects into the ear for purposes of cleaning and relieving irritation. Unskilled attempts to remove a foreign body from the ear may also result in damage to the membrane. Forceful changes of air pressure in the meatus, as might result from blast waves from loud noises or explosions, may cause the membrane to rupture. Finally, forcible syringing for various forms of therapy can result in a rupture.

 Assessment. An immediate, sharp pain and loud noises in the ear at the time of the injury are symptomatic. The pain usually subsides and is replaced by a slight hearing impairment and tinnitus. The hearing impairment is the result of a break in the continuity of the ossicular chain and possibly to the accumulation of exudate in the middle ear. Tinnitus may indicate damage to the cochlea; however, cochlear damage is most often associated with a blast injury. In such case, permanent deafness may result.

Clients should be encouraged to have an examination performed as soon as possible after these symptoms are experienced. Otoscopic examinations are generally performed to determine the extent of the injury. Audiometric hearing tests are also usually done.

 Data analysis
Data analysis may reveal nursing diagnoses of alterations in comfort and sensory perception alterations.

 Planning and implementation. Therapy is planned to prevent infection. Because infection causes the defect to enlarge and further impair hearing or cause mastoiditis, instructions about aural hygiene (for example, keeping water out of the ears during bathing or swimming) should be given. Antibiotics are prescribed. If the injury does not heal spontaneously, hearing may be enhanced by cauterization with silver nitrate to stimulate growth of the epithelium.

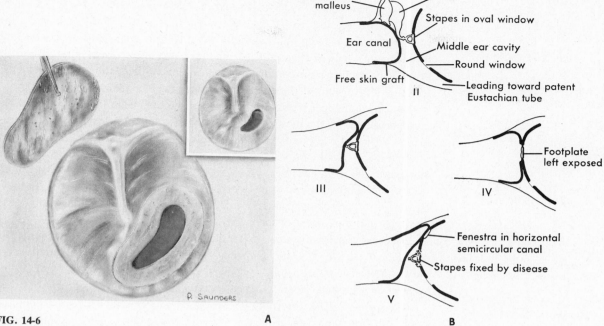

Remnant of malleus
Incus
Stapes in oval window
Ear canal
Middle ear cavity
Round window
Free skin graft
II
Leading toward patent
Eustachian tube

III

IV
Footplate
left exposed

Fenestra in horizontal
semicircular canal
Stapes fixed by disease
V

P. SAUNDERS

A   **B**

FIG. 14-6
Tympanoplasty surgical procedures. **A,**
Type I, or myringoplasty. **B,** Types II,
III, IV, and V. (From DeWeese, David
D., and Saunders, William H.: Text-
book of otolaryngology, ed. 4, St.
Louis, 1973, The C.V. Mosby Co.)

A myringoplasty may be performed when these therapies are not effective. *Tympanoplasty* refers to a group of operative procedures performed to restore hearing in clients with conductive hearing loss. There are various types of tympanoplasty procedures (Fig. 14-6). Type I, *myringoplasty,* is the simplest and is performed to close a perforated eardrum that is the result of trauma or infection. Type II is an extension of type I in which the malleus has been removed and the eardrum is replaced by a graft that makes contact with the incus. Type III is performed when only the stapes remain. The drumhead is replaced by a graft that contacts the stapes. Therefore sound is transmitted from the eardrum to the stapes. Type IV is performed with the ossicular chain has been destroyed by disease or therapeutic means. A graft attached to the tympanic orifice and middle ear space is used to create a small, air-containing cavity. In type V, an extensive skin graft is performed, and a small window is made into the horizontal canal.

Nursing care following tympanoplasty. When a tympanoplasty is performed, the client is hospitalized for approximately 4 days. A dressing is left in place; therefore the nurse should observe the dressing frequently for blood and drainage. The outer dressing may be changed as needed, but the inner dressing should remain intact.

Evaluation. The evaluation component of the nursing process is ongoing. Nursing care is planned around diagnoses such as alterations in comfort and sensory perception.

EXPECTED OUTCOMES
The client and/or family can:
1. Describe the causes of tympanic membrane rupture.
2. State plans for prevention, health maintenance, and care.
3. Describe plans for follow-up care.

743

Hearing impairment

Types of hearing loss. There are two general types of hearing loss: conductive and sensorineural. If an individual has elements of both, the condition is termed mixed hearing loss.[12]

Conductive hearing loss is present when there is damage to the conducting mechanism. It may be caused by any condition that interferes with the passage of sound waves through the external auditory meatus or the middle ear and with the transmission of stimuli through normal movement of the stapes. In children, otitis media and upper respiratory tract infections that result in obstruction of the eustachian tube are the most common causes of conductive loss. Impacted cerumen or a foreign body in the ear canal may obstruct the passage of sound waves through the external auditory canals. Abnormalities of the tympanic membrane and middle ear may interfere with sound passage to the middle ear. A congenital malformation of one of the ossicles may interfere with movement of the ossicles. Otosclerosis may cause a fixation of the stapes in the oval window and thus interfere with movement of the stapes.

Because the involvement in conductive hearing loss is in the external or middle ear, the client is able to analyze the sound once it reaches the inner ear. However, to accomplish this, sounds in the environment may have to be increased or amplified. Hearing aids are useful for this purpose.

Sensorineural hearing loss is caused by any condition that damages the organ of Corti, the cochlear nerve, or the acoustic branch of the auditory nerve (cranial nerve VIII). The causes are varied. Maternal infections such as syphilis may damage the auditory apparatus of the fetus and cause a hearing impairment. Viral infections (rubella, parotitis, rubeola) during the intrauterine period and bacterial infections (such as meningitis) during the postnatal period may be responsible for a sensorineural type impairment. Anoxia from any source, especially in the infant, may cause damage to the auditory apparatus and result in a hearing impairment.[13]

Ototoxic drugs (for example, streptomycin, kanamycin, neomycin, salicylates, or quinine) have been reported to injure or destroy the hair cells of the cochlea. Kanamycin and neomycin have been reported to be the worst offenders.[14] The use of these drugs during pregnancy may be dangerous because they cross the placental barrier and may cause congenital anomalies and deformities.[4]

Physical trauma (such as from a blow on the head) and acoustic trauma from high noise levels have been recognized as causative agents in all age groups. *Erythroblastosis fetalis* and presbycusis are other conditions responsible for causing sensorineural type hearing loss.

In a client with sensorineural loss, sounds are conducted to the inner ear, but they are not perceived. These clients also tend to speak loudly in situations where it is inappropriate.

Since there is no medical therapy for sensorineural hearing loss, clients should be encouraged to avoid factors that predispose them to this type of loss.

Mixed hearing loss is experienced when both conductive and sensorineural loss is present. Any of the states discussed under conductive and sensorineural loss may be a cause of mixed hearing loss.

Reactions to hearing impairments. Sound is an important aspect of our environment. When one becomes deprived of sounds, varied reactions may be noted. Clients with hearing impairments may feel uncomfortable and may become easily discouraged because of difficulty they may experience in understanding their family, friends, television, and radio. Many clients have a tendency to withdraw from conversations or social contacts or to limit contacts to family and friends with whom they feel comfortable. Withdrawal may particularly be observed in a noisy environment because much of what is said is missed by the hard-of-hearing client. He may give inappropriate responses to questions or statements rather than admit he did not understand. Such reactions indicate the need to avoid embarrassment from constantly asking others to repeat a statement. In less noisy surroundings where speech can be heard, withdrawal is less likely to be noted. The client may smile to cover up his inability to understand.

Many individuals with hearing impairment give the impression of being antisocial. Children may play alone, and adolescents or adults may refrain from participating in club or community activities. Older clients may sit alone and stare into space. They are often afraid of making an inappropriate response in interpersonal dialogue.[2] As a result, they may become depressed from lack of stimulation from the outside world.

The nurse should plan and instruct families to plan, so that the client remains a part of his environment (see suggestions opposite). The hard-of-hearing client should be encouraged to participate in activities with the family. Clients who are hospitalized or are in an extended-care facility should be visited frequently by family members and friends. Staff members should also plan visits periodically during the day to provide some form of stimulation.

Another reaction may be to the other extreme—the extremely aggressive client. Rather than withdraw from conversations, he may try to dominate them to cover up his hearing impairment.

The adult who is hard-of-hearing has a tendency to be paranoid. This is evidenced by the fact that on entering a room where others are laughing or talking and he cannot understand what they are saying, he often tends to think that they are talking about him or laughing at him. Therefore it is important to include hard-of-hearing individuals in conversations when they are around.

Coping with hearing impairment. The age of the client when impairment became evident and the suddenness of the impairment determine how well he will be able to cope with it. The child who is born deaf or who acquires deafness shortly after birth or before he learns to speak will possibly have defects in language development. Speech development may be arrested at the babbling or cooing stage. If this happens, he must be taught to recognize speech through visual cues. Some authorities contend that if the impairment is acquired under 4 years of age, speech will be lost entirely. If it is lost after the age of 10, the normal use of expression, speech, and articulation will remain although comprehension will be lost.[9] Another contention is that if the impairment is acquired after basic language concepts (expressive and receptive) are developed, the client's speech will not be lost but he will not develop speech beyond that point. As a result, these clients must be continually stimulated so that they do not lose the language already acquired. They must be taught and talked to. It is thought that the adult who acquires some type of hearing impairment usually has enough residual hearing present that speech can still be heard.[10]

The client who acquires a hearing impairment before speech develops is thought to have fewer adjustment problems than one who acquires the impairment after speech development. The client who suddenly experiences hearing

---

SUGGESTIONS FOR CLIENTS WITH HEARING LOSS

1. Initiate conversations rather than waiting for others to speak to you first.
2. Position yourself so that your better ear is toward the speaker.
3. Install a telephone amplifier at home. The amplifier is attached to the receiver and has a volume control.
4. Ask your spouse or a friend to tell you when the topic of conversation changes. Knowing the topic of conversation reduces the guesswork.
5. Always position yourself so that good light is on the face of the speaker.
6. When dining in a restaurant, give the waiter your complete order and thus avoid having to answer the waiter's questions, which may be difficult to understand.
7. If you rely on lip reading, avoid dining by candlelight. Better lighting is necessary for good communication.

From McCartney, James H., and Nadler, Gay: How to help your patient cope with hearing loss. Geriatrics **34**:69-76, March 1979.

impairment or deafness, as from trauma, is considered to have more adjustment problems than the one who loses his ability to hear gradually.

Aural rehabilitation. Some form of aural rehabilitation is essential for the client with a hearing impairment. The kind of rehabilitation used is based on the degree and type of impairment. Before any type of rehabilitation is started, speech audiometric tests are performed. The results of these tests provide the basis for prescribing rehabilitation therapy based on individual needs.

Aural rehabilitation may include sound amplification, auditory training, speech reading (lipreading), speech training, and language training. Each of these is designed to reestablish or maintain efficiency of oral communication.

Hearing and speech therapy may be started as early as 15 months of age. An early age is essential to prepare the child for school later. Such therapy may be carried out directly in the clinic by a professional therapist or in the home by parents, community health nurses, or teacher. When therapy is carried out in the home, it is essential that the family understand their role in the teaching process. Each form of aural rehabilitation is briefly discussed. For more detailed discussions of these, the student should consult the references at the end of the unit, related to aural rehabilitation.

Sound amplification. Sound amplification may be accomplished by hearing aids worn by the client or by amplifiers placed in the environment.

Hearing aids. Hearing aids are devices used to amplify sound. With amplified sound the client is able to protect himself from environmental dangers, learn language by hearing it, and as a result, enjoy the environmental pleasures of conversation and music.

Hearing aids are particularly useful in conductive hearing loss and may be worn by children as early as 6 months of age. When they are used during the growing years, parents should be encouraged to make periodic visits to the audiologist so that adjustments can be made in the receiver. Children should also be encouraged to wear the aid. Special instructions may be given by the audiologist on the care of the aid. For a sensitive, insecure individual, the use of a hearing aid may cause emotional problems because of the social impact it has. Such a reaction is more likely to be experienced during the adolescent period. The family and the nurse should be aware of problems that may be produced so that support can be given as needed.

TYPES OF HEARING AIDS. There are four types of hearing aids: postauricular, body, eyeglass, and in-the-ear models. The *postauricular type* (worn behind the external ear) and the *body type* (worn on the torso) are perhaps the most common. The body type resembles a small compact (Fig. 14-7). It is usually carried in the pocket, clipped to a piece of clothing, or placed into a holsterlike carrier that is strapped around the torso. It is especially useful for children and the elderly.

A third type, the *eyeglass hearing aid,* has the microphone and amplifier incorporated in the temple bows of the glasses. This type permits the entire unit to be worn in the temple piece for one ear or in both pieces for binaural use. The ear mold is incorporated into the bow(s) of the glasses and forms the association between the hearing aid and the parts of the inner ear that alert the brain to the sound.

The *in-the-ear model* is the latest type to be developed. This type fits directly into the ear without any dangling or obvious coils and resembles a large button. Because of the reduced size of the device and possibly its flesh-colored appear-

FIG. 14-7
Various types of hearing aids. Left, body type; top center, in-the-ear type; right, eyeglass type. (From Saunders, William H., and others: Nursing care in eye, ear, nose, and throat disorders, ed. 4, St. Louis, 1979, The C.V. Mosby Co.)

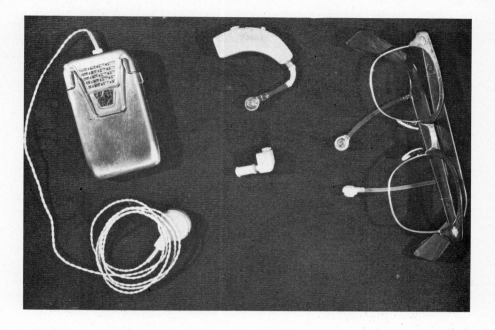

ance, the cosmetic effect is enhanced. Therefore more individuals are thought to be willing to wear this type of hearing aid. However, the in-the-ear type is not considered sufficient for severe hearing loss.

SELECTING A HEARING AID. Several factors are considered essential for hearing aid efficiency. Because questions may be raised by clients regarding the best type of aid, the nurse should be aware of the essential factors so that proper instruction can be given.

The nurse should be aware of the importance of the client's having a hearing aid that has a *controllable volume* and that is *properly fitted*. The client's ability to adjust to the hearing aid may be determined by how well it fits and how well the volume can be controlled. The receiver should fit well in the ear, and the amplifier should amplify sound without causing discomfort. Excessive noise is uncomfortable and painful and may damage the cochlear nerve if repeated excessively. Therefore many authorities recommend the use of an automatic volume control that "clips" the output of the amplifier if noise threatens to exceed the threshold of comfort. The automatic volume control is especially essential for children because they are often in environments of sudden and violent noises.

Sound should not leak from the receiver. When leakage occurs, a squealing sound is heard. As a result, the original sound becomes intolerable, intense, and distorted.

Knowledge of the factors just discussed enhances the nurse's ability to discuss pointers related to function rather than appearance. Since hearing changes with age, a hearing aid reevaluation, by an audiologist, is recommended periodically (for example, especially before purchasing a new one). The client should be referred to an audiologist whenever questions are raised that are beyond the scope of nursing.

CARING FOR A HEARING AID. Nurses and families of clients with hearing aids should be knowledgeable about the working of hearing aids. Thus in the event that the client is not able to assume care for the aid, care can be assumed by the family or the nurse until he is able to do so himself. To assume care, the family and nurse must be familiar with the following important points of care:

1. Turning the hearing aid off before the ear mold or receiver is removed from the ear.
2. Cleansing the case with a cloth dampened with water rather than alcohol or acetone. These substances may distort the shape of the ear mold, or affect the ear mold material.[5]
3. Washing the ear mold in warm soapy water. (A pipe cleaner may be used to remove wax from the opening.)
4. Checking the apparatus when squealing occurs. (Squealing may be caused by a loose-fitting ear mold, an improperly inserted mold, incorrect volume, or a defective transmitter.)
5. Avoiding exposure of the aid to radiation or ice. Excessive heat may distort the aid, and moisture may cause corrosion of the electrical contacts.
6. Removing the battery when the aid is not in use for extended periods.
7. Storing batteries in a cool, dry location, being careful not to place them on a metal surface.

When the client is hospitalized, the nurse should make every possible effort to gain assurance of the client. He should be permitted to wear the hearing aid while in the hospital. When it is necessary to remove the aid, it should be within the client's reach so he can reenter the world of sound at will. An extra set of batteries should also be on hand. When the client is admitted to the hospital, the nurse should question him or his family about particular peculiarities of the aid and what company to contact in case of malfunctioning.

A plan of care must be developed and directed toward enhancing cooperation, reducing confusion, and promoting comfort. The client should be informed on all procedures beforehand. He should be told when he will receive an injection or when and why other therapeutic measures are to be performed. The hearing aid should be removed during the night and during hygienic care. When the client is awakened from sleep, the nurse must avoid frightening him. One way of preventing this is to approach him frontally and from a distance; that is, awake him from the foot of the bed rather than from the head. If it is necessary to shake the client to awaken him, this must be done gently to avoid fright as he awakes into an environment whose sounds are blanked out.

The nurse should be familiar with possible reactions to hospitalization. As with clients with normal hearing, the client with a hearing aid may use the hospitalization to regress in the use of the aid. Signs of regression may include a refusal to use residual hearing, blaming others for speaking too low, or demanding them to raise their voices. Some clients, particularly older clients, have a tendency to withdraw from the environment by removing the hearing aid. An occasional removal to rest from the distraction of the environment generally does not indicate regression. The nurse must therefore be able to recognize behaviors that indicate regression and those that indicate the need to rest.

Amplifiers. The *table model* or *room model* amplifier uses headphones and is particularly useful in schools because it ensures that classroom sounds can reach the student. Portable auditory training units are also available for this purpose. These may be used individually or for group training in the home or school. Individual controls are provided so that sound adjustments may be made on the basis of individual needs and comfort. These controls are especially useful in group training.

Some telephones also have amplifiers for vocational as well as personal use. As a result, employment and social contacts are not hampered.

Cochlear implants. A new electronic device has been developed to facilitate the hearing of deaf clients. This device, known as the cochlear implant, has an internal part and an external part. The internal part is implanted surgically, whereas the external part is worn outside the body. The device has several intricate parts, which function to enable the client to hear sound.

Auditory training. Auditory training is designed to teach the client to use his residual hearing. This is accomplished by helping the client develop listening skills (Fig. 14-8). Such training is usually given with the help of amplification or hearing aids. However, some individuals have enough residual hearing to hear sound without amplification.

It is often recommended that auditory training be started early in life to provide adequate stimulation during the time when the child is normally becoming aware of the meaning of sounds and speech and when the neurological mechanisms for speech are developing. The cortical centers are thought to be able to readily discriminate between auditory stimuli during the first 3 years of life but tends to become less capable with increasing age. When started at an early age (2 to 3 years old), a great deal of the auditory training is informal and carried out within the home. Parents are instructed to talk to the child in a soft voice, but one that is loud enough to be heard. The child should be constantly exposed to, and encouraged to identify, sounds of daily living such as domestic noises, musical rhythms, bells, and street sounds. Efforts must be directed toward helping the

FIG. 14-8
Speech therapist helps child develop listening skills. (Courtesy National Foundation, March of Dimes.)

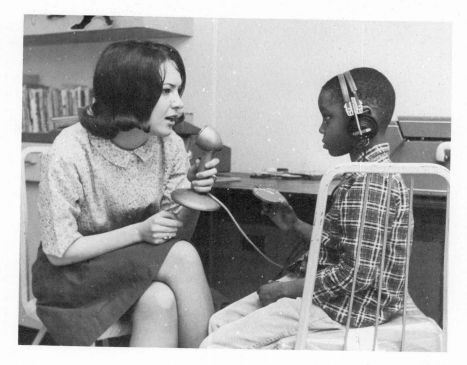

child differentiate sounds. When the child learns to grossly identify sounds, some authorities recommend prescribing a hearing aid.

When similar training is carried on outside the home, as in preschool clinics, some form of amplification is used. In some speech and hearing centers, both the child and his parents are permitted to attend classes. If adequate understanding is accomplished by school age, the child may be able to attend regular classes.

Speech reading. The client with hearing impairment tends to compensate by increasing his capacity to use his visual sensations. Speech reading capitalizes on this compensatory factor by enabling the client to develop maximally his ability to learn through his eyes. Thus speech reading (lipreading, visual communication) encompasses the observation and utilization of visual cues such as lip movements, gestures, and body movements as the client learns to understand speech. For the client to comprehend what is said to the fullest extent, training for speech reading is often combined with auditory training. Since adequate vision is essential for speech reading, the importance of periodic visual examination cannot be overemphasized.

For effective speech reading, programs are geared toward individual interest, experiences, and needs. In the preschool period, games in which a child has shown interest are often used, and lessons are often built around story telling and nursery rhymes of animals. As often as possible activities of daily living are associated with speech reading. For example, the statements "put on your pants" or "comb your hair" may be used.

In speech reading for the school-age child and adults, the client is instructed to watch the teacher pronounce words in which specific consonant sounds appear repeatedly. In this way, he becomes familiar with certain frequently repeated movements of pronunciation.

Speech training. Any degree of hearing loss is usually reflected in the client's voice pattern. Therefore speech training is an important part of aural rehabilitation.

Speech training involves teaching the child to speak correctly. It is generally started in the early preschool years. This is the period during natural development when speech is more readily acquired. Authorities feel that children 1 and 2 years of age can more readily learn new language than 4-year-olds. The general belief is that as age increases, the more difficult it is to acquire new language. To assist in the acquisition of speech, toys, frequently used household articles, and appliances should be called by name, and every encouragement should be given to the child when he attempts to repeat what he hears. Sign language should be discouraged unless the hearing impairment is such that language cannot be taught by the speech technique.

Education for the hard-of-hearing. Whenever feasible, children with a hearing impairment should be educated within their communities with children of normal hearing. Education may be started in nursery school. Simple modifications may have to be made regardless of the level of school. The child may remain in the classroom with children having normal hearing but may be permitted to sit at the front of the class and use lipreading to supplement hearing. The use of special portable amplification units, classroom amplifications, and desk-type hearing aids permit "heterogeneous education." Such units also enable the child to participate in other activities such as gymnastics.

Education for the deaf. Some communities have day schools that are a part of the public school systems. Children who attend day school participate in the same activities as children with normal hearing, but their education is specially supervised. One advantage of such day school is that these children are an integral part of the home environment after the school day.

Residential schools are a part of the state educational program for the deaf. These schools accept children of all age groups who require specific education and training through the use of amplified speech, hearing aids, speech reading, sign language, auditory training, and visual education.

The decision as to which school the child attends should be left to the parents. However, they should have ample knowledge on which to base their decision. An audiologist should be consulted because audiologists are familiar with educational facilities for the hard-of-hearing and the deaf. Pointers that should be discussed with parents as they make the decision are speech and language skills, the child's ability to compensate for the hearing impairment, and his ability to compete with children who do not have hearing impairments.

Before the child completes high school, consideration must be given to some type of vocation. The hard-of-hearing or deaf student may attend college with normal-hearing students. This, however, may be extremely difficult because of the increased emphasis on communication skills. Gallaudet College in Washington, D.C., is exclusively for deaf students. It is supported by the federal government. Nurses should be aware of this so that information can be given to parents and deaf clients when there is a need.

The child who is not able to attend college must be made aware of vocational opportunities. A vocational counselor should be consulted for such purposes.

Education for parents. Parents of deaf children may take an established correspondence course designed to guide and educate them regarding the deaf child. This service is provided by the John Tracy Clinic in Los Angeles, California.

Nurses may also be instrumental in informing parents of hard-of-hearing and deaf children and the public about organizations that are concerned with hearing. Some of these are The American Hearing Society and The American Speech and Hearing Association.

The management of the client with a hearing impairment is a team effort. The family must work closely with the client, educators, and health team members (physician, nurse, speech therapist, audiologist) to help the client remain as safe and secure in his environment as possible.

Speech

Overview of speech

Humans are social beings, and therefore characteristically have an intense desire to communicate. Such communication may be expressed by gestures, physical contact, posture, facial expressions, touch, pantomime, noises, crying, or through spoken or written words. It is through the spoken word (speech) that, for most of us, our thoughts are shared or communicated with others, interpersonal relationships are developed, and ideas are discovered.

Nursing process for common health problems

Unlike breathing, crying, or swallowing, speech is not developed at birth. It develops later in life. Before the linguistic revolution, the theory was commonly held that speech was learned by imitative tendencies. However, present linguists contend that speech is not learned by imitation. Those who support this argument point out characteristic changes in language during the early stage of speech development. It can be noted that during the early stages of language development, when the child is able to say two-word sentences, two classes of words are generally used, but in a manner different from that of the adult. One group includes a small number of commonly used words, which are referred to as "pivot words." These words may be used either in the initial position or final position of phrases. The second group comprises a larger group of uncommonly used words. These are referred to as "open-class words." For example, it is not uncommon to hear the toddler say "mamma *out,* dada *out,* doggie *out, see* baby, *see* dog, *see* mama." The *out* and *see* in these "sentences" are pivot words. The use of these and similar words is common in early childhood speech.

Another point that is used to discredit imitation as a basis of speech development is the characteristic use of inversions that are unlike those of the adult model.[16] For example, *all gone* is frequently used by the child in a number of instances. The child may use it to indicate a certain food has been eaten—"all gone bananas, all gone water, all gone candy." However, when using these two words, the adult would say "candy all gone," "the water is all gone," or "the bananas are all gone." Therefore if the child learned speech more on the basis of imitation, he would tend to follow the model of the adult who attempts to correct him.

FACTORS AFFECTING SPEECH DEVELOPMENT

Speech development follows a sequential pattern beginning with sucking, swallowing, and chewing and progressing to babbling, cooing, and finally to speaking. A spontaneous and steady improvement in speech is noted.

However, some children are slow in starting to use words and, as a result, are thought to have *delayed speech*. A meager and simplified vocabulary is characteristic of delayed speech. But even more characteristic is sentence structure that is much below the level expected of a child his age: for example, a child of 5 years has delayed speech if he uses only simple two- and three-word sentences. The child may also tend to use gestures for communicative purposes. Speech may be delayed because of physiological or psychosocial factors.

Physiological factors

For speech to develop normally, the movements of the lips, tongue, jaws, palate, larynx, and muscles of respiration must be coordinated. Any interference with these may affect speech development. The infant with cleft lip and palate may have difficulty making consonant sounds, or variations may also be noted in voice quality and articulation. A child with a gross malocclusion may find it difficult to produce certain sounds.

The child with central nervous system disorders may have the muscular coordination necessary for speech development, but because of damage to the higher faculties, speech may be delayed or defective. Paralysis or weakness of the muscles necessary for speech may be responsible for causing speech defects.

The child who has a hearing impairment may not develop speech because he does not hear sounds or he hears them incorrectly. The mentally retarded child generally has a short auditory memory span. As a result, he is not able to hear all the sounds in a word when it is stated.

14 Auditory system and speech

Psychosocial factors

Delayed speech may occur if there is no need to speak—the child gets all his needs and wants satisfied by using gestures.

Psychological trauma from severe emotional upsets such as fear and lack of attention during the stages of speech development may affect speech either temporarily or permanently. Lack of stimulation from the environment (for example, parents) may also affect speech development.

Another factor, which may become evident after the child starts school, is the hearing of a different type of speech in the two environments: one language at home and another at school. When this happens, the child may become confused, and this confusion may affect his ability to develop speech.

To help the child develop speech as normally as possible, therapy is generally directed toward the cause.

Assessment
NURSING HISTORY

The taking of a speech nursing history is essential to the development of an individualized plan of care. Information should be obtained about progression of the child's speech. For example, were the usual babbling sounds made during infancy? Was the babbling continuous, or did it stop when babbling was normally expected? How old was the child when the first words were stated? What were the first words? How many words can the child say now? Give examples of these words. Does the child have difficulty pronouncing words? What are they? Does the child use complete sentences when talking? Does the child imitate speech of those around him? How does the child indicate he wants something? For example, does he use sentences, gestures, sounds, or short phrases? If he uses gestures, is it in relation to sound or phrase?

Checklist for assessment of speech problems

The nurse should have knowledge about the sequence of speech development and factors that affect its development so that when deviations are noted, proper referrals can be made. Although this serves as a guide, the nurse must consider such factors as culture when assessments are made of speech development.

A list of danger signs follows, which may be used for assessing speech development. [8]

1. The child is not talking at all by age 2.
2. Speech is largely unintelligible after age 3.
3. Sounds are more than a year late in appearing, according to developmental sequence.
4. There are many omissions of initial consonants after age 3.
5. There are no sentences by age 3.
6. There are many substitutions of easy sounds for difficult ones after age 5.
7. The child uses mostly vowel sounds in his speech.
8. Word endings are consistently dropped after age 5.
9. Sentence structure is noticeably faulty at 5.
10. The child is embarrassed and disturbed by his speech at any age.
11. The child is noticeably nonfluent after age 5.
12. The child is distorting, omitting, or substituting any sounds after age 7.
13. The voice is a monotone, extremely loud, largely inaudible, or of poor quality.

14. The pitch is not appropriate to the child's age and sex.
15. There is noticeable hypernasality or lack of nasal resonance.
16. There are unusual confusions, reversals, or telescoping in connected speech.
17. There is abnormal rhythm, rate, and inflection after age 5.

Developmental history
Although characteristics of language development have been identified, one must not forget the part that maturational factors may play.

Neonate. Some observers contend that the first cry is an important part of language development because it indicates the beginning of speech. During the first 2 weeks of life, a similar cry is noted in response to all types of stimuli. However, by the latter part of the first month of life, different stimuli elicit a different cry. A cry in response to discomfort can be differentiated from one in response to pain. Crying therefore affords the infant a means of expressing himself.

Infant. Infancy is an important period in language development. Small throaty sounds or noises such as gurgling, sucking, cooing, and babbling appear during this period. Expressions of pleasure are also vocalized as laughing, and the infant seemingly develops an awareness of the new vocal experiences. These experiences elicit a kind of auditory stimulation. It is not uncommon to hear what is thought to be the infant imitating himself. For example, "la" may be followed by "la la la." Vocalizations may also be heard in his apparent attempt to repeat simple sounds made by the parents, siblings, or family friends. These sounds may be old ones (cooing or babbling) or entirely new "clicking" sounds. A "narrowing process" is thought to begin as the infant continues to explore and interact with those in his environment because parents do not repeat all the sounds he makes but selectively reinforce those sounds that are found in their own language.

During the latter part of the infancy period, the infant begins to integrate babblings and imitations into a sequential pattern, resulting in what sounds like normal speech. Expressions of the simple words *mama* and *dada* are common. Elements of emotional communication can be detected in the tone, loudness, and voice quality. It is during this period that adults engage in nonsense conversations with the infant. Such stimulations are of extreme importance in speech development.

The child begins to use one-word sentences that may have several meanings. The word *dog* may mean "see the dog" or "my dog." By the end of this period, the child can say two or three words. Between 12 and 18 months, a reduction may be noted in speech development. This is thought to be related to the fact that the child begins to direct his attention to exploring the environment and toward motor development. To reduce worry, parents should be informed about this aspect of development.

Toddler. This period is characterized by the development of rapid speech and language patterns. At the beginning of this stage, the child acquires coordination and muscular control of the larynx, palate, tongue, and lips and thus is able to express single two- and three-word sentences—"here doggie, there go car." He can also point to named objects or person (bottle or mama), which indicates comprehension of speech. His relinquishing a toy or some other object on request also indicates understanding of speech.

Later during this stage, the child uses a combination of words, phrases, and sentences. Pronouns are used for the first time. The pronoun *I* is widely used. The word *no* is often used by the child to control his environment and includes a number of meanings. The child's vocabulary continues to develop, longer sentences are used, and other parts of speech such as verbs, adjectives, adverbs, and prepositions become a part of the vocabulary. Appropriate responses to *on* and *under* are noted. The toddler may talk continuously if he is content and in a warm, happy, and reassuring environment.

Screaming, squealing, and yelling become common methods of expression. Nonfluent behavior similar to stuttering may also be experienced. Such behavior is thought to be related to an increase in the rate and speed of talking in contrast to earlier months. The nonfluency usually disappears within 6 months unless the parents become overly concerned. Parents should therefore be informed that nonfluent speech is a normal part of speech development. Any form of ridicule or correction should be discouraged. Problems develop only after the child pays strict attention to his pattern of speech.

Child. The preschool level is the stage of rapid speech development. This child shows a continued interest in learning new words. When a new word is heard, the child may ask for it to be repeated until he pronounces it correctly. Descriptive comments are often made about story book or comic book pictures. He obeys additional prepositional commands such as *in back, in front,* and *beside*.

As the child grows older, spoken responses become more structurally complete, as witnessed by the sentences that are used. The toddler of 2 will say "play car." At 3, he will say "I play car" or "me play car." By 4, the child will say "I play with car," and by the preschool period he will use a simple sentence such as "I play with the car."

The school-age child communicates with a group of individuals, especially children of the same age and sex. His mastery of speech greatly matures, and his vocabulary vastly increases from 1500 to 2100 words. He is able to use simple five- to seven-word sentences. As he grows older, the kind of sentence used and the length of the sentence greatly increase, and generally he enjoys speaking.

Adolescent. During the adolescent period, it is not uncommon for communications to take place with members of the opposite sex and "outgroups." Slang words may be an important part of the adolescent's vocabulary.

Young adult. The young adult converses with a multiplicity of people at home, on the job, and at social functions. Conversations are usually centered around employment, the family, and other outside interests.

Older adult. Many individuals in this stage of development spend a great portion of their time talking about memories of past experiences.

Planning

PLANNING FOR SPEECH PROMOTION

The early periods of childhood are important to speech development. Both reflexive vocalizations and actual simple use of language can be observed during the first 5 years of life. These periods are critical in speech development. The nurse should therefore make parents aware of the importance of these periods in speech development. Parents ought to be encouraged to stimulate speech development. The basic principle that should be stressed is to stimulate, encourage, and provide opportunity for speech.

TABLE 14-1

Pattern of normal language development in vocalization and response to vocal sound

Age (months)	Vocalization	Response to vocal sound
1	Crying, whimpering, produces some vowels and k, g, h; explosive sounds	
2 to 3	Pitch higher; different cries for pain and hunger; some repetition, such as gagaga; adds m and ng	May coo, sigh, gurgle, smile, or be soothed by pleasant adult voice; may cry in response to angry voice
4	Smiles, laughs, gurgles when comfortable; begins vocal play when alone; begins to use vowels and m, k, g, b, p, and ng	Imitation of other speech stops to reappear at 9 mo.; interruption of babbling causes child to stop vocalizing
5	Increase of above; occasionally responds to parents' babbling	Responds to voices by turning eye or head; responds to friendly or angry tones, shows displeasure
6	Increase in rhythm and intensity; more noncrying sounds; nasal tones and tongue tip activity begins	Gestures begin in response to pleasant or angry tones
7	More variety; some sounds repeated several days; adds d, t, n, and w	Mostly rejects demands to imitate sounds; responds to gestures plus voice
8	Begins to imitate own vocal play of mama and dada, but not in response to adults; pitch and reflection change	Calls for attention; babbles with gestures; imitates hand clapping and so on accompanied by voice
9 to 10	More variety in crying, pitch, and more vocalizing than crying; makes effort to imitate others; can imitate; may use one word correctly	Retreats from strangers and others by crying; begins to comprehend no-no and dada; may respond to bye-bye with gestures
11	Can imitate correct number of syllables and sounds heard; imitates some new sounds	Shows interest in words associated with objects or important activities
12	Accompanies vocalization with gestures; may acquire first true word or words; interested in isolated words connected with own needs and activities	May imitate animal sounds or adult exclamations; imitates the initial sound of adult words; often imitates two- and three-syllable words

Adapted from Lillywhite, Herold, and others: Pediatrician's handbook of communication disorders, Philadelphia, 1970, Lea & Febiger.

TABLE 14-2

Pattern of normal language development in articulation and general intelligibility

Age (years)	Articulation	General intelligibility
1 to 2	Uses all vowels and consonants, m, b, p, k, g, w, h, n, t, and d; omits most final consonants, some initial; substitutes consonants above for more difficult; much unintelligible jargon around 18 mo; good inflection and rate	Words used may be no more than 25% intelligible to unfamiliar listener; jargon near 18 mo almost 100% unintelligible; improvement noticeable between 21 and 24 mo
2 to 3	Continues all sounds above with vowels but use is inconsistent; tries many new sounds, but poor mastery; much substitution; omission of final consonants; articulation lags behind vocabulary	Words about 65% intelligible by 2 yr; 70% to 80% intelligible in context by 3 yr; many individual sounds faulty but total context generally understood; some incomprehensibility because of faulty sentence structure
3 to 4	Masters b, t, d, k, and g and tries many others, including f, v, th, s, and z and consonant combinations tr, bl, pr, gr, and dr, but r and l may be faulty, so substitutes w or omits; speech almost intelligible; uses th inconsistently	Speech usually 90% to 100% intelligible in context; individual sounds still faulty and some trouble with sentence structure
4 to 5	Masters f and v and many consonant combinations; should be little omission of initial and final consonants; fewer substitutes but may be some; may distort r, l, s, z, sh, ch, j, and th; no trouble with multisyllabled words	Speech is intelligible in context even though some sounds are still faulty
5 to 6	Masters r, l, and th and such blends as th, gr, bl, br, pr, etc.; may still have some trouble with blends such as thr, sk, st, and shr; may still distort s, z, sh, ch, and j; may not master these sounds until 7½ years	Good

From Lillywhite, Herold, and others: Pediatrician's handbook of communication disorders, Philadelphia, 1970, Lea & Febiger.

TABLE 14-3

Pattern of normal language development in expressive speech and comprehension of speech

Age (years)	Expressive speech	Comprehension of speech
1 to 2	Uses 1 to 3 words at 12 mo, 10 to 15 at 15 mo, 15 to 20 at 18 mo, about 100 to 200 by 2 yr; knows names of most objects he uses; names few people; uses verbs but not correctly with subjects; jargon and echolalia; names one to three pictures	Begins to relate symbol and object meaning; adjusts to comments; inhibits on command; responds correctly to "give me that," "sit down," "stand up," with gestures; puts watch to ear on command; understands simple questions, recognizes 120 to 275 words
2 to 3	Vocabulary increases to 300 to 500 words; says "where kitty," "ball all gone," "want cookie," and "go bye-bye"; jargon mostly gone, vocalizing increases, has fluency trouble, speech not adequate for communication needs	Rapid increase in comprehension vocabulary to 400 at 2½ years, 800 at 3 years; responds to commands using "on," "under," "up," "down," "over there," "by," "run," "walk," "jump up," "throw," "run fast," "be quiet," and commands containing two related actions
3 to 4	Uses 600 to 1000 words, becomes conscious of speech; three to four words per speech response; personal pronouns, some adjectives, adverbs and prepositions appear; mostly simple sentences, but some complex; speech more useful	Understands up to 1500 words by 4 years; recognizes plurals, sex difference, pronouns, adjectives; comprehends complex and compound sentences; answers simple questions
4 to 5	Increase in vocabulary to 1100 to 1600 words; more three- and four-syllable words; more adjectives; adverbs, prepositions, and conjunctions; articles appear; four-, five-, and 6-word sentences, syntax quite good; uses plurals; fluency improves; proper nouns decrease, pronouns increase	Comprehends from 1500 to 2000 words; carries out more complex commands, with two to three actions; understands dependent clause, "if," "because," "when," "why"
5 to 6	Increase in vocabulary to 1500 to 2100 words; complete five- and six-word sentences, compound, complex, with some dependent clauses; syntax near normal; quite fluent; more multisyllable words	Understands vocabulary to 2500 to 2800 words; responds correctly to more complicated sentences but is still confused at times by involved sentences

From Lillywhite, Herold, and others: Pediatrician's handbook of communication disorders, Philadelphia, 1970, Lea & Febiger.

In addition to pointers discussed regarding development, the nurse should use the content of Tables 14-1 to 14-3 as supplementary information.

Implementation

COMMON SPEECH PROBLEMS OF THE CHILD

Articulation disorders

Common speech disorders are those associated with articulation, rhythm, and voice.

Articulation disorders account for the majority of speech disorders and involve the omission of consonants or the substitution of wrong consonant sounds for the correct ones. Such omissions and substitutions interfere with the intelligibility of speech.

Defective use of certain consonants is common in children. The temporary use of defective articulation is often referred to as "baby talk." Children with normal speech may also omit or substitute consonants during times of emotional stress and excitement. Structural anomalies such as cleft palate, a hearing defect, or faulty neurological development may be responsible for articulatory disorders. Therefore, even in the absence of obvious pathological conditions, parents should be encouraged to seek a health care professional.

Articulation disorders are classified as nonfunctional and functional.

Nonfunctional disorders. Nonfunctional disorders include dysarthria and apraxia.

Dysarthria occurs when the individual experiences difficulty in moving, controlling, and coordinating the muscles and organs of articulation, phonation, or respiration. This may be the result of damage to the central nervous system.

757

Nursing process for common health problems

He may therefore have problems in making himself understood by others. At a slow speed of conversation, the problem may be less apparent, but at a speed of normal conversation, it is difficult for him to make himself understood by others. Nursing intervention is planned to enhance the client's communication. Whatever approach is used, it should be based on individual needs and planned so that continuity is maintained. The use of slate boards, pad and pencil, flash cards, pictures, and gestures has been suggested. Sufficient time should be provided for the client to speak. The use of short sentences should be encouraged. Only questions that require a yes or no answer should be used.

Apraxia, the inability to purposefully carry out movements or reproduce correct articulatory sounds in the presence of normal hearing, occurs when there is a disturbance at a higher level of the nervous system. The child with severe brain damage or a motor disability or the adult with a degenerative or traumatic cerebral lesion often experiences apraxia.

Functional disorder. *Dyslalia* refers to a defect of articulation that occurs in early childhood and usually resolves spontaneously as use of language progresses. [9] A defective use of the phonetic sounds of speech is a functional disorder. It is attributed to a functional condition rather than an organic one and usually occurs when the correct speech pattern is not learned. Failure to learn correct speech may be a result of persistent use of faulty speech patterns after early speech development, imitations of faulty speech patterns, or a hearing impairment. Children are often guilty of imitating faulty speech of other children or adults, either jokingly or as a means of gaining attention. Hearing or visual impairment, dental abnormalities, and a defect in mental development are also often responsible for the development of dyslalia.

Environmental factors are also likely to produce dyslalia. For example, dyslalia may persist in an environment where there is little encouragement for the use of speech or the improvement of speech or where the child's faulty speech is continually interpreted by an older family member.

Planning and implementation. Therapy is planned according to the cause of the disorder. If the defect is related to the environment, parents may be encouraged to send the child to a nursery school or to correct the environmental factor. A psychological evaluation may be made to determine possible reasons for retention of infantile speech patterns. Speech therapy may be prescribed if the child omits or substitutes sounds after 7 years of age. Audiological evaluations may be made, since omission of sound is often caused by an impairment in hearing.

The family should also be involved in helping the child develop normal speech patterns. Various approaches have been suggested. Family members are encouraged to speak distinctly and precisely. Special periods should be set aside for therapy. These periods should be enjoyable. A family member may read nursery rhymes or short stories, look through picture books while naming the objects or animals, or play games of imitating various animal sounds.

Disorder of rhythm: stuttering

Stuttering (stammering) is a disorder characterized by a repetition of syllables and words. Repetition of words is thought to be more common and is considered normal in young children around 3 years of age (nonfluent period). It is during this period when the child attempts to put words and phrases together. Immaturity of the speech center is also thought to produce stuttering in the nonfluent period, but persistence of stuttering is not considered normal.

Although stuttering may occur in the absence of emotional stress, often emotional problems and physical tensions are associated with it. When emotional factors are responsible, nonfluent stutter may become a primary, and possibly a secondary, stutter. [8]

Primary stutter occurs during the late preschool and early school-age periods. It is characterized by an increase in the degree of nonfluency rather than the expected decrease. As a result, the child becomes concerned about it and attempts to avoid it by using physical postures instead of words.

The secondary stutter develops as the fluency decreases. Varied facial grimaces, irregular respiratory patterns, and arm swinging characterize secondary stuttering. These reactions are described as being signs of avoidance struggles.

Planning and implementation. Therapy varies according to the age of the child and the degree of fluency disturbances. It aims to facilitate free speech and to allow the child to regain confidence in fluent speech. Various recommendations have been made. No attempt should be made to overprotect the child. Instead, he should be treated as other children within the family. Parents should be patient with the child and ample time should be permitted for speech. They should be instructed not to ridicule the child's speech pattern and to accept the hesitant speech as a temporary phase in speech development. The child must be made to feel secure and loved. He must be given ample opportunities to speak. Games involving speech, such as repetition of nursery rhymes and stories, are thought to be important forms of therapy.

Therapy for the school-age child, adolescent, and adult follows the same principle, but modifications are made, based on age. Often it may be necessary to refer the client to a speech pathologist.

Voice quality deviations

Disorders of voice are uncommon. Except for the prepuberty voice change, deviations in the quality of voice usually accompany some other disorder. For example, *hypernasality* often accompanies a cleft palate, although it may be functional. In either case, a speech therapist should be consulted to help the child develop nonnasal speech. For hypernasality of a functional nature, therapy is planned to teach the child how to use his soft palate. Blowing exercises (blowing bubbles, blowing at boats in a bathtub) are means by which this is accomplished. Exercise for the older child may include blowing a musical instrument such as a clarinet, flute, or trumpet.

Hyponasality most commonly occurs when a child has excessively enlarged adenoids. Characteristically the voice quality is hoarse and lacks adequate nasal tone, and the speech may be thick and indistinct. Usually removal of the adenoids results in disappearance of the disorder. If it persists after surgery, a speech therapist may be consulted to help the child relearn the correct use of his soft palate.

COMMON HEALTH PROBLEMS OF THE ADULT

Deviations of the normal quality of voice are often associated with laryngeal pathological conditions that may ultimately affect the voice.

Laryngitis

Laryngitis, inflammation of the larynx, most often occurs as part of inflammatory disorders of the throat or lower passages of the respiratory tract. It may also occur from overuse of the voice and is common in heavy smokers. Hoarseness, cough, and fever are the common symptoms. These manifestations usually disappear within a few days. Children tend to have alarming attacks of dyspnea, particularly at night. The attack is called *croup* and is considered to be the spasmodic form of acute laryngitis (see Chapter 21).

The *chronic* form of laryngitis is a result of long-continued irritation from any condition that causes acute laryngitis (such as smoking, irritating fumes, and voice overuse). Laryngitis from voice overuse is more likely to occur in public speakers and cheerleaders.

The acute form of laryngitis is usually treated with mist therapy, sedatives, and antibiotics. Fluids are encouraged. If the inflammation is from overuse, the client is instructed not to use his voice. If this is not possible, voice activity is limited. He is also instructed to stop smoking and to avoid sources of irritation.

Tumors
Tumors of the larynx may be benign or malignant. Growths of the larynx may occur as a result of irritation from excessive use of the voice as well as from irritating chemicals. Malignant tumors more likely result from longstanding irritation from smoking and air pollutants than from other causes.

Benign tumors. *Nodules* between the vocal cords, caused by prepubescent endocrine changes, allergies, and voice overuse from yelling, are often responsible for producing hoarseness in the child between 8 and 10 years of age. Cessation of activity (resting the voice) and removal of allergenic factors usually result in disappearance of the nodule, or it may disappear spontaneously when the voice changes.

Polyps of the larynx are perhaps the most common benign tumors of the larynx. They occur primarily in men. Chronic irritation is considered the chief factor in causation. Heavy smokers, singers, and persons who impose great strain on the larynx frequently develop polyps of the larynx. Progressive hoarseness is the characteristic symptom.

Carcinoma of the larynx. Carcinoma is the most common tumor of the larynx. It occurs ten to twelve times more often in men over 60 years of age.[17] Long-continued irritation from industrial chemicals, cigarette smoking, and continuous straining of the vocal cords are thought to be the predisposing factors. Avoiding these irritants may well be a prime factor in prevention.

Assessment. The symptoms that occur depend on the part of the larynx affected. Most carcinoma of the larynx occurs directly over the larynx, although it may also occur above (supraglottic) or below (infraglottic) the vocal cords.

Hoarseness, which is often the symptom responsible for the client's decision to consult a physician, occurs when the true vocal cord is involved.[15] Failure to seek health care results in development of symptoms such as pain, dysphagia, hemoptysis, and dyspnea. Dyspnea is a later symptom because of obstruction of the air passages from growth of the tumor.

A diagnosis of laryngeal carcinoma is established by direct visualization and is confirmed by biopsy obtained during a laryngoscopic examination. In some institutions, a laryngogram may be performed with the client under local anesthetic to help establish a diagnosis.

Data analysis
Data analysis may reveal nursing diagnoses of impaired communication, anticipatory grieving, and disturbance in self-concept.

Planning and implementation. The therapy planned for the client with carcinoma of the larynx depends on factors such as the site, the stage of the tumor, and the age and degree of regional neck involvement.[15] Irradiation or surgery (for example, partial or total laryngectomy) may be used as a form of therapy.

Partial laryngectomy is usually performed in early stages when only one vocal cord is involved and both cords are mobile. Several techniques may be used for a partial laryngectomy. The *laryngofissure* technique is most common. With this technique the larynx is split in the midline, and the diseased tissue is excised.

A tracheostomy is performed to ensure airway patency during the immediate postoperative period. The nursing care that is implemented during this period should be directed toward maintaining airway patency and promoting emotional support. The client should be assured that the tracheostomy is only temporary and that the necessary care for the tracheostomy will be provided. In the early postoperative period, dysphagia may be experienced; therefore nutrition may be provided either intravenously or by nasogastric feedings. If the client is permitted oral feedings, soft foods (gelatins, custards) should be encouraged. Care must be taken that the client does not aspirate. If some of the feeding is aspirated, the trachea should be suctioned through the tracheostomy tube.

The nurse should also observe the client closely for the development of subcutaneous emphysema, a common complication following laryngofissure and tracheostomy.[15] This complication occurs when air escapes under the skin of the neck and face. It is characterized by a crackling sensation on palpation of the skin. The physician should be made aware of the development of this complication.

A *hemilaryngectomy* (or vertical laryngectomy) may sometimes be performed. This surgery involves removal of one side of the thyroid cartilage.[15]

A *supraglottic laryngectomy* (or horizontal laryngectomy) involves the removal of the epiglottis and the structures above the level of the true vocal cords. The voice is maintained.[15] Usually a unilateral radical neck dissection is done with a supraglottic laryngectomy. Swallowing is a problem for 2 to 3 weeks postoperatively. Food and liquids especially have a tendency to flow into the trachea and produce a cough. Nursing care is similar to that planned for the client with a partial laryngectomy. One difference is that a cuffed tracheostomy tube is inserted to decrease chances of aspiration, which is not uncommon in the postoperative period. A second difference is that nutrition is provided by nasogastric feedings for approximately 2 weeks. When oral feedings are started, semisolid foods are prescribed (Jello, custards, ice cream, mashed potatoes, cooked cereals).

The client is frequently instructed on a technique to close the glottis during swallowing to prevent aspiration of foods and liquids. One such technique, described in Saunders,[15] involves having the client take a deep breath, hold it, place the food on the back of the tongue, swallow three times while holding his breath, and then cough. If foods have been aspirated, it is coughed up.

When feedings are begun, the nurse should support the client emotionally by providing as much encouragement as is necessary. Assessments and documentation should be made of the amount of food taken, any signs of aspiration, and signs indicative of aspiration pneumonia.

761

Chest assessments, weights, and intake and output should be monitored. If intake is inadequate, the client is usually supplemented with intravenous fluids.

Irradiation therapy. Irradiation therapy is usually used for clients who have carcinoma that involves only one cord or clients without cord fixation or extra-laryngeal extension.[3]

For advanced lesions, a *total laryngectomy* is performed. A total laryngectomy entails removal of the entire larynx, along with the epiglottis and cricoid cartilage. As a result, aphonia is experienced. When the larynx is removed, no connections exist between the trachea and pharynx. The lower end of the trachea is brought forward, sutured onto the skin of the neck and a permanent opening in the neck is created, which is referred to as a *tracheal stoma*. The operation may be combined with a radical neck dissection if the metastasis involves the neck glands.

A radical neck dissection involves removal of all contents of one side of the neck except the carotid artery; the vagus, hypoglossal, and lingual nerves with the sympathetic chain; the phrenic nerve; and certain muscle groups.

Preoperative nursing care. The client who is about to face a laryngectomy needs continued support. The nurse must spend as much time as possible with him, assessing his physical and mental status. Because of the impact of the surgery, this type of client has many fears—relating to his appearance once the larynx is removed, the diagnosis, the surgery, loss of voice, and possible loss of social relationships and his job. If the client raises questions, they must be answered honestly and in terms that are understood. He must be told about the surgery, what it involves, and the effects it will have on his communication. He will not be able to speak after surgery; however, he must be assured of the value of the surgery. The entire health team must work together to help minimize his fears by stressing the positive aspects of what can be done to gain a new method of communication. The nurse must be aware of the physician's explanation so that it can be reinforced.

Before surgery, it might be helpful for a laryngectomee who has been successfully rehabilitated to visit the client, to talk to him, and demonstrate the communication process. A speech therapist should also be consulted in the pre-operative period. Not only should the therapist and laryngectomee talk to the client, but they should talk to the family as well.

Postoperative nursing care. In the postoperative period, some psychological shock and subsequent depression are likely to be experienced by the client. He may withdraw. These reactions may be related to the inability to speak and to certain fears that may now appear more real. Although the health team should avoid sympathy and pity, they should support the client and restore confidence and hope for the future. The family should be encouraged to do the same. If the client is greatly depressed, a second visit by the laryngectomee who saw him in the preoperative period might be in order.

The client must be encouraged to communicate in the manner established in the preoperative period. Any attempts at speaking in the early period are discouraged in order to avoid injury and promote healing. A pad and pencil or slate should be available at the bedside at all times.

A tracheostomy tube will be in place, and therefore some of the approaches discussed under tracheostomy will be applicable. A nasogastric tube will be inserted for feeding. Gavage feedings may be started on the first postoperative day, and the tube removed in approximately a week. Sterile water may be administered first, and the diet progressively increased from a liquid to regular.

In addition to alterations in speaking, methods of breathing, and feeding, changes will be noted in other functions. The client will not be able to laugh or cry audibly. The client who is full of laughter or who likes to cry openly will be greatly affected. Smell, and subsequently taste, will be hampered because air no longer enters the nose. The nurse must support the client as he expresses concerns about these factors and inform him of ways of overcoming them.

COMPLICATIONS FOLLOWING LARYNGECTOMY. Potential complications following a laryngectomy include *fistula formation, rupture of the carotid artery,* and *stenosis of the tracheostomy.* Fistula formation is most common, and it tends to heal spontaneously, although it may take weeks. Rupture of the carotid is more likely to occur following a radical neck dissection and is especially likely in a client who has received irradiation.[3] Emergency care of this complication is essential. The neck wound should be compressed in an effort to stop the bleeding, and the physician contacted immediately. Stenosis of the tracheostomy, evidenced by shortness of breath, requires a surgical revision to enlarge the opening. The nurse should be aware of these potential complications and make assessments for them as care is implemented.

Voice production after surgery of the larynx. When only a partial laryngectomy is performed and one cord or the major portion of one cord is left intact, a useful voice can be produced. This occurs after healing takes place and after scar tissue replaces the destroyed area. The remaining cord now vibrates against the scar tissue to produce sound.

When a total laryngectomy is performed, new methods of speech must be developed. The surgeon makes the decision as to when speech therapy should start. Instructions to start speech therapy are usually delayed until the muscles and mucous membranes are well healed and are no longer tender. Esophageal speech, pharyngeal speech, or an artificial method of speech are used.

ESOPHAGEAL AND PHARYNGEAL SPEECH. The esophageal method is perhaps the most common and most effective method of speech. Esophageal speech is accomplished by swallowing air and holding it under the esophagus. When the air is forced up through the esophagus, it vibrates, and as a result a hoarse, low-pitched voice quality is produced.

The second, less commonly employed method is the pharyngeal method. This speech method is accomplished by locking air into the throat by using the tongue and its muscles. This eliminates the necessity of swallowing air deep in the esophagus. As speech therapy is continued, the family should be included. They should be counseled concerning the client's new voice and the importance of encouraging him to improve it through use. The family should be cautioned not to talk for the client, but should make him talk and should avoid responding to nonverbal communication.

ARTIFICIAL METHODS OF SPEECH. Artificial methods of speech are accomplished with mechanical or electronic devices. These devices provide functional communication and are generally used only by clients who are unable to learn esophageal speech. One disadvantage of these methods of speech is that the device may not always be handy when needed. The artificial larynx, although considered outdated, is the most commonly used mechanical device. The device is placed over the tracheal stoma whenever the client desires to speak.

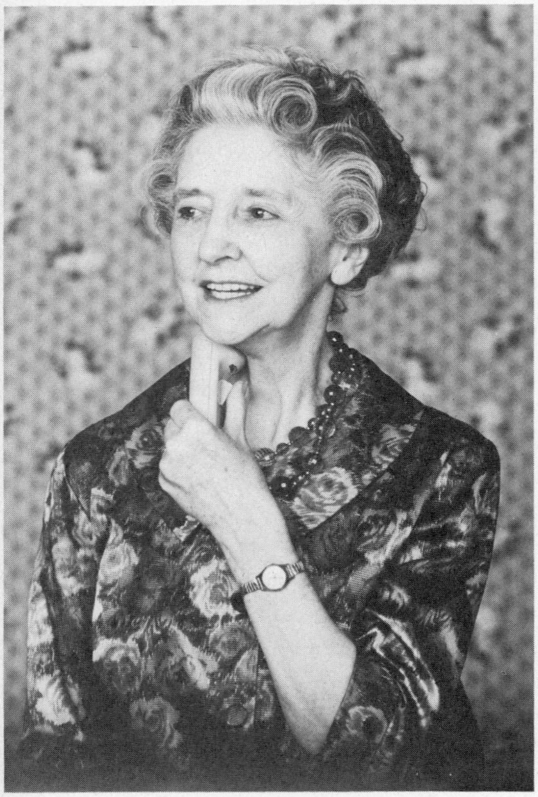

Nursing process for common health problems

FIG. 14-9
Artificial larynx is electronic device that permits laryngectomized client to speak. (Courtesy Indiana Bell Telephone Company, Indianapolis.)

There are several types of electrolarynges currently available. One type is similar in appearance to a flashlight. It contains batteries and a vibrator. The vibrator is placed against the side of the neck (submaxillary area), and a monotone speech is produced by the action of the buccal cavity, tongue, and lips (Fig. 14-9).

Research is currently being conducted toward the construction of a new larynx by surgical means using adjacent throat tissue. This experimentation offers hope for future clients with laryngeal carcinoma.

Discharge instructions. Preparation for discharge must be started early. Clients are likely to have concerns about the appearance of the scar. The nurse should inform them about special devices to cover the stoma. The male client may be encouraged to start wearing a shirt and tie as soon as possible after the operation. When a tie is worn, a knot should be placed above the neck opening. To facilitate reaching the opening, the second button on the shirt should be left open. Shirts might be altered to raise the collar so that the button and collar are above the opening. Bibs may also be purchased. Women can be encouraged to wear scarves or use specially designed jewelry to conceal the opening.

Because noxious fumes and dust may enter the trachea, the client should be instructed about special filters that may be purchased. The stoma should be covered when the client is coughing, since secretions escape through the opening.

The client should also be informed about amplifiers that can be used for business, social, and professional situations. These may be small enough to be carried in the pocket or large enough to be placed on a table. They are particularly useful when the client must talk before a large audience.

The client should be encouraged to engage in all his usual activities and hobbies. However, limitations may have to be made on activities such as swimming and strenuous exercise.

If it is necessary for the client to change jobs, a social worker or vocational counselor should be consulted. Employment in an industrial setting with irritating fumes and dust may necessitate a change in jobs. If the client's employment warrants continued verbal communication, whether he changes jobs depends on how well he adjusts to esophageal speech.

Before the client is discharged, the nurse must inform him of community resources. He should be made aware of the laryngectomy clubs, whose members are laryngectomized clients. These clubs may have various names—Lost Chord Club or New Voices Club. Pamphlets may be obtained from the American Cancer Society to assist the client in adjusting to his new manner of voice production. Some of these pamphlets have valuable information about locations of laryngectomee clubs and sources of supply of the special aids he needs, such as bibs, jewelry, and other devices. Medical identification cards and bracelets can be obtained from the International Association of Laryngectomees. These cards contain information regarding the stoma and how to provide assisted ventilation in an emergency.

Evaluation. The client having a laryngectomy has problems related to impaired verbal communication, disturbance in self-concept, ineffective airway clearance, ineffective breathing, ineffective coping, fear, and grieving. The nursing care plan must be evaluated on an ongoing basis.

EXPECTED OUTCOMES

The client and/or family can:

1. Describe laryngectomy.
2. Communicate feelings about the surgery and changes in life-style.
3. State plans for follow-up health care, including speech rehabilitation.
4. State community resources that may be used (for example, American Cancer Society, laryngectomee clubs).
5. State signs indicative of emergency health care (for example, bleeding, difficulty breathing).
6. Discuss strategies for enhancing self-concept.

Evaluation

Evaluation, the final stage of the nursing process, is ongoing. Clients with health problems of the auditory system and speech may have problems of sensory perception alteration, impaired verbal communication, ineffective coping, fear, disturbance in self-concept, grief, alteration in comfort, and potential for injury.

EXPECTED OUTCOMES

The client and/or family can:

1. State the health problem.
2. State plans for safety and protection of the auditory system.
3. Demonstrate proper care of devices such as hearing aids and laryngectomy tubes.
4. Discuss plans for follow-up care in relation to auditory and speech aids.
5. State plans for health maintenance.
6. Discuss appropriate community resources that can be used if the need arises.

Summary

The care of the client with problems of the auditory system is based on knowledge of physiological and pathophysiological states. Care for the client involves the use of the nursing process. As a basis for the care, information is taken from a nursing history. The nursing history includes health, development, social, and psychological elements. The physical skill used to acquire data is inspection. Screening tests and diagnostic tests are valuable in determining the presence or absence of a visual problem. Once information is obtained from these parameters, it is analyzed and used as a basis for planning and implementing care.

The nursing care planned for clients encompasses those strategies directed toward health promotion as well as maintenance and restoration.

Common health problems affect the neonate, including congenital anomalies (macrotia, anotia, polyotia, and congenital atresia). Otitis media is common among infants and children. This age group also commonly inserts foreign objects into the ear, which may cause varying degrees of hearing impairment. Otosclerosis and Meniere's disease affect young adults. Several problems may occur across the life span, including otitis externa, labyrinthitis, tympanic membrane rupture, and hearing loss (including conductive, sensorineural, and mixed). Aural rehabilitation involves the use of hearing aids, amplifiers, and auditory training. Varied approaches may be used for the education of clients with forms of hearing impairment.

A close relationship exists between hearing and speech. As a result, impairment in one area may affect the other. Physical and psychosocial factors may affect speech development and result in problems. Common speech problems are those associated with articulation (dysarthria, apraxia), rhythm (stuttering), and voice (hypernasality and hyponasality). Laryngitis and tumors are common among adults. Varied modes of therapy that may be employed for clients with auditory problems include medications, surgery, and speech and auditory training.

References

1. Blake, Roland P., editor: Industrial safety, ed. 3, Englewood Cliffs, N.J., 1963, Prentice Hall, Inc.
2. Clark, Christina C., and Mills, Gretchen C.: Communicating with hearing-impaired elderly adults, J. Gerontol. Nurs. 5:40-44, May-June 1979.
3. DeWeese, David D., and Saunders, William H.: Textbook of otolaryngology, ed. 6, St. Louis, 1982, The C.V. Mosby Co.
4. Hawkins, Joseph E.: Drug ototoxicity. In Stowe, Marshall: Differential diagnosis in pediatric otolaryngology, Boston, 1975, Little, Brown Co.
5. Hipskind, Nicholas M.: Aural rehabilitation for adults, Otolaryngol. Clin. North Am. 11:823-834, October 1978.
6. Illingsworth, Ronald S.: The development of the infant and young child: normal and abnormal, Baltimore, 1966, Williams & Wilkins Co.
7. Keefer, Chester S., and Wilkins, Robert W., editors: Essentials of clinical practice, Boston, 1970, Little, Brown Co.
8. Lillywhite, Herold, and others: Pediatrician's handbook of communication disorders, Philadelphia, 1970, Lea & Febiger.
9. Morley, Muriel E.: The development and disorders of speech in childhood, ed. 3, Baltimore, 1972, Williams & Wilkins Co.
10. Newby, Hayes A.: Audiology, ed. 2, New York, 1964, Appleton-Century-Crofts.
11. Nilo, Ernest R.: Hearing impairment. In Saunders, William H., Havener, William H., Fair, Carol J., and Havener, Gail, editors: Nursing care in eye, ear, nose, and throat disorders, ed. 4, St. Louis, 1979, The C.V. Mosby Co.
12. Newman, M. Haskell: Hearing loss. In Strome, Marshall: Differential diagnosis in pediatric otolaryngology, Boston, 1975, Little, Brown Co.
13. Nichols, Richard D.: Sensorineural deafness. In Strome, Marshall: Differential diagnosis in pediatric otolaryngology, Boston, 1975, Little, Brown Co.
14. Northern, Jerry L., and Downs, Marion P.: Hearing in children, ed. 2, Baltimore, 1978, Williams & Wilkins Co.
15. Saunders, William H., and others: Nursing care in eye, ear, nose, and throat disorders, ed. 4, St. Louis, 1979, The C.V. Mosby Co.
16. Smith, Frank, and Miller, George A.: Developmental psycholinguistics. In The genesis of language, Cambridge, Mass., 1968, The M.I.T. Press.
17. Walike, Joseph W., and others: Diseases of the upper respiratory tract. In Harrison's principles of internal medicine, ed. 9, New York, 1980, McGraw-Hill, pp. 1274-1275.

Additional readings

Brown, Marie S., and Grunfeld, Carol: Otitis media. Issues Compr. Pediatr. Nurs. **3:**35-53, August, 1978.

Daniels, William Andrew: Communications and rehabilitation. In The adolescent patient, St. Louis, 1970, The C.V. Mosby Co.

Davis, Hallowell, and Silverman, S. Richard, editors: Hearing and deafness, ed. 3, New York, 1970, Holt, Rinehart and Winston.

Dye, Beverly J.: Hearing conservation education program, Occup. Health Nurs. **27:**12-14, January 1979.

Ferry, Peggy C., and Cooper, Judith A.: Sign language in communication disorders of childhood, J. Pediatr. **93:**547-552, October 1978.

Goda, Sidney: Speech development in children, Am. J. Nurs. **70:**276-278, February 1970.

Goodhill, Victor, and others: Pathology, diagnosis, and therapy of deafness. In Travis, Lee Edward, editor: Handbook of speech pathology and audiology, New York, 1971, Appleton-Century-Crofts.

McCartney, James H., and Nadler, Gay: How to help your patients cope with hearing loss, Geriatrics **34:**69-76, March 1979.

Newman, M. Haskell: Conductive hearing loss. In Strome, Marshall: Differential diagnosis in pediatric otolaryngology, Boston, 1975, Little, Brown Co.

Payne, Peter D., and Payne, Regina L.: Behavioral manifestations of children with hearing loss, Am. J. Nurs. **70:**1718-1719, August 1970.

Snidecor, John C.: Speech without a larynx. In Travis, Lee Edward, editor: Handbook of speech pathology and audiology, New York, 1971, Appleton-Century-Crofts.

for clients with common health problems of the

15 Integumentary system

Assessment

Data analysis

Planning

Implementation

Evaluation

Common health problems involving the integumentary system occur across the life span. These problems are often the cause for disfigurement, but more commonly cause discomfort and embarrassment. For example, allergies are often annoying. Pruritus, a symptom that accompanies a variety of integumentary lesions, is also extremely annoying and may affect daily social relationships with others or the ability to sleep or engage in daily activities. The disfigurement that so often is experienced may be the result of tissue injuries. Disfigurement, too, is often the cause of social isolation and in many instances may be the cause of psychological changes.

Although problems may occur throughout the life span, some problems are more common in one age group than in others. For example, pigmentary changes and vascular lesions are common in neonates; rashes, inflammations, and infections are common in infants, children, adolescents, and young adults; and cancer is common in older adults.

The nurse can use this information in planning, implementing, and evaluating care of clients with common health problems of the integument.

Overview of the integument

The skin is a complex specialized organ that has various functions, the major function of which is protective. It maintains body equilibrium against harmful effects of the environment. For example, it contains sensory nerve endings, which are specialized in their response to temperature, pain, and touch. By means of these nerve endings, the skin is able to carry out its "perceptive-protective" role by protecting the individual from inherent dangers within the environment. Through the skin the individual is able to feel varying degrees of pressure, heat, and cold, as well as experience sensations of pleasure and pain.

The skin's ability to protect the body from entrance of microorganisms is made possible through the intact *corneum*. The acidity of perspiration is responsible for retarding the growth of most human pathogens by maintaining a skin pH of 3.0 to 5.0. An increase in sweat reduces the acidity and disinfectant properties.

The skin assists the body in temperature regulation in several ways. Cooling is accomplished by capillary vasodilation and evaporation of perspiration, whereas capillary constriction facilitates heat conservation. It acts as a barrier to prevent the loss of body fluids to the external environment, and provides for internal homeostasis (a prime function of the epidermis).

The skin contains glands and appendages that help perform its overall function. The sweat glands serve as a primary means of regulating body temperature by eliminating moisture through the skin. The pores in the skin permit the elimination of waste products. The oily secretions of sebaceous glands are essential in keeping the outer layer supple and preventing fissure formation.

Assessment
NURSING HISTORY

The nursing history should be obtained at first contact with the client and should complement the other assessments. During the taking of a nursing history, it is important to gather data regarding the client's health, development, and social and psychological states. The information obtained from the history should be evaluated and used as a basis for establishing a nursing diagnosis, and subsequently planning, implementing, and evaluating nursing care.

Health history

Assessing information about the health of the integument is an essential part of the nursing history. The history, in part, can be taken as physical assessments are made. The extent at which the nurse can do this will vary, depending on how well these skills have been mastered. Pertinent questions that will facilitate understanding of the client (child or adult) and his health problems should be asked. Focus questions should be related to those listed in the material on p. 770.

Developmental history

The character of the skin varies with the age of the individual. These variations should be evaluated according to the age of the client.

Neonate. The skin of the neonate is thin because of the lack of development of dermal papillae and appendages. It is covered with vernix caseosa, a cheese-like material and product of the sebaceous gland that protects the neonate from superficial infections, and with lanugo (fine hair) that is lost a few weeks after birth. This hair is displaced by new hairs that begin to grow in the follicle. Cilia, tiny white cysts that commonly appear scattered over the face, result from either faulty or partially occluded pilosebaceous follicles.[40] It is transient and usually

Nursing process for common health problems

disappears spontaneously a few weeks following birth. Nails are paper thin. Sweat and sebaceous glands are present but gradually become smaller and are functionless.[40] Reactions to tactile sensation are minimal. Crying and reflex withdrawal are the most characteristic responses to tactile stimuli.

Infant. During infancy, lubricating sebum is secreted. As a result, the skin does not peel as much as it does in the neonatal period. Sweat glands begin to function, thus facilitating regulation of body temperature. The thickness of subcutaneous fat increases throughout the first year and decreases during toddlerhood. Response to tactile stimuli is more delayed. By 7 to 9 months of age, the infant deliberately withdraws from stimuli. By the end of the first year, he carries his hand to the site of irritation.

Child. During the preschool and early school-age period, there is a gradual loss of adipose tissue. Between 7 to 10 years of age the sebaceous glands become active. This occurs in response to increasing adrenal androgens with a subsequent increase in sebum[1]; otherwise, few changes occur.

Adolescent. During the preadolescent period, growth of the apocrine glands begins. As they begin to function, a characteristic axillary odor is emitted. This odor arises from gram-positive bacteria degradation of the apocrine secretion.[50] The sebaceous glands, which gradually became inactive after birth, become reactivated. Subcutaneous fat begins to accumulate, with accumulation more common in girls than in boys.

FOCUS QUESTIONS FOR HEALTH HISTORY

A. *Data, duration, and nature of the problem*
1. What is the problem?
2. When was the problem (for example, rash, itch, lesion) first noticed?
3. Did it appear suddenly, gradually, or progressively? If gradual or progressive, over what period of time?
4. Were any other symptoms experienced when the problem was first noticed? Was there itching, pain, or a burning sensation?
5. Was the problem noticed after eating or drinking a specific food or beverage? If yes, what did you (or the child) eat or drink?
6. Does anything specific seem to precipitate the problem? If yes, tell me about it.
7. Are you (or is the child) on any special medication? If yes, what medication? What route was it taken? Was it prescribed? Was the problem noticed after taking the medication? Have previous reactions to medication been experienced? If yes, what? Would you describe the reaction?
8. Has the problem been experienced before? If yes, when? How similar is it with the previous occurrence? What caused the problem the last time it was experienced? Does it seem to be seasonal? Does it occur during the spring or summer? Or does it occur while you are in the presence of certain materials?
9. Was there a recent change in a detergent or cosmetic agent? When did the problem occur in relation to the change?
10. What do you think caused the problem?
11. Has the child been exposed to anyone with a communicable disease?

B. *Location*
1. On what part of the body was the problem first noticed?

C. *Appearance (including size, shape, distribution)*
1. What did the rash (or lesion) look like when it first appeared? Or could you describe what it looked like when it was first noticed?
2. Have any changes been noticed since it first appeared? If yes, describe the changes, or describe how the changes differ or compare with how it looks now.
3. Was this mark present at birth? If yes, how does it compare at this time in terms of its appearance at birth? Is it longer, larger, swollen? Has it spread?

D. *Therapy*
1. Has any form of treatment been used? If yes, what? Lotions, soaps, ointment? Did it seem to help?
2. How do you normally care for the problem? (This information could be helpful if it is a chronic problem.)
3. What seems to make the problem better or worse?

E. *Family and psychosocial elements*
1. Does anyone in your family (parent, sibling, significant other) currently have a skin problem? If so, tell me about it.
2. Has anyone in your family (parent, sibling, significant other) experienced a problem similar to this before?
3. Has the child (or have you) been exposed to anyone with a skin problem?
4. Is there anything else you would like to tell me about your health history?

During adolescence, activity of the sebaceous glands of the skin increases. This is brought on by the hormonal influence of androgens and estrogens. An increase in hair growth such as the beard and pubic hair also are the result of androgens. The increased sebum is the result of a marked increase in the lipid surface film of free fatty acids. The apocrine sweat glands begin to function and, as a result, sweating increases.

Changes in pigmentation during adolescence are also evident. Melanocytes (the pigment-producing cells of the skin), which are under the influence of hormonal and environmental factors, are the source of pigmentation. Subcutaneous fat continues to increase in girls, and boys tend to become thinner. With an increase in subcutaneous fat (especially among girls), it is not uncommon for striae to develop on various parts of the body.

Adult. During this period there are no significant noticeable changes in the appearance of the skin. However, many changes are taking place but are not evident until the years of older adulthood.

Older adult. As the individual ages, varied changes may be noted in the appearance and character of the skin. Dryness is increased, and scaliness becomes more noticeable. These characteristics are related to a reduction in sebaceous activity and diminished hydration of the horny layer of the skin. Changes (for example, decrease in number) that occur in fibrous connective tissue are responsible for the inelasticity of the aged skin. A reduction in the subcutaneous fat also contributes to loss of elasticity. As a result, sagging and wrinkling become apparent, the skin becomes thinner, and characteristically, a skin fold tends to persist after pinching. Folding of the skin is also thought to be related to a deposition of calcium salts in connective tissue. Because of these changes, the older client's skin becomes more vulnerable to trauma. There is increased difficulty in conserving heat. There is also an increase in the time it takes tissue repair to occur. A decrease is also noted in sweating ability because of partial atrophy of the sweat glands.

With age, changes occur in the pigmentation of the skin. A reduction in melanocytes, which are under the influence of hormones, will subsequently have an effect on pigmentation. Hence, age spots (senile lentigo) are not uncommon. These changes are especially common in exposed areas. The tiny dermal blood vessels become fragile and tear easily.

The number of active eccrine sweat glands are reduced, and subsequently their output is reduced. Apocrine sweat glands tend to atrophy. Sebaceous gland secretion decreases.

Characteristic changes may also be noted in the appendages of the skin as the client ages. Hair follicles decrease in size and number. As a result, growth is slowed, hair is lost, and the characteristic *baldness* may be observed. Usually, graying of the hair occurs because over the years the new hair follicles that replace the old ones contain less melanin pigment. However, in some instances hair pigment is retained; thus, no characteristic change in the color of the hair is noted. Hair growth accelerates, especially in the ears, nose, and eyebrows, and it tends to become coarser. The growth of nails is slowed; they become brittle, appear ridged, and have a tendency to flake (Fig. 15-1).

Social history

When a social history is obtained, factors to be considered include age and economics, especially as it relates to the length of time the problem has existed.[29] An evaluation of the data obtained will enhance development of an individual-

771

FIG. 15-1
Skin changes are characteristic of older adult. Note wrinkling of skin, graying and coarseness of hair, baldness, and prominent veins.

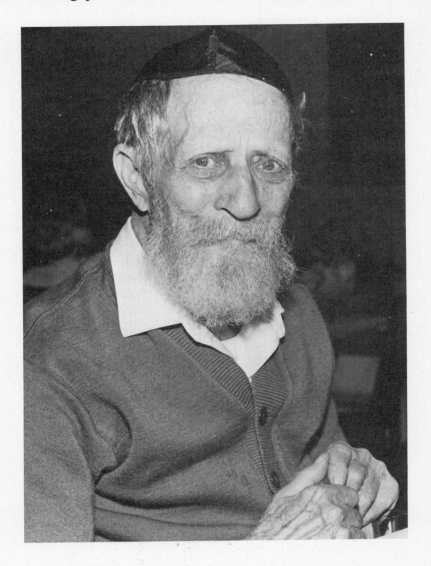

ized plan of care. For example, the cosmetic value of the skin is significant during the adolescent period. A number of skin problems are long-standing, often necessitating a large number of missed days from school or work. This may place an increased financial burden on the client and family. Therefore the following information should be obtained: The effect the lesion has on school or work activities. Is it necessary to miss several days from school or work? What effect does it have on school or employment? Is there difficulty in maintaining employment? How many days have been lost from school or work? How does the problem affect relationships with others at home, school, or work? What effect does it have on peer group relationships or any associates? Does it present any other problems? For the young child a question such as "Do you still play with your best friend?" might be in order.

Psychological history　　In obtaining a psychological history as it relates to the integument, the nurse must remember that the skin serves as a primary source of gratification across the life span. It is through contact with others that this gratification is

772

experienced. For example, the skin acts as a channel of communication. Emotions may be communicated by blushing with anger, shame, or excitement. It is through the skin that one receives a touch, slap, or pinch. According to Hecht,[27] the skin also carries emotional evidence of a person's inner state by reflecting feelings of health and self-respect as well as feelings of illness or lack of self-respect. Because of these psychosocial assets, a climate should be created so that the client is free to express feelings. Open-ended statements lend themselves to acquiring information that might not be acquired from specific questions. A statement such as "Tell me how you feel about this problem" may be helpful. Observe the client as the response is given, and follow up on responses. The nurse should also listen for cues that may be indicative of client concerns. For example, the way the lesion is described may provide information about the real meaning of the lesion to the individual. By using these techniques, the nurse can obtain enough information to develop an individualized plan of care.

Physical assessment

The nurse, through making assessments of clients with problems of the integument, establishes nursing diagnoses that are instrumental in formulating a plan of care. The nurse, often being the first health care person to see a client, can obtain valuable information by using the physical assessment skills—*inspection* and *palpation*. Some assessments require the simultaneous use of each modality.

Inspection. To obtain accurate data through the use of inspection, it is imperative that certain conditions be met. Proper illumination is a must. Daylight is considered the best transmitter of illumination. However, in the absence of daylight, a stand light or gooseneck light with a 60-watt bulb is usually adequate. To avoid a glare or shadow, the light should be placed close to the skin.

Regardless of the health care environment (home, clinic, hospital) complete inspection of the integument should include assessments of color of the skin, presence of moisture, state of the appendages, and presence of lesions.

Color of the skin. Assess *normal* coloration and discoloration.

Coloration: The nurse should obtain baseline data because the coloring of the skin varies among healthy individuals. Subsequently, this information can be used for later comparison. In whites, the skin has a pinkish hue, whereas in dark-skinned individuals (blacks, Mediterraneans, Hispanics, Indians) the color of the skin varies with the skin tone of the individual. For example, the color of the lips and gums may have a bluish hue.[43] Observe for the normal underlying red tones that are usually present in all persons.[37] Skin tones are best determined on non-sun-exposed areas.

Discoloration: Assess for paleness, cyanosis, redness, or flushing, jaundice, pigmentation.

Paleness: The nailbeds, conjunctiva, mucous membranes, and lips are excellent areas on which to make this assessment, especially in dark-skinned individuals.[43]

Cyanosis: Cyanosis is a bluish discoloration that occurs as a result of reduced hemoglobin in increased amounts in the subpapillary venous plexus of the skin. It is caused by factors such as an abnormal reduction of oxyhemoglobin in systemic capillaries, a disturbance in the gaseous exchange between alveolar air and pulmonary capillary blood, a contamination of arterial blood with venous blood, and hemoglobin abnormalities.[33]

The nurse should determine whether the cyanosis is transient. For example, does it appear more pronounced at one time than another? In full-term infants cyanosis tends to be transient. Is it central? During infancy, the blood vessel tone and vascular distribution are not fully functional.[40] Subsequently, blood tends to pool centrally, and the skin may have poor circulation. Often after the infant has been crying or if the environmental temperature is lowered, the skin appears cyanotic.

The lips, mucous membranes of the mouth, nail beds, and ear lobes should be observed in dark-skinned individuals. In addition, black clients who are heavily pigmented in these areas should have this assessment made in other areas such as hands, soles of the feet, and conjunctiva.

Redness or flushing: If either is evident, further assessments are in order. For example, assess for *flushing*. If flushing is evident, what is the client's temperature? Is he embarrassed? Is he excited? For *redness,* has he been exposed to sun or another heat source? Either of these conditions might be responsible for the discoloration.

Jaundice: Jaundice is yellowish discoloration of the skin and mucous membranes caused by staining by bile pigment. It is best detected in the sclera and can be seen in the mucous membrane of the lips and hard palate. In making this assessment, the nurse should determine the age of the client. Jaundice is common during the neonatal period and is usually classified as physiological jaundice. In other age groups, it is pathological. For example, in young adults it may be indicative of infectious hepatitis; in middle-aged or older individuals it may be indicative of common duct stone and neoplastic jaundice.[47]

Pigmentation: Assess for hyperpigmentation or hypopigmentation. *Hyperpigmentation* is excessive pigment caused by an increased production of melanin from either a normal or increased number of melanocytes.[40] Assess for localized areas of hyperpigmentation (for example, freckles) or for generalized areas (for example, darkening) that may be related to problems of the adrenal or pituitary gland. *Hypopigmentation,* a reduction in the amount of pigment, may occur as a result of genetic, endocrine, or nutritional problems; chemicals; or trauma, which may damage or destroy melanocytes. The nurse should assess for localized or generalized areas of hypopigmentation.

Presence or absence of moisture. Assess for dryness, oiliness, or perspiration. When assessing moisture (such as perspiration), the nurse should consider variables such as age, activity, emotional state, and environment. Infants usually begin to perspire around 1 month of age. Its occurrence earlier may be a result of a central or sympathetic nervous system disorder, or of a drug-addicted mother. Activities such as crying, exercising, reaction to a hot environment, or fear may normally cause a person to perspire. However, excessive moisture may also be disease related.

State of appendages. Assess color, shape, configurations of nails, and distribution and color of hair. Are nails well groomed? Thick? What color are they? Fungal infections may leave a yellowish color. Distribution of hair? Is facial hair present (especially in the female)? Is there evidence of bald spots? Color? What is the texture?

Presence of lesions. Assess the specific type, location, size, shape, color, surface characteristics or appearance, and distribution of lesions. The specific type of lesion can be evaluated in relation to the level of the lesion to the skin surface.[17,18] For example, is it flat, elevated, or depressed? The nurse should be able to accurately describe primary and secondary lesions. Knowledge of the meaning of each enables the nurse to make accurate assessments. Following are descriptions of primary and secondary lesions.

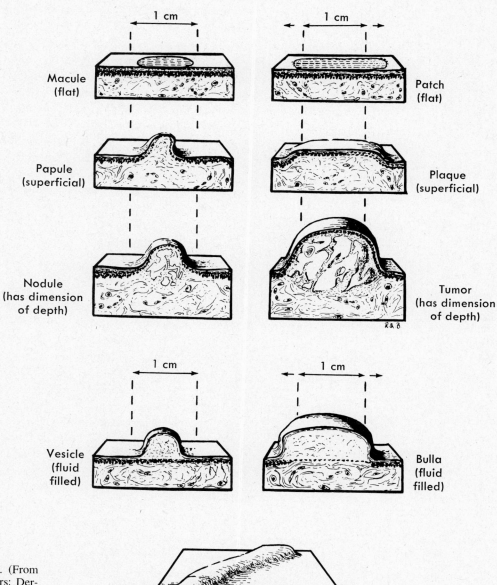

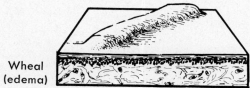

FIG. 15-2
Description of primary lesions. (From Stewart, William D., and others: Dermatology: diagnosis and treatment of cutaneous disorders, ed. 4, St. Louis, 1978, The C.V. Mosby Co.)

Primary lesions vary in elevation, size, shape, and color and include the following (Fig. 15-2):

A *macule* is a circumscribed discolorated area on the skin or mucous membrane that is neither elevated nor depressed. It is less than 1 cm in diameter and can be seen but not felt.

A *papule* is a solid elevation on the skin or mucous membrane that is less than 1 cm in diameter. A papule can be seen and felt and contains no fluid.

A *nodule* (tubercle) is a circumscribed solid elevation on the skin and mucous membrane less than 1 cm in diameter and deeper than a papule.

A *vesicle* (vesiculae, small blister) is a superficial elevation of the skin and mucous membrane that contains a clear fluid. It is less than 1 cm in diameter.

A *plaque* is a solid elevated lesion on the skin and mucous membrane larger than 1 cm in diameter.

A *pustule* is a vesicle or bulla that contains pus rather than a clear fluid.

A *bulla* (bleb, blister) is an elevation of the skin or mucous membrane that contains serous or seropurulent fluid. It is larger than a vesicle (for example, greater than 1 cm).

A *tumor* is a soft or firm mass of the skin, mucous membrane, or subcutaneous tissue that may be freely movable or fixed. It is usually greater than 1 cm and deeper than a nodule.

A *wheal* (hive) is a transient irregular-shaped elevation. It usually develops within seconds but disappears slowly. Usually itching and tingling accompany the wheal.

Secondary lesions include the following:

A *scale* is abnormal stratum corneum that has been separated from the skin and is characterized by flaking and thickening.

An *excoriation* (abrasion, erosion, scratch mark) is a superficial loss of epidermis that is produced by scratching, rubbing, or other means.

A *fissure* (crack) is a deep linear break through the epidermis into the dermis caused by disease or injury.

A *crust* (scab) is a dried mass of serum, pus, or blood on the surface of the skin. It may be mixed with bacterial or epithelial debris.

An *ulcer* is an opened wound that involves the epidermis and dermis. It is irregularly shaped and results from necrosis of tissue.

A *scar* (cicatrix) is a formation of new connective tissue. It is at first red and later turns pale. It occurs as part of the normal reparative and healing process. It may be elevated or depressed.

A *keloid* is a hyperplastic mass of fibrous tissue that develops at the site of a burn or skin wound.[5] Characteristically it is firm and elevated. Keloids are common in blacks (Fig. 15-3).

Lichenification is a dry, leathery thickening of the epidermis caused by chronic irritation.

Telangiectasia is a fine and often irregular red line produced by dilatation of a capillary.

Petechiae are tiny collections of blood outside of the capillaries. They are often reddish purple in color.

FIG. 15-3
Keloid. (From Stewart, William D., and others: Dermatology: diagnosis and treatment of cutaneous disorders, ed. 4, St. Louis, 1978, The C. V. Mosby Co.)

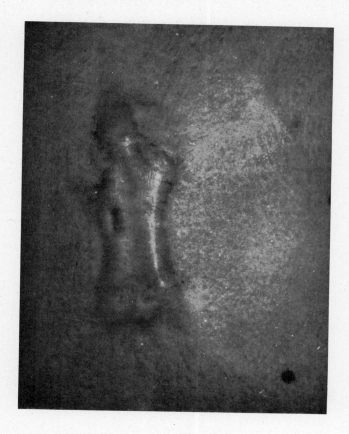

To assess the type of lesion, the nurse must obtain the following information.

Location. Are the lesions localized or generalized? If they are localized, what area of the body is involved? On what part of the body was it first noticed?

Size and shape. What is the actual or approximate size of the lesion? The lesion should be measured in its point of longest diameter. If a measuring device is not available, be as descriptive as possible in describing the size of the lesion in simple terms. When possible, use descriptive terms in describing shape. Are the lesions irregularly shaped, round, or oval?

Color. Are they red? If so, can a description be given as to the shade of red? Are they brownish red? Purplish red? Are they whitish?

Surface characteristics or appearance. Inspect the lesion for cleanliness, induration, or glazing. Are they scarred, vesicular, mascular, pustular, or bullous? Are they dry or weeping? If secretions are found in the lesions, are they scanty, profuse, purulent, or hemorrhagic? The presence of an odor should be noted.

Distribution. Do the lesions appear in clusters or are they grouped?

Palpation. The physical assessment skill of palpation is useful in defining the exact area of involvement. Palpation can be used in assessing temperature, texture, and the presence or absence of turgor.

Nursing process for common health problems

Temperature. Assess whether the skin is warm or cold to touch. It is useful to use the back of the hands to make this assessment because the skin is thinner and more sensitive to temperature change. The same hand should be used to palpate all areas.

Texture. Assess whether the area is smooth or rough. Is the hair coarse or fine? Body hair tends to be fine; facial hair tends to be coarse. Are the nails brittle?

Turgor and mobility. Assess for the presence or absence of turgor. To assess mobility, lift a fold of skin and note the speed of its return into place. Hydrated skin rises when pinched and returns to position when released. Dehydrated skin will remain in the pinched position. The specific area selected for this assessment should be an area where there is adequate subcutaneous fat. Sites commonly used for this assessment include the lower abdomen and calf, especially in the infant (Fig. 15-4), the forearm, sternum, and under the clavicle, where there is no excess tissue.

FIG. 15-4
Assessing for tissue turgor. **A,** Good tissue turgor. **B,** Bad tissue turgor. (From Prior, J.A., and Silberstein, J.S.: Physical diagnosis, ed. 5, St. Louis, 1977, The C.V. Mosby Co.)

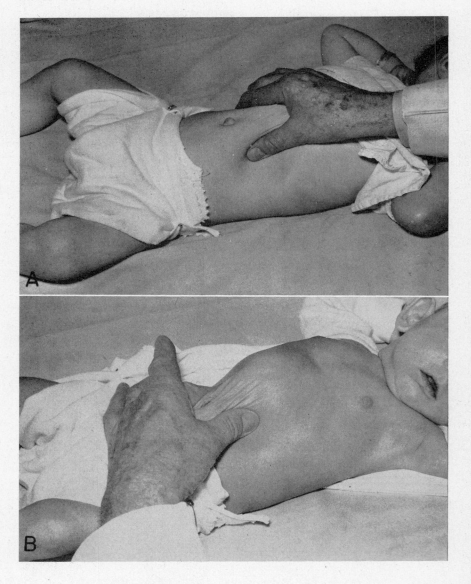

DIAGNOSTIC ASSESSMENT

A number of tests are used to diagnose skin disorders. Included among these are punch biopsy and sensitivity tests. Direct examination is also a useful diagnostic method. The nurse, to facilitate preparation of a care plan, must be familiar with these tests.

Punch biopsy

A punch biopsy involves removal of small sections of a cutaneous lesion, either by a scalpel or by a dermal punch followed by a histological examination of the specimen. The dermal punch, which is driven by electrical power, penetrates through the skin to a desired depth. In preparation for the biopsy, the area is cleansed with an antiseptic solution, and an anesthetic is injected into the skin lesion. A biopsy is useful in confirming the diagnosis of specific skin disorders such as tumors.

Sensitivity tests (allergy skin testing)

Three common methods used for introduction of the allergen in testing for sensitization include the cutaneous, pericutaneous, and intracutaneous methods.

Cutaneous method. A *patch test* is used to identify irritant substances to which a client is sensitive. A test material is placed on the skin surface and covered with a nonsensitizing and nonabsorbent dressing.[51] More than one test material may be used. In such instances, each area is numbered and identified. Unless marked irritation appears, the patch is usually left in place for 48 hours, then removed and left opened to air for 15 minutes, and a reading made. A positive reaction indicates an allergy or primary irritation (special measures are usually taken to eliminate primary irritation). Test results are graded on a scale of plus one through four, and reactions range from erythema to irritant reaction. For example, plus one is erythema; plus two is erythema, edema, and vesicle; plus three is erythema, edema, pseudopods, bullae, and ulceration; and plus four is irritant reaction.[51]

Covered parts of the body, such as the anterior surface of the thigh and lower back, are the areas most frequently used.

Pericutaneous method. A *scratch test* involves making a superficial scratch, approximately ½ inch (1.25 cm) long, through the epidermis without causing bleeding, and followed by placing a concentrated allergen on the scratched area. A control substance may also be used. The material is left in place for 15 minutes, after which the skin is rinsed and dried. Readings are made on both the control area and the tested area.

Intracutaneous method. The *intradermal test* is more sensitive and involves the injection of a minute amount (0.02 ml) of a dilute antigen within the epidermis.[25] Readings are made after 15 minutes. The inner surface of the arm is the most commonly used site. The abdomen, back, and thigh may also be used. Positive reactions for the scratch and intradermal test result in the formation of a wheal and suggest the presence of IgE in the skin. The more sensitive the individual, the larger the wheal at a lower concentration of test allergen. When a positive skin test correlates with the history, the allergen can possibly be identified as a causative agent.[25]

The pericutaneous and intracutaneous tests may result in the appearance of systemic symptoms such as nausea, chills, flushing, and dyspnea. Therefore epinephrine should always be readily available when these methods are used.

Radioallergosorbent test (RAST). RAST is a test that measures serum IgE antibodies to a variety of allergens. The technique involves labeling antibodies to a certain fragment of IgE that has been purified by an immunosorbent technique.[50]

779

Challenge test. Another useful modality in testing for allergy is the challenge test. This test involves identifying the offending substance and challenging the client with the substance in a quantity that the client would normally consume.

A strict elimination diet is used in an attempt to establish which foods may cause the reaction if food is considered the source. The diet is started by first eliminating milk. If this diet does not give relief within 2 weeks, meats, eggs, fish, and cheese may be eliminated. If no improvements are noted after this period, food is discredited as the cause of the allergy. At any point a specific food is identified, it is removed from the diet. The nurse should stress to the client the importance of adhering to the prescribed dietary regimen.

Evaluation of color changes. The nurse should evaluate the assessments of color in relation to variables such as position, environmental temperature, and emotional state. For example, position is particularly important when color changes of the extremities are assessed. Color changes may be indicative of a disease or illness. First, it is helpful to observe the part, such as an extremity, at heart level and then in an elevated or lowered position, barring contraindications. Assessing the part in the latter positions may produce a false color and mimic a pathophysiological state.

Consideration must also be given to the temperature of the environment and to the client's emotional state. A cold or air-conditioned environment may produce a bluish discoloration (for example, "cold cyanosis")[37] in areas such as the nailbeds or the lips in some individuals, whereas an extremely warm environment or embarrassment may produce a flushed appearance because of superficial vasodilation. Paleness may be also evident in an emotional state such as fright or when the environment is cold. The temperature of the assessment environment in which an assessment is being made should therefore be comfortable, and efforts should be directed toward eliminating embarrassment during the examination to decrease chances of a false assessment.

Direct examinations

Examination for the presence of fungi may be made by direct examination with the use of microscope, culture, and Wood's light. Tissue taken from *skin scrapings* may be used for microscopic and culture examination. More specifically, skin scrapings are used for identification of a fungus after the history suggests that a fungus might be present. After the area has been cleansed with an antiseptic and permitted to dry, a scalpel is used to obtain a scraping of the skin. The specimen is then collected in a container, cultured for 3 weeks, and studies made for the type of fungus present. Part of the scrapings may be placed on a microscopic slide and, after special preparation, analyzed for fungal elements. *Wood's light,* a selected wavelength of light, is used to examine the scalp for ringworms. Such examinations must be performed in a dark room. An ultraviolet light and a Wood's filter produce fluorescence of hair infested with human or animal fungus. Direct microscopic examination of the hairs confirms the diagnosis, and a culture is taken to confirm the type.

Data analysis

After the nurse has collected all pertinent data about the client, the information is compared with standards appropriate to the age, sex, development, and life-style of the individual. This phase of the process ends with an analysis of the data and the formulation of nursing diagnoses or problems. These diagnoses or problems will serve as a basis for development of an individualized plan of care. Potential or actual diagnoses that may be included are alterations in comfort, disturbance in self-concept, impairment of skin integrity, ineffective coping, fear, fluid volume deficit, anticipatory grieving, potential for injury, impaired physical mobility, and alterations in nutrition.

Planning

PLANNING FOR HEALTH PROMOTION

Health promotion is essential to preserving healthy skin. The nurse has an important role in teaching about the proper care of the skin and its appendages. The nurse should use the characteristics of the skin at various stages as guidelines for health teaching. In health the skin should be soft, supple, and moderately oily; it should not crack or scale and should be free of eruptions.

Cleanliness is essential for healthy skin in all stages of life, because it enables the skin to maintain its elimination function by removing bacteria, excessive oils, and dirt. Bathing is the primary means through which cleanliness is maintained. Daily bathing should be encouraged, because it not only cleans, but also serves to soothe, relax, and promote comfort. Bathing is particularly essential during stages when an excess amount of oil is being produced. During the stage of increased sebaceous activity, the sebaceous glands and pores are in danger of becoming clogged, which could result in infection.

Cleansing should be accomplished with the use of a good toilet soap and water. Antibacterial soaps can be used if there is danger of bacterial infection. After the bath, the skin should be rinsed thoroughly to prevent soap from accumulating on the skin and causing irritation, and then patted dry with a soft towel. The areas between the toes should be washed and dried thoroughly to prevent maceration and bacterial or fungal growths. Powder should be applied on those parts where two skin surfaces come in contact. The use of alcohol is to be discouraged because of its drying and defatting effect.

The nurse should encourage modification in the bath at specific periods during the life span. For example, young and middle-aged clients generally tolerate soap cleansing and maximum amounts of water; whereas older clients are less able to tolerate soap, especially during colder months. The skin of the latter has a tendency to peel and dry; therefore bathing for these clients should be limited to two or three times weekly, except for the face, neck, ears, axilla, hands, and groin. These areas should be washed daily. The use of superfatted soaps and bath oils should be encouraged. Superfatted soaps cause less irritation. Oils seal moisture into the skin and form a protective layer between the skin and air, thereby preventing dehydration of the corneum. Instructions should therefore be given as to the proper use of bath oils. They should be applied or added to water after the client has soaked for 15 to 20 minutes. This facilitates sealing the moisture into the skin.

The appendages must also be cared for. The hair should be kept scrupulously clean. The frequency of shampooing is individually determined. Those with oily hair should be encouraged to wash it at least weekly. Dry hair ought to be washed less frequently, and cream should be applied after washing to prevent it from becoming brittle and the ends from splitting. The nails must be kept clean and well groomed.

Nursing process for common health problems

The nurse should also instruct individuals on measures related to *environmental temperature, clothing, diet,* and *exposure to sunlight.* The environmental temperature should not be overheated, because high temperatures may lead to inflammatory disorders such as miliaria or other rashes. Such reactions are particularly likely to occur in infants.

Clothes must be properly cared for and rinsed to prevent accumulation of irritating soaps and detergents, which may result in inflammatory disorders such as diaper rash. The diet must also contain adequate nutrient substances. Vitamin A has been demonstrated to be effective in promoting healthy skin.

Extensive exposure to sunlight should be avoided. Instructions should be given to use some type of protective agent when it is necessary to be in the sun for long periods of time.

Immunization

The provision of information about immunization is another area in which the nurse can influence health promotion. Immunization can be defined as a means of preventing or modifying natural infection by the administration of antibody or antigen.[38] It is accomplished by passive immunization (administration of antibody) or by active immunization (administration of antigen as a killed microorganism, a component of a microorganism, or a live attenuated microorganism). It generally provides permanent immunity by stimulating the host to produce its own antibody. As a result, its aim is to help individuals maintain a state of health against various bacterial and viral illnesses. Active immunization is provided routinely for diphtheria, tetanus, pertussis (DTP), poliomyelitis (TOPV), measles, mumps, and rubella (MMR). Occasionally, immunization against typhoid may be administered. For overseas travel, immunization for cholera, yellow fever, or smallpox may be required. (The Center for Disease Control guidelines should be consulted for recommendations for specific countries.)

Immunization schedules. Immunization is usually begun during infancy, with booster doses administered at periodic intervals throughout the childhood, adolescence, and adulthood. The *Report of the Committee on Infectious Diseases (The Red Book),*[52] revised every 3 years, contains authoritative recommendations about immunization schedules (Tables 15-1 and 15-2). The Advisory Committee of Immunization Practices (ACIP) of the United States Public Health Service also makes recommendations regarding immunization. (See material on p. 783 for information regarding immunization abbreviations.) Table 15-3 describes communicable diseases.

Diphtheria, tetanus, pertussis. Active immunization with the triple preparation DTP is acquired by administration of the toxins (diphtheria and tetanus) and the killed pertussis vaccine in a series of three intramuscular injections, followed at intervals by a series of booster injections (Table 15-1). The series is administered in triplicate because the antibody titers are considered higher in combination than with one single agent. It is recommended that immunization be started at 2 months of age, with the remaining two dosages being administered at bimonthly intervals. Booster dosages are administered around age 18 months and again between the ages of 4 and 6 years. It is recommended that additional boosters of tetanus and diphtheria be repeated every 10 years after the initial five injections of DTP. If the series is not started until school age, the pertussis vaccine is not administered because the risk of hypersensitivity reactions is thought to exceed the need for protection.[28,38]

TABLE 15-1

Recommended schedule for active immunization of normal infants and children

Age	Immunization type
2 mo	DTP; TOPV
4 mo	DTP; TOPV
6 mo	DTP
1 yr	Tuberculin test
15 mo	Measles; rubella; mumps
1½ yr	DTP; TOPV
4-6 yr	DTP; TOPV
14-16 yr	Td (repeat every 10 years)

Adapted from The Report of the Committee on Infectious Diseases, ed. 19, Evanston, Ill., 1982, American Academy of Pediatrics.

TABLE 15-2

Primary immunization schedule for children not immunized in early infancy

Schedule	Immunization type
Under age 6	
First visit	DTP; TOPV; tuberculin test
Interval after first visit	
1 mo	Measles; mumps; rubella
2 mo	DTP; TOPV
4 mo	DTP; TOPV
10 to 16 mo or preschool	DTP; TOPV
Age 14-16 yr	Td (repeat every 10 years)
Age 6 and older	
First visit	Td; TOPV; tuberculin test
Interval after first visit	
1 mo	Measles; mumps; rubella
2 mo	Td; TOPV
8 to 14 mo	Td; TOPV
Age, 14-16 yr	Td (repeat every 10 years)

Adapted from The Report of the Committee on Infectious Diseases, ed. 19, Evanston, Ill., 1982, American Academy of Pediatrics, p. 11.

KEY TO IMMUNIZATION ABBREVIATIONS

DTP   Diphtheria and tetanus toxoid combined with pertussis vaccine

TOPV   Trivalent oral poliovirus vaccine

Td   Combined tetanus and diphtheria toxoids (adult type) in contrast to diphtheria and tetanus (DT) toxoids, which contain a larger amount of diphtheria antigen.

Polio vaccine. The trivalent oral polio vaccine (TOPV) consists of three types of modified and attenuated polioviruses. Usually, two oral doses of the vaccine are given at 4- to 6-week intervals, starting at approximately 2 months of age and administered again around 4 months. The third dose is administered about 1 year later.

Measles, mumps, rubella (MMR). Combinations of measles (rubeola), mumps, and rubella (German measles) vaccines, which are attenuated live virus vaccines, have proved effective. One injection produces lifetime immunity against these diseases. It is recommended to be administered around 15 months of age. Administration of the vaccine before this time is not recommended because it is thought the antibodies transmitted from the mother may interfere with the development of active immunity.

Nursing responsibilities. Nurses assume a great responsibility for immunizations, because they are often the health care professional administering the vaccine and frequently must make decisions about varied aspects of immunizations. One of the decisions that may have to be made is whether to administer a vaccine at the recommended time schedule or to delay administration for varied reasons. Whatever decisions are made, these can be enhanced by making detailed assessments about reactions and about health status.

Assessment. Assessment must be made before administration of the vaccine, the data evaluated, and a decision made regarding administration (see material on p. 787). A severe reaction after a previous vaccine, characterized by high temperature, convulsion, and shock, demands that the immunization schedule be discontinued.[30] When a moderate fever is evident, the child may only be given one-half the dose during the remaining visits. Subsequently, the total number of vaccines will be increased so that the total recommended amount of antigen is given. If it is necessary to delay a vaccine at a given time for reasons other than a severe reaction, subsequent vaccines are given on schedule until the series is completed.

During an initial visit, or during first contact with the child, additional information should be obtained about health status and therapy. There are certain conditions that contraindicate administration of vaccines (for example, acute febrile illness for DTP, and immune deficiency, either because of disease or therapy such as cancer chemotherapy for TOPV). For MMR, the list of contraindications is longer and includes severe febrile illness, immune deficiency disease, those receiving immunosuppressive therapy, malignancies (for example, leukemia and lymphoma), pregnancy (because of the risks to the fetus becoming infected, resulting in damage to it), and allergy to the vaccine or components of the vaccine.

On each visit the temperature should be taken and assessments made regarding the presence of an infection (for example, upper respiratory tract, throat, or ear infection). Some authorities recommend a delay if the data are positive.[31] However, for positive data (for example, an elevated temperature) the nurse must consider other possible causes for the elevation. Is the child fretful? Fretfulness and crying may be responsible for an elevated temperature. Is the child irritable or restless? This might be indicative of an early infection.[22]

Instructions. Once the vaccine is administered, an important aspect of care is to instruct the client and family about *what to expect.* Making them aware of expected reactions will lessen their anxiety. A slight fever and irritability within

TABLE 15-3

Communicable diseases

Disease	Etiological agent	Symptoms	Occurrence	Transmission	Reservoir of infection
Diphtheria: acute infectious disease characterized by edema and the formation of a membrane on the epithelial surface, usually the throat	*Corynebacterium diphtheriae*	Fatigue, headache, sore throat, slight fever, nasal discharge	Highest in school-age children who have not been immunized	Direct by inhaling infective droplets that were exhaled or coughed up by human carrier; or indirect by articles contaminated by infected individuals	Discharges from nose and throat
Pertussis (whooping cough): an acute infectious disease characterized by episodes of coughing that end with a whoop on inspiration	*Bordetella pertussis*	Sneezing, lacrimation, cough more severe at night, characteristic whoop, vomiting	Common in school-age children	Direct from an infected person through upper respiratory tract secretions; indirect by contact with articles freshly contaminated by an infected person	
Measles (rubeola): an acute infection characterized by fever, rash, and upper respiratory tract symptoms (Fig. 15-5)	Filtrable virus (paramyxovirus)	High fever, maculopapular rash, upper respiratory tract symptoms, cough, malaise, coryza, Koplik spots on the buccal mucosa of cheek (appear 24-48 hours before rash), photophobia, and conjunctivitis	More common among children before 10 years of age	Direct droplet contact of respiratory tract secretions	Active cases of measles
Chicken pox (varicella): an acute viral disease characterized by generalized eruptions of vesicles and papules, pustules, crusted lesions, and itching (Figs. 15-5 and 15-6)	Filtrable virus	Fever ranging from 101° to 105° F (38.3° to 40.6° C), rash distributed mainly on the trunk, malaise, headache, pruritus	Common among children	Direct person-to-person through droplets; indirect through discharges from skin lesions or nasal and pharyngeal secretions	
German measles (rubella): acute viral disease characterized by eruptions similar to those of rubeola	Filtrable virus (paramyxovirus)	Low-grade fever, malaise, headache, sore throat, coryza during first 5 days	Common among children and young adults	Person-to-person through droplets or air transmission, articles freshly contaminated with nasopharyngeal secretions, feces, and urine	
Mumps (epidemic parotitis): acute viral infectious disease characterized by swelling of salivary glands, especially parotid glands	Filtrable virus (paramyxovirus)	Fever, headache, earache, malaise, anorexia, swelling of parotid gland, and pain, especially on ingesting sour substances	Children between ages 5 and 15	Direct contact and droplet infection; indirect by secretions of oral cavity or respiratory tract	
Smallpox (variola): acute infection	Filtrable virus, pox virus variolae	Fever, headache, malaise, chills, vomiting, generalized eruptions	All age groups susceptible	Droplet infection from respiratory tract, infectious material (such as clothing and linen)	An individual who is ill with or convalescing from smallpox

Port of entry	Incubation period	Complications	Measures of control	Nursing intervention
Nose or mouth; occasionally through skin	2-7 days; average 3-5 days	Myocarditis; paralysis of the soft palate, pharynx, larynx; respiratory paralysis	Isolation until nasal and throat cultures are negative; bed rest; antibiotics	Explain importance of isolation; use principles of medical asepsis; maintain patent airway by suctioning as often as necessary; reduce exertion by assisting client in meeting basic needs; encourage bed rest; assist with meals; soft foods generally better tolerated; provide diversional activity that is not taxing on client; promote comfort; daily bath; cleanse and lubricate nose and mouth frequently (do not swab because bleeding may occur); protect client from chilling and drafts; observe for signs that indicate complications
Mucous membrane of respiratory tract	7-16 days; average 10 days	Bronchopneumonia	Isolation until paroxysmal cough ceases; rest; antibiotics	Maintain isolation; use tissue for nasal discharge and discard in proper container; maintain body resistance; protect client from persons with upper respiratory tract infections and from drafts; provide adequate nutrition and fluids; prevent coughing episodes by discouraging any activity that may precipitate coughing attacks, such as exercise, excitement (laughing, crying); avoid hot, cold, highly seasoned foods; give sedatives as prescribed
Nose and mouth	8-21 days; average 10-14 days	Otitis media; pneumonia; encephalitis	Isolated if possible for approximately 1 week after rash disappears; antibiotics if bacterial complications occur	Maintain respiratory isolation as closely as possible; use tissue for nasal discharge and discard properly; protect client from persons with upper respiratory infections; provide adequate rest, nutrition, and fluids; provide measures to control itching; protect clients from drafts and chilling; protect eyes from glare by use of dark glasses or placing bed so that client does not face light; promote relaxation; provide some means of relaxation
Nose and mouth	2-3 weeks; average 17 days	Secondary skin infection (i.e., impetigo, furuncles, cellulitis)	Isolation until skin heals; highly contagious (i.e., 24 hours before appearance of rash to scab for most)	Maintain bed rest; provide adequate hydration; prevent skin irritation; pat dry after baths; provide methods to control itching; daily bath with bran; use soothing lotions; keep fingernails short and clean; prevent scratching; use mittens, gloves, pajamas; linens should be cool and smooth; provide some form of diversion; explain to parents that marks gradually disappear
Nose and throat	14-21 days; average 16 days	Arthritis; rarely, encephalitis; if occurs during 1st trimester of pregnancy, offspring may develop congenital defects (cataracts, deafness, heart defects, mental retardation)	Isolation for duration of fever and rash; bed rest during febrile stage	Maintain respiratory isolation; provide adequate nutrition and fluids; provide measures to relieve itching
Nose and throat	2-3 weeks; average 18 days	Orchitis; oophoritis; meningoencephalitis	Isolation until swelling ceases; rest in bed; if mumps is developed after puberty, bed rest should be maintained until complete recovery to prevent gonadal involvement	Maintain isolation precautions; maintain adequate diet; mild, bland, semisolid foods usually better tolerated than sour or spicy foods; frequent mouth care; provide adequate rest; administer antipyretics
Nose and throat	7-17 days; average 12 days	Pulmonary edema; heart failure; abortion	Isolate until skin lesions disappear; antibiotics to prevent pyogenic complications; cardiotonic glycosides for cardiac problems	Maintain isolation precautions; all nasal, oral, fecal, and urinary discharges should be disinfected by high-pressure steam or boiling; encourage contacts to be vaccinated or revaccinated; maintain adequate hydration and nutrition; avoid bright lights; maintain adequate ventilation; assess vital signs frequently

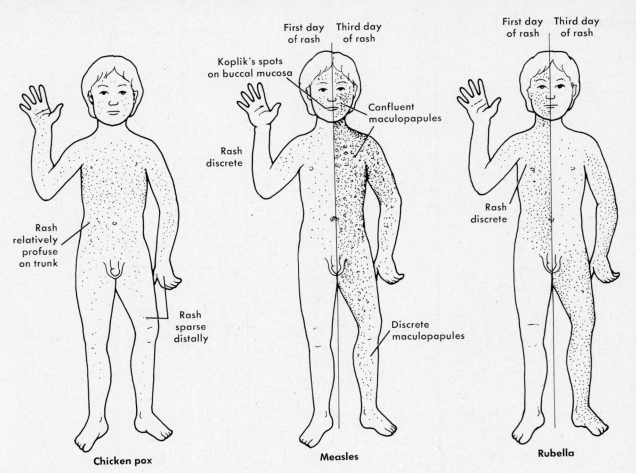

First day of rash | Third day of rash

Koplik's spots on buccal mucosa

Confluent maculopapules

Rash discrete

Rash relatively profuse on trunk

Rash sparse distally

Discrete maculopapules

First day of rash | Third day of rash

Rash discrete

Chicken pox   **Measles**   **Rubella**

FIG. 15-5
Distribution of rashes in three communicable diseases.

the first 24 hours are to be expected. However, persistence of a temperature beyond this period should be reported. Generally, parents are instructed to give the child acetaminophen for an elevated temperature.

More specifically, the nurse may wish to provide instructions about possible side effects. Side effects are generally transient and include fever and rash for measles and rubella. For the latter, arthralgia is often experienced by adults. These usually occur 1 to 2 weeks after the vaccine is administered. For DTP, erythema or pain at the injection site may occur within 1 to 2 days. Clients should be informed that any type of *systemic* or *unexpected reaction* should be reported.

There is a lack of agreement as to whether the child immunized with MMR should be around a pregnant woman during the first trimester because of the possibility of fetal damage.

Instructions should be given as to the importance of *completing the immunization series*. When the series begins, a schedule should be given to the parents with instructions as to when subsequent immunizations are to be administered. Many parents have become lax at returning with their children for booster injections. The importance of follow-up booster injections should be emphasized.

When the series is completed, parents should be given a record of all injections. The American Academy of Pediatrics has developed a personal immunization card that is useful in maintaining records (Fig. 15-7).

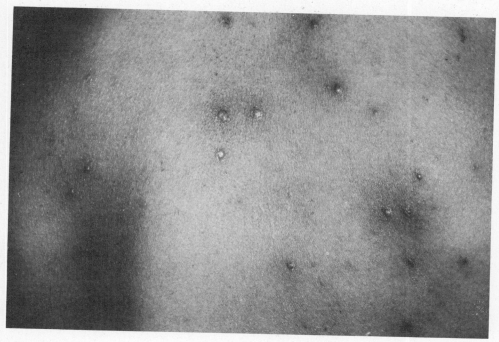

FIG. 15-6
Chicken pox. (From Stewart, William D., and others: Dermatology: diagnosis and treatment of cutaneous disorders, ed. 4, St. Louis, 1978, The C.V. Mosby Co.)

ASSESSMENT GUIDE FOR IMMUNIZATION*

A. *Assess prior health status.* (These questions are necessary to ascertain a health history).
　1. Has the child been fully immunized? DTP? MMR? Polio?
　2. At what age did the child receive his DTP, MMR, polio shot?
　3. Is the child on any special medications?
　4. Tell me about the child's health.
　5. Does the child have a chronic illness?
　6. Does the child have a problem involving the central nervous system? Is there a history of seizures? Tremors? Twitching? Blackout spells? (Obtaining information about neurological status is especially essential when the pertussis vaccine is to be administered, because it has been documented to cause central nervous system problems.[30]
　7. Is there a history of immunological deficiency (that is, cancer of the lymph system)?
　8. How did the child react after the last shot or vaccine?
　9. Did the child have a reaction after the last shot? If yes, was it severe? Tell me about the reaction.
　10. Did the child spike a temperature? What was the temperature?
　11. Did you notice any seizure activity? Did you see a physician?
　12. Was the child irritable? Fretful? Restless for a couple of days?

B. *Assess health status at the time of immunization.* (Answers to these questions may provide cues to a beginning infection or illness. Febrile illness or an active infection is generally considered a contraindication to immunization, because the immunization itself may cause an elevation.)
　1. Has the child been fretful, restless, or irritable for the last couple of days?
　2. Have there been any changes in his sleep pattern?
　3. How often does the child have a cold? How long does the cold last? (With a history of chronic cold, it is recommended that the immunization be administered.[38])
　4. Are there open skin lesions? (This assessment is particularly important before smallpox vaccinations. In addition to questioning about open lesions, the nurse should assess by observation.)
　5. Does anyone in close contact with the child have open lesions?

C. *Assess potential for hypersensitivity.*
　1. Is there a history of eczema?
　2. Does this child have any allergies? Is he allergic to any antibiotics? (Antibiotics are included in rubella and polio vaccines.[5])

*These questions can be used as general guidelines in obtaining data about an individual's immunization status. However, the nurse should generate a more specific list of questions from those presented so that the client will give information that will be useful in the process of implementing care.

FIG. 15-7
Immunization card.

IMMUNIZATION RECORD (give dates)					
	1	2	3	4	5
DPT					
DT					
Td					
TOPV					
Measles		Rubella		Mumps	
Flu		Other			

PLANNING FOR HEALTH MAINTENANCE AND RESTORATION

The nurse should consider the following concepts as care is planned for clients with problems of the integument: (1) humans are social beings and care about what others think; and (2) the appearance of the skin has meaning in terms of one's self-esteem and feelings of acceptability to others.

Skin lesions present a special problem because they can be seen by the client as well as by others. The client with a dermatological problem is usually a sensitive observer of reactions of others. Nurses must therefore recognize their own feelings about these problems. If nurses are aware of their feelings, their ability to control their expressions as care is given to the client will be enhanced. Nurses must not stare at the client's disfigurement, nor avoid the sight of it. Instead, they should observe the client as any other client. When caring for the client or changing dressings, nurses should not hesitate to touch the skin. Awareness of the nature of the lesion will enable them to use logical and necessary protective strategies. For example, infectious disorders with open lesions necessitate the use of gloves.

Many dermatological problems are long-standing. Therefore, as early as possible, the client with such a disorder should be encouraged to become independent in his care. He should be instructed on how to properly care for his skin. If compresses are needed, he should be instructed on how to properly apply them. When the client is admitted to the hospital, he should be allowed to assist in his care as much as possible. However, the nurse should demonstrate acceptance by assisting the client, even if he is physically able to care for himself.

Family members must not be forgotten. Ample opportunities should be provided for them to air their feelings. They must be instructed on how they can help with the care of the client.

A symptom common to a number of skin lesions is pruritus. It is so common that discussion of the symptom is needed. Knowledge of it and some of the factors associated with it will facilitate understanding of the care needed for these clients.

Pruritus: a model for planning and implementation

Pruritus (itching), a normal sensation, is perhaps the most common symptom that accompanies a variety of skin disorders. It is subjective, may occur in varied age groups, and may be triggered by internal or external factors. For example, factors such as perspiration, heat, cold, soaps, chemicals, and, to a sensitized person, various proteins or pollens. Physical changes in the skin, such as dryness from excessive bathing, chafing, and tickling from various fabrics (wool, nylon, and other synthetics), may also be responsible. It may also be trig-

788

gered by the ingestion of drugs, stress, and emotions, and it may be the first indication of a serious internal disease such as Hodgkins' disease or leukemia.

The presence of itching is antagonizing and may serve to prolong the healing of an initial skin disorder. When an individual itches, he tends to scratch to obtain relief. Trauma may result from scratching. Subsequently the skin may become open to bacteria, thereby becoming a primary source of infection.

Excessive warmth and heat, rough fabrics (for example, wool), fatigue, emotional distress, perspiration, and idleness tend to make itching worse. It generally occurs more commonly at night, possibly because at night the individual's attention is less likely to be distracted and thus he is more aware of the sensation. The increased intensity at night is also thought to be related to increased warmth of the skin from bed coverings.

Various forms of therapeutic measures may be used to assure a certain degree of relief. Local therapy, such as antipruritic lotions, wet dressings, and baths, has proved beneficial. Analgesics and sedatives are often used to increase the itch threshold. Antihistamine drugs (trimeprazine tartrate [Temaril] or methdilazine [Tacaryl]) and corticosteroids are also prescribed. When the latter are prescribed, they are used only for short periods because of the serious complications that may develop with long-term use.

An awareness of factors that intensify an itch will facilitate planning for relief of the problem. Measures to divert the client's attention and to avoid overheating and emotional upsets may be instrumental in accomplishing this. Medication should be administered before the patient becomes too uncomfortable.

Heat increases the symptom because the nerve endings concerned with pruritic sensations are more sensitive to increased capillary dilatation. Therefore the nurse should provide measures to prevent vasodilation. Enough bedding and clothing should be provided to keep the client comfortably warm but not overly heated. The environmental temperature must be comfortable. It should be checked frequently and adjustments made as necessary.

The nurse should be cognizant of the factors that tend to upset or irritate the client. Excitement, increased emotions, and fatigue lower the threshold for itching. The client should be encouraged to avoid these as much as possible. If the client is tense, providing a night snack or encouraging reading before bedtime may be instrumental in facilitating relaxation. Engaging the client in some form of diversional activity based on his interest may also be useful. The client should be assisted in performing daily activities. Reassurance should be given as needed. It is important to encourage him to resist the impulse to scratch. If he cannot resist, he should be instructed to press the areas with his fingers or hands rather than scratch. White gloves or mittens are helpful, particularly for the young child. Fingernails should be kept short to prevent trauma to the skin.

Other restorative therapies

Varied forms of therapy may be prescribed for lesions or problems of the skin. Dressings, baths, and preparations (lotions and creams) are discussed.

Wet dressings. Crust, scales, and debris that accumulate on the skin must be cleansed and removed gently. Wet dressings, perhaps among the most important form of local therapy used in dermatological problems, are used. They are beneficial in cleaning debris from wounds, loosening scales, promoting drainage, softening the skin, relieving itching, and soothing the inflamed skin. In addition, medication may be used in combination with wet dressings to enhance drainage.

Although wet dressings may be applied continuously for 1 to 2 days, they are more often applied intermittently several times per day. When they are applied intermittently, a cream may also be applied to the skin to prevent dryness. Dressings may be open or closed and may be used to facilitate application of heat or cold. Cold wet dressings produce vasoconstriction of the capillaries. As a result, an involved area is allowed to rest. On the other hand, hot or warm compresses produce dilation of the capillary walls and facilitate phagocytosis.

Throughout therapy, the temperature of the dressing should be maintained. Heating pads, used with care, are instrumental in maintaining the temperature of hot or warm dressings. In an effort to prevent evaporation, the compress should be covered with an impermeable material such as cellophane wrap. A covering also facilitates maintenance of the desired temperature. Closed wet dressings do not need frequent changes because closure prevents evaporation and facilitates retention of heat. Compresses should be changed approximately every 2 hours, or more often if they become dry.

When dressings are a form of therapy, the nurse should teach the client how to properly prepare and apply dressings. Absorbent gauze should be used. Kerlix, a type of gauze consisting of one to three layers, makes an excellent dressing and also has an elastic quality that enhances its use as a dressing. Towels and sheets may be used, although they are not as suitable as Kerlix. The nurse should discourage clients from using woolen material, because it irritates the skin, dries easily, and tends to shrink when wet. Rough or coarse materials stick to the skin and should not be used. Generally, when excessive dryness and cracks appear, dressings are discontinued.

When wet dressings are used for open lesions, measures should be taken to prevent introducing organisms into the lesions. Dressings should never be moistened by pouring a solution over a dry outer layer. Therefore when dressings are changed, the outer covering should be removed completely before the dressing is soaked. To prevent damage to the skin should the dressing adhere, the inner dressing should be soaked before attempts are made to remove it.

Solutions that may be used for dressings include water, saline, magnesium sulfate, Alpha-Keri, potassium permanganate, and silver nitrate.

The use of wet dressings demands that the nurse be cognizant of how to apply them to different parts of the body. Following are a few guidelines:

1. Body parts that come in contact with each other should be separated. For example, if dressings are placed on the fingers or toes, each finger should be wrapped separately. Commercial gloves are available for use as dressings.
2. A sock may be used to hold a foot dressing in place.
3. A dressing that resembles a face mask can be used for a face dressing.
4. A turban can be used for the head.
5. Material that has been folded like a diaper can be used to hold perineal or groin dressings in place.

Baths. Baths have the same effect as wet dressings and are useful therapy in conditions where the use of compresses would be impractical. In conditions where the dermatosis is generalized and extensive, baths may be used. The location of the involvement may also demand the use of a bath rather than dressings, as with involvement of the perianal area. The entire body may be immersed in water, or only the involved part may be immersed.

Tub baths and sitz baths may be prescribed, and various preparations may be added to effect cleansing irritated skin. Colloidal preparations, such as Aveeno and Soyaloid, are often prescribed. Tar baths are useful in treating psoriasis and eczema.

The nurse must be cognizant of safety factors. When baths are administered, the temperature of the bath solution should be comfortable. Clients should not be left in the tub for more than ½ hour and should be observed frequently during the bath. The timing for the dressing change or bath should be considered. They should be planned well in advance of meals or other specific activities to decrease fatigue and irritability.

Preparations. Raw, weeping surfaces must be coated to facilitate drying and to eliminate organisms. Water in *cream solvents* may be useful for these purposes.

Lotions cause evaporation. Many lotions contain astringents that cause surface proteins to precipitate, thereby producing a scaling and drying effect on the skin.

Creams are ointments that contain an emulsifying agent (lowering the surface tension) with water. When the water evaporates from the cream, a cooling effect is produced on the skin while the medicine is being absorbed. Steroid creams suppress inflammatory reactions and are frequently used. Prednisolone, prednisone, and hydrocortisone are often used. Various antibiotic creams are also used to combat infection.

Dry, scaly areas must be kept soft and protected from excessive drying and infection. *Ointments* are useful in these conditions because they tend to heat the skin by reducing radiation and evaporation.

Implementation

COMMON HEALTH PROBLEMS OF THE NEONATE

Hemangiomas

Skin problems common to the neonate are congenital vascular lesions (tumors) and problems associated with pigmentary changes. These changes are generally visible at or shortly after birth.

Hemangiomas, congenital vascular lesions of the skin, appear at birth or in the neonatal period. They are commonly referred to as birthmarks. The most common hemangiomas are discussed.

Assessment. *Port-wine stains* (nevus flammeus) consist of dilated mature capillaries in the upper dermis. They appear at birth and usually in various sizes and shapes. They are usually flat, although they may be irregular, slightly raised, and may vary in color from red to reddish purple. The color depends on which layer of the dermal vessel is involved.[51] Most stains appear on the face and neck and, unfortunately, produce a noticeable disfigurement. They may, however, occur on the buttocks (Fig. 15-8), occipital area, and extremities, and cause no cosmetic problems.

Strawberry hemangioma is a raised lesion that is characterized by bright red patches that resemble a strawberry (Fig. 15-9). It is usually present at birth, but may occur within a few months after birth. It may be found on any area of the body, tends to grow rapidly in the neonatal or infancy periods, but later disappears completely,[51] usually by age 7.[3]

Cavernous hemangiomas are raised bluish red lesions composed of dilated blood vessels and usually present at birth. They occur deeper in the dermis[51] and may occur on any part of the skin surface.

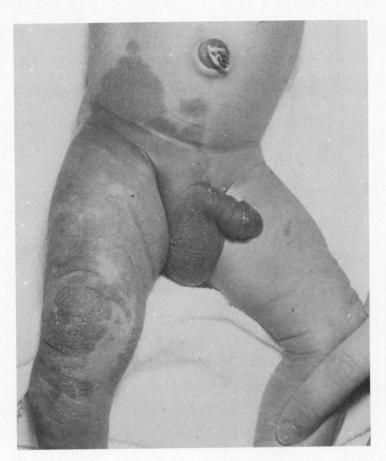

FIG. 15-8
Port-wine stain. (From Jensen, M., Benson, R., and Bobak, I.: Maternity care, ed. 2, St. Louis, 1981, The C.V. Mosby Co.)

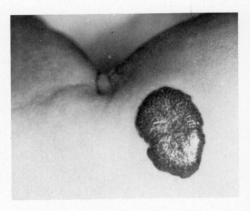

FIG. 15-9
Strawberry mark. (From Shirkey, H.: Pediatric therapy, ed. 6, St. Louis, 1980, The C.V. Mosby Co.)

Pigmented nevus is a benign tumor composed of nevus cells (benign tumor cells derived from melanocytes).[4] Characteristically these lesions are flat and range in size from a few millimeters to a centimeter or more. The color of the lesion may range from a slight discoloration to black.

Mongolian spots are areas of increased pigmentation, present at birth, that usually blend into surrounding normal skin. These bluish purple lesions usually appear on the lumbosacral region. They are common in Oriental infants and infants of dark-skinned races; they occur rarely in whites.[51] They usually disappear spontaneously during childhood.

Data analysis
Data analysis may reveal the following nursing diagnoses for infants with vascular lesions: impairment of skin integrity and potential disturbance in self-concept.

Planning and implementation. Stains that appear on the face may be a source of emotional trauma for the child as well as the family. A plan of care therefore must be directed toward the goal of removing the source of the problem. Forms of therapy that have been directed toward this end (for example, for port-wine stains) have included dermabrasion and freezing the lesion (that is, with carbon dioxide or slush). Such therapy usually results in paling of the lesion. Skin-colored cosmetic creams or powders have also proved useful in disguising the lesion. All health team members must provide as much emotional support to the family as is needed so as to reduce sensitive feelings about the lesion. For example, for strawberry hemangioma, no therapy is indicated unless it is located near a body orifice. The same is generally true for cavernous hemangiomas because no therapy is necessary unless the lesions are extensive. For these, plastic surgery may be indicated.

Evaluation. Evaluation of the nursing plan for the neonate with vascular lesions and pigmentary changes is an ongoing process. Because of the uniqueness of individuals and their families, expressions of concern and acceptance of the problem will likely be varied.

EXPECTED OUTCOMES

The family can:
1. Describe the hemangioma, nevus, or pigmentation change.
2. Indicate an understanding of the basis for the health problem.
3. Express feelings about the problem.
4. State plans for follow-up management and care.

COMMON HEALTH PROBLEMS OF THE INFANT AND CHILD

Diaper rash

Problems that occur during infancy and childhood include rashes and infections (bacterial, viral, and fungal).

Diaper rash, an erythematous rash that occurs in the diaper region, is the most common skin condition in infancy. It is caused by prolonged contact of the skin with urine and feces, and frequently occurs during hot months and most commonly in infants over 3 months of age—an age group more likely to wear wet diapers at night.

Pathophysiology. The skin beneath the diaper becomes irritated and erythematous. These symptoms may be caused by organic acids in the stool or by ammonia produced by bacterial decomposition of urine.

Assessment. The distribution of the irritated area corresponds to the spread of urine. The buttocks are more likely to be involved in infants who sleep on their backs. Infants who sleep face down are more likely to have involvement of the anterior abdomen.

Data analysis

Data analysis may reveal nursing diagnoses of alterations in comfort related to irritation of skin in the diaper area, and potential impairment in skin integrity.

Planning and implementation. The goals of therapy should be to promote comfort, control the rash, and prevent further development of the rash. Several strategies may be used to accomplish these goals. Mild protective ointments (containing vitamins A and D) and powders may be prescribed for comfort and to hasten the healing process. Exposing the area to air or heat enhances drying of the rash.

Prevention is an essential form of therapy. Measures should be directed toward the diaper area. Thorough cleansing after soiling is essential. The skin generally appears clean after urination; consequently the area may only be wiped with a dry section of the diaper and a clean diaper applied. This practice should be discouraged. The following suggestions will be helpful: (1) dress the infant as lightly as possible to reduce the hot, humid climate of the diaper region; (2) change diapers promptly; (3) cleanse the area with a nonalkaline soap and dry thoroughly; (4) avoid use of rubber or plastic pants; (5) wash diapers with a simple laundry soap and rinse thoroughly. The newer types of absorbent disposable diapers are considered useful in preventing diaper rash.

 Evaluation. Evaluation of the nursing plan for the child with a diaper rash is ongoing and an essential component of the nursing process.

EXPECTED OUTCOMES

The family can:
1. Describe diaper rash.
2. State the cause of the rash.
3. Describe measures for prevention.
4. State plans for health maintenance.
5. State plans for follow-up care.

Miliaria

Miliaria (prickly heat or heat rash) is a condition of the eccrine glands caused by a transient blockage of the sweat ducts. Infants, because of the immaturity of the skin, and obese individuals are predisposed to it. Excesses in perspiration, heat, clothes, and high humidity, or febrile conditions may precipitate miliaria.

 Assessment. Miliaria is characterized by mild eruptions of a tiny red rash with papules and by burning and itching. The rash may appear suddenly, primarily on covered body surfaces such as the body folds and bends of the elbows. The lesions may disappear after a few days but may reappear, particularly during the warm months.

> **Data analysis**
> *Data analysis may reveal nursing diagnoses of alterations in comfort and potential impairment in skin integrity.*

 Planning and implementation. The goals of therapy are to relieve irritating sensations and to prevent occurrences of miliaria. Measures to avoid perspiration are helpful. Lightweight clothing, frequent cold baths, dusting of the area with powder, and limited physical activity facilitate cooling and are therefore effective, preventive, and therapeutic measures. Calamine lotion or other forms of antihistamines are helpful in relieving the itch. If a secondary infection occurs, antibiotics are prescribed.

Evaluation. Evaluation of the nursing care plan for the client with miliaria is ongoing.

EXPECTED OUTCOMES

The family can:
1. Describe miliaria, including the cause and factors that precipitate it.

794

FIG. 15-10
Seborrheic dermatitis. (From Shirkey, H.: Pediatric therapy, ed. 6, St. Louis, 1980, The C.V. Mosby Co.)

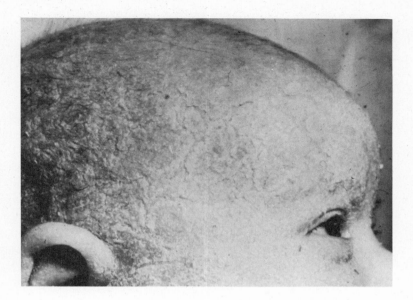

2. State plans for maintaining the integrity of the skin.
3. Describe plans for prevention.
4. Describe plans for follow-up care.

Cradle cap

Cradle cap is a form of seborrheic dermatitis of the scalp (Fig. 15-10). This is one of the areas where the number and the activity of the sebaceous glands are high. Although the scalp is the primary site, it may appear on other body areas such as the ears, eyebrow, axilla, and diaper area. It is common in infants under 6 months of age. During this period the sebaceous glands are functioning as a result of transplacentally derived maternal sex hormones.[40] It usually clears spontaneously.

Pathophysiology. Cradle cap represents a collection of vernix caseosa and shedding skin caught around the hairs of the scalp.

 Assessment. Characteristically, it is yellowish, greasy, and crusty.[46] Erythematous dry scaling eruptions are also common.

> **Data analysis**
> *Data analysis may reveal nursing diagnoses of alterations in comfort and potential impairment of skin integrity.*

 Planning and implementation. Therapy is planned to facilitate removal of the crusts. Strategies to accomplish this include frequent hair hygiene followed by removal with a soft brush and comb. A shampoo is used and should remain in contact with the scalp for 5 to 15 minutes to soften and loosen the scale. Rinsing with moderate rubbing facilitates this process. Topical medications (corticosteroids, antibiotics) may be prescribed when secondary infections develop. Prevention is essential. Therefore adequate cleansing of the scalp should be stressed.

 Evaluation. Evaluation of the nursing care plan for the child with cradle cap is ongoing as the health problem improves.

795

EXPECTED OUTCOMES

The family can:
1. Describe cradle cap.
2. Describe strategies for prevention and maintenance.
3. State frequency, duration, use, and side effects of prescribed medications.
4. Describe plans for follow-up care.

Intertrigo

Intertrigo (chafing) is an inflammatory disorder that occurs primarily in obese individuals. High environmental temperature and humidity tend to precipitate the inflammation.

 Assessment. Intertrigo usually affects those body areas where two surfaces remain in contact and irritate each other. Such areas include the axilla, upper part of the thighs, and folds of the groin, neck, and breast. On these areas the temperature is higher, thus causing more perspiration, retention of sebum, and more friction. As a result, the skin in these areas becomes erythemic and abraded because of the loss of the outermost skin layer. Burning and itching may accompany the inflammation. Usually the process is self-limiting and lasts only a few days. However, it can lead to a secondary bacterial or fungal infection.[40]

> **Data analysis**
> *Data analysis may reveal nursing diagnoses of alterations in comfort and impairment of skin integrity.*

 Planning and implementation. Proper hygiene is an essential preventive measure. The area should be kept dry to relieve the inflammation. Dryness may be accomplished by exposing the affected part to air, which facilitates evaporation of moisture. Clothing should be light. Materials that hold moisture should not be worn. The use of ointments and cornstarch is discouraged because ointments are occlusive and cornstarch encourages the growth of *Candida* organisms. Antibiotic powders may be prescribed to prevent infection. Steroid creams and lotions may be used because of their antiinflammatory effect.

 Evaluation. The nursing care plan is evaluated on an ongoing basis.

EXPECTED OUTCOMES

The family can:
1. Describe intertrigo, including precipitating factors.
2. State strategies for prevention.
3. State indication for and side effects of prescribed medical therapies.
4. Describe plans for follow-up care.

Impetigo

Impetigo contagiosa is a superficial skin infection caused by coagulase-positive staphylococci or by group A beta hemolytic streptococci (Fig. 15-11). Children are more susceptible than adults. Dirty fingernails and pets are the chief sources of infection in children. (In adults, barber and beauty shops, Turkish baths, and swimming pools are the chief sources.) It generally occurs most often during the spring and summer months. It is extremely contagious. Acute glomerulonephritis may develop because of a nephritogenic strain of beta hemolytic streptococci.[40,51] Rheumatic fever can also be a sequela.

 Assessment. Characteristically impetigo develops quickly and begins as an erythematous macule on which thin-walled vesicles develop. These lesions,

FIG. 15-11
Impetigo contagiosa. (From Stewart, William D., and others: Dermatology, ed. 4, St. Louis, 1978, The C.V. Mosby Co.)

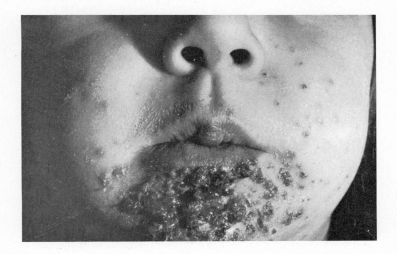

which appear most commonly on the face and extremities, usually rupture easily and their content, a sticky fluid, oozes. The exudate dries and forms a yellowish-brown crust. Satellite lesions may form and progress through the same sequence. Pruritus may be severe.

> **Data analysis**
> *Data analysis may reveal nursing diagnoses of alterations in comfort (for example, pruritus) and impairment in skin integrity.*

Planning and implementation. The goals of therapy are to prevent infection and promote comfort. A culture of the lesion is obtained so that appropriate antibiotic therapy can be prescribed. Systemic antibiotics commonly used are penicillin, oxacillin, and erythromycin. Topical antibiotic ointments (neomycin sulfate and bacitracin) may also be prescribed. Antiseptic soaps and wet compresses (with Burow's solution) may be used to facilitate loosening of crust and subsequently facilitate removal.

Strategies to prevent the "itch-scratch" cycle should be used. These strategies are useful in preventing the spread of infection. The child should not be permitted to scratch the involved areas. It may be necessary to restrain the very young child. Elbow restraints and mittens are useful for this purpose.

These children are usually not hospitalized unless the infection is severe; however, the nurse must teach parents important principles of care, specifically those related to preventing the spread of infection. Such measures include (1) maintaining extreme cleanliness by washing frequently with a soap containing an antibacterial agent (it may be helpful for the entire family to wash with the soap while the child is being treated); (2) using separate towels and washcloths; (3) proper disposing of waste materials; (4) changing linens frequently and washing them immediately. The nurse must also provide instructions about the removal of crust (for example, with compresses). Instructions should be provided about proper application of compresses.

Ecthyma. Ecthyma is a deep form of impetigo caused by beta hemolytic *Streptococcus* organisms. It involves both the epidermis and dermis and results in scarring. Neglect or lack of appropriate treatment of impetigo has been related to the development of ecthyma.[51]

Assessment. The lesions begin in the same manner as those of impetigo, but rapidly become covered with a crust that is surrounded by a slightly raised firm border and that develops into superficial necrotic ulcers. The arms and legs are most commonly affected.

> **Data analysis**
> *Data analysis may reveal nursing diagnosis of alteration in comfort.*

Planning and implementation. Frequent cleansing with soap and water is essential. Systemic antibiotics and compresses are prescribed to soften the crusts.

Evaluation. Evaluation of the nursing care plan for the child with impetigo and ecthyma is ongoing.

EXPECTED OUTCOMES

The child and/or family can:
1. Describe the impetigo or ecthyma, including sources that may cause the problem.
2. State plans for care.
3. Describe plans for preventing the infection.
4. Describe methods of protecting family members from the infection.
5. Demonstrate methods of therapeutic care.
6. State use, dosage, time, route, and side effects of prescribed medications.
7. Describe plans for health maintenance.
8. Describe plans for follow-up care and maintenance.

Warts

Warts (verrucae) are benign growths of the skin caused by a filtrable virus (Fig. 15-12). They are common in school-age children, contagious, and aggravated by irritation. Continued irritation causes the wart to enlarge. The various types of warts are named according to location. *Verruca vulgaris* (the common wart), *verruca plantaris* (wart on the sole), and *verruca plana juvenilis* (flat juvenile wart) are the common types. These lesions tend to occur at sites of trauma and may be seen along a scratch mark. The exact mechanism of spread is not understood.

Assessment. The lesion of *verruca vulgaris* is characterized by a well-circumscribed, papillomatous growth. It is commonly found on the dorsal and palmar surface of the hand, fingers, and surrounding nails.

Similar to the common wart is the *plantar wart.* However, because of the location on the sole, it is more subject to pressure and tends to be pushed inward into the dermis. There is a considerable amount of callus on the surface because of pressure. Pressure also greatly increases the pain.

> **Data analysis**
> *Data analysis may reveal nursing diagnoses of potential for injury and potential impairment of skin integrity.*

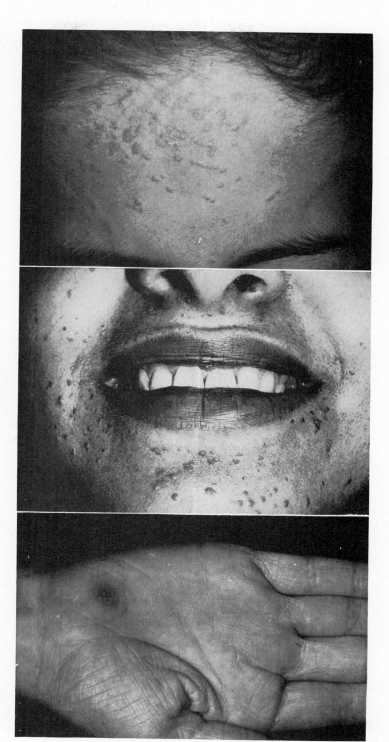

FIG. 15-12
Warts. (From Stewart, William D., and others: Dermatology: diagnosis and treatment of cutaneous disorders, ed. 4, St. Louis, 1978, The C.V. Mosby Co.)

Nursing process for common health problems

   Planning and implementation. Prevention is an important form of therapy. Children should be instructed to wear some type of footwear, especially when they walk in areas where there is an increased possibility of contracting the virus. Because of its location, children have a tendency to pick at them. This practice may permit the wart to transfer to other parts of the body. Therefore children should be instructed not to engage in this practice.

   Evaluation. The nursing care plan is evaluated on an ongoing basis.

EXPECTED OUTCOMES

The child and/or family can:
1. Describe the health problem, including the cause of the problem.
2. Describe strategies for prevention.
3. Describe measures for health maintenance.
4. State plans for follow-up care when problems arise.

Tinea

Tinea (ringworm, dermatophytosis) is caused by a fungus and may be manifested in different parts of the body. Scaling, erythema, and occasional vesicles characterize tinea. The organisms that cause these infections grow best in the presence of moisture and heat. Tinea capitis and corporis are the types that commonly occur in children.

   Assessment. *Tinea capitis* is ringworm of the scalp (Fig. 15-13). It occurs chiefly in children. It rarely affects infants and adults. *Microsporum canis* and *Trichophyton tonsurans* are usually responsible for the infection. A bald spot usually occurs on the occipital area of the scalp, but any area of the scalp may be involved. Erythema and scaling about the area are common.

When the body is involved, it is referred to as *tinea corporis* (Fig. 15-14). *Trichophyton mentagrophytes* and *Microsporum canis* are usually responsible.[3] Erythematous papules with scaling usually appear on the trunk and extremities. Small vesicles encircle the area. The diagnosis for tinea is made on examination with the Wood's light (a yellow-green fluorescence often is seen[3]).

> **Data analysis**
> *Data analysis may reveal nursing diagnoses of alterations in comfort and impairment of skin integrity.*

   Planning and implementation. Therapy is planned to control the infection and to prevent further irritation. Griseofulvin (Fulvicin), which is administered orally, and tinactin 1%, a topical antifungal agent, are the most widely used medications for dermatophytes. Since fungal infections increase in the presence of heat and moisture, the child should be instructed to wear clothing that is light and absorbent. Antibiotic therapy is usually prescribed only if there is a secondary infection. Instructions regarding hygiene practices (keeping combs clean and frequent shampooing) are essential.

   Evaluation. Evaluation of the nursing care plan for the child with tinea is ongoing.

EXPECTED OUTCOMES

The child and/or family can:
1. Describe tinea.
2. Describe methods of managing the problem.

FIG. 15-13
Tinea capitis. (From Stewart, William D., and others: Dermatology: diagnosis and treatment of cutaneous disorders, ed. 4, St. Louis, 1978, The C.V. Mosby Co.)

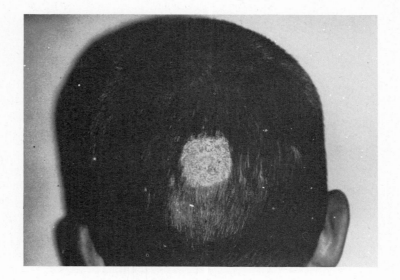

FIG. 15-14
Tinea corporis. (From Stewart, William D., and others: Dermatology: diagnosis and treatment of cutaneous disorders, ed. 4, St. Louis, 1978, The C.V. Mosby Co.)

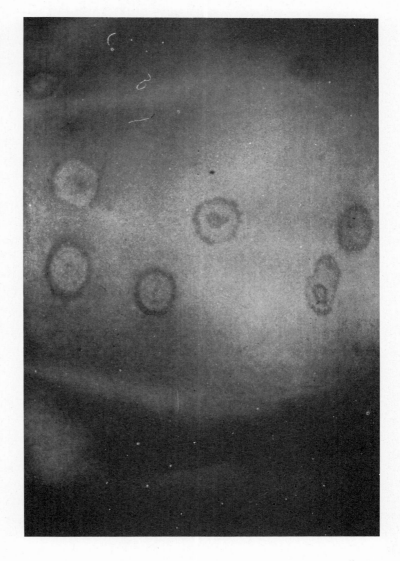

3. State measures for prevention.
4. Describe plans for health maintenance.
5. State use, dosage, time, route, and side effects of any prescribed medications.
6. State plans for follow-up care and management.

Pediculosis

Pediculosis is a condition characterized by infestation of the hairy areas of the body with lice. There are three varieties of pediculosis. These are named according to the area affected: *pediculosis capitis* (head), *pediculosis corporis* (body), and *pediculosis pubis* (pubic area). Pediculosis capitis and corporis are the types common in children.

Assessment. Itching is a common occurrence. Cues that may indicate that a child has head lice include a dermatitis around the nape of the neck and frequent head scratching.[22] Itching tends to be more intense at night. Scratching may result in secondary infection. Examination reveals ova firmly attached to the hairs of the host. Body lice cling to underwear, particularly woolen or flannel underwear. Each type of louse obtains nourishment from blood.

Data analysis
Data analysis may reveal nursing diagnoses of alterations in comfort, potential for injury, and potential impairment of skin integrity.

Planning and implementation. The goals of therapy are to prevent spread of the infestation and to destroy the ova. A benzene preparation such as Kwell shampoo is prescribed for washing the hair. The hair should be washed thoroughly, followed by removal of the nits by combing the hair with a fine-tooth comb. Tweezers may also be used in their removal. When shampoos are used, care must be taken not to get them in the eyes and mouth.

For body lice, the clothing, bedding, and pillows should be disinfected. An autoclave should be used if available. Pressing the seams with a hot iron is also useful in a home situation.

Prevention is an essential aspect of therapy. Children must be instructed to refrain from sharing or using combs, hair brushes, hats, scarves, or other personal items. The practice of good personal hygiene is extremely important, because infestation is associated with poor hygienic conditions.

Evaluation. Evaluation of the nursing care plan for the client with pediculosis is ongoing.

EXPECTED OUTCOMES

The child and/or family can:
1. Describe pediculosis.
2. Describe the plan for management.
3. State strategies for prevention.
4. State plans for health maintenance.
5. State plans for follow-up care and indicate follow-up health services.

Atopic dermatitis

Common cutaneous problems in childhood are related to the hypersensitivity state and include atopic dermatitis (eczema) and contact dermatitis.

Atopic dermatitis is an inflammatory skin disorder characterized by erythema, edema, pruritus, exudation, crusting, and scaling.[53] It tends to occur in individuals with a hereditary predisposition. These individuals tend to acquire immediate sensitization to allergens and develop asthma and hay fever. Individuals with atopic dermatitis tend to have a high serum concentration of IgE. However, it has not been demonstrated that atopic dermatitis is primarily caused by IgE-mediated allergy.

Pathophysiology. Certain changes have been demonstrated in individuals with atopic dermatitis. One such change is an alteration in peripheral cutaneous vasoconstriction of the involved skin. The skin temperature, especially of the extremities, tends to be low. Abnormalities in the rates of cooling and warming in response to temperatures are evident, especially in the flexural areas.[51,53]

There is also increased perspiration in the area of involvement. Individuals with atopic dermatitis have an increased tendency toward perspiring, which tends to intensify the itching; subsequently, scratching has directly been related to the development of dermatitis. A reduction in sebum has also been noted and is thought to be related to a decrease in the numbers of dermal glands, and may be responsible for the increased water loss.[42]

The vascular response noted in individuals with atopic dermatitis is the appearance of dermographism on pressure of the skin with a blunt instrument. This reaction is opposite the usual erythema reaction. These are considered changes that occur in response to acetylcholine, nicotinic acid esters, and histamine.[51]

Infantile eczema is a form of atopic dermatitis that usually begins in infancy between the ages of 2 and 3 months. The appearance of eczema frequently coincides with the introduction of certain foods in the infant's diet, such as milk, wheat, eggs, oranges, oats, and barley. Occasionally, contact with wool, cat and dog hair, pollens, and feathers is responsible.

Assessment. The earliest lesions appear as erythematous, weepy patches on the cheeks. The lesions may extend to the face, scalp, neck, and diaper area. Localized involvement may be noted on the extensor surfaces (for example, popliteal and antecubital) of the extremities (Fig. 15-15). During periods of exacerbation, which is characteristic, involvement may be evident in a large part of the body.[51]

Itching, which is intense, is evident when the infant continually scratches the skin by rubbing his face in bedclothes or against the crib. Trauma may occur from this activity and produce weeping, excoriation, and crusting, which may be the source of secondary infection.

Remissions tend to occur between 3 and 5 years of age. Usually by age 5 the disease is quiescent. However, a mild form of eczema may persist in the antecubital and popliteal fossae, behind the ears, and on the face and neck. During childhood, antecubital and popliteal involvement are common. The presenting symptoms (for example, pruritus), a family history of allergy, elevated serum IgE concentrations, demonstration of reaginic antibodies to a variety of foods and inhalants, and dermographism are used in establishing a diagnosis.

Data analysis
Data analysis may reveal nursing diagnoses of potential impairment of skin integrity, alterations in comfort related to pruritus, and ineffective coping.

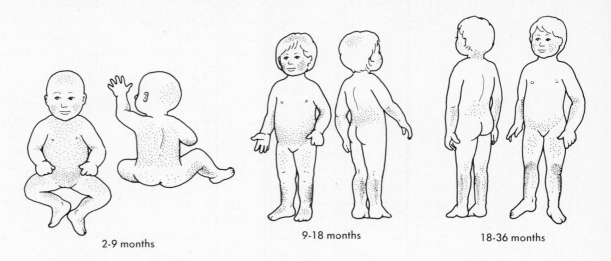

2-9 months   9-18 months   18-36 months

FIG. 15-15
Distribution of eczematous lesions according to age.

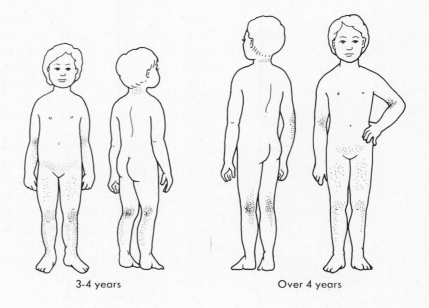

3-4 years   Over 4 years

☞ **Planning and implementation.** Therapy is directed toward controlling factors in the environment that precipitate the itch-scratch-itch cycle. This may include avoidance of ingestants, injectants, and contactants that produce itching.

Temperature extremes, high humidity, and other factors that enhance the itch-scratch cycle should be avoided. The environment (play or sleep) should be well ventilated. Sweating leads to itching and subsequent scratching.

The clothing of infants and small children should be light and soft. Clothing made of cotton and corduroy is *preferred*. All wool should be avoided because the fibers from wool have a tendency to irritate sensitive skin. For this reason, infants should not be allowed to crawl on wool carpet. In addition, any form of irritant should be avoided (for example, paints, cleansers, dust, chemical sprays).

The skin of individuals with atopic dermatitis tends to be dry. Therefore defatting soaps and detergents should be avoided. Bathing should be brief (for example, not exceeding 5 minutes) and in lukewarm water.

804

Other forms of supportive therapy include wet compresses, usually with Burow's solution because it has an antipruritic and antiinflammatory effect. Colloid or tar-type baths may be used for their soothing effects, and antipruritic agents (elixir of trimeprazine for infants) are frequently prescribed to control pruritus.

☞ **Evaluation.** Evaluation is an essential component of the nursing process.

EXPECTED OUTCOMES

The child and/or family can:
1. Describe atopic dermatitis.
2. Describe measures for health maintenance.
3. Demonstrate strategies of therapeutic care.
4. State use, dosage, frequency, route, and side effects of any prescribed medications.
5. State plans for follow-up care and management.

Contact dermatitis

Contact dermatitis is an acute inflammatory reaction of the skin that occurs as a result of one or two processes. The first process relates to direct damage of the skin cells by an agent (for example, strong acids or alkalis) and results in an irritant-type dermatitis. The second process, allergic contact dermatitis, is an acquired, cell-mediated, immune reaction (delayed type) that results from contact with allergens within the environment. There must be a previously sensitizing exposure to the agent.

Pathophysiology. Physiologically, the stratum corneum, especially the lower third and possibly the granular cellular layer, acts as a barrier to the entrance of most substances.[4] A variety of agents may disrupt the barrier. Subsequently, contact with the allergen (sensitizer) causes the sensitized lymphocytes to migrate into the area of contact and induce an inflammatory reaction.[39]

These two reactions are characteristically different. The reaction in the irritant form occurs on the exact area of contact, a few hours after contact, and is characterized by erythematous or bullous eruptions; the allergic type occurs 24 to 72 hours after exposure and is evidenced by the classic signs: redness, heat, pain, swelling. The reaction initially is confined to the site of contact.[39] Contact dermatitis is the most common type of dermatitis occurring in children between 2 and 12 years of age.[53]

Common causative agents include weeds and vines (usually poison ivy), cosmetics, chemicals in clothing, and medications.

☞ **Assessment.** *Poison ivy dermatitis* is a contact dermatitis caused by weeds or vines, such as poison ivy, sumac, and oak, that occurs commonly during the summer and is caused by contact with resin of the plant. The exposed surfaces of the body are often affected (for example, dorsal surfaces of the hands, forearms, face, and neck). The lesions appear as lineal streaks, which are produced as the plant brushes over the skin.

Ingestions of poison oak oleoresin and extreme skin involvement may induce nephritis.[39] Vicks VapoRub, a commonly used substance, contains plant substances that may irritate the skin.

Cosmetic dermatitis occurs as a result of contact with various cosmetic agents. It may be acquired either by contact with cosmetics worn by individuals with whom the child comes in contact, or by application of cosmetic in play (or in adolescent girls as they experiment with various cosmetic products such as lipstick, perfumes, nail polish, and hair dyes). The areas commonly affected are the forehead, eyes, face, and neck.

805

Nursing process for common health problems

Clothing dermatitis is not uncommon in children. Woolens are common offenders and usually produce irritation to the skin. The irritation may be a result of residue of soaps or laundry detergents. Flame-resistant clothing that contains formaldehyde resins may cause dermatitis.

Dermatitis from drugs, *dermatitis medicamentosa,* is caused by drugs that are ingested, absorbed through the skin and mucosa, or given by injection or inhalation. Some drugs reported to cause allergic dermatitis include acids, alkalis, antibiotics (especially penicillin and streptomycin), sulfonamides, serum, dyes, and barbiturates. Topical antihistamine, benzocaine, metycaine, and local anesthetics such as xylocaine and carbocaine are often responsible.

> **Data analysis**
> *Data analysis may reveal nursing diagnoses of potential for injury, alterations in comfort, and potential impairment in skin integrity.*

Planning and implementation. Therapy depends on the specific type of dermatitis. For example, the best form of therapy for dermatitis from weeds is avoidance of contact. Children should be taught to recognize weeds and vines that may produce problems. If contact with these occurs, the area should be cleansed with soap and water immediately after contact to prevent dermatitis. Steroids, topical and oral, may be prescribed for mild and extensive cases, respectively. Cosmetic products that produce reactions should be avoided. Clothing should be washed thoroughly, and residue of soaps or detergents should be removed. Flame-resistant clothing should be washed thoroughly before they are worn. Drugs identified to cause problems should be avoided.

Evaluation. The nursing care plan is evaluated on an ongoing basis.

EXPECTED OUTCOMES

The child or family can:
1. Describe dermatitis.
2. Describe possible sources of the problem.
3. Describe methods of preventing the problem.
4. Describe plans for care if contact is made with specific sources.
5. Describe plans for health maintenance.
6. Describe plans for follow-up care if problems develop.

COMMON HEALTH PROBLEMS OF THE ADOLESCENT

Acne vulgaris

Acne vulgaris is a chronic inflammatory disease involving the sebaceous follicles, primarily of the forehead and cheeks (Fig. 15-16). However, the chest and back may sometimes be involved.

The exact cause of acne is unknown; however, it is thought to be related to hormonal changes occurring during the time when secondary sex characteristics are developing. For example, reports have indicated higher plasma testosterone levels in boys at the onset of acne, as compared with those without acne; as well as higher levels 6 to 12 months before acne develops as compared with those who do not develop acne.[1] The cyclic exacerbations of acne during menstruation also tends to support the hormonal relationship.

Several factors have been reported to precipitate acne.[32]

1. The presence of *Propionibacterium acnes* (formerly called *Corynebacterium*) in the skin. A high concentration of this organism, which is an

FIG. 15-16
A, Acne vulgaris in 19-year-old client. **B,** Same client after 5 weeks of oral treatment with erythromycin stearate. (From Daniel, William A. Jr.: The adolescent patient, St. Louis, 1970, The C.V. Mosby Co.)

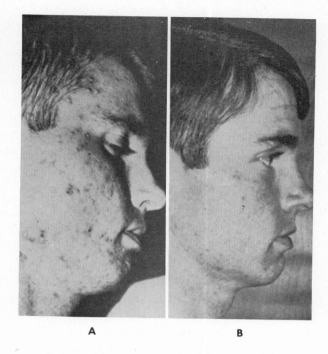

A   B

anaerobic inhabitant of the normal hair follicle, has been found in acne susceptible individuals.

2. Blockage of sebaceous follicles. The content of the sebaceous glands cannot be expelled to the surface and results in *comedone* formation.

3. An increased production of sebum. The production of sebum (a lipid containing triglyceride, cholesterol, and wax esters) is stimulated by androgens.

Emotional or physical stress, sleep loss, excessive heat, and occlusive cosmetics tend to aggravate already existing acne or initiate acne. The current thought is that diet has no relationship to the development of acne. No age is immune to acne.[32] It occurs chiefly during adolescence, but may persist in adulthood. All adolescents are thought to develop acne to some degree.[14]

Assessment. Acne occurs in varying degrees of severity and may exhibit a variety of lesions. Among these are comedones—whiteheads (closed comedones), papules, pustules, and blackheads (open comedones), cysts, and scars. Comedones, the primary lesion, are more common in the less severe types of acne.

The whiteheads, small white inflammatory papules that appear primarily on the cheeks and forehead, are thought to occur as a result of blocked pilosebaceous follicles. Accumulation of melanin in the follicle "mouth" is thought to be responsible for most of the blackheads. Papules are tender and are often responsible for the discomfort that is experienced. Pustules, tiny abscesses, white or yellowish in color, may appear either around comedones, papules, or on the normal skin. Cysts are least common, but most serious. Scars may occur in several forms and often are the cause of unhappiness in the adolescent. Common types of scars of acne are pock, pitted, and keloid. The latter is disfiguring.[35]

Nursing process for common health problems

> **Data analysis**
> *Data analysis may reveal nursing diagnoses of potential for disturbance in self-concept related to blemishes and potential impairment of skin integrity because of disfiguring scar development.*

Planning and implementation. Based on this diagnosis, the goals of therapy should be to promote health and maintain physical and psychosocial integrity. Client instructions should be an integral part of the care plan and should be based on precipitating factors and specific aspects of therapy.

Health promotion. Instructions should be directed toward hygienic practices, nutrition, rest and activity, and sunlight.

Hygienic measures. The skin must be kept clean. Daily bathing with soap and water is essential in removing dirt and bacteria. This measure also prevents oil from drying on the skin surface and thereby plugging the sebaceous glands. Soaps with antibacterial properties help keep the bacterial level down, thus preventing secondary infections. (Because of its antiseptic and drying effects, an alcoholic lotion or alcohol (70%) has been recommended for use when the skin is extremely oily.)

Clients should be encouraged to use only clean towels and pillowcases. The scalp should be kept clean by washing the hair at least twice weekly, avoiding oily hair preparations. Hair should be styled to keep it off the face. The client should be encouraged to practice good oral hygiene by properly cleaning and flossing the teeth.

To avoid damage to the skin, the fingernails should be kept short and clean. Blackheads should not be pricked or squeezed, because this further damages the skin. Cosmetics should be used only under guidance of a dermatologist.

Nutrition. The value of diet in controlling acne has been debated. At one time, one contention was that fats or carbohydrates and specific foods such as chocolate, nuts, fish, and sharp cheese be restricted or avoided. This is no longer considered significant, and a balanced diet is encouraged.

Rest and activity. The nurse should encourage the client to get ample rest and exercise. During exercise, excessive perspiring should be avoided because it stimulates the skin glands to produce more sebum. Worry and anxiety tend to make acne worse and therefore should be minimized.

Sunlight. Exposure to ultraviolet light or the sun is thought to be helpful because of the peeling effect. However, prolonged exposure to the sun should be avoided. Sunscreens should be used when it is necessary to be in the sun for prolonged periods.

Maintaining psychosocial integrity. The importance of early therapy should be shared with the client and his parents. Adolescence is a period of life when positive relationships are of extreme importance. Adolescents are concerned about appearance and the attractiveness of their skin. Subsequently they tend to dislike blemishes because of the feeling that such will affect their physical appearance, popularity, and relationships with others. Efforts should be directed toward trying to enhance maintenance of relationships. Therefore parents should be instructed not to take the ''let nature take care of it'' attitude, because early therapy will likely reduce chances of social and personality disturbance and disfigurement from scars.

Maintaining physical integrity. Therapy generally includes the use of medications that are useful in decreasing the process of pilosebaceous plugging, surgery, and x-ray treatment. Preparations that contain keratolytic agents and salicylic acid, speed drying, and scaling are often prescribed. Systemic and topical antibiotics may be prescribed to control infection. The tetracycline drugs and erythromycin are most widely prescribed. These broad-spectrum antibiotics, given in combination with topical agents or therapy, reduce the number of *Propionibacterium acnes* organisms in the fundibular portion of the hair follicles. Subsequently the amount of lipase available to catabolize the triglycerides in the sebum is reduced.[22] Strategies that will facilitate absorption of tetracycline should be used. These include not taking the medication on an empty stomach, with milk, or with divalent cation-containing antacids. Milk and foods containing calcium bind the drug and prevent absorption.

Topical antibiotics, in the form of lotions, may also be prescribed to reduce the organism count. Commonly prescribed topical agents include clindamycin, erythromycin, and tetracycline lotions. Topical agents that may be used in combination with systemic antibiotics are benzoyl peroxide, retinoic acid (retin A and vitamin C), and steroids.

Retinoic acid causes stinging. This can be minimized by *not* applying it directly after bathing. Hydration promotes penetration and a more prominent irritant reaction.

Estrogenic therapy is sometimes recommended for girls, particularly those prone to premenstrual flare-ups. If the acne is extensive, oral corticosteroids may be prescribed for their antiinflammatory effect.

Instructions should be given about the importance of adhering to therapy. Premature discontinuation of medications tends to cause relapse. Medications should be continued as long as the physician recommends, even though the acne may appear better.[14] It may take weeks, not days, for a response to be noted. The adolescent may tend to share medications with a friend because of the important peer relationship. This practice should be discouraged.

Acne surgery. Pustules and cysts may be removed by incision and drainage. Such surgery is seldom necessary.

Dermabrasion. Dermabrasion, a corrective plastic procedure involving the removal of the surface layers of the scarred skin, has been used to lessen the depth of the scars. A hand rasp, sandpaper, scalpel, or motor-driven winebrush are the instruments used to accomplish this.

Roentgen therapy. Roentgen therapy is generally only prescribed for extreme cases and usually not for adolescents. Such therapy suppresses sebaceous activity. The benefit from roentgen therapy is transient, and hazards are significant.[53]

Ultraviolet light. Ultraviolet light is effective because it produces peeling of the keratin layer and reduces obstruction of the sebaceous gland and comedone formation.[51] It is generally administered at weekly intervals.

Evaluation. Evaluation of the nursing care plan for the client with acne is continuous and provides information for making changes in the plan as the client's status changes.

EXPECTED OUTCOMES

The client and/or family can:

1. Describe acne.
2. Describe plans for implementing the prescribed therapy.
3. State plans for health maintenance.
4. Demonstrate sensitivity to change in body image.
5. State use, dosage, time, route, and side effects of any prescribed medications.
6. Describe plans for follow-up care and problems requiring health care services.

COMMON HEALTH PROBLEMS OF THE YOUNG ADULT

Furuncle

Common problems occurring during the young adult period are infections, mainly bacterial.

A furuncle (boil) is an acute localized infection of one hair follicle or sebaceous gland, usually caused by staphylococci. A furuncle usually develops as a small perifollicular abscess that produces destruction of the hair follicle. Residual scarring may result.

Most commonly, a furuncle occurs on the face, neck, axilla, forearm, buttocks, groin, or legs. Erythema, induration, pain, itching, and swelling, followed by pus formation, characterizes a furuncle. Gradually the infection approaches the surface and becomes extremely painful, especially on motion or pressure.[45] Within a few days the area becomes soft and forms a core.

Carbuncle

A carbuncle (boil) is an acute, circumscribed, cutaneous, and subcutaneous abscess usually caused by *Staphylococcus aureus*. It is often experienced by diabetics and is more common in men than women.

A carbuncle is larger and deeper than a furuncle and occurs at the nape of the neck and upper part of the back. The relative thickness and impermeability of the skin overlying these areas lead to lateral extension and location. Large areas of induration, swelling, and redness with multiple drainage sites are characteristic.[45] Generally carbuncles are extremely painful; however, in some instances, little discomfort is experienced. Malaise, chills, and pyrexia often accompany the infection.

Furunculosis is the term used to describe multiple or recurrent lesions. Lowered resistance (such as in debilitated individuals), chronic disease, malnutrition, and uncontrolled diabetes are the main predisposing factors to furunculosis. Systemic responses such as fever, anorexia, weakness, malaise, or toxemia often accompany it.

> **Data analysis**
> *Data analysis may reveal nursing diagnoses of alterations in comfort: pain and impairment of skin integrity.*

Planning and implementation. Therapy is similar for furuncles, carbuncles, and furunculosis. The nurse should encourage clients who have infections of the skin to practice principles of medical asepsis and to follow a general hygiene program. Frequent handwashing is extremely important. In addition, the face should be washed several times each day with an antibacterial liquid soap. Those containing hexachlorophene, povidone-iodine, or chlorhexidine have been suggested.[51] Family members should also be encouraged to follow these hygienic practices. Because dryness inhibits bacterial growth, the involved area should be kept dry with an alcohol-containing lotion. The lesion, especially while moist and while draining, should be kept covered with a dressing. The dressing should be changed as frequently as possible and properly disposed of. Any article contaminated with drainage from the area (for example, towels, linen, clothing) should be kept separate from other articles until properly laundered.

The practice of squeezing boils should be discouraged because it favors the spread of infection to surrounding tissue and the bloodstream and may result in septicemia.

An adequate diet and fluid intake should be encouraged. Adequate rest and relief of emotional stress are also essential.

The lesion may heal by discharging purulent material from the core. If not, the process may be speeded up with the use of antibiotics and by application of hot wet compresses. Antibiotics are administered orally or parenterally to prevent infection, promote healing, and relieve pain. Surgery (incision and drainage) is often indicated when the lesions become localized.

☞ **Evaluation.** Evaluation of the nursing care plan for the client with an infection such as a furuncle, carbuncle, or furunculosis is continuous and provides the necessary information for modification of the plan.

EXPECTED OUTCOMES

The client can:
1. Describe the health problem (furuncle or carbuncle).
2. Describe plans for preventing or managing the infection.
3. Describe methods of protecting family members from the infection.
4. Demonstrate methods of therapeutic care.
5. State use, dosage, time, route, side effects of prescribed medications.
6. Describe plans for health maintenance.
7. Describe plans for follow-up care.

Psoriasis

Psoriasis, a chronic inflammatory disease of the skin, occurs commonly in young adults. The exact cause of psoriasis is not known. It is thought to have a genetic basis, but the mode of inheritance has not been established. Some observers consider metabolic and dietary disturbances as factors in causation. For example, the mechanism of psoriasis has been explained as an abnormal epidermal protein metabolism and gene-linked psoriasis virus.[3] Remission and exacerbations are characteristic. Environmental changes (for example, exposure to cold), anxiety, tension, and fatigue are associated with psoriasis. It tends to regress during warm months and recur during cold weather. Exposure to sunlight tends to provide relief.

Pathophysiology. In psoriasis, changes occur in the keratinizing process. Normally the transit time from mitosis to the stratum corneum is 26 to 28 days.[51] In psoriasis the thickened epidermis proliferates at a rapid rate, having a cell turnover four to five times faster than normal. This results in a turnover time of approximately 7 days.[56] Although the exact factors responsible for the loss of epidermal growth have not been identified, a deficiency of cyclic nucleotides is thought to be responsible.[55] Prostaglandins are also thought to have an effect.

☞ **Assessment.** The lesions of psoriasis are characterized by thick, large, loose, dry, silvery plaques. The lesions are most often found on bony prominences such as the knees, elbows, and sacrum, and on the scalp, trunk, ears, and nails.

811

Nursing process for common health problems

> **Data analysis**
> *Data analysis may reveal potential nursing diagnoses of alterations in comfort, ineffective individual coping, impairment of skin integrity, and disturbance in self-concept.*

Planning and implementation. Therapy is directed toward removal of the scales. Proper hygiene is essential, and such measures facilitate removal of scales. Tub baths, the use of special soaps, or an oil such as Alpha-Keri is helpful. Primary forms of therapy include peeling agents such as ammoniated mercury, coal tar, and sulfur. These may be applied two to three times per day. Because mercury can be absorbed by the skin, vigorous rubbing should be discouraged. It must be rubbed only enough to distribute it on the skin.

Antimetabolites or folic acid antagonists (such as methotrexate) are used in several forms of psoriasis. Such drugs inhibit rapid cellular proliferation, thereby restoring skin to a more normal state. Methotrexate is rapidly absorbed from an empty stomach. Certain drugs (for example, aspirin, sulfonamides) increase the toxic effects by displacing it from albumin binding.[51] Therefore the use of these drugs with methotrexate is discouraged. Topical or systemic steroids may be prescribed. Exposure to sun or ultraviolet therapy has proved beneficial.

Other forms of therapy

Grenz radiation therapy. Grenz radiation is a form of ionizing radiation with a spectrum bordering between ultraviolet rays and roentgen rays.[51] It has proved useful on superficial lesions, especially those of the scalp, perianal, and genital regions. The treatments are divided and usually repeated at 6-month intervals.

PUVA therapy. PUVA therapy, a new treatment modality, is a form of photochemotherapy that involves the oral administration of 8-methoxypsoralen, which is photoactive, followed by exposure to a high-intensity, long-wave ultraviolet-light system (PUVA).[51] This form of treatment is increasingly used in larger centers.

Day-care centers. Reports have been made of the establishment of psoriasis day-care centers. Such centers are used for clients with severe generalized psoriasis. The treatment is extensive and is administered during the day. The client is free in the evening.

Evaluation. Evaluation of the nursing care plan for the client with psoriasis is continuous and provides information for modification of the plan as the client's status changes.

EXPECTED OUTCOMES

The client and/or family can:
1. Describe psoriasis.
2. State plans for following therapeutic plan.
3. Demonstrate methods of therapeutic care (baths, applications of peeling agents).
4. Demonstrate sensitivity to changes in body image.
5. State plans for health maintenance.
6. State use, dosage, frequency, route, side effects of any prescribed medications.
7. State plans for follow-up care and problems requiring health services.

15 Integumentary system

Lupus erythematosus

Lupus erythematosus is a multisystem disease affecting several organs. Its exact cause is not known; however, immunological mechanisms have been used to explain its occurrence.

Pathophysiology. Antinuclear antibodies (ANA), including antibodies to deoxyribonucleic acid (DNA), and nucleoprotein are found in the serum of clients with systemic lupus.[34] These antibodies form antigen-antibody complexes with their specific antigens.

There are two forms of lupus erythematosus: systemic lupus erythematosus (SLE) and discoid lupus erythematosus (DLE).

Systemic lupus erythematosus. Systemic lupus erythematosus is a disease of the connective tissue that primarily affects women between the second and fifth decades. Its occurrence in women versus men is a ratio of 9:1 and occurs at a rate of 2 to 3 per 100,000 population.[34]

Assessment. Systemic lupus erythematosus is characterized by involvement of a variety of organs, including the joints, skin, kidney, central nervous system, and cardiopulmonary system.

Joint involvement, especially arthritis and arthralgia, occurs most frequently and involves the hands, feet, or the larger joints. Characteristically, redness, warmth, and tenderness are common. The cutaneous lesion most commonly experienced is an erythematosus facial eruption with butterfly distribution over the malar area and bridge of the nose. These lesions are believed to occur for a short period of time.[51] Cutaneous lesions may also occur in other parts of the body, especially in those areas exposed to sun.

Involvement of the renal system is considered most serious. Such involvement may range from the development of proteinuria and hematuria to renal failure. Neurological involvement is often manifested by behavioral changes, peripheral neuritis, and seizures. Pericarditis and pleurisy are the problems that signify the cardiopulmonary system is involved. Systemic involvement is manifested by fever, weakness, anorexia, weight loss, fatigue, and malaise.

> *Data analysis*
> *Data analysis may reveal nursing diagnoses of disturbance in self-concept, impairment in skin integrity, and potential impairment of mobility.*

Planning and implementation. Nursing care, which is individualized, is an essential element of treatment. Nurses have the responsibility of being knowledgeable about the pharmacodynamics of the prescribed therapy, which primarily consists of the administration of drugs such as corticosteroids (cortisone, hydrocortisone, prednisone, prednisolone) to suppress the inflammatory process, and immunosuppressive therapy such as azathioprine (Imuran), which suppresses the immune response. Symptomatic therapy, including analgesics and rest, are prescribed for joint and muscle pain, salicylates for fever, antibiotics for infections, and specific therapy for the involved organ systems. The care plan must reflect an understanding of this therapy as well as an understanding of the disease process. Intake, output, weight, and vital signs should be monitored, and the nurse must be alert for signs and symptoms that indicate involvement of varied body systems. Measures must be planned to prevent complications associated with joint involvement and bed rest. Since depression may be experienced, emotional support should be given to both the client and the family. Therapeutic techniques (for example, listening and facilitating verbalization of fears and concerns) should be a part of the care. Client instructions should also be a part of the care plan. The client should be informed about the therapy (its use, side effects, and so on) and strategies given as to how to manage at home.

Discoid lupus erythematosus. Discoid lupus erythematosus is a chronic disease of the skin characterized by a scarring dermatitis occurring in exposed areas. It is thought to be of autoimmune origin.[51] However, enrivonmental factors such as sun, trauma, infection, and cold are thought to play a part in the disease.[4] For example, exposure to sunlight has been reported to precipitate the appearance of new lesions and cause older lesions to worsen.

Pathophysiology. The lesions progress through several phases, including a scaling phase that extends from the scale into the follicular opening. Scarring and pigmentary changes may precede the lesion. For example, the lesion may atrophy and appear pale and depressed.

Assessment. Discoid lupus erythematosus starts insidiously with a small lesion (for example, well-defined red, scaly, patchy macules usually appearing over the bridge of the nose, malar area, forehead, ears, and neck). The appearance of the rash over the nose elicits the characteristic "butterfly pattern." The mucous membrane of the oral cavity may be involved.

The diagnosis is based on laboratory findings that reveal leukopenia, thrombocytopenia, elevated sedimentation rates, and serum gamma globulin levels. A positive antinuclear antibody test (ANA) is essential in establishing the diagnosis. The LE cell test, which indicates the presence of circulating anti-DNA antibodies, is positive. Immunoglobulins IgG, IgA, IgM, properdin, and C_3 and C_4 fractions of complement have been demonstrated in active stages of the disease.[51] Additional lesions gradually appear and involve the scalp, arms, and back of hands. Symptoms characteristic of systemic lupus may also occur, including malaise, weight loss, and joint pains.

Data analysis
Data analysis may reveal nursing diagnoses of disturbance in self-concept and impairment in skin integrity.

Planning and implementation. Therapy is often individualized and symptomatic. Antimalarial therapy (drugs such as chloroquine, hydroxychloroquine, amodiaquine, and quinacrine) has been used to control skin lesions. Large dosages of the drugs are usually given during the acute stages, and maintenance dosages are given afterwards. The use of these drugs warrants close consideration of the risk of antimalarial drugs. Dosages exceeding 8 g/kg produces toxic effects on the retina, which may result in irreversible changes and subsequent blindness.[34,51] Clients using these drugs should be informed of the side effects (nausea, vomiting, headaches, corneal opacities) and instructed to get ophthalmoscopic examinations at regularly scheduled intervals.

Because of the effect the sun has on the problem, instructions should be given to avoid exposure to sun and to use sunscreen preparations when exposure is unavoidable.

 Evaluation. Evaluation of the nursing process for the client with lupus erythematosus is continuous and provides information for modifying the care plan as the client's status changes.

EXPECTED OUTCOMES

The client and/or family can:
1. Describe lupus erythematosus.
2. Describe plans for managing problems associated with lupus erythematosus.
3. Describe plans for health maintenance.
4. State use, dosage, frequency, route, and side effects of prescribed medications.
5. Demonstrate sensitivity to changes in body image.
6. Demonstrate sensitivity to behavioral changes.
7. Describe plans for follow-up care and use of health care services.

Injuries caused by cold

Cold injuries may occur as a result of exposure to either freezing temperature or high winds, such as in a blizzard when individuals have no way of keeping warm. Mountain climbers and winter sports enthusiasts are often affected. Persons exposed to ordinary cold but dressed inadequately, or alcoholics or other ill persons whose defense against cold is lowered, may also sustain cold injuries.

Exposure to extreme cold may affect a body part or the entire body and may result in varying degrees of tissue destruction. Frostbite and hypothermia are common examples.

Frostbite. Frostbite, or freezing of a part of the body, occurs when there is insufficient heat to counteract external cold. Variables that may predispose to frostbite include improper clothing, poor circulation (such as from arterial disease), fatigue, tight clothing (especially footwear), inadequate nutrition, and alcohol. Exposed areas and distal parts (fingers, chin, cheeks, ears, nose, and toes) are commonly affected.

Pathophysiology. The injuries that occur as a result of frostbite are the result of constriction of the dermal vessels in response to surface cooling. This is a compensatory effort to conserve body heat. Vasoconstriction is a direct effect of cold on the vessels and a response to cool blood reaching, via the afferent impulses, the vasomotor center (for example, the body attempts to maintain temperature to vital organs, such as the brain and lungs, by shunting blood away from the skin, muscles, and extremities). As a result, symptoms such as coldness, tingling, a burning sensation, hypoesthesia, reduction in temperature, numbness, and the redness-to-white waxy appearance are characteristic.

 Assessment. Two classifications used to describe frostbite are superficial and deep frostbite. *Superficial frostbite* usually involves the fingertips, nose, ears, or cheeks. The individual complains of a burning or tingling sensation, followed by numbness. Blanching, failure of the part to change to red after pressure is applied, is often experienced. Inspection of the skin reveals a change in color of the skin. The skin appears gray, and the underlying tissue remains soft.

Deep frostbite is more serious and often involves the hands and feet. The tissue is cold, white, and feels solid to touch. After it thaws, the color changes to pink to purplish blue. Pain is experienced, blisters may form, and gangrene may occur within a couple of days.

> **Data analysis**
> *Data analysis may reveal nursing diagnoses of impairment of skin integrity, fear, potential for injury, and alterations in sensory perception.*

Planning and implementation. Therapeutic measures are used to prevent trauma to tissue and to rewarm the tissue. Before tissue damage occurs, a number of measures may be implemented: applying firm, steady pressure to the area (a warm hand may be used); blowing warm breath on the spot; or placing fingers under the armpits. An essential aspect of these therapies is to maintain a motionless state of the involved part. Rubbing and manipulation are discouraged because such practice may damage the tissue. Placing clothing over the area will prevent deepening of the injury. Tingling is usually experienced as warmth and color (hyperemia) return. The appearance of blisters also indicates tissue recovery and is thus considered a good prognostic sign.

Another form of therapy involves thawing the involved part by rapid rewarming. Following are principles of rewarming:

1. Maintain temperature of water between 100° F to 105° F, or 37.8° C to 40.6° C (temperature agreed on by the International Medical Conference on Frostbite, 1964).
2. Maintain warmth of water by adding fresh hot water because water tends to lose its heat rapidly.
3. Surround body part with water and refrain from permitting body part (such as the foot) to rest on bottom of container.

After rewarming, the affected part should be cleaned and placed in a sterile sheet. A device (such as a cradle) might be used to prevent the weight of the covering from touching the part.

Preventing cold injuries. Possibly one of the most important aspects of cold injuries is prevention. Being aware of the hazards and symptoms that may occur is paramount to protection. The nurse should be knowledgeable of these hazards and symptoms and so must inform individuals who must be in cold temperatures to protect themselves against the cold. Ample clothing must be worn in cold weather. Gloves or mittens should be used to keep the hands warm. Actually, mittens are preferred because the heat given off by each finger serves to keep the others warm. It is important that the feet be kept dry during cold weather. Tight clothing, especially tight gloves and shoes, should be avoided, because such objects will interfere with circulation and increase the effect of the cold weather. Alcohol and tobacco should be avoided because they alter circulation to the peripheral vessels. Muscular activity should be increased (move about, exercise fingers and toes) to facilitate heat production. When possible, intake of carbohydrates should be frequent. It is a good practice to take snack foods such as raisins or other dried fruits when there may be exposure to cold outdoor temperature. These serve as a quick source of energy and are easy to carry. When it is impossible to abide by these preventive measures, exposure to cold should be brief.

Hypothermia. Hypothermia is general body cooling that occurs when the body loses heat at a rate faster than it can be produced. Exposure to low, rapidly falling temperatures, cold moisture, ice, or snow are conditions common to the development of hypothermia. A state of hunger, fatigue, or exertion often contributes to this injury. Accidental hypothermia has recently been documented to be a common entity in the elderly. If the temperature is below freezing, frostbite may accompany hypothermia.

 Assessment. The physiological effects indicative of heat loss include shivering (an involuntary contraction of the muscles to generate more heat), apathy, clumsiness, listlessness, slow reactions, confusion, and difficulty in speaking (that is, slurred speech). The latter symptoms indicate a reduction in the amount of oxygen being transported to the brain. They generally occur when the temperature falls below 95° F (35° C) rectally.[5] When the temperature falls below 90° F (32.2° C), shivering stops and muscle rigidity occurs. The individual becomes irrational, vital signs decrease, and unconsciousness results. A temperature below 78° F (25.5° C) usually results in death.[5]

Data analysis
Data analysis may reveal nursing diagnoses of alterations in comfort, alterations in cardiac output, fear, potential for injury, impaired physical mobility, and sensory perception alterations.

Planning and implementation. Because of the seriousness of generalized cooling, an acute emergency exists. The individual should be taken to a health care facility immediately. In the meantime, in preparation for transfer, first-aid measures should be implemented to prevent further heat loss, including removing the individual from outdoors, removing wet clothing, and keeping him dry. Other measures, such as applying external heat to the uninvolved part and supplying internal heat, are essential. Hot-water bottles or an electric blanket may be used as a source of external heat, and hot liquids (for example, hot sweet liquids such as syrup) may be given to increase the caloric value. If there is a delay in transferring the individual, and if he is in a warm environment, a warm bath may be administered.

Because ventricular fibrillation is a serious consequence, especially if the temperature approaches 81° F (27.2° C), it is generally not recommended to rewarm the client outside a health care facility. In the hospital the client is rewarmed under close observation. A whirlpool bath may be used. Reports have indicated the use of peritoneal dialysis[41] as a means of rewarming. The rewarming process is continued until the involved area becomes deep red or bluish. Thawing results in hyperemia because of a return of the blood into the large vessels. These changes occur because of the action of histamine that was released by the cells at the time of the original cell injury. Itching, a burning sensation, and pain may occur. Analgesics and sedatives might be prescribed for the pain.

Various forms of systemic therapy have been suggested. Many of these are controversial. Anticoagulants may be given to prevent thrombosis; vasodilators (such as papaverine, nicotinic acid, and alcohol) may be used to reduce vasospasms; and antibiotics may be used to prevent infections. Sympathectomy and administration of low-molecular dextran have been used.

Evaluation. Evaluation of the nursing care plan is a continuous process. The information obtained from the process of evaluation provides data for modification of the plan.

EXPECTED OUTCOMES

The client and/or family can:
1. Describe the health problem, including factors that can precipitate the problem.
2. Describe plans for preventing future problems.
3. Describe plans for health maintenance.
4. Describe plans for follow-up care.

COMMON HEALTH PROBLEMS OF THE MIDDLE-AGED AND OLDER ADULT

Skin cancer

Skin cancer, the most common type of malignant disease, is considered a disease of the middle-aged and elderly adult (occasionally it occurs in children). Both intrinsic and extrinsic factors may cause skin cancer. Intrinsic factors are those inherent within the cell, whereas extrinsic factors are those related to the external influences on the cell's environment, such as overexposure to sunlight, exposure to ionizing radiation, chemicals, industrial irritants, or trauma.

The most important single etiological factor responsible for carcinomas of the skin is chronic exposure to ultraviolet light of the sunburn wavelengths (290 to 320 nm), especially in individuals not protected by intense melanin pigmentation.[3] Hence, whites are afflicted more often than members of darker-skinned races. The incidence of skin cancer in blacks and orientals is low. The fact that darker-skinned individuals have less skin cancer is thought to be related to the pigment and increased keratinization. Individuals who are fair-skinned, blonde, redhead, have freckles, or burn easily are considered high risks. Sun-exposed areas are most commonly involved.

Chemical carcinogens, for example, inorganic arsenicals and some organic hydrocarbons, are also causes of skin cancer. Other carcinogenic agents are ionizing radiation, including x-rays, grenz rays, and gamma rays.[23]

Skin cancer occurs about twice as often in men as in women. The incidence in men is thought to be related to the personal habits of smoking or chewing tobacco, and possibly more significant is the fact that men are more likely to engage in work that exposes them to carcinogenic agents.

There is also an occupational relationship in skin cancer. Cancer is more common in farmers and sailors, possibly because of their outdoor work. Radiologists and radiology technicians are more often affected than other physicians and other technicians.

The most common types of neoplasm of the skin are basal cell and squamous cell carcinoma.

Basal cell carcinoma. Basal cell carcinoma (basal cell epithelioma), the most common type of skin cancer, arises from the epidermis.[24,25] Common among the sixth, seventh, and eighth decades, it occurs equally in men and women[7] and accounts for approximately 65% of all skin cancers.[51] Factors such as prolonged exposure to sunlight (for example, solar wavelengths between 290 and 320 nm,[26] radiation, thermal energy, mechanical energy, and chemicals have been indicated as possible causes. Pigmentation is thought to be a natural inherent protection and accounts for its rare occurrence in blacks and orientals. It frequently occurs in blondes and redheads.

Assessment. Basal cell carcinoma is characterized by a small nodular growth with a central ulceration, crusting, and discrete rolled borders.[27] If neglected, it tends to occur between the hairline and upper lip, is locally invasive, and tends to destroy underlying and adjacent tissue. It rarely metastasizes,[7,27,51] and pain is uncommon. Diagnosis is established by biopsy.

Data analysis
Data analysis may reveal nursing diagnoses of impairment of skin integrity, disturbance in self-concept, anticipatory grieving, and fear.

Planning and implementation. The goal of therapy is to destroy the lesion completely. This may be accomplished by curettage, electrodesiccation, x-ray therapy, and surgical excision.

Curettage is a therapeutic technique that involves the scraping away of diseased tissue with a dermal curette. A circular motion is used, and the process is repeated until all the desired tissue is removed.

Electrodesiccation is a superficial destruction of the skin using high-frequency electrical current. The current is delivered by an electrode. This therapy, often used in combination with curettage, is useful in removing lesions such as warts and keratoses.

Electrocoagulation is a deeper and more severe destruction of tissue. With this method, enough heat is created to coagulate the tissue. This method produces better hemostasis and more scarring. Skin tumors are often removed with this method. Heat produced by this method sterilizes this tissue; consequently, strict asepsis is not necessary.[40] Curettage is often combined to remove the coagulated tissue.

Cryosurgery is the method of removing skin lesions by freezing. Solid carbon dioxide and liquid nitrogen are substances commonly used to destroy tissue. The freezing point of these substances is well below the level necessary to destroy tissue.

Squamous cell carcinoma. Squamous cell carcinoma is a slowly growing neoplasm that arises from the epidermis. It most commonly arises from preexisting actinic (or solar) keratoses.[23] The age group most commonly affected are those in the sixth, seventh, and eighth decades of life. It is more common in men.

Assessment. Squamous cell carcinoma occurs mainly on the mucous membranes and on sun-exposed areas of the skin, such as the face, neck, ears, arms, and dorsum of the hands.[25] The majority occurs on the face and ears.[51] It usually arises on the mucous membranes from chronic irritation from pipe smoking, dentures, teeth, and on the glans penis of uncircumcised males.[51] It usually starts as a painless, flesh-colored papule, plaque, or nodule with visible scales, tends to enlarge, and develops necrosis with a central ulceration.[24] The diagnosis is confirmed by biopsy.

Data analysis
Data analysis may reveal nursing diagnoses of impairment in skin integrity, fear, disturbance in self-concept, and anticipatory grieving.

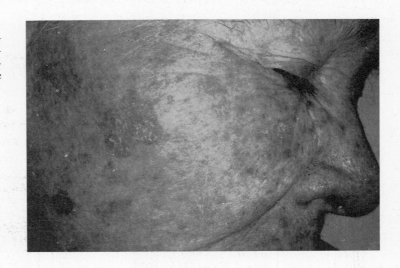

FIG. 15-17
Actinic keratosis. (From Stewart, William D., and others: Dermatology: diagnosis and treatment of cutaneous disorders, ed. 4, St. Louis, 1978, The C.V. Mosby Co.)

Planning and implementation. Forms of therapy include electrodesiccation and curettage for small lesions (less than 2 cm), and surgical excision for larger ones and those that tend to recur. Radiation therapy has been reported to be used for clients who either refuse surgery or cannot tolerate extensive surgery.

Precancerous lesions. There are certain precancerous lesions of the skin from which squamous cell carcinoma is likely to develop. Two of these include actinic keratoses and arsenical keratosis.

Actinic keratosis. Actinic keratosis (solar keratosis) is a precancerous lesion that commonly occurs on sun-exposed skin of fair-skinned individuals.[7,24,54] (Fig. 15-17). Approximately 13% develop into squamous cell carcinoma.[51]

PATHOPHYSIOLOGY. Chronic sun exposure damages the elastic fibers of the skin and causes wrinkling, telangiectasia, and accented skin folds.

ASSESSMENT. Considered the most common of the precancerous lesions,[7] it is characterized by well-defined macules, papules, or plaques that range in color from tan to pink to flesh-colored, with a surface that is rough and gritty. Sensations of itching, burning, or stinging of the lesion are common.[24] Because of their rough surface, they are reported to be easily palpated.

DATA ANALYSIS
Data analysis may reveal nursing diagnoses of impairment of skin integrity, fear, and anticipatory grieving.

PLANNING AND IMPLEMENTATION. The methods of treatment are electrodesiccation, curettage, and topical application of 5-FU (5-fluorouracil) in the form of lotions or creams; trichloroacetic acid, and use of cryotherapy.[7,27]

Arsenical keratosis. Arsenical keratosis, a precancerous lesion, commonly occurs in individuals who have received inorganic arsenicals as a form of medical therapy, or who have received them by accident. Arsenical compounds were at one time used for treating arthritis, asthma, and psoriasis. The lesions, characterized as multiple, hard, and wartlike, may not appear until 10 years after exposure.

820

Cancerous lesions

Bowen's disease. Bowen's disease is a slowly growing squamous cell carcinoma that has not broken through the basement membrane into the dermis.[24] Men and women are equally affected. Approximately 5% to 10% have been reported to invade the dermis and become squamous cell carcinoma.[24]

 Assessment. Bowen's disease occurs as a solitary lesion and has been characterized as being pink or red to light brown. Most lesions affect unexposed areas of the trunk, although any area can be involved. Chemical analysis of the lesion has shown an abnormal concentration of arsenic in the lesion.[51] Many of the clients have histories of having received inorganic arsenic preparations either by accident or for medicinal purposes a decade or more before.

> *Data analysis*
> *Data analysis may reveal nursing diagnoses of impairment of skin integrity, fear, and anticipatory grieving.*

 Planning and implementation. Therapy includes local excision, electrodesiccation, curettage, external beam radiation, and cryosurgery. The use of 5-FU is generally limited to those individuals in whom other forms of therapy cannot be used or in those who refuse other forms of therapy.

Malignant melanoma. Melanoma is a malignant tumor that is derived from melanocytic cells. It generally originates from a pigmented nevus.[16] It is more common in women and tends to occur earlier than basal cell and squamous cell carcinoma. Individuals in the fourth, fifth, sixth, and seventh decades of life are most commonly affected.

 Assessment. The color of the lesion may appear in shades of tan, brown, black, red, white, and blue.[24] The surface of the lesion appears irregular. The diagnosis of melanoma is confirmed by biopsy and histological examination of tissue.

Three types of melanomas have been described: lentigo maligna melanoma (LMN), superficial spreading melanoma (SSM), and nodular melanoma (NM).

Lentigo maligna melanoma, characterized by frecklelike lesions, is most commonly located on the chest and temple, but may occur in any sun-exposed surface. It usually develops around the seventh decade of life and is more common in women.[7]

Superficial spreading melanoma, a flat to slightly elevated lesion, is characterized by a variety of colors (for example, ranging from tan-black, brown, blue, gray, to pink).[21] It may occur on any area of the body, but most often appears on the head and neck. Individuals in the 40- to 50-year age group are more frequently affected. Its occurrence in men and women is about the same.

Nodular melanoma is characterized by shades of blue (for example, blue gray, reddish gray). It occurs on any location and is considered to occur twice as frequently in men than in women.

> *Data analysis*
> *Data analysis may reveal nursing diagnoses of disturbance in self-concept, fear, anticipatory grieving, and impairment of skin integrity.*

Nursing process for common health problems

 Planning and implementation. Prevention is an essential element in treatment. In addition to the danger signals of cancer, authorities have documented criteria that may be useful in evaluating changes that may be indicative of malignant lesions.[7,21,51] Use of this information can be beneficial to the nurse because instruction is provided about promoting and maintaining health of the skin.

Instructions should be given regarding the importance of observing the following changes in the skin:

1. Change in the surface area of a nevus (for example, a change from a previously flat nevus to a raised, palpable, nodular, or thick one).
2. A sudden change in color, either lighter or darker (for example, brownish to black).
3. A sudden change in size.
4. A change in the surface characteristics (for example, change from a smooth to scaly surface, or the appearance of a discharge [serous or bloody] from slight trauma, or ulceration).
5. A change in the sensation of the lesion (for example, the development of itching, tingling, or pain in the area of pigmentation).

Because lesions can be seen with the naked eye, their potential for cure has been documented to be over 90% if detected in the early stage. Therefore any significant changes, as noted in the mentioned criteria, or any type of skin or mucous membrane irritation or lesion warrants seeking health care assistance.

Instructions should be provided about the importance of avoiding conditions that encourage the development of skin cancer. Awareness of risk factors can facilitate pinpointing those individuals who are in need of specific instructions. Clients, especially those who are fair-skinned, redheads, and those who freckle or burn easily, should be encouraged to avoid unnecessary exposure to sun. They should be instructed to wear protective clothing and to curtail activity in the sun, especially during hours of peak ultraviolet light intensity (10 AM to 12 PM).[24,26] Protective lotions or creams should be used when it is necessary to be in the sun for long periods. Sunscreens containing 5% para-aminobenzoic acid (PABA) absorb the oncogenic 280 to 320 nm wavelength and prevent damage to the skin.[23,24]

Promoting psychosocial health. Nurses must be cognizant of the psychological impact the cancer as well as the surgical intervention (especially if the surgery is extensive and has the potential of causing disfigurement) might have on the client. If a disfigurement occurs, the nurse should suggest measures that will help the client cope with it. Depending on the location of the scar (or disfigurement), the nurse might suggest clothing to cover the area (that is, on the arm), makeup to improve cosmetic appearance, or a change in hairstyle.

 Evaluation. Evaluation of the nursing care plan for the client with skin cancer is continuous and provides information necessary for altering the plan.

EXPECTED OUTCOMES

The client and/or family can:
1. Describe melanoma.
2. Describe methods of managing the problem.
3. Understand the therapy and the need for follow-up health care.
4. State plans for health maintenance.
5. Express feelings and concerns freely.
6. Describe plans for follow-up care and use of community resources.
7. State use, dosage, time, route, and side effects of prescribed medications.
8. Discuss community resources that can provide assistance as needed.

Accidental hypothermia

Accidental hypothermia, an unintentional drop in body temperature below 95° F (35° C) occurs as a complication of exposure. Its development is considered to be related to exogenous factors such as low external temperature, as well as to unknown endogenous factors.[41] Its occurrence is usually in elderly individuals.

Assessment. The symptoms that occur have been documented to develop insidiously and may involve all body systems. The skin is usually cool to touch, pale, and the muscles are red, giving the appearance of rigor mortis. Tremors are not uncommon. Unconsciousness usually occurs when the temperature reaches less than 80° F (26.7° C). The pupils are miotic, the respiratory rate is decreased, and bradycardia and hypotension (reflecting myocardial depression) usually occur. There is often generalized edema.

Electrocardiographic changes often show abnormal patterns, including bradycardia, atrial fibrillation, and a J wave that occurs at the junction of the QRS complex and ST segment.[41] Varied changes may be noted in blood studies, including elevated serum amylase and low blood sugar. The blood is hemoconcentrated. Metabolic acidosis occurs.

> **Data analysis**
> *Data analysis may reveal nursing diagnoses of alterations in comfort, alterations in cardiac output, fear, potential for injury, impaired physical mobility, and sensory perception alterations.*

Planning and implementation. Therapy is generally instituted immediately and planned to expand blood volume and to maintain a patent airway.

Large volumes of fluid, including glucose, saline, and low-molecular dextran, may be used. Attempts may be made to restore the core temperature by using heated hemodialysis or warmed peritoneal dialysis fluid. External rewarming is contraindicated because of its tendency to dilate constricted peripheral vessels, which diverts blood from the visceral organs.[41]

As therapy is implemented, the nurse must make frequent assessments of vital signs and of signs indicative of complications (hypoxia, pulmonary edema, congestive heart failure, dysrhythmias, and renal failure).

COMMON HEALTH PROBLEMS THAT OCCUR ACROSS THE LIFE SPAN

Hypersensitivity reactions: allergy

Allergy is a form of immune reaction that differs from immunological reactions in that it causes harm to the tissues of the body. Allergic reactions are based on a state of hypersensitivity and may result when the client comes in contact with a substance to which he has become sensitized by previous exposure. The tendency to become allergic may be inherited. For example, if either parent has a history of allergy, one of the offspring may develop an allergic reaction at any age.

Numerous substances (antigens) are responsible for producing allergic reactions. The antigens may be external (inhaled, ingested, injected, or applied to the skin), internal, or intrinsic. Intrinsic responses are associated with infections and affect the respiratory tract.

Antigens that are inhaled are perhaps the most common offenders. These assume greater importance with increasing age. Allergens that contaminate the indoors generally produce sensitization at an earlier age, for example, animal danders, feathers, and house dust. Plant pollens, molds, and fungi are seasonal

823

and may take several exposures to produce a reaction. Cosmetic preparations, detergents, and drugs may also be inhaled and produce a reaction in the sensitized individual.

Ingested allergens are most often those related to foods. Food allergies are generally manifested early in life. Cow's milk, egg whites, fish, clams, lobster, nuts, various fruits, and wheat are food products that commonly are sensitizing, especially in infancy.

Certain drugs are also often responsible for producing allergic reactions. The drugs may be ingested or injected or merely come in contact with the skin. Salicylates, sulfonamides, and antibiotics (including penicillin and streptomycin) are common offenders.

Other reactions may occur from injection of various vaccines and irritants from bites or stings of mosquitoes, wasps, or bees. In many instances the lesions develop beyond the area of injury.

Planning and implementation. Once the allergenic factors are identified, the nurse should instruct the client about controlling them (see material on p. 825). This must be done in all environments—the home, hospital, or other health care facilities. Following are measures to control allergenic factors:

1. *The specific allergen must be removed from the client's environment.* In the home, if an individual is allergic to animal hair, animals must not be permitted inside. The family must also be encouraged to participate in eliminating offenders from the environment. If it is dust, the environment should be dusted daily with a damp cloth, but not while the client is in the room. Weekly cleaning of the environment is essential. Since air ducts often contain dust and molds and have a tendency to stir up room dust, they should be sealed off. Electrical radiators may be used as a substitute.

2. *Acceptable substitutes should replace nonacceptable items.* Application of this principle is particularly important when the client is admitted to the hospital. On admission, the nurse should assess whether the client has a known allergy. If so, notations should be made so that the fact can be readily noted by all health team members. If the client is allergic to feather pillows, he should be permitted to use his personal pillow, or the nurse should provide another form of pillow for him. If the client is allergic to flowers, plastic or paper flowers may be used instead. If the allergen is food, a substitute should be found, or the food should be eliminated from the diet entirely. Substitutions are more likely to be made in infancy, since milk substitutes are not uncommon.

Clients with food allergies must be encouraged to become keen observers of the content of packaged foods. They must be instructed to question the content of foods they eat outside the home.

If they are allergic to certain fabrics, they must also become closer label checkers.

Nurses should especially use their teaching role when drugs are used to control allergic symptoms. When these are used, the client should be informed about side effects and the importance of bringing them to the physician's attention. Therefore the nurse's major role in managing allergies is instructing clients and their families in ways they can best control the allergy.

Desensitization (hyposensitization). The nurse can also help the client *increase resistance to the offending allergens.* Desensitization is the means by which this objective is accomplished and is employed when it is not feasible for the client to avoid the allergen. It is accomplished by administering small, but successively increasing, dosages of a specific allergen subcutaneously over a period of time.

Because nurses are often the ones who administer the desensitization injections, they should be knowledgeable about all aspects of therapy.

A tuberculin syringe is used so that the antigen can be measured precisely. The solution must not be permitted to ooze out of the needle. The injection should be made slowly to prevent the tiny blood vessels from rupturing. Pressure should be applied over the area, but the area should not be rubbed. Injections should always be given in an extremity so that a tourniquet can be applied should

---

ASSESSMENT AND IMPLEMENTATION GUIDE FOR CLIENTS WITH AN ALLERGY

The nurse should make assessments of substances that may be related to the development of allergic disorders. Instructions should be given to eliminate, from the environment, those substances that may be responsible for precipitating an attack.

Source	Assessment	Implementation
Animal dander	Do attacks occur after being around animals?	Keep pets with fur outside, or remove them entirely from the home environment.
	Are animals kept in the house?	Select a suitable pet substitute, such as a goldfish.
	Do attacks occur after exposure to feathers?	Refrain from using feather pillows; replace with synthetic pillows.
Dust	What effect does dust have on allergic attacks?	Eliminate as much dust from the environment as possible.
		Remove items from the environment that tend to collect dust, such as unnecessary articles from top of furniture, wall pictures, and carpet.
		Floors should be wood or covered with linoleum; substitute throw rugs that can be washed frequently for carpet.
		Refrain from storing articles under the bed.
		Frequently damp dust woodwork, floors, wall pictures, and shades.
		Do not use venetian blinds.
		Keep drapes cleaned.
		Keep closet doors closed.
		Prevent dust accumulation: vacuum two to three times weekly; damp dust daily; keep air vents clean by washing two to three times per month; change filters at least monthly.
		It may be necessary to: refrain from dusting or vacuuming entirely, or wear commercial mask while carrying out household chores such as dusting and vacuuming.
Foods	Do certain foods precipitate attacks?	Eliminate the specific foods from the diet.
		Check food labels carefully.
Lint	What effect does being around lint have on development of symptoms?	Discard lint-producing items such as blankets and spreads; replace with nonlint-producing ones such as cotton.
Mold	What effect does being around mold have?	Since molds grow in moist areas: eliminate house plants from the environment; clean refrigerator at least twice monthly; refrain from storing foods that tend to grow mold quickly, such as cheese, more than 2 to 3 days in the refrigerator; empty drip pans weekly; clean showers, bathtubs, and shower curtains frequently; make weekly checks on damp areas for evidence of mold growth, such as around drain pipes and in basements; repair leaks; scrub away molds.
Plants	Does being around plants precipitate symptoms?	Remove specific plant from the environment.
		Substitute plastic plants/flowers but damp dust at least two to three times per week.
Pollens	Is the individual sensitive to seasonal inhalants?	Eliminate outside air from the environment.
		Keep windows closed.
		Use air conditioning.
		Install electrostatic air filters. (These are tax deductible.)
		Plan vacation during pollen season.
Smoke	What effect does smoking have on the development of attacks, such as asthmatic?	Eliminate smoke from the environment: refrain from smoking; do not remain in smoke-filled rooms; ask individuals not to smoke in your presence.

a severe reaction occur. If such a reaction occurs, the tourniquet should be applied proximal to the injection site to reduce the systemic reaction.

Skin testing always precedes desensitization. A small scratch is made on the flexor surface of the forearm, and the antigen is applied to the scratch. If the scratch test is negative, the intradermal test is started. The concentration of the antigen is increased until a positive test is obtained. A positive reaction is indicated by the appearance of a blanched wheal or a reddened area at the site of injection. Therapy may be altered throughout the course of desensitization, depending on the client's response. If the client experiences no reaction from a given injection, the next highest dose may be omitted to reach the maintenance dose more quickly. If a slight reaction is experienced from any injection, the same dosage is administered at the time of the next injection. If the client experiences wheezing or if a large wheal is noted, the following dose is reduced. Once the maximum tolerated dose is reached, injections at this dilution are repeated at regularly scheduled intervals. These may be continued for 2 to 3 years or indefinitely.

Urticaria

Urticaria, or hives, is a common skin disorder characterized by the appearrance of multiple erythematous, edematous wheals of various sizes and occurring throughout different parts of the body (Fig. 15-18). Certain ingestants, such as foods, drugs, inhalants, contactants, injectants, and infection, may be responsible for producing a urticarial response[12] (see material at left). Physical factors such as cold *(cold urticaria),* light *(solar urticaria),* heat, exertion, and emotional stress have also been reported to produce urticaria in some individuals. Such urticaria has been referred to as *cholinergic urticaria.*

Urticaria occurs more frequently in women than in men.[53] It may also occur in nonallergic as well as atopic individuals.

Pathophysiology. The hive is the dermal manifestation of interaction between antigen and IgE antibody fixed to mast cells. Histamine, the primary mediator substance implicated in urticaria, is released from mast cells through a variety of immune and nonimmune mechanisms. The lesion (hive) itself occurs as a result of dilation and increased permeability of the capillaries, which is caused by histamine.

CAUSES OF URTICARIA*

Ingestants

Foods: Eggs, nuts, berries, fish, shellfish (reaction occurs shortly after food is ingested.)

Drugs: Penicillin, sulfonamides, aspirin, vaccines, insulin (reaction may occur immediately or within an hour, hours, or days after exposure, depending on the mechanism involved.[49]

Inhalants: Pollens, molds, danders (reaction may occur following inhalation or after immediate contact.)

Contactants: Plants, drugs applied to skin, saliva (from cats and dogs)

Injectants: Drugs such as penicillin, insect stings and bites, transfused blood antiserum

Physical agents: Cold, light, heat, pressure

*Urticaria may also be associated with infectious diseases (hepatitis, mononucleosis), noninfectious systemic disease such as lupus, and hereditary and psychological factors (tension anxiety).

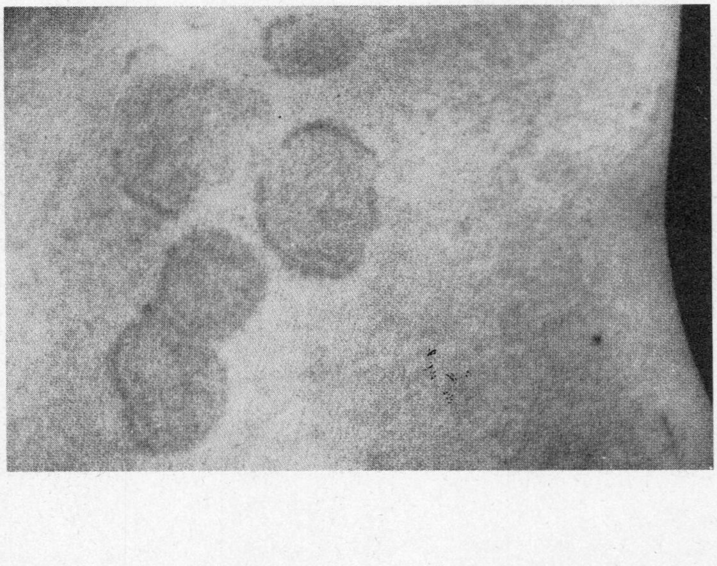

FIG. 15-18
Urticaria. (From Stewart, William D., and others: Dermatology: diagnosis and treatment of cutaneous disorders, ed. 4, St. Louis, 1978, The C.V. Mosby Co.)

Assessment. The involved areas become reddened because of dilation of the arterioles. Fluid leakage in the tissue causes the edema and large wheals. The lesions tend to blanch on pressure. Pruritus or a burning sensation generally accompanies the lesion.

The diagnosis is established with the history and physical examination, food-symptom diary, and varied laboratory studies such as complete blood count, sedimentation rate (to eliminate chronic diseases as a cause of the urticaria), and urinalysis to determine possibility of an infection or inflammatory disease. Other tests are performed to rule out specific problems (for example, complement assays for C_3; C_4 for rheumatic disease) such as lupus antinuclear antibody test for lupus erythematosus; monospot test for infectious mononucleosis; serum enzymes SGOT, SGPT for hepatitis and T_4 for hyperthyroidism.[49] Immunoglobulin (IgG, IgA, IgM) levels may also be obtained. In some instances a food elimination and challenge test may be used.

Data analysis
Data analysis may reveal potential nursing diagnoses of knowledge deficit, alteration in nutrition, and alterations in comfort.

Planning and implementation. Therapy is planned to relieve the symptoms. Epinephrine is prescribed in acute situations. Antihistamines such as diphenhydramine (Benadryl), cyproheptadine (Periactin), and hydroxyzine (Atarax) are frequently prescribed to lessen sensitivity reactions. Corticosteroids may occasionally be used in life-threatening situations for their antiinflammatory effects.

Anaphylaxis

Anaphylaxis is an immediate immunological reaction that may be mild or severe. It may occur suddenly (within seconds) and unexpectedly, is frequently iatrogenic, is potentially life-threatening, and is the result of massive outpouring of mediator substances into the cardiovascular system. It usually occurs in individuals who have become sensitized. A minimum of two exposures to the antigen is required to produce sensitization or antibody formation. A second exposure may result in the reaction (antigen-antibody combination).

A number of agents may cause anaphylaxis, including drugs such as antibiotics (penicillin and its semisynthetic derivatives), diagnostic contrast media (iodine preparations), biologicals (antitoxins, egg-based vaccines, tetanus toxoid), local anesthetics, intravenous narcotics, aspirin, and other injectables such as iron-dextran (Imferon) and nitrofurantoin. ACTH and insulin have also been reported causes. Insect stings, particularly those in the hymenoptera order (bee, wasp, yellow jacket, and hornet),[13] snake bites, certain foods (such as eggs, nuts, fish, shellfish), and skin-testing solutions are noted causes.

Pathophysiology. Anaphylaxis is considered to be mediated through IgE antibodies that bind to surface receptors of basophils and tissue mast cells.[20] The interaction of the antigen and the all-bound IgE antibodies results in the release of chemical mediators from the cells. The substances include histamine, slow-reacting substance of anaphylaxis (SRS-A), eosinophil chemotactic factor of anaphylaxis (ECF-A), serotonin, and the kinins such as bradykinin.

Chemical mediators bind to specific receptors on smooth muscle and blood vessels and produce generalized vasodilation, vascular permeability with resulting edema, increased mucus-gland secretion, and contraction of smooth muscles.

Assessment. As a result of the effects presented above, signs and symptoms are produced that may vary from mild flushing, urticaria, and itching, to severe respiratory distress. Acute anaphylaxis (anaphylactic shock) is characterized by sudden anxiety and a pounding headache. Signs and symptoms indicative of respiratory obstruction occur and include dyspnea, wheezing, chest tightness, coughing, stridor, and hoarseness. Vascular collapse follows quickly, as may be evidenced by rapid weak pulse, hypotension, dysrhythmias, and shock (for example, anaphylactic shock). The shock is primarily caused by increased size of the vascular bed with pooling of blood, thereby causing a greatly reduced venous return and ultimately reduced cardiac output. Gastrointestinal symptoms such as nausea, vomiting, diarrhea, and dysphagia may also occur. Generally the more rapidly the symptoms appear, the more severe the reactions are likely to be.[8]

> **Data analysis**
> *Data analysis may reveal nursing diagnoses of potential for ineffective breathing pattern, alterations in cardiac output, fear, and potential for fluid volume deficit.*

Planning and implementation

Preventing allergic reactions. There are a number of areas where preventive measures may be used. Nurses, being directly responsible for administering drugs, have a prime responsibility in prevention. A careful history regarding previous reaction and substances to which they are allergic should be obtained on all individuals seen in a health care facility. Before any medications or substances that may cause potential anaphylaxis are given, detailed assessments should be made as to whether the client is allergic to the specific substance. Any doubt in the client's mind warrants consulting the physician so that an alternative medication can be prescribed.

Clients should be encouraged to be alert to hidden sources and become conscientious label readers. For example, a number of cold and sinus relief preparations contain aspirin, to which they may be allergic. Encourage individuals to keep immunizations current to avoid the potential need for antisera.[13]

Those individuals who are known to be allergic to substances, especially those prone to develop anaphylactic reactions, should be instructed to wear a Medic Alert bracelet or necklace indicating the substance to which they are allergic.

In instances where skin testing is indicated, appropriate emergency drugs (epinephrine) and resuscitation equipment should be close at hand. Instructions should also be given about reactions that may occur outside a health care facility. It is not uncommon for clients with known previous anaphylactic reactions to be instructed on the proper administration of emergency medications, either by injection or inhalation. Prompt medical assistance should be strongly encouraged when a reaction occurs.

Nursing care during a reaction. When an allergic reaction occurs (especially an anaphylactic reaction), therapy must be started promptly, even when the symptoms are mild. Therapy is planned to accomplish maintenance of patency of airway, relief of the allergic response, and prevention of shock.

Maintaining a patent airway. In severe anaphylaxis, large areas of the skin (the face and extremities) and the larynx may become edematous; therefore clothing about the neck should be loosened, oxygen should be administered via positive pressure to relieve hypoxia, and mucus should be aspirated as often as necessary. Aminophylline may be administered intravenously if bronchospasms are evident. Endotracheal intubation equipment should be available, provided laryngeal edema is not relieved by medications.

Relieving the allergic response. Epinephrine 1:1000 (0.2 to 0.5 ml) is administered intravenously or intracardially. This may be repeated at 15-minute intervals.[13] An equal amount may be injected around the injection site or sting to decrease absorption of the antigen. A tourniquet may also be placed proximal to the injection site to retard venous return. The tourniquet should be removed temporarily every 10 to 15 minutes. An antihistamine such as diphenhydramine (Benadryl) or a corticosteroid such as hydrocortisone succinate (Solu-Cortef) may also be administered to lessen the sensitivity reaction.

Preventing shock. The client should be placed in a recumbent position. An intravenous fluid route should be established to deliver volume (usually isotonic saline) to combat shock and to administer vasopressor drugs such as metaraminol (Aramine). Vital signs must be assessed frequently, and significant changes should be communicated to the physician.

In addition, the client should be monitored carefully and a defibrillator should be readily available for immediate use in the event that cardiopulmonary resuscitation is required.

Evaluation. Evaluation of the nursing plan for the client with allergies is an ongoing process.

EXPECTED OUTCOMES

The client and/or family can:
1. Describe the allergy, including the cause.
2. Demonstrate plans for preventing allergic reactions.
3. Demonstrate plans for care during an allergic response.
4. State restrictions.
5. Describe reactions requiring emergency health care.
6. Indicate plans for follow-up care.
7. State emergency management for emergency reactions.
8. State use, dosage, route, method of administration, and side effects of drugs used for an allergic reaction.
9. Demonstrate knowledge of when to seek health care.

Burns

Burns are tissue injuries caused by thermal (liquid or flame), chemical, or electrical agents. Burns caused by each of these agents have many similarities. Radiant energy and friction may also cause burns.

Burns are a major contributor of accidents during the childhood years. The preschool years, in particular, are of highest vulnerability. (Statistics are presented later in relation to all age groups.)

Thermal burns: patterns of occurrence and prevention. At some stages of development, certain types of thermal burns are more likely to occur than others. The nurse should therefore use these stages as points of reference in providing instructions about the prevention of burns.

Nursing process for common health problems

Immersion scald burns. Perhaps the most dangerous burn injuries affecting the infant or toddler are immersion scald burns. Such burns are likely to occur during the bath. Often a family member prepares the bath water and proceeds with the bath, thinking that the water has been tested for temperature. However, because of some distraction such as a telephone call, one may have forgotten to test the water. As a result, the child is immersed in the water and is burned. In an effort to prevent immersion scald burns during baths, caretakers should always test bath water before immersing a child in a tub and should teach children to test bath water before stepping in. Another strategy in prevention is to always place cold water in the tub first and add enough hot water to bring the bath to a comfortable temperature.

Scald burns. Scald burns that result from overturned containers of hot liquids are frequently encountered during the toddler period. This is the stage when the child is curious and constantly tries to find out ''how things are made'' or ''what is in the pot.'' Adults are often scalded in the shower when they grasp the cold handle and inadvertently turn it off while taking a shower.

Scald burns can be prevented. Precautions that should be taken include turning pan and pot handles away and out of the child's reach and discouraging overhanging tablecloths, because infants and small children can easily tug on them and pull over hot food or beverages on themselves; and encouraging parents to watch for other potentially dangerous situations such as a cord dangling from a coffeepot or other electrical appliance. Another aspect of prevention is informing clients about the availability of devices that can be installed at the faucet or shower that automatically stop the flow of water if it reaches a scalding temperature.[57]

Flame burns. Flame burns, caused by ignited play clothing, occur most often in the preschool and early school-age child (4 to 8 years old). The use of flame-resistant material for clothing is especially thought to reduce the number of flame burns. Home heating units should be such that children's clothes cannot catch fire, and parents should be encouraged to purchase flame-resistant toys. The trash burn usually involves the school-age boy. Again, prevention is of key importance. Children should be instructed not to play in or around fire. They should not be permitted to burn trash in the absence of an adult, and they should particularly be closely observed during the leaf-burning season. School-age children are also likely to play with matches, and this practice should be discouraged. Matches and cigarette lighters should be kept out of their reach. Proper guards should be used around stoves, fireplaces, and lamps to prevent inquisitive children from burning themselves. Cooking utensils or other containers with hot liquids should be placed so that they cannot be easily overturned. Since 1972, all children's sleepwear (up to and including size 6X) is required by federal law to be flame resistant. As much as possible, children's clothing should be made of inflammable materials.[36]

Smoking. Smoking in bed and careless handling of cigarettes and fireworks and the misuse of combustible materials are often responsible for burns in the adolescent and adult periods. The practice of smoking in bed can potentiate a major fire accident and should be discouraged. Regulations regarding firearms and combustible materials should be adhered to. The community health nurse and school nurse can particularly teach children and families regarding fire hazards in and around the home. The occupational health nurse can provide instructions about fire safety in the work setting.

Burn wound classification. The classification of burns in all age groups is determined by the depth of the tissue injury and the extent of body surface involved. The depth gives a description of the physical appearance of the burn, and the extent indicates the percentage of the body surface that has been burned. More commonly, burns are classified as first, second, or third degree (Fig. 15-19). Sometimes a fourth-degree classification is used. Also, it is not uncommon to see only the terms *partial thickness* or *full thickness* used to describe a burn injury.

A *first-degree* burn is a partial-thickness burn that involves the superficial layers of the epidermis and is characterized by redness, pain, slight tenderness, and blanching on pressure. No blisters are present, and minimal systemic involvement occurs. First-degree burns are generally not serious unless large areas of the body are involved. A mild scald from steam and a sunburn are common examples of first-degree burns. Healing takes place within 1 to 2 weeks.

Second-degree burns destroy the epidermis and involve the dermis. They, too, are classified as partial-thickness burns. Injury to the deeper layers of the skin and capillaries accounts for the redness and blisters. As a result, fluid leaks from the blood into the tissue to produce blisters. Pain is present because the

FIG. 15-19
Classification of burns according to depth of burn. (From Warner, Carmen Germaine, editor: Emergency care: assessment and intervention, ed. 2, St. Louis, 1978, The C.V. Mosby Co.)

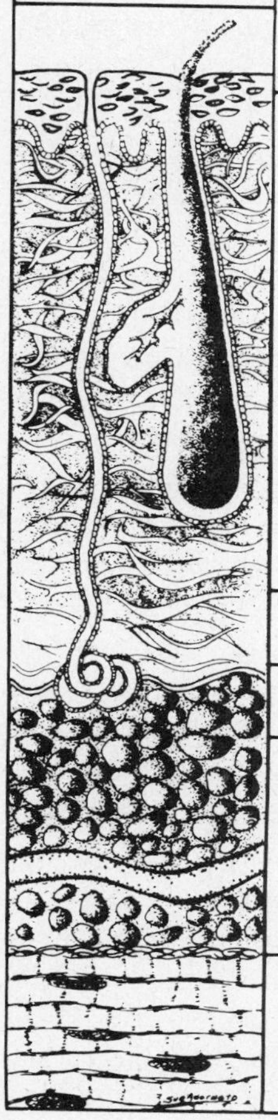

	Depth of burn		Pain and pinprick sensitivity	Appearance	Healing time	End result of healing	Treatment
		Detailed classification					
	1°	Erythema only, no loss of epidermis	Hyperalgesia	Erythema		Normal skin	Allow to heal by natural processes / Protect from further injury and infection
	2° Partial skin loss	Superficial, no loss of dermis	Hyperalgesia or normal		6-10 days		
		Intermediate / Healing from hair follicles	Normal to hypo- algesia	Erythema to opaque white blisters are characteristic	7-14 days	Normal to slightly pitted and/or poorly pigmented	
		Deep / Healing from sweat glands	Hypoalgesia to analgesia		14-21 days	Hairless and depigmented / Texture normal to pitted or flat and shiny	Elective skin grafting may save time and give better end result
	3° Whole skin loss	Deep dermal Occasionally heal from scattered epithelium	Analgesia	White opaque to charred, coagulated; subcutaneous veins may be visible	More than 21 days	Poor texture Hypertrophic Scar frequent	
		Whole skin loss Healing from edges only			Never if area is large	Hypertrophic scar and chronic granulations unless grafted	Skin grafting mandatory
	4° Deep tissue loss	Deep structure loss	May be some algesia				

protective coverings of the nerve endings are irritated. Second-degree burns are not serious or life-threatening unless 25% to 30% of the body surface is involved.[9,17] In the absence of infection and trauma, healing usually occurs in 14 to 21 days, and scarring is minimal or absent. Healing takes place by spontaneous epithelial regeneration from the base of the hair shafts and epithelial lining of skin glands.

Third-degree burns involve the full thickness of the skin, with destruction of the epidermis and dermis. Hence, they are frequently classified as full-thickness burns. There may also be involvement of the underlying tissue and organs. The appearance of the skin is leatherlike and may range in color from white to tan-brown-red-black.[10] Pain is uncommon after the initial acute pain because the nerve endings are destroyed. Edema, which results from increased capillary permeability, is present, and the area appears blanched or charred. Blanching is the result of contraction of the skin capillaries. Healing usually takes place after months of extensive treatment.

A fourth-degree burn involves the underlying fat, muscles, tendons, and bones. It is more likely to result from intense heat, from blazing chemical fires, and during war. These burns also require extensive management.

Four classifications have been described. However, more than one degree of burn may occur on the same general area. Hence the client may have painful partial-thickness burns and full-thickness burns as well.

Pathophysiology. The pathophysiological derangements that result from burns are multiple and result in alterations in normal skin function, alterations in the vascular system (including fluid shifts and alterations in blood elements), and alterations in metabolism.

Alterations in skin function. Thermal injury considerably decreases the skin's ability to curtail water loss from a burned area. As much as 6 to 8 liters per day may be lost from large burn wounds.[57] Because the protective covering is either partially or completely destroyed, the skin's ability to protect itself from the invasion of organisms is also affected.

Alterations in vascular system. Fluid shift, hemolysis, and sluggish blood flow are the vascular effects. Immediately after a burn injury occurs, the capillary permeability is altered throughout the body. Subsequently, *fluid shifts* occur readily and continue for approximately 48 hours.[6] Fluids containing water, sodium, electrolytes, chloride, and colloids (proteins) escape from the intravascular compartment into the interstitial spaces. This creates what is called burn edema, which is best demonstrated by extensive swelling of the involved area (third-degree burns) and sometimes of the surrounding areas (blisters formation in second-degree burns). However, the fluid may not always be readily seen because it may be deep or under the thick, leatherlike surface of a full-thickness burn. Potassium ions are transferred from the damaged cells to the bloodstream. (The high potassium level is often responsible for cardiac arrest in burned clients).

In addition to fluid shifts, destruction of the cells and tissue is also responsible for loss of electrolytes. For example, injury to the subcutaneous fat causes a chemical reaction and results in calcium loss. Protein, particularly albumin because of its small molecules, will be lost. This protein loss decreases the circulating volume as well as altering the albumin to globulin (A/G) ratio, which affects the osmotic pressure.

Another effect is the *sluggish blood flow*. The fluid portion of the blood (plasma) also escapes from the intravascular compartment. As a result, the blood becomes thick, or hemoconcentrated, and flows sluggishly. The hematocrit rises because there is less fluid to dilute the solid components of the blood. The sluggish blood flow results in a drop in cardiac output, decreased tissue perfusion, tissue hypoxia, metabolic acidosis, and, if therapy is not started to combat the changes, shock. A consequence of the sluggish blood flow is that it permits bacteria and cellular matter in the blood to precipitate to the lower parts of the vessels, particularly smaller vessels. As a result, thrombi develop and produce ischemia to the involved area.[6]

Hemolysis is another effect. If the wound is extensive, red cells leak from the damaged capillaries and become trapped and held in the wound. This results in hemolysis (destruction) of the cells. The kidneys attempt to filter out hemoglobin from the blood, resulting in hemoglobinuria. Consequently the accumulation of hemoglobin pigment in the tubules may produce renal failure in absence of adequate fluid. This is often the cause of the anemia in the severely burned client.

Anemia, another systemic effect, occurs as a result of loss of red blood cells from hemolysis at the burn site, damaged red blood cells with subsequent decreased life span, and from thrombi, which contain red blood cells. Red blood cells are lost at the injured site and may be lost if other body organs are involved (for example, liver, spleen).

Physiological compensation. The body attempts to compensate for the changes by constricting the blood vessels, by withdrawing fluid from other areas, and by causing the blood vessels in the splanchnic area and skin to contract. In this way an adequate supply of blood to the vital organs is maintained. However, therapy must be started to facilitate combating the changes.

Within 2 to 3 days after a burn injury, fluid shifts at a slower rate because the colloidal osmotic pressure gradient between the plasma and interstitial fluid decreases.

About 49 to 72 hours after the burn the fluid shift reverses, and fluid returns to the intravascular compartment from the burned area, resulting in an increase in sodium and chloride ions. At this time an increase may be noted in the urine output, the hematocrit level will decrease, and edema will be lessened. Large amounts of potassium are lost in the urine. During this period the client should also be observed closely for signs of pulmonary edema.

Alterations in metabolism. A *hypermetabolic response,* proportional to the extent of the burn, occurs in major thermal burns. The metabolic expenditure at rest has been reported to increase as much as 40% to 100% above normal in clients whose burns exceed 30% of the total body surface.[11] The elevated metabolic demands occur as a result of the neurohormonal control mechanism that regulates energy use. Reports indicate that increased rates of gluconeogenesis, decreased levels of insulin, and increased plasma concentration of glucagon are consistent with an increased flow of glucose to the wound where it is required for wound healing.[10]

Monitoring physiological reactions. Because of the hemodynamic changes that occur in an extensive burn, frequent laboratory determinations must include electrolytes (Na^+, Cl^-, K^+), hemoglobin and hematocrit, serum proteins, BUN, urinalysis, and glucose. Throughout the initial period, blood studies are usually made at least every 6 hours. The nurse must be aware of normal values so that any discrepancy can be promptly reported to the physician.

Psychosocial reactions to burn injuries. When a client sustains an extensive burn, he not only suffers from physical trauma but also experiences serious emotional trauma. The burn usually occurs so rapidly that the client does not have the opportunity to prepare himself. Within a matter of minutes, the independent individual becomes dependent on others. The burned client may be difficult to manage because he is not able to adjust to his physical incapacity. He may be faced with fears of disfigurement, physical discomfort, surgical procedures, and a long convalescence. Burn injuries are likely to result in a number of responses. Studies have indicated that in children, anxiety is by far the most pronounced response. The major sources of anxiety are fears of death, mutilation, pain, and abandonment. Separation from family and friends, a feeling of inadequacy and rejection, problems associated with the accident, and conflicts caused by dependency are other sources of problems.[53]

During the period of painful inactivity the client may relive the episode many times in an effort to attempt to find the reason why it all happened. He may believe that the burn was caused by his own negligence or that of someone close to him. The pain that is experienced may be interpreted as punishment. Guilt feelings may also arise if the client is the only survivor from the fire. The nurse should be prepared to help the client and his family deal with such feelings.

During the period of painful inactivity and recuperation the client undergoes a certain amount of regression and helplessness. This is seen most frequently in a client whose hands, face, or organs of excretion or reproduction are injured. The client who depends on the use of his hands for a living may be tremendously disturbed by burns of this area. The client who has facial burns is often terrified by the disfigurement and the idea of possible loss of vision. The state of helplessness and dependency may also be frightening, because the helplessness denies the client the pleasure of caring for himself. It may also deny certain comforts that make for small pleasures and dignities of life. For example, a client may not be able to scratch his nose, clean himself after toileting, change his position, or even smile without pain. In the child, regression may be manifested by thumbsucking, whimpering, crying, or demanding behavior. He may be both verbally and physically aggressive as a response to apprehension and frustration.

The client who is, by nature, independent may avoid making appropriate requests for help. It may be only through force of circumstances that he asks for help. These circumstances may also cause the client to do some limit testing to determine just how much aggression and dependency will be tolerated by the family and health care providers.

Because a burn injury may change the image a person has of himself, the burn client may withdraw from all social contacts. Clients who are severely burned are prone to a series of unique mental phenomena similar to those experienced by clients with debilitating conditions. The cycle starts with denial, which is followed by repression, suppression, and finally acceptance. It is only after acceptance that the client can take full advantage of the treatment program, help make plans, and take appropriate actions. The health team must understand the expected reactions and help him adjust to them. During the initial period the client may be too frightened to ask questions. After the acute effects have decreased, he may begin to ask questions. All avenues of communication must be kept open.

During the adjustment period the nurse and family can help by encouraging the client to engage in constructive activities. These may help remove the conflict over dependency, as well as make him feel that he is contributing directly toward his recovery. Stimulation beyond the hospital should be encouraged. This might be accomplished by providing television, radio, newspapers, and books, and even encouraging visits from the family and significant friends. These must be considerations not only while the client is hospitalized, but also after he returns home or to another health care facility. As often as necessary, the occupational therapist should be consulted to help plan activities for the client.

Visual evidence of the likelihood of uneventful recovery may be encouraging in the early phase of the hospitalization. Contact with clients who have had similar burns and have almost recovered is an important source of encouragement. The use of photographs before and after a burn might also be helpful.

Assessment. The dramatic nature of burns should not overshadow the fact that there may be other associated and threatening injuries. Therefore when a client is seen after a burn injury has occurred, the nurse should make complete assessments concerning the following factors.

Airway, breathing, circulation (ABCs)
1. *Airway* patency and signs that may be indicative of obstruction (dyspnea, stridor, hoarseness, prolonged expiration).
2. *Breathing* inadequacy or ventilation exchange. If the chest is involved, assess whether accessory muscles are used.
3. *Circulation,* that is, vital signs and signs indicative of the adequacy of peripheral circulation (color, temperature, peripheral pulses, sensorium).

Parts of body involved
1. *Face and neck.* Burns about the face and neck are more likely to result in inhalation of fumes and produce damage to the pulmonary tree and subsequent edema. *Edema* of these areas may result in *respiratory obstruction,* which may be characterized by dyspnea, stridor, hoarseness, and prolonged expiration. The color of the sputum and the presence of singed hairs in the nasal passages should be observed. Singed hair or sooty, carbonaceous, or bloody sputum demands that close assessments be made of respiratory status.
2. *Extremities* (hands and feet). Be alert for the presence of jewelry. Jewelry on an affected part should be removed. Skin on the inner arm is very thin; thus full-thickness burns are not uncommon in this area.
3. *Genitalia.* Burns of the genitalia have a high infection rate.

Weight of the client. Baseline measurements are essential because the quality of fluid administered is often determined according to weight.

Age of the client. The importance of age relates to the difference in surface area, character of the skin, poor antibody response, and degenerative changes at various stages of life. In the very young burned client (for example, those under age 2) a larger area per unit of weight is involved. The skin of the very young is thin and not fully developed in comparison with the skin of a young or middle-aged adult. Therefore application of intense heat for a given period of time will cause greater penetration than will occur under the same circumstances in adulthood. Subsequently the mortality rate is higher in those under age 2 and over age 60.[10,17]

Nursing process for common health problems

Young children have immature kidneys, and, as a result, they are less capable of regulating the excretion of water and electrolytes. Thus overhydration or underhydration may be a real problem in the management of the young client with a burn injury. The antibody response in children under age 2 is poor. As a result, they are prone to develop severe infections. A 60-year-old individual is likely to have degenerative changes that are aggravated by the stress of the burn injury.

Health history and pathological state. The health history is significant in that a prior pathological condition may become aggravated during the process of recovery. The status of tetanus immunization should be assessed. Tetanus is a hazard of extensive burn injuries. The client should receive tetanus toxoid intramuscularly, either as an initial immunizing dose or as a booster, unless an initial immunizing dose or booster has been administered within the past 10 years.[16] Passive immunization should be provided simultaneously with the use of tetanus immune globulin human (TIGH) or hyperimmune globulin (Hypertet) if no information can be ascertained about the status of tetanus immunization.[16]

Specific questions should be asked regarding other health problems. Obesity; respiratory, cardiac, renal, and metabolic diseases; arthritis; and injuries such as fractures will influence the response to injury.

Circumstances involving the burn injury. The type of agent involved in causing the burn is important. If caused by *thermal* agents: How long was the individual exposed to the agent? What type of material was involved? Was carpet involved? What type of flooring? Was vinyl furniture involved?

For *electrical* injuries, assess the voltage involved and duration of exposure.

Chemical injuries warrant assessing the agent, duration of exposure, and whether noxious fumes were given off and first-aid measures used.

Environment in which the injury occurred. It is essential that information be obtained as to whether the injury occurred in an open or closed environment? Indoors or outdoors? Indoor fires have the greatest risk of being associated with smoke inhalation or respiratory tract injury.

Prior therapy. Assessments should be made as to whether medications have been administered. If so, what type? The importance of assessing whether *pain* medication has been administered cannot be overemphasized. If the client has already received medication, subsequent pain medication may further depress the client's respiratory status. If pain medications have not been administered, the nurse should initially observe whether pain is a presenting symptom. If so, how severe? Assessing the degree of pain is extremely important because pain inhibits the vasomotor center, thereby increasing the capacity of the vascular bed and reducing venous return, which may result in shock. Therefore the assessment for pain should be an initial assessment.

Assessing extent of burn injury. An estimate of the body surface area involved can be made by applying several methods. The *rule of nines* is one method and is useful for the immediate appraisal of the burned area. The body is divided into regions, each representing approximately 9% or a multiple of 9% of the body surface. For example, the anterior of an upper extremity is 4.5%, the posterior is 4.5%; thus the entire extremity would be 9%. The anterior lower extremity is 9% and the posterior is 9%, making the entire extremity 18%. The perineum is 1%, resulting in a total body surface area of 100% (Fig. 15-20).

Berkow's method is calculated on the basis of the client's age and changes

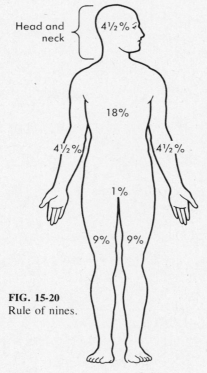

Head and neck

4½%

18%

4½%   4½%

1%

9%   9%

FIG. 15-20
Rule of nines.

that occur in proportion of the head and legs to the rest of the body as the individual grows.[19] The arms and trunk have fixed values in that they have a fixed proportion throughout life.

Another method for determining the extent of involvement is the *Lund-Browder chart* (Fig. 15-21). This method is thought to be more accurate because it takes into account changes in percentage of body surface at various stages of development. In children, a greater amount is allowed for the head and trunk and less for the lower extremities.

Data analysis
Data analysis may reveal nursing diagnoses of potential for ineffective airway clearance, alterations in comfort, fluid volume deficit, alterations in cardiac output, alteration in nutrition, self-care deficit, potential for infection related to impairment of skin integrity, fear, greiving, ineffective coping, and diversional activity deficit.

FIG. 15-21
Burn estimate diagram. (From Jacoby, F.G.: Nursing care of the patient with burns, ed. 2, St. Louis, 1976, The C.V. Mosby Co.)

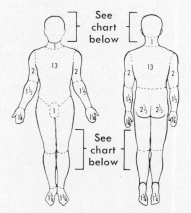

Age:_____
Sex: _____
Weight: _____
Height: _____

Area	Inf.	1-4	5-9	10-14	15	Adult	Part.	Full	Total	Donor areas
Head	19	17	13	11	9	7				
Neck	2	2	2	2	2	2				
Ant. trunk	13	13	13	13	13	13				
Post. trunk	13	13	13	13	13	13				
R. buttock	2½	2½	2½	2½	2½	2½				
L. buttock	2½	2½	2½	2½	2½	2½				
Genitalia	1	1	1	1	1	1				
R.U. arm	4	4	4	4	4	4				
L.U. arm	4	4	4	4	4	4				
R.L. arm	3	3	3	3	3	3				
L.L. arm	3	3	3	3	3	3				
R. hand	2½	2½	2½	2½	2½	2½				
L. hand	2½	2½	2½	2½	2½	2½				
R. thigh	5½	6½	8	8½	9	9½				
L. thigh	5½	6½	8	8½	9	9½				
R. leg	5	5	5½	6	6½	7				
L. leg	5	5	5½	6	6½	7				
R. foot	3½	3½	3½	3½	3½	3½				
L. foot	3½	3½	3½	3½	3½	3½				
						Total				

Planning and implementation. On the basis of the presented diagnoses, the goals of therapy should be to maintain vital functions and preserve body parts. These can be accomplished through maintenance of an adequate airway, relieving pain, maintaining fluid and electrolyte balance, maintaining nutrition, preventing infection and other complications, and caring for the burn wound.

Maintaining an adequate airway. Whenever there are signs that indicate respiratory involvement, maintenance of respiratory function takes priority. Such involvement is more likely to occur in burns that involve the face and head. If secretions are excessive, they should be suctioned. A tracheostomy or endotracheal intubation may be required if the respiratory tract is involved (Fig. 15-22). In the absence of overt respiratory involvement, a tracheostomy may be performed immediately rather than waiting until more obvious signs are present. This approach eliminates the procedure's being performed under less favorable conditions. An endotracheal tube may be inserted, and oxygen may be administered. The nurse must be familiar with all aspects of respiratory care. The care of the burned client with assisted ventilation does not differ from that of a client with other disorders.

Relieving pain. Medications are administered in small dosages to control pain. If sedation is necessary, morphine is usually administered because it provides cutaneous analgesia and sedation superior to that of meperidine (Demerol). Medications for pain are administered intravenously to ensure adequate absorption. They are not administered subcutaneously or intramuscularly because peripheral circulation is sluggish and may pool for a delayed period of

FIG. 15-22
Burns of head and neck require a tracheostomy. (Courtesy Shriner's Hospital for Crippled Children, Cincinnati.)

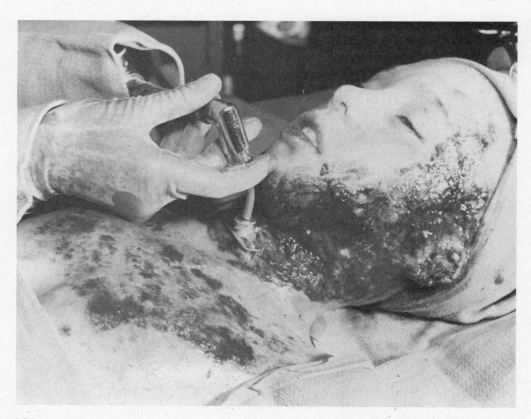

time. Subsequently the delayed effect may be confused with an inadequate dose. If the dose is repeated, a cumulative overdose may occur once the peripheral circulation improves. The client must therefore be observed closely for the effects of the drug and for signs of respiratory depression.

Maintaining fluid balance. Once the airway has been assured and pain is controlled, efforts are directed toward fluid replacement. Replacing fluid during the initial period is important because of the severe hemodynamic changes that are occurring. Fluid replacement is accomplished through the use of an intravenous cutdown method or the peripheral intravenous method. Generally a cutdown is required if more than 10% of a child's body surface is involved and more than 20% of an adult's.[17]

Electrolytes, colloids, and water are lost from the intravascular space as a result of burns. Red blood cells may also be lost. Therefore to restore hemodynamics, each of these must be replaced. Ringer's lactate is the initial fluid of choice to replace volume and to cover the loss of sodium and chloride in the burn injury. Dextrose solutions may be administered to cover insensible loss. Potassium is not administered because of its shift to the intravascular fluid. Colloids (such as dextran) are plasma expanders that maintain colloidal osmotic pressure.

Although there are several methods for determining the amount of fluid to be replaced, Brooke's formula (a modification of Evans' formula) is widely used. This formula recommends the use of 1.5 ml of fluid per kilogram of body weight per percent of body surface involved. It also suggests the use of colloid and electrolyte solution in a 1:3 ratio. The amount of water administered is calculated according to age. The water requirement for the adult is 2000 ml, and less for children. Fluid requirements are calculated up to 50% of surface involvement in adults, and 30% in children to avoid fluid overload.[48] However, individuals with a larger percentage of burns need more fluid. For a 24-hour period, half the calculated fluid is administered during the first 8 hours, one fourth during the second 8 hours, and one fourth during the third 8 hours. About half the amount of the first 24-hour colloids and electrolytes is administered in the second 24 hours. This regimen is followed because the ratio of fluid loss is greatest initially, and it progressively decreases 48 hours after the injury.

Assessing adequacy of fluid therapy. The most important responsibility of the nurse during the initial phase of therapy is to ascertain that the fluids are being administered and maintained in the manner and amount ordered. Although the amount and type of fluid are determined by the physician, they are controlled by the nurse. The importance of the client's receiving, on schedule, the amount of fluid ordered cannot be overemphasized.

To determine the adequacy of fluid therapy, careful assessments must be made of the vital signs, central venous pressure or pulmonary wedge pressure, urinary output, and level of consciousness.

Because plasma is lost through the burned area, the blood volume, blood flow, and cardiac output may be reduced. The nurse must therefore make frequent assessments of the vital signs and urinary output. These assessments should be made at least every hour or as often as necessary. If the upper extremities have been burned, it may be hard to obtain a blood pressure reading because of edema of the extremities. Therefore other means must be relied on to determine the state of the client. The blood pressure reading may be taken in the lower extremities or monitored by an indwelling arterial line. If the radial pulse is not accessible, the nurse might assess the temporal or popliteal or apical pulses.

Central venous pressure (CVP) reading is a reliable guide in determining the ability of the heart to tolerate large volumes of fluids. A CVP reading greater than 15 cm of water is an early sign of overhydration. A Swan-Ganz catheter will give an even more accurate assessment of the client's fluid status. It is a catheter placed in the pulmonary artery by way of the internal jugular vein or brachial vein.

Hourly urine output is an extremely valuable index in determining the adequacy of general circulation. To ensure accurate hourly readings, an indwelling catheter is inserted and connected to a drainage system. The catheter may be inserted in the emergency unit and maintained throughout the initial period. To evaluate the effectiveness or ineffectiveness of fluid therapy, the nurse must be aware of normal and abnormal urine volumes. The urine output in a child weighing less than 30 pounds should be between 1 and 1.5 ml/kg/hr. In the older child and adult the range should be between 0.5 and 1 ml/kg/hr.[15] These are possibly more reliable, although some general guidelines have been established to depict a volume compatible with good renal function: 10 to 20 ml/hr in the infant, 20 to 50 ml/hr in the child, and 30 to 70 ml/hr in the adult.

The rate of intravenous fluid administration is adjusted according to the hourly urinary output. If the fluid output falls below normal, the rate of intravenous fluid administration may be increased. Failure to increase the fluid rate may lead to renal failure. An output that exceeds normal levels usually indicates excessive fluid administration, and if the situation is not corrected, pulmonary edema may result. The physician therefore should be consulted as often as necessary. At the same time the nurse should observe the client for symptoms that indicate excessive or inadequate fluid replacement. Signs and symptoms indicative of *inadequate* fluid replacement are those of *impending shock:* excessive thirst, restlessness, disorientation, increased pulse, decreased blood pressure, and decreased urine output. Signs and symptoms indicative of *excessive* fluid replacement are those of *pulmonary edema:* dyspnea, venous engorgement, moist rales, and increased blood pressure.

Problems that may affect the administration of fluid must be carefully observed. For example, the intravenous cutdown site must be observed for evidence of fluid leakage. Venospasms and blood clots are often responsible for poor administration. Because of continuous intravenous administrations, thrombophlebitis may occur about the third or fourth day. With this in mind, the nurse should observe the site of infusion carefully for signs of thrombophlebitis, such as tenderness and the appearance of a red streak. Pain may be elicited by applying pressure over the area and above the cutdown site. If these adverse signs are observed, or if fluid therapy is not being maintained, the physician should be consulted.

As assessments are made of the urine output, the nurse should also assess specific gravity, pH, and glucose, as well as observe the character of the urine. These assessments are essential parameters in determining complications. The presence of blood (hematuria) or sediments and a change in specific gravity above and below normal values warrant calling the physician.

Assessment of the level of consciousness is important because information is provided regarding the adequacy of blood flow.

Maintaining adequate nutrition. Although thirst is a major symptom during the first couple of days, clients with major burns should not be given oral fluids for the first 48 hours or until peristalsis is present. A paralytic ileus and gastric dilations may result from splanchnic contractions. The administration of water may cause water intoxication. The nurse must be instrumental in explaining to the client why water must be withheld. Measures must be used to decrease the thirst. Frequent oral hygiene and allowing the client to rinse his mouth with cold water or hold a cold, moistened gauze in his mouth are helpful.

During the period immediately following the burn, large amounts of proteins and electrolytes are lost. Nitrogen is lost as a result of tissue catabolism. Therefore adequate proteins, calories, and vitamins must be provided to coincide with metabolic demands so that healing can take place. Special electrolyte solutions may be administered through a nasogastric tube. The tube is usually kept in place until the client can tolerate foods by mouth.

A high-protein diet may be prescribed after the fifth day. Generally an intake of 2 to 3 g of protein and 70 calories per kilogram of body weight is desirable. The amount of food is gradually increased to the client's needs. Failure to supply enough calories to meet body needs results in rapid consumption of endogenous fuel reserves, starvation, weight loss, delayed wound healing, and decreased resistance.

To ensure that the client receives the desired protein and calorie intake, he is placed on a high-protein, high-calorie diet with supplemental, between-meal, high-protein liquid feedings. The nurse should explain to the client the importance of maintaining an adequate nutritional intake. At the same time the nurse must use strategies to facilitate meeting the client's nutritional needs. When oral feedings are started, frequent small feedings may be more acceptable than one large feeding because the client's physiological need is generally greater than his appetite. The nurse should work closely with the dietitian and provide palatable supplemental feedings. Changing the flavor and color of feedings may be desirable. Variety may also be necessary and instrumental in helping the client consume the high-protein, high-calorie diet.

Children, more often than adults, express dislike for certain foods. As a result, no matter how often they are fed, they will refuse to eat these foods. When these circumstances arise, it is important that the child be fed foods he likes in double or triple amounts. Consultation with the parents may be necessary to determine the child's likes and dislikes. Permitting a parent to feed the child may also be helpful. The nurse should keep notes of the amounts and types of foods eaten. Having the mother or a relative bring food in from the outside may also be helpful if the client is lagging in his food intake. Milk, eggs, and meat are desirable and nutritious foods for children as well as adults.

Vitamin supplements such as vitamin B-complex (thiamine, riboflavin, and niacin) and vitamin C may be given regularly with meals. Vitamin C facilitates tissue regeneration, whereas vitamin B supplies oxidative enzyme systems to metabolize extra carbohydrates and proteins.

Other factors that influence a client's acceptance of foods must be identified. If the client is weak and if environmental disturbances or emotional or physical responses hinder him from eating, the nurse must plan to relieve these factors. If the client is weak or if dressings are applied about the hands, he may not be able to feed himself. The nurse must therefore feed the client or allow a family member to feed him. Whoever feeds the client should not appear rushed. Care must be maintained not to make the client totally dependent. He should gradually be encouraged to help with the process. As soon as the client can manage the meal by himself, he should be permitted to do so. Self-help devices may be important adjuncts to helping the client feed himself.

Dressing changes often cause much pain and discomfort. They also produce an unpleasant odor. Therefore dressing changes should always be carried out well in advance of mealtime. In this way, pain can be relieved and odors eliminated from the environment. Before mealtime, oral hygiene must be administered as often as necessary. If facial dressings interfere with chewing solid foods, ground foods may be substituted. Allowing the client to eat in a position that is near the normal eating position often will have a direct influence on his intake. Some form of diversion—watching television or listening to the radio—may provide stimulation and be instrumental in helping the client improve his intake. The nurse should not hesitate to try any strategies that will enhance maintenance of adequate nutrition.

Preventing and controlling infection and other complications. The most common complication of burn injuries is infection. Contaminating sources may be air, dust, other persons, hair, and clothing. Organisms can be harbored under burn tissue, and unless measures are taken to control them, they tend to multiply.

There are several methods presently being used to prevent contaminating sources from reaching the client. In some institutions the client is placed on strict isolation; other facilities use reverse isolation, isolation tents, positive air pressure units, and air circulation systems. Such systems push used air out of the room to keep a constant flow of fresh air into the rooms. In still others, only sterile equipment and supplies are used, and no isolation precautions are taken. The use of local antibacterial agents is particularly valuable in the latter. Provisions may also be made for administering antibiotics. Many physicians, however, prefer to treat the infections as they occur.

Cleanliness is essential, regardless of the method used. Proper handwashing is effective in preventing transfer of organisms to and from the client. The hands

---

WOUND AND SKIN PRECAUTIONS

Wound and skin precautions are taken for diseases that are spread either by direct contact with wounds or by indirect contact with articles contaminated with secretions from wounds. These precautions are taken for wound and skin infections caused by staphylococcal and streptococcal organisms, as well as those caused by gram-negative organisms (for example, *Pseudomonas, Escherichia coli, Proteus*). In addition, wounds with copious drainage require specific precautions. Following are precautions for wound and skin infections:

1. Use of a private room.
2. Use of a gown by all individuals coming in direct contact with the wound or skin area.
3. A mask during dressing changes.
4. Gloves by all individuals having direct contact with the wound or skin area.
5. Proper hand-washing techniques. The hands must be washed on entering and leaving the isolation room or area.
6. Double bag. All linens used in the room and all articles contaminated with secretions must be double bagged and labeled properly before being sent for cleaning, disinfection, or sterilization.

---

should be washed thoroughly under running water before and after treatments and after handling contaminated materials. Personnel caring for burned clients should wear gowns, masks, and gloves. When these are worn, they should be used properly and changed as frequently as necessary (see material on p. 842).

A number of topical agents are currently used to facilitate control of infection (Table 15-4). Specifically, these agents delay colonization and reduce the number of organisms. The use of these agents requires that sterile precautions and isolation be observed. A thin layer of the ointment or cream is placed over the burn area with a tongue blade or a sterile glove, or it may be embedded in gauze and placed over the area. When dressings are used, they may be changed daily or more frequently if necessary. When silver nitrate is used, the dressing is kept wet with the solution.

Burn wound sepsis. The burn wound is generally thought to be sterile for the first 24 hours after the burn. After this period, bacteria contaminate the surface and massively invade the burn wound and surrounding tissue.[44] Burn wound sepsis is present when organisms (cultured and measured quantitatively) total more than 100,000 per gram of involved tissue and invade the unburned tissue around and under the wound. There may also be visceral metastasis via the lymphatics, with perivascular and perineural involvement. Burn wound sepsis usually occurs in clients with full-thickness burns.

Staphylococcus and *Streptococcus* organisms are the primary offenders; however, *Proteus aeruginosa* and *Proteus vulgaris* are increasingly becoming major offenders. One of the earliest signs to indicate septic involvement is a gradual increase or sudden decrease in temperature. If the sepsis is caused by gram-negative organisms, leukopenia, hypothermia, and rapid wound deterioration occur. Bleeding tendencies such as petechiae, ecchymosis, and oozing may be manifest. If sepsis is caused by gram-positive organisms, the temperature rises sharply, and there is a marked increase in respiratory and pulse rates. Disorientation may also be a presenting symptom because of both gram-negative and gram-positive organisms. Treatment consists of intravenous fluids, blood transfusions, massive doses of antibiotics, and topical antibacterials.

TABLE 15-4

Commonly used topical agents for burns

Agent	How applied and adverse effects	Nursing responsibilities
Silver nitrate solution	Wet occlusive dressings or soaks; may cause electrolyte disturbances because of hypotonicity of the silver nitrate solution; treatment may be complicated by methemeglobinemia; stains clothing and floors	Frequent assessments usually made of sodium, potassium, chloride, and bicarbonate; abnormal values should be reported to the physician; protect clothing and floor
Mafenide acetate (Sulfamylon cream), a water-soluble cream base	Directly to wound or on mesh gauze strip; useful in *Pseudomonas* infections; may cause respiratory and acid-base disturbances because it is a carbonic anhydrase inhibitor and is absorbed throughout the wound in large amounts	Observe for symptoms of acid-base disturbances and allergic manifestations (rash, hives, and so forth); inform client that stinging sensation may be felt when agent is applied; give pain medication when necessary; give emotional support; emphasize importance of medication
Gentamicin sulfate (Garamycin), ointment or cream	Directly to wound or on mesh gauze; may cause renal and auditory nerve damage	Observe for symptoms that indicate damage to the auditory nerve and kidney
Furazolium chloride (Novofur)	Incorporated in wet occlusive dressing	
Silver sulfadiazine, a water-soluble ointment	Directly to wound by sterile glove and left exposed or a mesh gauze is placed over it; useful in *Pseudomonas* infections	Observe for rashes and signs of sensitivity; thoroughly wash area to remove film on subsequent applications

Nursing process for common health problems

As a preventive aspect, efforts should be directed toward keeping the bacterial count in the client's environment to a minimum. Fortunately the use of antibacterials has helped to decrease the incidence of burn wound sepsis in severely burned clients. The nurse must carefully monitor the client for signs and symptoms indicative of burn wound sepsis. The vital signs, CVP, and urinary output should be assessed. A sudden drop in these require immediate intervention.

Care of the burn wound. Once the initial therapy has been initiated, attention is directed to the care of the wound itself. Before actual therapy is started, care is taken to cleanse the wound and remove the detached epithelium and dirt because they provide an excellent medium for bacterial growth. The area may be washed with distilled water or normal saline and an antibacterial soap. This may be done in the emergency unit, or the client may be taken to the surgical suite. If the latter is the case, therapy is likely to be performed under general anesthesia. Some authorities do not advocate an initial excision. Those who advocate this practice believe that it is impossible to determine the depth of a burn wound in the initial period and that excision at this time may result in removal of normal tissue, resulting in increased blood loss.

LOCAL CARE OF THE BURN WOUND. There are varied techniques for treating burn wounds. Studies have shown that the results of many of these are similar. Common methods of local care are described.

The nurse should be familiar with the following terms that are used in relation to burn care:

debridement Removal of eschar at the interface of the living and dead tissue; only dead tissue is removed.
dermabrasion A means of "planing" down the eschar, thus minimizing the amount of material that can become a source of infection.
eschar Thick, dry, nonviable tissue that forms over second- and third-degree burn areas; it may be brownish or black.
escharotomy Surgical incision through the full depth of the skin to release pressure of eschar on central arteries and veins, resulting in restoration of circulation to the area.
granulation tissue A deep pink, fragile tissue that bleeds easily.

METHODS OF BURN WOUND CARE. The aims of local treatment can be achieved by use of either the open, semiopen, or closed methods. Use of these methods depend on the location and extent of the injury. There are differences in opinion about local treatment, and therefore the nurse must follow the therapeutic plan of individual physicians. Each method has certain advantages. They may be combined for the same client, depending on the extent and body part involved.

In the *open method* (exposure method), an antibacterial agent is applied, and the burned area is left open to the air. As a result, a protective eschar forms, which prevents bacterial invasion, hinders reproduction of bacteria, and enhances healing. It also makes assessment of the area easy. Burns of areas where dressings are hard to apply (face, neck, perineum, trunk, limbs, and back) lend themselves to this type of treatment. Clients who are hospitalized are more likely to be treated with this method than the closed method. The nurse should observe for the presence of eschar formation, swelling, and signs of infection. The area may be washed with an antibacterial solution under sterile conditions, and the eschar removed. Clients who are involved in civilian disaster and those who sustain deep, second-degree burns are usually treated with this method. Healing usually takes place within a couple of weeks. When this method is used, rigid isolation techniques are required. A private room should be provided. The client should be placed on sterile, dry sheets, and the entire burn surface exposed. Sterile linens are generally used until eschar develops, which may take from 24 to 36 hours. During exposure the client must be protected from drafts, and bed clothes must be kept off the body surface. Cradle and bed devices may be useful in keeping the bed clothes off the body surface. The CircOlectric bed or Stryker frame bed may be used to facilitate turning the client and exposing the burn wound.

The semiopen method involves covering the wound with a topical antimicrobial agent.[6] To keep the medication on the wound, a thin layer of dressing may be used. The medication is cleansed at prescribed times, the wound inspected, debrided if necessary, and followed by reapplication of medication.

In the *closed method* (pressure, or occlusive, method), sterile dressings are applied to protect the burn area from contamination, provide joint and limb immobilization, and promote drainage from the wound. Burns of the hands are best treated with this method. It is also useful for clients who do not require hospitalization. After the area has been cleaned and debrided, dressings are placed over the wound in layers. Fine-meshed gauze impregnated with an antibacterial ointment or petrolatum may be placed next to the skin to prevent the dressing from sticking as the exudate dries. Large, bulky dressings (such as abdominal pads or Kerlix) may be placed over the gauze and covered with an elastic bandage. The use of such dressings makes provisions for elevation, support, and compression. The nurse must keep the body part in proper alignment to prevent deformities. The skin surfaces must be separated and the part observed for signs of impaired circulation.

When *dressings* are used, they are generally changed daily or every 2 to 5 days by the physician. If the dressing change is painful, an analgesic should be administered before the procedure is started. The dressings should be changed under aseptic conditions. During the dressing change the wound is closely examined by the physician and debrided as necessary.

Jobst garments are commonly used. These resemble stretch stockings and are worn to hold burn scars flat in an effort to minimize them and make them softer.

Wet soaks are also useful vehicles for the removal of eschar. They keep the eschar soft and are useful when infection is present. Later, *hydrotherapy* may become the major source of debridement for eschar and debris. Hydrotherapy provides a means for softening the crust, which facilitates removal. It is also instrumental in keeping the area clean and promoting wound drainage.

Closure of the burn wound. Later management of the burn wound is accomplished through the use of skin grafts. *Skin grafts* are used to close an open wound and thus minimize the chance of infection, prevent fluid loss, and restore the appearance and function of the affected part. Grafts may be temporary or permanent and are generally classed according to the source of tissue.

If the graft is obtained from living persons or cadavers, it is referred to as *homograft* or *allograft*. These are used as temporary coverings for extensive burns until the client's own skin is available for grafting. Such grafts are performed early in the treatment period (2 to 3 days after the burn) to decrease the

845

loss of water, electrolytes, proteins, and body fluids. Pain is also decreased. Application of homografts also serves to control infection as well as hasten the development of granulation tissue. Rejection may not occur until 2 to 3 weeks after the graft. When a cadaver's skin is used, consent in writing must be obtained from the family of the deceased, and the skin must be removed within 6 hours after death. Amniotic membranes, considered to have bactericidal action, have proved to be beneficial as a means of covering burn wounds.

Heterografts or *xenografts* are coverings of animal skin or synthetic skin. Pigskin is frequently used; Teflon, nylon, and velour are common forms of synthetic grafts. These are also temporary coverings.

Grafts obtained from an identical twin and donated to the other twin are referred to as *isografts*. If the graft is obtained from the uninjured part of the client, it is referred to as an *autograft*. Isografts and autografts are used as permanent coverings.

Autografts may be classed on the basis of thickness. Full-thickness and split-thickness grafts are common. *Full-thickness grafts* are taken at the junction of the dermis and subcutaneous tissue. These grafts are used either over body areas that are subjected to friction or trauma or when good cosmetic results are essential. There are two types of full-thickness grafts, free grafts and pedicle grafts. The *free graft* is devoid of its own blood supply and therefore gets its nourishment from capillary growth from the granulating tissue. With the *pedicle graft* the blood supply from the subcutaneous vessels is preserved in the pedicle portion of the graft.

Split-thickness grafts may be thin, intermediate, or thick. The thin split-thickness graft includes all the epidermis and some of the dermis, whereas thick split-thickness grafts include a deeper portion of the dermis. The donor sites for these will heal spontaneously by regeneration unless they become infected. Among the varieties of split-thickness grafts are the following:

1. *Postage-stamp grafts* are the size of a postage stamp and are used when there is not enough autogenous skin to cover the raw recipient area.

2. *Mesh grafts*, which have been made possible with the development of skin meshes, cover irregular, contoured areas. The skin is stretched as a net. These also permit exudate to escape and increase the coverage of the skin area.

3. *Pinch grafts* are small cones of skin that are lifted and transplanted to the recipient site. The pieces of skin grow together to give a unified appearance once healing takes place. They are generally used on body parts that will be covered by clothing, since these grafts do not result in a smooth appearance.

The skin is removed by an instrument called a dermatome. Any area of the body may be the source of skin for grafts. However, the most frequently used sites are the upper thighs and lower trunk because these parts are covered by clothing, thereby eliminating visibility of the scars.

PREPARATION FOR GRAFTS. For grafting to be successful, the donor tissue must be healthy. Adequate nutrition is important in promoting tissue health. Therefore the client must be encouraged to take adequate proteins, vitamins, and fluids in the period preceding the skin graft. Antibiotics are prescribed to prevent infection. Wet soaks are usually prescribed to facilitate debridement and to reduce edema of the granulation tissue.

Psychological preparation must also be part of the therapeutic plan. Before surgery the nurse will institute some of the same measures that are carried out for other types of surgery. Surgery is usually performed in multiple stages. Generally the physician explains the surgery to the client, but the nurse should be available to answer questions and reinforce explanations. The nurse must be able to identify cues that indicate worry and concern and provide an atmosphere that facilitates expression of these concerns.

Before surgery, the donor area is to be judiciously cleansed with an antibacterial soap to help reduce the bacterial count on the skin. Such preparation may be carried out before the client goes to surgery and repeated after he arrives there.

POSTOPERATIVE NURSING CARE. Donor sites may be treated with the open or closed method. The client's age and the location of donor site usually determine which method will be used. Donor sites are usually closed in the young child and the incontinent adult. If the closed method is used, the client returns from surgery with dressings on both the recipient and donor sites. Dressings are applied onto the recipient site to maintain firm contact between the graft and the wound surface and onto the donor site to control bleeding and prevent infection. Scarlet Red, a bacteriostatic agent, may be used as a covering for donor sites. Heat lamps facilitate healing of tissue and, when used, should be placed 15 inches from the donor site. The Scarlet Red dries and is trimmed daily by the nurse or physician. Donor sites are usually healed within 7 to 10 days. The nurse must be aware of the location of donor and recipient areas. Neither of these should be disturbed without specific instructions from the physician. However, the part should be slightly elevated to avoid passive congestion of the venous blood, thereby reducing swelling. Often a pressure bandage is applied to help achieve these objectives.

During the first couple of days the client may complain of discomfort in the donor site. Usually ice bags are ordered to be applied to the area to provide comfort. The ice application also helps reduce bleeding. The nurse must be attuned to complaints of pain, particularly from the recipient site. Pain in the early postoperative period may indicate formation of a hematoma, whereas, in the later period it is more likely to signify an infection. Any complaint of a throbbing pain and an elevated temperature should be brought to the attention of the physician.

The nurse should be aware of the conditions that interfere with a successful graft. Common causes of failure are motion, trauma, and infection. Nursing intervention should thus be planned to prevent these. Unnecessary movement of the grafted area may cause the graft to become displaced. The part should therefore be immobilized to facilitate growth of the capillaries into the transplant. For children, the application of splints or circular casts will provide some means of immobilization. When grafts are applied to the face, talking should be discouraged. However, the nurse should provide some means of communication for the client, most commonly a pad and pencil. Excessive pressure, as from a tight bandage, may impair circulation and interfere with healing. The formation of a hematoma between the graft and recipient site will block the flow of blood and hinder healing. The nurse should observe for signs that indicate impaired circulation.

Because injury may affect the graft, the client must be encouraged not to lie on the graft and to avoid bumps. The nurse should anticipate the client's needs and assist him with care as often as necessary. To facilitate turning, the client may be placed on a CircOlectric bed, particularly if the graft has been applied to the trunk. Other special turning frames may also be used. It is helpful to plan

847

certain activities, such as deep breathing exercises, around the client's turning schedule. These, along with ambulation, assist in preventing pulmonary and circulatory complications.

Whenever dressings are changed, aseptic technique must be used. If moist dressings are ordered, the solution and all other equipment should be sterile.

With thin grafts, healing of the donor site may take place within 1 to 2 weeks. Thick grafts may take longer.

When the client is discharged, generally instructions are given to keep the site oiled because of absence of apocrine and sebaceous glands. Lanolized lotion is helpful for this purpose because it tends to minimize chafing and itching.

FORMATION OF ESCHAR. Full-thickness circumferential burns of the trunk and extremities usually result in the formation of a tight eschar that constricts and prevents adequate circulation. This results in ischemia in the extremities and an impairment in distal capillary filling. The formation of eschar on the thorax results in incomplete chest expansion.

If the burn area involves the chest, frequent assessment of chest movements must be made. Involvement of the extremities warrants assessing for signs of circulatory impairment. These include absent pulses (for example, radial, ulnar, palmar arch, and digital regions if upper extremities are involved, and pedal pulses if lower extremities are involved), changes in temperature from warmness to coldness, color changes (for example, normal color to pale or bluish discoloration), alteration in sensation (numbness, tingling), and impairment in movement (inability to move the part). The Doppler Flowmeter has greatly helped in the assessment of limb circulation.

When the nurse observes signs of circulatory impairment and notifies the physician, the client is usually taken to the surgical suite for an escharotomy. An escharotomy is the surgical release of pressure with the restoration of circulation to the area. It is accomplished by incising the skin down to the line of the subcutaneous fat in a longitudinal direction on either side. The incision resembles bivalving a cast on an extremity (Fig. 15-23). Since nerve endings are destroyed in full-thickness burns, an anesthetic is not needed. The immediate effect is pressure relief and a resultant restoration of circulation.

GASTROINTESTINAL COMPLICATIONS. Gastrointestinal complications frequently occur in clients with burns involving a large percentage of the body surface. Gastric dilation is a frequent complication. It may occur suddenly in the initial period after the injury and create a picture of hypovolemic shock. Burned clients should be observed closely for shock symptoms and abdominal distension. These symptoms demand the immediate passage of a nasogastric tube. Often nasogastric tubes are passed in the initial burn phase in an effort to prevent this complication. Paralytic ileus is also common in extensive burns.

Curling's ulcers (stress ulcers) usually develop in the stomach and duodenum. They are classically multiple, and the majority occur in the body or fundus of the stomach. They are more likely to occur at the end of the first week after the burn. The pathogenesis is unknown, but it is thought to be related to stress. High levels of circulating adrenal corticoids are found, which result from stimulation of the adrenal cortex by ACTH. An increase in gastric secretions that alters gastric microcirculation has been proposed as a possible cause.[44] Bleeding is the first symptom that indicates development of Curling's ulcer. The client may expectorate or vomit blood. Blood may appear in the nasogastric tube, or blood

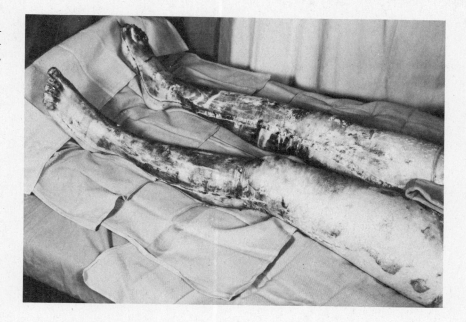

may be noted in the stool (melena). Increased anorexia in association with gastric distention is also thought to be significant. Often antacids are ordered as a preventive measure.

Rehabilitation. The responsibility for rehabilitation of the burned client in some hospitals rests on the physical therapist. In others the responsibility is placed on the nurse under the direction of the physician. In all situations the client should be evaluated in the acute phase, and therapy should be started as soon as he is physically able. The goals to be accomplished center around (1) prevention of contractures, (2) maintenance of joint motion, and (3) maintenance of muscle tone. These measures can be accomplished through proper positioning and active, passive, and assistive exercises.

Sometimes because of the extent of a burn, a significant deformity or disability may result. In these cases vocational counseling and retraining may be necessary. The nurse must be aware of the community resources to which the client can be referred, and he should be encouraged to resume his place in his family group and in the community.

First-aid intervention for thermal burns. The primary objective in first-aid intervention is to stop the burning process. For example, when clothing catches fire, the first thing to do is to smother the flames. This may be accomplished by having the client lie in a horizontal position. Lying in this position permits flames to burn up and away from the exposed parts of the body, such as the hands and face. Running should definitely be discouraged because it only serves to fan the flames and causes the clothing to burn faster. Standing should also be discouraged because of the greater chance of the flames' being inhaled. After the client assumes a horizontal position, a rug, coat, blanket, towel, sheet, or similar material should be thrown over him to shut off the oxygen supply to the flame. Water may also be thrown over the client to extinguish the flames, or the client may be rolled onto the ground or floor to smother the flame.

Once the flames are controlled—and before transporting the client to the hospital—the clothing should be pulled off, provided it is not stuck to the skin.

Nursing process for common health problems

In addition to clothing, metal objects (rings) and synthetic materials (wigs) should also be removed. Removal is important because cellular destruction occurs as long as cells of the body remain superheated. In an effort to end the burning process, the injured area should be immersed in cool water. In addition to destroying the heat, immersion also eliminates pain. The body should be covered with a clean sheet to prevent contamination of the burned area. This measure also prevents air from coming in contact with the burn injury and thereby reduces pain. Towels that have been soaked in cool water are useful. There once was a practice to use ice water. This practice is discouraged because of its detrimental effect. Excessive cold is thought to interfere with capillary perfusion and the viability of the injured area, and further increases the depth of the burn area. Application of cold to a large body surface area may also result in prolonged hypothermia and cardiac dysrhythmias from rapid lowering of body temperature.[32]

Instructions should be given about the use of home remedies such as ointment or baking soda. These applications should not be used. If the burn is extensive and if it involves the face and neck, oral fluids are contraindicated because of the danger of vomiting. Signs of respiratory involvement should be observed for during the initial period, especially if the burn involves the face or neck. The airway must be kept patent, and any secretions from the mouth must be removed. Constricting clothing should be removed from the neck and chest to facilitate breathing. Artificial respiration should be administered if necessary. The client should be transported to the hospital as quickly as possible after initial first aid is given. He should be kept warm but should not be overheated. Generally one blanket provides sufficient warmth.

When a *scald burn* occurs, the clothing should be removed from the body as quickly as possible, since clothing holds heat. If the burn is caused by grease, pour cold water over the victim to remove the grease and stop the burning process (do not use for other burns, because it may produce shock). The client should be comforted, because he is likely to be frightened. Otherwise the same general measures should be carried out to alleviate pain and protect the injury from contamination.

 Evaluation. Evaluation of the nursing plan for the client with a thermal injury is an ongoing component of the nursing process as the client is rehabilitated, depending on the extent of the injury.

EXPECTED OUTCOMES

The client and/or family can:
1. Describe burns.
2. Demonstrate plans for prevention.
3. Demonstrate plan for implementing therapeutic care.
4. Describe plans for pain management.
5. Describe plans for maintaining mobility (exercises) and self-care activities.
6. State limitations of activity.
7. Demonstrate sensitivity to changes in body image.
8. Describe plans for health maintenance, including diet, skin, care, and activity.
9. Describe plans for follow-up care and use of community resources.
10. State plans for following the therapeutic regimen.

Chemical burns. Acids and alkalis are frequently responsible for causing tissue injury. Injury from chemicals may range from slight irritation to extensive localized tissue destruction. According to Fitzgerald, such damage is the result of chemical coagulation of protein, precipitation of chemical compounds in the cells, severe cellular dehydration, protoplasmic poisoning, or complete dissociation of proteins.[30]

Alkaline substances tend to produce more difficulty because they are not neutralized by tissue fluids. Alkaline substances tend to bind to tissues, produce protein hydrolysis with liquefaction, and destroy tissue.[30]

Individuals who sustain chemical burns may, if they are extensive, lose large amounts of electrolytes. Inhalation injuries are not uncommon in some chemical burns (for example, chlorine). Such injuries occur because some chemicals, when heated, have a tendency to produce noxious substances.[28]

Planning and implementation. Burns that result from chemicals should be washed *immediately* with copious amounts of tap water to stop the burning action of the agent. Garments should not be removed until they have been soaked with water and there is some assurance that the chemical has been removed. It is best to use flowing water from a faucet or hose. If these are not available water should be poured over the area. Clothing should then be removed, because chemicals may remain on the clothing and come in contact with the skin and continue the burning process. The client should also be encouraged to take a shower. After some assurance is given that the chemical has been fully removed, the client should be transferred to a hospital for evaluation and treatment. Because fluid and electrolytes are lost in large chemical burns, fluid therapy similar to that used in thermal agent burns may be prescribed.

Electrical burns. When electrical energy is conducted through the body, it may have no effect, or it may cause injury or death. The extent of tissue involvement, which may result from exposure to electrical current, may vary from superficial burns to extensive deep injuries. Factors responsible for the degree of tissue injury include the intensity of the current, resistance of tissue, and duration of exposure. For example, the superficial damage that may occur when a low-intensity current comes in contact with moist skin may be nil.

Superficial burns that result from electrical energy may resemble the different degrees of thermal burns. One distinguishing characteristic is that the involved areas (entry point and exit point) are small. After the source of electricity has been removed, therapeutic intervention follows the same patterns as that for thermal burns.

The dreaded consequences of electrical currents are ventricular fibrillation, shock, severe metabolic acidosis (because of rapid loss of body fluid into the damaged tissue), and the release of myoglobin from muscles, which can threaten renal failure. Respiratory arrest may result from interrupting the function of the medullary center.

Planning and implementation. When an electrical burn is sustained, the client should be removed from the source of electric current as quickly as possible. Before an attempt is made to remove the victim, the current must be turned off. A nonconducting material (such as a dry stick) may be used to rescue the victim. The rescuer should stand on nonconducting material or wear rubber boots during the rescuing procedure. The importance of the rescuer's not coming in contact with the victim exposed to electrical charges is extremely important because such contact will cause the same amount of current to be conducted through the rescuer's body.

Nursing process for common health problems

Preventing electrical injuries. Every possible attempt should be made to prevent electrical burns. To prevent some of these injuries, especially in children, electrical cords should be kept off the floor, and outlets should be properly guarded. Special knobs that cannot be operated by the toddler are available for stoves and should be purchased.

Sunburn. Sunbathing often results in sunburn. Reactions to sun vary from person to person. Usually exposure in the sun for an hour may produce a sunburn; however, the condition of the person's skin and the wavelength of the sun are variables that closely relate to how fast a sunburn is likely to occur. For example, the skin of the infant and young child will burn more quickly than that of an older child or adult. Hence a sunburn is more serious in infants than in older children and adults. On exposure, the reaction may appear suddenly, or it may not occur until a day after exposure. The former reaction is characterized by redness, burning, and heat or by bleb formation.

The degree of involvement also characterizes the reaction. An uncomfortable dry feeling in the skin that disappears in approximately 24 hours characterizes a mild sunburn. Severe sunburn causes more discomfort, which is aggravated by the slightest movement. The skin becomes parched and reddened. The redness occurs as a result of dilation of the tiny blood vessels in the dermis. Severe sunburn may be accompanied by systemic symptoms (such as nausea, chills, fever, and tachycardia), which may last for a couple of days. Blisters may form over the exposed part.

 Planning and implementation. When a sunburn occurs, mineral and vegetable oils and topical anesthetics are forms of therapy that may be prescribed.

Preventing sunburns. Individuals who sunbathe should be encouraged to increase exposure to the sun gradually and to use sunscreen agents when sunbathing (for example, paraaminobenzoic acid). These agents primarily block carcinogens.

Since the infant's skin, because of its immaturity, cannot tolerate as much heat as older individuals, parents should be cautioned against exposing them to strong sunlight. Instructions should also be related to giving consideration to the time of day one sunbathes. Sunbathing should be done at a time other than the 2-hour period around noon. As much as two thirds of the ultraviolet light comes through during this time.[2] Large hats should be worn while out in the sun.

Evaluation

Evaluation is the final component of the nursing process. This process enables the nurse to evaluate plans for health promotion, maintenance, and restoration on an ongoing basis. Problems of the integumentary system frequently include impairment in skin integrity, alterations in comfort, impaired physical mobility, fear, grieving, disturbance in self-concept, ineffective coping, fluid volume deficit, potential for injury, and alterations in nutrition.

EXPECTED OUTCOMES

The client and/or family can:
1. Explain the specific integumentary problem.
2. State plans for implementing health promotion strategies.
3. Describe the prescribed therapies, including the purpose, route, dosage, frequency, duration, and side effects.

4. Describe the specific precautions to take in application of each prescribed therapy, including baths, compresses, and so on.
5. Safely implement the prescribed therapy.
6. State plans for health maintenance, including the management of self-care activities during periods of exacerbation.
7. Demonstrate satisfactory adjustments of life-style imposed by the problem.
8. State plans for health care, plans for follow-up care, and use of appropriate resources.

The nurse and client may determine when the problem has resolved as well as determine the appropriate time to terminate the nurse-client relationship. In other instances when the problem is not resolved, the nurse can facilitate continuity of care by referring the client to the appropriate agency. This is crucial to the attainment of an optimal level of wellness.

Summary

Caring for clients with problems of the integument can be a challenge. Basic to the care of these clients is a complete nursing history that encompasses a health, development, social, and psychological history. The information obtained from this history along with physical assessments (for example, obtained from inspection and palpation) and diagnostic tests (biopsies, sensitivity tests, allergy tests, and direct examinations) are analyzed and used in formulating individualized care plans.

Nursing care is planned to promote health as well as maintain and restore the integrity of the integument. Health teaching and instruction about skin care (cleansing, effect of environmental temperature, clothing, and diet) and the need for immunizations are significant to health promotion. As with assessment, considerations should be given to the client's age, sex, life-style, and education as health promotion strategies are planned.

Common health problems of the neonatal period are hemangiomas, pigmented nevi, and mongolian spots; whereas during childhood, rashes, infections, and inflammatory problems are common. Principles of medical and surgical asepsis are essential to the management of many of the problems occurring in this age group. From adolescence through the young adult years, inflammations, infections, and cold injuries are common, specifically, acne, furuncles, carbuncles, furunculosis, psoriasis, and lupus erythematosus. Accident hypothermia and skin cancer are common during the older adult years. Problems that occur throughout varied periods of development include allergies and thermal burns. Many of the integumentary problems are chronic. As a result, supportive care and ongoing instructions and care are integral to the care of clients with problems of the integument.

References

1. Anyan, Walter R.: Dermatologic conditions appearing in the adult patient. In Anyan, Walter, R.: Adolescent Medicine in primary care, New York, 1978, John Wiley & Sons.
2. Artz, Curtis P.: Changing concepts of electrical injury, Am. J. Surg. **128:**600-602, November 1974.
3. Behrman, Howard T., and others: Common skin diseases, diagnosis and treatment, ed. 3, New York, 1978, Grune & Stratton.

Nursing process for common health problems

4. Bluefarb, Samuel M.: Scope monogram on dermatology, Kalamazoo, Mich., 1974, Upjohn Laboratories.
5. Bowman, Warren, and Bunce, Gary: Injuries in the winter environment, Emerg. Product News, October 1975, pp. 478-479, 540.
6. Busby, Helen C.: Nursing management of the acute burn patient and nursing management of optimal burn recovery, J. Contin. Educ. Nurs. **10**:16-30, August 1979.
7. Close, Larry Garth, and Goepfert, Helmuth: Recognizing skin cancer of the head and neck, Geriatrics **34**:39-49, November 1979.
8. Committee on Drugs, American Academy of Pediatrics: Anaphylaxis, Pediatrics **51**:136-139, January 1973.
9. Committee on Trauma, American College of Surgeons: Burns. In The management of fractures and soft tissues injuries, Philadelphia, 1976, W.B. Saunders Co.
10. Curreri, William P.: Burns. In Schwartz, Seymour I., and others, editors: Principles of surgery, ed. 5, New York, 1979, McGraw-Hill Book Co.
11. Curreri, William P., and Luterman, Arnold: Nutritional support of the burned patient, Surg. Clin. North Am. **58**:1151-1156, December 1978.
12. Dunsky, Eliot: Common allergic disorders. In Kaye, Robert, and others, editors: Core textbook of pediatrics, Philadelphia, 1978, J.B. Lippincott Co.
13. Easton, James G.: Anaphylaxis. In Bierman, Warren G., and Pearlman, David S., editors: Allergic diseases of infancy, childhood and adolescence, Philadelphia, 1980, W.B. Saunders Co.
14. Esterly, Nancy B., and Furey, Nancy L.: Acne: current concepts, Pediatrics **62**:1044-1055, December 1978.
15. Fitzgerald, Robert T.: Prehospital care of burned patients, Crit. Care Q. **1**:13-24, December 1978.
16. Fitzpatrick, Thomas B.: Malignant melanoma of the skin. In Harrison's principles of internal medicine, ed. 9, New York, 1980, McGraw-Hill Book Co.
17. Fitzpatrick, Thomas B., and Haynes, Harley A.: Interpretation of alterations in the skin. In Harrison's principles of internal medicine, ed. 9, New York, 1980, McGraw-Hill Book Co.
18. Fitzpatrick, Thomas B., and Haynes, Harley A.: Skin lesions of general medical significance. In Harrison's principles of internal medicine, ed. 9, New York, 1980, McGraw-Hill Book Co.
19. Fitzpatrick, T.B., and Haynes, H.A.: Harrison's principles of internal medicine, ed. 9, New York, 1980, McGraw-Hill Book Co.
20. Freedman, S.O.: Anaphylaxis and serum sickness. In Freedman, S.O., and Goldy, P., editors: Clinical immunology, ed. 2, Hagerstown, Md., 1976, Harper and Row, Publishers.
21. Goldsmith, Harry S.: Melanoma: an overview, Ca—Cancer J. Clin. **29**:194-215, July-August 1979.
22. Harmon, Vera M., and Steele, Shirley M.: Nursing care of the skin: a developmental approach, New York, 1975, Appleton-Century-Crofts.
23. Haynes, Harley A.: Primary cancer of the skin. In Harrison's principles of internal medicine, ed. 9, New York, 1980, McGraw-Hill Book Co.
24. Haynes, Harley A.: The front line on skin cancers, Emerg. Med. **10**:131-135, October 1978.
25. Haynes, Harley A., and Fitzpatrick, Thomas B.: Cutaneous manifestation of internal malignancy. In Harrison's principles of internal medicine, ed. 9, New York, 1980, McGraw-Hill Book Co.
26. Heagerty, Margaret C., and others: Child health: basis for primary care, New York, 1980, Appleton-Century-Crofts.
27. Hecht, M.: Psychiatric aspects of dermatology. In Bellak, L., editor: Psychology of physical illness, New York, 1953, Grune & Stratton.
28. Jessen, R. Thomas, and Merwin, Charles F.: Identifying and treating skin malignancies, Geriatrics **34**:71-78, June 1979.
29. Kaye, Robert, and others, editors: Core textbook of pediatrics, Philadelphia, 1978, J.B. Lippincott Co.
30. Kempe, C.H., and others: Current pediatrics: diagnosis and treatment, ed. 4, Los Altos, Calif., 1976, Lange Medical Publications.
31. Langer, Robert, and Binnick, Steven: Treatment of acne vulgaris, Am. Fam. Phys. **20**:117-118, August 1979.
32. Lee, June M.: Emotional reactions to trauma, Nurs. Clin. North Am. **5**(4):577-587, December 1979.
33. Lukas, Daniel S., and Barr, David P.: Cyanosis. In Mitchell, Cyril Mitchell, editor: Signs and symptoms, ed. 4, Philadelphia, 1964, J.B. Lippincott Co.
34. Mannik, Mart, and Gilliland, Bruce C.: Systemic lupus erythematosus. In Harrison's principles of internal medicine, ed. 9, New York, 1980, McGraw-Hill Book Co.
35. Marks, Ronald: Common facial dermatoses, Bristol, England, 1976, John Wright & Sons.

36. McGurie, Andres: Prevention of burns, Crit. Care Q. **1:**1-10, December 1978.
37. Mitchell, Ann Chappell: Black skin: an historical, psychological and health care perspective, J. Contin. Educ. Nurs. **10:**28-33, 1979.
38. Moffet, Hugh L.: Principles of immunization. In Kaye, Robert, and others, editors: Core textbook of pediatrics, Philadelphia, 1978, J.B. Lippincott Co.
39. Parker, Frank: Contact dermatitis. In Bierman, Warren G., and Pearlman, David S., editors: Allergic diseases in infancy, childhood and adolescence, Philadelphia, 1980, W.B. Saunders Co.
40. Parrish, John A.: Dermatology and skin care, 1975, McGraw-Hill Book Co.
41. Petersdorf, Robert G.: Disturbances of heat regulation. In Harrison's principles of internal medicine, ed. 9, New York, 1980, McGraw-Hill Book Co.
42. Rachelefsky, Gary S., and Jacobs, Alvin H.: Atopic dermatitis. In Bierman, Warren G., and Pearlman, David S., editors: Allergic disease of infancy, childhood and adolescence, Philadelphia, 1980, W.B. Saunders Co.
43. Roach, Lora B.: Assessment: color changes in dark skin, Nursing 77 **49:**19-22, January 1977.
44. Robbins, Stanley L.: Pathology, ed. 4, Philadelphia, 1979, W.B. Saunders Co.
45. Rogers, David E., and Turck, Marvin: Staphylococcal infections. In Harrison's principles of internal medicine, ed. 9, New York, 1980, McGraw-Hill Book Co.
46. Saned, Gordon C.: Manual of skin diseases, ed. 4, Philadelphia, 1980, J.B. Lippincott Co.
47. Schiff, Leon: Jaundice. In Mitchell, Cyril, editor: Signs and symptoms, Philadelphia, 1964, J.B. Lippincott Co.
48. Schwartz, Seymour I., and others: Principles of surgery, ed. 3, New York, 1979, McGraw-Hill Book Co.
49. Shapiro, Gail G.: Urticaria and angioedema. In Bierman, C. Warren, and Pearlman, David S.: Allergic diseases of infancy, childhood, and adolescence, Philadelphia, 1980, W.B. Saunders Co.
50. Speer, Frederic, and Dockhorn, Robert J.: Allergy and immunology in children, Springfield, Ill., 1973, Charles C Thomas, Publisher.
51. Stewart, William D., and others: Dermatology: diagnosis and treatment of cutaneous disorders, St. Louis, 1978, The C.V. Mosby Co.
52. The report of the Committee on Infectious Disease, Evanston, Ill., 1977, American Academy of Pediatrics.
53. Vaughan, James, and others: Textbook of pediatrics, ed. 10, Philadelphia, 1975, W.B. Saunders Co.
54. Verbov, Julian: Skin diseases in the elderly, Philadelphia, 1974, J.B. Lippincott Co.
55. Vorhees, J.J., and Marcelo, C.: Molecular mechanisms and cyclic nucleotide cascade in psoriasis. In Farber, E.M., and Cox, A.J., editors: Psoriasis proceedings of the second international symposium, New York, 1977, York Medical Books.
56. Weinstein, G.D., and Frost, P.: Abnormal cell proliferation in psoriasis, J. Invest. Dermatol. **50:**254, 1968.
57. Yarbrough, Dabney, R., and Artz, Curtis P.: Managing the critically burned patient, Geriatrics **28:**81-85, December 1973.

Additional readings

Allyn, Patricia: Inhalation inquiries, Crit. Care Q. **1:**37-42, December 1978.

Blair, C., and Lewis, C.A.: The pigment of comedones. Br. J. Dermatol. **82:**522, 1970.

Burgoon, Carroll F., Jr., and Burgoon, Jane S.: Aging and the cutaneous system, Geriatrics **13:**391-401, June 1958.

Cahn, Milton M.: The skin from infancy to old age, Am. J. Nurs. **60:**993-995, July 1960.

Carney, Robert G.: The aging skin, Am. J. Nurs. **63:**110-112, June 1963.

Caudle, P.R. Kain, and Potter J.: Characteristics of burned children, Br. J. Plastic Surg. **23:**63-64, January 1970.

Committee on Trauma, American College of Surgeons: Early care of the injured patient: initial care of thermal burns, chemicals and electrical injury and cold injuries, Philadelphia, 1976, W.B. Saunders Co.

Forbes, Maureen: Communicable diseases and some infections of the skin, Issues Comprehensive Pediatr. Nurs. **1:**1-26, July-August 1977.

Freis, Peter C.: Nursing skills in the outpatient management of childhood inhalant allergy, Issues Comprehensive Pediatr. Nurs. **3:**24-34, August 1978.

Frye, Susan, and Lander, Julie: The initial management of the acutely burned child, Issues Comprehensive Pediatr. Nurs. **1:**39-59, July-August 1977.

Nursing process for common health problems

Fulginiti, Vincent A.: Immunization. In Bierman, Warren G., and Pearlman, David S., editors: Allergic disease of infancy, childhood and adolescence, Philadelphia, 1980, W.B. Saunders Co.

Genovesi, Michael G., and others: Transient hypoxemia in firemen following inhalation of smoke, Chest **71:**441-444, April 4, 1977.

Gleich, Gerald J., and Yunginger, John W.: The radioallergosorbent test: its present place and likely future in the practice of allergy, Advanced Asthma Allergy **2:**1-9, April 1975.

Grosch, Elizabeth, and Lambert, H.E.: The treatment of difficult cutaneous basal and squamous cell carcinomas with electrons, Br. J. Radiol. **52:**472-477, June 1979.

Haburchak, David R., and Pruitt, Basil A.: Use of systemic antibiotics in the burned patient, Surg. Clin. North Am. **58:**1119-1132, December 1978.

Hersperger, Joan E., and Dahl, Lynnette M.: Electrical and chemical injuries, Crit. Care Q. **1:**43-49, December 1978.

Holter, Robert F., and Burgoon, Carroll F. Jr.: Psychological consideration sof the skin in childhood, Pediatr. Clin. North Am. **8**(3):719-736, August 1961.

Howard, William A.: Allergy in infancy and childhood, Pediatr. Ann. **8:**474-478, August 1979.

Hurwitz, Sidney: Signals from the skin, Emerg. Med. **11:**91-115, July 15, 1979.

Jarratt, Michael: Viral infection of the skin, Pediatr. Clin. North Am. **25:**339-355, May 1978.

Kaplan, David, and Sadovsky, Richard: Diagnosis and management of systemic lupus erythematosus, Am. Fam. Phys. **17:**133-138, January 1978.

Kjaer, George C.: Psychiatric aspects of thermal burns, Northwest Med. **68:**537-541, June 1969.

Marvin, Janet: Acute care of the burn patient, Crit. Care Q. **1:**25-35, December 1978.

Murphy, Wilma L.: Skin coverage for burn injury, Assoc. Oper. Rm. Nurs. J. **20:**794-801, November 1974.

Ninam, Carolyn, and Shoemaker, Priscilla: Human amniotic membranes for burns, Am. J. Nurs. **75:**1468-1469, September 1975.

Paxton, P., and others: Nursing assessment and intervention: providing safe nursing care for ethnic people of color, New York, 1976, Appleton-Century-Crofts.

Rasmussen, James E.: A new look at old acne, Pediatr. Clin. North Am. **25:**285-303, May 1978.

Rubin, Anne: Black skin: here's how to adjust your assessment and care, RN **42**(3):31-35, March 1979.

Shoemaker, W.C., and others: Burn pathophysiology in man. I. Sequential hemodynamic alterations, J. Surg. Res. **14:**64-73, January 1973.

Soroff, H.S., and others: The relationship between plasma sodium and the state of hydration in the burned patient, Surg. Gynecol. Obstet. **102:**472-482, 1956.

Thompson, June M., and Bowers, Arden C.: Clinical manual of health assessment, St. Louis, 1980, The C.V. Mosby Co.

Treating cold exposure injury, Emerg. Product News, November-December 1974, pp. 30-32.

Trunkey, Donald D.: Inhalation injury, Surg. Clin. North Am. **58:**1133-1140, December 1978.

Trunkey, Donald, and Parks, Steve: Burns in children, Current Problems Pediatr. **6:**3-51, January 1976.

Wagner, Mary M.: Emergency care of the burned patient, Am. J. Nurs. **77:**1788-1791, November 1977.

Williams, Barbara P.: The problems and life-style of severely burned man. In Bergersen, Betty S., and others, editors: Current concepts in clinical nursing, vol. 2, St. Louis, 1969, The C.V. Mosby Co.

Zurier, Robert B.: Systemic lupus erythematosus, Hosp. Pract. **14:**45-54, August 1979.

NURSING PROCESS

for clients with common health problems of

16 Fluid and electrolyte balance

Assessment

Data analysis

Planning

Implementation

Evaluation

Growth, development, and life maintenance depend on a dynamic pattern of fluid and electrolyte balance. The purpose of this chapter is to discuss common fluid and electrolyte problems, such as fluid deficit and excess; extracellular fluid volume deficit and excess; changes in fluid distribution; and major electrolyte imbalances of potassium, sodium, calcium, and magnesium. The nurse assesses the client's fluid and electrolyte status, analyzes data to compare with age-appropriate norms, and makes nursing diagnoses of actual or potential fluid volume deficits or excesses, alterations in nutritional status, or urinary or bowel elimination patterns resulting from electrolyte imbalance. Plans, developed to restore fluid and electrolyte balance, are implemented according to the client's unique needs for age and body size and evaluated according to established criteria for expected client outcomes.

Overview of fluids and electrolytes

The cell is bathed in an environment of blood and tissue fluid, which hold the potential for cellular survival by providing a dynamic source of oxygen, nutrients, and water. Because of their capacity for storage, cells are able to survive for brief periods of time without taking up chemicals and nutrients from the blood, but oxygen must be constantly available.

Nursing process for common health problems

The nurse must understand fluids and electrolytes and their relationship to cellular life in order to assess and manage client problems. Knowledge of factors of fluid location and movement are essential to this understanding.

BODY WATER COMPARTMENTS

The body consists of lean tissue, fat, and water. The lean portions are primarily muscle mass and contain about 75% water. Fatty tissue is essentially anhydrous (without water). The total body water (TBW) of an adult varies with gender, age, and the relative amounts of muscle and fat mass. Up to 80% of newborns' weight is water. Young, muscular men tend to have a higher proportion of water weight (up to 60%); women, obese individuals, and older adults have a smaller proportion of their weight representing water (about 50%).

The total body water content is divided into two major compartments: intracellular and extracellular.

Intracellular fluid

Intracellular fluid (inside the cell wall) is found in cells of muscles, organs, glands, bone marrow, and red blood. It is relatively stable in its behavior and makes up about 37% of the weight of an adult and 40% of a child. Intracellular fluid is an abundant source of protein. Its major cation is potassium, and its anion, phosphate.

Extracellular fluid

Extracellular fluid includes the water within the interstitial spaces, the intravascular fluid (plasma), and transcellular fluid (pleural, peritoneal, intraocular, joint and cerebrospinal fluid). Composition of body weight representing extracellular fluid is also variable, depending on gender, age, and body proportion of fat and lean mass (Fig. 16-1). The major cation is sodium, and the major anion, chloride.

FIG. 16-1
Comparative fluid composition of an infant and adult according to body weights.

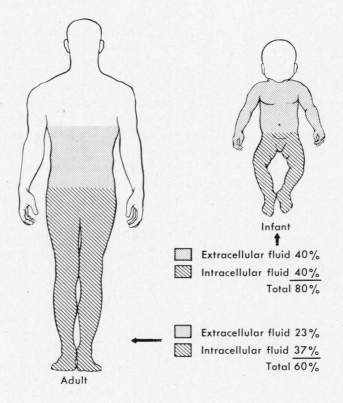

Infant
- ▨ Extracellular fluid 40%
- ▧ Intracellular fluid 40%
- Total 80%

- ▨ Extracellular fluid 23%
- ▧ Intracellular fluid 37%
- Total 60%

Adult

Interstitial fluid. Interstitial fluid is between tissue cells, but not within the vascular bed. Although it represents a relatively small percentage of the TBW, it is dynamic and the first line of defense when the body is confronted with increased or decreased demands for fluid. Because water imbalances are initially adjusted by shifts involving the interstitial fluid, individuals who have greater proportions of their TBW in this compartment are most prone to problems created by sudden or prolonged physiological demands. For example, an infant (with water intake needs three times greater than those of an average adult) who experiences loss of body fluids or a major reduction in intake will have a drastic change in overall fluid status as compared with a healthy adult with a lesser proportion of body weight composed of interstitial fluid. Reasons for this include factors of metabolic rate and renal function, as well as the TBW percentage of this unstable fluid. Adults have a low metabolic rate, mature kidneys that selectively conserve fluids and electrolytes, and a low percentage of interstitial fluid. Infants and young children have a high metabolic rate (three times greater than the adult) with rapid fluid turnover, immature kidneys that excrete a high volume of dilute urine because of their inability to concentrate and selectively resorb fluid, and a high percentage of interstitial fluid in their body.

Intravascular and transcellular fluid. The total blood volume, or intravascular fluid, represents about 8% of an adult's body weight. Plasma comprises more than half of this quantity.

The transcellular fluid is formed by cellular activity. Glandular secretions, mucous membrane secretions, and contents of certain body cavities make up its ultimate volume, which is approximately 1 liter for the average adult. The quantity in the intestinal tract will normally rise (up to 2 to 3 liters) after eating, however, and remain high for an hour or so.

MAINTENANCE OF WATER COMPARTMENTS

Forces that maintain the TBW within the various compartments are also responsible for the dynamic fluid adjustments. In order to understand various fluid and electrolyte imbalances, it is essential to review these factors that control TBW shifts or fluid losses from the compartments.

Hydrostatic and osmotic forces

Plasma volume is maintained by a balance between the net hydrostatic filtration pressure and the colloidal osmotic pressure exerted by the plasma proteins. At the arterial end of the capillary there is a high hydrostatic pressure, which is a product of the cardiovascular mechanisms (pumping force of the heart, blood volume, and peripheral resistance). This hydrostatic pressure *pushes* water and other substances out of the blood stream into the cellular beds. At the venous end of the microcirculatory unit, the blood is more concentrated with colloids and thus exerts an osmotic pressure that *pulls* water and the waste products of the cell back into the bloodstream for venous return. Any factor that interferes with this process (such as low blood volume, cardiovascular failure, or protein deficit) will affect this interrelated mechanism and result in fluid imbalances. For example, if the hydrostatic pressure falls and filtration fails, fluid moves into the capillary and dilutes the colloids in an attempt to regain a satisfactory hydrostatic-osmotic gradient.

Neurohormonal factors

Several hormones influence body fluid balance. Among these are the antidiuretic hormone (ADH), the mineralocorticoids (aldosterone, desoxycortiocosteroids), and glucocorticoids. These hormones help conserve water and sodium and enhance potassium excretion. Working with the chemical mediators (such as the catecholamines), which are released into the bloodstream by the nervous system, they also alter energy transformation by inhibiting insulin release and stimulating glucagon release (see Chapter 9). Volume receptors in the left atrium and great veins respond to overdistension by increasing urine output and to volume depletion by inciting the release of ADH. Baroreceptors react to low arterial (hydrostatic) pressure by constricting the afferent artery in the kidneys, thus conserving fluid by limiting urine output.

Other factors

The kidneys, lungs, and skin also interact in response to changing fluid demands. Because they serve as organs of excretion, they control fluid loss and help in the regulation of acid-base balance. The rate of electrolytes in fluid compartment maintenance is considered in detail because electrolytes exert considerable influence over homeodynamic mechanisms.

ELECTROLYTES

Electrolytes are dissolved chemical substances that possess electrical potential. Positive electrolytes (cations) are sodium, potassium, calcium, and magnesium. Negative electrolytes (anions) are chloride, bicarbonate, phosphate, sulfate, organic acids, and protein.

The concentration of electrolytes within body water compartments influences fluid balance and cellular functioning. The concentration of dissolved particles per liter of solution determines the osmolarity (osmotic pressure). *Osmolarity* is expressed in terms of concentration of solute per unit of a *total volume*. *Osmolality* is a similar term, but identifies the concentration of the solute *per given unit* of solvent.

The normal osmolarity of body fluids is 275 to 295 mOsm/L of water because of the dynamics of water compartments. The designation milliosmol (mOsm) ($1/1000$ of an osmol) is derived from calculating osmotic pressure exerted by a mole of an un-ionized substance. (A mole is the quantity of a substance equal to its molecular weight in grams.)

Electrolytes are usually expressed in milliequivalents (mEq, $1/1000$ of an equivalent) per liter. An equivalent is the gram molecular weight of a substance divided by its valence or number of charges per molecule. It represents the quantity (weight) of a substance that would chemically replace or react with 1 g of hydrogen.

The dominant ion within a fluid compartment is the primary determinant of the osmolarity for that compartment. Potassium and sodium are the dominant ions for intracellular and extracellular spaces, respectively.

The regulation of osmolarity is controlled largely by intake and output of water and salt. Small discrepancies in the balance of these substances within spaces may be responsible for stimulating the neurohormonal responses described earlier.

Assessment

NURSING HISTORY

Assessment of the client's fluid and electrolyte status is often determined during the nursing history. A balanced state of fluids and electrolytes is influenced by the intake of water, body requirements, and efficacy of regulatory systems, especially the kidneys. Each individual has a unique demand for daily replacements that is determined by age and body surface area, metabolic rate, activity, environmental temperature and humidity, physiological losses, and the integrity of intrinsic regulatory mechanisms. Because all body secretions and excretions contain both water and electrolytes, reciprocal effects are created among the various compartments in any adjustment process. These can be assessed by gathering and interpreting the following data.

Age and body surface area

Infants and children have proportions of body water, fat, and surface area that differ appreciably from adults. The TBW in infants, for example is about 750 ml/kg of body weight as compared with 550 ml/kg for an average adult. Although it would seem that an infant would be protected by a high reserve of water, the contrary is true because much of it is in the unstable extracellular spaces and subject to a high turnover.

The infant and young child also have a relatively greater surface area and experience twice the insensible losses per 1 kg of body weight when contrasted with an adult. Metabolic rate is also high and thus results in an increased water expenditure.

Calculation of body surface area. The nurses must be familiar with modes of calculating body surface area (BSA), because such data are essential for determining drug dosages and fluid requirements. Fig. 16-2 demonstrates one method of determining body surface area when the height and weight are known. Because the ratio of BSA to weight varies inversely to length, a short, small infant has relatively more BSA than an adult. When the BSA is known (usually ex-

FIG. 16-2
Nomogram for estimation of body surface. (From Shirkey, H.C.: Drug therapy. In Vaughan, V.C. III, and McKay, R.J., editors: Nelson's textbook of pediatrics, ed. 10, Philadelphia, 1975, W.B. Saunders Co.)

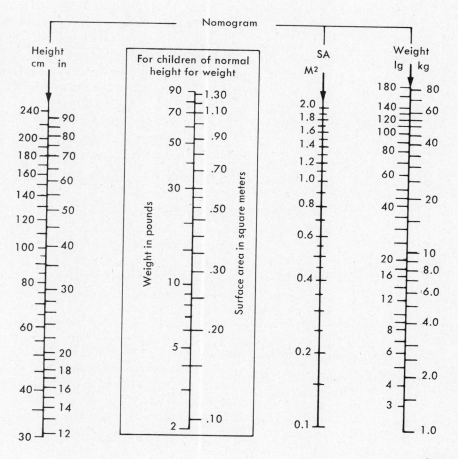

pressed in meters squared $[m^2]$), it can be used in a formula to calculate a pediatric dosage.

$$\frac{\text{BSA of child}}{\text{BSA of adult}} \times \text{Adult dose} = \text{Estimated child dose}$$

or

$$\text{BSA of child } (m^2) \times \text{Dose}/m^2 = \text{Child dose}$$

Activity and environmental influences

The insensible water losses of the body (water lost through evaporation from the skin or through the lungs) is greatly increased in the presence of excessive heat and low humidity. On a daily basis, adults lose up to 15 ml/kg of water through their skin and lungs. Fever and rapid respirations accelerate such losses.

Urine output

Urine output reflects blood volume and pressure as well as other factors of perfusion, and is ordinarily 0.5 to 1.0 ml/kg/hour. A 70-kg man would be expected to produce at least 1000 to 1500 ml of urine per day. Women and the elderly often have only a 500 to 800 ml daily output. Small children have renal losses per kilogram of body weight that are essentially twice the adult rate. In order to eliminate waste products of metabolism, it is estimated that approximately 500 ml of urine must be produced daily in the average adult. If the individual has renal insufficiency or an overwhelming infection, this obligatory output is considerably increased, perhaps up to 2000 ml of urine, in order to prevent renal failure. Quantities of sodium and potassium, as well as other substances, are excreted in the urine.

Others factors of loss

Stress, both emotional and physical, can create the tendency for the body to retain water and sodium. In the presence of cardiovascular, neurological, renal, or hormonal pathological conditions, this tendency is exaggerated. Unusual losses such as those that may accompany hemorrhage, vomiting, diarrhea, burns, wound drainage, or a gastrointestinal suctioning procedure demand special attention when one is planning to meet daily fluid and electrolyte needs.

DIAGNOSTIC ASSESSMENT

Serum levels of electrolytes are commonly used to identify deficits or excesses. These are identified in Table 16-1. Hemoconcentration or hemodilution can be monitored with hematocrit levels.

Data analysis

After the nurse has collected information about the client's fluid and electrolyte balance, the information is compared with norms for age, gender, and development. The data can be analyzed and nursing problems or diagnoses identified. Potential or actual nursing diagnoses may include alterations in fluid balance, alterations in cardiac output, sensory perceptual alterations, impairment of skin integrity, alterations in tissue perfusion, and alterations in urinary elimination.

Planning
PLANNING FOR HEALTH PROMOTION

As a care plan is developed for clients with problems that relate to fluids and electrolytes, consideration should be given to strategies that will promote a balance, as well as those specific to restoration and maintenance. A number of problems may be responsible for causing a fluid and electrolyte imbalance. The nurse's awareness of these causes will facilitate the development of a plan of care that has a two-fold focus—promotion, in addition to restoration and maintenance.

16 Fluid and electrolyte balance

Fluids and electrolytes are essential for the functioning of the organs of the body. The intake of these substances must be adequate in order to meet daily requirements. The nurse should therefore encourage clients to maintain a normal intake of foods and fluids to facilitate a balance. In addition to planning to meet daily requirements, consideration must be given to clients with preexisting deficits such as those that occur from vomiting, diarrhea, restricted intake of food and fluids, excessive perspiration, suction, and drainage, as well as to those clients being fed intravenously, those with severe burns, or those with adrenal, cardiovascular, and renal diseases. Certain medications also have an effect on fluid and electrolyte status.

A variety of problems must be anticipated and a plan of care developed to maintain a closely normal state. For example, normal gastric juice is abundant in chloride and contains a relatively high amount of potassium and some sodium. Therefore whenever vomiting occurs, the intake of fluids should be discouraged, particularly if vomiting is persistent. The amount and character of fluid loss should be documented. A complete documented description of the fluid loss facilitates replacement. The same applies to intestinal losses as may occur from diarrhea or intestinal drainage. In addition, medications for both vomiting and diarrhea should be administered as required. Intravenous fluids are likely to be ordered for persistent vomiting; these should be maintained as prescribed. When oral fluids can be taken and retained, the foods offered should be those high in potassium, such as milk and orange juice.

Another common example in which the nurse can be instrumental in promoting balance is in the use of physiological saline for irrigations of gastrointestinal tubes. Other fluids such as plain water, in addition to injuring the mucosa, promote increased secretion of intestinal juice and cause electrolytes to be withdrawn from the extracellular fluid.

Careful records must be kept of intake, output, and body weight. These measures are beneficial in detecting alterations in fluid balance.

A wide range of symptoms may be experienced when an electrolyte imbalance develops. The nurse should be alert to these so that they can be reported at their earliest occurrence. The reader is referred to the pages that follow for specific symptoms and nursing considerations for fluids and electrolytes.

PLANNING FOR HEALTH MAINTENANCE AND RESTORATION

Fluid intake is largely a direct function of the ingestion of water and food substances. Water is also produced within the body as an end product of oxidation. It is estimated that adults produce 300 ml of water in this way. This is augmented by a wide range of secretions produced by organs and glands.

The nurse should be aware that clients who are consistently using ventilators or ultrasonic humidifiers (especially with warmed nebulization) can absorb up to a liter of fluid per day as a result of such devices. Any use of respiratory adjuncts deserves special consideration, especially when in use for small children or debilitated clients (see Chapter 21).

Planning for client hydration

An infant requires approximately 180 to 200 ml of fluid per kilogram of body weight daily. Adults need 2500 to 3000 ml of fluid, or less than 60 ml/kg of body weight. This amount is approximately one third of a child's requirement per unit of weight. This amount is usually supplied by ingested food and water. If there are no pathological conditions, these respective amounts of fluid will adequately hydrate the client each day.

Nursing process for common health problems

Infants and young children who are healthy take fluids readily in the form of milk, water, and juice. Active adults who eat a balanced diet and ingest beverages in amounts of 1500 to 2000 ml normally have sufficient intake when these amounts are added to the fluid produced in the metabolic process. Elderly individuals usually require considerable encouragement to take fluids. Tea and coffee are preferred beverages for many. Others prefer juice or perhaps beer. Whatever the fluid of choice, daily intake should be high enough to maintain dilute urine, which is less irritating to the delicate lining of the urinary tract. The kidneys of the aged individual are less efficient in concentrating urine while at complete rest, and thus care should be taken to avoid high evening intake that might result in nocturia. Because older individuals have less fluid reserve, considerable caution should be observed regarding fluid intake in order to assure that adequate amounts are provided to meet maintenance needs. Elderly clients do not have a keen thirst mechanism, and forgetfulness or confusion as well as general weakness may contribute to low fluid intake. Low intake and the output of a dilute urine both contribute to a dehydrated state. Care should be taken to ascertain that fluid intake is sufficient. Intake records should be maintained for reference. One method to encourage fluids capitalizes on the elderly client's concern for regular bowel functioning. The nurse can explain that increased fluid intake enhances bowel regularity.

When planning for client hydration, the nurse must remember that basal fluid needs are appreciably altered in the presence of any stressors (mentioned previously) that increase the demand for water intake.

Fluid therapy   Fluid therapy to meet maintenance needs or replace losses may be accomplished by the administration of substances orally, rectally, or intravenously. Oral replacement is the safest method of administering fluids and electrolytes. It is relatively free from immunological reactions and depends on normal channels for distribution of components to tissue areas. If normal mastication and swallowing mechanisms have been impaired by neurological damage or are contraindicated by injury or illness or if a client has anorexia, a nasogastric tube can be used to introduce fluids, nutrients, and even medication. A protoclysis is sometimes employed to introduce fluid and sodium chloride into the colon where it can be absorbed. The bowel, however, is incapable of absorbing nutrients.

Parenteral fluid replacement, especially intravenous therapy, is a common procedure in the hospital. It does not depend on an adequately functioning gastrointestinal tract and takes effect immediately; the body can still adjust levels of fluid in body compartments in the same way as when intake is oral. Substances with high molecular weight and medications normally destroyed by gastric juices can be introduced in this way. Levels of fluids and electrolytes in the vascular system can be controlled with considerable precision. Therapy can be instituted to replace actual circulating volume and can be maintained for a long period of time. See discussion of hyperalimentation in Chapter 17; see Chapter 8 for discussion of administration of intravenous fluids.

Hypodermoclysis, or subcutaneous infiltration of fluid, is useful for very young or very old persons whose veins are small or difficult to enter. Tissue areas commonly employed are the abdomen, lateral thighs, lateral chest, and the buttocks. An enzyme such as hyaluronidase is usually administered concurrently to increase the spread and absorption of the fluid. This method of replacement is contraindicated in the presence of edema.

The intradermal, intraosseus, intraarterial, and intraperitoneal routes are others useful in unique circumstances.

Regardless of the route, the administration apparatus must be sterile. The fluid must be free of pyrogens and of approximately the same chemical tonicity as plasma and contain plasma ions.

Implementation

COMMON HEALTH PROBLEMS THAT OCCUR ACROSS THE LIFE SPAN

Major fluid imbalances

Fluid deficit and excess. *All body fluids contain water and electrolytes.* Therefore any disturbance in body functioning that results in a loss of body fluid also results in a reduction of essential electrolyte substances. Fluid balance can be assured only when intake approximates output. As soon as levels of loss exceed levels of intake, disequilibrium occurs, resulting in a cycle of events in which the body attempts to compensate for the loss.

Dehydration. True dehydration is a deficit of water without salt or an unusual excess of salt. It is characterized by hemoconcentration. There is a rise in hematocrit, osmolality, and protein and electrolyte concentration. Weight loss from 2% to 6% is typical for mild to severe dehydration, respectively. The condition is most likely to be encountered in infants, the elderly, or individuals having recent surgery or severe burns.

Usual causes include: (1) a decrease in fluid intake, (2) an acute loss of secretions and excretions such as vomitus, diarrhea, or fistulous drainage, (3) fever, and (4) intestinal obstruction. Therapy involves giving balanced fluids such as Ringer's lactate. Some physicians prefer 5% dextrose in water.

Pathophysiology. The clinical course of dehydration may be insidious or acute in its development. As water and electrolytes are lost, the extracellular fluid becomes hypertonic, thus drawing water from the cells. Consequently, there is ultimately a resulting deficit in intracellular, as well as extracellular, fluids. As hypovolemia becomes pronounced, it creates a stimulus for the release of ADH. This occurs primarily because intracerebral osmoreceptor cells are sensitive to an increase in serum osmolality (concentrated plasma). There are also volume receptors in the left atrium that react to a decreased cardiac output and are thought to signal ADH release in an attempt to conserve body fluid. (Pain, opiates, barbiturates, and nicotine also produce this fluid-conserving response.) During this compensatory response several things may be clinically evident, and the nurse needs to understand these signs and symptoms that signal dehydration.

Assessment. The nurse can observe the dehydrated client and gather information significant to the care plan. Following are significant indicators of dehydration.

THIRST. In volume depletion, there is a rise in the osmolarity of extracellular fluid, and a resultant shift of water from intracellular to extracellular spaces in an attempt to restore a balanced state. As soon as body fluid loss reaches 2% or more, the thirst center in the hypothalamus is activated as a result of the excess of sodium in relation to water. The cerebral cortex is stimulated, evoking a desire to drink.

Because responding to thirst requires a recognition of the stimulus and an activity of drinking, its value is essentially negated in clients who cannot either express thirst in a meaningful way or obtain fluid. The very young, the elderly, and those who are lethargic, comatose, depressed, or debilitated are prone to dehydration. Others who require assistance in eating, such as clients who are visually impaired, handicapped, paralyzed, taking sedatives, tranquilizers, diuretics, or cathartics, or experiencing unusually high fluid losses are also among those prone to water deficits. Caretakers of these individuals must be especially alert to the importance of facilitating hydration.

CONCENTRATED URINE AND OLIGURIA. Urinary mechanisms play a crucial role in the maintenance of fluid and electrolyte balance. Individuals with healthy kidneys will respond with increased tubular resorption. Urinary output is thus a valuable indicator of fluid volume status. If the output falls below 25 ml/hr in an adult, for example, there is invariably dehydration. The specific gravity will rise above 1.025. When urine sodium falls below 10 to 20 mEq/L, especially if intake is restricted, hypovolemia exists. Serum sodium on the other hand is not valuable in assessing depleted fluids. In most low-volume states (except acute hemorrhage) the hematocrit will rise, perhaps in association with a concurrent rise in hemoglobin and BUN.

Nurses may assess indirectly that the urine output is low. For example, fewer requests for a bedpan, infrequent diaper changes, and dark urine may be indicative of dehydration. Because concentrated urine is irritating to the skin, prolonged low urine output may be accompanied by skin excoriation at the urinary meatus or over the perineum and buttocks if the individual is incontinent.

WEIGHT LOSS. Body weight is a reliable index of fluid loss. A loss of 1 L of fluid will yield a loss of 1 kg of weight. It is important that the weight be evaluated at the same time each day with the same clothing on and, preferably, immediately after the bladder is emptied. Body weight is considered by many authorities to be the most reliable index of hydration status.

POOR SKIN TURGOR. When body fluid levels are adequate, skin is plump and resilient. In dehydration, elasticity and firm appearance are lost. Dehydration can be detected by gently pinching the skin together in a fold and observing its behavior. If the fold remains adherent for several seconds, poor skin turgor is said to exist (see Chapter 15). (In well-hydrated clients, the skin returns immediately to its prepinched state.)

When one deals with elderly clients, skin turgor should be evaluated on the anterior chest wall because skin on extremities may appear severely dehydrated, even when there is fluid excess. Skin turgor is assessed most readily in infants and young children by using the abdominal area. It is important to note that false or misleading results from the skin turgor test may occur in the presence of excess subcutaneous fat (may seem well-hydrated despite low volume) or in conjunction with malnourishment (may seem dehydrated despite normal fluid volume).

RISE IN BODY TEMPERATURE. The body depends on water to conduct heat outside the body. When water is not present in adequate amounts in the tissue, it no longer assists in heat elimination and fever results. (The nurse should be aware that even though the core temperature of the body may be high, the extremities and superficial trunk areas may be cool and pale as a result of collapsed peripheral circulation that accompanies a severe dehydration episode.) Fever induces increased respiration and diaphoresis, thus aggravating fluid loss. However, if the diaphoresis continues until the dehydration is profound, there will be a failure of perspiration activity. It is therefore useful to assess the axilla of the severely ill client because an absence of moisture may be a vital clue to dehydration.

PULSE RATE AND BLOOD PRESSURE ALTERATIONS. A normal pulse rate usually indicates normal hydration, but tachycardia may not necessarily indicate hypovolemia. An increased heart rate accompanies many stressors, and may be unrelated to a change in cardiac output. However, if the peripheral pulses are easily obliterated or if they are barely perceptible, the nurse should suspect significant volume depletion.

The blood pressure, on the other hand, is a better indicator of hypovolemia. Although the systolic pressure is seldom affected until volume losses of blood reach 20% to 25% of the total, the pulse pressure may decrease earlier because of the marked rise in peripheral resistance, or a decrease in stroke volume and cardiac output, or both. This phenomenon can be assessed early by performing a simple test to determine if blood pressure is affected by changes in posture, that is, *postural vital signs*. Individuals with normal volume who possess good vascular tone respond readily to changes in posture by rapidly constricting blood vessels returning pooled blood in capacitance veins in the trunk and extremities to the central circulation. This adjustment is not operant in the severely volume-depleted client because vasoconstrictor potential has been exhausted. Therefore, when the body must adapt to a sitting or standing position, an exaggerated hypotensive effect is created from blood volume shifts, and the systolic pressure cannot be sustained.

The following procedure should be followed when assessing for this orthostatic drop in blood pressure caused by low volume.

1. Record the blood pressure and pulse with the client in a supine position.
2. Sit the client upright (90 degrees), and record the blood pressure and pulse again.
3. Assist the client to a standing posture, and record the blood pressure and pulse again.
4. Compare the three readings. If either of the following results from the position changes, the client is hypovolemic.
   a. Decrease of 20 mm Hg or more in the systolic or diastolic blood pressure or
   b. Increase of 20 beats or more per minute in the pulse rate

Because postural changes can result in dizziness, fainting, and visual disturbances when occurring with low volume states, the nurse must carefully support the client during the test to prevent injuries. The initiation of the test is not advised if there are precluding conditions that would make it unsafe to perform (for example, clients who are having problems with balance and coordination).

STOOL NUMBER AND CONSISTENCY. Stools that are dry and hard indicate a dehydrated state because additional water is absorbed in the large intestine to compensate for total body fluid deficits. Frequent loose, watery stools reflect a mechanism for high body fluid loss and thus need to be noted and recorded. Obtaining information on the number and character of stools is often left to the discretion of a nursing assistant and may not be clinically interpreted unless there is an obvious reason to expect dehydration or constipation. Diarrhea and constipation are unfortunately too frequently considered "elimination problems," and

Nursing process for common health problems

their significance to hydration and electrolyte status may therefore go undetected unless they are specific factors in the nursing assessment plan.

SKIN AND MUCOUS MEMBRANES. The skin of a well-hydrated client is warm and elastic, and mucous membranes glisten. However, skin and mucous membranes must be evaluated along with other factors to prevent misleading conclusions. For example, a dry mouth and lips that are dry and cracked may result from dehydration, or in some instances, merely reflect that the individual is a mouth-breather and that the humidity is low. Dry skin may occur with low volume states or in conjunction with febrile states. Certain drugs also have dry mouth and dry mucous membranes as side effects, for example, atropine.

The tongue may be swollen in early dehydration and later will become dry and longitudinally wrinkled if volume is not restored. Dry, sticky oral secretions reflect dehydration, too. The nurse may note this telltale sign while providing oral hygiene or administering oral medications. Offering additional fluids at this point may make the client considerably more comfortable and contribute to correcting fluid depletion.

Eyes that are well hydrated are sparkling and bright. If eyes lack luster and appear dull, the client may have a low volume state. Organ atrophy (for example, sunken eyeballs or fontanels) reflect severe states of water deficit.

DIMINISHED RATE AND DEGREE OF VEIN FILLING. Vein filling is a significant factor in assessing hydration. To check for rate and degree of vein filling, select an easily visible vein in the hand or foot that is not in a dependent position. Occlude the vein distally and empty it by stroking proximally. Release the occlusion and immediately note how rapidly the vessel fills. In adequate hydrational states, the vein fills at once. In dehydration, the vein fills slowly and may even remain unfilled.

BEHAVIORAL CHANGES. In cases of severe low volume, the client's level of consciousness may decline and behavioral changes may be noted. Anxiety, agitation, and disorientation are not uncommon, especially among the elderly who are fluid depleted.

Data analysis
After gathering information about the client's hydration status, data are compared with norms appropriate for age and weight. Data analysis may reveal actual or potential diagnoses of alteration in bowel elimination, fluid volume deficit, ineffective breathing pattern, alteration in nutrition, impairment of skin integrity, alteration in tissue perfusion, or alteration in patterns of urinary elimination.

Planning and implementation. Because dehydration places added burdens on the various body systems and can lead to electrolyte imbalances, shock, renal failure, and other critical complications, the nurse and client must establish goals to (1) restore fluid balance, (2) maintain hemodynamic balance, and (3) maintain skin integrity.

RESTORING FLUID BALANCE. The client's fluid needs are based on age, weight, and replacement requirements, which are the result of special circumstances, such as draining wounds, suctioning, diarrhea, and fever. Fluid administration should be scheduled as carefully as medications or other therapeutic measures. The nurse should ensure that the individual has a choice in the selection of fluids to the extent that the condition allows, and that selected beverages are served at the appropriate temperature. The nurse may need to help the client take fluids, or family members may be enlisted to participate in the program of hydration.

Opportunities for elimination, handwashing, oral hygiene, and proper positioning should precede fluid administration. Time should be taken to make this nurse-client contact positive. The fluid intake should not be rushed because it may create frustration and discouragement and perhaps even result in accidental pulmonary aspiration. Praise delivered along with a beverage also may induce subsequent positive interactions with fluid administration.

Infants and young children are especially prone to dehydration and may deteriorate rapidly without an adequate fluid intake. Although juices may be more nutritious, the nurse may need to offer whatever liquid the child will take including carbonated beverages, fruit punch, or oral electrolyte solutions. Caloric content, electrolyte composition, or other factors may need to be considered; therefore, the physician, nurse, and dietitian should collaborate when planning for hydration.

Combining socialization or play with fluid administration is a useful technique that nurses and family members may employ to encourage adequate liquid intake. Although fluids should be offered and the client urged to drink, threats of punishment for failure to comply should be avoided.

Critical dehydration problems may demand alternate modes of fluid therapy. For example, if oral intake is vomited, if swallowing is prohibited, or if a client is in a coma, intravenous therapy will be necessary to facilitate fluid administration. Antiemetics may be used to manage vomiting. Nasogastric tube feedings may be indicated in other instances.

Careful intake and output records and daily weights cannot be stressed enough for clients at risk of dehydration. Nurses should recognize that these records are crucial determinants in the evaluation of the client's responses to fluid therapy and serve to guide therapeutic management. These records should be maintained by the nursing staff with the same care used for others, such as the record for medication delivery. Selected intake and output recordings may be delegated to nursing assistants in some institutions, but the resultant worksheets or records must be carefully and frequently monitored by professional personnel for evaluation of a client's response to therapeutic plans.

MAINTAINING HEMODYNAMIC STABILITY. Dehydration may produce shock and concomitant changes in blood pressure, heart rate, and stroke volume (see Chapter 20). Rapid infusions of fluids may be required to restore cardiovascular status. These may be given at rates higher than normal, and large-bore intravenous catheters may be used.

MAINTAINING SKIN INTEGRITY. It is essential to maintain skin integrity and prevent tissue breakdown. The client should be turned and repositioned frequently and the skin and mucous membranes lubricated as needed.

Evaluation. Changes in the client's hydration status can be evaluated by specific gravity of urine, changes in body weight, improved skin turgor, increased intake and urinary output, improved venous filling and full pulse volume, and normal blood pressure.

869

Nursing process for common health problems

EXPECTED OUTCOMES

The client and/or family can:
1. Describe dehydration.
2. State plans for prevention of dehydration.
3. State plans for compliance with plans for rehydration.
4. State plans for follow-up health care.

Water intoxication. This condition is manifested by excess water in all compartments. Electrolyte disturbance is absent because all compartmental volumes increase concurrently.

Severe stress, with excess production of ADH, can be the cause. Other endocrine pathological conditions may contribute to such a condition. Occasionally the renal blood flow is drastically impaired to the point that excess water cannot be excreted.

 Assessment. Clinical signs are weakness, drowsiness, loss of muscular control, and behavioral changes including disorientation. Weight gain is evident. The skin is flushed and moist, but excess sweating seldom occurs. Moist respirations may be present. In uncompensated episodes, the terminal stage is marked by extreme hemodilution, absent deep tendon reflexes, and oliguria.

Planning and implementation. Therapy primarily depends on water restriction.

Solute-loading hypertonicity. Hypertonicity occurs when clients are subjected to a load of solutes in excess of water required for excretion. This entity can be caused by parenteral hyperalimentation or nasogastric feedings when such feedings are not supplemented by water. It can occur in unconscious clients or infants who are being fed solutes but who cannot complain of thirst. Individuals on milk and cream regimens for ulcer management or infants who are fed undiluted milk, not supplemented with water, are prone to solute-loading hypertonicity.

When the body is confronted with a heavy load of solutes, it responds by a maximal renal absorption of water. However, when the renal reabsorption threshold of a solute is exceeded, an osmotic diuresis is induced. Thus, additional water is lost by urinary output. When large quantities of glucose or amino acids are consumed and they cannot be completely metabolized or resorbed by the renal mechanisms, obligatory water excretion occurs.

 Assessment. Solute overloading can be noted clinically by symptoms of dehydration with a few exceptions. Unlike true dehydration, there is an increase in weight and a good urinary output. The blood plasma exhibits an elevated osmolality and a sodium concentration out of proportion to the red blood cell hemoconcentration. The treatment involves giving water without solutes. Insulin is sometimes employed to prevent diuresis induced by inadequately metabolized glucose.

 Planning and implementation. Nurses should be cautious to ensure that clients receiving solute-rich feedings have supplemental water. Many clients with nasogastric tubes have no water restrictions; thus fluids should not be restricted unless there are specific clinical indications for fluid restriction. Infants need water as well as regular feedings, especially if they receive undiluted cow's milk.

Extracellular fluid volume deficit and excess

Extracellular fluid volume deficit. Extracellular fluid volume deficit is characterized by a deficit of both water and electrolytes in extracellular fluid in relatively the same proportions. The conditions commonly responsible for producing the deficit are a drastic decrease in intake of water, vomiting, diarrhea, fistulous drainage, and intestinal obstruction. Symptoms characteristic of this deficit include dry skin and mucous membranes, decrease in urine output (for example, oliguria or anuria), elevated temperature, weight loss, and lassitude. Intravenous infusions of isotonic saline are generally used for treatment.

Extracellular fluid volume excess. This imbalance involves excesses of water and electrolytes in plasma as well as in interstitial fluids. Cellular volume is not generally affected.

The causes of extracellular fluid volume excess include (1) excessive infusion of normal saline, which contains more milliequivalents per liter of sodium and chloride than normal extracellular fluids, (2) congestive heart failure, (3) portal hypertension, and (4) chronic renal disease. Furthermore, any disease that is characterized by low plasma protein (cirrhosis, nephrosis, or malnutrition) has less effective osmotic pull at the venous end of the capillary, thus permitting water and salt to remain in extracellular spaces. In certain forms of stress, including trauma and surgery, overactive adrenal hormones may result in salt and water retention. Therapeutic use of adrenal cortical hormones in large amounts may produce the same response.

In disease in which there is a reduction of renal blood flow (such as congestive heart failure), aldosterone is activated, which stimulates the renal retention of sodium in response to the excretion of potassium and hydrogen ions. As sodium is retained, ADH is released to aid in water reabsorption in distal renal tubules. These factors all contribute to excesses in extracellular fluid.

 Assessment. The signs and symptoms are (1) weight gain (more than 5%), (2) edema, (3) moist rales, (4) puffy eyelids, (5) dyspnea, and (6) a bounding pulse (because of plasma volume increase). Laboratory values for hematocrit, hemoglobin, and red blood cell count are subnormal.

Planning and implementation. Therapy is aimed at removing water and sodium from interstitial fluid and plasma without altering osmolality or composition of the extracellular fluid. Diuretics, paracentesis, thoracentesis, or phlebotomy are among the modes of treatment.

Changes in fluid distribution

Third space syndrome. The third space syndrome is essentially a form of dehydration because there is a deficit of fluid available for the extracellular pool, although the total body fluid is not reduced. This phenomenon occurs when there is a local reservoir of fluid immobilized such as in ascites, cellulitis, intestinal obstructions, crush injuries, or vascular occlusions.

 Assessment. There are signs of a decrease in plasma volume with hypotension. Tachycardia, peripheral vasoconstriction, and oliguria complete the classical picture. Most clinicians agree that a rising hematocrit value in the absence of external fluid loss is diagnostic of this third space dehydration syndrome. There is no weight loss because the fluid is not lost outside the body.

 Planning and implementation. Therapy consists of administration of plasma, salts, and water while judiciously monitoring the hematocrit, vital signs, and urinary output.

Edema. Edema refers to the accumulation of excess interstitial fluid in the tissues. In edema, fluid is abnormally shifted from the various body compartments. Although the fluid is not lost outside the body, it cannot be used to meet obligatory water requirements. Thus dehydration can actually exist, because serum sodium levels are not elevated and, in fact, may be subnormal.

Pathophysiology. Edema is a result of positive pressure in interstitial spaces. It may be caused by (1) an increase in capillary hydrostatic pressure from venous obstruction or heart failure, (2) decreased plasma proteins because of insufficient protein intake or excessive loss by kidneys, (3) increased interstitial fluid protein resulting from obstructed lymphatics (lymphedema), or (4) porous capillaries created by forces (such as a toxin) that allow abundant amounts of protein to escape. The last condition is referred to as *inflammatory edema.* Fluid retention by kidneys is also a cause of edema formation.

Assessment. Edema is clinically evident when the interstitial fluid volume increases at least 10% or 15% and is noted by weight gain. It is first observed in areas with low tissue tension, such as the eyelids. It may be aggravated by inactivity, because normal muscle movement helps fluid reenter the capillaries. Fatty tissue, varicose veins, or even constricting clothing such as garters and girdles can interfere enough to deter fluid movement out of the interstitial areas. The presence of edema not only creates an imbalance in water and electrolyte levels but may also inhibit movement of limbs and alter arterial blood flow to vital organs (especially in a confined space such as the cranial vault). Ultimately, it may be extensive enough to affect the lungs and internal and external respiratory exchange. Specific effects of edema related to the urinary, cardiovascular, and respiratory systems are discussed in Chapters 19, 20, and 21.

The nurse and client can observe for the presence of edema. Edema is initially noted in dependent areas such as the ankles, fingers, or if the client is supine, in the sacral area. The extent of edema can be assessed by measuring the circumference of the involved part with a tape measure. Edema can also be detected by palpation. Special terms are often used to describe edema.

pitting edema Areas where fluid has accumulated to the extent that when pressure is applied to a given point, a depression remains temporarily (see Chapter 20).
ascites Excessive fluid accumulation in the peritoneal cavity.
dependent edema Fluid accumulation in areas that are influenced by gravitational forces, such as the feet, ankles, hands, or sacrum.
anasarca Generalized edema.
hydrothorax Excessive fluid accumulated in the pleural cavity.

Data analysis
Data analysis may reveal actual or potential nursing diagnoses of alterations in cardiac output, fluid volume deficit, alterations in nutrition, disturbances in self-concept, alterations in tissue perfusion, and alterations in patterns of urinary elimination.

Planning and implementation. Objectives of nursing care for the client with edema depend on the cause of edema, but may include objectives to (1) decrease interstitial fluid in the tissues, (2) promote circulation, and (3) maintain skin integrity. Plans should be implemented as soon as edema is evident.

DECREASING INTERSTITIAL FLUID. Edema is managed by a low-sodium diet and by the administration of diuretics, intravenous salt-poor albumin, or exchange resins. Water intake may be restricted as well. The client should be observed for dehydration, however, because interstitial fluid is trapped in tissue and is not available for maintaining hydration.

PROMOTING CIRCULATION. In order to assure unobstructed circulation, the nurse and client must plan to avoid constricting clothing and positions. The client should be encouraged to wear loose clothing and obtain active and passive exercise. Bedfast clients should be turned and repositioned frequently and an alternating pressure mattress used as needed. Elastic stockings or sleeves may be used to promote circulation in dependent areas.

MAINTAINING SKIN INTEGRITY. Edematous tissue is fragile and vulnerable to infection. The skin must therefore be kept clean and dry and protected from injury. A high-protein diet may be encouraged to provide adequate nutrition.

Evaluation. The nurse can evaluate changes in the distribution of fluid and reduction of edema by monitoring changes in the client's weight. Intake and output records and observation of edematous parts also provide evaluative data.

EXPECTED OUTCOMES
The client and/or family can:
1. Describe edema.
2. Describe plans to prevent edema with diet, exercise, and medication.
3. State plans for maintaining skin integrity.
4. State plans for compliance with diuretic therapy, low-sodium diet, and fluid restrictions.
5. Describe signs indicative of impending edema, such as weight gain, increasing size of body parts, or swelling in dependent areas.
6. State plans for follow-up health care and use of community resources.

Major electrolyte imbalances

All cells of the body are surrounded by fluid and electrolytes. The relative concentration of these substances in various tissues remains stable if the individual is in a homeodynamic state.

Pathophysiology. Electrolytes are obtained from the diet and absorbed through the gastrointestinal tract. Excretion occurs through the skin (perspiration), urine, and feces. Any factor of intake or excretion may contribute to imbalances. Furthermore, some electrolytes require vitamins or minerals to facilitate absorption; for example, vitamin D is essential for the uptake of calcium or phosphorus. Disease or dysfunction of the gastrointestinal tract, endocrine system, skin, or kidneys and the effects of selected medications can contribute to major electrolyte imbalances.

Assessment. The signs and symptoms that occur when electrolytes are in concentrations that are too low or too high depend largely on the physiological role of the electrolyte affected. Disturbances of potassium, sodium, calcium, and magnesium must be anticipated and promptly recognized by the nurse (Table 16-2).

Data analysis
Nursing diagnoses related to electrolyte imbalances are varied and depend on the physiological changes produced by the imbalance. Data analysis may reveal nursing diagnoses of alteration in bowel or urinary elimination, impairment of skin integrity, alteration in cardiac output, alteration in thought processes, ineffective breathing patterns, sensory perceptual alteration, and potential for injury.

TABLE 16-2

Fluid and electrolyte imbalances

Imbalance	Clinical signs and symptoms	Therapy	Anticipate in
Dehydration	Thirst, anxiety, weight loss, poor skin turgor, slow vein filling, elevated temperature, tachycardia, dry mucous membranes, decreased level of consciousness, increased hematocrit, increased BUN, increased RBC concentration	Volume replacement	Any condition in which water output exceeds intake; vomiting, diarrhea
Edema	Weight gain exceeding 5%; rales; dyspnea; puffy eyelids, swollen ankles, and so on; bounding pulse	Salt-poor albumin, exchange resins, diuretics	Protein deficiency, venous obstruction, heart failure, obstructed lymphatics, toxin ingestion, liver disease, renal disease
Third space syndrome	Hypotension, tachycardia, peripheral vasoconstriction, oliguria, no weight loss, increased hematocrit with no evidence of fluid loss	Plasma, salts, water replacement, diuretics, paracentesis, thoracentesis	Ascites, cellulitis, crush injuries, vascular occlusion, intestinal obstructions
Hypokalemia	Weakness, flaccidity; diminished reflexes; weak pulse, hypotension; ECG changes—increased P wave amplitude, flat or inverted T waves, ST segment depression, prominent U wave, prolonged PR interval; dyspnea; nausea, vomiting; mental depression	Oral or IV potassium therapy	Long-term diuresis (that is, thiazides), vomiting, diarrhea, draining fistulas, heat stroke, diabetic acidosis, alcoholism, malnutrition
Hyperkalemia	Muscle cramps; nausea, diarrhea, vomiting; weakness; hyperactivity; dizziness; paresthesias; ECG changes— early, high-peaked T waves, ST segment depressed, P wave disappears, later—QRS widens, T waves taller, premature ectopic beat; escape beats, ventricular flutter, fibrillation, standstill	$NaHCO_3$: 45 mEq IV over 5 min, may repeat in 10 min NaCl: IV Calcium gluconate: 0.5 ml/kg of 10% solution over 2-4 min (do not give in central line) Infuse $D_{50}W$ over 30-60 min with insulin Exchange resins: Kayexalate 20-50 g in 100-200 ml of 20% sorbitol orally (repeat every 3-4 hr) or 50 mg with 50 g sorbitol and 200 ml water as retention enema over 30-60 min Steroids Perioneal dialysis or hemodialysis Glucose-insulin infusion: 2-4 g glucose and 20-30 units insulin IV in 200-700 ml $D_{20}W$ over 30-60 min; or 1000 ml $D_{10}W$ with 90 mEq $NaHCO_3$ (infuse 300 ml over 30 min and remainder over 2-3 hr; give 25 units regular insulin SC at beginning of infusion)	Adrenal cortical insufficiency, acidosis, burns or other major tissue trauma, renal failure; overshooting IV or oral potassium
Hypocalcemia	Abdominal and muscle cramps, tetany, tingling of fingers and circumoral area, hyperactive reflexes, impaired mental functioning, laryngeal stridor, local or generalized seizures, ECG changes: prolonged QT interval caused by lengthened ST segment	IV calcium; 20-30 ml of 10% calcium gluconate IV over 10-15 min	Infections, burns, diarrhea, excessive use of citrated blood, pancreatitis, parathyroid malfunction
Hypomagnesemia	Positive Chvostek's sign,* hyperactive reflexes, coarse tremors, seizures, disorientation, gait disturbances, choreiform or athetoid movements, stupor	Magnesium sulfate: 2 mEq/kg body weight IV over 4 hr at rate not exceeding 150 mg/min	Vomiting, diarrhea, enterostomal drainage, cirrhosis, diuretic therapy, delirium tremens

*Unilateral contraction of facial muscle on facial nerve percussion (anterior to ear).

TABLE 16-2, cont'd

Fluid and electrolyte imbalances

Imbalance	Clinical signs and symptoms	Therapy	Anticipate in
Hyponatremia	Heat cramps; general weakness and fatigue; decreased cardiac output; hypotension; fainting; lip and nailbed cyanosis; cool, clammy skin; scant urine output; elevated intracranial pressure with headache, confusion, agitation, etc.; seizures; coma	Hypertonic saline (do not give more than 300 ml in 4 hr; monitor plasma chloride and bicarbonate levels cautiously)	Salt deficit, cirrhosis, diabetic ketoacidosis, heart failure, hormonal disturbances (such as ADH, ACTH), poorly managed diuretic therapy; diarrhea, perspiration
Hypernatremia	Irritability, lethargy, coma, seizures, delirium, weakness, signs and symptoms of dehydration, high-pitched cry in infants	Balanced IV solution	Perspiration, fever, failure of thirst mechanism, inadequate water intake with high-protein feedings

   Planning and implementation. The client and nurse can develop a nursing care plan relevant to the specific electrolyte imbalance. General goals may include (1) restoration of normal serum electrolyte levels and (2) management of related symptoms.

Potassium disorders. The major physiological roles of potassium encompass the maintenance of cellular osmotic pressure, the facilitation of neuromuscular activity (especially the skeletal and myocardial fibers), glucose uptake, and the regulation of acid-base balance.

Potassium must be ingested on a daily basis. (It is not stored.) The normal diet supplies this need. Although some potassium is excreted through the skin and stools, the overwhelming route of elimination is the urine. The kidneys possess the ability to excrete potassium from a high intake, but cannot selectively retain the electrolyte when the intake is deficient. The kidneys resorb, secrete, and excrete the ion in order to maintain an appropriate serum concentration. Aldosterone plays an important role by enhancing water and sodium retention, thus encouraging potassium excretion. Acid-base balance is strongly associated with potassium excretion, too, because the behavior of potassium and hydrogen ions is closely linked to an exchange with sodium ions. If excess hydrogen must be eliminated, less potassium will be lost because both ions require exchange with a sodium ion for excretion.

Hypokalemia. A deficiency in potassium is invariably accompanied by a deficiency in fluid volume. In the body's attempt to conserve water, aldosterone levels are elevated. Although water and sodium are retained, potassium loss is accelerated in the process. Conditions that are likely to result in hypokalemia include insulin therapy, which facilitates potassium entry into the cell (depleting extracellular fluids); long-term diuretic therapy (especially with thiazides); any gastrointestinal fluid loss such as vomiting, diarrhea, suctioning, or draining fistulas; heat stroke; diabetic acidosis; and alcoholism. Steroid administration, which causes sodium retention, is also responsible for producing hypokalemia. Clients who receive digitalis should be especially observed for hypokalemia (see Chapter 20).

   Assessment. Signs and symptoms of hypokalemia include paresthesias, diminished reflexes, cramping, muscle weakness and flaccidity, dyspnea, mental depression, and ECG changes (that is, flat or inverted T wave, ST segment depression, prominent U wave, and prolonged PR interval). Lower extremities are usually the first zone of symptoms. Many clients experience low bowel motility with anorexia, nausea, vomiting, and constipation.

Planning and implementation. The treatment for hypokalemia is the administration of potassium. The lost ion is replaced over several days by intravenous infusion, dietary intake, or combinations with pharmaceuticals, depending on the severity of the problem.

Potassium depletion in conjunction with diuretic therapy can be controlled by intake of foods known to be high in potassium but low in sodium. Among these are dried fruit (peaches, apricots, raisins, prunes), molasses, bananas, avocados, cola drinks, salt-free milk, grape juice, bitter chocolate, and instant coffee.

Potassium depletion caused by gastrointestinal suction can be curbed by proper precautions in irrigating the tubing, continuous measurement of the products of suctioning, and good judgment in general nursing care. If a client has continuous suctioning of the gastrointestinal tract, water and electrolytes are removed. Usually there is a concurrent order for "nothing by mouth." This means that no fluids should be introduced orally—not even to rinse the mouth, because even this can stimulate the production of secretions that will be merely suctioned outside the body. Ice chips yield water, which will be swallowed and stimulate secretions as the water takes up chlorides. If irrigations are done, it is important that normal saline is used to prevent the phenomenon of pulling out electrolytes. Irrigating fluid should be measured to ascertain differences between how much is introduced and how much is withdrawn. Other electrolytes lost in varying amounts, depending on the placement of the tube, include chloride, hydrogen, and bicarbonate.

Repeated tap water enemas can result in a similar imbalance.

PRECAUTIONS. Potassium therapy requires careful monitoring of the client and the replacement regimen. Potassium is excreted chiefly by the kidneys; thus adequate renal functioning is imperative. Urinary output should be within normal limits before the potassium is administered.

Potassium is best replaced by the oral route in the form of potassium chloride. Enteric-coated tablets are seldom used over an extended period of time because of their tendency to damage the lining of the gastrointestinal tract. Complications that can occur include ulcerations, bleeding, distension, nausea, vomiting, and severe pain. Giving the potassium with large amounts of water (at least 6 ounces) will help alleviate such distress.

When intravenous potassium is administered, it must be well diluted. It is *never* given "push," because high abrupt serum levels will induce cardiac arrest. All intravenous solutions containing potassium must be well mixed and given slowly. Usually the maximum amount of potassium is 40 mEq/L, and no more than 30 mEq should be given in an hour.

When an initial intravenous infusion is established, the line should be placed and proper functioning assured *before* adding the potassium to the flask. (If an accidental infiltration occurs while the venipuncture is being performed, a severe local reaction could ensue, because the agent is irritating to the tissue.) Always rotate the flask several times when adding potassium to prevent its tendency to settle in the flask. When the IV is being administered, frequent site checks are recommended to guard against infiltration or phlebitis. Because all veins receiving potassium are irritated somewhat, local tenderness or pain may be expected. This can be managed by slowing the rate.

Clients with renal pathological conditions, adrenal insufficiency, or heart disease require extraordinarily close clinical supervision during IV potassium therapy. This may include constant ECG monitoring in some settings.

Hyperkalemia. An excess of free potassium usually results from a malfunctioning excretory organ for potassium, such as renal failure or gastrointestinal obstruction. Trauma in which cells are crushed (burns, soft tissue injuries) also releases sodium stores. Adrenocortical insufficiency and excess IV potassium administration (even with aqueous K penicillin) are among other causes of hyperkalemia. *False hyperkalemia* can occur as a result of a hemolyzed blood sample, too.

Assessment. Signs and symptoms may be subtle and include many of those common to hypokalemia. Muscle cramps, nausea, vomiting, paresthesias, dizziness, and hyperactivity may be present. Early changes in the ECG that signal hyperkalemia are high-peaked T waves and ST segment depression. Later the P wave may disappear, the QRS widens, and the T waves become even taller. Finally, in severe excess states, premature ectopic beats, ventricular flutter, fibrillation, and standstill are likely to ensue.

Planning and implementation. The treatment for hyperkalemia may be done on an emergent basis because of the life-threatening nature of the problem. Therapy is aimed at counteracting potassium, reducing the serum level of potassium, preventing additional intake and uptake of potassium, and increasing the serum pH. Calcium counteracts the effect of potassium on the heart and is frequently given as an emergency measure. Insulin and dextrose may be given intravenously to reduce extracellular levels by transformed glycogen entering the cell linked to potassium. Intravenous sodium chloride is useful in encouraging the renal secretion of potassium. Sodium bicarbonate increases the serum pH and also lowers serum potassium through positive ion exchange. Exchange resins, steroids, and dialysis are other measures to reduce the serum level, especially in the event of severe ECG changes that suggest ensuing myocardial failure.

Sodium disorders. Sodium is the principle active solute in the extracellular space, determining the volumes of both the intravascular and interstitial spaces. It also influences the size of the cell mass because of its role in controlling water flow across the cell membrane. Conduction of neuromuscular impulses involves sodium, as well as potassium and calcium. Finally, sodium regulates certain chemical reactions in the cell and helps regulate acid-base balance.

Hyponatremia. Hyponatremia is a term usually used to indicate a salt deficit, but there are at least some exceptions worthy to note that do not involve a salt deficit but are hyponatremic states, such as cirrhosis, diabetic ketoacidosis, heart failure, and inappropriate secretion of antidiuretic hormone.[1] This section is concerned with clinical problems in which there is a sodium loss in excess of water. These include (1) renal salt wasting, (2) inappropriately managed diuretic therapy, (3) adrenocortical insufficiency, and (4) losses from intestinal drainage or diarrhea, surgical drainage, and perspiration.[1]

Hyponatremia results from sodium losses that exceed concurrent water loss. The consequent hyposmolality of extracellular fluids causes water to move inside the cells until a balanced osmolality of intracellular and extracellular fluid exists. The most common cause in hospitalized clients is excessive water consumption without sufficient salt intake.

 Assessment. Signs and symptoms of hyponatremia range from mild heat cramps to critical illness and collapse. Cardiovascular indices result essentially from the effects of concomitant plasma volume loss, not merely from the loss of sodium. There is a reduction in cardiac output and a tendency for arterial hypotension. Lips and nailbeds appear cyanotic, and the skin may be cool and clammy if depletion is marked (that is, less than 100 mEq/L). Fainting may occur because of postural hypotension, and the individual may complain of generalized weakness and fatigue. Urine output is scanty, and hyaline and granular casts may be present. Nocturia may be experienced (even though daily volume is low) because the normal diurnal variation is seemingly reversed. Thirst is generally not felt, and there is a loss of appetite, nausea, and vomiting. These clues are especially important if the client has been administered diuretics or is on a low-salt diet while having impaired renal function. Neuromuscular manifestations vary depending on the rapidity of hyponatremic development. Signs of elevated intracranial pressure (caused by overhydration of brain cells) are apparent, and confusion, lethargy, and delirium are common. Ability to perform simple mental tasks is reduced. Seizures may be precipitated in severe cases. It is important to note that these neurological signs and symptoms closely parallel those of other central nervous system disorders; thus even focal indices should be evaluated in view of sodium deficit before engaging in definitive therapy.

 Planning and implementation. Therapy is aimed at correcting the sodium deficit, thus reestablishing normal osmolality. Fluid restriction is the first line treatment aimed at correcting the hemodilution and reestablishing a normal osmotic gradient. A hypertonic saline infusion given cautiously over an extended time interval is a common treatment modality.

Nursing responsibilities include ensuring that (1) plasma chloride and bicarbonate levels are determined, at least midpoint in therapy, and (2) that no more than 300 ml of hypertonic saline solution is given in any 4-hour period.

Hypernatremia. This electrolyte imbalance is characterized by an excess of sodium in extracellular fluid that results from either unusual losses of water or failure to ensure adequate hydration. The resulting hypertonicity creates an osmotic pull of water from the cells into extracellular spaces.

Among the common clinical causes are: (1) large urinary losses of water when intake is restricted, such as postoperatively or in febrile states, (2) heavy evaporative losses from the skin, and (3) failure to respond to sense of thirst, for example, clients who are comatose or who have neurological pathological conditions. Hypernatremia is seldom seen in normal individuals because the sense of thirst is a natural drive to maintain fluid-electrolyte balance. However, when clients are unable to respond to thirst, hypernatremia will result unless needs are anticipated and met by others. A common cause of this problem is administration of high-protein feedings, especially by gavage, without accompanying water intake. Large doses of carbenicillin can also create hypernatremia because of its high sodium content. Infant feedings of undiluted milk, and milk and cream ulcer diets are also potential precursors of salt excess unless water intake is assured. It is a common misunderstanding that persons having a naso-gastric tube in place are automatically not allowed anything by mouth except for ordered feedings. Nurses must assume responsibility for calculating and administering water to meet basal body requirements of such persons.

☞ *Assessment.* Early signs and symptoms are caused by central nervous system depression. Irritability (accompanied by a high-pitched cry in infancy), lethargy, and finally coma are seen. Delirium, seizures, and EEG changes may be noted. Muscular weakness, fever, and signs of blood volume deficit often occur secondary to the dehydrating phenomenon of hypernatremia.

☞ *Planning and implementation.* Therapy is aimed at diluting the sodium excess by a balanced intravenous solution that provides free water and electrolytes essential for stabilizing the fluid compartments.

Calcium disorders. Although calcium is important to the support of bones and teeth, it also has other responsibilities that are vital to health. Calcium affects the permeability of cell membranes and has a specific role in the coagulation of blood. Finally, this ion is responsible in part for neuromuscular irritability.

Hypocalcemia. Hypocalcemia can occur as a result of parathyroid malfunction or destruction, or accidental removal of the parathyroid gland in surgery, but more commonly occurs when calcium is immobilized by infections or burns. Diarrhea, the use of citrated blood (which binds calcium), dietary deficiencies of calcium or vitamin D, renal failure, pancreatitis, and severe tissue destruction are among other causes of hypocalcemia.

☞ *Assessment.* Signs and symptoms include abdominal and muscle cramps, tetany, tingling of fingers and the circumoral area, hyperactive reflexes, impaired mental functioning, laryngeal stridor, and local or generalized seizures. The characteristic ECG pattern is a prolonged QT interval caused by a lengthened ST segment. Dysrhythmias and even cardiac arrest may occur.

☞ *Planning and implementation.* The therapy for hypocalcemia is directed toward correcting the plasma level of the electrolyte while concurrently treating the underlying cause. Special care must be given to a client taking digitalis because a low serum calcium reduces the sensitivity of the heart to digitalis. However, when calcium replacement is given, the sensitivity to the drug is greatly enhanced and digitalis toxicity can result (see Chapter 20).

Intravenous administration of calcium requires caution because the drug is irritating to tissues and can cause sloughing if extravasation occurs. The agent must be given slowly and the patient monitored cautiously, with special attention to ECG pattern changes.

Hypercalcemia. Calcium excess, or hypercalcemia, is usually found in conjunction with overactive parathyroids but may also be caused by excessive ingestion of milk or vitamin D (which increases calcium absorption), or it may be an accompaniment of multiple myeloma and other malignancies, pathological fractures, renal disease, or prolonged inactivity or bed rest (which mobilizes calcium.)

The plasma level rises above 5.8 mEq/L, and the x-ray films of bones reveal cavitation. Urine may show a heavy calcium precipitate.

☞ *Assessment.* Clinical signs and symptoms include anorexia, nausea, weight loss, thirst, polyuria, bone and flank pain, renal stones, lethargy, and azotemia. The ECG will reveal a shortened QT interval and prominent U waves. Dysrhythmias will ensue. Extremely high levels may cause death by stoppage of the heart in systole.

Planning and implementation. The management involves saline hydration to encourage diuresis of calcium. Phosphates may be employed to promote calcium excretion. Loop diuretics (such as furosemide) are used to enhance urinary output, thus the output of calcium. Mithramycin, an antineoplastic drug, is currently used to control hypercalcemia in selected individuals because it has been noted that the agent causes hypocalcemia in clients undergoing treatment for malignancies.

Magnesium disorders. Currently the clinical importance of magnesium is poorly understood, but it seems that magnesium is essential for enzyme activation and serves as a medium for certain neuromuscular functions. There is an estimated 2000 mEq of magnesium in the body, almost half of which is in the bones. Structures rich in blood (liver, heart, and skeletal muscle) have high cellular concentrations of this cation and yield it readily if intake is reduced. Magnesium is chiefly excreted by the feces (60%) and secondarily by urine (40%). The parathyroid is responsible for renal conservation of magnesium. Other regulatory agents include the adrenal gland, vitamin D, and the absorptive behavior of upper gastrointestinal mucosa.

Hypomagnesemia. Magnesium deficiencies are predictable in the presence of diarrhea, vomiting, enterostomal drainage, pathological conditions of malabsorption, cirrhosis, diuretic therapy, acidosis, and chronic alcoholism with delirium tremens. The plasma level falls below 1.4 mEq/L. (The normal level is 1.5 to 2.5 mEq/L). Like potassium, serum levels do not always reflect a true state of deficiency or excess.

Assessment. Signs and symptoms include a positive Chvostek's sign (unilateral contraction of facial muscles on percussion of facial nerve anterior to the ear), seizures, disorientation, hyperactive reflexes, coarse tremors, gait disturbances, choreiform or athetoid movements, and stupor.

Planning and implementation. Therapy consists of administration of magnesium sulfate in intravenous solution or by intramuscular injection. Correction is rapid, often within an hour or two.

Hypermagnesemia. This condition usually results from renal insufficiency. Individuals who cannot excrete magnesium may obtain an excess by repeated use of magnesium in enemas, cathartics, or antacids. Rarely, overdoses of therapeutic magnesium can induce hypermagnesemia.

Assessment. Signs and symptoms include neuromuscular depression and paralysis, dyspnea, and cardiac dysrhythmias. The CNS depression includes an effect on medullary centers, thus incuding hypotension.

Planning and implementation. Clinical management is aimed at hydration to promote renal excretion because the kidneys are the only exit route for this electrolyte. Diuretic therapy (including dialysis in severe cases) is indicated to hasten magnesium elimination. In the meantime, many clients will receive calcium to antagonize the depressing effects of the excess magnesium on neuromuscular tissue.

Evaluation. The outcome of the care plan is evaluated according to the client's response to the specific electrolyte imbalance. Objective criteria include monitoring of serum electrolyte levels as well as subjective data related to the nursing problems associated with the imbalance.

16 Fluid and electrolyte balance

EXPECTED OUTCOMES

The client and/or family can:
1. Describe the electrolyte imbalance.
2. State plans for preventing electrolyte imbalances.
3. State plans for compliance with therapeutic plans such as diet and use of medications.
4. Describe plans for follow-up care and use of community resources.

Evaluation

Evaluation is an ongoing process as the nurse and client plan to maintain fluid and electrolyte balance. Nursing problems resulting from fluid and electrolyte imbalances are complex and may include alterations in fluid balance, alterations in cardiac output, sensory perceptual alterations, impairment of skin integrity, alterations in tissue perfusion, and alterations in urinary elimination.

EXPECTED OUTCOMES

The client and/or family can:
1. State plans for health promotion, including maintenance of adequate fluid intake and electrolyte balance.
2. State plans for health maintenance or restoration for specific fluid and electrolyte disorders. These may include therapeutic diets and use of medications.
3. Describe the significance of fluid and electrolyte disorders in younger and older individuals.
4. State indications for health care and plans for follow-up care and use of community resources.

Summary

All body cells contain and are surrounded by water and electrolytes. These substances create a dynamic environment that supports life processes of tissues. Oxygen, nutrients, and chemicals are transported through this medium. The nurse must understand the physiology of fluids and electrolytes and their relationship to cellular activity in order to make clinical assessments and plan, implement, and evaluate nursing care for clients with nursing problems involving either fluid balance or electrolyte disturbances.

The principal body water compartments are the intracellular and extracellular spaces. The latter encompass interstitial fluid, intravascular fluid (plasma), and transcellular fluid (pleural, peritoneal, intraocular, joint, and cerebrospinal fluid). Forces that maintain these compartments and enable adjustments are hydrostatic and osmotic pressure gradients, the several neurohormonal influences, and organs of excretion.

The nurse has an important role in assessing the client's fluid and electrolyte status. Many disturbances in fluid and electrolyte balance relate to dehydration and its subsequent effect on cellular activity. Major imbalances of potassium, sodium, calcium, and magnesium have been addressed because they produce life-threatening complications if unchecked.

Plans for fluid and electrolyte imbalances often include the administration of oral, nasogastric, or intravenous fluids and electrolytes. Understanding the rationale for fluid orders, preparing the client for the procedure, and observing for adverse local and systemic responses are responsibilities of the nurse.

881

Nursing process for common health problems

It is imperative that the nurse appreciate the unique needs of clients, based on their age, size, and physical status and incorporate these into the plan of care.

Evaluation of the care plan is determined by goals and objectives specified in planning for restoration of fluid and electrolyte balance. Client expected outcomes relate to fluid and electrolyte status appropriate to the client's age and unique needs; data gathered from intake and output records, daily weights, and laboratory analysis of serum and urine can be used to determine the success of the nursing plan.

Reference

1. Maxwell, Morton H., and Kleeman, Charles R.: Clinical disorders of fluid and electrolyte metabolism, ed. 2, New York, 1972, McGraw-Hill Book Co.

Additional readings

Boylan, Ann, and Marbach, Bernard: Dehydration: subtle, sinister . . . preventable, R.N. **42:** 36-41, August 1979.

Felver, Linda: Understanding the electrolyte maze, Am. J. Nurs. **80:**1591-1596, September 1980.

Grant, Marcia M., and Kuby, Winifred M.: Assessing a patient's hydration status, Am. J. Nurs. **75:**1306-1311, August 1975.

Lander, Julie Davis: Nursing care of children with fluid and electrolyte disorders, Issues compr. pediatr. nurs. **4:**41-52, April 1980.

McGrath, Barbara Jo: Fluids, electrolytes, and replacement therapy in pediatric nursing, M.C.N., **5:**58-62, January/February 1980.

Menzel, Linda K.: Clinical problems of electrolyte balance, Nurs. Clin. North Am. **15:**559-576, September 1980.

O'Brien, D.: Fluid and electrolyte therapy. In Kempl, C.H., Silver, H.K., and O'Brien, D.: Pediatric diagnosis and treatment, ed. 4, Los Altos, Calif., 1976, Lange Medical Publications.

Scipien, G.: Comprehensive pediatric nursing, New York, 1979, McGraw-Hill Book Co.

Shoemaker, William C.: Hemodynamic and oxygen transport patterns of common shock syndromes, proceedings of a symposium on recent research developments and current clinical practice in shock, The Upjohn Co., 1975.

Weil, W.: Fluid and electrolyte metabolism in infants and children, New York, 1977, Grune & Stratton.

Winters, R.W.: The body fluids in pediatrics, Boston, 1973, Little, Brown and Co.

17 Upper gastrointestinal system

Assessment

Data analysis

Planning

Implementation

Evaluation

The upper gastrointestinal system facilitates nutrition with mechanisms for ingestion and digestion necessary to support growth and maintain metabolism throughout the life span. Common health problems, however, may interfere with these mechanisms. Some problems are unique to a specific age group, others recur across the life span. Neonates and infants, for example, have difficulty obtaining nutrition if there is a congenital defect of the mouth such as a cleft lip or palate, metabolic defects such as phenylketonuria, or environmental disorders such as low birth weight or failure to thrive syndrome. Common health problems during the adult years include cirrhosis, hepatitis, peptic ulcer disease, and gallbladder disease. Throughout the life span individuals may experience the hazards of malnutrition (obesity, emaciation), alcoholism, hernias, caries, and periodontal disease. The purpose of this chapter is to provide the nurse information about skills for identifying actual or potential nursing problems in order to develop, implement, and evaluate plans for health promotion, maintenance, and restoration for clients with common health problems of the upper gastrointestinal system.

Overview of the upper gastrointestinal system

The gastrointestinal system includes organs of ingestion and digestion (the mouth, esophagus, stomach, and small intestine), as well as the accessory organs of the gallbladder, liver, and pancreas. The gastrointestinal system is an open system sharing feedback components with the central nervous system, autonomic nervous system, metabolic pathways, hormonal tracts, and sensory organs.

Ingestion and digestion begin in the mouth where sucking reflexes and, later, controlled movements of the *mouth* and *tongue* enable the individual to ingest food. From infancy throughout the life cycle the *teeth* are accessory organs of ingestion for grinding and mastication of food. Digestion in the mouth is initiated by *ptyalin,* an enzyme secreted by the salivary gland for metabolic breakdown of starches.

By means of swallowing and peristalsis, food is transported through the *esophagus* and *cardiac sphincter* to the *stomach*. The stomach is a distensible organ that serves as a reservoir for partially digested foods, liquefies the food, absorbs water and alcohol, and secretes additional hormones and enzymes for digestion. Digestion in the stomach is primarily aided by gastric juice containing hydrochloric acid, pepsin, and renin. Hydrochloric acid and pepsin initiate protein digestion, whereas renin acts specifically to facilitate milk digestion.

Food from the stomach passes through the *pyloric sphincter* to the *duodenum* for continuing digestion. Here, metabolic enzymes and hormones supplied by accessory organs complete digestion and prepare the food for absorption or elimination.

The *pancreas* produces the digestive enzymes *trypsin* (for protein digestion), *amylase* (for carbohydrate digestion), and *lipase* (for fat digestion), which empty through the pancreatic duct into the duodenum. The pancreas also produces the hormones *insulin* and *glucagon,* which are necessary for carbohydrate metabolism, usage, and storage. Interferences in production of these enzymes or hormones result in nutritional deprivation.

The *liver* produces *bile* for fat emulsification. Bile is also necessary in absorption of fat and fat-soluble vitamins from the intestine. Bile is transmitted from the hepatic duct to the *gallbladder* for storage and released to the small intestine through the common bile duct.

The liver is a vital organ that regulates use and storage of end products of metabolic activity. The liver converts carbohydrates into usable glucose or stores them as glycogen, and it deaminizes protein and prepares the waste product, urea, for elimination by the kidney. The liver stores vitamins A, B_{12}, D, and K, and the minerals iron and copper, and synthesizes cholesterol, phospholipids, and lipoproteins. The liver conjugates bilirubin, the breakdown product of red blood cells, and makes it water soluble for elimination in bile. Additionally, the liver controls a balance of formed elements of the blood by breaking down hemoglobin and red blood cells and synthesizing prothrombin, fibrinogen, and other coagulation proteins. The liver also has detoxifying properties. Poisons, certain chemicals, and some drugs are detoxified by the liver. Blood supply to the liver comes directly from the mesentary by way of the portal vein, before circulation in the body. The hepatic artery carries oxygenated blood to the liver, and the hepatic vein carries deoxygenated blood to the vena cava.

The process of conversion of nutrients to energy is referred to as metabolism. Following ingestion and digestion of foods, potential energy in chemical bonds is released as kinetic energy to be used or stored. The ATP molecule facilitates energy use by the cell and metabolic pathways, including catabolic activity (release of energy) and anabolic activity (storage).

The rate of energy exchange is referred to as the *basal metabolic rate* (BMR). The BMR varies with age, sex, physiological changes, and extrinsic factors such as drugs, illness, culture, and climate. The BMR decreases with age, although it does increase during periods of growth such as adolescence or pregnancy. The BMR is generally higher in men. The BMR in women decreases during menstruation.

Regulation of food intake occurs in the hypothalamus, the appetite center. The ventromedial nucleus is referred to as the *satiety center,* and stimulation diminishes the appetite. The ventrolateral area is the *feeding center,* and stimulation here produces sensations of hunger. Connections with the autonomic nervous system and the hypothalamus have been demonstrated, and catecholamine levels may influence hunger and satiety.

Nutrition to the cells is provided by sufficient intake of food to maintain health and support growth. The need for calorie intake depends on the client's age, stage of growth, body size, energy expenditure, and metabolic rate. Daily dietary allowances of protein (20%), carbohydrates (40%), and fats (40%) form the basis of a diet that is calculated to supply calories for the individual's needs.

Extrinsic variables influence food intake and metabolism. Availability of food and appetite may be related to economic factors, cultural and religious beliefs, sensory capabilities to taste and enjoy food, and feelings of well-being that may increase or decrease the desire for food.

Assessment
NURSING HISTORY

The nurse can gather information about the client's nutritional patterns and the integrity of the gastrointestinal system in order to plan nursing care. The nursing history facilitates systematic data collection, and the information obtained can be related to the client's stage of development, and social, psychological, and physical health.

Health history

The nursing history should be obtained at the initial contact with the client. The nutrition component of the nursing history focuses on the client's patterns of eating, problems with digestion, and identification of health problems that might interfere with nutrition.

Initial data collection should include the client's age, height, weight, and body size, and these should be compared with norms (see Appendix A). The nurse should determine if there has been weight gain or loss during the last year. Changes of more than 10% are significant, particularly if the loss or gain has occurred within a short period of time.

The nurse can obtain information about the client's nutrition patterns by taking a diet history. The nurse can ask the client to describe his usual eating habits and specifically all foods eaten in the last 24 hours. The nurse can order this information in terms of calories and nutrients appropriate to the client's age and compare this with recommended daily dietary allowances.

The nurse can also obtain information about the client's food preferences and eating habits. Questions to elicit this information include: What foods do you like? Dislike? How is your appetite? What are your usual mealtimes? How do your work and life-style affect your eating? Who buys the food? Who prepares the food? With whom do you eat?

How the client obtains his nutrition depends on his level of maturation and varies across the life span. For instance, newborns and infants nurse from the breast or bottle, but as they grow older, they are more independent in feeding. The nurse should assess what feeding skills the client has acquired. Is the infant weaned? Can he hold finger foods? Can he feed himself with eating utensils?

If there is interference with the digestive organs, the client may obtain his nutrition by alternative feeding patterns, such as parenterally or by nasogastric or gavage feedings. The nurse should determine what alternative feeding patterns are used and how they satisfy the client's need for nutrition.

What the client eats is also determined by his ability to chew and digest foods. Solid foods are included in the diet when the client can chew, and the nurse can ascertain how well food is tolerated. Does he regurgitate his feedings? Is there nausea, vomiting, or diarrhea after eating? Does the client have heartburn? Does he eructate (belch) or have abdominal distension? Is the client allergic to any food? Does the client have anorexia or dysphagia? Has there been a change in appetite? Has there been a change in bowel elimination? Color? Frequency? What does the client do if he does have these symptoms? Does it bring relief?

Assessment should also be made relative to the client's digestive processes. Does the client complain of indigestion or abdominal pain? Does it occur before or after eating? Is it associated with a particular food? Is it related to emotional stress? Is there vomiting? Does the emesis contain blood or bile? Is the client jaundiced? What does the client do for these problems? How does it help?

The history should include questions about past or current health problems that might interfere with nutrition. These may include problems with mobility, sensory losses, limited self-care activities, pain, anxiety, confusion, allergies, injuries, nutritional deficits, metabolic problems, and self-concept related to body size and weight.

The nurse can also determine the risk for health problems that interfere with nutrition. A health hazard appraisal (see Chapter 5) can be used to acquire this information.

Developmental history

Neonate. Eating is one of the first activities of the neonate, and he obtains nutrition from his mother's breast or a bottle by reflexes that enable him to find the nipple (rooting), grasp it (sucking), and swallow. Because the stomach capacity is small, the neonate will need to be fed every 3 to 4 hours. Peristalsis is not firmly established, and regurgitation of the feeding is not unusual.

Feeding patterns. When it has been established that the neonate possesses intact swallowing reflexes and respiratory passages, the nurse or mother may offer the neonate his first feeding. Sterile water may be given 4 to 6 hours after feeding, although some advocate a 10% glucose-water solution for the first feeding because it is easy to swallow, and should the neonate aspirate, it is not irritating to respiratory mucosa. Others permit breast- or formula-feeding.

Breast-feeding. Most authorities currently recommend breast feeding up to 12 months, unless there are special problems.

The first supply of breast milk, *colostrum,* is thin and watery and contains carbohydrates to nourish the newborn until the supply of true breast milk appears on the third of fourth day after delivery. Breast milk contains more carbohydrates and vitamins A and C than cow's milk, as well as antibodies to protect the neonate from allergies, pathogenic strains of *E coli,* and possibly mumps, influenza, and other diseases.

The nurse may need to help the mother with the first few feedings, especially if this is her first experience with breast-feeding. The mother should be relaxed and comfortable; some women prefer a side-lying position, but others are more comfortable supported in Fowler's position. The newborn should have a full grasp on the nipple, but the mother's breast should not press against his nostril (Fig. 17-1).

The baby should empty both breasts during the feeding. Most of the milk is obtained during the first 5 to 10 minutes of nursing, and although additional nursing time is pleasurable for the baby, the feeding time should not exceed 20 to 30 minutes.

The baby should be bubbled midway during the feeding to allow swallowed air to be expelled. To bubble the baby, he may be held in a sitting position on the mother's lap while she gently pats his back. This position allows the mother to observe the baby and prevents aspiration of regurgitated feedings. Some mothers may prefer putting the baby across one shoulder and patting him on the back. If the mother bubbles the baby in this manner, she should observe him frequently.

Formula-feeding. Feeding the neonate with a cow's milk formula is an alternative to breast-feeding. Because the digestive tract is immature, most physicians recommend a diluted cow's milk formula, but others may prefer undiluted whole or skim milk. Cow's milk formulas contain three times as much protein and calcium as breast milk, but both types of feeding meet nutritional needs of the neonate.

Several types of commercial formulas are available, and the physician will usually suggest one for the mother to use. These formulas may be prepackaged and need only to be warmed and fed to the baby; others come in a powdered form

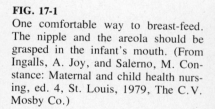

FIG. 17-1
One comfortable way to breast-feed. The nipple and the areola should be grasped in the infant's mouth. (From Ingalls, A. Joy, and Salerno, M. Constance: Maternal and child health nursing, ed. 4, St. Louis, 1979, The C.V. Mosby Co.)

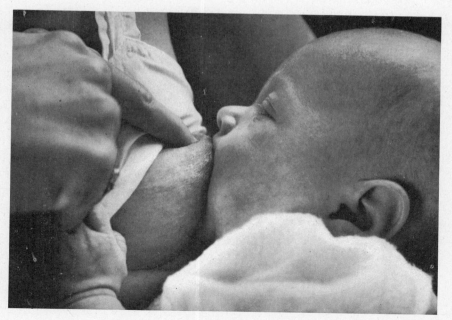

and are prepared by adding water. Commercial formulas, although slightly more expensive than preparing the formula from canned, evaporated, or dried milk, are simple, safe, and convenient to use.

Some families, however, may wish to prepare a formula from evaporated milk. Because the cow's milk protein is difficult for the neonate to digest, the milk is usually diluted with water. A source of carbohydrate must be added to the milk to furnish sufficient calories for growth. There are several ways to prepare the formula, but all are done to avoid contamination and all must be refrigerated to prevent bacterial growth.

If the client has an uncontaminated water supply, it is possible to use a clean technique for formula preparation. The bottles can be cleaned with soap and water and the can of milk or formula washed. Before formula preparation the preparer should wash the hands. To make one 4-ounce bottle of formula, 2 ounces of milk or formula is poured into the bottle and 2 ounces of water added. This bottle must be used in 30 minutes. Some parents prefer to make a day's supply of formula, and several bottles can be prepared at one time and refrigerated.

Although rarely done, formula can be prepared and then sterilized. The terminal method of sterilization is described.

The contents of a 13-ounce can of evaporated milk are added to 26 ounces of water and 2 tablespoons of corn syrup. The formula is mixed in a clean bowl and poured into clean bottles, which are topped with a nipple and nipple guard. The bottles are placed in a sterilizer or a large covered pot with a rack in the bottom. The bottle tops should be put on tightly and then unscrewed one-quarter turn to allow escape of air that accumulates during sterilization. The sterilizer should be filled halfway with water and brought to an active boil for 25 minutes. When the formula has cooled, it is refrigerated until time for use. The mother should plan to make enough formula for 1 day plus an extra feeding that can be used until the next formula is prepared. The average newborn consumes about 2 to 3 ounces of formula per pound (0.5 kg) of body weight each day.

Bottle feedings are usually offered to the baby at body temperature, although some physicians advocate the feeding of milk as it comes from the refrigerator. After warming the bottle in a pan of water, the mother should shake a few drops of the feeding on the inner aspect of her wrist to test the temperature. At this time the mother can check the holes in the nipple for the ease with which the formula comes from the bottle. When the bottle is shaken gently, a few drops of formula should appear. Nipples with holes that are too small or too large make feeding frustrating and should be changed.

Feeding techniques for the baby who is formula-fed are similar to those for the breast-fed baby. The baby should be held in an upright position next to the mother to promote closeness and security, as well as to prevent otitis media, which occurs more frequently if the baby is fed in a recumbent position. At no time should the bottle be propped and the baby left alone to feed; the baby could choke and aspirate the formula into his lungs. The baby should be bubbled after every 1 to 3 ounces of formula. Many fathers enjoy feeding their babies and should be given an opportunity to participate in this experience.

Weight gain. Weight gain is a useful measurement of nutrition in the neonate. Normally the neonate loses 5% to 10% of his birth weight because of limited initial feedings and loss of meconium, but he should regain this weight in 2 weeks and continue to gain 6 to 8 ounces a week. Some parents believe that fat babies are cute or healthy and may tend to overfeed their child. The parents should be encouraged to keep the baby within a normal range of weight gain.

Infant. During infancy the need for nutrition is particularly crucial to support periods of rapid growth and maturation. The gastrointestinal tract is able to handle more complex forms of food, and solid foods can be included in the diet to provide proteins, vitamins, and calories for growth. In the middle of the first year, teeth begin to erupt, and the infant is able to eat foods that must be chewed. The infant also becomes more coordinated in his motor abilities and will indicate a desire to be more independent in his feeding by holding his bottle and food.

Infancy is a critical period of lipocyte (fat cell) development. The diet should contain nutrients and calories for growth, but emphasis must be given to avoid overfeeding and creating an environment for obesity. Most infants are not developmentally ready for solid foods until about 3 months and will push the food out of their mouths. Furthermore, the gastrointestinal tract is immature, and allergy is likely.

Feeding patterns. Each physician has his own preference for including foods in the diet and using vitamin and mineral supplements to provide essentials for growth, but solid foods are usually offered after the first 3 to 6 months of life. The foods that will be added to the infant's diet can be prepared by blenderizing and straining cooked table foods, or they may be purchased in prepared form at the grocery store. Sugar or salt should not be added to the foods.

Cereal is usually the first solid food offered. The cereal should be prepared by diluting it with formula or milk and fed to the infant on a small spoon that is placed at the back of the tongue. The infant will make many movements with his tongue while he is learning to swallow solid foods, and much of the feeding may be spit out. This does not mean that he does not like the food, and parents must be patient while the infant gains the muscle control necessary to swallow easily. The cereal should not be given in the bottle, since this will not give the infant an opportunity to learn to eat from a spoon. For the first feedings, 1 to 2 teaspoons of cereal are sufficient, and the amount is increased to ¼ cup by the time the infant is 1 year old.

Other solid foods are added gradually and may include meats, fruits and vegetables, and egg yolk. Egg whites are not offered until the child is 1 year old because many children are allergic to the complex protein in egg white. A teaspoon of each new food should be introduced at the beginning of the meal so that the infant can become used to a new food taste. If the infant refuses the food the first time, it should be offered on another day. Refusal does not usually mean the child does not like the food. The mother should wait about a week between the offering of each new food so that she can observe the infant for intolerance such as diarrhea or a skin rash.

Fluids are important in the infant's diet, and water or juices should be offered frequently. Orange juice, which is offered at 4 to 6 months, is a good source of vitamin C and should be given daily. The juice should be strained and diluted with water. When fluids are given with meals, it is best to give the solid foods first so that the infant does not become sated with fluids. Fluids are particularly important in conditions of excessive perspiration, fever, or fluid loss from diarrhea.

Nursing process for common health problems

When the infant is 6 to 9 months old, he begins to show interest in self-feeding. At this time he can grasp objects, and hand-to-mouth coordination improves. Parents should encourage this activity by giving the infant finger foods such as crackers or soft raw fruits and vegetables. Initial attempts at self-feeding are usually messy, and the parents may wish to put newspapers or a sheet of plastic under the infant's chair.

Weaning from the bottle or breast begins when the infant is 6 to 9 months old and can hold a cup. Weaning is a gradual process and should be comfortable for the parents and baby. At this time the infant is usually given homogenized milk, and the cup should be offered in the morning when the infant is rested and interested in a new activity. Some mothers may wish to purchase training cups that have spouts or special lips to make the transition from sucking to drinking easier. Soft plastic cups may also be used, and they should be filled with a small amount of milk to avoid spilling. The mother should be prepared for spills and accidents while the infant is mastering this skill. As the infant gains proficiency in using the cup, the bottle or breast feedings are gradually omitted, and by the time the child is 12 to 18 months old, he should drink all fluids from a cup.

Weight gain. The weight gain of the infant can be used as a guide for the amount of food served to him. Generally the infant doubles his birth weight in 6 months and triples it in a year. If the muscles are firm and the infant appears alert, he is probably receiving adequate nutrition. Parents should be more concerned with safety than weight gain and must be cautioned against overfeeding and worrying about weight gain.

Dentition. Teeth begin to erupt when the infant is about 6 months old. Usually the lower incisors are the first to appear and are followed by the upper incisors. Teething may be accompanied by drooling, painful swelling of the gums, nausea, vomiting, diarrhea, or a slight fever. Often, chewing on teething crackers or clean, soft rubber toys will ease the eruption of the teeth. If there is unusual pain or a fever, the physician may prescribe topical anesthetics, aspirin, or acetaminophen (Tylenol) to alleviate these discomforts.

Toddler and preschooler. Metabolism and growth needs slowly diminish during early childhood. The toddler and preschooler are more interested in mastering their environment than in eating. Parents should not be concerned with this decrease in appetite and lack of interest in food. When the lateral incisors, cuspids, and molars erupt, additional chewing surfaces are provided, and the variety of foods the child eats can be expanded. The child is also more coordinated and able to feed himself.

Feeding patterns. The young child usually enjoys a variety of foods and may be fed simple foods that are prepared for the rest of the family. The child may exhibit food preferences, but if he is consistently offered a well-balanced diet, he should obtain adequate nutrition.

As finger dexterity improves, the child is able to use tableware to feed himself. When the child is about 15 months old, he can hold a spoon (Fig. 17-2). Using a knife and fork require more skill and should not be expected until the child is 4 or 5 years old.

Young children are great imitators and can learn table manners by observing their parents. Mealtime should be pleasant for the family, and even though accidents may happen, the young child can learn to be a part of the family at mealtime.

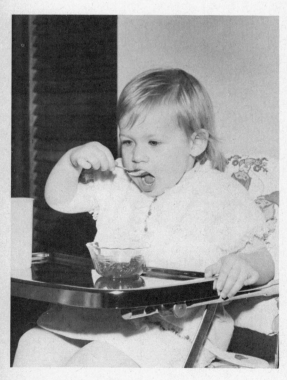

FIG. 17-2
Toddler gains skill in self-feeding.

Dentition. The teeth of the young child continue to erupt in an orderly pattern, but variations are not unusual, and the parents should not be concerned over differences between children. When the child is about 1 year old, his first molars appear; at age 18 months the canines or eyeteeth appear; and at age 2 the second set of molars will begin to come in. The total set of deciduous teeth (baby teeth) includes eight incisors and eight molars, and the first dentition is completed when the child is from 2 to 3 years old.

School-age child. During the school-age years, eating is one of the less important activities in the child's busy life. Eating at school or with friends may expose the child to new forms of food, and the variety in the diet and the complexity of the food increases. The school-age child goes through periods of losing the primary dentition, which is replaced with permanent teeth, and his appetite may diminish during these times.

Feeding patterns. Most school children obtain nutrition from three main meals during the day. Some of these meals may be eaten at school where lunch and/or breakfast programs are offered. The meals that are served at school are planned to provide one third of the daily food needs, and the parent should be aware of the need for meals served at home.

Dentition. The permanent teeth begin to erupt when the child is about 6 years old, with the first permanent molars appearing. Other teeth usually fill the mouth in the same way the primary dentition did, with incisors being replaced first and molars erupting later. Usually the deciduous teeth are lost by age 10, and the permanent teeth gradually complete the secondary dentition.

Adolescent and young adult. Adolescence is marked by an increase in metabolism and growth. Extra calories and protein are required to meet these changing needs. The diet during adolescence provides the basis for adult health and should include food from the basic four food groups. The diet should be supplemented by nutritious snacks rather than empty calories such as are found in colas, french fries, and sweets.

The diet of the teenage girl is particularly important because it must provide iron that is lost during menstruation as well as lay the foundation for pregnancy and lactation. Some girls will become pregnant during adolescence and early adulthood, and they should be prepared for this experience by obtaining a well-balanced diet throughout adolescence.

Feeding patterns. The adolescent may seem to eat all the time; his appetite is good, and he needs the nutrition to support growth. Eating may take on social significance, and the teenager likes to eat out and snack with his friends. Parents should provide plenty of nutritious snacks and not deny food to the growing adolescent.

Most adolescents are concerned with their appearance and are not inclined to overeat. Girls who control their weight by various forms of dieting should be sure that they are not eliminating essential food elements as they count calories. The adolescent may also be concerned with the appearance of his complexion, and since the sebaceous glands are overactive at this time, some recommend limiting the fat content in the diet.

Dentition. In addition to the permanent teeth that erupted during the school-age years, two more sets of molars fill the mouth. These molars appear early in adolescence and later as a young adult. These last molars are called "wisdom teeth" and complete the set of 32 permanent teeth.

Nursing process for common health problems

Adult. Metabolism decreases 5% to 8% every 10 years during the adult years, and the need for calories is not as great as it was during adolescence and young adulthood. The adult may find it difficult to adjust to the need to reduce caloric intake, and many adults become overweight.

Feeding patterns. Eating is a social activity for many adults, and the meals may be planned around employment hours or may be a form of relaxation for the adult. It is still important to have three or more meals a day, and the adult who misses a meal on a busy day is not meeting his needs for nutrition.

Older adult. Gastrointestinal activity slows with age; fewer gastric juices are produced, and peristalsis is slowed. The sense of taste and smell may become less acute, and many older persons must have carious teeth extracted. These physiological changes, combined with chronic illness or living alone, may make eating unappealing. Although metabolism continues to decrease each decade, the older person still must be assured of an intake of basic nutrients to support cell life.

Feeding patterns. Mealtime may be more flexible for the older person who is retired and does not have deadlines to meet. It is often an effort, however, for him to prepare adequate meals. He may be on a limited budget or unable to go out and shop for groceries. Many older persons live alone and simply do not prepare meals for themselves. Because it is important to maintain nutrition during the aging years (particularly to meet the need for protein, vitamins A, C, and D, and calcium), older persons may consider using community agencies, grocery stores, and food services that deliver hot and cold meals to the home.

Dentition. Many older persons have teeth that are carious or loosened by diseased gums and must be extracted. The extracted teeth should be replaced with partial or complete dentures so that digestion is aided by the ability to chew. The alveolar bone may atrophy, and if the older person has dentures, they should be refitted periodically so that they do not irritate the gums.

Social history   Eating and nutrition patterns are highly influenced by social factors of economic status, religious beliefs, eating habits and food preferences, and cultural or ethnic traditions. The nurse should ascertain to what extent these factors influence the client's nutritional status.

Economic influences. Economic factors are the most significant variable impinging on eating habits and food preferences.[20] The client's economic status not only dictates the money available for food purchases, it also determines membership in a socioeconomic class where values for nutrition influence the type of food eaten. Persons in lower economic groups, for example, often eat foods to satisfy physiological needs, whereas to those who are more affluent, food represents social status, and eating is an activity to be shared and enjoyed. In lower income brackets the food budget may represent as much as one fourth of the total income, whereas families with larger incomes generally spend proportionately less income on food purchases. Value for nutrition in lower socioeconomic groups is often oriented toward high carbohydrate diets of snack foods, and obesity is not considered a detriment to physical attractiveness or health. Individuals in middle and upper socioeconomic class on the other hand tend to value leaness, even though the diet may be higher in alcohol and fats that may contribute to cardiovascular disease and cirrhosis.

Religious influences. Religion also plays an important factor in food consumption. Holidays are often times for eating traditional foods and celebrating

892

TYPICAL FOOD CUSTOMS AND METHODS OF COOKING USED BY VARIOUS RACIAL AND NATIONAL GROUPS

Greek

Frying is a common method of cooking. Vegetables are often fried or baked in oil. No gravy is served.

Hearty main dishes are:

Lamb, vegetables, rice, or cracked wheat.

Soup containing meat or legumes and other vegetables.

Vegetables such as eggplant, green pepper, or squash stuffed with ground meat, rice, or cracked wheat.

Green salads served with oil dressings are popular.

Lemon is often added to soup.

Fruit is a common dessert.

Italian

Vegetables are often cooked in oil. Olive oil is preferred though some Italians mix it with other oils or use olive oil for salad dressings only.

Parboiled vegetables are often fried in oil or simmered in tomato sauce.

Meat is frequently fried or served with tomato sauce.

Cheese, legumes, tomatoes, greens, and oil are the foundation of many dishes.

Creamed soups are not common.

Minestrone is a nourishing soup made with legumes and a variety of fresh vegetables such as cabbage, onions, peas, and string beans.

Milk puddings and custards are seldom used.

Fruit is a common dessert.

Jewish (Orthodox)

No pork, ham, or bacon may be used.

Meat must be killed and cooked according to kosher law. Meat is boiled, cooked with vegetables, or roasted. Orthodox Jews do not use meat and dairy products at the same meal. The hind quarter of any animal is never used. Meat soups are used.

Poultry is usually eaten on Sabbath eve.

Any fish without scales or fins is prohibited. Fish is fried or boiled. Gifilte fish is chopped fish, seasoned and boiled. No gravy is served.

Vegetables are usually cooked with meat and soups.

Borscht, a beet soup containing sour cream, is common.

Meat must be soaked ½ hour, be drained and salted once, and be allowed to drain on a perforated board 1 hour to remove any remaining blood.

Milk may not be taken 3 to 6 hours after meat has been eaten. This means that children may have to take half of their milk in the middle of the morning or afternoon.

Sweet butter is commonly used.

Sour cream is used on cottage cheese and vegetables. To reduce cost, evaporated milk clotted with lemon juice may be recommended.

Mexican

Chili peppers, both green and red, are frequently used to season vegetables and meat. Hot vegetable sauces are used on meats, beans, and eggs.

The common form of bread is the tortilla made from corn meal or wheat flour; it is a broad, flat cake cooked on top of a stove or hot plate and served at every meal. A tortilla is used as a spoon or ladle to scoop up a chili dish.

Enchiladas are commonly used. Cheese and chopped onion are sprinkled on tortillas and then a thickened hot chili sauce is poured over them.

Frijoles or pinto beans are cooked with salt pork and oregano.

Chili con carne served on rice is well liked.

Eggs are scrambled with tomatoes, minced onion, minced green pepper, and chili powder.

Lentils, tomatoes, onions, and eggs furnish a hearty hot dish.

Black

Vegetables are cooked with salt pork, ham, or bacon; the liquid in which they are cooked (called potlikker) is served with the vegetables, thus conserving vitamins and minerals.

Fat is used very liberally in the diet.

Crisp diced salt pork is often served with cream gravy.

Bacon is used often.

Hot breads are very popular.

Since rice is a favorite food, the use of brown rice or restored rice should be encouraged.

Sweets are used frequently, often to the exclusion of other health-protecting foods.

Canned fruit cocktail and canned peaches are favorite fruits.

Polish

Milk and sour cream are used in soup. Sour cream is served on potatoes and other vegetables.

Cottage cheese is used in dumplings and cheese cakes.

Vegetables are overcooked. Frequently they are served in soup or boiled and served with hot milk.

Meat is usually cooked in soup or with vegetables or put into dumplings. Meat is sometimes tied in cabbage leaves and simmered in tomato sauce.

Soups and one-dish meals are popular.

Few desserts are prepared.

Many bakery goods such as sweet rolls, coffee cake, doughnuts, and cookies are used.

Chinese

Vegetables are not eaten raw; they are cut into bite-size pieces and cooked quickly, only long enough to sterilize them, and then they are served immediately. Little water is used, but the water in which vegetables are cooked is not discarded. Vegetables are often steamed.

A large amount of vegetable is frequently combined with a small amount of pork, chicken, fish, or eggs.

Young green peas in pods are cooked. The whole pod is served.

The favorite methods of meat cookery are steaming, braising, roasting, and frying.

Sweet-and-sour pork is a favorite food. Vinegar added to meat extracts calcium from the bones. The liquid is consumed along with the meat.

Meat is cut into small pieces and never served in large pieces.

Green peppers are often stuffed with fish.

Japanese

Japanese methods of cooking are similar to Chinese methods. Meat is cut in thin slivers and fried with onion. A small amount of water and a large amount of vegetables are added. It is then cooked a short time.

Sometimes raw egg is dropped on rice. It is then seasoned with soya sauce.

Very few sweets are used. Cakes made of soy beans or lima beans are colored and sweetened with sugar.

Adapted from You're you . . . and that's beautiful! Copyright © 1973 by the American National Red Cross. Reprinted with permission.

893

Nursing process for common health problems

TABLE 17-1
Cultural food patterns

Food group	Mexican/Spanish	Black	American Indian	Puerto Rican	Chinese
Milk	Milk (fresh, dry, evaporated) Cheese (not all kinds) Flan (sweet custard) Ice cream	Milk (homogenized, dry, evaporated) Buttermilk Ice cream Pudding (bread, rice, chocolate) Cheese	Milk (fresh, evaporated) Ice cream Cream pies	Milk Cheese	Milk (usually flavored until taste develops)
Meat Poultry Eggs Legumes Fish/seafood	Beef Lamb Pork (salt pork often) Chicken Fish/seafood Eggs Tripe Frankfurters Nuts Dry beans (black, pinto) Chick peas Lentils	Beef Lamb Fat meat Salt pork Bacon Pork Chitterlings Neck bones Pigs' feet and tails Tripe Chicken Turkey Duck Goose Fish (fresh and canned) Eggs Nuts Peas (black-eyed, cow, chick) Beans (navy, red, pinto) Peanut butter Game (rabbit, venison)	Beef Pork Lamb Chicken Duck Turkey Goose Fish (fresh and canned) Shellfish Eggs Legumes—beans (red, white, black), black-eyed peas, sunflower seeds Walnuts Acorns Pine nuts Peanut butter Rabbit	Pork Ham Bacon Chicken Eggs Codfish/shellfish Beans (navy, kidney, and dry) Pigeon peas	Pork Fish/shellfish Duck Chicken Organ meats Eggs Soy beans Nuts (almonds) Beans (red, black) Split peas Bean curd (tofu) Pork sausage Bean sprouts
Vegetable and fruit	Leafy greens (fresh): Spinach Wild greens Green beans Peas Green peppers Cactus leaves Lettuce Cabbage Celery Onions Corn Sweet potatoes Carrots Pumpkin Summer squash Tomatoes Beets Red peppers Radishes Garlic Melon Plums	Leafy greens (fresh): Wild greens Spinach Mustard greens Beet tops Collards Chard Turnip greens String beans Peas Green peppers Cabbage Pumpkin Yellow squash Carrots Corn Turnips Potatoes (sweet and white) Onions Beets Tomatoes Radishes	Leafy greens (fresh): Dandelion Mustard Watercress Green beans Peas Lettuce Cucumber Yellow squash Pumpkin Carrots Eggplant Onions Cabbage (raw and cooked) Turnips (cooked) Potatoes (sweet and white) Beets Tomatoes Oranges Grapefruit Melons	Leafy greens (fresh): Mustard greens Turnip Spinach Collards Broccoli Lettuce Okra String beans Kale Peppers Cabbage Celery root Celery Eggplant Onions Potatoes Squash Sweet potatoes Pimiento Beets Tomatoes Oranges	Leafy greens (fresh): Bok choy (Chinese mustard) Others Green peppers Peas in pod Green beans Cucumbers Watercress Chinese cabbage Okra Celery White turnips Mushrooms Eggplant Bamboo shoots Soybean sprouts Summer squash Tomatoes Fruits (not often): Oranges Melons Papaya

Adapted from You're you . . . and that's beautiful! Copyright © 1973 by The American National Red Cross. Reprinted with permission.

Japanese	Jewish	Italian	Greek	Polish
Milk—younger generation	Milk Sour cream Cottage cheese Cream cheese Swiss cheese Other cheeses	Milk—young people primarily Italian cheeses Cottage cheese	Milk—sweet fermented Goat's milk cheese	Milk—sweet fermented Sour cream Cottage cheese
Pork Beef Fish/shellfish Chicken Soy beans Soy cake Red beans Lima beans Tofu Eggs Nuts Bean sprouts	All meats (no pork if Orthodox) Liver Chicken Turkey Duck Goose Eggs Fish/shellfish (no shellfish for Orthodox) Split peas Kidney beans Lentils Chick peas Nuts	Lamb Pork Beef Veal Organs Sausage Veal loaf Chicken Duck Eggs Fish/shellfish Split peas	Lamb Some beef Pork (little) Chicken Duck Eggs Fish/seafood Split peas Beans (navy, pinto) Chick peas Nuts	Lamb Sausage Other meats Organs Tongue Tripe Chicken Duck Eggs Fish Pigeon peas

Leafy greens (fresh):
  Spinach
String beans
Cabbage
Cucumber
Celery
Potatoes (limited amount)
Eggplant
Mushrooms
Yellow squash
Carrots
Tomatoes
Radishes
Pickled vegetables (as dessert)
Oranges
Tangerines
Grapefruit
Plums
	Green peppers
	Peas
	Endive
	Lettuce
	Cabbage
	Turnips
	Sauerkraut
	Onions
	Eggplant
	Garlic
	Carrots
	Corn
	Tomatoes
	Oranges
	Lemons
	Grapefruit
	Limes
	Berries
	Other fruits
		Leafy greens (fresh):
		  Spinach
		  Escarole
		  Chicory
		Green peppers
		String beans
		Broccoli
		Okra
		Zucchini
		Eggplant
		Cabbage
		Onions
		Celery
		Garlic
		Tomatoes
		Oranges
		Lemons
		Grapefruit
		Raisins
		Other fruits and berries
			Leafy greens (fresh):
			  Spinach
			  Turnip greens
			  Chicory
			  Dandelion greens
			Broccoli
			String beans
			Parsley
			Green peppers
			Leeks
			Eggplant
			Tomatoes
			Onions
			Potatoes
			Garlic
			Oranges
			Lemons
			Others
				Leafy greens (fresh):
				  Spinach
				  Kale
				Broccoli
				Green peppers
				String beans
				Cabbage
				Lettuce
				Turnips
				Sauerkraut
				Onions
				Carrots
				Squash
				Beets
				Potatoes
				Some citrus
				Other fruits and berries

Continued.

TABLE 17-1, cont'd

Cultural food patterns

Food group	Mexican/Spanish	Black	American Indian	Puerto Rican	Chinese
	Apricots	Oranges	Strawberries	Lemons	
	Peaches	Melon	Grapes	Grapefruit	
	Guava fruit	Lemons	Bananas	Canned pears	
	Oranges/lemons/limes	Strawberries	Peaches	Canned fruit cocktail	
	Fruit cocktail	Grapes	Pears	Bananas	
	Papaya	Bananas	Apples		
	Cactus fruit	Peaches	Pineapple		
	Zapote (a fruit)	Pineapple	Fruit cocktail		
	Bananas	Apples			
	Apples	Fruit cocktail			
	Fruit juices (other than grapefruit/orange)				
Cereals	Cornmeal	Rice	Cream of Wheat	Rolled oats	Rice
	Oatmeal	Hominy/grits	Oatmeal	Rice	Millet
	Rice	Cornmeal	Rice	White bread	Oats
	Spaghetti/macaroni	Farina	Dry cereals		Wheat
	Noodles	Oatmeal	White bread		Noodles (egg/rice)
	Biscuits	Spaghetti	Whole wheat bread		Macaroni
	Sweet bread	Cream of Wheat	Cornbread		Rice cakes
	Tortilla	Dry cereals	Biscuits		White bread
	Bread (white and cornmeal)	Hot breads	Pancakes		Rice flour
		Sweet rolls			
		Biscuits			
		Cornbread			
Fats	Olive oil	Bacon		Lard	Lard
	Chicken fat	Salt pork		Bacon fat	Peanut oil
		Lard			
		Butter			
Sweets	Custard type cooking	Syrup/molasses		Sugar in coffee	Preserved fruits
		Sweets		Fruit paste	Candied fruits
		Fried pies		Ice cream	Almond cakes
				(Few desserts)	
Beverages	Black coffee	Tea		Coffee	Tea
	Wine	Coffee			
		Carbonated drinks			
		Powdered drink mixes			
		Lemonade			

occasions with festive eating. For some, religious traditions determine foods that cannot be eaten. Orthodox Jews, for example, do not eat pork. Catholic dietary laws are becoming more liberal, but some still prefer to abstain from meat on Fridays and other religious occasions. Consideration should be given to the client's religious preferences when meals are planned, particularly where diet modification is required.

Eating habits and food preferences. Individuals' attitudes or values about nutrition influence what is eaten and when. Some individuals may eat three meals a day, with the main meal at noon; others prefer the main meal in the evening or prefer to eat several small meals. Clients who work may have a variable

Japanese	Jewish	Italian	Greek	Polish
Rice	Oatmeal	Cornmeal	Cornmeal	Rice
Rice cakes	Rice	Farina	Oatmeal	Hominy
Crackers	Barley	Spaghetti	Cornbread	Cornmeal
Noodles	Farina	Whole wheat bread	White bread	Farina
White bread	Buckwheat (kasha)	Italian white		Oatmeal
	Wheat cereal	bread		Spaghetti
	Noodles			Cornbread
	Breads (rye, white, egg)			Hot bread
	Matzo			Sweet rolls
	White rolls			
	Butter	Olive oil	Olive oil	Bacon fat
	Vegetable fats/oil	Butter	Chicken fat	Salt pork
	Chicken fat	Margarine		Lard
		Others		Butter
Soybean cakes	Honey	Few sweets	Custard type puddings	Syrup/molasses
Pickled vegetables	Cheesecake	Puddings		Sweets
(instead of desserts)	Strudel	Spumoni		Fried pies
	Honey cakes			
Tea	Coffee	Coffee	Black coffee	Tea
	Tea	Dry wine		Coffee
	Carbonated drinks			Carbonated drinks
				Prepared drink mixes
				Lemonade

schedule and difficult access to food. Many eat in cafeterias or at fast-food restaurants, and the nurse should interview the client as to his eating habits during these times.

Food preferences are also important in meal selection. Some prefer vegetarian meals; others may have dislikes of certain foods. The nurse, when taking a diet history, should elicit this information and determine if the diet contributes to adequate nutrition. Of particular concern are individuals who eat strictly vegetarian diets, food faddists, or those who give a history of *pica* (habitual, compulsive eating of nonfood substances), because these individuals may not be obtaining adequate nutrients.

Nursing process for common health problems

Cultural and ethnic influences. Selection and preparation of food is learned in the context of a social environment and is therefore tied to the client's culture and ethnic heritage. The nurse should be cognizant of the client's cultural or ethnic menus and use these as a basis for diet counseling and meal planning; several are identified in the following material and Table 17-1.

Psychological history

The client's psychological state and coping patterns are often intricately tied to eating and nutrition, and therefore the nurse should determine the client's mental status, level of understanding about nutrition, coping patterns that may relate to food intake, as well as the presence of anxiety or illness that might interfere with nutrition.

Throughout the nursing history the nurse should determine the client's mental status. Alertness or lethargy exhibited by the client may relate to adequacy of nutrition. Lethargy and inappropriate cognition can be caused by malnutrition.

The nurse should also determine the client's understanding about nutrition and the components of a well-balanced diet, and the meaning food has to the client. This information is useful in determining the potential for nutrition instruction for maintaining wellness.

The psychological history can also be used to determine the client's coping patterns. Some use food and alcohol as coping resources and may eat compulsively or drink to excess. Others, in depression, may not eat sufficiently. Weight loss in adolescent girls, for example, may be indicative of *anorexia nervosa,* extreme weight loss from refusal to eat.

Anxiety or illness as influences on nutrition. Persons who experience temporary or chronic anxiety or who are in varying states of illness may have disruptions of hunger or appetite. Anxiety may increase or decrease hunger sensations, and there may be increases or decreases in salivation, production of gastric juices, and gastric motility. Individuals who are ill may be in pain, may have nausea, or may be required to abstain from food before diagnostic studies or surgery. Ill persons may have interferences with olfactory inputs or oral structures that further inhibit the desire to eat. Nursing interventions such as caring for the mouth before meals, arranging food attractively, serving favorite foods, modifying the social milieu at mealtime, and removing displeasing sights and odors are appropriate to encourage these individuals to obtain optimal nutrition.

Physical assessment

Physical assessment includes *inspection, auscultation, palpation,* and *percussion* of the client's abdomen and inspection and palpation of the mouth to determine deviations from normal mechanisms of ingestion and digestion. Data from the client's history, developmental stage, and social and psychological histories are used with information obtained from the physical assessment to determine the client's actual or potential health problems.

Before the physical examination the nurse should review data obtained from the nursing history and the results of relevant biochemical studies. The nurse should note the client's weight and height. Weight loss or gain of 10% in 1 year is significant, and even more significant if it has occurred in a shorter period of time. The nurse should ascertain that the weight gain is not edema, or that edema is not masking weight loss.

Anthropometric measurements provide estimates of muscle mass, protein and fat stores, and nutritional status[14,16,25] (Table 17-2). Using the nondom-

TABLE 17-2

Anthropometric measurements

Test	Gender	Normal values	Values showing malnutrition
Tricep skinfold (TSF)	Male	11-12.5 mm	7.5-11 mm
	Female	15-16.5 mm	10-15 mm
Mid upper arm circumference (MUAC)	Male	26-29 cm	20-26 cm
	Female	26-28.5 cm	20-26 cm
Arm muscle circumference (AMC)	Male	23-25 cm	16-23 cm
	Female	20-23 cm	14-20 cm

$$AMC = MUAC - 0.314 \times TSF$$

inant arm, the triceps skinfold thickness (TSF) can be measured to determine fat stores over the triceps. The skin is lifted at the midarm circumference and measured 1 cm below. The fold can be measured with calipers (Fig. 17-3) and compared with norms. The mid upper arm circumference (MUAC) represents fat and protein stores. With the arm hanging freely, the circumference is measured at the midpoint of the arm. The arm muscle circumference (AMC) reflects protein stores and is calculated by the following formula $AMC = MUAC - 0.314 \times TSF$. Measuring the head circumference of the neonate or infant indicates brain development, another parameter of nutritional health. The circumference is measured with the infant on his back, encircling the head with the tape measure at the largest circumference at the supraorbital ridges anteriorly and at the occiput posteriorly. Ranges are compared with norms for age and weight, with 31 cm to 37 cm considered normal.[16]

Biochemical studies of the blood and urine can be used to monitor nutritional health (see biochemical parameters, p. 900). Visceral protein status reflects the depletion of protein stores and is measured by serum albumin and serum transferrin levels. The total lymphocytic count can be obtained to determine immune competence, because lymphocyte synthesis depends on adequate nutrition. Nitrogen metabolism is assessed with the creatinine height index and the urinary urea nitrogen levels. These studies are particularly useful if malnutrition is suspected or if clients have health problems that impair nutrition.

Inspection. Inspection includes systematic observations of the client's appearance as it relates to nutritional health as well as inspection of the mouth and abdomen to differentiate normal appearance and health problems.

The general appearance of the client is a reflection of the nutritional health of the tissues. The hair should be shiny and thick. Hair that is dull, dry, sparse, stringy, or falls out easily may indicate nutritional deficiencies. The skin on the face should have normal turgor. Skin that is scaling or flaking may be caused by vitamin deficiencies. The lips should be moist and free of swelling or fissures. The nurse can inspect the client's hands and nails. Nails that are brittle, ridged, cracked, or clubbed may indicate long-standing malnutrition. The skeleton should be normal shape for the client's age; bow legs or beading on the costrocondral junction indicates rickets. Muscles can be inspected for tone and strength. Weakness or muscle wasting (the decreased proportion of muscle to subcutaneous fat) may reflect malnutrition. The general activity of the client should also be noted in terms of energy and attention span. Lethargic, apathetic individuals with reduced attention span may have nutritional anemias.

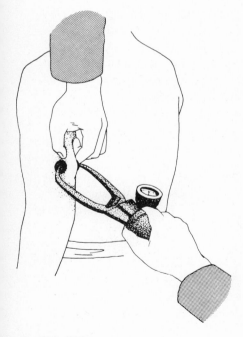

FIG. 17-3

Measuring triceps skinfold with calipers. (From Guthrie, Helen: Introductory nutrition, ed. 4, St. Louis, 1979, The C.V. Mosby Co.)

BIOCHEMICAL PARAMETERS OF NUTRITION

Studies	Values showing malnutrition
Visceral protein status	
Serum albumin	<3.0 g/100 mg
Transferrin	<150 mg/100 mg
Immune competence	
Total lymphocyte count	<1000/ml
PPD skin test	Delayed or absent response
Nitrogen metabolism	
BUN	<2 to 6
Creatinine height index	Decreases
UUN	24 hr. urine/determined by calorie intake

Inspection of the mouth should be done with a flashlight and tongue depressor to visualize the structures within the mouth. The mouth of the neonate should be inspected shortly after birth. The nurse should observe the neonate's lips and palate for clefts and ascertain that the tongue is freely movable. In subsequent appraisals the nurse should examine the tissues of the oral cavity for color, lubrication, bleeding, or presence of leukoplakia or lesions. The gums and mucous membranes should be pink and firm. In infants, white nodules on the alveolar margin are known as *Epstein's pearls* and are normal. The teeth, when they appear, should be observed for location and presence of caries. The gingiva should be attached to the tooth and firm. Receding, spongy, bleeding, or inflamed gingiva may be signs of malnutrition or poor oral care. The nurse can also note if the client has dentures or partial plates. The tongue should move easily and be free of swelling, rawness, lesions, or color changes indicative of disease. A shiny, smooth tongue, for example, is associated with niacin deficiency or pernicious anemia, whereas a tongue, palate, or inner aspect of the cheek with patches may be caused by a monilia infection (thrush).

Inspection of the abdomen is a part of the complete physical assessment. The client should be supine and the abdomen exposed. The abdominal muscles will be more relaxed if the client bends his knees. The abdomen can be demarcated for ease of description into four or nine sections. To mark the abdomen in quadrants, a horizontal line is drawn through the umbilicus; then a vertical line from the xiphoid to the symphysis pubis marks the left lower quadrant, the left upper quadrant, the right upper quadrant, and the right lower quadrant (Fig. 17-4).

The nurse inspects the skin on the trunk for color and surface characteristics such as contour and symmetry, noting the presence of distension or ascites. Abnormal color includes redness or inflamed areas, jaundice, pallor, bruises, or discolorations. The abdomen should be free of lesions or rashes. Distended veins, dilated blood vessels, or petechiae may indicate obstruction of portal circulation. Striae (stretch marks) occur when the abdomen is stretched and indicate weight gain followed by weight loss.

The nurse should also observe the abdomen for visible peristalsis. Strong peristaltic waves may be indicative of bowel obstruction or in infants of pyloric stenosis. The nurse can inspect the abdomen for hernias, which are likely to occur at the umbilicus or in the inguinal area.

Auscultation. Auscultation of the abdomen is performed to listen for the presence of peristaltic bowel sounds and vascular sounds. Auscultation precedes palpation or percussion, because these maneuvers increase gastrointestinal motility.

Bowel sounds are caused by air mixing with fluid during peristalsis, and the nurse listens for frequency, intensity, and pitch. Bowel sounds usually occur at a rate of 5 to 35 per minute. They increase if the client has diarrhea and decrease in the presence of paralytic ileus or obstruction. The intensity of the sounds describes the strength of peristalsis. The pitch of the sounds reflects the amount of tension in the intestinal wall. Normal sounds in the small intestine are described as high pitched and gurgling, whereas those in the large intestine are generally lower pitched and rumbling. Changes in pitch are caused by mechanical or physical obstruction.

To listen for bowel sounds, the nurse uses the diaphragm of the stethoscope

900

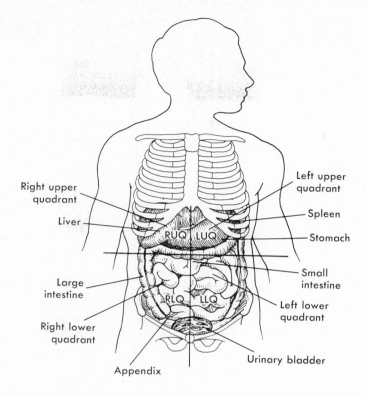

FIG. 17-4
Quadrants of the abdomen. Note organs
underlying each quadrant.

Right upper
quadrant

Liver

Large
intestine

Right lower
quadrant

Appendix

RUQ   LUQ

RLQ   LLQ

Left upper
quadrant

Spleen

Stomach

Small
intestine

Left lower
quadrant

Urinary bladder

to listen in each quadrant of the abdomen for 2 to 5 minutes starting at the lower left quadrant and moving counterclockwise. Because bowel sounds increase after eating, the examination is more accurate 1 to 2 hours after the meal.

Auscultation is also used to identify arteriovascular sounds around the epigastrium. *Bruits* (murmurs) may be heard using the bell of the stethoscope and are usually normal in the young, but may indicate arterial changes such as aneurysms in adults.

Percussion. The next step in the physical assessment is percussion of the abdomen. This is done to determine presence of air or fluid in the abdominal cavity and to identify the size and location of the organs, particularly the liver and spleen. A light tapping movement is used systematically in each quadrant. The sounds of percussion are tympany or dullness. Tympany is the sound made by a gastric bubble or air in the abdomen. Increases in fluid sound dull or flat. Percussion may reveal ascites or fluid-filled tumors, noted by flatness, or intestinal obstruction and paralytic ileus, noted by tympany. A full bladder produces dullness on percussion.

Palpation. Palpation of the abdomen is done to determine muscle tone, tenderness, size of organs, and the presence of masses. The nurse begins palpation by using a light touch with the pads of the finger tips and increases pressure in each of the four quadrants to note size and location of organs. Bimanual palpation techniques may be used to further identify the size and shape of the liver. The inguinal area and femoral areas should be palpated to identify hernias. The reader is referred to texts on physical assessment for further information on palpation of abdominal organs.

DIAGNOSTIC ASSESSMENT

Radiological assessment

Radiological examinations are used to determine location, size, and shape of the organs of the gastrointestinal system. They are usually performed before endoscopic procedures.

Teeth and mouth. Dental x-ray examinations are made to evaluate the carious lesions of the teeth, position of the teeth under the gums, surrounding soft tissue, and obstructions of the salivary glands. A topical anesthetic may be used if the gag reflex causes discomfort to the client.

Esophagus, stomach, and intestines. Radiopaque barium, which is swallowed by the client, can be used to locate inflammations, ulcerations, and obstructions in the esophagus, stomach, and intestines. Peristaltic activity can be observed under fluoroscopy while the barium is swallowed.

The client prepares for a gastrointestinal x-ray examination by abstaining from food or fluids for 8 hours. The client should also be instructed not to smoke or chew gum, because these can increase the amount of air in the stomach and intestines.

After swallowing the barium, the client is turned from his side to his back to promote gravity flow of the barium. Roentgenograms are taken at various intervals as the barium passes to the intestines. An *upper gastrointestinal series* includes x-ray films of the esophagus, stomach, and duodenum and usually takes 2 to 3 hours. A *lower gastrointestinal series* may be done 6 to 8 hours later, when the barium has passed to the small and large intestines.

Because these x-ray examinations take several hours, the client may be exhausted and should be permitted to rest. His diet should be ordered immediately; fluid loss, electrolyte imbalance, and dehydration may be serious in clients who eat nothing for 16 hours.

A cathartic is usually given when the examination is completed to promote expulsion of the barium. The client may notice that his stools have a chalky white color as the barium is eliminated and should not be alarmed. If the client does not defecate within 2 or 3 days, an enema may be ordered to prevent impaction.

Gallbladder and bile ducts. A *cholecystogram* (gallbladder series) is used to detect stones, tumors, or inflammation in the gallbladder. This examination depends on the radiographic dye's being concentrated by the gallbladder; if there is impairment of liver function and the bile is not released, a cholecystogram is not effective.

The evening before, the physician may order a low-fat or clear-liquid meal. Approximately 2 hours later the client takes a series of oral tablets (determined by his weight) that contain dye. Commonly used dyes are iopanoic acid (Telepaque), ipodate (Oragrafin) sodium, and iodoalphionic acid (Priodax). If the client vomits the dye, the physician may request that the tablets be given again, or he may give the dye intravenously immediately before the cholecystogram. After taking the dye, the client should not have anything more to eat. Fluids are usually not restricted unless other diagnostic studies are being performed at this time.

The morning of the examination, an enema may be given to stimulate expulsion of gas, which would obstruct visualization of the gallbladder. After an initial x-ray film, the client may be requested to consume a high-fat meal. The fat stimulates the gallbladder to release bile along the ducts, and if stones are present, they appear as densities. The common bile duct can also be ob-

902

served during the procedure. X-ray procedures vary in each facility, and the nurse should be cognizant of specific preparations for cholecystograms.

After the cholecystogram, the client may resume his usual activities. The dye is excreted in the urine, and the client should be instructed that he may experience temporary burning on urination until the dye is excreted. Some clients also experience abdominal cramping and diarrhea.

A *cholangiogram* is done to detect obstructions in the bile ducts. The dye is given intravenously or inserted through a needle, catheter, or T tube, which has been inserted in the common bile duct during surgery. An iodine dye is used for this examination, and the client may have an allergic reaction or experience chills and hot flashes and should be prepared for these sensations.

A *transhepatic percutaneous cholangiogram* is done to differentiate intrahepatic jaundice from extrahepatic jaundice. A needle is inserted through the abdomen into the main bile ducts of the liver. The bile is withdrawn, and the dye, which is inserted through the needle, perfuses the liver. The filling of the ducts is observed by fluoroscopy, and x-ray films are taken. After the procedure, the client is observed for signs of bleeding or bile leakage.

Endoscopic retrograde cholangiopancreatography. The pancreatic and bile ducts can also be directly visualized. The ducts are connected at the ampulla of vater. A flexible fiberscope is passed to the duodenum at the point of the ampulla. Dye may also be injected for radiographic examination.

Ultrasound. Ultrasound procedures (use of reflected sound waves) can be used to obtain an image of the liver, gallbladder, or pancreas. The client is prepared by evacuating the bowel by means of laxatives or enemas, and a sonar probe passes over the abdomen to record images.

Scans. A *liver scan* is a radionuclide procedure used to detect obstructions in the liver. A radioactive isotope such as colloidal technetium (^{99}Tc) or gallium citrate (^{67}Ga) is administered, and 30 to 60 minutes afterward, a scanner is passed over the liver. Obstructions appear as areas of increased uptake. No special radiation precautions are necessary, because only diagnostic doses of the isotopes are used. If gallium is used, the client should receive a laxative or enema after the test to clear the gastrointestinal tract and prevent absorption of the isotope.

A scan may also be done to detect obstructions in the *pancreas*. The procedure is similar to that for a liver scan.

Direct visualization procedures: endoscopy

Esophagoscopy, gastroscopy, duodenoscopy. The esophagus, stomach, and duodenum can be visualized by inserting a lighted tubular instrument (esophagoscope, gastroscope, fiber gastroscope, or duodenofibroscope) into these body cavities for the purpose of observing the mucosa, removing foreign bodies, or obtaining tissue or secretions for biopsy and analysis. Although these procedures are not painful, the client may be frightened by the size of the equipment, and the nurse can offer explanations about the procedure.

The visualization of the esophagus, stomach, and duodenum is done 6 to 8 hours after the client has fasted. Before the tube is passed, the client is given an anticholinergic drug to decrease oral and gastric secretions, and a sedative or narcotic may be given if the client is apprehensive. Dentures should be removed, and the client may be more comfortable in a hospital gown. Immediately before the instrument is passed, a topical anesthetic is sprayed onto the oral cavity to inhibit the gag reflex. The client should expectorate the anesthetic into an emesis basin so that it is not swallowed. As the tube is passed, the client can be encouraged to take deep breaths to overcome the urge to gag.

Immediately before the procedure the client should be properly positioned. If the esophagus is to be visualized, the client is recumbent on the examination table and his head and shoulders extend slightly over the table. If the stomach and duodenum are to be examined the client may lay on his right side.

When the procedure is completed, the client should not have anything to eat or drink until the gag reflex returns, in about 4 hours. The nurse can test for the return of the gag reflex by touching the back of the throat with a cotton swab or tongue depressor. Ice packs, saline gargles, throat lozenges, and aspirin may be ordered to relieve discomfort from local trauma. The procedure is exhausting, and the nurse and client should plan for rest.

Peritonoscopy. A peritonoscopy is a special procedure that permits direct visualization of the anterior surface of liver, gallbladder, and parts of the mesentery. In this procedure tumors and obstructions can be identified and a biopsy specimen taken without exploratory surgery. After the abdomen has been cleansed and a local anesthetic given, an instrument is inserted through an incision in the abdomen to permit visualization of the abdominal organs. When the procedure is completed, the nurse must observe the client for bleeding for 24 hours, and the vital signs should be taken every 15 minutes for the first 4 hours and then every 4 hours thereafter.

Biopsies

Biopsies are performed to obtain tissue for microscopic examination. They may be obtained during direct visualization procedures, at the time of exploratory surgery, or by passing nasogastric or gastrointestinal tubes with special attachments to obtain the specimen.

Liver biopsy. A liver biopsy is a procedure that is used to obtain a specimen of hepatic tissue. Before the biopsy is obtained, the client should receive nothing by mouth for 2 to 4 hours and may be given an injection of vitamin K to prevent bleeding and a sedative to relax him. The abdomen is prepared with an antiseptic, and the client is positioned on his back with his arms extended over his head. After a local anesthetic has been injected, an aspiration needle is inserted between the eighth and ninth intercostal spaces. At this time, the client is instructed to inhale and hold his breath to elevate the rib cage. The aspiration is accomplished in a few seconds, and the client may relax. A bandage is put over the entrance site to maintain asepsis.

The liver is a vascular organ, and both hemorrhage and leakage of bile caused by perforation of a bile duct are not infrequent complications. Furthermore, a chemical peritonitis could result if there is persistent bile leakage from injury to the ducts. To prevent these dangers, the client should be positioned on his right side to compress the liver against the ribs to control bleeding. The client usually remains on his right side for 4 hours and in bed for 24 hours. Vital signs should be recorded every 15 to 30 minutes during the first 4 hours and every 4 hours for 48 hours.

Oral exfoliative cytology. Oral exfoliative cytology is performed to obtain loosened cells in the mouth for examination of unusual cellular growth. A moistened tongue blade is used to scrape the area in question to obtain loosened cells. The cells are then spread on a slide, placed in a preservative, and sent to the laboratory for cytological examination.

Gastric exfoliative cytology. Tumor cells in the stomach are easily loosened and may be aspirated for pathological examination. After the client has fasted for 8 hours, a nasogastric tube is inserted, and saline is washed through it to loosen the cells of the gastric mucosa. When the specimen has been obtained, the nurse may remove the nasogastric tube and assist the client with mouth care.

Analytical examinations

Excretory functions of the gastrointestinal tract and accessory organs can be determined by analyzing gastrointestinal contents or stimulating digestive organs to produce hormones or enzymes. The tests involve collection of samples of gastric juices, urine, or blood.

Gastric analysis. A gastric analysis is done to determine the presence and amount of hydrochloric acid and undigested food in the stomach. The client should receive nothing by mouth for 6 to 8 hours before the test. After that time the nurse, technician, or physician will pass a nasogastric tube and obtain a fasting specimen of gastric contents. A gastric stimulant such as histamine (histamine phosphate) is then given to stimulate the production of hydrochloric acid. The client may feel flushed and have tachycardia or a headache after the injection of histamine. These are normal reactions, and the client should not be alarmed, but the nurse should monitor the vital signs in anticipation of an allergic reaction. If a severe histamine reaction is precipitated, epinephrine (Adrenalin) can be given as an antidote. Betazole (Histalog), an analog of histamine, is preferred by some physicians as a gastric stimulant because the systemic reactions are fewer and milder.

Specimens of gastric contents are aspirated every 15 to 20 minutes until three to five specimens have been obtained. A dye such as Topfer's solution or blue litmus paper can be added to the gastric specimens to detect the presence of hydrochloric acid. These dyes turn red if hydrochloric acid is present. Quantitative as well as qualitative analysis is completed in the laboratory.

When the analysis is finished, the nasogastric tube is removed. The nurse should assist the client with mouth care and observe him for nausea or vomiting.

Tubeless gastric analysis. The Diagnex Blue, or Azuresin, test can be used to indirectly measure the presence of hydrochloric acid in the stomach. Urinary excretion of a dye causes a measurable substance to be eliminated from the kidneys when hydrochloric acid is present in the stomach. The client should not take any medications for 24 hours before the test and should abstain from food and fluid for 6 to 8 hours. He is then given a packet of dye crystals (Azuresin, or Diagnex Blue) to swallow with one glass of water. The urine is saved for 2 hours and measured for the amount of dye excreted. A blue color in the urine indicates the presence of hydrochloric acid. This test does not determine the amount of hydrochloric acid, only its presence. The client should be instructed that his urine will continue to be blue for 2 or 3 days until the dye is completely excreted.

Duodenal analysis (biliary drainage). Samples of secretions in the duodenum can be obtained by passing a gastrointestinal tube into the duodenum. The tube is in the duodenum when clear brown liquid appears. The contents of the duodenum are then aspirated to determine the presence of pancreatic enzymes, blood, tumor cells, or bile. Magnesium sulfate or olive oil may be given through the tube to stimulate the flow of bile. Duodenal secretions are aspirated for several hours to obtain sufficient fluid for analysis.

When the test is completed, the gastrointestinal tube is removed. The nurse should assist the client with mouth care and order his next meal.

Liver function studies

Liver function studies are based on assessing the various functions of the liver to determine damage or disease process in the liver. They usually involve collecting blood or urine samples to assay the excretory, metabolic, or detoxifying abilities of the liver (Table 17-3).

Bilirubin assay. Bilirubin is a product of hemoglobin breakdown and is excreted with bile into the duodenum where most of the bilirubin is excreted as stercobilin, the substance that gives the dark brown color to stools. A smaller amount of bilirubin is eliminated by the kidneys as urine urobilinogen. Increased bilirubin in the blood indicates obstruction of the liver or biliary system and is observed clinically as jaundice, a yellow color of the skin and sclera. When there is an obstruction, the stools become white and the urine darker as bilirubin output is blocked.

Serum bilirubin (total) is measured quantitatively by the van den Bergh reaction, which gives a measurement of the bilirubin in the blood. The normal level is 0.2 to 1.4 mg/100 ml.

Icterus index indicates the amount of bile pigment in the bloodstream. Four to 6 units is normal.

Urinary urobilinogen measurement indicates the amount of urobilinogen in

TABLE 17-3
Liver function studies

Test	Description	Normal values
Tests to determine excretory function		
Bilirubin assay	Measures liver's ability to conjugate and excrete bilirubin	Serum bilirubin: 0.2-1.4 mg/100 ml
		Icterus index: 4-6 units
		Urinary urobilinogen: 0.5-4.0 Ehrlich units in 24 hours
Serum alkaline phosphatase	Measures amount of alkaline phosphatase excreted by liver; increases in destructive jaundice	2-5 Bodansky units, adults; 3-13 Bodansky units, children
Enzymes	Measures amount of enzymes present in liver tissue; increases noted in liver disease	SGOT 10-40 units/ml
		SGPT 5-35 units/ml
		LDH 80-120 Wackar units
Tests to determine metabolic function		
Serum proteins	Evaluates liver's ability to synthesize proteins	Total protein 6.6-8 g/100 ml
		Albumin 3.5-5.5 g/100 ml
		Globulin 2.5-3.5 g/100 ml
		A/G ratio 3:1
Serum ammonia	Measures ability of liver to convert ammonia to urea	20-150 μg/100 ml (diffusion)
Serum cholesterol	Measures synthesis or blockage of cholesterol	Total 50-250 mg/100 ml
		Esters = 60%-75% of total
Serum amylase	Measures carbohydrate metabolism	4-25 U/ml
Serum lipase	Measures fat metabolism	2 U/ml
Cephalin-cholesterol flocculation	Measures changes of serum proteins in a colloidal suspension	1+ after 24 hr
Prothrombin time		12 to 15 sec
Tests to determine detoxifying function		
BSP	Measures rate BSP dye is removed from the blood by parenchymal cells.	3%-7% dye remaining after 45 min

906

the urine. Urine specimens are saved for 24 hours. Normal 24-hour output is 0 to 4 mg. The specimen can also be obtained during a 2-hour period in the afternoon when excretion of urobilinogen is the highest.

Bromsulphalein (BSP) excretion. The BSP test measures the rate at which the dye BSP is removed from the bloodstream by the liver parenchymal cells. The client should not eat or drink after midnight. A fasting blood sample is obtained in the morning, and a measured amount of dye, based on body weight, is injected. A sample is withdrawn from the vein in the opposite arm exactly 45 minutes later, at which time less than 3% to 7% of the dye should remain in the bloodstream.

Serum alkaline phosphatase. Alkaline phosphatase is formed in bone and liver cells and excreted with bile. The serum alkaline phosphatase levels are increased in obstructive liver disease because the alkaline phosphatase is returned to the bloodstream. For adults a level of 2 to 5 Bodansky units is normal; for children, 3 to 13 Bodansky units.

Proteins. Measurement of serum proteins and the ratio of albumin to globulin (A/G ratio) indicate the ability of the liver to synthesize protein. The latter test is not as accurate and may be used less frequently. Serum protein levels are decreased in liver disease. Normal values are: total protein, 6.6 to 8 g/100 ml of blood; albumin, 3.5 to 5.5 g/100 ml of blood; globulin 2.5 to 3.5 g/100 ml of blood; A/G ratio, 3:1.

Serum ammonia. Serum ammonia levels increase during liver disease because the liver is unable to deaminize protein. A level under 75 μg of ammonia nitrogen/100 ml of blood is normal.

Cephalin-cholesterol flocculation. A sample of the client's serum is added to a colloidal suspension of cephalin-cholesterol solution. Flocculation and sedimentation occur if there is liver disease. Normal value is 1+ after 24 hours.

Galactose tolerance. The galactose tolerance test is done to measure the ability of the liver to convert galactose to glycogen. If free galactose remains, liver ability is impaired.

This test can be done with either oral or intravenous administration of a measured amount of galactose. For the oral galactose tolerance, the client is given nothing by mouth after midnight. In the morning he voids and is given a measured amount of galactose, by body weight. Hourly urine specimens are obtained for 5 hours. Excretion of more than 3 g of galactose is indicative of liver disease. If an intravenous galactose tolerance test is used, 0.5 mg/kg of body weight is given, and blood specimens are collected at 15 minutes and 45 minutes. No galactose should be apparent in the bloodstream after 75 minutes.

Data analysis

After collecting relevant subjective and objective data, the client and nurse determine potential or real nursing problems. The nursing diagnoses can be listed and placed in priority order. Although nursing diagnoses are derived from data collected and are unique to each client, common nursing diagnoses associated with alteration in nutrition may include alterations in comfort, ineffective family coping, fluid volume deficit, knowledge deficit, noncompliance, alterations in parenting, self-care deficit, disturbance in self-concept, and sleep pattern disturbance.

TABLE 17-4
Basic four food groups

Food group	Food	Major nutritional value
Meats	Meats, fish, eggs, legumes	Protein, calcium, fat
Milk	Milk, cheese, cottage cheese, ice cream, yogurt	Protein, carbohydrate, fat, calcium, vitamins A and D
Fruits and vegetables	Fruits and vegetables, fresh, frozen, canned	Carbohydrates, vitamins, minerals
Breads and cereals	Breads, cereals, rice, potatoes, pasta	Carbohydrates, vitamin A and B-complex

Planning

PLANNING FOR HEALTH PROMOTION

Nutrition for health

Health promotion for nutrition involves eating a well-balanced diet and protecting the teeth and gastrointestinal structures from inflammation or injury. The nurse has a significant role in health teaching and may work with other health team members, the dietitian, physician, or dentist to ensure high-level wellness for individuals and groups.

Nutrition adequate to support growth and metabolism is an essential foundation of physical and mental health. Evidence from a variety of studies attributes many health problems in the United States to faulty dietary habits.[13] The major causes of death in the United States—cardiovascular disease, cancer, diabetes mellitus, and liver disease—are associated with nutrition habits. It is imperative, therefore that health professionals assume responsibility for teaching clients food practices that contribute to wellness.

TABLE 17-5
Lifetime needs for nutrition

	Infant	Toddler-preschooler	School-age child	Adolescent	Adult	Older adult
Calories						
Per pound*	50	45	32-41	23-32	18	16-18
Total daily†	480-900	1-2 yr: 1100 2-3 yr: 1250 3-4 yr: 1400	6-8 yr: 2000 8-10 yr: 2200 10-12 yr: boys: 2500	12-18 yr: girls: 2300-2400 boys: 2700-3000	Men: 2100-2800 Women: 1850-2000 Women: 1850-2000	Men: 2200 Women: 1800 Women: 1800
Meats and eggs	3 servings 2-3 mo: egg yolk, strained meats 12 mo: whole egg	2 or more	2 or more	2 or more	2 or more	2 or more
Milk	Formula or breast milk	2-3 cups	3 cups	4 cups	2 cups	2 cups
Fruits and vegetables	Dilute orange juice, strained fruits and vegetables	4 servings	4 servings	4 servings	4 servings	4 servings
Bread and cereals	1-2 mo: cereal 5-8 mo: toast, teething biscuit 7-12 mo: mashed potato, pasta	4 servings	4 servings	4 servings	4 servings	4 servings
Fats and carbohydrates			To meet caloric needs			

*Data from Nelson, W.E., editor: Textbook of pediatrics, ed. 8, Philadelphia, 1964, W.B. Saunders Co.
†Calorie adjustments based on weight and age from Recommended dietary allowances, a report of the Food and Nutrition Board, revised 1968, Washington, D.C., National Academy of Sciences–National Research Council.

Proteins, carbohydrates, fats, vitamins, and minerals are needed to provide nutrition to the cells. These essential food elements are obtained when a well-balanced meal is eaten. For convenience in meal planning, foods can be classified in four food groups—meats, milk, fruits and vegetables, and breads and cereals—to provide a daily dietary of intake of proteins (approximately 20% of the daily diet), carbohydrates (40%), and fats (40%) (Table 17-4). Selecting foods from these groups assures minimum daily requirements of basic nutrition.

The number of servings from each food group depends on the age, size, and metabolic needs of each person (Table 17-5). Infants will need fewer total calories than adolescents, for instance, because their stomach capacity is smaller and the number of calories needed to support their metabolism and activity patterns is less. The four food groups provide basic nutrition, and added calories may be obtained from snacks.

The United States Department of Agriculture and the United States Department of Health and Human Services have issued dietary guidelines for Americans, shown below. These guidelines can provide a basis for meal planning.

Meal planning is an important aspect of ensuring adequate nutrition, and the nurse may be involved in instructing individuals and families about food

---

DIETARY GUIDELINES FOR AMERICANS

Eat a variety of foods.
Maintain ideal weight.
Avoid excess fat, saturated fat, and cholesterol.
    Choose lean meat, fish, poultry, dry beans and peas as protein sources.
    Moderate use of eggs and organ meats (such as liver).
    Limit intake of butter, cream, hydrogenated margarines, shortenings and coconut oil, and foods
        made from such products.
    Trim excess fat off meats.
    Broil, bake, or boil rather than fry.
    Read labels carefully to determine both amount and types of fat contained in foods.
Eat foods with adequate starch and fiber.
    Substitute starches for fats and sugars.
    Select foods that are good sources of fiber and starch, such as whole grain breads and cereals,
        fruits and vegetables, beans, peas, and nuts.
Avoid too much sugar.
    Use less of all sugars, including white sugar, brown sugar, raw sugar, honey, and syrups.
    Eat less of foods containing these sugars, such as candy, soft drinks, ice cream, cakes, cookies.
    Select fresh fruits or fruits canned without sugar or light syrup rather than heavy syrup.
    Read food labels for clues on sugar content—if the names sucrose, glucose, maltose, dextrose,
        lactose, fructose, or syrups appear first, then there is a large amount of sugar.
Avoid too much sodium.
    Learn to enjoy the unsalted flavors of foods.
    Cook with only small amounts of added salt.
    Add little or no salt to food at the table.
    Limit intake of salty foods, such as potato chips, pretzels, salted nuts and popcorn, condiments
        (soy sauce, steak sauce, garlic salt), cheese, pickled foods, cured meats.
    Read food labels carefully to determine the amounts of sodium in processed foods and snack
        items.
If you drink alcohol, do so in moderation.

Adapted from: Nutrition and your health, U.S. Dept. of Agriculture and U.S. Dept. of Health and Human Services, February 1980.

TABLE 17-6

Mean heights and weights and
recommended energy intake

Age and sex group	Weight		Height		Energy		
					Needs		Range in kcal
	kg	lb	cm	in	MJ	kcal	
Infants							
0.0-0.5 yr.	6	13	60	24	kg × 0.48	kg × 115	95-145
0.5-1.0 yr.	9	20	71	28	kg × 0.44	kg × 105	80-135
Children							
1-3 yr.	13	29	90	35	5.5	1300	900-1800
4-6 yr.	20	44	112	44	7.1	1700	1300-2300
7-10 yr.	28	62	132	52	10.1	2400	1650-3300
Males							
11-14 yr.	45	99	157	62	11.3	2700	2000-3700
15-18 yr.	66	145	176	69	11.8	2800	2100-3900
19-22 yr.	70	154	177	70	12.2	2900	2500-3300
23-50 yr.	70	154	178	70	11.3	2700	2300-3100
51-75 yr.	70	154	178	70	10.1	2400	2000-2800
76+ yr.	70	154	178	70	8.6	2050	1650-2450
Females							
11-14 yr.	46	101	157	62	9.2	2200	1500-3000
15-18 yr.	55	120	163	64	8.8	2100	1200-3000
19-22 yr.	55	120	163	64	8.8	2100	1700-2500
23-50 yr.	55	120	163	64	8.4	2000	1600-2400
51-75 yr.	55	120	163	64	7.6	1800	1400-2200
76+ yr.	55	120	163	64	6.7	1600	1200-2000
Pregnancy						+300	
Lactation						+500	

From Recommended Dietary Allowances, revised 1980, Food and Nutrition Board, National Academy of Sciences–National Research Council, Washington, D.C. The data in this table have been assembled from the observed median heights and weights of children, together with desirable weights for adults for mean heights of men (70 in) and women (64 in) between the ages of 18 and 34 years as surveyed in the U.S. population (DHEW/NCHS data).

Energy allowances for the young adults are for men and women doing light work. The allowances for the two older age groups represent mean energy needs over these age spans, allowing for a 2% decrease in basal (resting) metabolic rate per decade and a reduction in activity of 200 kcal per day for men and women between 51 and 75 years; 500 kcal for men over 75 years; and 400 kcal for women over 75. The customary range of daily energy output is shown for adults in the range column and is based on a variation in energy needs of ±400 kcal at any one age, emphasizing the wide range of energy intakes appropriate for any group of people.

Energy allowances for children through age 18 are based on median energy intakes of children of these ages followed in longitudinal growth studies. Ranges are the tenth and ninetieth percentiles of energy intake, to indicate range of energy consumption among children of these ages.

selection. Food should be prepared in a palatable form for each person. Infants and edentulous persons, for example, should have a diet of soft or pureed foods, which are easy to ingest and swallow. Meals should be planned according to the family's economic resources, individual preferences, and cultural and religious values.

The Food and Nutrition Board establishes standards for recommended daily allowances (RDAs) of nutrients that guard against deficiencies (Tables 17-6 to 17-8). The standards are revised every 5 years and can be used to plan for food needs of individuals and groups, to plan public assistance and education programs, and to evaluate adequacy of food supplies.[17]

Food labeling provides information about contents of prepared foods. Foods that are restored (one or more nutrients lost in processing is replaced), enriched (cereal products with iron and B vitamins added), fortified (nutrients added that are normally not present or present in limited amounts), or foods that have claims made about them in advertising must so state on the label. Furthermore, food

TABLE 17-7

Estimated safe and adequate daily dietary intakes of additional selected vitamins and minerals

Age group	Vitamins			Trace elements*						Electrolytes		
	Vitamin K (μg)	Biotin (μg)	Pantothenic acid (mg)	Copper (mg)	Manganese (mg)	Fluoride (mg)	Chromium (mg)	Selenium (mg)	Molybdenum (mg)	Sodium (mg)	Potassium (mg)	Chloride (mg)
Infants												
0.0-0.5 yr	12	35	2	0.5-0.7	0.5-0.7	0.1-0.5	0.01-0.04	0.01-0.04	0.03-0.06	115-350	350-925	275-700
0.5-1.0 yr	10-20	50	3	0.7-1.0	0.7-1.0	0.2-1.0	0.02-0.06	0.02-0.06	0.04-0.08	250-750	425-1275	400-1200
Children and adolescents												
1-3 yr	15-30	65	3	1.0-1.5	1.0-1.5	0.5-1.5	0.02-0.08	0.02-0.08	0.05-0.1	325-975	550-1650	500-1500
4-6 yr	20-40	85	3-4	1.5-2.0	1.5-2.0	1.0-2.5	0.03-0.12	0.03-0.12	0.06-0.15	450-1350	775-2325	700-2100
7-10 yr	30-60	120	4-5	2.0-2.5	2.0-3.0	1.5-2.5	0.05-0.2	0.05-0.2	0.1-0.3	600-1800	1000-3000	925-2775
11+ yr	50-100	100-200	4-7	2.0-3.0	2.5-5.0	1.5-2.5	0.05-0.2	0.05-0.2	0.15-0.5	900-2700	1525-4575	1400-4200
Adults	70-140	100-200	4-7	2.0-3.0	2.5-5.0	1.5-4.0	0.05-0.2	0.05-0.2	0.15-0.5	1100-3300	1875-5625	1700-5100

From Recommended Dietary Allowances, Revised 1980. Food and Nutrition Board, National Academy of Sciences–National Research Council. Because there is less information on which to base allowances, these figures are not given in the main table of the RDAs and are provided here in the form of ranges of recommended intakes.

*Since the toxic levels for many trace elements may be only several times usual intakes, the upper levels for the trace elements given in this table should not be habitually exceeded.

TABLE 17-8

Recommended Dietary Allowances, Revised 1980 (Designed for the maintenance of good nutrition of practically all

Age and sex group	Weight		Height		Protein (g)	Fat-soluble vitamins				
	kg	lb	cm	in		Vitamin A (µg RE†)	Vitamin D (µg‡)	Vitamin E (mg αTE#)	Vitamin C (mg)	Thiamin (mg)
Infants										
0.0-0.5 yr	6	13	60	24	kg × 2.2	420	10	3	35	0.3
0.5-1.0 yr	9	20	71	28	kg × 2.0	400	10	4	35	0.5
Children										
1-3 yr	13	29	90	35	23	400	10	5	45	0.7
4-6 yr	20	44	112	44	30	500	10	6	45	0.9
7-10 yr	28	62	132	52	34	700	10	7	45	1.2
Males										
11-14 yr	45	99	157	62	45	1000	10	8	50	1.4
15-18 yr	66	145	176	69	56	1000	10	10	60	1.4
19-22 yr	70	154	177	70	56	1000	7.5	10	60	1.5
23-50 yr	70	154	178	70	56	1000	5	10	60	1.4
51+ yr	70	154	178	70	56	1000	5	10	60	1.2
Females										
11-14 yr	46	101	157	62	46	800	10	8	50	1.1
15-18 yr	55	120	163	64	46	800	10	8	60	1.1
19-22 yr	55	120	163	64	44	800	7.5	8	60	1.1
23-50 yr	55	120	163	64	44	800	5	8	60	1.0
51+ yr	55	120	163	64	44	800	5	8	60	1.0
Pregnancy						+30	+200	+5	+2	+20	+0.4
Lactation						+20	+400	+5	+3	+40	+0.5

The allowances are intended to provide for individual variations among most normal persons as they live in the United States under usual environmental stresses. Diets should heights by individual year of age and for suggested average energy intakes.

†Retinol equivalents; 1 retinol equivalent = 1 µg. retinol or 6 µg. β-carotene.
‡As cholecalciferol: 10 µg. cholecalciferol = 400 IU vitamin D.
#αtocopherol equivalents: 1 mg d-α-tocopherol = 1 αTE.
¶1 NE (niacin equivalent) = 1 mg niacin or 60 mg dietary tryptophan.
||The folacin allowances refer to dietary sources as determined by *Lactobacillus casei* assay after treatment with enzymes ("conjugases") to make polyglutamyl forms of the
**The RDA for vitamin B₁₂ in infants is based on average concentration of the vitamin in human milk. The allowances after weaning are based on energy intake (as recom-
††The increased requirement during pregnancy cannot be met by the iron content of habitual American diets or by the existing iron stores of many women; therefore, the use
tion of the mother for 2 to 3 months after parturition is advisable in order to replenish stores depleted by pregnancy.

processors must include nutrition information about size of serving, number of servings in each container, number of calories, and amount of each nutrient, with percentages of protein and seven selected vitamins and minerals in recommended daily allowances. This information is useful in meal planning and in shopping for special diets.

Food that is ingested should be clean, safe, and inspected for disease. Fresh fruits and vegetables should be washed before eating to remove microorganisms or chemicals and sprays that have been used to preserve freshness. Certain foods require refrigeration to prevent microbial growth. Milk, custards, eggs, and mayonnaise are common examples of foods that can cause *Salmonella* food poisoning and should be stored in the refrigerator. Foods that are not heated for a sufficient time before canning can harbor anaerobic *Clostridium botulinum*. Cans that are bulging, cracked, or dented should not be purchased, because contamination may have occurred. Meat products should be inspected for disease in the healthy people in the USA. Food and Nutrition Board, National Academy of Sciences–National Research Council)

Water-soluble vitamins					Minerals					
Riboflavin (mg)	Niacin (mg NE‖)	Vitamin B₆ (mg)	Folacin‖ (µg)	Vitamin B₁₂ (µg)	Calcium (mg)	Phosphorus (mg)	Magnesium (mg)	Iron (mg)	Zinc (mg)	Iodine (µg)
0.4	6	0.3	30	0.5**	360	240	50	10	3	40
0.6	8	0.6	45	1.5	540	360	70	15	5	50
0.8	9	0.9	100	2.0	800	800	150	15	10	70
1.0	11	1.3	200	2.5	800	800	200	10	10	90
1.4	16	1.6	300	3.0	800	800	250	10	10	120
1.6	18	1.8	400	3.0	1200	1200	350	18	15	150
1.7	18	2.0	400	3.0	1200	1200	400	18	15	150
1.7	19	2.2	400	3.0	800	800	350	10	15	150
1.6	18	2.2	400	3.0	800	800	350	10	15	150
1.4	16	2.2	400	3.0	800	800	350	10	15	150
1.3	15	1.8	400	3.0	1200	1200	300	18	15	150
1.3	14	2.0	400	3.0	1200	1200	300	18	15	150
1.3	14	2.0	400	3.0	800	800	300	18	15	150
1.2	13	2.0	400	3.0	800	800	300	18	15	150
1.2	13	2.0	400	3.0	800	800	300	18	15	150
+0.3	+2	+0.6	+400	+1.0	+400	+400	+150	††	+5	+25
+0.5	+5	+0.5	+100	+1.0	+400	+400	+150	††	+10	+50

be based on a variety of common foods in order to provide other nutrients for which human requirements have been less well defined. See preceding table for weights and

vitamin available to the test organism.
mended by the American Academy of Pediatrics) and consideration of other factors, such as intestinal absorption.
of 30 to 60 mg supplemental iron is recommended. Iron needs during lactation are not substantially different from those of nonpregnant women, but continued supplementa-

animal, and all home-canned or home-cured food, especially nonacid fruits and vegetables and pork, should be cooked thoroughly before eating. Drinking water should come from approved sources and, if its safety is in doubt, should be boiled for 20 minutes or treated with water purification tablets.

Oral hygiene The teeth have an important role in ingestion and digestion of food, and the client should be instructed in principles of oral hygiene that will preserve these functions. Oral hygiene begins as soon as the teeth begin to erupt. At this time the parents can swab the teeth and gums with a cotton-tipped applicator to remove accumulation of food particles and massage the gums. Later, when most of the teeth are erupted and the child can manipulate a toothbrush, the child may be instructed in one of several methods of brushing the teeth (see material on p. 914).

Infants and preschoolers who obtain milk formula or juice from a bottle may develop *bottle mouth syndrome* if they are permitted to go to sleep with the bottle

SUGGESTED METHODS OF BRUSHING TEETH AND DENTURES

Teeth

1. Use a clean, soft toothbrush. The brush should be selected for the size of the client's mouth. The brush should be stored so that the bristles are clean and dry.
2. Use water and toothpaste, salt, or baking soda.
3. Brush the teeth within 30 minutes after eating, in one of two ways:
   a. The upper teeth and gums should be brushed from the gum line downward (Fig. 17-5, *A*). The lower gums and teeth should be brushed from the gum line to the biting surface of the tooth. Each tooth should be brushed on the inner and outer surfaces (Fig. 17-5, *B*). The biting surfaces should be brushed in a back-and-forth motion (Fig. 17-5, *C*).
   b. In another method, a soft, bristled brush is held at the gum line and vibrated at a 45-degree angle along the gum line (Fig. 17-6, *A* and *B*). The crowns are brushed in a back-and-forth motion (Fig. 17-6, *C*).
4. Use dental floss after brushing to remove particles between the teeth (Fig. 17-7).

Dentures

1. Dentures may be brushed with a toothpaste or soaked in a denture cleanser.
2. Plastic dentures should be stored in a dry container; vulcanite dentures should be stored in a solution.
3. Dentures should be assessed periodically for fit.

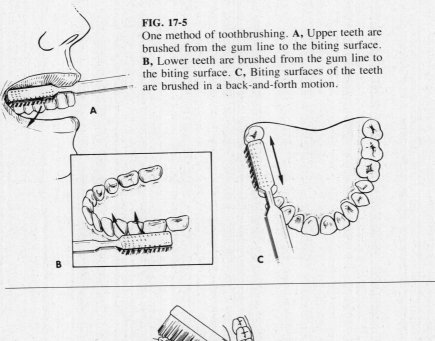

FIG. 17-5
One method of toothbrushing. **A,** Upper teeth are brushed from the gum line to the biting surface. **B,** Lower teeth are brushed from the gum line to the biting surface. **C,** Biting surfaces of the teeth are brushed in a back-and-forth motion.

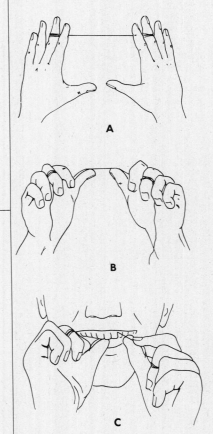

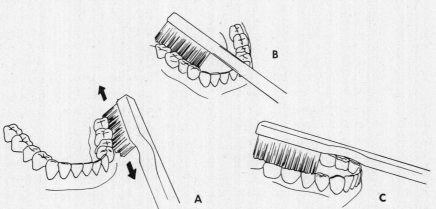

FIG. 17-6
Alternative method of toothbrushing. **A,** Toothbrush held at 45-degree angle to the gum line to brush outer aspect of teeth. **B,** Brushing inner aspect of teeth. **C,** Brushing biting surfaces.

FIG. 17-7
Tooth flossing. **A,** Wrap floss around fingers. **B,** Support with thumbs. **C,** Insert floss between each tooth.

propped against their teeth. The milk or juice is in continuous contact with the teeth and precipitates decay. Parents should be instructed not to allow children to go to sleep sucking on a bottle.

Tooth brushing and flossing are done to remove tooth deposits and prevent caries. Pellicle (a film that forms on the teeth) and materia alba (a combination of protein, bacteria, and necrotic cells) adheres to the teeth and gums; materia alba contributes to breath odors. Plaque is an accumulation of decomposed foods, mucus, and bacteria. If the plaque is not removed, the bacteria produce acids that destroy tooth enamel and cause decay. Finally, a calculus deposit (tartar) can build up from the plaque and hold additional food particles, furthering the decay process.

Oral hygiene also contributes to the prevention of periodontal diseases, gingivitis, loosened teeth, and bone destruction. If plaque and calculus are not adequately removed, bacteria accumulate on the teeth, releasing irritating substances that cause the gums to swell, be tender, bleed easily, and eventually draw away from the teeth. Finally, teeth can become loosened and supporting bone destroyed.

Oral hygiene is particularly important for persons who are unconscious or are not receiving oral intake of food.[21] It should be given at least every 4 hours. The nurse or family can help the client brush his teeth and massage the gums. If the client is unable to swallow, a suction catheter can be used to remove fluids used in oral care. Mouthwashes and astringents may be used to freshen the mouth and stimulate the oral mucosa. Dilute hydrogen peroxide, mouthwash, or lemon and glycerine swabs may be used to stimulate salivation and soften crusts. Antimicrobial mouthwashes should be used for clients who have gastrointestinal tubes in place because ascending infections can occur. When the oral care is completed, a lubricant may be applied to the lips to prevent drying or cracking.

The client should be encouraged to visit his dentist on a regular basis. The first visit should be planned when the child's teeth have erupted, at about age 2 or 3 years. At this time the dentist observes the position of the teeth and the health of the gums and oral tissues. Since no painful procedures are done during this visit, the child can become acquainted with the dentist and equipment in his office in a relaxed atmosphere. Some parents may prefer taking their children to a *pedodontist,* a dentist who specializes in pediatric dentistry. The pedodontist's chair is usually smaller, and he or she may have toys to amuse the child while dental work is performed.

Visits to the dentist should be continued on a regular basis, usually every 6 to 12 months. In the school-age child the dentist evaluates the growth and position of the permanent teeth as they erupt. Teeth that are not aligned properly can contribute to dental decay, poor speech, and difficulty in chewing. The child with malpositioned teeth should be referred to an *orthodontist,* a dentist who specializes in aligning teeth. Braces and other appliances may be used by the orthodontist to bring the teeth into proper alignment.

PLANNING FOR HEALTH MAINTENANCE AND RESTORATION

Planning for health maintenance or restoration may involve short-term or long-term goals with specific objectives for meal planning. Special solutions such as intravenous fluids, enteral hyperalimentation, total parenteral nutrition (TPN), elemental diets, or fat emulsion solutions may be used as a substitute or supplement to the regular diet. Alternative routes may be established for the client who is unable to obtain food orally. Nutrition may then be provided by intravenous infusions, gavage feedings, transpyloric or duodenal feedings, esophagostomy feedings, or gastrostomy feedings. The nurse can assist the client and family as they adapt to these temporary or permanent changes in nutritional sources and routes.

Alternative feeding patterns

The client's usual diet provides the most satisfying source of nutrition. During acute illness or chronic disease, however, the diet can be modified to increase or decrease calories or to add or eliminate specific nutritional components. These diets are discussed where appropriate throughout the text. Additionally, solutions and formulas such as intravenous infusions, enteral hyperalimentation, TPN, elemental diets, or fat emulsions may be used to substitute for or supplement the client's usual diet.

Intravenous infusion. Intravenous infusions are given when the client may have nothing by mouth for a short period of time, such as after surgery, or when the client is dehydrated and requires infusion of fluids, electrolytes, or medications. Most infusions contain dextrose in water and are used to provide carbohydrates for protein sparing or prevent starvation ketosis. These feedings are not nutritionally complete; an infusion of 1000 ml D_5W, for example, contains only 200 calories. Thus an adult client receiving 3000 ml of D_5W in 24 hours obtains only 600 calories per day, and once nutritional reserves are depleted (about 10 days) will rapidly lose weight. Although vitamins and electrolytes may be added to the intravenous feedings, more nutrients are needed to maintain nutrition in the cells over a long period of time.

Enteral hyperalimentation. Undernourished clients may receive supplemental sources of nutrition from prepared formulas. The formulas are used when the client does not obtain adequate nutrition from his regular diet or is unable to swallow. The feedings can supplement the diet or provide total nutritional support. The formulas may be given orally or through nasogastric, duodenal, nasojejunic, cervical esophagostomy or gastrostomy tubes.

Commercial formulas provide complete nutrition in a variety of bases. Most provide 1 to 2 calories per ml of feeding, and the nurse should be familiar with the specific ingredients and the calories provided.

Most formulas are concentrated and should be diluted to half strength for the first few feedings and increased gradually as the client tolerates. Hyperosmolar coma is a potential hazard to clients receiving enteral hyperalimentation feedings, and the nurse can provide fluids along with the formula to prevent dehydration.

Formulas given orally to clients can be offered in an attractive manner. A glass is preferable to a can, for example. If the client finds the formula unpalatable, it can be flavored or offered frozen. Some prefer the formula through a straw or after having the mouth numbed with ice to minimize the flavor. If possible a mint can be offered after the feeding to remove the aftertaste.

When the client is receiving enteral hyperalimentation, the nurse should evaluate the client's response to the feeding. Weight gain and signs of adequate nutrition are useful parameters for monitoring the client's response. The nurse should also observe the client's stools, because many of the formula bases cause diarrhea and may need to be changed.

Total parenteral nutrition. Total parenteral nutrition (TPN), or parenteral hyperalimentation, offers a way of providing nutrients that support tissue growth by means of intravenous infusion. The solution contains water, concentrated glucose (15% to 25%), amino acids (4%), vitamins, and electrolytes in sufficient amounts to support cellular growth, and is planned for the needs of a specific client. The solution usually provides 1 calorie/ml fluid. The solution is used for clients who lose nutrients through diarrhea or vomiting, for neonates with congenital anomalies that interfere with nutrition, or for any person with debilitating nutritional losses such as colitis, burns, infections, anorexia nervosa, failure to thrive, or anorexia caused by chemotherapy or radiation therapy. The solution is also used to promote nutrition in clients receiving cancer chemotherapy, because it is believed that the improved nutrition enhances cellular proliferation, reducing the number of cells in the resting stage and making cells more responsive to therapy.

The solution is usually administered through an indwelling catheter in the superior or inferior vena cava (Fig. 17-8). The increased amount of blood there dilutes the solution in the bloodstream and prevents venous thrombosis.

Sterile technique with gloves and mask should be used to insert the catheter and change the dressing. When the infusion catheter is inserted, the nurse should explain the procedure to the client and assist as the catheter is being inserted. The client should be positioned in the Trendelenburg position with a pillow under the shoulders to hyperextend the shoulder and produce venous dilation. The site should be shaved, defatted with acetone, and scrubbed with an antiseptic. The insertion site is then infiltrated with a local anesthetic. Immediately before insertion, the client should be instructed to inhale and hold his breath, bearing down with his mouth closed (Valsalva maneuver), to prevent air entry into the vein while the catheter is inserted.

Once the infusion catheter is inserted, the nurse should observe the infusion site for signs of infection or thrombosis. An antibiotic dressing may be used at the point of entry of the catheter and should be changed daily using aseptic technique. Medications should not be infused through this line.

The feeding should be infused with an infusion pump to ensure a constant infusion rate. If the infusion rate is behind schedule, it is possible to recalculate

FIG. 17-8
Infusion of total parenteral nutrition. Infusion catheter is inserted in the superior vena cava, and the drip rate is regulated by an infusion pump.

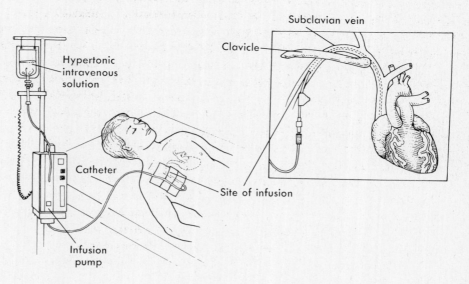

the rate for the remaining feeding, although the faster rate should not exceed the original rate by more than 10%.

The nurse must also keep accurate intake-and-output records when the client is receiving parenteral hyperalimentation fluids. Oral intake should be recorded as well as output from nasogastric tubes, colostomies, and the urinary tract. Daily weights are useful parameters to evaluate weight gain, and the client should gain about ¼ lb (0.55 kg) each day.

Fluid overload and dehydration should be monitored closely for clients receiving TPN fluids. Since the TPN solution contains electrolytes, the nurse should also observe the client for clinical and laboratory indications of excess or deficit (Table 17-9).

Continuous feeding of concentrated glucose may cause osmotic diuresis and glucosuria. To detect these phenomena, the urine should be tested for glucose with the Clinitest method and measured for specific gravity four times a day.

The client may also exhibit a protein allergy. Headache, fever, nausea and vomiting, abdominal pain, or seizures may indicate this allergy, and the nurse should report these observations.

If the client is not receiving any oral fluids, he should be given mouth care at least every 4 hours to prevent crusted secretions in the oral cavity. Neonates should also be permitted to suck on a nipple to provide oral satisfaction and strengthen the muscles that will later be used in nursing.

In some instances, clients may receive parenteral hyperalimentation fluids at home.[1] The individual who is instructed on the mechanical aspects of the feeding, and with the assistance of family members, may be able to improve his nutritional status without hospitalization. This is particularly beneficial to clients with chronic nutritional losses who can otherwise maintain normal life-styles by being treated at home.

Elemental diets. Elemental diets are used to provide easily digested nutrients in an elemental form for individuals who may have interferences with the digestive process as might occur with gastrointestinal fistulas, food allergies, malabsorption syndromes, or gastrointestinal upsets from radiation or chemotherapy. The diet may also be used as preparation for gastrointestinal surgery because it is low in residue. The diet is often used as a transition diet from hyperalimentation therapy.

The diet, which may be given orally or through nasogastric or gastrostomy tubes, contains protein in an elemental form (usually protein hydrosylate and synthetic amino acids), carbohydrates, and fats. Vitamins and minerals may be added as needed.

The nurse should observe the client for changes in stools that might result from the dietary modification and for abdominal distension caused by overfeeding.

Fat emulsion feedings. Clients who require adjustments in their caloric and lipid requirements may be offered intravenous feedings of a 10% intravenous fat emulsion. One solution contains 10% soybean oil, 1.2% egg yolk, and 2.25% phospholipids in a glycerin and water solution, giving a total caloric value of 1.1 calories per 1 ml of feeding. It is recommended, however, that no more than 60% of the total diet come from this source. (Carbohydrates and amino acids are provided by other sources.)

One advantage of this feeding is that it can be administered in a peripheral

TABLE 17-9

Potential metabolic complications associated with TPN

Complication	Characterized by	Usual cause	Treatment
Hyperglycemia	Elevated blood glucose	Carbohydrate intolerance; too rapid initiation of TPN Infection Diabetes mellitus	Decrease rate Search for infection Consider insulin
Hyperosmolar nonketotic dehydration	Hyperglycemia Dehydration Increase in serum osmolality and serum sodium Somnolence Seizures Coma	Failure to recognize initial hyperglycemia and increased glucose in urine	Give insulin to correct hyperglycemia Give 5% dextrose and hypertonic saline (¼ to ½ strength) rather than TPN solution to correct free water deficit Continue to monitor serum glucose, osmolality, sodium, and potassium
Hypoglycemia	Hypothermia Somnolence or lethargy Peripheral vasoconstriction	Usually caused by interruption of TPN solution infusion	Immediately begin appropriate dextrose infusion Monitor serum glucose and potassium
Hyperchloremic metabolic acidosis	Decrease in blood pH Decrease in serum (HCO_3^-) Decrease in blood (base excess) Increase in serum (Cl^-) Increase in serum (Na^+)	Excessive renal or gastrointestinal losses of base Infusion of preformed hydrogen ion Cationic amino acids greater than the concentration of anionic amino acids in TPN solution	Decrease chloride excess in TPN solution by exchanging chloride ion with acetate ion Improve balance between cationic and anionic amino acids in TPN solution
Hyperammonemia	Elevated blood ammonia levels Somnolence Lethargy Seizures Coma	Hepatic dysfunction Deficiency in urea cycle amino acids	Slow infusion rate Discontinue infusion
Hypophosphatemia	Paresthesia Mental confusion Hyperventilation Lethargy Decreased RBC function	Usually caused by inadequate inorganic phosphate in TPN solution (concentrated glucose infusion may precipitate syndrome)	Add phosphate to TPN solution In an emergency give potassium slowly, mixed well with peripheral 5% dextrose solutions (Rapid correction of hypophosphatemia may cause hypocalcemic tetany)
Hypokalemia	Muscular weakness Cardiac arrhythmias Altered digitalis sensitivity	Excessive gastrointestinal or urinary potassium losses; deficit of potassium in TPN solution	Increase potassium concentration in TPN solution based on patient's requirements
Hyponatremia	Lethargy Confusion	Excessive gastrointestinal or urinary sodium losses; water intoxication	Increase sodium concentration in TPN solution based on patient's requirements; limit free water intake to treat water intoxication
Hypomagnesemia	Vertigo Weakness Distension Positive Chvostek sign Convulsive seizures with or without tetany	Insufficient magnesium in TPN solution Excessive gastrointestinal or renal losses	Increase magnesium in TPN solution In an emergency, give $MgSO_4$ solution intramuscularly
Prerenal azotemia	Lassitude	Dehydration (possible hyperosmolar type) Calorie:nitrogen imbalance	Correct free water deficit Give insulin if patient is hyperglycemic Increase nonprotein calories to achieve calorie:nitrogen ratio of about 185:1

From Insights into parenteral nutrition. Reprinted with permission of Traverol Laboratories, Inc., Deerfield, Ill.

vein. Filters should not be used in administration, because breakdown of the emulsion could occur; nor should the solution be mixed with electrolytes or other additives, although a Y connector can be used at the infusion site to add intralipid fluids.

Fat emulsion feedings are contraindicated for clients with hyperlipemia, lipoid nephrosis, and acute pancreatitis and should be used with caution for clients with liver disease, anemia, blood coagulation interferences, pulmonary disease, or in instances in which fat embolism (see Chapter 11) would be likely. When such feedings are used over a period of time, liver function studies and serum cholesterol levels should be monitored.

The first infusion should not be greater than 500 ml for the first 24 hours so that the client's reaction to the fat emulsion can be observed. Allergic reactions are manifested by nausea, vomiting, headache, dyspnea, and chest pain and warrant discontinuing the feeding. If tolerated, the feedings can be increased gradually.

Alternative feeding routes

Clients who have interferences with ingestion or have special dietary needs may use alternative feeding routes to meet the needs for nutrition to the cells. Clients who are unable to swallow (such as a premature infant or an unconscious individual) may be fed through a nasogastric or esophagostomy tube, and clients who have gastric or esophageal obstructions may be fed directly into the stomach by gastrostomy feedings. The client who can have nothing by mouth or who is debilitated may require intravenous feedings or parenteral hyperalimentation feedings to support cellular growth while oral intake is restricted.

Nasogastric (gavage) feedings. Introducing feedings into the stomach by means of a nasogastric tube is called gavage feeding. Gavage feedings may be necessary for clients who have difficulty swallowing. Premature infants have poorly developed sucking and swallowing reflexes and are often fed by gavage feedings. Clients who are unconscious or unable to swallow may also receive their dietary requirements by this method. Some believe that feedings introduced into the stomach preserve intestinal mucosa integrity and are used more efficiently when absorbed from the portal circulation.[19]

The procedure for gavage feeding is similar for infants, children, and adults except for the size of the feeding tube and the length it is passed as well as the amount of feeding given to support metabolism. The procedure for passing a nasogastric tube follows.

1. The client is positioned comfortably in Fowler's position.
2. The (feeding) tube is selected by size for the client (infants: size 6 to 8; children: size 8 to 12; adults: size 12 to 16). The tube is measured before inserting. For infants and children, the tube is either measured from the tip of the nose to a point midway between xiphoid process and umbilicus[29] or from the tip of the nose to the earlobe and from the earlobe to the xiphoid process (Fig. 17-9, *A*); for adults, from the tip of ear to the nose and then from the nose to the end of the xiphoid process (Fig. 17-9, *B*). These measurements provide estimations of placement in the fundus. It is important to place the tube in the stomach, not the duodenum to avoid iatrogenic dumping syndrome of nausea and vomiting caused by osmotic shifts of fluids to the intestine.[12]
3. Rubber tubes may be chilled in ice to make them rigid and easier to pass. Polyethylene tubes usually do not need to be iced. All tubes are lubri-

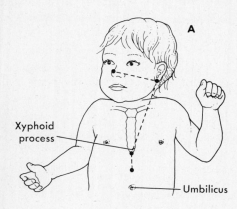

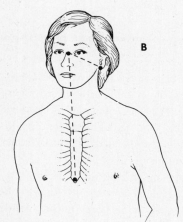

FIG. 17-9
Measuring nasogastric tube for insertion. **A,** Infants and children. **B,** Adults.

cated with a water-soluble lubricant and checked for patency by running sterile water through them before insertion.

4. The client can be instructed to hold head up and keep his eyes open as the tube is passed through the nares and pharynx toward the ear (Fig. 17-10, *A*). Then the client bends his head toward his chest, and the tube is passed into the nasopharynx, esophagus, and stomach (Fig. 17-10, *B*). If the client is able to cooperate, he should take shallow breaths when the tube stimulates the gag reflex to minimize gagging. The tube is passed more easily if the client can swallow or take sips of water. Swallowing closes the epiglottis and prevents the feeding tube from passing into the trachea. If nasal obstruction is met when first passing the tube, the other nostril may be used.

5. The nurse checks to be sure that the tube is in the stomach. The tube is in the stomach when (a) gastric contents return when aspirated, and (b) air can be heard with a stethoscope over the stomach as air is introduced into the feeding tube with a bulb syringe (Fig. 17-10, *C*). If there is respiratory distress, the tube is in the lungs.

6. When the nurse has verified the position of the feeding tube in the stomach, it is secured with tape. the tube should be taped to avoid obstructing vision or breathing (Fig. 17-10, *D*) and with a rubber band around the tube pinned to the sheet or the client's clothing.

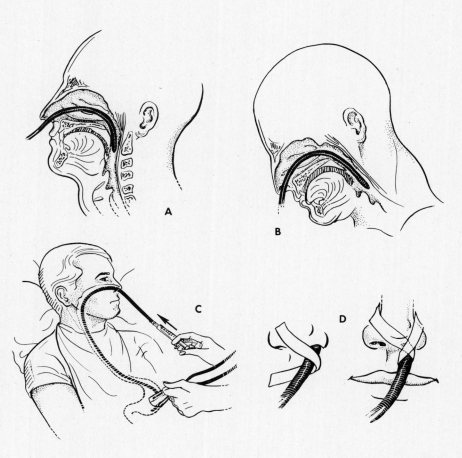

FIG. 17-10
Insertion of a nasogastric tube. **A,** Nasogastric tube is inserted through the nares with the head upright. **B,** Client is instructed to flex his head as the nasogastric tube passes through the pharynx and esophagus. **C,** Verifying placement of the tube by inserting air and listening with a stethoscope. **D,** One way of fixing the nasogastric tube to the nose. (From Dison, Norma Greenler: Clinical nursing techniques, ed. 4, St. Louis, 1979, The C.V. Mosby Co.)

921

GAVAGE FEEDINGS

Purpose	1. Provide calories and nutrition when oral ingestion of food is not possible.
	2. Provide nutrition when sucking and swallowing reflexes are weak or absent.
Meats and eggs	Strained liver, egg, ground meat.
Milk	Whole milk, skim milk, powdered nonfat dry milk.
Fruits and vegetables	Applesauce, cooked and strained vegetables, orange juice, apple juice.
Breads and cereals	Cooked farina, white bread (no crusts).
Suggestions	1. Select food from basic four groups; plan for age and size of client.
	2. Add water to liquefy foods.
	3. Mix in blender to the consistency that will pass through the feeding tube.
	4. Add pectin if client has diarrhea.
	5. Refrigerate to prevent spoilage.

Various feedings may be given by gavage. Neonates may be fed breast milk or cow's milk formula. Table food can be mixed in a blender with water to make a feeding that will pass easily through the feeding tube (see gavage feedings above). Commercial formulas may also be used, but they tend to be less filling and may cause diarrhea. Elemental diets may also be used. Water and other liquids may be given at any time as long as the diet permits.

When a gavage feeding is given, it is important to establish a pleasant, relaxed atmosphere. The environment should be clean and attractive, and the feeding served in a pitcher or teapot. Neonates and infants may be held while they are fed, and the child and adult should be in an upright position. This is not only a natural position for eating but also promotes gravity flow of the feeding as the gavage feeding enters the stomach. Neonates and infants should be bubbled frequently during gavage feedings.

Since there is a possibility that the feeding tube will become dislodged between feedings, the nurse should verify its position before each meal. The nurse should also aspirate gastric contents before beginning to feed the client. If more than 30 to 50 ml (depending on the client's age) of feeding is obtained, the stomach may become distended with further feedings. The nurse should check with the physician before feeding any client who has abdominal distension or nausea.

The feeding may be given intermittently or continuously. Intermittent gavage feedings are given by pouring the warmed feeding into a funnel of the barrel of an Asepto syringe that is attached to the feeding tube. The tubing should be pinched as the feeding is poured into the funnel to avoid entry of air into the tubing. The feeding is then given by gravity flow, about 10 ml/min to prevent the nausea and distension that may occur when peristalsis is stimulated. A small amount of water should be used after the feeding to clear the tubing.

After the feeding the client should be made comfortable and positioned to prevent aspiration. The client should be encouraged to brush his teeth after each meal, because the absence of food to stimulate salivation and massage of gums may cause plaque formation on the teeth. The nares should be cleansed, and a water-soluble lubricant applied to prevent irritation of the nose. Infants and unconscious clients are usually positioned on their side to prevent aspiration, and if the client is nauseated, the feeding tube should not be clamped (to provide an outlet for regurgitated or vomited feedings).

Gavage feedings can also be given, and are better tolerated, by continuous infusion. A gravity flow infusion pump connected to the feeding tube can be used to ensure constant flow rates. Initial feedings for adults should be infused at a rate of 50 ml/hr and increased 25 ml/hr each day as the client tolerates.[10] The rate for infusions for infants and children must be adjusted for the client's gastric capacity.

The nurse should disconnect the feeding tube from the infusion pump every 4 to 6 hours and aspirate gastric contents to verify tube placement and absorption of feedings. If more than 100 ml is aspirated, the feedings should be stopped and restarted in 2 hours.[19] The infusion can be slowed if the client complains of cramping, nausea, or vomiting. The tubing should be flushed every 6 hours and fluids offered as needed. To aid gravity and prevent reflux, the head of the bed should remain elevated 30 degrees while the client is receiving gavage feedings. The fluid container should only be filled with fluid for 3 to 4 hours so the formula does not spoil.

Clients receiving gavage feedings should be monitored for fluid and electrolyte imbalances.[15] The most common is dehydration caused by the hyperosmolarity of many commercial feedings. Conscious clients may complain of thirst, but the nurse should observe the unconscious client and infant for signs of dehydration (see Chapter 16). Fluids can be offered through the tube following the feeding and at other times if the client has a fever, is hot, or is diaphoretic. Clients with renal disease or alterations in cardiac output should be observed for fluid overload.

Transpyloric (nasojejunic) feedings. Feeding special formulas through a feeding tube positioned in the jejunum can be used for small pregestational-age neonates, full-term neonates, infants who require alternative approaches to feeding, or adults after surgery—because the small intestine is not immobilized by the ileus after anesthesia.[19] Formulas to maintain nutritional requirements given this way are better tolerated, complications of intravenous therapy are avoided, and anabolic states are achieved early. Furthermore, the jejunum can accommodate an increased volume of feeding.

To insert the transpyloric feeding tube in the *neonate,* the client is positioned on his right side. The tube is measured from the bridge of the nose to the heel and marked with tape. The tube is then lubricated and inserted through the nares to the stomach. Permitting the neonate to suck on a pacifier may facilitate tube passage. During insertion the client should be observed (usually by monitor) for bradycardia, which might occur as a result of vagal stimulation. Position of the tube in the stomach can be verified by aspirating gastric contents and/or inserting 1 to 2 cc of air through the tube and listening with a stethoscope. From this point, with the neonate still on his right side, the tube should pass into the jejunum by natural peristaltic activity. Expectorated mucus can be removed by aspiration with a bulb syringe in the nares and posterior pharynx. Placement of the tube in the jejunum is observed when bile appears in the tube or when the pH of aspirated contents is 7.5. Finally, x-ray films are taken to ascertain the exact location of the feeding tube. At this time the tube can be taped to the forehead and feeding offered.

Feedings should be offered at room temperature, but no more than 6 to 8 hours of feedings should be prepared at one time to prevent bacterial growth. The feeding is generally administered with a reservoir regulated by an infusion pump.

The formula should have an osmolarity of less than 370 mOsm/L, and great care should be taken to prevent dumping syndrome or hypovolemic shock, which is caused by the difference in the concentration of the feeding and the isotonic nature of the fluid in the jejunum. Serum and urine osmolarities should be monitored frequently. Urine specific gravity should also be determined in order to assess adequate hydration.

During the feeding the nurse observes the infant for dyspnea, bradycardia, regurgitation, distension, nausea, or vomiting. If the abdomen does become distended and reflux is noted, a nasogastric tube can be inserted in the other nostril to aspirate gastric contents and air. The transpyloric feeding tube can be irrigated with 0.45% normal saline every 8 hours to maintain tube patency and usually need not be changed for 30 to 80 days, thus minimizing trauma and likelihood of infection. If the tube becomes dislodged, it should not be repositioned, however, because perforation or necrotizing enterocolitis could result.

During the feeding, attention should also be given to developing sucking mechanisms and stimulating sensory experiences of taste and smell. A pacifier as well as a bottle with a small amount of formula can be used to stimulate sucking. Later, as the infant gains skill in feeding, the bottle can be used to stimulate preistalsis by giving part of the feeding by bottle. To do this, the transpyloric infusion can be stopped for ½ hour to stimulate hunger. As the client's capacity for bottle formula increases, the amount of transpyloric feeding is decreased.

Mouth care should be given with lemon and glycerin. This not only loosens crusted secretions but also stimulates saliva and taste. The neonate should also be allowed to smell the formula in an attempt to develop sensory acuity and stimulate peristalsis.

FIG. 17-11
Keofeed tube. (Courtesy Health Development Corp., Mountain View, Calif.)

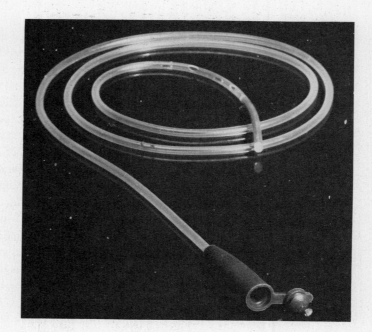

FIG. 17-12
Cervical esophagostomy.

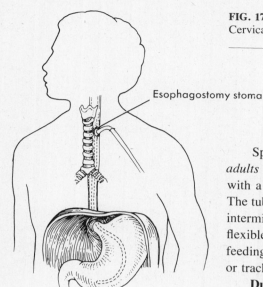

Esophagostomy stoma

Special feeding tubes such as the Dobbhoff or Keofeed tube can be used for *adults* (Fig. 17-11). These are longer than nasogastric tubes and may be passed with a gastroscope, by peristalsis, or by using a J wire under fluoroscopy.[10,19] The tubes may be passed to the lower duodenum or jejunum and can be used for intermittent or continuous feeding. Since the tubes are smaller, softer, and more flexible, there is less oropharyngeal irritation, and they can be used for long-term feeding routes. Esophageal necrosis is also minimized if used with endotracheal or tracheostomy tubes.

Duodenal feedings. Feeding tubes can also be placed in the duodenum for purposes of offering formula feeding. It is believed that this approach reduces perforation and necrotizing entercolitis in low birth weight neonates.[23] Before the feeding tube is inserted, a gastric catheter is passed to the stomach and the gastric contents aspirated. The duodenal tube is measured for placement from the neonate's eyebrows to his heels and inserted through the mouth. Passing of the tube is facilitated by positioning the neonate on his right side during insertion; gravity and peristalsis carry the tube to the duodenum. The nurse can aspirate duodenal contents and determine the pH to verify position. A pH of 6.5 indicates tube placement in the duodenum, and the client can be fed.

Cervical esophagostomy feedings. An alternative feeding route for clients who have difficulty swallowing is to create a stoma below the cervical esophagus to allow passage of a feeding tube.[6] This route minimizes trauma and irritation of the nasogastric feeding tube and averts the need for abdominal surgery to create a gastrostomy. The stoma is created below the cervical esophagus (Fig. 17-12), and when healing takes place, in about 10 days, feeding can begin. The client or family is instructed how to insert the feeding tube, aspirate the feeding tube for residual contents before each feeding, and give the feeding. Blenderized or commercial feedings can be used and, as with other alternative feedings, fluids should be offered and mouth care given every 4 to 6 hours.

A cervical esophagostomy can also be created to drain saliva or chewed food if the client has an esophageal atresia. This congenital defect may not be repaired until the infant is able to tolerate surgery; in the meantime a gastrostomy can be used as a route for feeding, and the esophagostomy is used to drain saliva and formula or food. The advantage of this procedure is that it permits development of sucking and swallowing skills even though esophagogastric continuity is not yet established. Since the stoma is not used for feeding, but rather is an outlet for fluids, an absorbent gauze square can be placed over the stoma to collect drainage.

Gastrostomy feedings. Clients who have obstructions in the mouth or esophagus or those for whom long-term alternative feeding is anticipated may receive feedings directly into the stomach. A gastrostomy feeding tube can be inserted into the stomach through a surgical incision and held in place with purse-

925

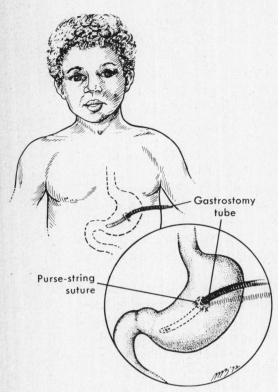

FIG. 17-13
Gastrostomy tube sutured in position.

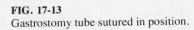

string sutures (Fig. 17-13). This feeding tube is used to give elemental diets, liquefied or blenderized feedings (see suggested diet plan for gavage feedings on p. 922), or formula directly into the stomach.

The feedings are given by pouring the warmed feeding into a funnel and permitting the feeding to enter the stomach by gravity. This is best accomplished when the client is in an upright position. When the feeding is completed, water or other liquids can be used to clear the gastrostomy tube.

Since no food enters the mouth, the salivary glands are not stimulated, and there is no oral pleasure from sucking or swallowing. Infants may be permitted to suck on a nipple to stimulate salivary flow and satisfy the need for sucking. Adults may wish to chew the food in preparation for feeding into the gastrostomy tube. While not esthetically pleasant, this provides the client with a taste for food, stimulates the oral tissues, and increases the flow of gastric juices.

Immediately after the feeding, the client should remain in an upright position while the stomach empties. If the client appears to be nauseated, the tubing should remain unclamped to provide an outlet for the feeding if vomiting occurs.

The skin around the gastrostomy tube should be cleansed frequently with soap and water. If gastric juices seep from the gastrostomy, the skin may become excoriated. Aluminum paste or karaya powder may be applied to the skin around the gastrostomy to prevent skin breakdown.

Implementation

COMMON HEALTH PROBLEMS OF THE NEONATE AND INFANT

Low birth weight

Low birth weight infants are defined as those weighing 5½ pounds (2500 g) or less, regardless of gestational age. Most, however, are preterm neonates. More black infants than white fall into this category, and the mortality of the former tends to be higher. Chinese- and Japanese-Americans have less infant mortality than either the white or black groups. Despite highly sophisticated systems of health care in the United States, of the 14/1000 infant death rate, two thirds are from low birth weight infants.[13] Many questions regarding these statistics have been raised but remain unanswered. Although health care of superior quality is available, a gap appears to exist in the delivery of these services to persons in need. Suspected causes of incongruence include socioeconomic factors and educational levels of potential clients.

Low birth weight infants are ten times more likely to develop cerebral palsy, seven times more likely to have anomalies, and five times more likely to have mental deficiencies than their counterparts of a normal-term birth weight. Because low birth weight causes considerable morbidity and mortality, medical and nursing management is extremely important to consider.

One method of management is to take action during obstetrical care to lengthen gestational age before birth. Mortality and physical and mental morbidity can be reduced up to two thirds by increasing the fetal age from 28 to 32 weeks.

Steps also can be taken to decrease factors that contribute to unwanted pregnancies among teen-agers (who tend to produce low birth weight offspring), to increase the quality of prenatal care, and to educate potential mothers about the hazards of pregnancy and childbirth under known adverse conditions.

Nursing care. When the infant of low birth weight is admitted to the nursery, the nurse should review the delivery room record carefully to determine the infant's immediate response to extrauterine life and should take steps to institute a comprehensive plan of care that gives special attention to oxygen needs, thermal regulation, nutrition and metabolism, and the prevention of complications from adverse physiological processes or infections.

Oxygen needs. In the infant with low birth weight, oxygen consumption and use is closely linked to the immaturity of the cardiovascular system. Constant monitoring of color, breathing, and heart rate should be undertaken. Assisted ventilation or respiratory therapy is often necessary and may be accomplished by several methods including self-inflating bag resuscitation (via mask), respirator, or nasotracheal intubation. Apnea should be anticipated, because of either the immaturity and malfunctioning of the central nervous system control or metabolic disturbances. Electrodes placed on the chest or a mattress that sounds an alarm if breathing stops help alert the nurse to apneic episodes so that immediate intervention can be performed. Monitoring of arterial blood gases is an important part of management of an infant with oxygenation problems. Oxygen concentrations of inhaled air as well as liter flow should be sampled and recorded. Because an infant can be subject to permanent damage and death from too little or too much oxygen, the nurse must be skilled in observational and therapeutic techniques relating to oxygen administration.

Thermal regulation. Temperature control is a critical factor in the care of low birth weight infants, because regulatory centers are immature and metabolic consumption levels are unstable. Chilling or overheating of an infant causes increased oxygen and glucose use and exhausts critical reserves of the struggling child as he fights to keep warm or keep cool. Incubators, radiant heat hoods, or even hot water bottles can be employed to provide warmth. Since infants are often apneic during rewarming, this provides an additional incentive for the nurse to avoid chilling the infant. A common way in which heat loss can occur is by the baby's coming in contact with colder objects such as a scale pan, linens, or an attendant's hands. Persons who work with high-risk infants must constantly strive to prevent such unnecessary heat losses and to promote a warm, stable thermal environment that does not require constant adjustments by the infant.

Nutrition and metabolism. Hypoglycemia often occurs in low birth weight infants because of inadequate regulatory mechanisms, low liver reserves of glycogen, and poor oxygen utilization. A high-pitched cry, apnea, twitching, cyanosis, or listlessness gives the nurse clues that such a condition may exist.

The premature infant has little liver glycogen, because these reserves are not built up significantly until the last months of gestation. Inability to make physiological adjustments such as controlling heat loss or decreasing metabolic losses of glucose makes the situation worse. Nutrition may be limited in the first day or two of life, because of delayed feeding regimens or problems in feeding. Although an adequate sucking response is usually present, it is often not well coordinated with the swallowing reflex in the premature infant. If feeding is done by an altered route because of anomalies or other clinical indices, a gavage procedure or parenteral fluids via an umbilical catheter are commonly used.

Nursing process for common health problems

Dextrostix, a small test tape designed to demonstrate glucose levels of blood in proportion to color changes induced by a drop of blood on the tape, can be employed as a screening device. The absence of a light blue color means a low blood glucose level and the necessity for a laboratory determination of blood glucose. A glucose level of less than 45 mg/100 ml is indicative of hypoglycemia in neonates larger than 2500 g, whereas a glucose level of 20 mg/100 ml is considered hypoglycemic in low birth weight infants.

Hypocalcemia is also a hazard to a low birth weight infant. Seizures, hyperirritability, and tremors are classic symptoms. The usual therapeutic approach is the administration of calcium gluconate. Careful observation of heart rate is necessary after the drug is given, because it may cause bradycardia.

Whatever the intervention necessary to maintain nutrition and metabolic homeodynamics, it must be carefully controlled. For example, if an infusion of glucose is stopped by infiltration or obstruction, the infant can be plunged into a crisis with considerable speed. Infusion pumps that ensure a well-regulated and continuous flow by a patent route are extremely desirable for the low birth weight child's safety and survival.

Other stress factors. Complications from adverse physiological processes and infections must be constantly guarded against. Strict aseptic technique, including frequent handwashing, cannot be overlooked. Any child in the high-risk nursery is greatly endangered when subjected to the added trauma of an infectious process. The low birth weight infant is also likely to have anomalies or regulatory disturbances, so that the attending nurse should be ever alert to adverse or changing physiological functioning. Stress should be kept at a minimum. For example, circumcisions should be avoided until the infant is well stabilized.

Emergency preparedness. Equipment should be at hand for emergency intervention, especially aspiration and cardiopulmonary resuscitation, and the nurse must be familiar with its use. Of special importance is the necessity for all personnel who work with neonates to be skilled in mouth-to-mouth and nose ventilation for managing asphyxia or apnea. These have the advantages of not requiring any special equipment and of controlling the volume and pressure of air. See Chapter 20 for resuscitation techniques.

Transportation of low birth weight infants to the sophisticated high-risk centers can be accomplished with expediency for clients by means of a specially equipped ambulance or helicopter. The infant transporter must be equipped to provide oxygen, warmth, suctioning, and parenteral fluid infusion and must have equipment for resuscitation. In addition to these devices, a skilled nurse or physician should accompany the neonate.

Parental responses to the infant. Parents tend to expect the same responses from premature infants as would be elicited from a full-term one, and when these responses do not occur, there is disappointment and a feeling of failure. Nurses must help them understand how the infant's responses differ because of an immature cortex and subcortical functioning.

The premature infant often appears emaciated and may not be as "cute and cuddly" as a full-term infant. The cry may be brief, high-pitched, and even feeble sounding, which can be annoying to an already frustrated mother whose infant requires special care.

Many early parent-infant satisfactions are derived from the feeding process;

therefore, when the premature infant requires gavage feeding, the mother may feel that she is unable to be important to the child and that others (such as the nurses) are achieving the satisfactions that are rightly hers. When parents do feed premature infants, they are usually frustrated, however, because the infant feeds slowly, sucks poorly, and tires easily, because of uncoordinated reflexes of sucking and swallowing. Unswallowed formula may be pushed out of the mouth, and there may be fears of gagging and choking. Without reassurance and encouragement of nurses, the parent may develop unusual concerns about feeding and the success of "parenting."

Respiratory reflexes are inconsistent in the premature neonate, and such infants periodically are apneic. This is understandably frightening unless the mother understands that, with maturation, these periods of apnea will cease.

The Moro reflex (see Chapter 10) is exaggerated in the premature neonate, and when the parent startles the infant when picking him up, he may cry, jerk, and seem frightened. This may be interpreted by the parent as rejection. It may even cause parents to avoid picking the child up and produce feelings of inadequacy in their ability to comfort.

It should be a specific part of a nursing plan to instruct parents about reflexes of the premature neonate, so that the infant's lack of ability, as opposed to the parents' behavior, is responsible for dissatisfaction in feeding and comforting approaches. For a parent who has had earlier experiences with a full-term infant, the differences may be less readily accepted than by first-time parents who do not possess certain expectations of responses from the infant. The trend to encourage parent-infant contact during hospitalization and to release these infants as early as possible for home care makes this nursing responsibility extremely important.

Necrotizing enterocolitis

Necrotizing enterocolitis (NEC) is an inflammation of the gastrointestinal tract that occurs occasionally in high-risk neonates, particularly low birth weight neonates. Mortality rates are high, and as many as 75% of neonates with NEC die.

The cause of NEC is unknown, but probably related to perinatal hypoxia and shunting of blood from the gastrointestinal tract to the vital organs. Bacterial invasion by *E coli,* Salmonella, or *Klebsiella* organisms cause inflammation and ultimate necrosis of the mucosa and submucosa. High-solute feedings are also implicated as providing a medium for bacterial growth.

The nurse, during periodic health assessments of the neonate, can detect changes indicative of NEC. There may be increased residual feedings remaining in the stomach after feeding and a distended abdomen. Bowel sounds are diminished, and there may be blood in the stools and diarrhea. The neonate may appear lethargic. There may be an increased temperature and decreased urinary output.

Nursing care is planned to provide rest to the gastrointestinal tract. Oral or gavage feedings are discontinued, and fluids and nutrients provided intravenously with lipids and total parenteral nutrition. A nasogastric tube may be inserted to relieve distension; antibiotics are used to treat the inflammation. In some instances surgery may be performed to remove the necrotic bowel and a permanent or temporary colostomy created as needed.

Hospitalization of the neonate is a distressing event for the parents and family. As discussed for the low birth weight infant, parental bonding may be disturbed as the neonate remains in the care of health professionals. The nurse must, therefore, plan to include parents and allow as many opportunities for physical contact as possible.

Cleft lip and cleft palate

A cleft lip and/or cleft palate is the most common congenital defect of the neonate that interferes with the need for nutrition. A cleft lip occurs when there is a failure of the fissure of the lip to close, and it may be unilateral or bilateral. A cleft palate results from an incomplete closure of the maxillary process; the soft and hard palate may be involved, or the soft palate alone. The cleft palate may be unilateral or bilateral, and a cleft lip usually occurs along with it (Fig. 17-14).

Clefts of the lip or palate are congenital defects of embryonic development, some caused by mutant genes, others by chromosomal abnormalities. Cleft lip, with or without cleft palate, occurs when the maxillary processes fail to fuse, an event that occurs during the sixth week of gestation. The hard and soft palates fuse during the seventh or twelfth weeks of gestation, and failure of fusion then causes cleft palate.

Cleft lip or cleft palate occur in about 1 in 1000 births. The incidence of cleft lip is higher in boys, whereas cleft palate occurs more frequently in girls.

 Assessment. The nurse performing a neonatal appraisal can easily identify the cleft lip or palate by inspecting the neonate's mouth and oral structures and observing the neonate as he obtains his first feedings. Feedings that spurt through the nose as the liquid enters the maxillary sinus may indicate the presence of a cleft palate. The nurse can also assess parent-infant bonding as the parents interact with their newborn.

> **Data analysis**
> *Data analysis may reveal nursing diagnoses of alterations in nutrition and disturbances in self-concept.*

Planning and implementation. The neonate with a cleft lip or palate has difficulty obtaining nutrition because he is unable to suck, and much of the feeding is lost through the cleft. Ensuring adequate nutrition is the most immediate concern for a newborn with a cleft lip or palate, and the nurse and mother should find a satisfactory way to feed him. Later the defect is corrected surgically.

Feeding. If the baby has a cleft lip, the nurse or mother may try to feed him by propping the baby on a pillow, gently holding the lip together with one hand, and holding a bottle with a soft nipple with the other hand. Breast milk can be pumped and fed by bottle until the lip is repaired. The baby can also be fed with a spoon, cup, or a nipple with a special flap that prevents loss of the feeding.

The baby with a cleft palate may be fed with a spoon, cup, or a rubber-tipped Asepto syringe, which is placed at the back of the tongue. Special nipples that cover the cleft and permit easier sucking may also be tried. If the cleft is unilateral, the mother may wish to try breast-feeding. Some surgeons use a maxillary prosthesis, which covers the cleft and prevents milk from entering the sinus as the baby swallows. The prosthesis should be removed and cleaned daily, and the parents should be instructed in its care.

930

When the baby with a cleft lip or palate is fed, he should be held and supported in an upright position to prevent aspiration and promote gravity flow of the feeding. The baby should be fed in a relaxed manner, because he is very responsive to maternal anxiety. It is important to bubble the baby to promote expulsion of air, which is swallowed in large quantities. When the feeding is completed, the baby should be offered water to clear his mouth of the milk that adheres to the tongue and mucous membranes. Parents should be encouraged to participate in feeding and other care activities so that infant-parent bonding can be promoted.

When the infant is ready to take solid foods, they should be offered in the same manner as they are for other infants. The foods should be given with a spoon, taking care to offer small bites and having the infant supported in an upright position. Several small feedings may be better than two or three large meals, and the feedings should be given slowly. Acid foods may be irritating to the mucous membranes around the cleft and should not be included in the diet.

Nursing care of client having cleft lip and palate repair. Surgical intervention is instituted to provide functional and cosmetic correction of the cleft lip and palate. Surgery for lip repair is performed during the first few weeks after birth (Fig. 17-15). Hard palate repair can be done when the infant is 10 months old, and soft palate repair when the maxillary structures are more developed, usually about 18 to 24 months of age. Additional operations may be needed to ensure proper closure of a cleft palate, particularly during adolescence when the oral structures increase in size.

Preoperative nursing care. The infant must be in good health before surgery. Dehydration and poor weight gain can be problems for infants with cleft lips and palates, and most surgeons prefer to wait until the child weighs at least 10 pounds (4.5 kg) and is able to withstand surgery. Upper respiratory tract infections and otitis media are common because microorganisms enter the cleft lip and palate, and the child should be free of colds or other respiratory tract infections before surgery.

The infant should also be prepared to obtain adequate nutrition after surgery. The newborn who is to have a lip repair may be taught to feed from an Asepto syringe in preparation for postoperative feedings. The older child who will have palate repair should be able to feed himself and hold a cup.

Postoperative nursing care. Postoperative nursing care objectives are to (1) prevent complications, (2) ensure adequate nutrition, (3) provide safety for the suture line, and (4) instruct the family in care of their child.

PREVENTING COMPLICATIONS. Excessive bleeding is the most serious postoperative complication. The client should be positioned on his side to prevent aspiration. Airway obstruction from laryngeal edema is not uncommon and the nurse must take measures to ensure an open airway. Oral suctioning may be ordered to remove mucus, but care should be exercised to avoid trauma to the palate. The client should be kept away from persons with known upper respiratory tract infections. The client may be turned frequently to either side, and antibiotics may be given to prevent respiratory tract infections.

ENSURING NUTRITION. After surgery the feedings must be given carefully to avoid damage to the suture line. The infant with a cleft lip repair is fed with an Asepto syringe so that he does not have to exert pressure on the suture by

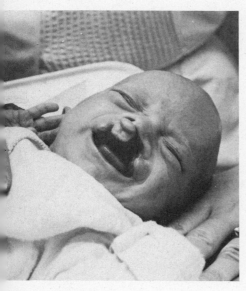

FIG. 17-14
Infant with cleft lip and palate. (Courtesy March of Dimes Birth Defects Foundation.)

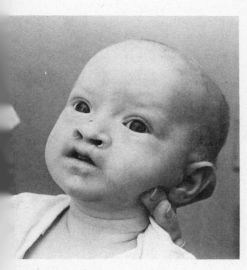

FIG. 17-15
Cleft lip is repaired soon after birth. (Courtesy March of Dimes Birth Defects Foundation.)

sucking. Intravenous feedings may be given to prevent dehydration while feeding is temporarily limited. When the suture line has healed, the infant may resume normal breast- or bottle-feedings, unless he also has a cleft palate.

The child who has had a cleft palate repair takes his liquids from a cup until the suture line is healed. The nurse or mother can assist him so that he does not traumatize the suture line. Sucking and sipping with a straw are discouraged because this creates tension on the sutures. As the palate heals, the diet is advanced to a soft diet and then to a regular diet that is appropriate for the child.

CARING FOR SUTURES. The suture line in cleft lip or cleft palate repair is delicate, and the nurse should plan to prevent the young clients from interfering with it. Elbow restraints are used to prevent handling or rubbing the surgical site. The restraints should be removed one at a time every 1 to 2 hours to exercise the arms. The client is also restrained so that he does not turn on his face, and at no time should the child be permitted to turn on his abdomen following cleft lip repair.

Infants with a cleft lip repair may have a Logan bar applied to prevent damage to the sutures (Fig. 17-16). This bar is applied with tapes and bridges the cleft. The tapes must be kept dry and secure. The suture line may be cleansed with saline after every feeding and more often if needed, and antibiotic ointment may be used to prevent infection. Sedatives may be used to prevent crying and stress on the sutures, and the nurse and mother should talk reassuringly to the infant so that he is not frightened or tearful.

INSTRUCTING THE FAMILY. The parents are encouraged to visit their child and participate in his care. Rooming-in adds to the security of the child and familiarizes the mother with his needs. If any special feeding techniques are to be used or medicines are to be given, the nurse should demonstrate and give the parents an opportunity to perform the task under supervision. Arm restraints are usually worn several weeks after the client is discharged, and the nurse should show the parents how to remove them and exercise the arms.

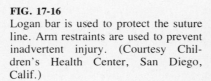

FIG. 17-16
Logan bar is used to protect the suture line. Arm restraints are used to prevent inadvertent injury. (Courtesy Children's Health Center, San Diego, Calif.)

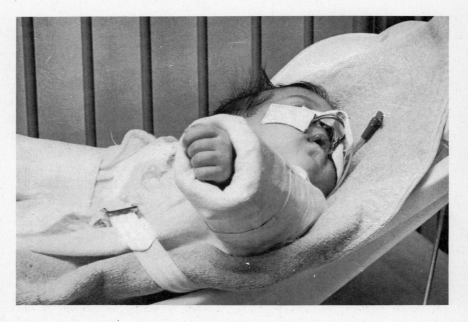

Discharge instructions. Plans for continuing care demand a multidisciplinary effort. A community health nurse may visit in the home if the mother needs assistance in feeding the infant. Speech development is often delayed in children who have cleft palates, and the parents should encourage speech by permitting the child to talk. If the child appears to have difficulty forming vowels or consonants, the physician may refer the child to a speech therapist. Dental structures may have been realigned during surgery, and it is important for the family to visit an orthodontist when the child is 4 to 6 years old.

The child may continue to have frequent upper respiratory tract infections and otitis media because of the disruption in the eustachian tube if the child has a cleft palate. The parents can be instructed to use health promotion strategies for prevention of upper respiratory tract infections (see Chapter 21). They should also be instructed to report infections or signs of hearing impairment to the physician.

The child's self-concept may be altered by his initial appearance and subsequent changes during reconstructive surgery. The parents can be sensitive to their own reactions as well as their infant's reaction and attempt to facilitate a positive body image. Cosmetic repair surgery may be required when the child is older and even more aware of his appearance, and family support is crucial to self-concept and development.

Evaluation. The nursing care plan is developed to ensure nutrition and enhance parental bonding and self-concept as functional and cosmetic repair of the cleft lip and/or palate is achieved.

EXPECTED OUTCOMES

The client and family can:
1. Describe cleft lip and cleft palate.
2. Demonstrate feeding techniques and use of feeding devices.
3. Describe methods of preventing upper respiratory tract infections.
4. Describe patterns of normal growth and development for a neonate, infant, and child.
5. Demonstrate parent-infant bonding and acceptance of infant with a congenital defect.
6. State indications for health care, including inadequate weight gain, upper respiratory tract infection, and otitis media.
7. State plans for follow-up health care.

Esophageal defects

Several defects may occur in the esophagus of the newborn. The esophagus may end in a blind pouch or be open into the trachea in several ways (Fig. 17-17). The most common is esophageal atresia with a tracheoesophageal fistula. The esophagus terminates in a pouch, and there is a fistula between the esophagus and the trachea. The defect is noticed in the nursery as the infant drools saliva, chokes, becomes cyanotic, and is in respiratory distress. Often, the first feeding of glucose and water will evoke choking and spitting. The diagnosis is confirmed by roentgenograms.

Until surgery is performed to correct the fistula, the infant is put in an incubator with high humidity to liquefy secretions. The client should be positioned on his back with his head and chest elevated, to prevent regurgitation of gastric juice into the lung. Aspiration of saliva is a common problem, and the newborn is suctioned frequently with a bulb syringe or a pliable suction catheter. Antibiotics may be given to prevent respiratory tract infection, and

933

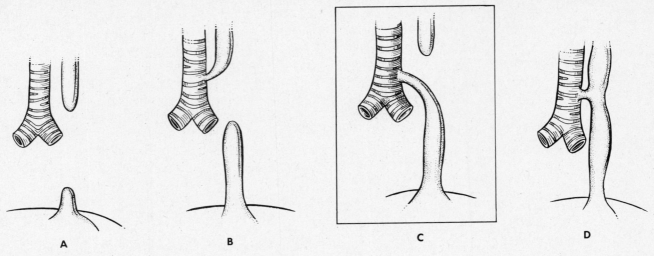

FIG. 17-17
Esophageal defects. **A,** Esophagus ends in blind pouch. **B,** Upper end of esophagus opens into trachea, and lower part ends in blind pouch. **C,** Upper part of esophagus ends in blind pouch, and lower end enters trachea. **D,** Fistulous tract between esophagus and trachea.

intravenous feedings or parenteral hyperalimentation by an infusion pump is given to maintain hydration and nutrition. A cervical esophagostomy may also be created.

Surgical intervention, often in several stages, is imperative to meet the need for nutrition as well as the need for oxygen. The defective esophagus is anastomosed, and the fistula closed. If the segments are far apart, distant tissue such as the colon may be used to bridge the gap. A gastrostomy tube is inserted in the stomach so that the infant can be fed while the esophagus heals and gastric distension can be relieved.

Postoperative nursing care is planned to provide nutrition, maintain respirations, and help the family care for their newborn. Intravenous feedings are used initially to prevent dehydration. Several days later the infant is fed through the gastrostomy tube until adequate esophageal blood supply is assured and he can tolerate oral feedings. The formula should be given slowly at room temperature, and the infant should be held during and after the feeding. During the feeding the infant should suck on a nipple to strengthen oral muscles in preparation for oral feedings. The first oral feeding is given about 2 weeks after surgery, and glucose-water is given through an Asepto syringe to be sure the infant can swallow the feeding. When the client is advanced to formula feedings, the parents may wish to feed their child.

Because a thoracic approach is often necessary, the nurse should plan to assess chest drainage frequently (see Chapter 21). Respirations are made easier by the use of high-humidity oxygenation. The head of the bed should be elevated, and endotracheal suctioning may be done as needed to keep the airway clear. Antibiotics may be used prophylactically to prevent respiratory tract infection.

The nurse should help the parents learn how to care for their child. If this is the first baby, it may be helpful to explain formula preparation and care of the newborn. When the baby is at home, the parents should observe him for adequate respirations during feeding. Sneezing, choking, or turning cyanotic while he feeds may indicate respiratory tract distress. Follow-up care may be long-term, because the esophagus may require periodic dilation.

Biliary atresia

Biliary atresia is a rare congenital defect in which the bile ducts fail to develop and bile accumulates in the liver. Bilirubin, the bile pigment, is absorbed by the bloodstream, and the infant becomes jaundiced. As previously mentioned, bile pigments are normally excreted in the stool, giving it a dark color, but when bile flow is blocked, the stool is white, and the urine becomes darker. The newborn may have ascites as fluid backs into the abdominal cavity. Liver function soon becomes impaired, and defects in blood-clotting appear. The diagnosis is based on clinical symptoms, liver function studies, and radiographic evidence of biliary atresia.

The prognosis is generally poor, but surgery may be attempted to restore the bile ducts. On several occasions, liver transplants have been attempted. If surgery is not considered, the client is given a low-fat diet with increased calories and vitamin K to provide nutrition and minimize the demands on the liver.

Pyloric stenosis

Pyloric stenosis is caused by hypertrophy of the pyloric sphincter. It occurs most frequently in firstborn white boys. Often, it is not diagnosed until the second to eighth week of life when the infant has projectile vomiting, visible reverse peristaltic waves, weight loss, and constipation and the hypertrophied sphincter can be felt in the abdomen as a mass the size of an olive. Dehydration follows rapidly when the infant vomits the feedings. The infant who is dehydrated will have poor skin turgor, depressed fontanels, sunken eyes, and metabolic alkalosis if dehydration is not reversed. The diagnosis is made by observing the infant after feeding and by radiographic studies of the hypertrophied sphincter.

The therapeutic plan depends on the nutritional status of the infant. Conservative therapy may be tried if the infant can retain some food. The infant is given antispasmodics and anticholingeric drugs 20 minutes before feedings so that the sphincter will be relaxed. Formula thickened with cereal may pass through the sphincter more easily. The formula may be given on a spoon or through a nipple with enlarged holes. Small, frequent feedings are more easily tolerated, and the feedings should be given in a relaxed manner, because the mother's anxiety can be easily transmitted to the infant.

If the infant is unable to retain any feedings, it is necessary to revise the hypertrophied sphincter. A *pylorotomy* (release of the pyloric muscle) or a *pyloroplasty* (total reconstruction of the sphincter) may be performed.

When the client returns from surgery, the nurse should observe him for bleeding, shock, and adequate nutrition. See discussion later in this chapter for nursing care of the client with gastric surgery. When peristalsis resumes, the infant is given oral glucose-water to ascertain that he can tolerate feedings. Formula- or breast-feedings can be resumed along with the infant's regular diet.

Phenylketonuria

Phenylketonuria (PKU) occurs in newborns when there is faulty utilization of the amino acid phenylalanine, which is present in all protein.[22] This rare disease is carried as an autosomal recessive trait, and there appears to be an increased incidence in blue-eyed, blond children. Phenylalanine, which is spilled in the bloodstream, causes brain damage and mental retardation if it is permitted to accumulate. The client may also have anemia, vomiting, and foul-smelling urine. The presence of phenylalanine can be detected in the blood or urine within 2 to 4 days after the neonate has been fed, and it is diagnostic of PKU.

If phenylalanine is detected, a special diet with a low protein content is instituted. One formula, Lofenalac, is made commercially and is given until the child is about 6 years old. This formula contains protein for growth but is limited in phenylalanine. The diet can be supplemented with pure carbohydrates and fats as well as with foods that have minimal amounts of phenylalanine. The nurse can suggest that the parents use a nutrition book or diet manual with a listing of the phenylalanine content of foods to plan a daily diet of not more than 20 mg of phenylalanine per kg of body weight. As the child matures, the Lofenalac can be prepared as a pudding or frozen and served as a dessert to provide variety in the meals. The diet should be continued until the child is 6 to 8 years old and blood levels of phenylalanine are satisfactory.

It is generally felt that the client will have no residual brain damage if the diet is followed. If the child is not treated until some brain damage has occurred, however, retardation will not be reversed but will be prevented from progressing. Because the effects of untreated PKU are so devastating, all family members should be encouraged to have genetic counseling.

Failure to thrive   Failure to thrive is a symptom rather than a diagnosis. The term is used to describe infants or young children who are two standard deviations below the mean for their age and sex or who fail to maintain appropriate development.[27] Sexual development delay may be a part of the syndrome.

Failure to thrive is a nutritional problem in which the client does not obtain adequate nutrition because of feeding problems. The syndrome may be simply the result of inadequate feedings, but more often is related to neglect. The problems are often associated with maternal deprivation and in essence may be a form of child abuse, that is, physical or emotional neglect. Undernutrition may be attributed to insufficient feedings or decreased infant-maternal bonding that allows satisfying feeding. Another theory is that intestinal absorption and metabolism are altered by emotional disorders transmitted from the hypothalamus, pituitary gland, and autonomic nervous system. Hyperactivity of these centers may contribute to growth suppression.

Because the syndrome is closely associated with maternal deprivation, it is important to assess potential risk in the mother-child relationship. It has been observed that risk factors include a mother who is immature, who has difficulty accepting the child as her own, whose own dependency needs are great, and who is receiving little support from the father or significant others.

The infant who is undernourished looks sick. He has not gained adequate weight and is physically underdeveloped. He may have anorexia, vomiting, or diarrhea, and be irritable or apathetic. Social responses may not be appropriate, and if observed during feeding, the infant does not relate to the person feeding him. The diagnosis is based on weight gain and development. Organic causes for malnutrition should be ruled out, however, before confirming the diagnosis of failure to thrive.

The goal of nursing care is to improve the infant's nutritional state. This may involve intensive instruction and counseling by the nurse and health team members such as the dietitian, social worker, physician, and community health nurse.

The care plan depends on the cause of the inadequate feeding patterns. If the mother or parents simply do not understand what or how to feed the child, instruction is appropriate. More often, however, the parent-child-family feeding system is more complex, and counseling is required. The care plan should be developed with the family with the nurse modeling parenting behaviors.

If the child has not gained weight within 2 weeks he may be hospitalized. At this time the nursing care should be directed toward stimulating a positive interest in food and pleasurable associations with feeding. Nursing actions may include limiting distractions from the environment, using behavior modification approaches, feeding the infant favorite foods, and following feeding schedules preferred by the infant.

Growth acceleration usually occurs over an extended period when the child has deprivation factors eliminated from his daily life. Protective care away from his parents, by placement with a foster family, is sometimes necessary until certain home conditions can be corrected.

Celiac disease

Celiac disease (gluten-induced enteropathy) is a rare disorder of absorption of nutrients. Infants and young children are most affected by this disease; the incidence is highest in whites. The disease is characterized by remissions and exacerbations, although clinical symptoms disappear in adulthood.

Celiac disease is believed to be an inborn error of metabolism in which the client is unable to digest gluten or protein portions of wheat or rye flour. Malnutrition and wasting are final outcomes of the disease if it is not treated. Diagnosis depends on clinical evidence and lowered serum protein levels, as well as loss of serum electrolytes such as calcium and iron.

The onset of celiac disease is usually not noted until 6 months and is signalled by episodes of diarrhea with bulky, foul-smelling stools. There may be anorexia and abdominal distension. Weight loss is marked and is evident in the limbs, buttocks, and groin where wrinkled skin hangs in folds. Behavioral changes such as irritability often accompany the disease. Growth retardation is common.

A *celiac crisis* can be caused by an intercurrent respiratory tract infection. The child passes large watery stools and has episodes of vomiting. The fluid and electrolyte loss leads rapidly to dehydration and acidosis.

Modification of the diet by omitting wheat, rye, and oat flours and reducing fat results in improvement of the child's nutritional status. Fluid balance should be maintained by offering fluids frequently. During acute episodes antibiotics or steroids may be prescribed.

The most important aspect of client teaching is explaining the gluten-free diet and helping the child and his parents plan suitable meals. Dietitians are helpful resource persons during the initial instruction period. Foods with wheat or rye flour must be eliminated from the diet. Other foods may also contain gluten and must also be eliminated. Some of these are meat loaf, puddings, gravies, processed meats (cold cuts), creamed soups, some candies, malted milk drinks, cakes, and biscuits. Food labels should be read for indication of rye or wheat products.

The diet, particularly in young children, may also be limited in starches and fats. This may mean, initially, a diet of skim milk, simple sugars, and banana flakes. Later, foods are added, singly, to determine their effect, until most foods, with the exception of wheat and rye, can be eaten. Supplemental vitamins A and D in a water-miscible base should be used. The diet is usually continued through adolescence.

The diet restrictions may be difficult for the child to follow. The nurse should encourage the parents to use a positive approach when planning menus and offer the child treats from allowed foods. Parents should also be prepared to expect variances in appetite and eating behavior. These should be approached calmly; the child should not be forced to eat.

Other teaching includes information about protecting the child from infections, particularly respiratory tract infections, that could precipitate a celiac crisis. The child should be kept warm, dressed sensibly, and away from individuals with known infections.

The nurse has an important role in assessing changes of nutritional status and encouraging the client to obtain medical attention. The nutritional changes resulting from celiac disease are distinctive and should receive early attention. Early correction of malnutrition enables the child to maintain health and achieve normal developmental tasks.

COMMON HEALTH PROBLEMS OF THE ADULT

Cancer of the mouth

The structures of the mouth—the lips, maxilla, mandible, and tongue—are infrequent sites for cancer, but they have the potential to severely impair the nutritional status of involved clients. Cancer of the mouth accounts for about 5% of all cancers in men and 2% in women.[30] Risk increases for those who smoke, those who are chronic alcohol abusers, or those who have chronic mouth irritation from food or impaired dentition.

Cancer of the lip. Cancer of the lip is primarily an epidermoid cancer that is believed to occur from a source of irritation such as pipe smoking or exposure to sun and wind. This cancer usually occurs in men. Any sore or lesion on the lip that does not heal within a few weeks should be examined by a physician. The lesion can be excised or treated with radiotherapy. Interruption to nutrition is minimal when the area involved is confined and treated early.

Cancer of the maxilla or mandible. Cancer of the maxilla or mandible presents more complicated problems. The tumors usually begin as small lesions on the roof or floor of the mouth. Early mouth cancer may be recognized by painless, velvetlike areas in the floor of the mouth, back of the tongue, or soft palate. Often, dentists are the first to identify these lesions. They are usually noticed in middle-aged adults. Surgery is indicated to prevent the spread of the malignant cells.

Removal of the maxilla or mandible involves extensive surgery. In addition to the interruption of nutrition, speech is impaired, and the appearance of facial features changes. Skin grafts and prostheses may be inserted during surgery to maintain form and function of the mouth.

Immediately after surgery the client may receive nutrition from intravenous infusions or by gavage. When healing has occurred, the client may have a liquid diet. It may be difficult for the client to swallow, and the nurse should offer encouragement and give the client plenty of time when he is eating. Obtaining sufficient nutrition may be a slow process, and the client becomes easily discouraged until he develops skill with swallowing.

Mouth care should be given frequently to prevent infection and freshen the mouth. Special orders are usually given by the physician, prescribing the mouth care preparations to be used so that they will not disrupt the suture line and healing.

Speech is made difficult when the oral cavity is altered. Speech therapy may be needed to help the client learn to reshape certain letters and improve his speech. The nurse should give the client opportunity to speak and not anticipate his needs. Family members are also vital in speech rehabilitation by listening to the client and giving him reassurance.

Cancer of the tongue. Cancer of the tongue occurs primarily in men and is most often a squamous cell carcinoma. The cancer is noticed as small ulcerated areas that do not heal. Ulcerations may be precipitated by irritation from tobacco, food, chronic alcoholism, and poorly aligned teeth. As the tumor grows, there is rapid metastasis to the floor of the mouth and lymph nodes in the neck.

The tumors may be treated by radiation or by removing the involved portion of the tongue. Interstitial or mold applications of radioactive substances may be applied to the tongue. They are usually left in the mouth for several days, and the client is fed by gavage. The client also should not attempt to talk, because the implant might become dislodged. Suction may be used to remove saliva, or a gauze wick to an emesis basin may be devised to prevent accumulation of saliva. Mouth care performed per physician's instructions during and after radiation is important to freshen the mouth, control odors, and loosen necrotic tissue. Special mouthwashes may be ordered by the physician. A suction source should be available in event of choking or aspiration.

If the tumor is small, only part of the tongue need be removed *(hemiglossectomy)*. If the metastasis is not contained, the entire tongue will be removed *(glossectomy)*. A radical neck dissection may also be done to remove metastases in surrounding tissue. When the tongue is removed, there is difficulty with swallowing and speaking. Liquid diets sufficient to support nutritional needs are offered frequently; gavage feedings may also be used.

Mouth care is essential to promote healing and hygiene. Mouthwashes and lemon and glycerin swabs may be used to loosen necrotic tissue, and lanolin or mineral oil may be used on the lips to prevent drying and cracking.

Speech is greatly altered by surgery on the tongue, and the client may be embarrassed by poor communication. The client may be referred to a speech therapist so that he is more easily understood. The family can offer much support by giving the client an opportunity to speak and not depending on written communications.

Esophagitis

Esophagitis may be an acute or chronic inflammation of the esophagus, caused by bacteria, trauma, or irritation from food or tobacco. It is most common in middle-aged adults. The client may experience heartburn, reflux of digestive juices as he bends over or is recumbent, or bleeding if there is severe mucosal ulceration. The diagnosis is made by biopsy, esophagoscopy, and barium swallow.

Esophagitis is treated by reducing the source of irritation. The client may be given a diet of bland foods (p. 944) and antacids to neutralize digestive juices. The client should also avoid smoking.

Cancer of the esophagus

Cancer of the esophagus invades the esophagus and ultimately obstructs food passage. The cancer is primarily an epidermoid carcinoma. The cause is not known, although it is believed that untreated achalasia, hiatal hernia, or lye stricture may be predisposing factors.

Cancer of the esophagus usually occurs in individuals over 60, but the incidence is rare, about 1 in 10,000.

The client with a tumor of the esophagus first notices that he has *difficulty in*

939

swallowing and, because food intake is limited, there is associated *weight loss*. Additionally there may be malaise and anorexia. The diagnosis is confirmed by x-ray studies, esphagoscopy, and biopsy.

Management of cancer of the esophagus may be curative or palliative, and surgery or radiation therapy or both may be used. Generally by the time diagnosis is made, the disease is advanced. Five-year survival rates are not favorable.

Radiation therapy may be used as an attempt at cure if the tumor is an epidermoid carcinoma. Radiation is also used as a palliative measure and produces relief of symptoms in most instances.[24]

Surgical approaches may be used to resect the tumor or to provide relief of the obstruction. Surgical removal and anastomosis of the esophagus provide the best esophageal continuity. Resection and use of a prosthetic esophagus also have been successful. Colon transplants may also be attempted to anastomose a portion of colon to the resected esophagus. If the tumor is inoperable, a gastrostomy may be created, and the client receives nutritional support from gastrostomy feedings.

Nursing care is based on the client's needs and the type of surgery. (See discussion of gastric surgery later in this chapter and discussion of thoracic surgery in Chapter 21.) Plans should include goals for maintaining optimum nutrition because the client is likely debilitated. The client and family must also deal with impending death. They may choose hospice or home care, and the nurse provides instructions and support in these settings.

Peptic ulcer disease

A peptic ulcer is an inflammation of the mucosa and submucosa of the lower esophagus, stomach, duodenum, and jejunum. The inflammation may be acute or chronic. In an acute inflammation the mucosa and occasionally the submucosa are involved, whereas a chronic inflammation erodes deeper tissues of the submucosa and muscular layers. Gastric and duodenal ulcers are the most common, and their similarities and differences are discussed here.

The incidence of peptic ulcer disease is estimated at 10% of the American population. Gastric ulcers affect adults 50 to 60 years old, whereas duodenal ulcers are more common in the 40- to 50-year age group. Twice as many men have peptic ulcer disease, although the incidence in women increases after menopause. The incidence is also higher in urban areas and in those with diets of high protein intake and decreased refined carbohydrates. The incidence of peptic ulcer disease in children is considerably less; the 12- to 18-year age group is primarily involved. In children under 6 years of age the incidence of gastric and duodenal ulcers is comparable, and the cause is usually attributed to toxins or sequelae of other illness. In children over 6, duodenal ulcers are more common than gastric ulcers.

Pathophysiology. The cause of peptic ulcer disease is not known, but seemingly there is an imbalance of acid production and mucosal resistance.[9] There may be either a source of irritation or a mucosa that is highly susceptible to irritation. Normally slightly alkaline mucus present in the stomach and duodenum along with food and saliva protect the mucosa from irritation of gastric juice, hydrochloric acid, and enzymes. If the mucus is insufficient or if the blood supply to the mucosal cells is inadequate, the gastric juices may cause ulceration.

Several theories have been proposed to explain the onset of ulceration.[11] One is that the ulcer is induced by irritants such as smoking, alcohol, or certain drugs (salicylates, adrenocorticosteroids, phenylbutazone). Increased secretion of acid in duodenal ulcers may be attributed to an increase in mass of parietal cells or excessive vagal stimulation. Psychological and physical stresses may also increase gastric secretion and motility by long-term vagal stimulation. There may be personality traits that lend themselves to causing peptic ulcers. Persons who are unhappy and perfectionistic often have peptic ulcers. Hormonal imbalances may aggravate peptic ulcers, because it is noticed that women after menopause have an increased incidence of ulcers. Finally, there may be an inherited basis for peptic ulcers, because there seems to be a familial tendency. Individuals with type O blood also seem to have a higher incidence of peptic ulcer.

The role of stress in the etiology of ulceration is becoming more evident, because individuals who are subjected to long-term physiological stress tend to have multiple gastric ulcers. Two special types are Curling's ulcers, and Cushing's ulcer. *Curling's ulcer* occurs after severe burns, whereas *Cushing's ulcer* coincides with prolonged central nervous system stress. The ulcers may be precipitated by transient decreased gastric blood supply and ischemia, disruption of the protective mucosa, or stimulation of the hypothalamic nuclei, which increases gastric secretion and blood flow. Clients who have nothing by mouth for prolonged periods of time or who have sepsis, burns, trauma, acute lung or kidney disease, and are in intensive care units should be assessed for stress ulcers and managed accordingly.

Assessment. The nurse can use the nursing history to obtain information about the client's life-style, nutrition patterns, and physical signs associated with peptic ulcer disease and impaired nutrition.

The symptoms of peptic ulcers are related to mucosal inflammation. There is *pain* when the stomach is empty and gastric juices are active. The pain usually begins 1 to 3 hours (gastric ulcers) or 3 to 4 hours (duodenal ulcers) after eating. The pain is described as being gnawing, aching, or burning. The pain in a gastric ulcer is felt in the left epigastric region, whereas the pain of a duodenal ulcer is felt in the right epigastric area. Pain appears to increase in the fall and spring. The pain also intensifies as the day progresses and may even radiate to the back. Gastric activity does not slow during sleep, and for this reason the client may be awakened with pain. Pain is further aggravated by nicotine. In addition to the pain, there is *dyspepsia* and *eructation* before eating. *Vomiting* is a late symptom and may indicate an obstruction from an ulcer that has become filled with scar tissue. The medical diagnosis is based on direct visualization of the mucosa, roentgenograms of the stomach and duodenum, biopsy, and gastric analysis that reveals increased amounts of hydrochloric acid.

Data analysis
Data analysis may reveal nursing diagnoses of alterations in nutrition and alterations in comfort.

Planning and implementation. Therapy is planned to heal the ulceration. Initial medical therapy is conservative and involves modifications in stress and diet as well as use of drug therapy to reduce gastric hyperacidity and hypermotility. If the ulcer does not heal or complications of obstruction, perforation, or hemorrhage occur, surgery may be required.

Nursing process for common health problems

Acute ulcers may respond to simple therapy and heal within 6 to 8 weeks. Chronic ulcers usually require modification of the activities that aggravate the ulcer or surgical removal of the ulcerated portion of the stomach or duodenum.

Nursing care objectives are to (1) provide rest for healing, (2) protect the mucosa, and (3) help the client comply with the therapeutic plan.

Providing rest. Physical and mental rest promotes healing of the ulcer. Decreased motor activity minimizes the stress on body, and reduction of stress from career and home pressures contributes to mental rest.

The nurse can provide stress counseling (see Chapter 8) and help the client develop a stress management plan. The client may be hospitalized so that he can obtain this needed rest, and sedatives or mild tranquilizers may be used to help the client relax. The nurse should understand the feelings of clients who must be suddenly hospitalized. Most clients are involved in home and career responsibilities and may resent having to stay in bed. The nurse should provide a quiet atmosphere by screening visitors and providing quiet diversional activities for the client.

TABLE 17-10

Common antacids

Drug	Dose/route	Side effects	Client instructions
Magnesium compounds			
Milk of magnesia	5 to 30 ml q.4h.	Diarrhea	Alternate with calcium carbonate or aluminum hydroxide to prevent diarrhea
Magnesium carbonate	500 mg to 2 g		
Magnesium hydroxide	300 mg to 600 mg		Use with caution in presence of renal disease
Magnesium oxide	250-1500 mg	Diarrhea	Report lethargy and drowsiness as signs of hypermagnesemia
Magnesium trisilicate	500 mg tablet or 1 g powder q.i.d.		
Aluminum compounds			
Aluminum hydroxide gel		Constipation	Alternate with Maalox or milk of magnesia to avoid constipation
Amphogel	5 to 40 ml	Interferes with absorption of other drugs	
Cremolin	4 to 8 ml q.2-4h.		Do not use if taking anticholinergics or barbiturates
Alkagel	15 to 30 ml q.1h.		Contains sodium; do not use if on sodium restricted diet
Aluminum phosphate gel			
Phosphagel	4% suspension, 15 to 45 ml q.2h.		
Aluminum carbonate			
Aluminum and magnesium compounds			
Magnesium hydroxide and aluminum hydroxide gel	5 to 30 ml q.1-4h.	Diarrhea	Contains magnesium; do not use in presence of fluid and electrolyte imbalances or malabsorption syndromes or renal disease
Maalox	200-400 mg		Alternate with aluminum compound and calcium carbonate
Magnesium trisilicate and aluminum hydroxide gel Gelusil	300 to 600 mg tablet or liquid, 4 to 8 ml q.2-4h.	Constipation	
Aluminum and magnesium hydroxide Riopan	400 to 800 mg liquid or tablet q.i.d.		Do not use in presence of renal disease; can cause hypermagnesemia
Calcium compounds			
Calcium carbonate	Precipitated chalk 1 to 2 g q.1h.	Constipation; hypercalcemia	Alternate with magnesium oxide to avoid constipation; monitor calcium levels, especially if milk intake is increased; use with caution in presence of renal disease

Protecting the mucosa. The mucosa is protected by neutralizing or reducing the acid content, eliminating sources of irritation, and slowing gastrointestinal motility. Medicine and diet modifications are used to protect the mucosa.

Antacids are used to neutralize hydrochloric acid. Systemic antacids should not be used for clients with peptic ulcer who require long-term use of the drug because frequent use of a systemic antacid such as baking soda disrupts the acid-base balance and cause metabolic alkalosis. Furthermore, use of a systemic antacid with milk can cause a *milk-alkali syndrome* of hypercalcemia and renal insufficiency.

Nonsystemic antacids are most often used to manage hyperacidity. There are many products available in liquid or tablet form. These antacids contain combinations of aluminum and magnesium as a base, and the drugs can be selected to comply with the client's dietary or health needs (Table 17-10). Side effects of the nonsystemic antacids are minimal. Diarrhea, constipation, and electrolyte imbalance are not unusual, but can be avoided by alternating several antacids.

The antacids may be taken as often as every hour during acute inflammation. If the antacid is in tablet form, the client should be instructed to chew it slowly. Liquid antacids may be diluted with a small amount of water and sipped slowly to provide continuous gastric coating or followed by a glass of water to avoid stasis in the esophagus.

Antacids given before a meal provide acid neutralization for about 30 minutes, whereas those taken after a meal may be effective for 2 to 3 hours. Occasionally the antacid may be given continuously in a drip through a nasogastric tube.

The gastrointestinal mucosa is further protected when gastric motility is slowed by anticholinergic and antispasmodic drugs. Anticholinergic drugs also decrease gastric secretions and motility and are usually given 30 minutes before the meal. These drugs inhibit basal or nocturnal gastric secretions and are therefore useful for nighttime use. The medications should be given on time and, if possible, left with the client to administer himself. Propantheline (Pro-Banthine) is a commonly used anticholinergic drug. Side effects of this and similar drugs are decreased urine output, tachycardia, and blurred vision. These drugs are contraindicated for individuals with glaucoma or benign prostatic hypertrophy. Clients who use these drugs should be observed for their side effects.

Histamine type II receptor antagonists such as cimetidine (Tagamet) are used to reduce gastric secretion. When taken on an empty stomach, they reduce the gastric acid secretion 90% to 100% for 4 hours or if taken after a meal 50% in the first hour and 75% in next.[26] Side effects are minimal.

Managing diet. The mucosa can also be protected by dietary management. Food acts as an irritant and a digestive stimulant, as well as protecting the mucosa. Carbohydrates and fats are the least stimulating but provide minimal neutralizing properties. Proteins neutralize effectively but stimulate gastric secretions. There are, therefore, varying approaches to diet.

During periods of acute inflammation some physicians initiate conservative therapy and prescribe a continuous intake of milk to coat the stomach. The protein in the milk is retained in the stomach and buffers gastric acid, and the fat delays gastric emptying. The milk can be taken orally, ½ cup every hour, or may be given through a nasogastric tube as a continuous drip into the stomach. If continuous milk drips are used, the nurse must refill the drip chamber frequently with refrigerated milk so that the milk does not sour.

When the inflammation has subsided somewhat, bland food is added to the diet (see bland diet below). Soft-cooked eggs and strained cereal are given first, followed by creamed soups, toast, and gelatin as tolerated. Other bland foods are added gradually. This diet is referred to as the Sippy diet for the physician who developed it.

Other physicians feel that the client should avoid only foods that are irritating to him. A bland diet is usually acceptable to most clients. Spicy foods, alcohol, and known irritants should be avoided. Meals should be eaten slowly. Small frequent meals provide food in the stomach, reduce gastric motility, and prevent rapid emptying into the duodenum. A bedtime snack should be taken to buffer the acid during the night. The atmosphere during the meal should be pleasant so that psychological stress does not upset the client and increase gastric motility.

Other irritants such as nicotine and drugs should be eliminated. The client is encouraged to stop smoking, a difficult task to accomplish. The client should also inform his physician if he is taking other medication that might be acting as an irritant. Nonirritating forms of analgesics and antipyretics, such as acetaminophen (Tylenol) may be used as a substitute for aspirin.

Instructions about the therapeutic plan. Coping with a peptic ulcer may require modifications in the client's life-style. The nurse should help the client and his family plan to follow the therapeutic plan. If the client is on a modified diet, the nurse and dietitian may instruct the client and his family on how to follow the diet. It is especially important that the person who prepares the family

---

BLAND DIET

Purpose	1. Reduce mechanical, chemical, and thermal irritation of the gastrointestinal tract.
	2. Slow the gastrointestinal motility by continuous presence of food.
	3. Neutralize acid secretions in peptic ulcer disease.
	4. Prevent hunger spasms.
Meat and eggs	Eggs, except fried; most meats prepared by baking, broiling, or boiling; lean ham, crisp bacon.
Milk	Regular milk, skim milk, cottage cheese, cream cheese, mild cheese.
Fruits and vegetables	Cooked or canned applesauce; peeled, baked apple; peaches, pears, peeled apricots, bing cherries, ripe banana; cooked vegetables; fruit juices (orange juice strained and diluted).
Breads and cereals	Oatmeal, Cream Of Wheat, soda crackers, noodles, macaroni, dry cereals, baked potato, white bread.
Foods to avoid	Pork, processed meats, extremely hot or cold foods, spices, concentrated sweets, alcohol, fried foods, whole-grain cereals and breads, condiments, coffee, iced tea, cold drinks, raw fruits and vegetables, rich desserts, gravies, nuts, raisins, coconut.
Suggestions	1. Eat slowly, chew food well.
	2. Eat small, frequent meals.
	3. Eat in a relaxed atmosphere.
	4. Serve foods at room temperature.
	5. Remain sitting for 20 minutes after the meal.

---

meals be present during dietary instruction. It is helpful if the foods are prepared and served in a bland form and those who wish to add more spices do so at the table. The client may find it difficult to eat regular meals because of his work schedule. The dietitian can suggest foods that are easily carried, such as snacks, and foods that may be eaten in a restaurant or packed in a lunch. The regularity of mealtimes is important in healing an ulcer.

The client also learns to cope with stresses in his life that may precipitate anxiety and increased gastric secretions. Avoiding situations that upset the client or learning to adjust to the stressful situations are two useful approaches in coping with stress. The nurse can help the client anticipate these stresses so that he will be prepared to cope with them.

The nurse should also help the client see the need for compliance with the therapy as long as it is prescribed. There is a tendency to terminate medications or diet once the pain is relieved or the client feels better; it is important, however, that the therapy be continued until healing has occurred.

Complications of peptic ulcers. If the medical therapy is not followed or if inflammation persists, there may be serious complications, the four most common of which are perforation (5%), obstruction (20%), hemorrhage (20%), and continuous pain or nonresponsiveness to conservative therapy (40%).[5] These complications pose threats to the nutritional status of the individual, and therapeutic intervention is required immediately.

Perforation. Perforation occurs when the submucosa becomes ulcerated and the gastric contents empty into the peritoneal cavity. Perforation occurs more frequently with bleeding duodenal ulcers. The client has severe pain, which causes him to draw his legs up for relief. The abdomen is tense, boardlike, and painful to touch. When fluid shifts to the peritoneal cavity, the client goes into shock, there is a rapid weak pulse and hypotension, and the client is diaphoretic. The perforation is diagnosed by the symptoms and a roentgenogram that shows air under the diaphragm.

Gastric decompression by the insertion of a nasogastric tube for the removal of gastric contents is used to prevent further spilling of gastric contents into the peritoneum. The perforation may heal if it is small; if the perforation is large, however, the opening may be sutured or reinforced with an omental graft. Intravenous fluids are used then to maintain fluid and electrolyte balance until gastric surgery is performed. Massive doses of antibiotics are given to combat peritonitis.

Obstruction. An obstruction can occur if scar tissue forms over the ulcer and food is not emptied from the pylorus. Edema from tissue inflammation around the ulcer may also cause an obstruction. There is fullness, abdominal distension, pain, gastric dilation, and, later, projectile vomiting.

Gastric decompression using a nasogastric tube is used initially to remove the gastric contents. The client should not have any oral intake for several days until the symptoms are reversed. Gradually, the client is tried on oral liquids to see if these are absorbed. If they are well tolerated, the nasogastric tube is removed. Surgery is usually necessary to release the obstruction permanently.

Hemorrhage. Hemorrhage results when the ulcer perforates a blood vessel. The bleeding from a duodenal ulcer is usually slow and manifested in tarry stools; gastric ulcers usually produce hematemesis and have a more sudden onset. The client is weak from the blood loss and may exhibit signs of anemia

945

and shock. It is imperative to stop the blood loss, and if the client is vomiting blood, to prevent aspiration into the lungs. Nasogastric suction may be used to remove blood from the stomach, and iced saline may be ordered to be inserted through the nasogastric tube to cause vasoconstriction of the perforated vessel. Vasoconstrictor drugs such as vasopressin (Pitressin) or epinephrine may be used to facilitate clot formation at the site of bleeding. The client is also treated for shock with replacement of blood and fluids as necessary. When bleeding has stopped, antacids may be administered per nasogastric tube. Surgery is indicated when the bleeding has been controlled to locate the source of bleeding. When the source of bleeding is located, the vessel is ligated. Additionally, it may be necessary to resect the ulcerated portion of the stomach or intestine.

Nursing care of the client having gastric surgery. Surgical intervention is necessary if the chronic ulcer does not respond to medical management, if there is a complication that interrupts nutrition to the cells, or if there is intractable pain. Various types of surgery can be performed, but the principles of preoperative and postoperative nursing care are similar for all types of surgical approaches.

The following are the types of surgery employed:

gastrectomy Total removal of the stomach (Fig. 17-18, *A*). The esophagus is anastomosed to the duodenum. There are no gastric juices for digestion, and malnutrition, anemia, and weight loss are common postoperatively. A thoracic approach to the surgery is usually used.

subtotal gastrectomy Removal of a part of the stomach, usually the ulcer and the acid-secreting mucosa. The remaining stomach is anastomosed to the duodenum.

gastroenterostomy Removal of a portion of the stomach, with anastomosis to the intestine.

gastroduodenostomy (Billroth I) Removal of the distal one third to one half of the stomach, with anastomosis to the duodenum (Fig. 17-18, *B*).

gastrojejunostomy (Billroth II) Removal of the lower stomach and antrum, with anastomosis to the jejunum (Fig. 17-18, *C*).

vagotomy Resection of the vagus nerve. Inhibition of vagal stimulation decreases motility and gastric secretions. Pain perception is not interrupted. This may be done at the time of a subtotal gastrectomy.

pyloroplasty Enlargement of the pyloric sphincter to permit passage of chyme.

Removal of any part of the stomach or duodenum produces loss in digestive ability, and problems may result with digestion of food, rapid emptying, abdominal distension, and fullness after eating. The surgery is performed to provide maximum nutrition while correcting the interference with adequate nutrition to the cells.

Preoperative nursing care. Preoperative preparation includes ensuring that the client is in the best nutritional health for gastric surgery. Blood or fluid loss may be replaced with intravenous infusions. A nasogastric tube may be inserted before surgery, and antibiotics given prophylactically.

The client may not be feeling well before surgery, and the nurse should approach each client individually. It is important that he understand his surgery and what will happen after surgery. The nurse should instruct the client in turning, coughing, and deep breathing and may inform him of the possibility of a nasogastric tube and intravenous feedings. Clients who will have a thoracic approach to their surgery should have the use of chest drainage tubes (see Chapter 21) explained to them.

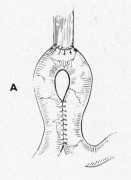
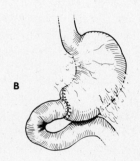
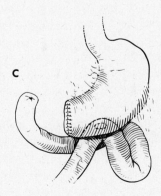

FIG. 17-18
Types of gastric surgery. **A,** Total gastrectomy. **B,** Gastroduodenostomy (Billroth I). **C,** Gastrojejunostomy (Billroth II).

946

Postoperative nursing care. After gastric surgery, nursing care is planned to (1) prevent complications, (2) prevent distension, (3) promote comfort, and (4) maintain nutrition.

PREVENTING COMPLICATIONS. Immediately on the client's return from the recovery room, the nurse should assess the vital signs on a regular basis. The nurse should observe the nasogastric tube and suction bottle for the amount and color of the drainage. Bloody drainage is normal for the first 12 hours and is followed by a dark green color indicating the presence of bile and intestinal secretions. Later the drainage may be dark brown as old blood is aspirated from the stomach. Any bright red drainage after the first 12 hours is indicative of bleeding and should be reported to the physician immediately. The amount and color of drainage are recorded on the intake-output record.

The dressing should be observed for any unusual bleeding. Dark red blood is indicative of old bleeding, but bright red blood is from fresh bleeding and should be reported to the physician. An abdominal binder may be used for clients who are obese to help support the incision. The binder should be changed daily and as needed so that the nurse can observe the dressing and give back care. Dehiscence and evisceration are rare complications, but the nurse should observe the suture line when changing dressings or assisting the physician with a dressing change.

The client must turn, cough, and breathe deeply every 2 to 4 hours to prevent atelectasis and hypostatic pneumonia. Coughing and deep breathing may be painful for the client, and the nurse can offer pain medication before helping the client, as well as splint the incision with a towel, draw sheet, or the hands. To assist venous return, the client should move in bed and exercise his legs. On the second postoperative day he may dangle his legs from the side of the bed and ambulate by the third day after surgery. Elastic hose may also be used to prevent phlebitis and embolus formation.

Nerves to the intestines may be temporarily injured during surgery and adynamic ileus may occur. This complication is usually prevented by gastric decompression and limiting oral fluids, but the nurse should observe the client for absence of flatus and feces and abdominal distension, all of which indicate ileus.

PREVENTING DISTENSION. Gastrointestinal distension may be prevented by gastric decompression with intermittent suction to remove secretions from the stomach so that accumulation of fluids does not impair healing or cause infection. A nasogastric tube such as a Levin tube or Salem sump tube is inserted during surgery, and the tube should be attached to the suction source immediately. The physician usually orders an intermittent suction source, but the Salem tube must be used with continuous suction. If distension does occur, the abdomen becomes hard and increases in size, and there are no bowel sounds or flatus expelled. These signs should be reported immediately to the physician.

The physician may order the nasogastric tube to be irrigated with 30 ml of normal saline to keep the tube patent. Hypotonic solutions such as distilled water should not be used for this purpose, since fluids and electrolytes could thereby be withdrawn. Levin tubes must be disconnected from the suction source to be irrigated, but the Salem sump tube should not disconnected, because it is a double-lumen tube and the irrigation solution is drawn through the tubing by suction (Fig. 17-19). If no returns are obtained when irrigating the tube,

FIG. 17-19
Salem pump tube. This nasogastric tube is irrigated by inserting irrigating solution into protruding section of tube; the suction source should not be disconnected, nor should tubing be aspirated. (Courtesy Sherwood Medical Industries, Inc., St. Louis.)

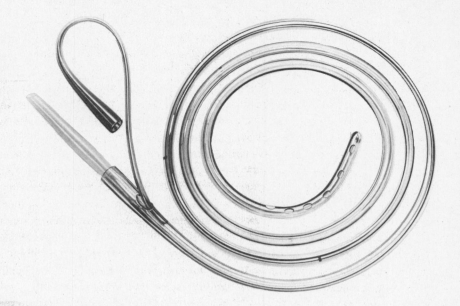

several mechanical interferences may be impeding irrigation. The nasogastric tube may be pressing against the gastric mucosa. Instructing the client to turn or cough, or withdrawing the tube slightly may facilitate irrigation. The air vent on the Salem sump tube reduces negative pressure and the pull on the mucosa. Occasionally gastric drainage is drawn through the air vent. In this instance, the vent should be gently irrigated. If no returns are obtained when these measures are taken, the physician should be notified. Fluid that is not withdrawn should be recorded as intake on the intake-output record.

The nostril may become irritated by the presence of the nasogastric tube and should be cleansed with a cotton-tip applicator and lubricated frequently with a water-soluble lubricant. The nurse should also observe that the tapes are secure (so that the tube does not become dislodged or cause pressure on the nostril) and change them as needed.

PROMOTING COMFORT. Abdominal surgery is painful and exhausting. The client may not wish a complete bath for the first few days after surgery. A sponge bath and frequent back rubs are usually sufficient to make the client comfortable for the first few days. Pain medication should be offered frequently. Visits from the family are reassuring but should be judiciously limited.

The client should be positioned in Fowler's position to make respirations easier. This position also promotes gastric drainage. The nurse should help the client be comfortable in this position with the use of pillows, and if necessary, a footboard should be used to prevent the client from sliding to the foot of the bed.

MAINTAINING NUTRITION. Nutrition is maintained by intravenous infusions during the first 24 to 48 hours. Electrolytes and vitamins may be added to the intravenous solutions to prevent nutritional imbalances caused by gastric suction and limited dietary intake. Although the client cannot have oral fluids, it is important to give mouth care every 4 hours to prevent parotitis and to refresh the mouth. The teeth and gums may be brushed, or the client may use lemon and glycerin swabs.

Oral fluids are permitted when peristalsis returns, usually in 2 to 3 days. Water may be given, 30 ml every hour, but the nasogastric tube is usually not removed until the client can tolerate oral fluids. It is important therefore to keep a very accurate record of intake and output. If the liquids are tolerated, the client is given a full liquid diet and then advanced to a bland or regular diet. The nurse should observe the client for his reaction to these diet changes and report any signs of nausea, vomiting, or abdominal distension.

Discharge instructions. The nurse helps the client prepare for discharge by evaluating his understanding of the diet, activity, and medications, and offering instructions as needed. Anemia, reflux gastritis, and the dumping syndrome are several problems the client should be prepared to manage.

By the time the client is ready to be dismissed, he is taking the foods that he will eat at home. Some physicians prefer a bland diet; others limit only those foods that are irritating to the client. The gastric capacity is smaller, and the client should be instructed to eat small, frequent meals, to eat slowly, and to avoid liquids with meals in order to avoid reflux gastritis, which causes pain, vomiting, and ultimately weight loss.

Clients who have had most of the stomach removed may have pernicious anemia as a result of the loss of intrinsic factor production. Vitamin B_{12} must then be given intramuscularly to assure body requirements of this vitamin.

If the client has had most of his stomach removed, he may experience the *dumping syndrome*. This syndrome occurs 1 to 3 weeks after surgery and is believed to be caused by the rapid emptying of food, especially concentrated carbohydrates, into the duodenum. The food is hypertonic and draws fluid from the bloodstream causing a transient hypovolemia. This shift of fluids produces faintness, dizziness, sweating, palpitations, nausea, vomiting, and flatulence, which can occur 5 to 30 minutes after eating. The client becomes hesitant to eat if he knows that these symptoms will occur. Fifty percent of persons with gastric resections may experience the dumping syndrome during the first year. Eating small meals, chewing food carefully, eating slowly, avoiding highly concentrated carbohydrates, avoiding liquids with meals, and lying down after meals may prevent the symptoms. Anticholinergic drugs are often given before meals to slow motility. The symptoms of dumping syndrome usually disappear after the first year.

The client is usually dismissed from the hospital within 2 to 3 weeks after surgery. He may take some time to adjust to modifications in his diet and regain his strength. The client should avoid strenuous activity until he becomes stronger. Weight loss, dehydration, nausea, and vomiting should be reported to the physician.

 Evaluation. The client with peptic ulcer disease may have problems of alterations in nutrition, and the nurse and client evaluate plans developed to maintain or restore nutrition.

EXPECTED OUTCOMES

The client and/or family can:
1. Describe peptic ulcer disease.
2. Describe plans for maintaining nutritional status, including diet modification, pharmacological therapy, and stress management.
3. State limitations of activity, if any.

4. State use, dosage, time, route, and side effects of prescribed medications (antacids, anticholinergics, antispasmodics, analgesics).
5. State diet modifications (bland diet, avoidance of irritating drugs and foods, and management of dumping syndrome if gastric resection is performed).
6. State indications of health problems requiring health care (pain, infection, fatigue, weight loss, nausea, and vomiting).
7. State plans for follow-up health care.

Cancer of the stomach

Cancer of the stomach is primarily an adenocarcinoma. Most (50%) are located in the pyloric area, whereas fewer are found in the lesser curvature (25%), or cardia (10%). The cause is not known, but is suspected to be precipitated by polyps or degenerative changes in gastric ulcers. The tumor may metastasize to lymph nodes, liver, spleen, pancreas, or esophagus.

About 24,000 individuals a year are diagnosed with cancer of the stomach.[30] Middle-aged adults (50 to 60) are most affected, men twice as frequently as women. The disease occurs more frequently in lower socioeconomic groups and those whose diets contain high starch and inadequate amounts of fresh fruits and vegetables. There is also a correlation observed between persons with pernicious anemia, although no causal relationship has been established.

The clinical indications of cancer of the stomach are varied, and in some instances no symptoms of the tumor are evident until metastases occur. Generally there is *weakness, anorexia, weight loss,* and *indigestion.* There may be ulcer-type pain that does not respond to therapy, although pain is a late symptom. Invasion of the gastric mucosa may cause *bleeding* in the stools or hematemesis. The tumor is diagnosed by x-ray studies (GI series) gastroscopy, biopsy, and gastric analysis that reveals lack of hydrochloric acid production.

The tumor is removed surgically. A partial or total resection of the stomach is done. Nursing care is similar to that for clients having gastric surgery and thoracic surgery. Radiation therapy and chemotherapy are rarely used adjuvants. The prognosis is poor, and much support for the client and family is needed from the health team.

Cholelithiasis

Cholelithiasis is an inflammation of the biliary tract associated with the presence of gallstones. The stones may lodge at the neck of the gallbladder (in the cystic duct or common bile duct) and obstruct bile flow or cause pressure and necrosis or inflammation of the mucosa.

Pathophysiology. Cholelithiasis is caused by stones formed from cholesterol, calcium, and bile salts and proteins in the gallbladder.[28] Stone formation may be precipitated by metabolic changes, inflammation of the gallbladder, or biliary stasis. It is believed that chemical alterations in the bile actually precede stone formation. This bile, saturated with cholesterol or containing cholesterol crystals, is described as *lithogenic bile*. Formation of stones seems to occur when bile acid and lecithin secretions decrease, lowering the capacity of the bile to dissolve cholesterol. The excess cholesterol precipitates as crystals, which aggregate to form gallstones. Precipitation of gallstones is encouraged by abnormal bile pigments, mucoproteins, or bacteria. Gallstones can also be precipitated by inflammation of the lining of the gallbladder. The bile concentration changes with inflammation, and stones are formed from the excess mucus production. Finally, biliary stasis may contribute to stone formation as stagnant bile remains in the gallbladder, causing inflammation or precipitation.

Cholelithiasis occurs more frequently in obese, middle-aged women, and

950

the incidence increases with age. Between 10% and 20% of the population has cholelithiasis. Gallstones appear to be more prevalent in the American Indian and in siblings of persons with cholelithiasis, but the role of genetics has not been identified. Others at risk are those with recurrent gallstones, multiparous women, and individuals who have had a gastrectomy and/or vagotomy. Because stagnation precipitates stones, it is believed that individuals who are immobilized for long periods or who lead sedentary lives are also at risk. Two thirds of clients with cholelithiasis also have chronic cholecystitis.

Assessment. During the nursing history the nurse has an opportunity to appraise the client's nutrition habits and digestive patterns. *Pain* is the most common symptoms of cholelithiasis. The pain is generally located in the epigastrium or right upper quadrant and may radiate to the right scapula. The pain may cause *nausea, vomiting,* or *diaphoresis.* There may be pain after eating. Severe pain may occur when the stones move and cause spasm of the duct.

Because bile is not available for digestion, there may be intolerance to fatty foods, occasionally accompanied by *indigestion, flatulence,* or *belching.* Blockage of bile causes bile pigments to be excreted in the blood and urine. The client becomes jaundiced, and the stools turns clay-colored because of the absence of bilirubin. If the inflammation is acute, there may be fever and leukocytosis.

The medical diagnosis is based on clinical symptoms, cholecystograms, cholangiography, and analysis of duodenal drainage. Laboratory data reveal elevated serum conjugated bilirubin, a rise in hepatic alkaline phosphatase, and increases in serum transaminase.

> **Data analysis**
> *Data analysis may reveal nursing diagnoses of alterations in nutrition and alteration in comfort.*

Planning and implementation. Cholelithiasis is treated by removing the gallbladder and exploring the duct for stones. Some surgeons prefer to wait until the acute attack has subsided and treat the client symptomatically before surgery.

Supportive management includes limiting fat intake in the diet, preventing dehydration, and controlling pain.

Smooth muscle relaxants such as papaverine or nitroglycerin are used to reduce spasms of the ducts and permit passage of bile. Synthetic narcotics are used to relieve pain. Narcotics such as morphine are not suitable analgesics, because they produce biliary spasm and only increase the pain.

If the inflammation is acute, or the client is a poor risk for surgery, the gallbladder may be opened and drained in a procedure known as a *cholecystotomy.* Later, when the inflammation has subsided, the gallbladder is removed in an operation known as a *cholecystectomy.* If stones are obstructing the ducts, the duct may be entered and the stone removed, a *choledocholithotomy.* The surgical approaches are similar, and nursing care planning is based on the needs of the individual client.

Nursing care of the client having gallbladder surgery
Preoperative nursing care. The client should be in good health before the

gallbladder is removed. Antibiotics may be used if the gallbladder is infected, but most important, the client should be in good nutritional health. Vitamin K and other fat-soluble vitamins are not absorbed when bile flow is obstructed. It is necessary therefore to give vitamin K intramuscularly several days before surgery to avoid complications of bleeding during and after surgery. Phytonadione solution (AquaMephyton), menadione, and menadione sodium bisulfite (Hykinone) are several preparations of vitamin K that can be given intramuscularly. If the client has been vomiting before surgery, he may receive intravenous infusions to replace lost fluids and electrolytes.

Before surgery the nurse should instruct the client in turning, coughing, and deep breathing. This may be painful after abdominal surgery, and the client should practice coughing and supporting his abdomen as he coughs before he goes to surgery. The nurse should also prepare the client for the use of special equipment such as a nasogastric tube and the T tube for biliary drainage or intravenous infusions, which may be used after surgery.

Postoperative nursing care. Objectives for postoperative care are to (1) prevent complications, (2) provide for bile drainage, (3) prevent distension, (4) minimize pain, and (5) maintain nutrition.

PREVENTING COMPLICATIONS. Immediately after surgery the nurse should assess the client's vital signs to detect bleeding. Internal bleeding can be detected by shock; external bleeding is manifested on the dressing. Some bile-tinged drainage is normal and frequently appears on the dressing, but evidence of fresh bleeding should be reported to the physician.

The client should be encouraged to turn, cough, and breath deeply every 2 to 4 hours to prevent cardiorespiratory complications. The client may be reluctant to move, and pain medication should be offered as often as permitted for the first few days. The nurse should plan nursing care to have the client turn and breathe deeply at intervals of pain relief. Splinting the incision with a towel, binder, or even the hands may make coughing less painful. Intermittent positive pressure breathing treatments may be ordered to aerate the lungs and prevent atelectasis and pneumonia. The client should be encouraged to cough after these treatments, because trapped mucus is loosened by mucolytic drugs used with this treatment.

Thrombophlebitis is a complication that can result when venous stasis occurs. The physician may order elastic hose to be worn, which will facilitate venous return by compressing the muscles against the veins to improve circulation. The nurse should also encourage the client to flex and extend his legs while he is in bed and to ambulate when he is permitted out of bed.

Wound evisceration and dehiscence are rare complications, but the nurse should observe the sutures when dressings are changed to detect weakening of the suture line. If the abdominal organs do eviscerate, the nurse should cover then with a moist, sterile dressing and notify the physician. No attempt should be made to reposition eviscerated organs.

PROVIDING FOR BILIARY DRAINAGE. Bile that was formerly stored in the gallbladder must escape to prevent distending the bile ducts or causing infection. Backflow of bile into the liver is prevented by providing a temporary outlet for the bile. A tube in the common bile duct or a Penrose drain in the peritoneal cavity may be used for this purpose.

The tube that is inserted into the common bile duct is referred to as a T

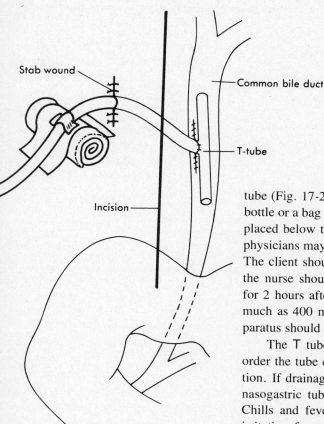

Stab wound

Common bile duct

T-tube

Incision

FIG. 17-20
T tube is inserted into common bile duct for biliary drainage. (From Given, Barbara A., and Simmons, Sandra J.: Gastroenterology in clinical nursing, ed. 3, St. Louis, 1979, The C. V. Mosby Co.)

tube (Fig. 17-20). The T tube is connected to gravity drainage, and a collection bottle or a bag can be used to collect the bile. The collecting apparatus is usually placed below the level of the bile duct for efficient gravity drainage, but some physicians may prefer the collection bag to be elevated to collect only overflow. The client should be placed in Fowler's position to promote bile drainage, and the nurse should observe the amount of drainage. Bloody drainage is normal for 2 hours after surgery, at which time a greenish brown color is normal. As much as 400 ml of drainage can be produced in 1 day, and the collection apparatus should be emptied before it becomes full, to prevent possible backflow.

The T tube is usually clamped as healing occurs, and the physician may order the tube clamped before meals so that bile can be accumulated for digestion. If drainage is excessive, the bile may be given to the client orally or per nasogastric tube. The bile can be mixed in juice to make it more palatable. Chills and fever may result when the tube is first clamped, indicating local irritation from the bile. When the drainage is diminished and the client can tolerate the presence of the bile, the tube is removed. Some clients may have drainage for 6 weeks to 6 months and may be dismissed from the hospital with the tube still in place.

When the Penrose drain is used, the dressing should be changed frequently to prevent odor and skin irritation from continuous biliary drainage. Montgomery straps can be used so that the dressing can be removed without removing the tapes each time the dressing is changed.

When the T tube or Penrose drain is removed, the nurse should observe the client's stool and urine for color changes that indicate a return to normal bile metabolism. If these color changes are not observed, it may be an indication that biliary flow is obstructed.

PREVENTING DISTENSION. Postoperative distension is avoided by providing an outlet for gastrointestinal fluids and flatus. A nasogastric tube may be used to decompress the stomach until peristalsis returns, and a flatus bag or rectal tube may be used to hasten the expulsion of flatus. An enema is usually given on the third or fourth day after surgery to stimulate peristalsis and the release of flatus.

MINIMIZING PAIN. Incisional pain can be lessened by positioning the client in Fowler's position to prevent tension on the suture line. Abdominal binders may be ordered to give additional support to the abdominal muscles and prevent tension. The binder should be changed and reapplied as needed.

Pain medication should be given as often as needed during the first few days after surgery. Some physicians may order 1% or 2% mepivacaine (Carbo-

953

FAT-RESTRICTED DIET

Purpose	1. Reduce gallbladder contractility and avoid pain.
	2. Reduce need for bile in absence of gallbladder function.
Meats and eggs	Lean meat, eggs limited to three a week.
Milk	Skim milk, nonfat dry milk, buttermilk, dry cottage cheese.
Fruits and vegetables	All except avocado.
Breads and cereals	All except hot breads.
Fats	1 to 2 pats of margarine or butter per day.
Foods to avoid	Whole milk, ice cream, cream, butter, margarine, cheeses, chocolate, gravies, sauces, pastries, nuts, fried foods, potato chips, fish canned in oil, goose, duck, pork, salad dressings, cooking oil, mayonnaise, lunch meats.
Suggestions	1. Select lean meats; cook meats on a rack so that the fat drips out.
	2. Use lemon juice and spices to season meats.
	3. Use lemon, vinegar, and seasonings to flavor salads.
	4. Use bouillon instead of creamed soups.

---

caine) to be injected in the T tube to relieve ductal spasms and associated pain. Postoperative pain decreases markedly by the third or fourth day after surgery, when the client ambulates and peristalsis returns.

MAINTAINING NUTRITION. Intravenous fluids may be used for the first 12 to 48 hours to provide for adequate fluid and electrolyte balance. Clear liquids are given when peristalsis has returned and the client can tolerate them. A fat-restricted diet (see above) is usually given until biliary drainage is reestablished; at that time, the client may follow a diet that is tolerated by him.

Discharge instructions. The client is usually dismissed 7 to 10 days after surgery. As with any abdominal surgery, the client is instructed to avoid heavy lifting and exertion until he has been examined by the physician, usually 4 to 6 weeks after surgery.

Cholecystitis

Cholecystitis is an inflammation of the gallbladder that may or may not result in gallstones. The disease may be acute or chronic. The inflammation is usually caused by a bacterial infection: *Staphylococcus* or *Streptococcus* organisms, *E coli,* or *Typhoid bacillus.* The wall of the gallbladder becomes inflamed. If the inflammation is chronic, the gallbladder becomes distended, and if the mucosa is damaged there may be outpouchings of the wall in which bacteria may lodge and continue to incite chronic inflammation. Stones may or may not be present.

Cholecystitis is more common in women and usually occurs in women 50 to 60. The disease occurs more frequently in obese individuals.

Assessment. The client may have *intolerance* to *fatty foods* accompanied by nausea and vomiting. In an acute attack the onset of pain is abrupt. The pain is located in the right upper quadrant of the abdomen and is severe. The gallbladder is usually palpable. The symptoms of chronic cholecystitis are similar although less severe and tend to occur several times before the individual seeks medical attention. The disease is diagnosed by the symptoms, elevated white count, and gallbladder x-ray studies.

Planning and implementation. Cholecystitis is managed conservatively with a low-fat, reducing diet or more commonly with surgery. The therapeutic

954

plan and nursing care are similar to a client with cholelithiasis and having gall-bladder surgery.

 Evaluation. The nursing care plan for the client with cholelithiasis or cholecystitis is developed for alterations in nutrition and nursing management of pain.

EXPECTED OUTCOMES

The client and/or family can:
1. Describe the health problem (cholelithiasis or cholecystitis).
2. State plans for maintaining nutritional status, including diet modifications such as fat-restricted and calorie-restricted diet.
3. Manage pain with use of analgesia, relaxation exercises, smooth muscle relaxants.
4. Describe care of incision and drains if surgery performed.
5. State use, dosage, time, route, and side effects of prescribed medications.
6. State limitations of activity.
7. State indications of problems requiring health care (pain, indigestion, flatulence, incisional drainage, temperature, weight loss, nausea, and vomiting).
8. State plans for follow-up health care.

Hepatitis

Hepatitis is an acute or chronic inflammation of the liver caused by a virus or toxins. Three types of viral hepatitis have been identified: type A (infectious hepatitis), type B (serum hepatitis), and non-A, non-B (posttransfusion hepatitis) (Table 17-11). Although undistinguishable clinically or morphologically, each has different causes, routes of transmission, incubation periods, and treatment, and is discussed individually. Toxic hepatitis, on the other hand, is caused by drugs or chemicals not toxified by the liver. The unique aspects of this form of hepatitis are also discussed.

Types of hepatitis

Hepatitis A. Hepatitis A (infectious hepatitis, IH) is an inflammation of the liver caused by type A virus (HAV). The virus is found in blood and feces and is transmitted primarily by the fecal-oral route or indirectly by ingestion of contaminated water, food, or shellfish (oysters or clams) that have grown in polluted water. Transmission by the parenteral route is rare. The incubation period of this virus is 2 to 7 weeks. The virus is present in the blood and feces at this time, and the infected individual, referred to as a *carrier,* is a major source of disease spread.

TABLE 17-11
Viral hepatitis

	Hepatitis A	Hepatitis B	Non-A, non-B hepatitis
Causative organism	Type A Virus	Type B Virus	Other Viruses
Specific antigen	$HA_s Ag$	Acute form: $HB_s Ag$ Chronic form: $HB_e Ag$	
Primary mode of transmission	Fecal/oral	Parenteral	Parenteral
Incubation period	2-7 weeks	6-26 weeks	6-9 weeks
Immunity	Passive: gamma globulin prophylaxis	Passive: Hepatitis B immune globulin; experimental vaccines approved for use	Immune serum globulin of limited value
Precautions for hospitalized clients	Blood precautions	Blood precautions	Blood precautions

Nursing process for common health problems

The incidence of hepatitis A is difficult to determine because many infected individuals are not aware of the disease, or the disease is not reported. The incidence increases in the fall and spring. Young adults are most often affected. The disease is spread rapidly in heavily populated areas such as dormitories, barracks, or low-income housing areas with inadequate sanitation. Consequently, persons living in these environments are at risk. Others at risk are those under 25, perhaps because they have not had opportunity to acquire immunity, and the elderly and debilitated. The incidence of hepatitis A is higher than for hepatitis B or non-A, non-B.

Hepatitis B. Hepatitis B (serum hepatitis) is an acute or chronic inflammation of the liver that is ultimately more severe than hepatitis A. Hepatitis B is caused by hepatitis B virus (HBV). HB_sAg antigens are associated with the acute form, whereas HB_eAg antigens are associated with the chronic form. The virus is transmitted via blood, mucous membranes, sexual contact, or sharing of food. The primary routes are by percutaneous inoculation with contaminated serum or plasma in blood transfusion or skin cuts, tattooing, or use of contaminated needles or instruments. The virus may also be contained in blood, saliva, semen, nasal secretions, and menstrual fluid of asymptomatic carriers; less common routes for spread are, therefore, mucosal invasions, sexual contact, or sharing of contaminated food or eating utensils. The incubation period of hepatitis B is 50 to 150 days, during which time the virus can be identified in the blood.

The incidence of hepatitis B is less than that of type A, but the course of the disease is more severe and the mortality rate higher. Those at risk are persons who use needles that are likely to be contaminated by blood such as health personnel who work in dialysis or oncology units, or drug users. Sexual partners of contagious individuals are also at risk, and homosexual populations have been found to have a high incidence of chronic hepatitis.

The clinical symptoms follow a course similar to those for type A, although the symptoms occur after a longer incubation period and are likely to be more severe. The diagnosis can be confirmed by the identification of the hepatitis B surface antigen (HB_sAg) in the blood.

Prevention of spread of the disease is imperative, and blood precautions are instituted. Hepatitis B immune globin (HBIG) may be used to confer passive immunity to exposed individuals, although it is not entirely effective. An effective vaccine has recently been approved for use. Clients with hepatitis B are immune to recurrences of the disease for 1 year, but immunity to hepatitis A is not conferred.

Non-A, non-B hepatitis. Other agents have been identified as causing hepatitis, although not one is isolated to be identified as hepatitis "C." The incidence of posttransfusion hepatitis is attributed to non-A, non-B agents, which are presumably viruses. The diagnosis of non-A, non-B hepatitis is primarily one of exclusion, and little is known about the epidemiological characteristics. The virus is more like hepatitis B than hepatitis A and is transmitted in the blood, primarily in blood transfusions or through percutaneous routes, particularly in illicit drug users or persons in dialysis units. The incubation period is about 6 to 9 weeks.

The incidence of non-A, non-B hepatitis is believed to be decreasing with mandatory screening of blood donors, although the incidence remains high with

BLOOD PRECAUTIONS

1. Private room: not necessary.
2. Gowns: not necessary.
3. Masks: not necessary.
4. Hands must be washed before and after patient contact.
5. Gloves: necessary for contact with blood or blood-soiled items.
6. Linens: need not be double-bagged before being sent to the laundry unless contaminated with blood.
7. Disposable needles, syringes, and other equipment should be used where possible.
8. Articles contaminated with blood must either be discarded or double-bagged and labeled before being sent for disinfection or sterilization.
9. Blood or blood-contaminated laboratory specimens must be labeled ''BLOOD PRECAUTIONS'' and appropriately bagged before being sent for laboratory analysis.

From Isolation techniques for use in hospitals, ed. 7, U.S. Dept. of Health, Education, and Welfare, 1975, Public Health Service.

commercial blood donors. Those at risk are individuals who receive blood transfusions and those health care personnel who are employed in dialysis units.

The clinical course of the disease is similar to that of hepatitis A. The disease is, however, more similar to type B in severity, although less acute as measured by SGOT.

Blood precautions (left) are instituted to prevent spread. Spread of the disease is minimized by exclusion of blood donated from commercial sources. Immune serum globulin is of limited value in preventing the disease in contacts.

Toxic hepatitis. Toxic hepatitis results from the misuse of chemicals or drugs that are detoxified by the liver. Arsenic, carbon tetrachloride, morphine, chlorpromazine, and barbiturates can induce toxic hepatitis. The symptoms are similar to those of infectious hepatitis. The treatment is to remove the cause and provide rest, nutrition, and comfort for liver regeneration. The nurse should be aware of the extent of liver disease when giving any drugs that are detoxified by the liver.

Pathophysiology. Pathophysiological changes occur in the liver as it becomes infiltrated by mononuclear cells, and hepatic necrosis and autolysis result. The symptoms of hepatitis are related to the degree of liver involvement and follow four stages: preicteric, icteric, precoma, and posticteric.

During the *preicteric* stage (prodromal phase) the client experiences nausea, vomiting, anorexia, low-grade fever, headache, malaise, fatigue, and weight loss. There may be a dull aching in the right upper quadrant caused by liver infiltration. Distaste for cigarettes is a unique sign in those who smoke. There also may be intolerance for alcohol or food. The stools may be clay-colored and the urine dark because of obstruction of bile flow into the small intestine. The liver and spleen are enlarged, reflecting the inflamed state of the liver. This stage lasts about a week.

The *icteric* stage is characterized by jaundice, which occurs as the liver is unable to excrete bilirubin that is now absorbed in the blood and appears in the sclera and skin. The jaundice occurs within 1 week of the onset of the preicteric stage and lasts for 6 to 8 weeks. Not all individuals manifest jaundice, however; some never do throughout the course of the disease. The client complains of pruritus associated with the jaundice. The stools are clay-colored because of the absence of pigment effects of bilirubin. The gastrointestinal symptoms decrease during this stage, and the liver becomes less tender and enlarged, although the spleen may remain enlarged.

If liver damage becomes severe, *precoma* signs such as asterixis, confusion, or mental changes may be noticed. With early management, however, most clients do not reach this stage unless other liver damage is also present.

The *posticteric,* or recovery, stage occurs in 2 to 24 weeks and lasts 3 to 4 months as liver regeneration occurs. Jaundice, fatigue, and gastrointestinal symptoms subside, and the liver returns to normal size. Recovery is faster in younger individuals and those with minimal liver damage.

Assessment. The nurse is responsible for assessing clients and assisting with early identification of potential carriers or individuals with the disease. The nurse can obtain a nursing history and note changes in the client's pattern of nutrition and bowel elimination during various stages of hepatitis.

The diagnosis of hepatitis is based on clinical symptoms and liver function studies such as SGOT and SGPT that are used to monitor the course of the disease. Fecal shedding of hepatitis A serum antigen (HA$_S$Ag) can be identified before the onset of jaundice and is useful to differentiate the causative organism or monitor the course of the disease. This test is not considered practical, however, because the virus is not present in the feces when clinical symptoms become evident. Hepatitis B can be diagnosed by the antigen in the blood. Direct and indirect bilirubin levels are elevated in the icteric stage, and the prothrombin time may be prolonged because of decreased use of vitamin K and abnormalities of prothrombin and fibrinogen production. Urinary urobilinogen increases for 2 or 3 days before the onset of jaundice and is useful to determine liver damage.

Data analysis
Data analysis may reveal nursing diagnoses of alterations in nutrition and bowel elimination as well as disturbances in sleep patterns. Plans are then developed according to individual client needs.

Planning and implementation. The nursing care plan is developed to support the client during recovery and prevent further liver damage. Common objectives are to (1) prevent the spread of the disease, (2) rest the liver, (3) assure adequate nutrition, and (4) provide symptomatic relief. Each nursing care plan is developed for the individual client, based on his needs, his age, and the severity of hepatic inflammation.

Preventing spread of the disease. The client may be treated at home or in the hospital, depending on the severity of the disease, age of the client, and facilities for nursing care. Precautions for spread of disease are instituted depending on the type of hepatitis. Because only low levels of HAV are secreted in the stools of clients with hepatitis A, once clinical manifestations are evident it is not necessary to institute enteric precautions. The major emphasis of preventing spread of the disease is, therefore, to use blood precautions (see p. 957), because the virus is present in the serum at this time.

Family members and others who have been exposed to hepatitis A may receive immune serum globulin (gamma globulin), 0.02 to 0.05 ml/kg of body weight, to reduce their chances of acquiring the disease. The nurse can help the client list those individuals who might have been in close contact with him during the incubation period when he was contagious as a carrier. The client who has had infectious hepatitis is immune to this particular virus. Immunity is not conferred, however, for serum hepatitis. Effective prophylaxis for hepatitis B and non-A, non-B has not been established.

Resting the liver. The client is placed on bed rest to promote liver regeneration. More blood is filtered through the liver when there is less demand for circulation elsewhere. Bed rest may be necessary for 4 to 6 weeks, and the client should be made comfortable and given quiet diversion to keep him in bed. Initially the client does not feel well and welcomes the rest. Activity is increased gradually as the liver recuperates and the infection runs its course.

Assuring adequate nutrition. To ensure adequate nutrition and minimize metabolic stress on the liver, a diet that is high in protein, calories, and vitamins is given to the client (see high-protein diet, p. 959). The diet may also be re-

---

HIGH-PROTEIN DIET

Purpose	1. Promote liver regeneration.
	2. Promote healing and tissue regrowth.
	3. Provide for needs during increased metabolism, such as fever and certain diseases.
	4. Provide protein during protein loss such as in ulcerative colitis, cystic fibrosis, nephritis, burns or during malabsorption.
Meats and eggs	All; two eggs a day.
Milk	All; use cheeses, ice cream, and snacks.
Fruits and vegetables	All.
Breads and cereals	All.
Suggestions	1. Protein should be 1½ to 2 times as much as normal servings per day.
	2. Use animal protein as source of protein.
	3. Provide sufficient calories so that protein will not be used to meet energy needs.
	4. Add powdered dry skim milk to sauces, gravies, custard, cooked cereal, potatoes, and milkshakes, to supplement protein.
	5. Offer between-meal snacks of custard or milkshakes.
	6. Consider expense of diet and suggest economical sources of protein, such as organ meats, meats on sale, use of powdered milk.

---

stricted in fat and contain a moderate amount of carbohydrate. Protein is necessary for tissue repair and anabolism. Although the client is eating a high-protein diet, it is also necessary to have sufficient carbohydrates so that the protein is not used to meet energy needs.

The appetite may be poor, and at first the diet may appear overwhelming. Small, frequent meals are more easily tolerated, and they should be given in a pleasant, attractive manner. If the client is nauseated, the nurse may give an antiemetic before eating. Mouth care may also stimulate the appetite. If the client is unable to eat, alternative feeding plans such as intravenous infusion or parenteral hyperalimentation feedings may be given.

Comfort measures. During the initial course of hepatitis the client does not feel well. The nurse or family member can help the client feel more comfortable by a daily bath and straightening the bed linens. The skin may be dry and itch as a consequence of jaundice. Lotions or a baking soda bath may soothe the skin. Antihistamines may be ordered if severe itching persists. Antipyretics are used to reduce the fever, and a sponge bath may help the client feel cool and comfortable. Fluids should be offered to the client with dry skin to prevent further dehydration. Later, when the client feels better, he may ambulate several times a day to prevent hazards of immobility and circulatory stasis.

Recovery from hepatitis A may take several months. The client will need to be encouraged to obtain a balance of rest and activity and follow a well-balanced diet to prevent further damage to the liver.

Evaluation. The client with hepatitis may demonstrate varying degrees of illness and exhibit nursing problems of alteration in nutrition and altered sleep patterns.

Nursing process for common health problems

EXPECTED OUTCOMES

The client and/or family can:

1. Describe hepatitis.
2. Describe methods for preventing transmission of the specific type of hepatitis.
3. Describe plans for health maintenance, including rest and adequate nutrition with a high-protein, high-calorie diet.
4. Describe plans for managing manifestations of liver damage such as pruritus, bleeding, jaundice, dehydration, and fluid retention.
5. State use, dosage, time, route, and side effects of prescribed medications.
6. State indications of problems requiring health care (infection, bleeding, nausea, vomiting, weight loss, changes in sensorium).
7. State plans for follow-up health care.

Cirrhosis

Cirrhosis is an inflammation of the liver that can be caused by several processes, infection, malnutrition, or obstruction of the biliary system. Regardless of the source of the inflammation, the end result is parenchymal cell death, regeneration, and scarring. The scarring diminishes blood flow and causes fibrosis, fatty degeneration, and later, obstruction of the portal vein.

Cirrhosis can be described by the cause or by morphological characteristics. Cirrhosis that occurs after an infection such as hepatitis is called *postnecrotic cirrhosis*. Malnutrition, as is often associated with alcoholism, can cause a special type of cirrhosis, *portal cirrhosis* (Laennec's cirrhosis). An obstruction of the biliary system that causes hepatic inflammation is called *biliary cirrhosis*. Morphologically, cirrhosis is described as micronodular (portal, associated with alcohol abuse), macronodular (postnecrotic cirrhosis), or mixed micronodular/macronodular, characterized by cellular necrosis, regeneration, and fibrosis. Laennec's cirrhosis (micronodular cirrhosis) is the most common and typifies pathological changes in the liver; nursing care for this type is typical, too, and is discussed here.

Pathophysiology. Laennec's cirrhosis is a degenerative disease of the liver preceded by fatty infiltration of hepatic cells. The decrease is probably caused by a defect in lipid metabolism, secretion, or storage. Lipids containing triglycerides and free fatty acids become sequestered in cellular compartments that enlarge and cause increased cellular concentration of lipids. Ultimately there is necrosis, regeneration, and fibrosis. Alcohol appears to stimulate the increased liver triglycerides and the process of liver degeneration. There may also be a relationship with a diet low in protein that stimulates fatty infiltration. The infiltration is potentially reversible, particularly with discontinued use of alcohol.

Cirrhosis is a common disease of middle-aged adults and is the seventh most common cause of death in the United States.[30] The incidence is slightly higher for men and nonwhites. Risk for cirrhosis is associated with alcoholism. Individuals with chronic alcohol abuse of 5 to 20 years are at greater risk, and even though they remain well nourished, the incidence of cirrhosis is increased. Malnutrition further increases the risk.

 Assessment. The degree of liver inflammation is evidenced by clinical symptoms related to destruction of hepatic cells, necrosis, regeneration, and scarring. Initially the client has vague *gastrointestinal* symptoms of nausea, anorexia, vomiting, weight loss, flatulence, fatigue, and headache. These are caused by metabolic changes of the liver associated with metabolizing proteins, carbohydrates, and fats. There may be abdominal pain that can be dull or sharp, steady or intermittent, at the site of the liver or referred.

As the disease progresses, the liver size increases as a result of inflammation and stretching of the capsule. The liver is usually palpable. *Ascites* results from obstruction of the portal vein, and can be determined by palpation and percussion. Continuing liver damage produces *jaundice* as a result of failure of parenchymal cells to metabolize bilirubin. Venules become distended, producing *spider angiomas* (red, pulsating arterioles on the skin surface). There may be *palmar erythema*. *Endocrine disorders* such as menstrual disorders, gynecomastia, loss of pubic hair, and impotence may result, because the liver is unable to metabolize hormones of the adrenal cortex, ovaries, or testes. *Hematological problems* resulting from liver failure include anemia, leukopenia, thrombocytopenia, and coagulation defects. Progressive *portal obstruction* by fibrosis may lead to portal hypertension, splenomegaly, hemorrhoids, or esophageal varices.

Hepatorenal syndrome (renal failure without renal disease) may result from decreased renal blood flow. There is high urine concentration with low urinary sodium excretion, oliguria, and azotemia.

The *cardiovascular system* is disrupted by the inflamed liver, and microscopic arteriovenous shunts develop. The cause is not known, but the effects are to decrease oxygen saturation and shift the oxyhemoglobin dissociation curve to the right. There may be an increased cardiac output and decreased peripheral resistance. The fingers may be clubbed as clinical evidence of these changes.

End stage cirrhosis is manifested in complications that may be death producing. These include hepatic coma, portal hypertension, and bleeding esophageal varices.

> **Data analysis**
> *Data analysis may reveal nursing diagnoses of alteration in nutrition, sleep pattern disturbances, noncompliance, and fluid imbalance.*

Planning and implementation. The goal of nursing care for a client with cirrhosis is to prevent continuing liver damage and provide supportive measures for cellular regeneration. Since many individuals have concurrent alcoholism, management of the behavioral aspects as well as the physiological results of alcoholism is imperative (see Chapter 4).

Supportive care is accomplished by (1) providing rest, (2) improving nutrition, and (3) reducing ascites. The nursing care plan should reflect the special needs of the client.

Providing rest. The client is placed on bed rest to limit the demands on the liver and promote tissue regeneration. Bed rest is usually more accepted if the client is comfortable. If the client is jaundiced, skin may be dry and itch. Soothing lotions should be applied frequently. Back care should be given several times a day, and the nurse can observe the coccyx for areas of breakdown.

Improving nutrition. The diet is designed to meet dietary needs in the absence of a properly functioning liver. A diet that is high in protein, vitamins, and calories is given to decrease metabolic stress on the liver (see p. 959). Bile salts are usually given with meals to facilitate the absorption of vitamins A and K.

There may also be bleeding when the liver is no longer able to synthesize prothrombin, and the nurse should take care that the client does not injure himself. His nails should be cut short so that he does not scratch himself, and after giving an intramuscular injection, the nurse should hold a cotton wipette over the site for hemostasis.

If the appetite is poor, the nurse may use supportive measures to stimulate it. A pleasant environment, small frequent meals, mouth care before eating, and antiemetics may be helpful.

No drugs or chemicals that must be detoxified by the liver are given when liver function is impaired. The metabolic by-products of these drugs may accumulate in the body and cause further damage.

Reducing ascites. Ascites, the accumulation of fluids in the abdomen from portal vein obstruction, may be limited by reducing sodium content of the diet, using diuretic drugs, and if necessary, removing the fluid through paracentesis (abdominal tap). The nurse should observe the progress of fluid reduction by accurate intake and output records and by weighing the client daily. The client should be weighed on the same scales, at the same time each day, and with the same amount of clothing.

A *low-sodium diet,* 200 to 500 mg per day (see Chapter 20), may be used to limit sodium, which causes fluid retention. The client should be instructed about his diet so that he does not obtain food other than that which is ordered for him. Low-sodium diets are not palatable to some clients, but the nurse should check with the physician before using a salt substitute.

Diuretics are also used to promote fluid loss. Thiazide diuretics, mercurial diuretics, or spironolactone (Aldactone) are usually used. Intake and output records should be kept carefully, and the nurse should observe the client for signs of excessive sodium loss, such as abdominal cramping and muscle pain.

A *paracentesis* may be done if ascites is severe. Proteins that are necessary for cellular repair are lost during the paracentesis, and this procedure is usually done if the fluid retention causes severe dyspnea. Before the procedure begins, the client should urinate to avoid trauma to the bladder. In the procedure 1000 to 1500 ml of fluid may be withdrawn, and the nurse should observe the client for hypovolemic shock. The nurse should also observe the dressing for drainage or bleeding.

Discharge instructions. When liver function is restored, the client needs continuing modification of his diet to support liver activity. The client who is an alcoholic must resolve that problem before healthy nutrition can be maintained. Community resources such as the social worker, community mental health clinics, Alcoholics Anonymous, and religious counselors may be used by the medical team to assist the client in his return to health.

Complications of cirrhosis. There are several complications of cirrhosis that may occur if liver degeneration persists; hepatic coma, portal hypertension, and esophageal varices are the three most common. The nurse should observe the client with cirrhosis to detect changes in his behavior and vital signs that may indicate impending complications.

Hepatic coma. Hepatic coma (hepatic encephalopathy) occurs as a result of metabolic changes associated with liver failure. A primary cause is ammonia excess. Ammonia is normally present in the blood from protein deaminization, muscle cell contractility, bacterial action on protein in the intestines, deaminization of protein by the kidney, or during intestinal bleeding when there is increased protein in the intestine. Protein is normally converted to ketoacids and ammonia, and urea (the end product of ammonia metabolism) is excreted in the urine. When the liver is unable to deaminate protein, there is an increase in serum ammonia. The brain cells are most affected by this excess ammonia, and coma and death result if the process is not reversed. Other precipitating factors are decreased cerebral perfusion resulting from fluid loss from diuretic use, potassium insufficiency and metabolic alkalosis, hypoxia, depressant drugs, analgesics, and infections.

The changes brought about by the rising ammonia levels are often subtle, and the nurse should become familiar with the clients usual behavior and make assessments of changes. Early signs are confusion, inappropriate behavior, drowsiness, yawning, restlessness or insomnia, decreased concentration, and delayed response time. Slurred speech and illegible writing are more overt changes. Later the client may manifest stupor and decreased level of consciousness (see Chapter 10).

As the coma becomes imminent, the client has liver flap *asterixis* (which is noted when the client is recumbent and dorsiflexes the foot or as an inability to hold the hands extended when the arms are outstretched), liver breath, *fetor hepaticus* (a fruity odor of the breath), and *spider telangiectasia* (dilated capillaries that extend on the skin surface). Once comatose, the client may not be responsive to any stimuli. The body temperature may rise, and rapid pulse and respirations are evident. Renal failure may result from hypovolemia. The client should be monitored for impending dysrhythmias (see Chapter 20) and fluid and electrolyte changes (see Chapter 16). The client is usually in an intensive care setting where these observations can be made continuously. The mortality rate for clients in hepatic coma is high, and if the level of consciousness does not improve, death usually occurs within 24 hours.

Hepatic coma may be prevented by reducing available protein that must be converted to ammonia. The diet is limited in protein, and the client is placed on strict bed rest to limit muscular activity. Furthermore, intestinal antibiotics such as neomycin (4 g/day), cation exchange enemas, or cathartics may be used to eliminate the bacterial flora in the intestines and thereby prevent the conversion of protein to ammonia in the intestines. Lactulose, a disaccharide that is not metabolized in the gastrointestinal tract, is used because it alters the bacterial flora and thereby prevents the production of ammonia; because it causes diarrhea, it facilitates excretion of nitrogenous wastes in the stool.[7]

Other approaches to treatment of hepatic coma may be exchange transfusion to remove toxins and allow cell regeneration,[18] or colon-bypass surgery to prevent absorption in the intestines, and in rare instances liver transplant. These approaches are not common; they are used primarily in medical centers where specialized staff and equipment are available.

Nursing care of the client in coma is supportive. Food and fluids are given intravenously or by gavage. The client should be turned frequently and the skin bathed and massaged regularly. If the client survives the coma, the care plan is developed to promote nutrition by increasing the protein gradually to 40 g daily, and to observe for changes that signal hepatic encephalopathy.

Portal hypertension. Portal hypertension is an elevated pressure in the portal vein caused by increased resistance to blood flow in the liver. There is increased splanchnic artery inflow and decreased outflow of blood in the hepatic vein. The overload of blood stimulates development of collateral circulation, particularly in the veins of the lower esophagus, abdominal wall (paraumbilical veins), and the hemorrhoidal veins. The ultimate danger of portal hypertension is rupture and hemorrhage of the distended veins. Since those in the esophagus are under greater pressure, they are most likely to rupture. Management is directed toward preventing bleeding or diverting the portal blood flow with surgically created shunts.

Bleeding episodes are prevented by minimizing chances for bleeding, such as limiting aspirin intake. The client should also avoid trauma from coughing, blowing, yelling, or using the Valsalva maneuver. Rough or spicy irritant foods should also be avoided.

Permanent reversal of portal hypertension may be achieved by surgical shunt procedures that reduce portal pressure by diverting blood from areas of high pressure to low pressure. A *portacaval shunt* can be done by anastomosis of the portal vein to the inferior vena cava. Another approach is to perform a *spleno-renal shunt,* an anastomosis of the splenic vein to the left renal vein, with the removal of the spleen.[8] Both surgeries involve thoracic approaches (see Chapter 21 for nursing care). The surgery is performed only for clients who are able to withstand extensive surgery, because many clients are too debilitated and are not operative risks. The shunts decrease chances of bleeding, but increase the risk of encephalopathy, because nitrogenous wastes in the blood are diverted from the liver and at best do not appreciably increase the client's life expectancy.

Esophageal varices. Esophageal varices are the third complication of cirrhosis. The veins of the esophagus become distended with venous blood as a result of portal hypertension. Increased abdominal pressure from coughing, nausea, vomiting, or the Valsalva maneuver from straining to defecate may cause the varices to bleed. Ingestion of alcohol, rough or irritating foods, acid regurgitation, stress, or medications such as aspirin may also aggravate bleeding. The varices may be diagnosed by esophagoscopy, but the physician may be hesitant to examine the esophagus and cause pressure on the distended veins.

When the varices bleed, an emergency exists. Profuse bleeding must be stopped to prevent blood loss and aspiration of blood into the lungs. Initially a nasogastric tube or an Ewald tube (a large lumen [30 fr] gastric tube inserted through the mouth) may be used to aspirate blood and instill iced saline to constrict arterioles.

To control the bleeding, an esophagogastric tube (Sengstaken-Blakemore tube) is inserted through the nose to the stomach (Fig. 17-21). One lumen is used to provide an outlet for the bleeding and is connected to a suction apparatus. The other two lumina open to inflatable balloons. The esophageal balloon is inflated to maintain pressure on the bleeding varices, and the gastric balloon is inflated to keep the tube in the stomach while slight traction is used to exert pressure on the esophagus. The traction may be provided by use of a football helmet and attaching the tube to the mouth piece or by use of a nasal cuff, a foam rubber pad that fits between the nares and the tube. The gastric balloon is inflated first, and if bleeding continues it is most likely from an esophageal site. The esophageal balloon is then inflated to a pressure greater than the client's portal pressure. Iced saline may be rinsed through the tube to constrict superficial bleeding vessels. When bleeding has been stopped for 24 hours as evidenced by absence of blood aspirated from the stomach, the balloons are deflated and the tube removed. If the tube must be used for several days, the esophageal and gastric balloons may be deflated periodically to prevent ulceration and necrosis.

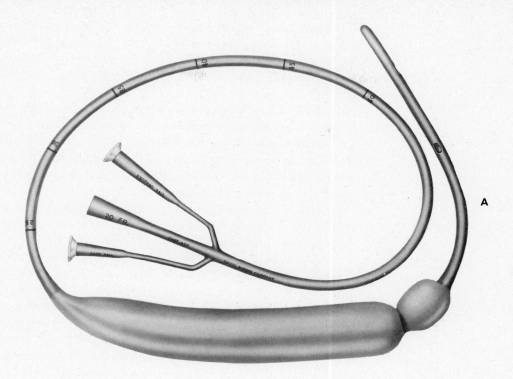

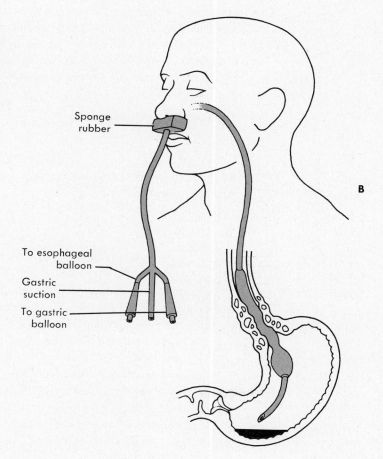

FIG. 17-21
Sengstaken-Blakemore tube. Note gastric balloon used to hold tube in place and esophageal balloon used to provide pressure on varices. The third lumen is used to aspirate gastric contents. **B,** Esophagogastric tube in position. Note foam cuff protecting nares. (**A** Courtesy Davol Inc., Providence, R.I.)

Sponge rubber

To esophageal balloon

Gastric suction

To gastric balloon

Nursing process for common health problems

Vasopressin (Pitressin) may be used as a continuous infusion to control bleeding. The drugs act to lower splanchnic pressure and splanchnic blood flow by constricting splanchnic arterioles. The nurse should monitor the client for signs of arteriole spasm of other organs (coronary artery spasm) and water retention.

Blood loss presents serious problems. The client may be in shock from blood loss and should be kept warm. Oxygen may be given if the hemoglobin levels are low and oxygenation is not adequate. Blood transfusions with fresh whole blood are often used to replace the blood loss. Fresh blood is preferred because it has more clotting factors, less ammonia content, and does not have the preservative sodium citrate, which is metabolized by the liver.

Nursing care during this critical time involves evaluating the client for response to hemorrhage control. The client is in a critical care setting where vital signs and fluid balance can be monitored continuously.

The nursing care plan also includes measures to promote comfort and prevent complications. Oral hygiene should be given frequently, particularly during bleeding, when the esophagogastric tube is in place. The nares should be cleansed and lubricated. When the client is confined to bed rest, he should be turned from side to side to prevent pressure areas and skin breakdown. If the client is nauseated, he should be turned on his side to prevent aspiration.

Surgical intervention may be considered when the bleeding has stopped. The surgeon may attempt to ligate the varices or perform bypass procedures to reduce the portal hypertension that is the original cause of the bleeding varices. Long-term prognosis is generally not favorable.

 Evaluation. Evaluation of the nursing care plan for the client with cirrhosis is ongoing as the client's health status changes. Nursing problems may include alterations in nutrition, alterations in fluid volume, disturbances in sleep, and noncompliance.

EXPECTED OUTCOMES

The client and/or family can:
1. Describe cirrhosis.
2. Describe plans for maintenance or restoration of nutrition, including a high-protein, high-calorie diet, sodium-restricted diet, and avoidance of toxic substances and alcohol.
3. State plans for compliance with the therapeutic plan.
4. State indications for health care including bleeding varices, changes in sensorium indicative of hepatic coma, fluid retention, and hypertension.
5. State plans for follow-up health care and use of community resources for nutrition and alcohol abuse.

Cancer of the liver

Cancer of the liver is a rarely occurring cancer that may be the primary site, or more likely a site of metastasis. Hepatic carcinoma is associated with cirrhosis; 70% of individuals with this tumor have cirrhotic livers. The tumors may originate in the parenchymal cells (hepatoma) or in the bile duct cells (cholangioma).

Cancer of the liver is a disease of the middle-aged and older adult (60 to 70 years), and accounting for less than 2% of all carcinoma. The incidence is higher in men; those at risk are individuals with cirrhosis.

The symptoms of liver cancer are vague and insidious in onset. There may be anorexia, weight loss, weakness, abdominal fullness and bloating, and abdominal pain. As the tumor grows, the pain becomes more severe and radiates to the back. The liver may be enlarged; obstructive jaundice occurs in about 50% of the clients and ascites occurs in most. The diagnosis is determined by liver scans, biopsy, and liver function studies.

If the tumor is solitary and localized and no metastasis is evident, surgical removal is attempted. A *total hepatic lobectomy* is the surgical procedure used, and because liver tissue regenerates, up to 90% of the liver can be removed without endangering liver function. In research centers total hepatectomies with liver transplants have also been attempted. Nursing care is similar to a client having abdominal surgery.

Most often, however, therapy is palliative. Chemotherapy with antimetabolite drugs provides temporary remission. Prognosis is generally poor despite surgery or chemotherapy, and 5-year survival rates are less than 1%.[24] Nursing care is planned with the client and family for supportive management.

Pancreatitis

Pancreatitis is an inflammation of the pancreas that may be acute or chronic. Pancreatitis is caused by a variety of toxins that incite the inflammation. *Acute* pancreatitis can be precipitated by alcohol use, biliary tract disease, duodenal obstruction, infections, trauma, or nutritional deficiencies. *Chronic* pancreatitis is more likely to be caused by alcohol ingestion or gallbladder disease. Autoimmune factors are also being considered as causes of pancreatitis.

Regardless of the cause, the pathological changes that occur during *acute* pancreatitis are related to an obstruction of the pancreatic ducts, causing rupture and release of digestive enzymes. The toxic enzymes cause inflammation of the pancreas, edema, enlargement of the pancreas, obstruction of the pancreatic duct, and ultimately necrosis. Necrosis of arteries results in bleeding into the pancreas and causes suppuration and tissue destruction. Destruction may be localized or involve the entire pancreas.

Chronic pancreatitis is caused by repeated attacks of acute pancreatitis. Eventually the pancreas becomes nodular, and there is calcification of vital tissue. There is pancreatic insufficiency, and because the islet cells are destroyed, diabetes mellitus. Pancreatitis is a disease of middle-aged adults and occurs in individuals with gallstones; alcohol users also tend to have greater risk for pancreatitis. The symptoms of pancreatitis are related to organ destruction and are as varied as the causes and extent of the disease. There may be back pain, nausea, vomiting, fever, leukocytosis, and occasionally jaundice.

An *acute* attack is characterized by severe midepigastric pain that may radiate to the back. The pain is accompanied by vomiting, which increases rather than relieves the pain. There may be abdominal tenderness, decreased bowel sounds, and paralytic ileus. Fluid loss may cause shock syndromes.

In *chronic* pancreatitis the symptoms are more diffuse and include weight loss (in spite of adequate diet), epigastric distress, pain, and foul-smelling stools. If islet cell destruction has occurred, the client will have symptoms of diabetes mellitus (see Chapter 9).

The diagnosis of pancreatitis is made on the basis of the symptoms, liver function studies, x-ray studies, and elevated serum amylase and lipase. It is also possible to visualize the pancreatic duct to determine if there is biliary tract disease or chronic or acute pancreatitis.

Therapeutic intervention for pancreatitis is primarily symptomatic. Drug therapy and diet modifications are used to treat chronic pancreatitis and prevent exacerbations. If symptoms become severe during an acute attack, the client may be hospitalized. Surgical approaches are rarely used, although partial pancreatectomy or vagotomy to reduce stimulation of pancreatic secretions may be attempted. Pancreatic transplants are in research stages.

Relief of *pain* is planned to provide the most relief with least amount of medication. Narcotics may be required for acute pain, but morphine should not be used because it causes spasms of the sphincter of Oddi. Heat, relaxation, and positioning may also help.

If the client is in *shock* from fluid and electrolyte loss, he may be admitted to an intensive care unit. Blood transfusions and plasma expanders may be used to replace lost volume. The nurse must monitor fluid and electrolyte status carefully at this time.

The *diet* is planned to meet nutritional needs. The client should avoid caffeine and alcohol, which stimulate pancreatitis. Small, frequent feedings of bland, easily digested food reduce the pancreatic secretions. Pancreatic extracts such as pancreatin (Viokase or Cotazym) may be used to supplement pancreatic enzymes. Bile salts are used to facilitate digestion of fat-soluble vitamins. Vitamin supplements may be prescribed. Antacids can be used to reduce gastric secretions that would stimulate pancreatic enzyme release. During acute attacks of vomiting, nutritional support is given with intravenous infusions. The client should be observed for *infection,* because the pancreas is susceptible to bacterial invasion. Vital signs should be recorded regularly. Antibiotics are used to prevent or treat infections.

After recovery from an acute attack the goal of management is to prevent further attacks. The client should be instructed about his diet and medications.

If islet cell destruction has occurred, the client will also be treated for hyperglycemia. Diet, oral antidiabetic agents, or insulin may be used. The nurse plans with the client how to incorporate these changes into his life-style and provides necessary instructions.

Cancer of the pancreas

Cancer of the pancreas is primarily an adenocarcinoma that may involve the head, body, or tail of the pancreas. Islet cells may be involved as well. The cancer metastasizes readily to the lymph, stomach, colon, and bile duct. The cause is unknown. Although there are correlations with chronic pancreatitis and alcoholism, no etiological significance is documented.

Pancreatic tumors are rare and account for 2% to 3% of all cancers. The disease affects adults age 60 to 70, men more often than women. As with other tumors of the gastrointestinal system, the symptoms of cancer of the pancreas are vague and insidious in onset. There may be anorexia, weight loss, weakness, and nausea. Pain is usually a late sign, and there may be jaundice, ascites, and a palpable abdominal mass. Recent onset of diabetes mellitus may indicate cancer of the pancreas. The diagnosis is based on x-ray studies, scans, transhepatic cholangiography, liver function studies, elevated fasting blood sugar, and exploratory surgery and biopsy.

At the time of diagnosis the tumor may be invasive and metastasized, and the prognosis is not favorable; death may occur in 3 to 6 months. Surgery may be done if the tumor is localized. A *Whipple procedure* includes the removal of the head of the pancreas, distal stomach, common bile duct, and duodenum. Palliative surgery such as a choleycystojejunostomy, gastrojejunostomy, or choledochojejunostomy may be done to restore output of bile and pancreatic enzymes.

Functioning islet cell tumors may be excised locally. Chemotherapy with antimetabolite drugs (see Chapter 6) may be offered palliatively.

Nursing care should be supportive and symptomatic. If surgery is performed, the nursing care plan should be developed to support nutrition. Pancreatic enzymes may be given as supplements.

COMMON HEALTH PROBLEMS THAT OCCUR ACROSS THE LIFE SPAN

Inflammations of the mouth

The mouth of a client of any age is a likely port of entry and site for inflammations such as stomatitis, herpes simplex, parotitis, monilial infections, caries, and periodontal disease. The nurse can assess the mouth of clients during health appraisal or when assisting the client with oral hygiene. Plans are made to prevent oral cavity inflammations in individuals who are debilitated or restricted in fluid intake and to maintain oral hygiene for those with actual inflammatory disease.

Stomatitis. Stomatitis, an inflammation of the oral mucosa, can be caused from systemic diseases, trauma, teething, poor hygiene, debilitation, lowered resistance to infection, or by allergic or toxic reactions to chemotherapy. Eating is painful when there is an infection in the mouth; foods may irritate the mouth, and the appetite is poor. Stomatitis can occur at any age and is diagnosed by culture and appearance of the mouth. Antibiotics or antifungal drugs may be used if the causative organism is cultured; otherwise, the inflammation is treated symptomatically. Mouth rinses, good oral hygiene, and anesthetic sprays may be used to provide comfort.

Aphthous stomatitis. Aphthous stomatitis (canker sore) is a painful ulceration of the mucous membranes of the mouth or lip. It appears spontaneously and usually disappears in a few days. Mouthwashes and topical anesthetic gargles can be used to limit the temporary discomfort.

Herpes simplex. Herpes simplex (type 1) (fever blister) is a viral infection that causes blisters in the mouth and on the lips. This infection occurs most often in persons who are debilitated or very young and is aggravated by stress or sunlight. Symptomatic relief is obtained from mouthwashes and anesthetic sprays.

Vincent's stomatitis. Vincent's stomatitis (trench mouth) is caused by a spirochete and fusiform bacillus. Swelling, bleeding, and a foul odor in the mouth are evident. Antibiotics are used to control the infection. Half-strength hydrogen peroxide mouthwash may be used to cleanse the mouth.

Parotitis. Parotitis is an infection of the parotid glands. This infection is more prevalent in clients who have not had oral intake for long periods of time. There is usually pain and swelling. Antibiotics are used to combat the infection. Good mouth care is essential in preventing parotitis, and all persons who do not have an oral intake should brush their teeth several times a day.

Thrush. Thrush is a monilial infection, found most commonly in the newborn whose mother has a monilial infection of the vagina or nipple. The infection is also common in adults who are taking antibiotics or who have poor oral hygiene. The tongue and mouth are covered with white patches (Fig. 17-22). Gentian violet or nystatin (Mycostatin) mouthwash is used to control the infection and is applied to the newborn's mouth with a swab. Adults may gargle with the mouthwash so that it is applied to all areas of the mouth.

Leukoplakia buccalis. Leukoplakia buccalis is a white placque on the tongue and oral mucosa of adults, caused by sclerosing of mucous membranes.

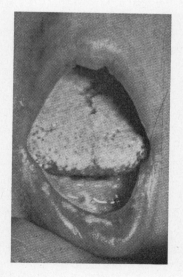

FIG. 17-22
Thrush. (Reproduced with permission from Potter, E.L., and Craig, J.M.: Pathology of the fetus and infant, ed. 3. Copyright © 1975 by Year Book Medical Publishers, Inc., Chicago.)

969

from constant irritation such as smoking or eating spicy foods. Dietary control and abstinence from smoking will minimize this irritation.

Caries. The enamel of the tooth can become eroded when food combines with normal oral bacteria *(Lactobacillus acidophilus)* and forms decay-producing lactic acid. The erosion is not visible initially but can be discovered by the dentist when he uses a probe to detect the weakened enamel. Later, the cavity may be noticed, particularly if there is pain.

Caries can be prevented by brushing the teeth after eating and limiting the carbohydrate in the diet. Many also recommend prevention of caries by *fluoridation,* which makes the tooth more resistant to decay acids. Fluoridation may be accomplished by adding fluoride to the drinking water. Fluoride can also be applied to the tooth in a toothpaste or in a concentrated form used by the dentist. Caries should be treated in early stages before extensive drilling and filling or extraction of the decayed tooth is necessary. Carious teeth that are extracted should be replaced by bridge work to maintain alignment of remaining teeth. Full-mouth extractions may be done if periodontal diseases cause severe inflammation of the gums and supporting structures.

Periodontal disease. Periodontal disease is an inflammation of the gums caused by poor oral hygiene and perhaps by lowered resistance to infection, as observed in individuals with diabetes mellitus. The gums become inflamed, bleed, and loosen from the teeth. Ultimately the tooth itself becomes loose and may require extraction. It is estimated that over 90% of adults over 40 have some form of periodontal disease.

Periodontal disease is best prevented by good oral hygiene and periodic prophylaxis (cleaning) by the dentist. Oral surgery and tooth extraction may be necessary if the inflammation becomes severe.

Overweight and obesity

Obesity is a condition of being overweight according to norms based on ideal weight for sex, age, and body build (see Appendix A). A person who is 10% to 19% heavier than the ideal weight is described as *overweight* (mildly obese), whereas a person 20% to 50% above the ideal weight is *obese* (moderate obesity), and those 50% over their ideal weight are *severely obese,* or morbidly obese.

Obesity is caused by an imbalance of caloric intake and energy expenditure, the result of either exogenous or endogenous factors. Exogenous causes account for the greatest incidence of obesity and may include cultural influences that value eating and obesity, cultural or ethnic diets high in fat and calories, economic factors that favor poor quality nutrition, or psychological conditions that reinforce poor eating habits. Physical inactivity and sedentary life-styles also contribute to obesity. Genetic backgrounds may influence obesity, because children of obese parents tend to be overweight. Eating patterns are known to determine weight gain; infants on demand feeding schedules, for example, are satisfied earlier, whereas those on scheduled feedings eat more than necessary. Endogenous causes of obesity include diseases (such as hypothyroidism, Cushing's syndrome, diabetes mellitus, or ventromedial hypothalamic injury) that cause metabolic disturbances of ingestion and digestion.

Pathophysiology. Excess calories consumed beyond energy needs are stored as fat, and long-term calorie excesses tend to increase the proportion of fat to lean body mass. This phenomenon occurs particularly at critical points of growth: the first half of pregnancy, birth through 2 years, childhood (7 to 11), and adolescence. According to the adipose cell theory, nutrition during these critical periods determines the number and size of adipocytes (fat cells).[20] If nutrition is provided beyond the need for metabolism and growth, the number of adipocytes increases (hyperplasia) or the fat cells become stretched from overeating (hypertrophy), setting the stage for obesity. There are two types of obesity. Childhood- or adolescent-onset obesity is caused by adipocyte hyperplasia, and adult-onset obesity by adipocyte hypertrophy.

Obesity presents a hazard to physical and mental health. Increasing demands are put on the body systems to support excess weight. The need for oxygen increases, stress is placed on the digestive organs and metabolism, and there is added weight to the musculoskeletal system. Body image and self-esteem are often poor in individuals who are overweight. Finally, there is an increased incidence of illness and slower healing in persons who are obese.

It is estimated that as many as 30% to 50% of Americans are obese. Obesity is a national health concern because of its effects on health and the causal relationship associated with hypertension, heart disease, and diabetes mellitus. Persons at risk for obesity are those with faulty feeding/eating patterns at critical times, sedentary life-styles, and genetic backgrounds that predispose to obesity.

 Assessment. The obese client is recognized by the disproportion of weight to height and body size. The client also exhibits excess weight as examined by skin folds that reveal excess subcutaneous fat. Tests of metabolic function are done to rule out endogenous obesity.

> **Data analysis**
> *Data analysis may reveal actual nursing diagnoses of alterations in nutrition and potential nursing diagnoses of noncompliance and disturbances in self-concept.*

Planning and implementation. Obesity can be managed by diet and exercise, behavior modification, and in selected individuals by surgical approaches such as intestinal bypass. Weight loss may occur over a long period of time and the nurse helps the client follow a therapeutic plan until weight loss has been achieved and maintained.

Diet and exercise. The goal of dietary management is to reduce weight as well as fat in a healthy manner that promotes continued maintenance of weight loss. The caloric intake should be reduced and activity increased. It is important to institute dietary controls when the person first becomes overweight; preventing obesity is easier than controlling it.

Diet instruction should begin during the antepartal period, particularly for those families with overweight parents where the infant is at risk. If the infant is being breast-fed, the parents should rely on weight gain to judge adequacy of feeding; bottle-fed infants should not be forced to finish each feeding. Later, as the child develops his eating habits and preferences, he should be offered well-balanced diets but encouraged to eat at his own pace. Requiring children to eat more than they desire may encourage food habits that later contribute to overeating. Food should not be used as a reward or punishment, because this may later cause compulsive eating patterns. Finally infants and children should be encouraged to lead active lives—to play outside instead of watching television, for example.

If the individual does exceed weight for age and height, he should seek medical assistance immediately. Weight reduction should be done with the supervision of the physician. Dieting with pills, fad diets, and gimmicks is expensive and hazardous to health, and is not advised.

A sensible plan of modifying dietary patterns is established with the client. Because adipose tissue has the energy potential of 3500 calories, it is necessary to decrease the calories by 500 each day in order to lose a pound a week. The diet should be planned so that weight loss is gradual and the hazards of protein catabolism and nitrogen loss from starvation approaches to dieting are averted.

The client is usually permitted three or four meals a day. The exchange lists (see Chapter 9) may be used as a basis for the diet so the client does not have to count calories. In another approach the client may simply reduce the total intake of food while eating nutritious foods. Compliance with a diet plan may be increased if the diet does not deviate drastically from the client's usual eating patterns.

Exercise is a significant component of a weight reduction plan. The client should be instructed to increase his usual activity and plan for 20 to 30 minutes of exercise daily. Walking is one simple exercise that can be tolerated by clients of all ages and health states. Bicycling, jogging, swimming, and other sports activities may be undertaken on the advice of health care personnel.

Behavioral modification. The source of the problem of overeating often lies in behavioral patterns and motivations of the client to eat. If the motivation factors are identified, it may be possible to modify these aspects of eating.[2] Approaches may include behavioral self-management, support groups such as Weight Watchers or Take off Pounds Sensibly (TOPS), or psychological counseling. The nurse may refer the client to these groups as appropriate. Compliance increases with group and family support.

When clients begin to lose weight, they can anticipate changes in self-concept. Problems of readjustment to a new image may be difficult not only for the client, but also for the client's spouse, family, or friends. The nurse can help the client cope with these changes by providing anticipatory guidance and support.

Gastric and intestinal bypass. For those individuals for whom dietary modification is unsuccessful in controlling obesity and the obesity is a threat to health, surgical approaches may be considered. An intestinal bypass (jejunoileal bypass) can be performed to decrease the absorptive surfaces of the jejunum.[4] A segment of the jejunum is removed, and the food bypasses directly into the ileum. Weight losses of 100 to 200 pounds (45.4 to 90.8 kg) may occur in 6 to 36 months.

Clients who are considered for this surgery must meet several criteria. The client must be morbidly obese (two to three times ideal weight) for 5 years of unsuccessful attempts at dieting. The client must be a good surgery risk, free of cardiovascular, respiratory, or endocrine disease, and, finally, must have a stable personality.

Preparation for a client having an intestinal bypass is similar to that of any individual having bowel surgery (see Chapter 18). Special modifications may be needed to accommodate the size of the client. Beds, chairs, and monitoring equipment such as blood pressure cuffs may need to be adapted for this individual.

Following surgery, nursing assessments and interventions are focused on maintaining fluid and electrolyte balance. Rapid emptying in the intestinal tract, which now occurs, causes severe diarrhea lasting up to 2 to 4 months after surgery. The nurse should assess intake and output accurately. Paregoric may be ordered to control diarrhea. Later, a low-fat diet may be used to prevent severe diarrhea.

Nutritional intake should be observed because decreased absorptive surface may lead to anemia, lowered carbohydrate tolerance, and vitamin A and C loss. Medications that are absorbed in the jejunum may also be less effective.

Gastric bypass, or gastric partitioning (stapling) is an alternative surgical approach for morbid obesity.[3] Surgical staples are inserted in the upper 10% of the stomach, creating a smaller reservoir for ingested food. A hole is created in the staple line through which food passes slowly, thereby increasing satiety while curtailing intake of food. After surgery the client consumes small quantities of liquified food (30 to 60 ml) and gradually increases consumption to capacity (regular diet) of 4 to 6 ounces. Calorie restriction and diet modification are required until weight loss is achieved. Like intestinal bypass surgery, clients who are candidates for this surgery must be morbidly obese for 5 years and good surgical risks without concomitant health problems. This procedure has advantages of less surgery time and preserving gastrointestinal continuity. Side effects include nausea, vomiting, and constipation. Follow-up behavior modification and diet modification are required for life-time control of obesity.

 Evaluation. The client who is overweight has problems of alterations in nutrition (more than body requirements). Evaluation of the nursing care plan focuses on objectives for weight loss and changes in self-concept.

EXPECTED OUTCOMES

The client and/or family can:
1. Describe overweight and obesity.
2. State plans for weight loss, including diet modification, exercise, and behavior modification.
3. Anticipate changes in self-concept.
4. State plans for follow-up health care and use of community resources for weight control.

Underweight and emaciation

Individuals who are underweight are more than 10% under their normal weight for height and body build according to norms (see Appendix A). The *primary* cause of weight loss is insufficient supply of nutrients to meet metabolic needs. *Secondary* factors influence the availability and utilization of food for adequate nutrition. These may include economic resources, social and cultural values, psychological needs, and disease states.

Economic factors are often related to weight loss. A direct source of food may not be available. In overpopulated areas the edible foods may be insufficient for each person to obtain nutrition. In other areas families do not have economic resources to buy adequate food supplies. Persons who receive welfare monies often find that they are unable to purchase food that will provide a diet to meet the needs of all the family members.

Social and cultural values also play a part in determining nutritional adequacy. Some societies value leaness, and starvation may be popular.

Psychological needs may influence nutrition. A person's appetite may be diminished by fear or anxiety, and the consequence is poor nutrition to the cells.

Nursing process for common health problems

Disease states also interfere with ingestion, digestion, or metabolism. These can include inflammations, tumors, or trauma of the gastrointestinal system, hyperthyroidism, diabetes mellitus, malabsorption syndromes such as celiac disease, or nontropical sprue. Other conditions such as fever, side effects of chemotherapy or radiation therapy that cause anorexia, nausea and vomiting, or diarrhea also affect the nutritional state, and contribute to weight loss and underweight. Clients who have surgery may be required to have nothing by mouth for several days and represent a potential for weight loss. The nurse should monitor the nutritional needs of these clients and plan for hydration and nutrition as necessary.

Regardless of the cause of inadequate food intake and use, the physiological changes result in depletion of body reserves or nutrition, tissue wasting, biochemical alterations in metabolism, and ultimately the physical signs of cachexia (wasting) and failures of growth and development. The process occurs over a period of time, and the nurse should be alert to observing incipient signs.

Weight loss is a significant health problem in the United States. Persons in the lower socioeconomic groups are particularly vulnerable. Others at risk are the elderly, persons living alone, pregnant women, food faddists, adolescents with anorexia nervosa, and the chemically dependent client.

 Assessment. The person who is underweight exhibits specific signs associated with depletion or nutritional reserves. Most obvious is weight loss or, in infants and children, the failure to maintain appropriate weight gain. The client has a general appearance of pallor and lethargy. The skin may be dry and reddened or swollen. The hair is dry, dull, and falls out easily. The eyes may be reddened and dry. Inspection of the mouth reveals cracked lips, swollen tongue, and pale, easily bleeding gums. There is obvious muscle wasting and weakness. Reflexes may be weak or absent and the client may be irritable or confused.

The diagnosis is based on height and weight norms for age and chemical laboratory studies for ketones, glucose, hemoglobin, and hematocrit. The latter tests are done to identify secondary causes of underweight. Starvation is indicated by the presence of ketones in the urine and blood. Anemia can be detected by hemoglobin and hematocrit levels.

Data analysis
Data analysis may reveal nursing diagnoses of alteration in nutrition (less than body requirements) and disturbance in self-concept.

Planning and implementation. The goal of nursing intervention is to restore the client to normal weight by supplying adequate nutrition and correcting nutritional deficiencies. This is accomplished by providing food and fluids as well as instruction about nutrition. Health teaching, dietary counseling, and antipoverty programs contribute to preventing and correcting malnutrition in individuals and groups.

Initially the client who is severely underweight may be hospitalized to provide nutrition and allow rest. Nutrition may be given by gavage or intravenously as hyperalimentation fluids or intralipid feedings. At this time nursing care is planned to provide a balance of nutrition to energy requirements. Attention is given to the physical effects of malnutrition by providing skin care and oral hygiene as necessary.

Long-term goals for correction of nutrition are initiated to provide instruction about proper nutrition and economic sources of food. The dietitian, social worker, and community health nurse help the client and family achieve these goals.

☞ **Evaluation.** Clients who are underweight have problems of alterations in nutrition (less than body requirements). The evaluation component of the nursing process is used to estimate outcomes as specified in objectives for restoration of nutritional status.

EXPECTED OUTCOMES
The client and/or family can:
1. Describe underweight and emaciation.
2. State plans for restoring nutrition, including use of foods, fluids, and nutritional supplements, and balance of activity and rest.
3. State plans for follow-up health care and use of community resources for meal planning and food procurement.

Gastritis
Gastritis may be an acute or chronic inflammation of the stomach caused by bacteria, toxins, or drugs. Children and elderly clients are more sensitive to ingestants and often experience acute gastritis.

An *acute gastritis* is a reaction to the toxic substance, usually food, alcohol, or drugs such as salicylates, and its symptoms include nausea, vomiting, diarrhea, stomach cramping, belching, and occasionally fever. If the symptoms persist for longer than a day, medical attention should be sought.

Treatment involves removing the toxic substance from the diet and giving fluids that are easily *digested*. Dehydration is a hazard in young children who have vomiting and diarrhea, and fluids are encouraged to prevent electrolyte loss. The parents or nurse should watch for poor skin turgor, lethargy, and muscle twitching, which indicate serious fluid and electrolyte loss.

Symptomatic support for the client with nausea, vomiting, or diarrhea is helpful. Mouth care, a cold washcloth to the forehead, a comfortable bed, and bed rest promote comfort. Persistent symptoms may be treated with antiemetics, antidiarrheal drugs, and smooth muscle relaxants.

Chronic gastritis occurs over a longer period of time. Exacerbations are precipitated by food or alcohol consumption. Gastric secretions are diminished, and the stomach wall atrophies. Nausea, belching, anorexia, and weight loss accompany an aching feeling in the stomach. The diagnosis is confirmed by gastroscopy and x-ray examination to rule out ulcerations or malignancy.

Treatment of chronic gastritis involves observance of a mechanical and chemical nonirritating diet (see bland diet, p. 944). Antacids may be used to give symptomatic relief from excess acidity brought on by dietary indiscretion. Vitamin B_{12} may be given if the intrinsic factor is destroyed and there are indications of pernicious anemia.

Traumatic injuries
Fracture of the jaw. The mandible, maxilla, or teeth may be chipped or fractured in an industrial accident or by the impact from an automobile, motorcycle, or human fist. The fractured bones may protrude through the skin or oral mucosa, causing bleeding and pain. The diagnosis is confirmed by x-ray examination.

Nursing process for common health problems

Immediate treatment involves immobilizing the jaw and controlling the bleeding; loose teeth should be saved in the event implantation is possible. Permanent reduction of the fractures is maintained by applying bands around the teeth and immobilizing the jaw with wires or rubber bands attached to the banded teeth.

While the jaw is healing, the client must obtain nutrition without disturbing the wired jaw. A liquid diet is usually given through a straw or Asepto syringe. If the client has difficulty swallowing, gavage feedings may be used. The diet should be varied to provide sufficient nutrients for tissue repair. After each meal the client should rinse his mouth with a mouthwash and rest in a sitting or side-lying position to prevent aspiration.

The nurse should observe the client for vomiting and respiratory distress such as dyspnea, wheezing, choking, or cyanosis, which can result if the client aspirates feedings or emesis. Suction equipment and wire cutters should be kept at the bedside at all times for use if the client aspirates. The nurse should not hesitate to cut the wires or rubber bands to permit removal of food or emesis that could obstruct the airway.

Stab wounds. Stab wounds may occur at any point in the gastrointestinal tract and may be caused by gunshot penetration, automobile accidents, direct stabbing of the gut, or by swallowed objects that irritate the lining of the gastrointestinal tract from within. The source of irritation is removed surgically, and the wound closed to permit gastrointestinal continuity. Alternative methods of feeding may be necessary while the wound heals.

Hernias

A hernia is the protrusion of an organ through the wall of the cavity that contains it. Hernias occur when there is increased stress on the cavity wall that has been weakened by trauma, age, obesity, pregnancy, or congenital deformity. Straining such as coughing, lifting heavy objects, sneezing, or forcing at stool causes increased intracavitary pressure and may precipitate herniation.

A hernia may be *reducible* (that is, able to be returned to its original position by manipulation) or *irreducible* (that is, unable to be returned to its body cavity). A hernia is *incarcerated* when the intestinal flow is obstructed. The hernia is *strangulated* when the blood supply is cut off. Immediate surgical intervention is performed when a hernia strangulates, to prevent anaerobic infection.

Umbilical hernia. Umbilical hernia occurs more often in neonates and obese women. The rectus muscle is weak, and the bowel protrudes through the umbilicus. The protrusion is easily noticed when the client cries or strains to defecate.

If the hernia occurs in the neonate, some physicians believe that the muscle may strengthen with growth and advise using tape or trusses to support the abdominal muscles. A truss is a device of straps with leather or felt padding that is applied to hold the hernia in a reduced position. Others prefer to do a herniorrhaphy when the child is about a year old, to prevent incarceration or strangulation. Umbilical hernias in adults are usually repaired as elective surgery.

Inguinal hernia. An inguinal hernia occurs when there is a weakness of the abdominal wall in which the spermatic cord (in men) or the round ligament (in women) enters. With an *indirect* inguinal hernia, the intestines protrude through the posterior inguinal wall. Most inguinal hernias occur in men and, if they become incarcerated, lead to bowel obstruction, vomiting, constipation, and abdominal distension.

The hernia can be reduced by manual replacement and use of a truss or by surgical repair. If the client is unable to withstand surgery he may be instructed to reduce the hernia by lying down with the feet elevated and pressing the hernia gently toward the abdominal cavity. A *truss* may be applied to maintain the hernia in a reduced position.

Most often however, surgical reduction (herniorrhaphy) is required to assure permanent reduction. An incision is made and the herniating tissue returned to the abdominal cavity. If the herniated area is not large, sutures are used to repair the defect.

Before surgery the client should be in optimal health. It is particularly important for the client to be free of cough or respiratory tract infections that would cause sneezing or straining after surgery.

Postoperative care is planned for the individual needs of the client, and depends on the type of anesthesia and surgery. If a spinal anesthetic is used, the client can usually resume a regular diet; if general anesthesia is used, he should wait until peristalsis returns. It is imperative to avoid abdominal distention and stress at the incision site. If necessary a nasogastric tube may be inserted. Cathartics and stool softeners can be used to prevent increased intraabdominal pressure caused by straining to defecate.

The nurse should observe the male client for hemorrhage into the scrotum. An ice bag may be used to control edema and minimize pain, and an athletic support can be used to support the edematous scrotum.

Men may have difficulty voiding after the surgery and are encouraged to stand at the bedside to use the urinal for the first voidings. The nurse should observe the client for urinary retention and abdominal distension.

The client is usually dismissed from the hospital in 3 to 7 days. He is instructed not to do heavy lifting for 3 to 6 weeks and to resume activities gradually. If the client is returning to a job that requires heavy lifting, he should further discuss activity limitation with the physician.

Hiatus hernia. A hiatus hernia (esophageal hernia or diaphragmatic hernia) results from a weakness of the diaphragm. The proximal portion of the stomach slips through the diaphragm into the thoracic cavity. This type of hernia is common in persons over 50 and is aggravated by increased abdominal pressure. The client complains of a feeling of fullness after eating and may have an esophagitis from reflux of digestive juices into the esophagus. There may be bleeding if ulceration of the esophageal mucosa has occurred, as well as flatus and regurgitation of food. The symptoms increase when the client bends forward or lies down with his feet elevated. The diagnosis is based on clinical symptoms, x-ray films of the upper gastrointestinal tract, and esophagoscopy.

The hiatus hernia may be treated symptomatically or surgically. With conservative treatment the client follows a diet that will prevent regurgitation of gastric juices and foods (bland diet, see p. 944). The client is instructed to eat slowly and remain sitting for 30 minutes after the meal. Antacids may be given between meals. Increased intraabdominal pressure can be avoided by wearing loose clothing, losing weight if obese, preventing constipation, and using good body mechanics when lifting heavy objects. The client may need to elevate the head of the bed on 6-inch blocks to help gravity maintain the stomach in the abdominal cavity while he sleeps.

If conservative approaches are unsuccessful, surgical intervention is indicated. A thoracic or abdominal approach may be used to reposition and anchor the esophagus. A vagotomy may also be done at this time to reduce acid reflux.

Incisional hernia. An incisional (ventral) hernia occurs when any organ protrudes through a surgical incision. The area is repaired surgically to prevent intestinal obstruction.

Femoral hernia. A femoral hernia occurs when the intestines protrude through the femoral ring into the femoral canal. This hernia is more common in pregnant women. It is repaired surgically.

Evaluation

The nursing care plan for the client with health problems of the upper gastrointestinal system is evaluated continuously as the nurse and client establish objectives for specific nursing problems or diagnoses. Common nursing problems often include potential or actual alterations in nutrition, alterations in comfort, ineffective family coping, fluid volume deficit, knowledge deficit, noncompliance, alteration in parenting, self-care deficit, disturbance in self-concept, and sleep pattern disturbance.

EXPECTED OUTCOMES

The client and/or family can:
1. State plans for health promotion, including components of a well-balanced diet appropriate to client's stage of growth and development, weight control, and plans for oral hygiene.
2. Describe changes in nutritional patterns related to growth and development throughout the life span.
3. State plans for health maintenance or promotion, including use of therapeutic diets and alternative feeding routes.
4. Describe plans for health restoration, including alternative feeding routes and diets, medications, or surgical interventions.
5. State indications for health care and plans for follow-up care and use of community resources.

As plans are evaluated, the nurse and client may discover that the problem has been resolved or that the plan can be modified or continued. Ultimate objectives are for the client to attain his optimal level of nutrition.

Summary

The nursing process for the client with common health problems of the upper gastrointestinal system provides a systematic mechanism for gathering data, identifying actual or potential nursing problems, developing appropriate plans, implementing them, and evaluating client outcomes. The relationship of the nurse and client changes as clients achieve independence in meeting their own health care needs.

During the assessment stage of the nursing process the nurse gathers information about the client's usual health habits for nutrition across the life span and relates the impact of sociocultural and psychological factors on the ability to meet needs for nutrition. Nursing diagnoses may include actual or potential alterations in nutrition, alterations in comfort, ineffective family coping, fluid volume deficit, knowledge deficit, noncompliance, alterations in parenting, self-care deficit, disturbances in self-concept, and sleep pattern disturbances.

Plans are developed for health promotion, maintenance, or restoration for specific nursing problems. Particular attention is directed toward attaining optimal nutritional status either with the client's usual diet or with alternative diets or feeding routes.

Health problems of the upper gastrointestinal system occur across the life span. Health problems of the neonate may include low birth weight, necrotizing enterocolitis, or congenital defects such as cleft lip, cleft palate, or esophageal atresia, or others such as PKU, failure to thrive, or celiac disease. Peptic ulcer disease has its greatest incidence in adulthood; other problems of this age group include gallbladder disease, hepatitis, cirrhosis, and pancreatitis. Of significant concern throughout the life span are those individuals who are overweight or underweight. Plans for these problems may be implemented by the nurse, client, or family and facilitated by resource persons such as the dietitian.

Evaluation, the final stage of the nursing process, is used to determine client's response to objectives specified during planning stages. The problem may be resolved or require modification or continuation of the plans in order for the client to attain his optimal level of wellness.

References

1. Baker, Dorothy: Hyperalimentation at home, Am. J. Nurs. **74**(10):1826-1829, 1974.
2. Berg, Nancy, and others: Behavior modification in a weight-control program, Family Comm. Health **1**(4):41-51, 1979.
3. Bolinger, Jeanne, and others: Gastric bypass for morbid obesity, Nurs. 81 **11**(1):55-59, 1981.
4. Brill, A.B., and others: Changes in body composition after jejunoileal bypass in morbidly obese patients, Am. J. Surg. **123:**419, 1972.
5. Brunner, Lillian: What to do (and what to teach your patient) about peptic ulcer, Nurs. 76 **6**(11):27-34, 1976.
6. Bush, James: Cervical esophagostomy to provide nutrition, Am. J. Nurs. **79**(1):107-109, 1979.
7. Dolan, Patricia O'Connor, and Greene, Harry: Conquering cirrhosis of the liver and a dangerous complication, Nurs. 76 **6**(11):44-53, 1976.
8. Ellis, P. Diane: Portal hypertension and bleeding esophageal and gastric varices: surgical approach to treatment, Heart Lung **6**(5):791-798, 1977.
9. Given, Barbara, and Simmons, Sandra: Gastroenterology in clinical nursing, ed. 3, St. Louis, 1979, The C.V. Mosby Co.
10. Griggs, Barbara, and Hoppe, Mary: Update: nasogastric tube feeding, Am. J. Nurs. **79**(3): 481-485, 1979.
11. Groër, Maureen, and Shekleton, Maureen: Basic pathophysiology: a conceptual approach, St. Louis, 1979, The C.V. Mosby Co.
12. Hanson, Robert: New approach to measuring adult nasogastric tubes for insertion, Am. J. Nurs. **80**(7):1334-1335, 1980.
13. Healthy People, The Surgeon General's Report on Health Promotion and Disease Prevention, Washington, D.C., 1979, U.S. Dept. H.E.W.
14. Keithley, Joyce: Proper nutritional assessment can prevent malnutrition, Nurs. 79 **9**(2): 68-72, 1979.
15. Kubo, Winifred: Fluid and electrolyte problems of tube-fed patients, Am. J. Nurs. **76:**912-916, June, 1976.
16. Malasanos, Lois, and others: Health assessment, ed. 2, St. Louis, 1981, The C.V. Mosby Co.
17. Munro, Hamish: Nutritional requirements in health, Crit. Care Med. **8**(1):2-8, 1980.
18. O'Brien, Kathleen: Cross circulation for hepatic coma, Am. J. Nurs. **77**(9):1459-1462, 1977.
19. Orr, Geoffry, and others: Alternatives to total parenteral nutrition in the critically ill patient, Crit. Care Med. **8**(1):29-33, 1980.
20. Overfield, Theresa: Obesity: prevention is easier than cure, Nurse Pract, **5**(5):25, 1980.
21. Reitz, Marie, and Pope, Wilma: Mouth care, Am. J. Nurs. **73**(10):1728-1730, 1973.
22. Reyzer, Nancy: Diagnosis: PKU, Am. J. Nurs. **78**(11):1895, 1978.
23. Rothfeder, Barbara, and Tiedeman, Mary: Feeding the low-birth-weight neonate, Nurs. 77 **7**(10):58-59, 1977.
24. Rubin, Philip, editor: Clinical oncology for medical students and physicians, a multidisciplinary approach, Rochester, N.Y., 1979, American Cancer Society.
25. Salmon, Susan: How to assess the nutritional status of acutely ill patients, Am. J. Nurs. **80**(5):922-924, 1980.
26. Samborsky, Veronica: Drug therapy for peptic ulcer, Am. J. Nurs. **78**(12):2064-2066, 1978.
27. Stephenson, Christina: non-organic failure to thrive, Nurse Pract. **5**(3):16, 1980.
28. Thorpe, Constance, and Caprini, Joseph: Gallbladder disease: current trends and treatment, Am. J. Nurs. **80**(12):2181-2185, 1980.
29. Ziemer, Mary, and Carroll, Jane: Infant gavage reconsidered, Am. J. Nurs. **8**(9):1543-1544, 1978.
30. 1981 Cancer Facts and Figures, New York, 1980, American Cancer Society, Inc.

Additional readings

Altshuler, Diane, and Hilden, Dolores: The patient with portal hypertension, Nurs. Clin. North Am. **12**(2):317-329, 1977.

Baranowski, Karen, and others: Viral hepatitis, Nurs. 76 **6**(5):31-38, 1976.

Belinsky, Irmgard: Visualizing the pancreatic and biliary ducts, Am. J. Nurs. **76**(6):936-937, 1976.

Block, Philip Lloyd: Dental health in hospitalized patients, Am. J. Nurs. **76**(6): 1162-1164, 1976.

Borgen, Linda: Total parenteral nutrition in adults, Am. J. Nurs. **78**(2):224-228, 1978.

Bossone, M. Christine: The liver: a pharmacologic perspective, Nurs. Clin. North Am. **12**(2): 291-303, 1977.

Boyer, Carol, and Oehlberg, Susan: Interpretation and clinical relevance of liver function tests, Nurs. Clin. North Am. **12**(2):275-290, 1977.

Caly, Joan: Assessing adults' nutrition, Am. J. Nurs. **77**(10):1605-1609, 1977.

Choi, Monica: Breast milk for infants who can't breast-feed, Am. J. Nurs. **78**(5):852-855, 1978.

Conevay, Alice, and Williams, Tamara: Parenteral alimentation, Am. J. Nurs. **76**(4):574-577, 1976.

Corcoran, Marya: Nursing role and management of failure-to-thrive clients, Comp. Pediatr. Nurs. **3**(4):29-40, 1978.

Cupoli, J.M.: Failure to thrive, Current Probl. Pediatr. **10**(11), 1980.

Daly, Katherine: Oral cancer, Everyday concerns, Am. J. Nurs. **79**(8):1415-1417, 1979.

Daniel, Evelyn: Chronic problems in rehabilitation of patients with Laennec's cirrhosis, Nurs. Clin. North Am. **12**(2):345-356, 1977.

Dyer, Elaine, and others: Dental health in adults, Am. J. Nurs. **76**(7):1156-1159, 1976.

Fauero, Martin, and others: Prevention and control of infections in specialized areas—viral hepatitis, Crit. Care Q. **3**(3):43-55, 1980.

Fields, Bessie: Adolescent alcoholism: treatment and rehabilitation, Fam. Comm. Health **2**(1): 61-90, 1979.

Genero, Susan: Necrotizing enterocolitis: detecting it and treating it, Nurs. 80, **10**(1):53, 1980.

Griffith, Rachel, and others: Care of the low-birth-weight infant, Perinatology-Neonatology, **5**(1):19-27, 1981.

Isolation Techniques for Use in Hospitals, U.S. Department of Health, Education, Welfare, Public Health Service, Washington, D.C., 1974, U.S. Government Printing Office.

Long, Gail: GI bleeding: what to do and when, Nurs. 78 **8**(3):44-50, 1978.

McConnell, Edwina: 10 Problems with nasogastric tubes . . . and how to solve them, Nurs. 79 **9**(4):78-81, 1979.

McElroy, Diane: Nursing care of patients with viral hepatitis, Nurs. Clin. North Am. **12**(2): 305-315, 1977.

Mojzisik, Cathy, and Martin, Edward: Gastric partitioning: the latest surgical means to control morbid obesity, Am. J. Nurs. **81**(3):569-572, 1981.

Oser, Jacob: Oral cancer, coping with the changes, Am. J. Nurs. **79**(8):1418-1419, 1979.

Penn, Israel: Management of the perforated duodenal ulcer, Heart Lung **7**(1):111-117, 1978.

Pierce, Lauretta: Anatomy and physiology of the liver in relation to clinical assessment, Nurs. Clin. North Am. **12**(2):259-273, 1977.

Sherman, Deborah, and others: Realistic nursing goals in terminal cirrhosis, Nurs. 78 **8**(6):43-47, 1978.

Shahinpour, Mayereh: The adult patient with bleeding esophageal varices, Nurs. Clin. North Am. **12**(2):331-343, 1977.

Slattery, Jill: Dental health in children, Am. J. Nurs. **76**(7):1159-1161, 1976.

Sweet, Karen: Hiatal hernia, what to guard against in post-op patients, Nurs. 77 **7**(8):36-43, 1977.

Tennant, Forest, and LaCour, Jean: Children at high risk for addiction and alcoholism: identification and intervention, Pediatr. Nurs. **5**(1):26-27, 1980.

White, Jane, and Schroeder, Mary Ann: When your client has a weight problem: nursing assessment, Am. J. Nurs. **81**(3):550-553, 1981.

18 Lower gastrointestinal system

Assessment

Data analysis

Planning

Implementation

Evaluation

The lower gastrointestinal system (small intestine, large intestine, rectum) provides for absorption of fluids and outlet for solid wastes. Disruptions of the system occur across the life span and are manifested by alterations in bowel elimination such as diarrhea and fluid loss or intestinal obstruction. The majority of common health problems occur in adulthood and are often attributed to the effects of diet, stress, and aging. The infant and the older adult are particularly vulnerable to the effects of fluid loss, and interventions must be instituted immediately to prevent dangerous complications of water and electrolyte imbalance. The purpose of this chapter is to acquaint the nurse with assessment skills for determining actual or potential nursing problems of bowel elimination and provide information necessary to plan for health promotion, maintenance, or restoration and implement and evaluate appropriate nursing care.

Overview of the lower gastrointestinal system

The process of elimination begins in the proximal portion of the small intestine, the *duodenum,* where the nutrients from the stomach are absorbed and waste products and water are propelled through the intestinal tract to the rectum. This process is aided by *peristalsis,* a rhythmic contraction of the intestines, and *villi,* fingerlike projections that greatly increase absorptive surfaces whereby nutrients can enter the lymphatics for distribution in the circulation. Peristaltic waves continue to propel products of ingestion and digestion to the *jejunum* and *ileum* and through the *ileocecal valve* where undigested foodstuffs, largely cellulose and bacteria, are passed to the large intestine as fecal matter.

The large intestine is composed of the *cecum,* the *ascending, transverse, descending* and *sigmoid colon,* and the *rectum.* Peristalsis here is much more forceful, and fecal matter (which is watery in the ascending and transverse colon) is propelled, while water is absorbed, into the descending colon. Fecal matter in the distal colon is largely formed stool and accumulates in the rectum until eliminated.

Defecation refers to the expulsion of fecal matter from the rectum and has a voluntary and involuntary phase. The presence of fecal matter in the sigmoid colon causes distension and stimulation of motor and sensory nerves surrounding the rectum. It should be recalled, however, that these nerves are not fully mature until 12 to 18 months of life (see Chapter 2). In the older individual the sensation of fecal matter stimulates the internal anal sphincter, and feces are propelled into the rectum. The external anal sphincter is under voluntary control, and with appropriate internal and environmental cues, defecation is accomplished.

Assessment
NURSING HISTORY

The nurse uses the nursing history to determine the client's usual bowel elimination patterns and to identify past, current, or potential health problems. The nurse must obtain the history and physical assessment in relation to the client's age and developmental stage, considering the impact of the client's social and psychological state.

Health history

When evaluating the elimination patterns of the client, the nurse should determine what is normal for each client. The nurse should know how often the client has bowel movements each day and what time they are most likely to occur. Significant information includes a change in bowel elimination habits or use of medication that might increase or decrease stooling. Some clients may use special measures to promote elimination; others may have alternative modes of elimination and require certain equipment. If the client is a young child, the nurse should ask the parents whether he is toilet trained and what word the child uses to indicate his need to defecate. The nurse should also note the presence of *encopresis* (fecal incontinence not from organic causes) or *tenesmus* (painful, ineffectual defecation).

The color, consistency, amount, and odor of the stool can provide important information, and the nurse should ask the client to describe the stool. Stools with fat content (greasy, pale, yellow) are described as *steatorrhea* stools. Stools with blood may be described as *melanin* stools (iron medications and red meats can cause the stool to become dark); *tarry* stools, if the occult blood is dark and sticky; or *currant jelly,* if bloody mucous is observable. Stools that are white, indicating absence of bile, may be described as *acholic.*

The nurse should relate other data from the comprehensive nursing history that might influence bowel elimination. Current or past health problems that cause inflammation of the bowel, obstruction of the intestines, or disruption to the nerve or blood vessel supply to the intestines, for example, may alter elimination patterns.

The nurse should also determine the client's risk for health problems of bowel elimination. Cancer of the colon, for example, is the second most common cause of cancer for middle-aged men and women, and risks include diets low in residue and high in carbohydrate and inflammatory gastrointestinal diseases.

Developmental history

Neonate. The first stool of the newborn is passed within 12 to 24 hours. This dark green stool is composed of dried intestinal secretions and is known as *meconium.* When the newborn begins breast- or formula-feeding, the stools become lighter in color. Newborns who are breast-fed usually have stools that are yellow and loose, whereas the stool of a formula-fed baby is darker yellow and firmer. The newborn normally passes 4 to 6 stools each day.

Infant. The bowel movements of the infant begin to pass formed contents and are fewer in number as solid foods are introduced into the diet. Even though bowel movements may appear to be regular, the infant is not able to control elimination of fecal wastes until he is older and the sensory nerves around the rectum have matured.

The older infant is interested in the waste products that come from his body, and as he does with everything else, he may want to play with his stool and even taste it; at other times, he may smear it on his clothing or crib. Parents should be aware of the meaning of this behavior and should not scold the infant for his curiosity. Cleaning up the stool in a calm manner will convey to the infant approval of him and the products of his body.

Toddler and preschooler. When the child is between 12 and 18 months of age and the nerve pathways to the rectum have developed, the child becomes aware of the presence of stool in the rectum. Also, at this time the child is beginning to communicate with his parents and is able to express his need to defecate. When these behaviors are noticed, the child is ready to be taught to defecate in the toilet.

Toilet training. Toilet training is a process extending over a period of years, and it may be upset by illness or stress within the family. Parents should not be discouraged with relapses to earlier patterns of elimination but should continue to help the child gain control of his bowels.

To begin toilet training, the parents should establish a simple word that the child will use to indicate the need to defecate. At first, the child may be taken to the bathroom at a regular time each day until he associates the word for the need to have a bowel movement with the appropriate sensation.

Several types of toilet seats may be used to make toilet training easier. Small training chairs that sit on the floor are comfortable for the child and are not associated with fears of flushing toilets. Other types of seats may be placed on the toilet to give support to the child. These seats simplify disposal of fecal material and avert the need to retrain the child to the toilet.

When the child indicates the need to have a bowel movement by saying the word his parents have taught him, he should be taken to the bathroom and given

984

sufficient time to defecate. Toys and other distractions should be eliminated so that the time in the bathroom is not prolonged. When the child has gained some skill in going to the bathroom by himself, he should have clothes that are easy to remove so that he can undress independently.

School-age child, adolescent, and adult. By the time the child enters school, he should have control of his bowel movements. The regularity of elimination is an individual habit that depends on the diet and exercise, but generally a consistent pattern of defecation is maintained through adulthood.

Older adult. Peristaltic activity slows as the individual ages, and in later maturity it is not abnormal for defecation to occur only every 2 to 3 days. Lack of exercise, inadequate dentition, and poor nutrition may further contribute to infrequency of stooling and irregular bowel habits.

Social history

Social and environmental cues influence the need for elimination by dictating socially approved times and places for fecal elimination. In the United States great emphasis is placed on privacy and cleanliness associated with defecation. Individuals learn early that modesty is required, that regular elimination is valued, and that cleanliness in disposal of fecal wastes and hand-washing techniques are to be observed. The nurse should be aware of these cultural values and include them in nursing care planning.

Cultural rituals also surround the initiation of the young into controlling elimination. Toilet training begins early in the United States, and to have trained the child early is often labeled as a virtue of successful parenting. The nurse should identify stages of development and appreciate cultural values in this aspect of the care plan.

Psychological history

Bowel elimination habits can be influenced by the client's psychological state, and the nurse should assess the client's coping resources and current mental health. Anxiety or stress, for example, may cause diarrhea or constipation requiring nursing intervention. Regressive coping mechanisms may cause the client to return to more comfortable stages and there may be involuntary stooling.

Physical assessment

The physical assessment of the intestines and rectum includes *inspection* and *palpation* of the abdomen, sacrum, anus, and rectum to detect changes in color, size, or shape of the structures. The examination is often performed with the physical assessment of the abdomen; techniques of inspection, auscultation, palpation, and percussion are discussed in Chapter 17.

Inspection. With the patient lying on his side (lateral position) or kneeling on the examination table with his shoulders and head resting on the table (knee-chest position), the nurse can inspect the sacrum and rectal areas. The sacrum should be observed for lumps, rashes, pilonidal dimpling, inflammation, and fissures. The skin of the pilonidal sinus is hairy, and accumulations of secretions here may cause cyst formation (pilonidal cyst). The anus is best observed by spreading the buttocks and looking for skin tags, fissures, external hemorrhoids, tumors, swelling, abscesses, or excoriation. The client should be instructed to perform Valsalva's maneuver (straining against a closed glottis) to elicit rectal prolapse or internal hemorrhoids.

Palpation. The nurse can palpate the rectum for 6 to 10 cm of the rectal canal. Using a gloved and lubricated finger, the nurse palpates the four rectal walls for nodes, masses, or presence of stool. In the man, the prostate can be palpated and the client asked to report tenderness. In the woman, the cervix can be felt in the anterior wall of the rectum.

DIAGNOSTIC ASSESSMENT

Direct visualization procedures

Anoscopy, proctoscopy, sigmoidoscopy, and colonoscopy. The mucosa of the anus, rectum, or sigmoid colon can be visualized or a biopsy can be performed with the use of a lighted sigmoidoscope or a colonoscope. The client is prepared for the procedure with clear liquid diets, cleansing enemas, and a laxative suppository, all of which are given the evening before, and/or the morning of the procedure to clear the rectum and colon of fecal material.

Before the examination the physician and nurse should explain the purpose of the procedure and what is expected of the client. The client should wear a hospital gown.

During the examination the client is positioned on a special examining table, which can be tilted so that the client is resting on his arms while his buttocks are elevated (Fig. 18-1). The nurse should observe the client for dizziness or shortness of breath while he is in this position. If the client is elderly or a young child, he may be supported in the knee-chest or Sims position (see Chapter 10) so that the examination can be completed with minimum discomfort.

After digital examination of the anus and rectum, the sigmoidoscope is lubricated and passed gently into the area to be observed. At this time the client should be instructed to breathe deeply to relax the abdominal muscles. If fecal material is present in the rectum or colon, it may be removed with large cotton swabs or suction, and air may be inserted to distend the colon for easier visualization.

The procedure is exhausting for most persons, and they should be permitted to rest when it is completed. Tissue should be provided to remove lubricant, and fluids offered if possible.

Sigmoidoscopy is recommended as a part of physical examination to detect colorectal cancer.[2] Men and women over 50 should have a sigmoidoscopic examination every 3 years after two negative examinations and more frequently if findings are positive.

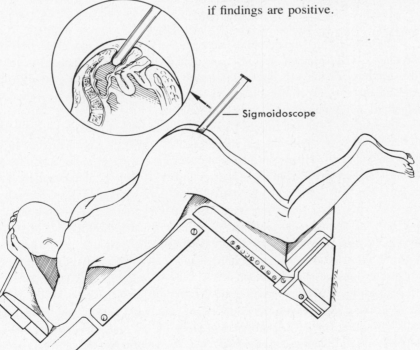

Sigmoidoscope

FIG. 18-1
Proctoscopic table is used to position the client for a sigmoidoscopy.

Radiographic examination: barium enema

A barium enema (lower GI series) introduces barium into the rectum to serve as a radiographic contrast medium in the diagnosis of polyps, tumors, or spasms of the rectum and sigmoid colon. The client is prepared for the x-ray examination with cleansing enemas or cathartics and laxatives and should have nothing to eat for 6 to 8 hours before the procedure. Barium is then introduced into the rectum, and its passage is observed by the radiologist under fluoroscopy. The client may experience a feeling of pressure as the barium fills the rectum, but he should attempt to retain it. When the procedure is completed, laxatives such as milk of magnesia or an oil-retention enema may be given to help expel the barium. Chalky stools will be evident until all the barium is expelled. The nurse should determine that the client has had a bowel movement after the barium enema, because the barium may cause him to become constipated or impacted.

Cultures and stool specimens

Anal cultures. Anal cultures may be obtained from the anus by placing cellophane tape on a tongue depressor and applying the sticky side to the anus. Larvae, which may have been deposited by pinworms, can then be obtained for culture. The hands should be washed carefully after this culture is obtained.

Stool specimen. Samples of stools may be obtained to detect the presence of pathogens, blood, and end products of digestion. The specimen should be obtained immediately after defecation and placed in a specimen container.

Special precautions may be needed for individual procedures. Stools that are to be examined for parasites or amoebae should be taken to the laboratory immediately for examination; a warmer or hot water bottle may be used to keep the specimen warm. If enemas are used to obtain specimens, only tap water should be used because soap or hypertonic solutions may alter the specimen. If the stool is to be examined for occult blood, the client should not eat red meats for 24 hours before the test. *Hemocult, Hematest,* or *guaiac examination* are three such tests that involve placing stool specimens on a filter paper, adding reagents, and observing color changes indicating the presence of occult blood. Instructions accompany each product. The nurse should observe handwashing procedures and aseptic technique when handling fecal material.

Data analysis

When all data are collected, the nurse compares the information with norms or standards; deviations reflect the client's actual or potential problems, which may be identified as nursing diagnoses. Accumulation of data and diagnosis is unique for each client. Diagnoses related to health problems of the lower gastrointestinal tract may include alterations in bowel elimination: constipation, diarrhea, or incontinence; alterations in comfort: pain; ineffective coping; fluid volume deficit; alterations in nutrition; and disturbances in self-concept. Using the diagnosis as a basis for the care plan, the nurse plans to help the client maintain health or cope with health problems.

Planning
PLANNING FOR HEALTH PROMOTION

The nurse has frequent opportunities to provide information about health and use health counseling and instruction skills. When discussing health promotion activities for bowel elimination, the nurse should stress the importance of exercise, diet, and fluids to maintain bowel habits as well as the need for sanitation of food and water consumed by the client.

987

**Promoting regular
elimination habits**

Exercise, fluids, and diet. Exercise, fluids, and a balanced diet help promote regular elimination. Simple exercise such as walking is necessary to maintain tone in the abdominal muscles that are used in defecation. Drinking 6 to 10 glasses of water each day provides lubrication and moisture for stools. For those clients who have difficulty defecating regularly, it may be helpful to drink a glass of cold water before breakfast and a cup of hot beverage with breakfast to stimulate defecation and then to sit on the toilet at a regular time. Regular bowel habits are further promoted by a well-balanced diet that contains bulk. The client who has irregular bowel habits is encouraged to eat cereals, brans, and fresh fruits to provide bulk in the diet (see high-fiber foods, below).

Sanitation. Disturbances in elimination can be caused by inadequate attention to external environment and by ingestion of contaminated foodstuffs. A common cause of diarrhea in certain areas is infestation by worms (see discussion later in this chapter). Prevention of this occurrence can be assisted by wearing shoes, hand-washing techniques, and eating only properly prepared and cooked foods. Water should be obtained from approved sources and, if from questionable sources, boiled or sanitized (see Chapter 17). Canned foods should be pur-

---

FOODS WITH HIGH FIBER CONTENT

Proteins	Vegetables	Fruits
Peanut butter	Artichoke	Apple
	Asparagus spears	Applesauce
Fats	Asparagus	Apricots
Nuts	Avocado	Banana
Olives	Green or wax beans	Blackberries, fresh
	Beets	Blueberries
Breads	Beet greens	Cantaloupe
Pumpernickle bread	Broccoli	Cherries
Bran muffins	Brussels sprouts	Fruit cocktail
	Cabbage, raw and cooked	Gooseberries
Cereals	Carrots, raw and cooked	Grapes with skins
All Bran	Cauliflower, raw and	Grapefruit
Bran Buds	cooked	Honeydew
Bran Chex	Celery	Nectarines
Bran Flakes	Collards	Orange
Cracklin' Bran	Kale	Peaches, canned and fresh
Total	Lentils	Pears, canned and fresh
Wheat Chex	Lettuce	Pineapple, canned and
Shredded Wheat	Mushrooms	fresh
Wheaties	Mustard greens	Plums
	Okra	Prunes
Starchy vegetables	Green pepper	Raisins
(bread exchange)		Rhubarb
Corn		Strawberries
Popcorn		Tangerines
White beans		Watermelon
Lima beans		
Peas		
Potatoes, potato chips		
Sweet potatoes		
Squash, winter		

chased without bulges or dents, which could provide a source of microbial entry. Home-canned foods should be packed according to canning instructions and boiled for 5 to 7 minutes before eating to prevent *botulism,* which can be caused by toxins in contaminated canned foods.

PLANNING FOR HEALTH MAINTENANCE AND RESTORATION

Maintaining elimination

The nursing care plan for clients with altered bowel elimination may include objectives for managing constipation and impaction or helping the client cope with an altered mode of elimination. The plans should be developed with the client and/or family and appropriate for age and developmental stage.

Constipation and impaction. Constipation is the retention of fecal material, delay in excretion, or deviation from usual elimination habits. Impaction, on the other hand, is the result of constipation that is not relieved and involves accumulation of fecal wastes in the rectum. Constipation may be *functional* (that is the result of dietary changes, increasing age, pregnancy, bed rest, drugs, muscle atony) or *organic* (related to changes in nerve or blood supply to the colon). Examples of the latter are strokes, paraplegia, quadriplegia, and cancer of the colon or rectum.

Constipation in children is unusual and often related to similar causes in adults. Constipation in the neonate is rare and may be caused by medications used by the mother during pregnancy. Metabolic diseases and congenital anatomical alterations of the intestinal tract account for constipation, but more often constipation results from a dietary change, frequently as the child is weaned to cow's milk.

Constipation may occur when the urge to defecate is ignored. The rectal mucosa then becomes insensitive to the defecation response, and defecation becomes increasingly irregular. Liquid continues to be absorbed from the fecal wastes, leaving hard, firm stools. Constipation may also result from an irritable bowel syndrome, in which colonic contents are delayed in passage to the rectum. Stools are hard and small and often covered with mucus.

Indications of constipation are observed when bowel movements are retained or delayed. There is a feeling of fullness in the rectum, and abdominal distension. Pressure on the sacral nerves may produce sacral pain. Headache and anorexia often result from prolonged constipation. Fever may be noted as a result of bacterial accumulation. Stools are hard, dry, and may contain mucus shreds.

Impaction is noted when watery stool passes around the unevacuated formed stool in the rectum. This should not, however, be confused with diarrhea. Manual palpation reveals a hardened mass.

Nurses should be familiar with common measures used to prevent constipation and impaction. These include encouraging fluids, increasing bulk in the diet, and obtaining exercise, or at least strengthening abdominal muscles by doing leg raises, sit-ups, or muscle-setting exercises. Additionally, the nurse should ascertain the client's usual habits and make every effort to comply with his routine during hospitalization. The client should be reminded to respond to the defecation urge and assume the most comfortable and natural position. If these measures are inadequate, stool softeners, laxatives, cathartics, or enemas may be necessary.

Bowel training, enemas, removal of impaction. If methods of health maintenance are not sufficient to cause elimination of stool, the nurse may plan to institute a bowel training program, give the client an enema, or if necessary,

GUIDELINES FOR BOWEL TRAINING

1. Offer 2½ ounces of prune juice each evening (increase or decrease as necessary).
2. Serve a hot and cold drink with breakfast.
3. Twenty minutes after breakfast, insert one to three glycerine suppositories.
4. Position client comfortably until defecation occurs. A toilet or commode offers the most natural position. Provide a warm, quiet, private environment.
5. Encourage the client to stimulate peristalsis (if necessary) by:
   a. Bending forward
   b. Exerting slight manual pressure downward on the abdomen
   c. Digital stimulation of the external sphincter.
6. Establish a daily routine. This plan is suggested for morning defecation but can be altered to the client's convenience.

Nursing process for common health problems

remove the impaction. The plans should be determined for the individual client and simulate his usual patterns of elimination.

Bowel training programs can be instituted for clients with chronic constipation, such as the elderly, or for individuals with cord injuries or sensory impairment. One program is described in the guidelines on p. 989. This routine, if followed conscientiously, will usually prevent problems of constipation.

In instances of severe constipation or when the rectum must be emptied for diagnostic procedures or surgery, an enema may be given to stimulate rectal emptying. Various solutions may be used, such as tap water, normal saline, or soap suds, and they are generally introduced into the rectum with the client lying on his left side so that the curvature of the sigmoid colon can be followed. Warm solutions (105° F or 40.5° C) and a large volume of fluid inserted into the rectum increase peristalsis. Other solutions may be given at room temperature and in lesser amounts to soften and lubricate the stools to promote evacuation. Adults are usually able to hold the fluid in the rectum until positioned on the bedpan or toilet, but infants and young children do not have sensory control in the rectum and should be propped on a bedpan with pillows under their backs while the enema is given and expelled.

Clients who wish to administer the enema themselves may do so in the Sims position or, if desired, lying supine with the legs raised. Clients with respiratory

FIG. 18-2
Types of gastrointestinal tubes.

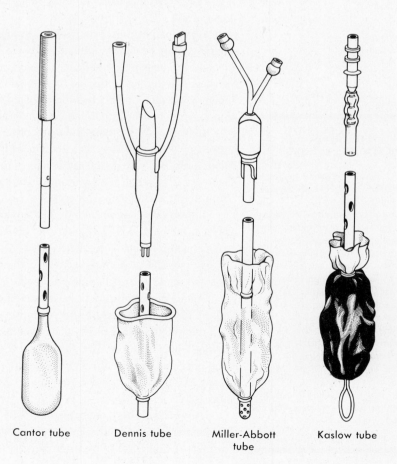

Cantor tube   Dennis tube   Miller-Abbott tube   Kaslow tube

distress may be given an enema while sitting up on a bedpan or toilet seat, although this position is not as effective.

If the client is unable to expel the fecal material after using laxatives, cathartics, or enemas, it may be removed digitally. Impactions may be removed by inserting a lubricated, gloved finger gently into the rectum and loosening impacted feces.

When the outlet for fecal waste is obstructed, alternative routes for elimination may be established. These may include intestinal decompression or the creation of a temporary or permanent opening into the bowel.

Intestinal decompression. Fluids, flatus, or undigested food that obstruct elimination may be removed from the intestines by inserting a gastrointestinal tube through the nose and stomach into the intestine. These double-lumen tubes (Fig. 18-2) are weighted with mercury to facilitate passage into the intestine. The physician usually inserts the tube, but after it has passed through the pyloric sphincter, the nurse may be instructed to advance the tube 2 to 3 inches (5.0 to 7.5 cm) every hour to help gravity and peristalsis promote passage of the tube. The nurse can also turn the client from side to side every 2 hours as the tube advances. When the position of the tube has been verified by x-ray examination and by testing the pH of aspirate (pH greater than 7 indicates intestines; less than 7, stomach), a low-suction source is attached to remove the obstruction.

When the client has a gastrointestinal tube inserted, the nurse should offer mouth care, using an antibiotic mouthwash to prevent growth of colonic bacteria, and cleanse and lubricate the nostril every 2 to 4 hours. The physician may leave orders for the tube to be irrigated with normal saline to maintain patency. The nurse should identify the lumen that is used for irrigation, because inserting irrigating fluid into the lumen for mercury could cause the mercury-containing balloon to rupture. Intake and output should be recorded accurately to indicate fluid loss or fluid retention. Irrigating solution that is not returned should be recorded as intake, to avoid confusion with fluid loss through the gastrointestinal tube.

Ileostomy. When an obstruction or disease is present in the small or large intestine, an opening may be created in the ileum to permit an outlet for feces (Fig. 18-3, *A*). The opening is usually permanent and necessitates wearing a special bag to collect the continuous drainage of watery fecal material. See discussion later in this chapter for related nursing care.

Colostomy. A colostomy is a temporary or permanent opening into the colon (Fig. 18-3, *B*), which may be created if there is an obstruction in the colon or if the colon becomes severely inflamed or diseased. Fecal material is eliminated through a stoma, and because fecal material is more formed in the colon, it may be necessary to irrigate the colostomy to stimulate evacuation of solid wastes. See discussion later in this chapter for related nursing care.

Cecostomy. A cecostomy is an opening in the cecum for temporary relief of an obstruction by providing an outlet for fecal material (Fig. 18-3, *C*). After the client has been given a local anesthetic, an opening is made through the abdomen. A catheter is advanced to the cecum, sutured in place, and connected to suction or gravity drainage. The skin around the cecostomy should be kept clean and dry and strengthened with tincture of benzoin or karaya powder to prevent it from becoming excoriated by fecal drainage.

Altered modes of elimination

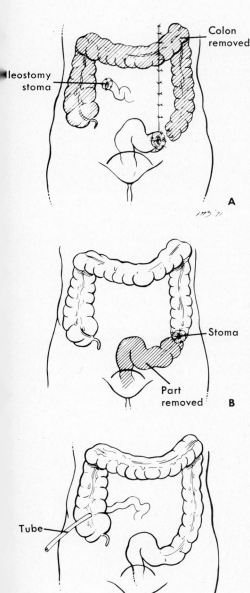

FIG. 18-3
Alternative modes of elimination: **A,** ileostomy; **B,** colostomy; **C,** cecostomy.

Implementation

COMMON HEALTH PROBLEMS OF THE NEONATE AND INFANT

Imperforate anus

In the rare congenital defect of imperforate anus, fecal elimination may be obstructed by (1) a thin membrane over the anus, (2) a rectum that ends in a blind pouch, or (3) an imperforate anus and a rectum that ends in a blind pouch located some distance from the anus (Fig. 18-4). This defect may occur with a fistula to the bladder or vagina, in which case there is an outlet for fecal wastes. If there is no outlet for the waste products, the abdomen becomes distended, and the neonate may vomit meconium. Often the obstruction can be detected in the nursery when the nurse takes the first rectal temperature. The diagnosis is based on clinical observations, digital examination of the rectum, and roentgenograms of the intestines and rectum.

Treatment must be instituted promptly to provide an outlet for feces. When the only problem is an imperforate anus, the thin membrane may be excised and the physician may order rectal dilations for several months to maintain an open passage for the feces. For this procedure the nurse or parent should lubricate the gloved little finger and gently dilate the anal opening.

When the rectum ends in a blind pouch or when there is an imperforate anus and a rectum ending in a blind pouch, a temporary colostomy (see discussion later in this chapter) is created until the neonate can withstand corrective surgery. The colostomy usually does not need to be irrigated because the infant is able to pass stool spontaneously. The parents should be instructed to keep the skin around the stoma clean and dry and change the collection bag or dressing frequently. The skin of the infant can easily become excoriated, and aluminum paste or karaya powder can be applied to prevent skin breakdown.

The congenital defects of the anus and rectum are usually corrected when the client is 3 to 6 months old. An abdominoperineal approach is used (see discussion later in this chapter) to reconstruct the anus and rectum. After surgery the infant should be positioned so that there is no pressure on the perineum. He may be placed in Bryant's traction (see Chapter 11) with his buttocks raised off the bed, or the nurse may position him on pillows with the perineal area exposed.

Nursing care should be directed toward promoting healing and preventing infection of the surgical site. Perineal cleanses may be ordered to stimulate circulation and cleanse the area. Since fecal wastes are now eliminated from the rectum, the nurse must change the diapers frequently to prevent irritation of the skin and subsequent infection.

FIG. 18-4
Imperforate anus. **A,** Imperforate anus with membrane covering anus. **B,** Imperforate anus with rectum ending in blind pouch. **C,** Imperforate anus with fistula between rectum and vagina. **D,** Normal anus with rectum ending in blind pouch.

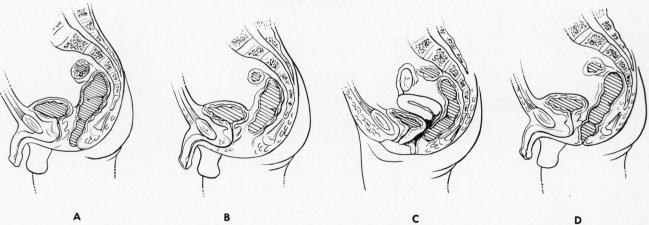

A   B   C   D

A regular diet is resumed when peristalsis returns, and fluids should be encouraged by offering formula and juices between meals. The nurse should observe the effect of the diet on the stool, because constipation may produce pain, and diarrhea could cause electrolyte loss and poor healing.

The parents should be involved in the care of their infant so that they will be able to take care of him when he is dismissed from the hospital. The parents should be instructed to observe the infant for free passage of stool and to inspect the perineal incision for inflammation or infection. If this is the family's first child or if they have not had the child at home, the nurse may also instruct them on aspects of growth and development.

Congenital megacolon (Hirschsprung's disease)

Congenital megacolon is a mechanical obstruction of the colon caused by an absence of nerve ganglia to a segment of the bowel (Fig. 18-5). Peristalsis does not occur in that area, and the bowel becomes hypertrophied and distended. There is also failure of the internal rectal sphincter to relax, and stool, liquids, and gas accumulate and further distend the bowel.

The disease occurs in neonates but may not be diagnosed until infancy or childhood. Boys are affected four times more often than girls.

Clinical evidence is noted by constipation and distension. In the neonate the primary indication is failure to pass meconium. There may also be bile-stained emesis. Dehydration, weight loss, and shock follow if the obstruction is not corrected. In infancy the client may have constipation, distension, diarrhea, and vomiting. Fluid loss, fever, and electrolyte imbalance are serious consequences and increase the risk of fatality. Symptoms noticed in childhood tend to be evidence of chronic obstruction such as constipation, distension, presence of fecal masses, and passage of ribbonlike stools.

Diagnosis is based on clinical evidence and by roentgenograms taken after a barium enema that reveal the atonic segment of the bowel. Rectal biopsy may also be used to demonstrate aganglionic cells.

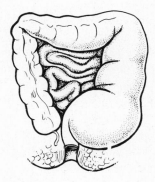

FIG. 18-5
Congenital megacolon.

Treatment of congenital megacolon depends on the age of the client and the severity of the obstruction. The child with chronic obstruction may be treated symptomatically with enemas, laxatives, and low-residue diet. Most often, however, a temporary colostomy is preferred to rest the bowel and permit return to normal caliber and tonicity. The megacolon can be permanently corrected by a pull-through anastomosis, which may be done at the time of the colostomy. In this surgery, the end of the intact bowel is pulled to a point near the rectum and anastomosed. A sphincterotomy of the internal sphincter may also be done to improve sphincter control. The colostomy is then closed within 3 months to a year.

Nursing care is planned to help the client and parents cope with altered elimination and reestablish gastrointestinal continuity. These are discussed later in this chapter.

Meconium ileus

Meconium ileus occurs when meconium is impacted in the intestinal tract of the neonate (Fig. 18-6). The meconium blocks the small intestine at or near the ileocecal valve, and peristalsis is insufficient to evacuate the stool. Intestinal obstruction follows, noticed by abdominal distension, vomiting, dehydration, and electrolyte imbalance.

The intestine must be entered immediately to remove the meconium. Depending on the area involved, a resection of the intestine with reanastomosis may be necessary.

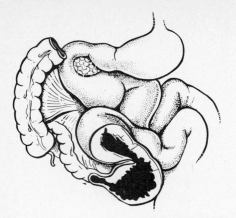

**COMMON HEALTH
PROBLEMS OF THE CHILD**

Parasitic infections

FIG. 18-6
Meconium ileus.

Meconium ileus may be one of the first signs of cystic fibrosis (see Chapter 21), because absence of pancreatic enzymes may cause thick meconium. The nurse should, therefore, urge further assessment of the neonate with meconium ileus.

Pinworm infection. Pinworm infection (oxyuriasis, enterobiasis) is a common parasitic infection of children, which is transmitted by ingesting the pinworm eggs. When the pinworm eggs are swallowed, they hatch in the intestine, and the females travel to the anus to deposit their eggs; the cycle is repeated in 6 to 8 weeks when the child reinfects himself by the rectum-to-hand-to-mouth route (Table 18-1).

Pinworms may be suspected if the child is irritable, loses his appetite, loses weight, picks his nose, or has vaginitis or anal itching. Anal itching increases at night when the females migrate to the anus to lay the eggs. The diagnosis can be made by collecting the eggs for microscopic examination.

Pinworms can be treated with piperazine citrate (Antepar) and pyrvinium pamoate (Povan), which are specific drugs for parasitic infections. Pyrivinium may stain the teeth or cause the stool, urine, or emesis to be red, and the nurse should instruct the parents about this harmless phenomenon. All children in the family are treated if one child has pinworms, because the worms are easily spread, and the child under treatment could become reinfected.

While the child is under treatment, the linens should be isolated and boiled twice a week. The underwear should also be washed carefully, and clean underwear should be used each day. The mother may wish to put gloves on the child to prevent his collecting the eggs under the fingernails if he scratches himself during the night, and the child should observe careful hand-washing habits. If the child is in school, the nurse or teacher should be aware of the incidence of pinworms and encourage hand washing and frequent cleansing of the toilets.

Ascariasis. Ascariasis occurs primarily in southern and rural areas where the clay soil provides a medium for growth and outdoor toilets are used. The life cycle of the roundworm *Ascaris lumbricoides* has several stages. The eggs are found in the excreted stool, and if the contaminated fecal material is ingested, the eggs enter the duodenum and hatch. The first-stage larvae develop, which molt within a week. The second-stage larvae may migrate to the liver, but usually they enter the lungs, where they molt and are expectorated and swallowed. The adult worms then attach to the small intestine to lay eggs, and the cycle is repeated in 4 to 6 weeks (Table 18-1).

The client who has roundworms may have vague symptoms of restlessness, weight loss, abdominal pain, colic, or anorexia. There may be an atypical pneumonia if the worms enter the pleural cavity, or there may be a bowel obstruction if worms accumulate in the intestines. The diagnosis is based on clinical symptoms and identification of the worms or ova in the stool.

When the roundworm is identified, it can be treated with piperazine. All infected members of the family should be treated at the same time so that the

TABLE 18-1

Common parasitic infections

Infection	Portal of entry	Clinical evidence	Usual treatment	Prevention of spread
Pinworms (oxyuriasis, enterobiasis)	Ingestion of pinworm eggs; eggs deposited on rectum; hand-to-mouth infection	Irritability, anal itching, anorexia, weight loss, nose picking	Piparazine citrate (Antepar); pyrvinium pamoate (Povan)	Treat all family members, boil linens twice a week; isolate infected child; change underwear daily; hand washing; wear gloves at night to avoid anal scratching
Roundworms (ascariasis)	Ingestion of eggs; hand-to-mouth from contaminated stool.	Restlessness, weight loss, anorexia, abdominal pain, bowel obstruction, atypical pneumonia (if worms enter pleural cavity)	Piperazine (Antepar)	Treat all family members; instruct family on proper disposal of fecal wastes; hand washing
Hookworm (uncinariasis)	Entry through skin (bare feet); larvae pass to lungs, are expectorated and swallowed	Anemia, anorexia, weight loss, fatigue	Hexylresorcinol; tetrachlorethyline	Instruct on disposal of fecal material; wear shoes in infested areas; hand washing
Trichinosis	Ingestion of uncooked pork	Abdominal pain, fever, diarrhea, nausea, vomiting, muscle pain, swelling around eyes	Thiabendazole	Cook pork products thoroughly
Beef tapeworm	Ingestion of uncooked beef	Vague symptoms; portions of worms noticed in stool	Quinacrine (Atabrine)	Cook beef products thoroughly

parasites are totally destroyed. Along with pharmacological intervention, the family should be instructed in proper disposal of fecal wastes and hand-washing procedures.

Hookworm infection. Hookworm (causing uncinariasis) enters the body in larva form by passing through the skin, particularly that of barefoot children. The larvae pass to the lungs and bronchi through the bloodstream where they molt and are expectorated and swallowed. From the stomach the larvae pass to the small intestine, attach themselves, and produce eggs. The child may become anemic, anorexic, fatigued, and malnourished. The diagnosis is made by detecting the eggs in the stool (Table 18-1).

Hookworm is treated with hexylresorcinol or tetrachlorethylene. The nurse should stress hand washing and the necessity of sanitary disposal of fecal material in the prevention of hookworm. Shoes should be worn in areas of warm climate and poor sewage, where hookworm is common.

Trichinosis. *Trichinella spiralis* is a roundworm that infects uncooked pork, particularly pork from garbage-fed hogs. The larvae in the encysted pork hatch in the client's intestine, mate, and release embryos into the bloodstream. The embryos are carried to muscle tissue where they become embedded. The client has fever, abdominal tenderness, muscle pain, nausea and vomiting, diarrhea, and swelling around the eyes. If the larvae infect the myocardium, there may be myocarditis. The diagnosis is made by a muscle biopsy (Table 18-1).

Thiabendazole, an oral anthelmintic drug, may be given to terminate the life cycle of the worm. Other supportive measures are used while the client is receiving treatment. The client is encouraged to obtain adequate nutrition and drink plenty of fluids. Aspirin may be given for pain. Trichinosis can be prevented by cooking pork thoroughly before eating it, and the nurse should instruct the family to cook all meats, because the worm can be present on cutting blocks and equipment used to grind any meat.

Beef tapeworm infection. Infection by beef tapeworm *(Taenia saginata)* is contracted from eating infected, uncooked beef. The larvae mature and attach in the intestine where they can grow as long as 12 feet. The symptoms are minimal, and the worm may be noticed as segments separate and are passed in the stools. The tapeworm is treated with quinacrine (Atabrine), which is given after the client has had a purgative and abstained from eating for 8 hours. Divided doses of the drug are given, followed by a cathartic to purge the intestines of the worm (Table 18-1).

COMMON HEALTH PROBLEMS OF THE YOUNG ADULT

Ulcerative colitis

Ulcerative colitis is a chronic ascending inflammation of the rectum and colon, which is characterized by periods of remission and exacerbation. The cause of ulcerative colitis is not known, although several theories have been offered. The most common is that an autoimmune factor produces the inflammation. There is a correlation between the disease and personality traits of perfectionism, rigidity, insecurity, and dependence on mother, but the relationship of these traits to the disease has not been proved causal. Stress may also have a bearing on inciting the inflammation.

Ulcerative colitis is a disease of adolescents and young adults. The onset occurs between ages 15 and 49, with the highest incidence at age 20 to 40. Men and women are affected equally. Blacks tend to have a low incidence, whereas there is a high incidence in Jews.

Pathophysiology. The inflammation of ulcerative colitis begins in the rectum or sigmoid colon as superficial ulcerated areas in the mucosa that bleed. The lesions of inflammatory infiltrate contain polymorphonuclear leukocytes, lymphocytes, and red blood cells and are referred to as crypt abscess. The disease progresses up the colon, and areas enlarge, causing an edematous and thickened bowel. The ulcers may perforate and cause abscesses. As the ulcers heal and fill with fibrotic tissue, the absorptive surface of the bowel is reduced.

Assessment. The nurse can assess the client's usual elimination patterns and during the history elicit information pertinent to inflammatory bowel disease. Diarrhea is the primary symptom of ulcerative colitis. The client may have as many as 20 to 30 stools a day, accompanied by cramping pains and flatulence. The stools contain blood, pus, and mucus. As scarring of the mucosa progresses, there may be loss of elasticity of the bowel, causing decreased sensation of the urge to defecate and consequent involuntary stooling.

Reduction of absorptive surfaces causes fluid and nutrient loss. Plasma proteins, prothrombin, fluids, and potassium are lost, and intestinal hypermotility shortens absorption time. The nurse should assess the client for dehydration, weight loss, and electrolyte intolerance. Severe electrolyte loss may cause metabolic acidosis. The client becomes weak, debilitated, and cachectic. The medical diagnosis is made by evaluating stool specimens, sigmoidoscopy, and x-ray examination of the lower gastrointestinal tract.

Data analysis
Data analysis may reveal nursing diagnoses of alterations in bowel elimination, fluid volume deficit, alterations in nutrition, and sleep pattern disturbances.

Planning and implementation. Initial treatment for ulcerative colitis is medical support for the inflamed bowel. The disease is characterized by remissions and exacerbations; most exacerbations respond to medical therapy. Surgical removal of the inflamed bowel may be required if the inflammation is severe or perforates to the intestines. About 20% of clients with ulcerative colitis ultimately require surgical intervention.

The nurse develops a care plan consistent with medical therapy. Nursing goals are established with the client and are directed to (1) reduce the inflammation, (2) reduce intestinal motility, (3) maintain nutrition and hydration, and (4) provide rest for healing. The clients are usually young, and illness at this time is seen as an interruption of important school and career activities. The client is also striving to establish independence, and illness may impair that goal. The nursing care plan should be developed to reflect these needs.

Reducing inflammation. Antiinflammatory steroids such as prednisone may be used during acute exacerbations to minimize inflammation and promote a sense of well-being. The use of these drugs over a period of time can precipitate changes in body systems, and the nurse should observe the client for signs of electrolyte imbalance, gastric hyperacidity, mood changes, osteoporosis, and changes in fat deposition. Steroids are usually used only during the acute inflammatory period. Azathioprine (Imuran) may be used as an immunosuppressive agent.

Local inflammation may be controlled by antidiarrheal drugs (such as kaolin) that coat the intestinal mucosa and reduce stooling. When the inflammation is severe, the incidence of infection increases, and sulfonamide drugs, particularly sulfasalazine (Azulfidine), may be used to prevent or treat intestinal infection.

Slowing intestinal motility. Absorption of nutrients is facilitated when the gastrointestinal motility is slowed; anticholinergic and antispasmodic drugs such as belladonna are given for this purpose. Diphenoxylate (Lomotil) is used to control diarrhea by decreasing gastrointestinal motility. This drug is an opiatelike drug, and the nurse should observe the client for effects of sedation. The nurse should also evaluate the effects of these drugs on the motility by noting the number and frequency of stooling. Heat from warm soaks or a tub bath may also be used to reduce colonic spasms.

Maintaining nutrition. A diet high in protein and calories is used to assure sufficient nutrients for growth and healing. Metabolic needs are increased during adolescence, and if nutrients are lost in diarrhea, they must be supplemented in the diet. Certain high-residue foods may be eliminated from the diet if they produce colonic spasms. For a low-residue diet see p. 1007. The environment should be conducive to eating, and mealtime should be a pleasant experience for the client. Often, clients may eat better in a small group and can be encouraged to eat in an ambulatory client dining room or in a social room on the nursing unit.

Fluid balance is difficult to maintain in clients with severe diarrhea, and intravenous fluids may be given during an acute exacerbation. The nurse should record the intake and output and observe the client for dehydration. Parenteral hyperalimentation may be used if the client loses excessive weight and becomes debilitated. This infusion supplies not only additional fluids but also amino acids to support anabolic activity.

Promoting rest. Physical and mental rest are necessary to healing. The client is usually hospitalized to control the pressures of home, school, or career that upset him. Sedatives and tranquilizers may be used at this time to ensure rest.

Prolonged illness increases anxiety. The anxiety can be reflected in increased intestinal motility, and the nurse should incorporate psychotherapeutic measures that will allay anxiety. The client may wish to express his feelings about his illness or hospitalization, and the nurse should provide opportunity for him to discuss these.

Anxiety may also be produced by family relationships that threaten the achievement of developmental tasks. The adolescent may be concerned about his adult responsibilities, and the young adult may be concerned with career decisions and increasing family responsibilities. Social workers and psychiatrists on the health team may be able to help the client resolve these conflicts.

When the acute inflammation has been controlled, the client is usually able to resume his normal activities. Remissions may be maintained for varying lengths of time, but in spite of the client's attention to medical therapy and adjustments in life-style, the inflammation may once again become acute.

Nursing care of the client having an ileostomy. If ulcerative colitis does not respond to medical therapy or if the ulcerations hemorrhage or perforate the intestines, it may be necessary to temporarily rest or remove the inflamed colon. A temporary ileostomy can be performed to permit fecal wastes to be eliminated through a stoma created in the ileum. A second stoma is made at this time, and when the colon is healed, the ends of the ileum are anastomosed. Most often, however, a permanent ileostomy is created. The inflamed colon and, if necessary, a part of the ileum or jejunum are removed, and fecal wastes are eliminated from the ileal stoma.

Several surgical approaches can be used, depending on the extent of involved colon.

1. An *ileostomy* with *partial colectomy* is the removal of part of the colon and creation of an ileal stoma. Two stomas are created so the remaining rectum may be anastomosed at a later time. The proximal stoma is the ileostomy, which drains fecal material, whereas the distal stoma opens to the remaining bowel.

2. A *total proctocolectomy* involves removal of the entire colon. An ileal stoma is created for fecal outlet.

3. A *pouch ileostomy* (Koch ileostomy), or continent ileostomy (Fig. 18-7), may be created by making a reservoir from the distal ileum. A nipple valve is created by the intussusception of the ileum, and the stoma placed on the abdomen. The client can drain the reservoir with a catheter and will not need to wear an appliance. The capacity of the pouch increases gradually after surgery and in about 6 months holds 500 ml.

The part and amount of the intestines that must be removed determine nutritional loss. When the entire colon is removed, fluids are not resorbed; if the ileum or jejunum is also removed, the client may lose fat, protein, and fat-soluble vitamins that are normally absorbed from that part of the intestine.

The ileostomy, unlike the colostomy (see discussion later in this chapter), drains continuously and cannot be regulated. Unless a pouch ileostomy is created, a drainage collection bag must be worn at all times to contain the products of elimination and prevent excoriation of the skin.

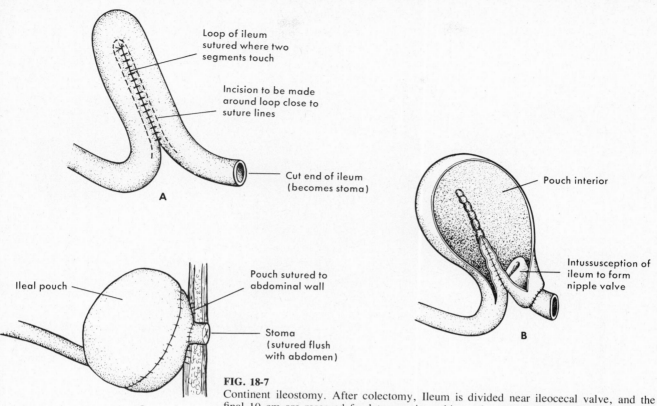

Loop of ileum
sutured where two
segments touch

Incision to be made
around loop close to
suture lines

Cut end of ileum
(becomes stoma)

A

Pouch interior

Intussusception of
ileum to form
nipple valve

B

Ileal pouch

Pouch sutured to
abdominal wall

Stoma
(sutured flush
with abdomen)

C

FIG. 18-7

Continent ileostomy. After colectomy, Ileum is divided near ileocecal valve, and the final 10 cm are reserved for later use in making valve and ileostomy. **A,** The next 30 to 35 cm proximal to this are folded in half into shape of letter U, and two adjacent loops are sutured together. **B,** An incision is made into each loop of U, close to suture, and ileum is laid open. A built-in valve mechanism called the nipple valve is fashioned out of terminal ileum, which is just distal to pouch. **C,** U is then folded in half to bring top of U to base, and sides are sutured together to create a pouch. Pouch is then sutured to abdominal wall and stoma to abdominal skin. When fecal material fills pouch, pressure shuts nipple valve and prevents leakage. (From Given, Barbara, and Simmons, Sandra: Gastroenterology in clinical nursing, ed. 3, St. Louis, 1979, The C. V. Mosby Co.)

Preoperative nursing care. Adjustment to changes in elimination and body image are difficult for the client, and he may have periods of depression and grief. The nurse should be understanding during this preoperative adjustment and encourage the client to express his feelings. If the client is agreeable, a person who has an ileostomy may visit and answer questions about the impending surgery. Some hospitals have enterostomal therapists who are skilled in helping the client cope with the ileostomy, giving nursing care before and after surgery, and planning care with this client.

It is advantageous if the client can become accustomed to wearing the ileostomy drainage bag before surgery. If the client does wear the bag, the ideal location for the stoma can be identified, and the surgeon can plan to locate the stoma for the client's convenience.

Before surgery the client should be in good nutritional health. If he has lost weight, he is encouraged to increase his caloric intake. Lost fluids may be replaced by intravenous infusions. Blood transfusions may be necessary if there has been blood loss from diarrhea.

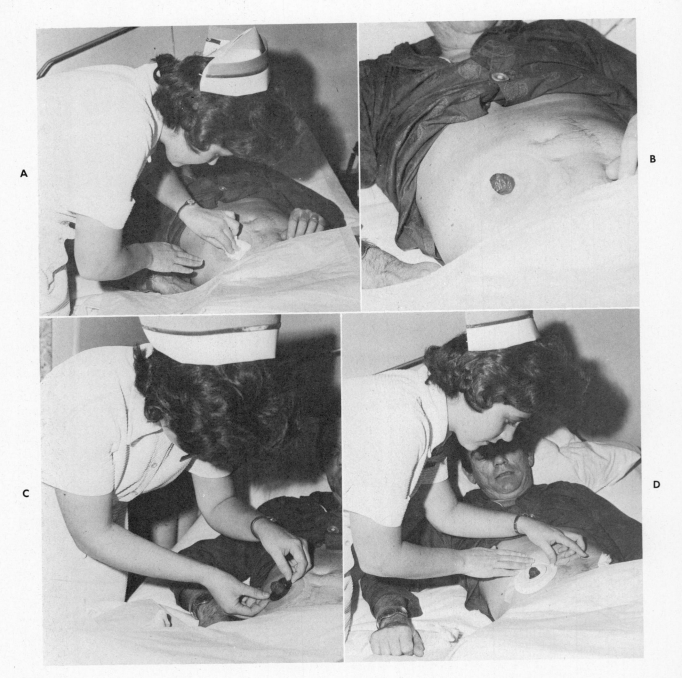

FIG. 18-8
A, Nurse is removing ileostomy pouch to wash skin around stoma with soap and water. **B,** Skin around stoma should be dry before collection pouch is reapplied. **C,** Karaya ring is used to protect the skin. **D,** Face plate is applied and made more secure with adhesive tape. **E,** Collection pouch is stretched over rim of face plate. **F,** Collection pouch applied. Note additional support from elastic waistband. (Courtesy Methodist Hospital of Indiana, Inc., Indianapolis.)

Immediately before surgery the client is prepared in a manner similar to that for clients having intestinal surgery (see discussion later in this chapter). The residue in the diet is decreased, cathartics and enemas are used to empty the colon, and intestinal antibiotics are given to reduce the microbial flora.

Postoperative nursing care. After surgery the nursing care plan should be developed to (1) prevent complications, (2) maintain nutrition, (3) provide for collection of drainage from the ileostomy, and (4) help the client cope with a new mode of elimination.

PREVENTING COMPLICATIONS. Immediately after surgery the client is encouraged to turn, cough, and breathe deeply to prevent cardiopulmonary complications. Young clients tend to move in bed and are out of bed the day after surgery, but older individuals may need encouragement.

A nasogastric tube is used to prevent distension. The physician may order irrigations of 20 to 30 ml of saline every 2 to 4 hours to keep the tube patent. The nurse should assist the client with oral hygiene and apply a water-soluble lubricant around the nares while the nasogastric tube is in place. The nasogastric tube is removed in 3 to 4 days when peristalsis returns.

Peritonitis is a complication that may occur if the digestive juices leak into the peritoneum. The nurse should note an increase in temperature, boardlike abdominal rigidity, and abdominal pain and report them to the physician.

MAINTAINING NUTRITION. Clients with ulcerative colitis are often debilitated, and it is important to encourage a diet that supports growth and healing. Nutrition is maintained by intravenous infusion until peristalsis returns, but when oral intake is permitted, the diet should include high-protein and high-carbohydrate foods. At this time, foods should be added to the diet individually so that the client can determine tolerance to each food. Because the products of digestion are eliminated in 4 to 6 hours, fresh fruits and foods of high fiber content may cause diarrhea or flatus and should be avoided. If foods with high fat content are not absorbed, it may be necessary to give supplemental fat-soluble vitamins.

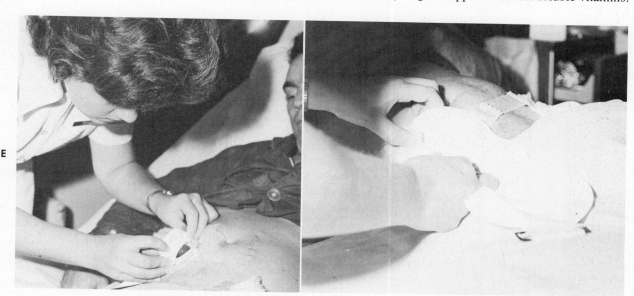

E

F

FIG. 18-8, cont'd
For legend see opposite page.

Fluids are lost through the ileostomy, and the client must consume sufficient fluids to offset this loss. Juices with high potassium content, such as orange juice, are helpful in replacing electrolytes that might be lost through the ileostomy.

COLLECTING ILEOSTOMY DRAINAGE. Depending on the type of ileostomy, provision must be made to collect the fecal drainage. Fecal wastes from the ileostomy contain digestive enzymes that, when in contact with the skin around the stoma, cause excoriation. A temporary ileostomy pouch is applied during surgery. This pouch should be emptied periodically, but it need not be removed unless fecal contents come in contact with the skin. At that time, the pouch may be removed, and the skin around the stoma washed with soap and water (Fig. 18-8, *A* and *B*). A protective coating of powders, gels, or Stomahesive pads or a karaya ring (Fig. 18-8, *C*) may be used to protect the skin before the ileostomy pouch is reapplied. Because the drainage is continuous, a ring of facial tissue paper put around the stoma or a small medicine cup placed over the stoma will collect drainage while the skin is being washed.

When the ileostomy has healed, in 2 to 3 weeks, a permanent drainage appliance is fitted. The physician, nurse, enterostomal therapist, or surgical supply salesperson who is trained in fitting the appliance helps the client select the appropriate equipment. The permanent collection pouches of rubber or plastic are secured to a metal or rubber face plate, which is attached to the skin with a special adhesive (Fig. 18-8, *D*). When the face plate is secured to the skin, the collection pouch is fitted over the stoma and put on the face plate by stretching the lip of the pouch over the rim of the face plate (Fig. 18-8, *E* and *F*). A belt may be used with the collection pouch for additional support.

The face plate should be changed every 3 to 7 days. An adhesive remover is used to loosen the cement that holds the appliance to the skin. At this time the skin is cleansed with soap and water and dried carefully. Karaya powder or a similar product may be used to protect the skin before the face plate is reapplied to the skin.

Deodorant powders or two crushed aspirin tablets can be used in the pouch to minimize odors during use. The pouch should be emptied each time the client goes to the bathroom so that fecal contents do not accumulate and produce an odor.

The client usually buys two collection pouches so that one can be cleaned and drying while the other is in use. Dilute chlorine bleach or soap and water are suitable cleansing agents.

If the client has a *pouch ileostomy,* the reservoir needs to be drained every 4 to 6 hours. Immediately after surgery the pouch is drained with a catheter attached to low-pressure suction. Ileal drainage is initially liquid but will thicken (although it is never formed) when the client begins to eat. Bloody discharge may be noticed for several days after surgery. More than 100 ml in 24 hours, however, should be reported to the physician. The client should be instructed to observe the drainage and report if the catheter becomes plugged, noted by a feeling of fullness in the pouch and absence of fecal drainage. If the catheter does become plugged it can be irrigated with 30 to 40 ml normal saline.

In preparation for removal of the catheter, the catheter is clamped for 3 to 4 hours to allow the pouch to distend. The catheter is usually left unclamped when the client sleeps.

When the catheter is removed, the client learns to insert a lubricated Silastic ileostomy catheter to drain the pouch. Most clients find it easiest to sit on the toilet and drain the catheter into the toilet. If the fecal drainage is thick, the client may irrigate the catheter with 20 to 40 ml water. Periodically the client may irrigate the pouch with water to remove fecal shreds. The pouch should be drained frequently initially, because the pouch only holds 70 to 100 ml. As the pouch capacity increases, the client need only drain the pouch every 4 to 6 hours. The stoma should be washed with soap and water and covered with a gauze square to protect clothing from drainage.

The client should be instructed to report difficulties of drainage or suture line leakage that could cause local or generalized peritonitis. Abdominal pain, fever, tachycardia, tenderness, or decreased bowel sounds should be reported immediately.

COPING WITH A NEW MODE OF ELIMINATION. When the client has worked through initial feelings about his ileostomy, he is ready to become more independent in its care. The nurse gradually instructs the client how to change the drainage pouch and prevent skin breakdown. Often, the individual is feeling better and willingly assumes responsibility for his own care.

The client will need special support from his family and friends as he adjusts to his ileostomy. Children and adolescents should feel comfortable with their family, and the nurse can help the parents understand the client's adjustment to this new mode of elimination. Peer acceptance is important to the adolescent, and he should be encouraged to participate in his usual activities. Married clients may fear the reaction of their spouse; it is helpful if the husband or wife can observe the ileostomy, its functioning, and its care during the hospital stay.

Discharge instructions. When the client goes home, he will be able to participate in all activities except sports that involve body contact. Children and adolescents may need parental guidance in selecting activities, but they need not be restricted in any other area. Clients should know that sexual intercourse and childbearing are possible even though they have an ileostomy.

Many communities have an Ostomy Club, in which persons who have had an ileostomy or colostomy meet regularly to discuss mutual problems. Often the client can obtain helpful suggestions and encouragement from this group.

Evaluation. Evaluation of changes in the client's behavior as a result of nursing actions is an ongoing process for the client with ulcerative colitis. Evaluation of specific objectives occurs at time periods appropriate to individual needs of the client and depends on medical or surgical management of the health problem. Nursing diagnoses often include altered bowel elimination, fluid imbalance, and altered self-concept.

EXPECTED OUTCOMES

The client and/or family can:
1. Describe ulcerative colitis (and surgical intervention if performed).
2. Verbalize acceptance of altered bowel elimination (if an ileostomy is performed).
3. State plans for health maintenance, including physical and emotional rest.
4. State plans for maintaining fluid and nutrition status with high-protein, low-residue diet and increased fluid intake.
5. State use, dosage, time, and route of prescribed medications (steroids, antidiarrheals, anticholinergics, antispasmodics).
6. Manage ostomy care, if necessary.
7. State plans for follow-up care and use of community resources for individuals with an ileostomy.

1003

**COMMON HEALTH
PROBLEMS OF THE ADULT**

Cancer of the colon and rectum

Cancer of the colon and rectum is a common health problem. Cancers of the rectum and large intestine are primarily adenocarcinomas, whereas cancer of the anus is of epidermoid origin. Of the tumors found in the lower gastrointestinal tract, 16% are in the cecum and ascending colon, 8% in the transverse colon, 6% in the descending colon, 20% in the sigmoid colon, and 50% in the rectum.[3]

Pathophysiology. The cause of the cancer is not known. Lesions in the lower gastrointestinal tract, particularly polyps and chronic ulcerative colitis, are known to undergo malignant changes, but they have no direct causal relationship.

Colorectal cancer is the second most common primary site for cancer and the second most frequent cause of cancer mortality in men and the third in women. Middle-aged adults are most affected, men and women in equal numbers.

It is believed that the increased incidence of colorectal cancer may be caused by frequent ingestion of low-residue diets. Such diets contain increased amounts of refined carbohydrates, minimal unabsorbable cellulose, and have longer transit time for fecal wastes. For this reason high-fiber content diets are urged. Other risks may include familial polyposis, ulcerative colitis, and diverticulitis.

Assessment. The nurse has a significant role in assessing clients with colorectal cancer. Participation in screening programs and instruction about warning signs of cancer such as change in bowel habits are two opportunities for facilitating early detection of this cancer.

Early signs of cancer of the rectum or colon are vague and may even be absent. The symptoms depend on the location of the tumor, but are related to the tumor invasion in the intestinal mucosa and extension around the bowel to ultimately cause stricture and *bowel obstruction*. If the tumor is in the rectum, the client may have rectal *pain*, rectal *bleeding*, and *tenesmus*. Tumors in the sigmoid colon have a "napkin ring" growth pattern and may produce bleeding. The client may be constipated and the stool ribbon-shaped. Tumors located in the right colon present gastrointestinal bleeding, anemia, and occasionally a nagging lower abdominal pain. There may be alternating diarrhea and constipation. The tumors can spread directly and attach to the abdominal wall or genitourinary tract, producing further symptoms of obstruction of these organs. Metastasis to liver and other organs can occur via lymphatics.

The tumor can be detected in its early stages by digital rectal exams, stool guaiac tests, and sigmoidoscopic or colonoscopic examination, and for this reason these examinations should be included in health appraisals of middle-aged individuals at risk. The diagnosis is confirmed by x-ray examination with barium enema and by tumor biopsy. The carcinoembryonic antigen (CEA) is found in the serum of some clients with colorectal cancer but, because it can be elevated in other cancers and benign inflammatory diseases, it is not as diagnostic as once believed. The tumor can be staged to plan and evaluate therapy (see staging of cancer, opposite page).

Data analysis
Data analysis may reveal nursing diagnoses of alterations in bowel elimination, alterations in comfort, fear, and disturbances in self-concept. Plans are developed for actual and potential nursing diagnoses.

STAGING OF CANCER OF THE LARGE INTESTINE AND RECTUM

TNM CLASSIFICATION (4)
Primary tumor (T)

TX   Depth of penetration not specified
T0   No clinically demonstrable tumor
TIS Carcinoma in situ
T1   Clinically benign lesion or lesion confined to the mucosa or submucosa
T2   Involvement of muscular wall or serosa, no extension beyond
T3   Involvement of all layers of colon or rectum with extension to immediately adjacent structures or organs or both, with no fistual present
T4   Fistula present along with any of the above degrees of tumor penetration
T5   Tumor has spread by direct extension beyond the immediately adjacent organs or tissues

Nodal involvement (N)

NX   Nodes not assessed or involvement not recorded
N0   Nodes not believed to be involved
N1   Regional nodes involved (distal to inferior mesenteric artery)

Distant metastasis (M)

MX   Not assessed
M0   No (known) distant metastasis
M1   Distant metastasis present
         Specify _____
         Specify sites according to the following notations:
           Pulmonary—PUL   Lymph nodes—LYM
           Osseous—OSS   Hepatic—HEP
           Other—OTH   Skin—SKI
           Brain—BRA   Pleura—PLE

From Rubin, Philip, editor: Clinical oncology for medical students and physicians, a multidisciplinary approach, Rochester, N.Y., 1979, American Cancer Society.

Planning and implementation. The nursing care plan for a client with colorectal cancer is initiated when the client seeks health care services. When the diagnosis is confirmed, the nurse plans with the client and family, depending on the type of intervention and the client's age and stage of development.

The diagnosis of cancer presents a significant emotional impact on the client and family, and the nurse can provide supportive care as the client and family work through acceptance. Support groups such as Families Facing Cancer, sponsored by local units of the American Cancer Society, Inc., are often valuable resources.

Surgery is the primary method of treatment for colorectal cancer, and radiation therapy or chemotherapy may be used palliatively or before surgery to reduce the tumor mass. Colorectal tumors are moderately radiosensitive, and some believe radiotherapy to be as curative as surgery.[3]

Colostomy. Tumors in the large intestine and rectum obstruct fecal elimination, and an outlet for waste products must be created. If the obstruction is acute, a gastrointestinal tube may be inserted to remove accumulating wastes and flatus. Removal of the tumor is necessary, however, to maintain intestinal elimination.

Tumors that are small and confined can be removed, and the remaining bowel anastomosed *(colectomy).* When the tumor is large and invasive, more bowel is resected, and a colostomy is created to provide an outlet for waste products. There are several types of colostomies, and the location and size of the tumor determine the extent of removal of colon, the type of colostomy, and whether the colostomy is temporary or permanent.

Types of colostomies

SINGLE-BARREL COLOSTOMY WITH ABDOMINOPERINEAL RESECTION. Tumors that invade the rectum and colon require more extensive surgery. The sigmoid colon is removed through an abdominal incision, and the rectum is removed through a perineal incision. A permanent, single-barrel colostomy is then formed to provide an outlet for fecal wastes (Fig. 18-9, *A*). Male clients may be rendered impotent if parasympathetic nerves are resected.

Nursing care is directed not only at establishing fecal elimination but also toward healing of the abdominoperineal incisions. During surgery the perineum is sutured, and the area is covered with dressings, which must be changed frequently to prevent accumulation of drainage and odor. A T binder may be used to hold dressings in place so that the dressings can be changed easily. The perineal area may be irrigated with sterile saline to promote healing. Healing is slow, and recovery may take several months.

LOOP COLOSTOMY. When the bowel is inflamed, a segment of the bowel may be brought to the abdomen and sutured for a temporary colostomy (Fig. 18-9, *B*). This loop of bowel is held in place with rubber tubing connected to a glass rod or a plastic bridge. Several days later, when peristalsis returns, the loop of bowel is cauterized to make an opening for fecal wastes, and the glass rod is removed. The client should be instructed that there are no nerve endings in the loop of intestine and the procedure is not painful. The odor of burning flesh and evacuation of feces, however, may be unpleasant. The nurse should be prepared to help the physician collect fecal material and flatus with a dressing or drainage pouch when the loop colostomy is opened.

Fecal material drains from the proximal opening of the loop colostomy. The physician may order routine irrigations to stimulate evacuations of wastes, and the nurse should identify the proper stoma before beginning the irrigation. When the inflammation subsides, the loop is sutured and replaced within the peritoneal cavity.

DOUBLE-BARREL COLOSTOMY. If the tumor is located in the ascending or transverse colon, the tumor is resected, the remaining ends of bowel are sutured through an incision in the abdomen and a stoma for fecal elimination is created (Fig. 18-9, *C*). This approach is known as a double-barrel colostomy, because there are two stomas. The proximal stoma evacuates fecal material, and the distal stoma leads to the rectum.

Drainage from the proximal stoma is normally liquid, because little water is absorbed. This stoma is usually irrigated to stimulate fecal evacuation. Fecal drainage does not occur through the distal stoma, but the physician may order an irrigation to loosen mucus shreds that accumulate in the colon and rectum. The client should sit on the toilet for these irrigations, because the fluid often escapes through the rectum.

CECOSTOMY. An opening into the cecum, cecostomy may be made to provide temporary outlet for fecal waste. This surgery is usually performed if the tumor cannot be resected or if there is total obstruction. The cecostomy may be temporary until the obstruction is relieved.

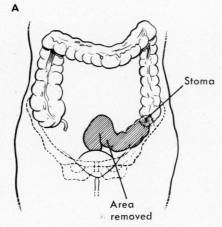

A

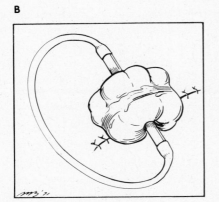

B

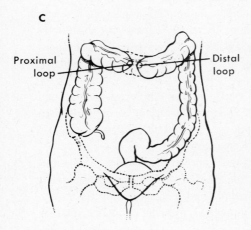

C

FIG. 18-9
Types of colostomies: **A,** single-barrel; **B,** loop; **C,** double-barrel.

1006

Preoperative nursing care. Preparation for intestinal surgery may take as long as 1 week, and the client is usually hospitalized several days beforehand. At this time the nursing care should include plans for (1) helping the client prepare for altered elimination, (2) promoting nutrition, (3) preparing the bowel for surgery, and (4) giving the client preoperative instructions.

PREPARING FOR ALTERED ELIMINATION. Regardless of the age of the client or the reason for relieving intestinal obstruction, there is an adjustment to a new mode of defecation. When the usual process of elimination is changed, the client may experience depression, regression, and changes in body image. Nurses should understand that many feelings are aroused when the client faces a change in his elimination pattern, and they should draw on his preoperative emotional strength to help him cope with surgery.

After explaining the surgery to the client, the physician may suggest that a person who has a colostomy visit the client. Talking with someone who has been through the surgery can be reassuring to the one facing it.

If the client expresses further interest, the nurse can demonstrate how evacuation will be accomplished and how the colostomy will be irrigated to stimulate defecation. If the client is familiar with the equipment and procedure for irrigating the colostomy, his postoperative recovery will be easier. Not all clients initially accept the need for a colostomy, and the nurse should respect the feelings of these persons but gently help them accept the need for surgical intervention.

PROMOTING NUTRITION. Clients who are to have intestinal surgery may be anemic, debilitated, or dehydrated, and nutritional supplements may be used to prepare them to withstand surgery. A diet high in protein and iron may be given along with necessary fluids and electrolytes. Blood transfusions may be given if the client is anemic.

PREPARING THE BOWEL FOR SURGERY. Since the intestinal tract will be entered, it is necessary to remove fecal contents and reduce the number of microorganisms that are normally present in the intestine. Cathartics, a low-residue

---

LOW-RESIDUE DIET

Purpose	1. Reduce the bulk in the diet and reduce the formed stool before intestinal surgery.
	2. Reduce irritation to the bowel when the bowel is inflamed with ulcerative colitis, colitis, or diverticulitis.
Meats and eggs	All meats. Prepare by roasting, broiling, or baking. Pork may be omitted in severely restricted diets. Eggs, except fried. Mild cheeses.
Milk	No milk if severely restricted; boil milk before serving if moderate restriction.
Fruits and vegetables	Cooked or canned fruits and vegetables such as carrots, beets, chopped spinach, green beans; strained fruit juices.
Breads and cereals	Refined breads and cereals, strained oatmeal, mashed, baked, scalloped potatoes, macaroni, noodles, spaghetti.
Foods to avoid	Alcohol, fried foods, spices, raw fruits and vegetables, whole-grain breads and cereals, pastries, nuts, dried fruits, vinegar, salad dressings, jams, marmalades, relishes, chocolate.
Suggestions	Eat slowly, chew food well.

diet (see p. 1007), and intestinal antibiotics are used to prepare the bowel for surgical intervention.

1. *Catharsis.* Cathartics and laxatives may be given as early as 1 week before surgery to stimulate peristalsis and emptying of fecal wastes. Immediately before surgery, normal saline enemas may be given until the returns are clear, to ensure complete emptying of the rectum and sigmoid colon. Because this may involve several enemas, the client may be fatigued and should be permitted to rest when the procedure is completed.

2. *Diet.* A low-residue diet or an elemental diet is used to reduce the amount of fecal wastes in the intestines. The absence of bulk in the diet causes less fecal waste and slows peristalsis. The day before surgery, the client is usually given a clear liquid diet to further reduce the accumulation of fecal wastes and slow intestinal peristalsis.

3. *Intestinal antimicrobials.* Surgery of the bowel is complicated by the number of normally occurring microorganisms in the intestines, and antimicrobials are used to reduce them. Succinylsulfathiazole (Sulfasuxidine), phthalylsulfathiazole (Sulfathalidine), neomycin, kanamycin, or polymyxin are commonly used antibiotics. Since these drugs may be given in doses higher than normal, the nurse should observe the client for side effects of diarrhea, skin rash, and nausea.

PREOPERATIVE INSTRUCTION. In addition to information about the colostomy and irrigation procedures, the client should be instructed about his responsibilities after intestinal surgery. He should be instructed in and practice turning, coughing, and deep breathing. The nurse should also explain the use of heavy abdominal dressings and other equipment that might be used after surgery, such as a nasogastric tube or intravenous infusion apparatus.

Postoperative nursing care. Postoperative nursing care goals include: (1) prevent complications, (2) maintain nutrition, and (3) help the client cope with a new mode of elimination. The care plan is based on the needs of the individual client, his preoperative acceptance of his colostomy, and his readiness to return to his optimum state of wellness.

PREVENTING COMPLICATIONS. The client is encouraged to turn, cough, and breathe deeply every 2 to 4 hours to prevent circulatory and respiratory complications. The client may receive intermittent positive pressure breathing therapy to prevent atelectasis and pneumonia. Elastic hose are used to assist venous return and prevent thrombophlebitis. The client usually ambulates on the second or third postoperative day. Ambulating not only improves circulation but also stimulates peristalsis and bowel evacuation.

MAINTAINING NUTRITION. Intravenous fluids may be given for the first 12 to 24 hours to prevent dehydration and electrolyte imbalance. When peristalsis returns, the client is given a liquid diet as tolerated and then is advanced to a low-residue diet. The nurse should assess the client's reaction to these diet changes, because it is important that the client not become dehydrated when fluid is lost through the colostomy.

COPING WITH AN ALTERED MODE OF ELIMINATION. Because feces are no longer eliminated through the rectum and are evacuated through the colostomy, the client must wear an appliance over the colostomy to collect the fecal material. A temporary collection pouch is applied immediately after surgery to collect any wastes. When peristalsis returns, usually on the second or third postoperative day, fecal wastes and flatus are expelled through the stoma. At this time, the stoma appears red and edematous, but eventually it will shrink and become flush with the skin.

There are several approaches to regulating the elimination of fecal wastes through the colostomy. Some clients will be able to establish regular elimination habits naturally; others may irrigate the colostomy with water on a regular basis to promote evacuation of fecal material. The location and permanence of the colostomy determine irrigation procedures.

Individuals with uncomplicated colostomies located in the descending colon may be able to develop regular elimination habits with diet, fluids, and exercise alone.[5] A collection pouch or gauze square can be used and changed as needed. If the colostomy is temporary, the client usually does not irrigate. Irrigation is not possible for colostomies in the ascending colon, because the stool is liquid and drains continuously. A collection pouch must be worn at all times.

COLOSTOMY IRRIGATIONS. Colostomy irrigations are used to control evacuation of fecal wastes. Warm (105° F or 40.5° C) tap water, normal saline, or other solutions are introduced into the stoma in sufficient quantity to stimulate peristalsis. Since regular irrigations promote bowel control, the client should select a time to begin irrigations that will be suitable for his schedule when he returns home. Initially, the irrigations are done daily, but later the client may find that irrigating the colostomy every other day or every third day may stimulate regular evacuation of fecal wastes, depending on the location of the colostomy, the diet, and the amount of activity.

The irrigation is best accomplished with the client in the position that promotes defecation—sitting on the toilet or commode. If the client is too weak to sit up, the irrigation may be done in bed, with the client positioned comfortably on his side.

One of two methods of irrigating the colostomy may be used. The principles of irrigation are similar in both methods, but the technique and equipment are different.

In the *conventional* irrigation method, an irrigation bag, lubricant, tubing with a clamp, a catheter, and an irrigation sheath with an elastic belt are used.[4] This equipment may be purchased from a pharmacy or surgical supply house, or it may be improvised with household materials such as plastic bags and soft tubing.

To begin the irrigation, the irrigation sheath, which is used to provide a trough for fecal materials and irrigating fluid, is worn over the stoma. The elastic belt is used to maintain a tight seal. The irrigation bag is then filled with 50 to 1000 ml of warm solution (depending on the size of the client), and a catheter (16 to 18 fr for children, 24 to 26 fr for adults) is attached to the irrigation bag. The catheter is lubricated and flushed with the irrigating solution. Before insertion of the catheter, the stoma should be dilated gently with a gloved and lubricated finger. Usually the little finger is used initially until the stoma can be dilated easily with other fingers. The catheter is then inserted 2 to 6 inches (5 to 15 cm) into the stoma. The catheter should not be forced into the colon, because it could perforate the bowel. Some advocate the use of an irrigating cone. This plastic cone-shaped device (Fig. 18-10) can be added to the irrigating catheter and inserted into the stoma, maintaining dilation and making installation of the irrigating solution easier. Backflow of the solution is thereby minimized, and

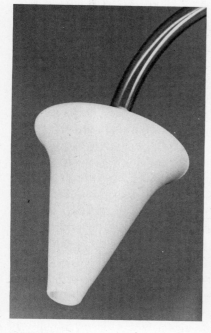

FIG. 18-10
Plastic irrigating cone. (Courtesy Marlen Manufacturing and Development Co., Cleveland, Ohio)

FIG. 18-11
Colostomy irrigations: **A,** conventional technique; **B,** bulb syringe technique.

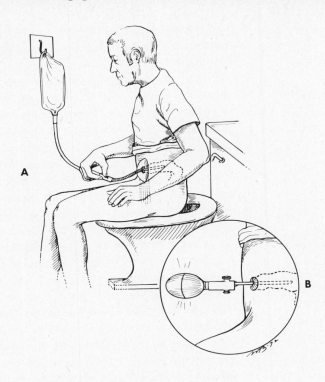

trauma to the bowel is less likely to occur. The irrigation bag should be held 12 to 18 inches (30 to 45 cm) above the stoma to obtain gravity flow of the solution. In the hospital an intravenous stand may be used, but at home the client may place a hook on the wall in the bathroom or use a coat hanger on the shower curtain rod to hold the irrigation bag at the appropriate height.

When all the equipment is assembled and the client is positioned comfortably (Fig. 18-11, *A*), the irrigating solution is slowly introduced into the colon. If the client complains of cramping, the flow is discontinued, and he is permitted to rest. When the cramping ceases, more solution can be permitted to enter the colon until fecal wastes begin to evacuate.

The client should be given enough time to evacuate fecal wastes; as long as 1 hour may be needed during initial irrigations. Gently massaging the abdomen may facilitate the expulsion of the feces. Drinking hot or cold liquids or pouring warm water over the stoma may also aid peristalsis and fecal evacuation. The client should be positioned comfortably while waiting for the results of the irrigation. Some clients may wish to have a bedside stand to rest their head on; others may wish to read while the irrigation is being completed. When all fecal material has been expelled, the client should wash his hands and apply a gauze square or clean collection pouch over the stoma.

In the *bulb syringe method* of irrigation, only an 8-ounce bulb syringe, a pitcher for irrigating solution, and an irrigation sheath and belt are needed to accomplish the procedure (Fig. 18-11, *B*). A special bulb syringe with a flexible nozzle has been made for this purpose, but regular bulb syringes may also be used. Both can be purchased at a pharmacy or surgical supply house.

In this method of irrigation 200 to 500 ml of irrigating solution is drawn into the bulb syringe and introduced through the stoma to stimulate peristalsis.

The solution should be introduced slowly to prevent cramping, and the client may massage his abdomen to facilitate elimination of fecal wastes.

USE OF COLLECTION POUCHES. When the irrigation is completed, a plastic pouch is used to collect fecal drainage that might appear between irrigations. This is particularly necessary when the colostomy is first being regulated and expulsion of fecal material is erratic. Later, especially if the colostomy is in the descending colon, the client may find that fecal elimination is controlled by regular irrigations, and he may need only a gauze square that can be held in place with a girdle, an elastic extension on undershorts, or a specially made elastic waistband.

There are several types of collection pouches, and the client should select one that keeps him dry and prevents fecal drainage from contacting the skin.[4] One type of pouch has an adhesive backing, which sticks to the skin. An opening is cut in the backing to correspond to the size of the stoma, and the pouch should adhere tightly to the stoma. Other collection pouches have a karaya ring to which the collection pouch may be attached. The karaya ring need not be changed with each removal of the collection pouch, and skin irritation is minimized. This type of pouch is useful when the colostomy is new, and the collection pouches must be changed frequently.

Before the collection pouch is applied, the skin and stoma should be cleansed gently with soap and water. The skin around the stoma can be shaved, if necessary, to enhance adhesiveness and prevent infection of hair follicles. If at first the drainage from the colostomy appears to be continuous when the pouch is changed, a collar of facial tissue can be applied around the stoma to prevent drainage from irritating the skin. A wick of tissue can also be inserted in the stoma to absorb drainage and decrease peristalsis while the collection pouch is being applied. Others use a sponge or a stoma drain.

To apply the pouch, the stoma should be measured and the opening in the pouch cut to fit the stoma. A skin preparation should be applied to the skin to strengthen the skin and prevent breakdown, and then the pouch is applied, pressing from the stoma outward to secure the pouch to the skin. The pouch should be applied in the direction of gravity flow to facilitate drainage. Additional security can be obtained by taping the edges of the pouch to the skin with Micropore tape.

The collection pouches should be emptied or changed before they become full and begin to separate from the stoma. If at all possible, the pouch should be emptied, thus saving the client from skin irritation caused by frequent changing of collection bags. Pouches with open bottoms that can be rolled up should be selected for initial use. In the removal of the pouch, adhesive remover should be used to loosen the adhesive, and the bag should be removed in the direction of hair growth. A small pinprick may be made in the top of the pouch to permit escape of flatus, which causes the bag to become distended and to separate from the skin. Most pouches are made to be disposable, but if necessary, they may be cleansed with soap and water, dried, and reused.

SKIN CARE. In spite of attempts to apply the collection pouch securely, there may be times when the fecal drainage may come in contact with the skin. The skin around the stoma is sensitive to the enzymes and fluid in the drainage, and this area should be protected from excoriation. The skin should be washed with soap and water and dried carefully each time the collection pouch is changed.

Nursing process for common health problems

Preparations to protect and strengthen the skin may be used before the skin becomes broken. Stomahesive plates applied to the skin around the stoma are effective barriers and also strengthen the skin.

If the area does become reddened, an antacid such as aluminum hydroxide gel (Amphojel) may be applied to the area and permitted to dry, to provide a protective coating and dry the excoriated area. If the skin is broken and weeping, one way to promote skin healing is to expose the skin to air and heat using a heat lamp for 8 to 10 minutes. The area can then be covered with antacid or dusted with karaya powder. Applying collection pouches securely and changing them before they are full provide the best insurance against skin breakdown.

CONTROL OF ODOR. Odor from the colostomy may be a source of embarrassment to the client. The nurse can use room deodorizers and deodorant sprays to control the odor in the room. A wick deodorant or drops of deodorant on paper near the client's bed are also helpful for the client and those who come near the bedside. Most odor can be controlled by cleanliness, and the collection pouches should be emptied frequently; the client should never be permitted to have a soiled gown or bed linen.

Certain foods may also produce unpleasant odors from the colostomy. Nuts, fish, eggs, onions, and asparagus tend to cause flatulence and odor. Avoiding these foods may minimize some of the odor.

To control the odor in the collection pouch, two crushed aspirin can be placed directly in the bag to absorb odors. If odor continues to be a problem, the physician may order an oral bismuth compound to be taken with meals, to control the odor internally.

CONTROLLING REGULARITY. Regular elimination is promoted not only by irrigating the colostomy but also by diet and exercise. The client is permitted to have a regular diet but should learn how foods and drugs affect his elimination habits. Foods that produce constipation or diarrhea should be eliminated from the diet. Certain drugs may also alter bowel habits, and the client should not use any medication without his physician's approval. The client should be encouraged to drink fluids, because some fluids are lost during irrigation and in drainage from the colostomy.

Because activity stimulates peristalsis, regular exercise should be encouraged. The client may participate in recreational activities and should obtain exercise from walking or bicycling daily.

Some clients may find that irrigating daily is not necessary to achieve regularity and may learn to irrigate the colostomy every second or third day. If the client can go for 24 hours without spilling, he can try to irrigate every other day. If he is not successful, he should return to daily irrigations.

Not all clients are able to achieve control of elimination either naturally or by irrigation. Individuals likely to have difficulty are those who have diarrhea, who have an inflamed bowel, who have had radiation therapy, and persons who are anxious about irrigating the colostomy or who do not do it on a regular basis. Older persons may also have difficulty because peristaltic activity and mucus production are slower, and regularity may not be possible. The nurse should plan with these clients to set more realistic goals for establishing elimination patterns and direct the plans to frequent emptying of collection bag and skin care.

Discharge instructions. Learning to irrigate the colostomy and observe regular bowel habits is an important task for the client. When the client has accepted the altered mode of elimination, he is ready to learn about the care of his colostomy. The nurse should be alert to clues of readiness, such as asking questions about the colostomy, the ability to look at the stoma, or willingness to participate in the irrigation.

The nursing care plan for client instruction should be developed and shared with all personnel so that teaching can be consistent. It is helpful if the same nurse can be with the client on a regular basis as he learns to irrigate the colostomy.

Family members should be included in the instruction, particularly if they will be assisting the client or doing the irrigation for him. Married persons may feel more comfortable if the spouse observes the colostomy in the hospital and is aware of the time and equipment involved in irrigating the colostomy.

Many clients have concerns about resumption of sexual relationships.[6] Concerns may center around personal attractiveness as well as ability to achieve erections. The nurse should be alert to clues indicating these concerns and be able to provide clients with additional understanding about their surgery.

Generally, sexual relationships after surgery resume presurgery patterns. Individuals with stable relationships with a spouse or others are more likely to reestablish these relationships. In instances in which no trauma to perineal nerve supply has been incurred, erection can be achieved. However, in some radical surgeries and in perineal resection in which parasympathetic nerves have been removed, the man may be impotent. The nurse can refer the client to the surgeon for discussion of penile implants for impotence.

If the client has difficulty in adapting the irrigating procedure to his home life-style, a community health nurse may visit to make suggestions for care. The client may wish to join the local Ostomy Club and thus obtain useful ideas from members who have had a similar experience.

Evaluation. The nursing care plan is evaluated continuously as the client prepares for surgery, recovers during the immediate postoperative period, and prepares to manage his own care before discharge from the hospital. The client who has had surgery for cancer of the colon or rectum may have nursing diagnoses associated with alterations in bowel elimination and disturbances in self-concept.

EXPECTED OUTCOMES

The client and/or family can:
1. Describe cancer of the colon or rectum and the surgical intervention.
2. Verbalize acceptance of altered mode of elimination (ostomy).
3. Manage colostomy care, including irrigation if necessary.
4. State plans for health maintenance, including diet, exercise, and rest.
5. Anticipate changes in self-concept and sexuality and utilize appropriate coping resources.
6. State indications for health care, including bleeding, change of elimination habits, pain, and fever.
7. State plans for follow-up care and use of community resources for individuals with cancer of the colon or rectum.

Crohn's disease

Crohn's disease (regional enterocolitis) is a nonspecific inflammatory disease of the small or large intestine. The cause of Crohn's disease is unknown, but the inflammation is characterized by ulcerations of the mucosa and submucosa and thickening of the intestinal wall that ultimately form scar tissue. The ulcerations occur in segments separated by normal mucosa, unlike the diffuse involvement of ulcerative colitis (see discussion earlier in this chapter). The ulcers may perforate and form fistulas with the abdominal wall or hollow organs such as the colon, bladder, or vagina. Scar formation impairs absorption of nutrients, and if there are strictures, there may be intestinal obstruction.

Crohn's disease affects middle-aged individuals. Two peaks of incidence are noted at age 20 to 30 and at 40 to 50.

The client with Crohn's disease has severe abdominal pain and cramping located in the lower right quadrant. Cramping is accompanied by three or four semisoft stools containing mucus, pus, and, if the ulcerations occur high in the small intestine, fat. The disease may have an acute form with mild symptoms or chronic form with a long history of diarrhea. In the chronic form nutritional loss is of concern, and the client experiences weight loss, anemia, fever, and fatigue.

Medical therapy is supportive and includes use of analgesics and anticholinergic drugs for abdominal pain and cramping and intestinal antibiotics such as phthalylsulfathiazole (Sulfathalidine) for local infection. A well-balanced, high-calorie, high-protein diet is used to offset nutritional losses. Fats and high-fiber foods may be eliminated if the client demonstrates intolerance to these.

Nursing care is planned for problems of alterations in nutrition and bowel elimination. The nurse can help the client learn about the therapeutic plan and offer support for compliance.

The course of the disease may include exacerbations. In some instances the diseased intestine may be surgically removed and the proximal portion anastomosed to the colon.

Diverticulosis
Diverticulosis is an outpouching of the mucous lining of the muscular layer of the intestine. The diverticula may be caused by congenital weakness of the bowel or by bowel distension. Recent evidence suggests that diets that are low in fiber content may predispose to diverticula formation. Diverticula also result from the normal slowing of the intestinal tract that occurs in later maturity. Diverticulosis is generally asymptomatic but can be diagnosed by barium enema or colonoscopy.

Diverticulosis is managed to prevent inflammation of the diverticula. Intestinal antibiotics such as neomycin or phthalylsulfathiazole (Sulfathalidine) are often given to prevent infection. The client is encouraged to prevent constipation by drinking fluids, obtaining adequate bulk in the diet, and getting sufficient exercise. Laxatives and enemas are discouraged because they only increase irritation of the bowel.

Diverticulitis
Diverticulitis occurs when the diverticula become infected or obstructed. Fecal material and gas are retained in the diverticula, and pressure causes the mucosa to herniate through the muscularis.

Diverticular disease (diverticulosis, diverticulitis) is common in middle-aged adults. Thirty percent of individuals over 60 may have the disease. The client may experience colicky abdominal pain. There may be fever, leukocytosis, constipation, or diarrhea, and in some instances hemorrhage. Complications may include rupture or perforation with resultant peritonitis.

The acute inflammation is treated by resting the bowel, eliminating oral intake of foods, and antibiotic therapy. Meperidine (Demerol) may be used to relieve the pain by reducing colon spasms. Antispasmodics may be used as well.

If the inflammation is not cleared, it may be necessary to resect the inflamed bowel or create a temporary colostomy until the inflammation subsides.

Hemorrhoids

Hemorrhoids are varicosities or outpouching of the veins of the hemorrhoidal plexus. Hemorrhoids that occur above the anal sphincter are referred to as *internal* hemorrhoids, whereas those outside the sphincter are known as *external* hemorrhoids.

The cause of hemorrhoids is not known, but the varicosities are aggravated by rectal congestion such as occurs with increased abdominal pressure, standing, or sitting. There may be an inherited predisposition for hemorrhoids as well. Hemorrhoids are a common problem, and most adults and older individuals experience the effects of these varicosities to some extent. Since the condition is precipitated by increased abdominal pressure and gravity, those at risk are obese individuals, pregnant women, individuals with intestinal tumors, persons who are constipated, and those who spend long hours sitting or standing.

The symptoms of hemorrhoids differ depending on location. Internal hemorrhoids are generally painless but bleed on defecation. Small but continuous bleeding results in iron-deficiency anemia. External hemorrhoids tend to cause intense rectal itching. Bleeding is rare, and pain may occur on defecation or if a vein ruptures and thromboses.

Hemorrhoids are usually treated conservatively by symptomatic control or by injection of sclerosing agents. Ligation or surgical removal may be attempted if the pain is severe and bleeding is frequent.

Conservative measures are used to minimize painful defecation. The client should avoid becoming constipated by eating a diet with sufficient bulk, drinking fluids, and obtaining exercise. Pain can be lessened by using warm compresses, taking sitz baths, and using topical anesthetics. Care should be taken when giving an enema or suppository to a client who has hemorrhoids, because they are painful and easily irritated.

If the pain becomes severe or if there is frequent bleeding, other supportive measures are needed. The physician may attempt to shrink the hemorrhoids with sclerosing solutions such as 5% phenol oil, which provides temporary, symptomatic relief. The hemorrhoids can also be ligated with a rubber band, which constricts circulation, and eventually the tissue becomes necrotic and sloughs.

Most commonly, however, the hemorrhoids are removed surgically in an operation known as a *hemorrhoidectomy*. The surgery involves excising the hemorrhoids and tying the pedicle with a ligature. Preoperatively the client receives laxatives and stool softeners and instructions about postoperative care.

When the client returns from surgery, the rectal area should be observed for bleeding. The vital signs are taken frequently to detect internal bleeding manifested as shock, and the dressing should be inspected for external bleeding. Bleeding may be apparent again 7 to 10 days after surgery when the sutures slough and should be monitored and reported to the surgeon.

The client should void within 6 to 8 hours after surgery. Voiding may be more difficult for a man, and he should be permitted to stand at the bedside to use the urinal if he cannot void in a prone position. Some physicians prefer that women void on the bedpan in a prone position so that urine does not contaminate the surgical site.

Moist heat may be used to increase circulation and promote healing. The client may take a sitz bath several times a day, or the physician may order warm soaks to be applied to the rectum. Care must be taken to prevent infection in the surgical area; antibiotics may be used as a prophylactic measure, but the area should be dried with cotton after each stool to minimize irritation and the presence of microorganisms.

Pain is not uncommon after rectal surgery, and analgesics and analgesic ointments should be offered as ordered to promote comfort. The client may be more at ease when comfortably positioned on his side or stomach, and he should use a flotation pad when he is sitting in a chair.

Because defecation is so painful, stool softeners are usually ordered to make the first few defecations less painful. A regular diet is usually given the day after surgery to provide bulk in the diet, and the nurse should encourage the drinking of fluids to prevent constipation. The client can be out of bed after surgery, and the exercise of walking stimulates peristalsis. The nurse should observe and record the elimination of the first stool, which usually occurs on the third or fourth postoperative day.

When the client returns home, he should continue a diet with adequate roughage and fluids to prevent constipation. Stool softeners may be used to prevent painful defecation.

Rectal abscess

A rectal abscess is an infection of the fatty tissue surrounding the rectum caused most often by a rectal infection. Rectal abscesses begin as inflammations of rectal crypts and proceed to cyst formation, extending into the submucosa. Microorganisms can also enter an abraded area and cause abscess formation.

Signs and symptoms relate to the inflammation. There may be redness, swelling, and pain. Pain is more severe on defecation and in sitting positions.

The abscess is usually treated by incision and drainage. After surgery, the nurse should observe for urinary retention. Male clients may void more easily standing. Healing by granulation is usual. A wet-to-dry gauze packing may be used to aid healing by removing necrotic tissue and stimulating healing. The packing should be removed gently, soaked loose with hydrogen peroxide, rinsed with saline, and repacked. The client with rectal abscess or other rectal surgery is often most comfortable positioned on his stomach. When the client is sitting, a flotation pad may be used to cushion the chair. Use of rubber rings should be avoided because they cause undue pressure on the area.

Pain should be managed with analgesics. The first defecation is often painful, and analgesia should be provided at this time.

Anal fissure

An anal fissure is an ulceration of the tissue surrounding the anal canal, usually caused by straining to evacuate hard stools. The fissure is a longitudinal ulceration of the rectal canal evidenced by torn skin at the anal canal.

Signs and symptoms are related to the tearing of tissue as formed stool is passed. There is severe pain and burning on defecation. Rectal bleeding may also be observed. Spasms of the sphincter irritate the fissure and contribute to rectal pain. The fissure is removed surgically. During healing stool softeners may be used, and sitz baths are encouraged to promote circulation and aid healing.

COMMON HEALTH PROBLEMS THAT OCCUR ACROSS THE LIFE SPAN

Diarrhea

Diarrhea is characterized by an increased frequency of stools or increased fluid content or quantity of stool passed. Diarrhea usually is a symptom of an enteric infection such as food allergy, ingestion of contaminated foods, and viral or bacterial infections, particularly *Escherichia coli*, *Staphylococcus aureus*, *salmonella*, and *Shigella*. Anxiety, drugs, and foods, however, may also cause diarrhea.

Diarrhea can affect individuals of any age, although infants, young children, and the elderly are more susceptible to infections and the consequences of fluid loss and therefore are at risk. Infants and young children are also susceptible to diarrhea caused by overfeeding or increased carbohydrates in the diet because of their immature gastrointestinal tracts. Cleanliness in food handling and proper formula preparation should be emphasized in health teaching about feeding practices.

Signs and symptoms of diarrhea depend on the severity and onset of the stooling. Accurate records of onset of symptoms, amount of diarrhea, and changes in diarrheal patterns should, therefore, be made. Diarrhea is usually described as mild or severe. *Mild diarrhea* is indicated by change of consistency, frequency (2 to 10 per day), and fluid content of stools. There may be irritability or a low-grade temperature. Vomiting occurs occasionally. Weight loss is about 10% of body weight. *Severe diarrhea* with *gradual onset* is manifested by increasingly frequent, loose, mucous-containing stools, often green or blood-tinged. Weight loss may be as high as 25%. Vomiting, abdominal cramps, and elevated temperature occur. *Severe diarrhea* with *rapid onset* is characterized by temperature elevations of 104° to 106° F (40° to 41.1° C), severe prostration, irritability, and possibly convulsions. The client has frequent explosive stooling. This type of diarrhea is usually caused by a viral or bacterial infection, often from food poisoning.

Secondary symptoms reflect the fluid and electrolyte loss and state of acidosis. Dehydration usually accompanies severe diarrhea and is noted by dry, flushed skin, dry mucous membranes of the lips and mouth, poor skin turgor, sunken eyes, depressed fontanels, rapid, weak pulse, and decreased urine output. Collapse indicated by flaccidity and pallor is an inevitable consequence of uncorrected dehydration.

Metabolic acidosis develops as bicarbonate is lost in the diarrhea and, because of decreased urinary output, acid-producing metabolites are retained. The respiratory rate may increase or decrease, but the depth increases. The carbon dioxide level may be less than 10 volumes per ml. Diagnosis is based on examination of the stool for causative agents and laboratory studies of fluids and electrolyte balance.

Intervention must be instituted immediately in order to reverse fluid and electrolyte losses and prevent dehydration or acidosis. When diarrhea is mild, dietary modification and increase in fluid intake may compensate for losses. In neonates, infants, and young children this may be accomplished by reducing carbohydrate and fat content of formula feedings and offering a 5% glucose in saline solution orally every 3 to 4 hours. Others prefer a half-strength skimmed milk formula or other fluid replacement such as Pedialyte. Fluids with electrolytes may be offered to older infants, children, and adults. Gatorade, boullion, and soft drinks are examples.

In severe diarrhea, the objective of treatment is to replace fluid loss and correct electrolyte imbalances. Initially fluid and electrolyte solutions may be given parenterally, and as vomiting and diarrhea decrease, they may be offered orally. The concentration of the oral fluids is increased gradually.

Absorption of nutrients is improved when the motility of the intestinal tract is slowed. Antispasmodic and antidiarrheal drugs may be used to control colonic spasms and reduce the number of loose stools. The nurse should record the num-

---

ENTERIC PRECAUTIONS

1. Private rooms: necessary for children who are able to move about and possibly share contaminated articles with others; private rooms are optional for adults.
2. Gowns: must be worn by all persons having direct contact with the patient's feces or with potentially contaminated objects such as bedpans, bedside commodes, and soiled linens.
3. Masks: not necessary.
4. Hands: must be washed on entering and leaving the isolation room or cubicle and as indicated during patient care activities.
5. Gloves: must be worn by all persons having direct contact with the patient's feces or with potentially contaminated objects such as bedpans, bedside commodes, and soiled linens.
6. Articles and linens: if contaminated with feces, must either be discarded or double bagged and appropriately labeled before being sent for disinfection or sterilization.

From Isolation techniques for use in hospitals, ed. 2, U.S. Dept. of Health, Education, and Welfare, 1975, Public Health Service.

ber and character of the stools to evaluate the client's reaction to pharmacological therapy.

The client who is admitted to the hospital with diarrhea should be isolated until the cause of the diarrhea is determined (see enteric precautions, p. 1017). Neonates with diarrhea should not be in the same nursery as well newborns, because diarrhea of bacterial origin can spread rapidly. Nurses should take precautions to prevent the spread of microorganisms and must observe scrupulous hand-washing procedures after handling diapers or bedpans and before caring for each client.

When the client has severe diarrhea, the nurse should make every effort to keep the buttocks clean and dry and prevent skin breakdown. The perineum should be washed after each stool, and a protective ointment applied around the anus. Linens should be changed as needed. Turn sheets and protective pads under the client may be used so that the bed need not be completely changed when soiled.

Salmonellosis

Salmonellosis (gastroenteritis or food poisoning) is an infection of the gastrointestinal tract that is caused by ingesting food or water contaminated with the *Salmonella* bacillus. Flooding and other natural disasters are occasions for *Salmonella* infections. Foods that are not properly refrigerated, particularly dairy products or eggs, are also sources of salmonellosis. The microbial infection produces an inflammation of the mucosa of the stomach and small intestine.

Symptoms of the *Salmonella* infection include nausea, vomiting, fever, anorexia, and diarrhea, and occur within 2 to 72 hours of infection. Children and older persons are more affected by this gastrointestinal upset and should be observed for fluid loss and dehydration. The diagnosis is confirmed by isolation of the microorganism in the stool or blood.

Treatment of salmonellosis is symptomatic. Antiemetic and antidiarrheal drugs may be used, and the client is encouraged to take fluids as tolerated. When the appetite returns, the food intake should be sufficient to meet the client's needs.

Typhoid fever, which is caused by *Salmonella typhi,* is a special type of *Salmonella* infection transmitted by contaminated food and water. The client may have symptoms similar to salmonellosis, but the onset may be slower. Some persons, however, may have a subclinical typhoid infection and are carriers of the disease. They are able to transmit the infection if poor hand-washing techniques are used after defecation. Antibiotics such as ampicillin and chloramphenicol (Chloromycetin) may be used to treat typhoid fever. Persons who have been exposed to typhoid fever or who travel in areas where the disease is prevalent can obtain immunization against the disease. Typhoid vaccine is given in two doses 4 weeks apart. The dose for adults is 0.5 ml and for children under ten is 0.25 ml. A booster injection can be given every 3 years.

Dysentery

Dysentery (amebiasis) is an enteric infection caused by the protozoan *Entamoeba histolytica.* The protozoan exists in two stages: the cyst and trophozoite. The cyst (the inactive form) is passed in the stool and is easily transmitted in contaminated food or water. Once the cyst has been ingested, the trophozoite (the active form) enters the intestinal wall and causes ulceration of the mucosa. Secondary amebiasis can result when the parasites migrate to other organs, commonly the liver, spleen, and lungs where abscess may develop. This disease usually occurs in the tropics but may also exist in the United States in areas where sanitation is poor. As many as 10% of the population in the United States may have acute or asymptomatic forms of the disease.

The disease is characterized by remissions and exacerbations. In the acute stage, which occurs in 2 to 4 days after exposure, the client notices pain in the right lower quadrant of the abdomen, has nausea and vomiting, becomes weak, and expels foul-smelling stools, containing pus. Some clients remain asymptomatic but are carriers of the protozoan and can transmit the infection to others if careful hand-washing and food handling procedures are not observed. The diagnosis is confirmed by identifying the cysts or trophozoites in the stools. This disease should be reported to the state board of health so that its cause and location can be determined and eradicated.

The client is usually isolated at home to prevent the spread of the infection. The client should be instructed to dispose of his stools by flushing them in a toilet that has sewer drainage or to disinfect the stools before disposing of them. Of utmost importance in controlling the spread of dysentery is the attention given to washing the hands after defecation and before preparing and eating food.

Amebicidal drugs such as emetine hydrochloride, chloroquine (Aralen) phosphate, diiodohydroxyquin (Diodoquin), and glycobiarsol (Milibis) are used to treat dysentery. Emetine hydrochloride and chloroquine are used primarily for extraintestinal amebiasis, whereas glycobiarsol and diiodohydroxyquin are used for intestinal amebiasis. Diodoquin is given orally 650 mg (adults) or 40 mg/kg (children) three times a day for 20 days. The side effects of this drug (which are rare), include diarrhea, dermatitis, and itching.

While being treated for amebiasis, the client should eat a balanced diet and obtain sufficient fluids to offset loss from diarrhea. Stool specimens may be examined after therapy to ascertain drug effectiveness.

Appendicitis
Appendicitis is an inflammation of the vestigial organ, the appendix. There is no specific cause of appendicitis, although the inflammation can occur spontaneously from an infection or from fecal wastes that have been trapped in the lumen of the appendix. The appendix can also become kinked, obstructing circulation. Abscess formation generally occurs, and the danger of rupture is omnipresent.

Appendicitis occurs most commonly in children, adolescents, and young adults, but individuals of any age may have appendicitis. Men are more frequently affected than women.

Appendicitis is characterized by a sharp abdominal pain that may be localized at McBurney's point (halfway between the umbilicus and right iliac crest). Palpation of the abdomen causes pain in the right lower quadrant. The client has a rigid abdomen and may draw his legs up to relieve the pain. There may be vomiting, diarrhea or constipation, or anorexia. Fever and leukocytosis are usual. If the inflamed appendix is not removed, it can rupture and cause peritonitis or abscess, or the infection can spread through the portal circulation and cause hepatitis. The diagnosis is based on symptoms and laboratory studies that indicate an acute infection.

Surgical removal of the appendix is usually done as an emergency procedure. Attempts are made to remove the inflamed appendix before it ruptures, and preoperative care is directed toward resting the colon. No enemas, heating pads, or laxatives should be used before surgery, because they could stimulate peristalsis and cause a rupture of the appendix. If an enema is ordered before surgery, it should be given very slowly and low in the rectum. A nasogastric tube may be used to prevent ileus and remove fluids from the intestines to prevent rupture.

Nursing care after the removal of the appendix is aimed at preventing spread of infection in the abdominal cavity. The client should be positioned in Fowler's position. If there has been a rupture of the appendix, a drain may remain in place for several days to localize the infection. Antibiotic therapy is used in massive doses until the inflammation subsides. Nursing care is similar to a client with abdominal surgery (see Chapter 17).

Peritonitis

Peritonitis is an acute inflammation of the peritoneal cavity that may be caused by a ruptured appendix, perforated ulcer, pelvic inflammatory disease, or other infections of the digestive or reproductive organs. The client has severe abdominal pain, a rigid abdomen, nausea, vomiting, an elevated temperature, and leukocytosis. Shock may occur as fluids are lost into the peritoneal cavity. Peristalsis slows as a result of the toxins, and there may be a paralytic ileus and a temporary slowing of gastrointestinal motility.

The treatment varies with the cause of the infection and is directed at eliminating the source and providing continuity of digestion and elimination. The client is positioned in Fowler's position to localize the infection, and a decompression tube may be used if there is intestinal obstruction, or ileus. Intravenous fluids are necessary for fluid replacement to combat shock and to provide nutrition to the cells. High doses of antibiotics are given to prevent systemic spread of the infection.

When the infection is localized, the symptoms begin to subside. At this time it is possible to perform surgery if necessary to drain the infection or remove the inflamed organ.

Intestinal obstruction

Intestinal obstruction is a multicausal clinical entity that produces slowed intestinal peristalsis and obstruction of fecal elimination. The ultimate hazard of obstruction is the fluid and electrolyte loss resulting in irreversible shock.

Intestinal obstruction can be caused by tumors, inflammations, mechanical obstructions such as hernias, adhesions, diverticulosis, volvulus, intussusception, neurogenic obstruction such as paralytic ileus, or vascular disease of vessels supplying the intestine. Fifty percent of obstructions are caused by strangulated hernias. Those at risk are individuals who have decreased gastrointestinal motility that might provide the potential for obstruction.

 Assessment. The onset and course of symptoms depend on location of the obstruction, with earlier symptoms occurring in upper intestine obstruction. The initial symptom of obstruction is *pain,* which is caused by stretching of the intestine. Obstruction higher in the intestine causes more severe pain.

Nausea and *vomiting* occur in the face of reverse peristalsis. The vomiting may be abrupt in onset, particularly if the obstruction is located in the small intestine. Emesis may contain fecal contents. Vomiting results in loss of water, hydrogen, and chloride, causing metabolic alkalosis, but as vomiting of alkaline fecal material occurs, the client experiences metabolic acidosis.

Obstructions caused by twisting of the intestines cause local ischemia. Ischemia lasting more than 2 hours causes irreversible damage because bowel permeability is increased, proteins are lost into the gut, and septic shock follows.

Obstruction results in *increased peristalsis* above the obstruction. Bowel sounds are markedly increased and can be heard on auscultation. Increased movement injures the intestinal wall, causing edema and resultant distension.

Distension above the obstruction causes large amounts of gas to collect. The gas contains nitrogen from swallowed air and is absorbed from the intestine. Pressure from collection of gas and fluid may obstruct circulation, allowing leakage of bacteria and toxins, and ultimately causing gangrene.

Dehydration is a further outcome of physiological changes produced by the obstruction. This is caused by fever, fluid shifts, and vomiting and contributes to hypovolemic shock.

☞ **Planning and implementation.** The aim of therapeutic management is to relieve the obstruction and establish gastrointestinal tract continuity. This is accomplished by intestinal decompression, restoration of fluid and electrolyte balance, treatment or prevention of shock, and surgery to remove the obstruction.

Gastrointestinal decompression. A gastrointestinal tube may be inserted to remove fluids and fecal material. The nurse should record the color, odor, and amount of fluid removed from gastrointestinal decompression and provide comfort measures for the client, including frequent mouth care.

The tube is removed when intestinal continuity is established and bowel sounds are heard. The tube is removed gradually (2 to 3 cm at a time) to avoid trauma and inducing vomiting from reverse peristalsis. The nurse should assist the client with mouth care and offer gargles or lozenges if the throat is irritated.

Fluids and electrolytes. Fluids and electrolytes are used to correct deficits and treat or prevent hypovolemic shock. Intravenous infusions are used, and the nurse should record intake and output, observe the client for clinical signs of fluid or electrolyte problems (see Chapter 16), and monitor vital signs that indicate impending shock.

Surgical approaches. Depending on the cause of the obstruction, surgery may be required to relieve or remove the obstruction. A cecostomy or temporary colostomy may be created to provide immediate opening for fecal wastes. Intestinal surgery may also include removing a portion of the bowel, repairing a hernia, or correcting a volvulus or intussusception. Nursing care is similar to a client having intestinal surgery.

Specific obstructions

Intussusception. Intussusception is the invagination or telescoping of a portion of the bowel, in which the upper intestine slides into the lower portion of the intestine (Fig. 18-12). This rare interference with elimination is one of the most common causes of intestinal obstruction in infants. The client has sudden cramping pain and abdominal distension and may vomit fecal material if the obstruction persists. The temperature may go as high as 106° F (41.1° C), and the stools may contain blood (currant-jelly stool). If the intussusception is not repaired, gangrene may result from the absence of circulation to the intestine; it is considered a life-threatening situation.

The invagination may correct itself spontaneously or be corrected by hydrostatic reduction with a barium enema. Most often, however, the condition is treated surgically by manually reducing the invagination or more frequently by resecting the involved segment of the intestine. After surgery, nutrition is provided by intravenous infusion until glucose-water and full-formula diets are tolerated. The presence of bowel sounds and the passing of the stool are noted as indications of the free movement of the gastrointestinal tract.

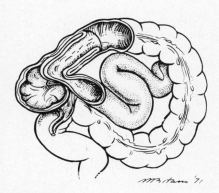

FIG. 18-12
Intussusception.

Nursing process for common health problems

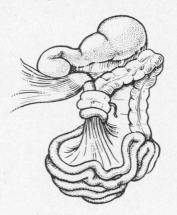

FIG. 18-13
Volvulus.

Volvulus. Volvulus is a twisting of a segment of the bowel (Fig. 18-13). It occurs spontaneously, perhaps the result of inadequate mesentery support. Volvulus occurs most frequently in children and older persons and produces a bowel obstruction. There is abdominal distension, vomiting, and pain. Surgery is required to untwist the bowel and reestablish gastrointestinal continuity.

Paralytic ileus. Paralytic ileus is an intestinal obstruction that occurs when peristalsis decreases because of toxins or trauma to the nerve endings in the intestines or in states of hypokalemia. Paralytic ileus is not uncommon after surgery as a result of the manipulation of the bowel and irritation of the nerves. There is no propulsive force to facilitate the elimination of flatus and feces, and the client experiences abdominal distension and severe pain. The nurse can, therefore, auscultate for bowel sounds in clients who have had surgery to detect potential or actual paralytic ileus.

The obstruction is relieved by gastrointestinal decompression and the use of a rectal tube to provide an outlet for flatus until the toxins or trauma has been eliminated and normal peristalsis returns. If the bowel is gangrenous, surgical removal is necessary.

Mesenteric vascular occlusion. The arteries or veins of the mesentery may become occluded by atherosclerosis, thrombosis, sickle cell disease, and pancreatic diseases. Older individuals and those with recent abdominal surgery are more likely to have occlusive disease.

When the circulation is occluded, the blood supply to the intestine is disrupted and the intestinal mucosa becomes edematous and ultimately gangrenous. The occlusion may be slow in onset or sudden, causing severe abdominal pain. There is abdominal distension, and bowel sounds are absent.

The occlusion is treated by surgical removal of the clot (endarterectomy), or if necessary, removal of the infarcted bowel. Anticoagulant drugs are used to prevent extension of thromboembolic disease.

Evaluation

Evaluation of nursing care for clients with common health problems of the lower gastrointestinal system is an ongoing component of the nursing process. The nurse and client make judgments about changes in the client's behavior as a result of nursing action. The primary nursing problem or diagnosis is often altered bowel elimination; others include alterations in comfort: pain, ineffective coping, fluid volume deficit, alterations in nutrition, and disturbances in self-concept.

EXPECTED OUTCOMES

The client and/or family can:
1. State plans for promoting health of the lower gastrointestinal system including exercise, fluids, and diet.
2. Describe patterns of growth and development as they relate to bowel elimination across the life span.
3. Describe plans for health maintenance and restoration, including use of laxatives, cathartics, enemas, and altered routes of elimination (intestinal decompression, ileostomy, cecostomy, colostomy).
4. Describe plans for health restoration, including surgical intervention, ostomy care, special diets, or prescribed medications.

5. Maintain nutrition and hydration with use of appropriate intake of foods and fluids.
6. State indications for health care and plans for follow-up care and use of community resources.

As plans are evaluated, the nurse and client can determine if problems are resolved or require modification or continuation. The nurse-client relationship is therefore altered appropriately so that the client attains expected outcomes for his own optimal level of health.

Summary

The nursing process is a systematic method for collecting and analyzing data about the client's health problems of the lower gastrointestinal system. The process directs the nurse and client to formulate plans, which are implemented and evaluated. Goals of nursing care are to assist the client with health promotion, maintenance, or restoration.

During the assessment stage the nurse collects data about the client's patterns of bowel elimination across the life span and relates these to information obtained from developmental, social, and psychological histories, and physical assessment. Data analysis may discover nursing problems of altered patterns of bowel elimination, pain, or altered self-concept.

During the planning stage the nurse and client establish goals for health promotion, maintenance, or restoration. Goals may include promoting or maintaining elimination or adjusting to altered routes of elimination.

Health problems of the lower gastrointestinal system occur across the life span. Health problems of the neonate and infant may include congenital defects such as imperforate anus, congenital megacolon, or meconium ileus. Ulcerative colitis occurs during young adulthood, whereas cancer of the colon is a significant health problem of adults. Diarrhea and intestinal infections occur across the life span, but are particularly hazardous in the infant or older adult. Plans are implemented for each problem as appropriate for the client's age and stage of development.

Evaluation is an ongoing component of the nursing process and helps the nurse and client estimate changes in the client's behavior as a result of nursing actions. Criteria established during planning are used to measure client expected outcomes, which are ultimately planned to enable the client to attain his maximum level of wellness.

References

1. Amar, Rose Ann: Treating the patient, not the constipation, Am. J. Nurs. **80**(9):1634-1635, 1980.
2. Guidelines for the Cancer Related Checkup, Recommendations and Rationale, CA **30**(4): 194-240, 1980.
3. Rubin, Philip, editor: Clinical oncology for medical students and physicians, a multidisciplinary approach, Rochester, N.Y., 1979, American Cancer Society.
4. Vukovich, Virginia, and Grubb, Reba: Care of the ostomy patient, ed. 2, St. Louis, 1973, The C.V. Mosby Co.
5. Walt, Rosemary: Colostomy irrigation yes or no? Am. J. Nurs. **77**(3):442-444, 1977.
6. Woods, Nancy: Human sexuality in health and illness, ed. 2, St. Louis, 1979, The C.V. Mosby Co.

Additional readings

Bass, Linda: More fiber—less constipation, Am. J. Nurs. **77**(2):254-255, 1977.

Broadwell, Debra C., and Jackson, Bettie S.: Principles of ostomy care, St. Louis, 1982, The C.V. Mosby Co.

Copeland, Lucia: Chronic diarrhea in infancy, Am. J. Nurs. **77**(3):461-463, 1977.

Cullen, Phyllis Palka: Patients with colorectal cancer: how to assess and meet their needs, Nurs. 76 **6**(9):42-47, 1976.

Dericks, Virginia, and Donovan, Constance: The ostomy patient really needs you, Nurs. 76 **6**(9): 30-33, 1976.

Given, Barbara, and Simmons, Sandra: Gastroentenology in clinical nursing, ed. 3, St. Louis, 1979, The C.V. Mosby Co.

Habeeb, Marjorie, and Kallstrom, Nina: Bowel program for institutionalized adults, Am. J. Nurs. **76**(4):606-608, 1976.

Hogstel, Mildred: How to give a safe and successful cleansing enema, Am. J. Nurs. **77**(5):816-817, 1977.

Hyman, Eleanor, and others: The pouch ileostomy, Nurs. 77 **7**(9):44-47, 1977.

Lamanske, Jacqueline: Helping the ileostomy patient to help himself, Nurs. 77 **7**(1):34-39, 1977.

Literte, Jean: Nursing care of patients with intestinal obstruction, Am. J. Nurs. **77**(6):1003-1006, 1977.

Schauder, Marilyn: Ostomy care: cone irrigations, Am. J. Nurs. **74**(8):1424-1427, 1974.

Stahlgren, Leroy, and Morris, Nicholas: Intestinal obstruction, Am. J. Nurs. **77**(6):999-1002, 1977.

Wentworth, Arlene, and Cox, Barbara: Nursing the patient with a continent ileostomy, Am. J. Nurs. **76**(9):1424-1428, 1976.

19 Urinary system

Assessment

Data analysis

Planning

Implementation

Evaluation

The urinary tract has significant functions of removing metabolic waste products and regulating fluid and electrolyte balance. Health problems that occur across the life span, however, may interfere with normal urinary elimination. Congenital defects such as renal agenesis, polycystic kidney, or exstrophy of the bladder are examples of health problems of the neonate and infant. Poststreptococcal acute glomerulonephritis and nephrosis are typical health problems of children. The urinary tract is affected by the aging process and tumors. Strictures and renal calculi occur in adults, whereas stress incontinence may be evident in older adults. Urinary tract infections, neurogenic disorders, and renal failure are likely to occur across the life span.

Overview of the urinary system

The urinary system is composed of the kidneys, ureters, bladder, and urethra. The two kidneys filter the circulating blood and retain or discard water and chemical substances as needed to maintain fluid and electrolyte balance. The ureters transport these substances in the form of urine to the bladder, which serves as a reservoir. The urethra is the channel by which urine is eliminated from the body.

There are approximatley 1 million nephrons in each kidney. These microscopic structural units are composed of (1) a *glomerulus* (network of capillaries encased in Bowman's capsule) whose function is to filter the blood, and (2) *tubules* where the filtrate is processed further. Some water and solutes are resorbed. The remainder is converted to urine and sent to the kidney pelvis.

The nephron clears the blood of excess sodium, potassium, chlorides, and the end products of metabolism, especially urea, creatinine, and urates. The normal glomerular filtration rate is 110 to 125 ml/min in adults. The rate in infants is one fourth to one half that of adults. All but about 1% of this quantity is resorbed by the tubules.

The renal blood flow is fairly constant despite changes in arterial blood pressure. Hypotension as low as 70 mm Hg or hypertension as high as 200 mm Hg does little to alter the rate of the flow because of a poorly understood phenomenon termed *autoregulation*. The eventual rate of urinary output is not similarly controlled, however, and tends to rise significantly as arterial pressure increases. Such increase is a result of the complex *overflow* mechanism in which substances the tubules cannot resorb quickly enough spill into the kidney pelvis as urine. Even though there may be only slight changes in the glomerular filtration rate, significant changes in urinary output may occur. Ordinarily the kidneys are highly sensitive to wide variations in diet and fluid intake and compensate by altering the consistency and volume of urinary output.

The efficient functioning of the genitourinary system depends on cardiovascular (see Chapter 20) and endocrine (see Chapter 9) mechanisms that regulate blood flow through the kidneys and determine which substances are to be resorbed and which are to be eliminated. For the renal mechanisms to perform well, there must be adequate intake, a blood pressure level that will ensure glomerular filtration, and unobstructed collecting and elimination organs that are neurologically competent.

Assessment
NURSING HISTORY
Health history

When genitourinary functions are assessed, a thorough history and physical examination are essential because many urinary tract problems can be traced to dysfunctions of other systems. Included in this should be a review of the client's daily habits regarding elimination and hygiene, and an accurate account of diet and medications consumed. For women, it is especially important to obtain a menstrual, pregnancy, and pelvic history. All individuals should also be provided an opportunity to discuss any experience with venereal disease, streptococcal infections, diabetes, and other conditions that can be precursors to genitourinary problems.

Developmental history

Neonate and infant. The fetus begins producing urine in the third month of intrauterine life, and at birth there is normally some urine in the bladder. However, voiding may not occur until the second day following birth. The neonate may void as few as 5 or as frequently as 40 times a day, depending on liquid intake, body temperature, and nervous system activity. The infant is capable of diluting urine but has limited ability to concentrate it until the second month of life. At this point the average infant will void about 400 ml/day. This output increases gradually until 1000 ml/day is likely to be eliminated by the time the child is 8 years old. By adolescence the daily output reaches 1500 ml and remains at about this level throughout adult life.

The urine of the neonate and infant is typically dilute and without characteristic odor. Occasionally the diaper may appear pinkish after voiding. This color is usually the result of normal urates in the urine and is not to be confused with blood. The older child's urine as well as the adult's is more highly colored and aromatic.

Adult. Adults void voluntarily four to six times a day, largely depending on their fluid intake. This pattern is fairly typical until after 60 years of age when the effects of aging create new considerations.

Older adult. The renal capacity diminishes with age because of an actual loss of functioning nephrons. The cardiovascular system is also less efficient. As changes in the central nervous system accompany the aging process, the visceral reflex that helps control elimination may become impaired. If the cerebral cortex has been affected, the control of voiding is likely to be maintained merely by the visceral reflex. When voluntary control declines and the bladder is controlled primarily by reflexes, it loses its tone and becomes smaller. Thus it is more active, and the client experiences both frequency and urgency. With the loss of bladder tone, there is a shortening of the warning period. Spontaneous contractions occur early in the filling stage. Retention is not uncommon and is one of the most typical causes of restlessness among elderly clients. It is often aggravated by fecal impaction and prostatic hypertrophy, which produces a mechanical obstruction to voiding.

Social history

Many important clues to urinary tract problems, especially in infancy and early childhood, can be found while eliciting a developmental history of the infant or child. Toilet-training patterns are especially important in early childhood urinary phenomena. Since continence is considered crucial by our society, social and psychological implications are closely tied to toilet training. The nurse should be alert to interaction patterns of the family during this crucial period. Undue stresses on the child from toilet training should be noted. How soon did the toilet training begin? What problems were encountered? Has continence been achieved? (If not, how does the historian feel about this?) Has punishment been tied to ''accidents''? Answers to these and other questions will help the nurse determine nonphysically based problems of urinary dysfunction.

Because urination is considered a personal part of life, some individuals may be reluctant to openly discuss problems or permit examinations of the genitalia. Dysfunctions may lead to perineal discomfort, odor, or incontinence, all of which are uncomfortable entities. Sexual intimacy may be even adversely affected because of urinary tract problems.

The nurse can facilitate open and frank discussions by displaying sensitivity to the client and providing reassurance during the data-gathering process.

Psychological history

The client's mode of handling any major life problem largely depends on his educational level, financial status, ethnic background, and perhaps religious preference. A knowledge of the characteristic coping style of an individual is useful in planning care. It is also valuable to understand relationships and interaction modes within the client's primary environment, because the ability to accept and adjust to health-related problems is largely influenced by such factors. This is particularly true if there are potential life-style or occupational limitations, long-term hospitalization, or life-threatening entities. Clients and their significant others who must face decisions about surgery, transplants, intrafamily organ donation, urinary diversion, dialysis, or other major problems require

Physical assessment

careful psychological assessments by the nurse and other resources on the health team.

The genitourinary examination should include an assessment of genitalia and the rectum as well as the structures of the urinary system. This, of course, requires that the client must be completely undressed and draped in a comfortable recumbent position to facilitate *inspection, palpation,* and *percussion* of structures. It is usually desirable to have the client void before this examination, because it tends to enhance comfort during procedures. Exceptions may be when it is necessary to inspect the genitalia for discharge (which might be washed away by urine) or when there is need to check for stress incontinence.

The nurse should be prepared to help the client assume varied positions for the examination, including lateral Sims, lithotomy, and knee-chest. Provision should be made for warmth and privacy by adequate draping.

All urological assessments must include a rectal examination to evaluate bladder placement, contour, and tissue consistency of related or adjacent structures. A rectal examination of a man permits a thorough assessment of the prostate as well as the bladder.

It is important that the external genitalia be thoroughly inspected for lesions, discharges, or other abnormalities. The bladder is also palpated and percussed to detect structural abnormalities. The lower kidney border is at the level of L3; the upper border at T12. Ordinarily the left kidney is located slightly superior to the right one. Assessing for kidney pain and tenderness requires that the clinician gently strike the costovertebral angle (angle made by rib 12 and the spinal column).

The presence of anatomical or physiological phenomena that interfere with normal urinary tract function should be noted. Deviations in the amount or character of urine or unusual voiding patterns are important factors to consider in client care.

Observation of the client's voiding, especially of a neonate, may assist in the discovery of mechanical obstructions or neurological impairment, which affect urination efficiency or predispose to infection.

Oliguria is the secretion of urine in scanty amounts. *Anuria* is absence of urinary secretion. *Retention* denotes that the bladder is unable to expel its reservoir of urine. *Pyuria* means that there is pus in the urine. *Dysuria* is local pain that accompanies urination (or micturition). *Polyuria* is the secretion of a large quantity of urine. *Pollakiuria,* or *frequency,* is excessive urination. *Enuresis* usually describes bedwetting but may denote any involuntary discharge of urine. *Hematuria* refers to blood in the urine. Several other prefixes (such as galactose, albumin, acetone, lipid, and hemoglobin) may precede "uria" to denote the presence of these substances in the urine in unusually large quantities.

DIAGNOSTIC ASSESSMENT

A series of laboratory examinations may be performed to assess the functioning status of the urinary tract. They include urine examination (especially urinalysis), instrumentation, and radiological studies.

Examination of urine (urinalysis)

Urinalysis is a valuable tool to assist in the assessment of renal function. Normal urine contains metabolic wastes of protein metabolism and excess electrolytes. Substances that are not present in normal urine in significant amounts include glucose, protein, erythrocytes, leukocytes, pus cells, and casts.[3] When

NORMAL URINE VALUES

Specific gravity	1.003-1.030
pH	4.6-8.0 (avg. 6.0)*
Osmolality	38-1,400 mOsm/kg water
Protein	10-150 mg/24 hr
Red blood cells	0-130,000/24 hr (Addis count)
White blood cells	0-650,000/24 hr (Addis count)
Casts	0-2,000/24 hr (Addis count)
Bacteria (clean, voided)	Less than 100 colonies/cc
Potassium	25-100 mEq/24 hr*
Sodium	130-260 mEq/24 hr*
Calcium	Less than 250 mg/24 hr*
Chloride	110-250 mEq/24 hr*
Phosphorus	0.9-1.3 g/24 hr*

*Influenced by intake.

any of these are present in significant amounts, there may be some malfunction in the body. However, some elevations occur because of functional influences. For example, proteinuria may be the result of glomerular disease or merely the result of dehydration, high dietary protein intake, or vigorous exercise. When abnormalities in urinary constituents are found, specific follow-up with detailed renal function tests may be indicated (see normal urine laboratory values opposite).

Types of specimens. *Voided* specimens without special preparation of the urinary meatus are usually satisfactory for routine purposes but have limited value in specific tests because they are highly contaminated with periurethral flora.

Clean catch, or *midstream,* specimens require that the periurethral area be cleansed before voiding and that the urine be caught for the specimen in midstream (after the client has voided a small amount) to ensure a minimum of urethral contaminants. Occasionally the physician may desire a "two-glass test," in which the initial urine is collected in one container and the midstream specimen in another. A "three-glass test" involves a third specimen that contains the final contents of the bladder expelled at the cessation of voiding (Fig. 19-1).

Adaptations for infants and children. Several methods are useful in obtaining specimens from the infant and young child. Infants can be suspended over a collection pan covered by a porous nylon sheet that allows urine to flow through readily but contains any fecal excreta. The sheet can be changed with ease, and it protects the infant from any skin trauma related to attaching other collecting devices. Fig. 19-2 illustrates ways to obtain specimens from young girls or boys by external collection devices. However, when they are used, cleansing remains an important consideration. If specimens are not obtained within an hour, the receptacle should be removed, the skin cleansed once again, and a new apparatus secured. As soon as voiding occurs, the device must be removed. This is especially important when a culture is to be done. Culturing must be done within 30 minutes of the voiding unless the urine is refrigerated, because warm temperatures enhance bacterial growth.

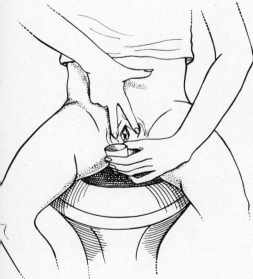

FIG. 19-1
Collecting clean-catch urine specimen. After thorough cleansing of urinary meatus, labia are held apart, and collecting receptacle is held so that it does not touch body. Sample is obtained while client is urinating.

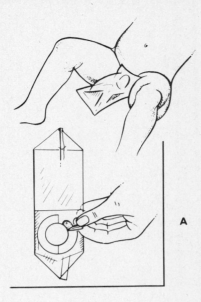
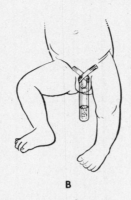
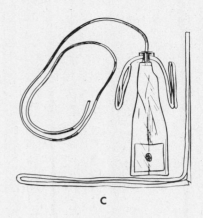

FIG. 19-2
Pediatric urine collection. **A,** Disposable urine collector in place. Note adhesive plate shown in detail. **B,** Test-tube method of collecting specimen from boy. **C,** Apparatus for 24-hour collection.

Some urologists and nephrologists prefer to collect specimens by use of the *percutaneous bladder tap,* which involves introducing a sterile needle into the bladder and aspirating urine for analysis. This procedure is safe and painless when performed by a skillful physician (Fig. 19-3).

A technique that is helpful in stimulation of urination in infants and young children is the *Perez reflex.* After the penis or pudendum is cleansed, the client is held face down over a sterile receptacle, pressure is applied over the suprapubic area, and the paraspinal muscles are stroked firmly (Fig. 19-4). The Perez reflex results in crying, extension of the back, reflexion of the legs and arms, and urination.

Catheterized specimens are usually obtained whenever there is a need to have a sterile urine sample for culture, although clean-catch samples are some-

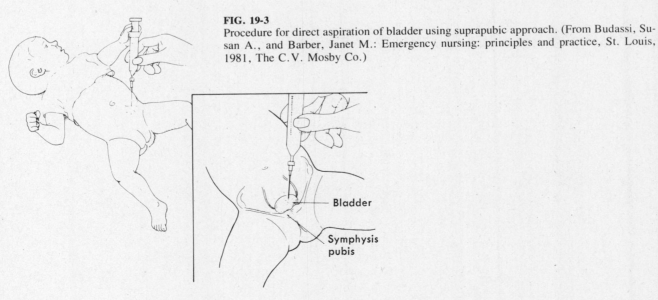

FIG. 19-3
Procedure for direct aspiration of bladder using suprapubic approach. (From Budassi, Susan A., and Barber, Janet M.: Emergency nursing: principles and practice, St. Louis, 1981, The C.V. Mosby Co.)

Bladder

Symphysis
pubis

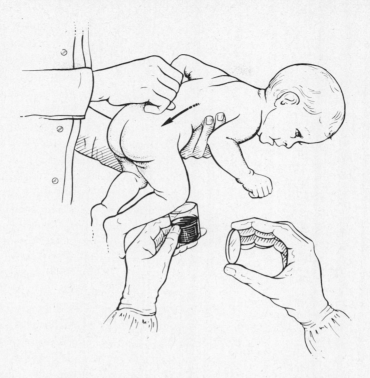

times used to reduce the trauma and infection potential inherent in catheterization.

Other collections
Urine may be collected from catheters already in place by entering the tubing aseptically and withdrawing a sample with a needle and syringe. These specimens are suitable for culture. Urine in drainage bags, however, should not be used. Chemical changes occur soon after the urine is discharged from the body, resulting in fermentation, precipitation, and disintegration. All these processes interfere with analysis. Ideally the specimen should always be examined soon after it is voided. Following are special examinations of urine.

Cultures for sensitivity. Urine is collected and sent to a laboratory where culture media are inoculated so that any organisms in the urine can grow and be identified along with their sensitivity to various drugs that may be selected for treatment.

Residual urine determination. Following voiding, a catheter is introduced into the bladder to detect the quantity of urine that remains after emptying by inherent reflex.

Cytological studies. An initial morning specimen is collected in an alcohol-prepared bottle for cell study and Papanicolaou examination.

Specific gravity and pH determinations. A specimen is assessed for pH and specific gravity by using nitrazine paper and a urinometer, respectively. The normal pH is 4.6 to 8.0, depending on dietary intake; normal specific gravity is 1.003 to 1.030.

Sugar and acetone. Urine can be tested for the presence of sugar and acetone by using special laboratory test tapes and chemicals.

Hematest. Assessing for the presence of blood in the urine is accomplished by using a laboratory test tape or by special papers and other chemical reagents designed for the purpose.

Nurses are frequently responsible for determining pH, specific gravity, and for detecting sugar, acetone, or blood through special test procedures that can be simply accomplished at the client's bedside or in a clinic setting.

Instrumentation: cystoscopy

Cystoscopy is an examination of the bladder by using an instrument (cystoscope) that illuminates and magnifies the interior of the bladder. The procedure is useful for detecting hemorrhage, inflammation, lesions, and mechanical-physical problems. Cystoscopy is also used to facilitate prostate resection and removal of calculi, and to introduce catheters and dye for contrast study of the urinary tract. An anesthetic may be used, especially for male clients.

The client should be instructed regarding the purpose and nature of the procedure. He should be told that he will sense a need to void as the scope is introduced and that his bladder will be distended with fluid during the examination to facilitate visualization. Oral fluids may be forced before the procedure if specimens are to be collected from the ureters or the kidneys, or they may be withheld if a general anesthetic is planned. Intravenous fluids may be used for some clients. Sedatives are usually given about 30 minutes before the examination to promote relaxation.

Cystoscopy is done in a lithotomy position, and the client is draped to expose only the perineum. Considerable care should be taken to avoid circulatory impairment from prolonged popliteal pressure.

It is anticipated that the client will have some discomfort after the procedure, especially when voiding. Urine will probably be pink-tinged for the first few voidings, but bright red bleeding should be reported. If dyes have been used, it is important to explain to the client that unusual coloring of urine is to be expected. Heat applications to the lower abdominal area, mild analgesics, forced fluids, and urinary antiseptics may be prescribed in the postprocedure orders.

Accidental trauma, especially perforation of the bladder or ureters, has occurred during cystoscopy, so the nurse should be cognizant of the potential hazard of peritonitis.

Some clients will have a catheter anchored after the cystoscopy, especially if an operative procedure has been done. Drainage patency should be assessed frequently, and notations made regarding the characteristics of the urine. The nurse should inform clients without catheters that they should use a urinal or bedpan for the first few voidings to permit inspection of the urine for blood or particulate matter.

Radiological assessment

A series of special studies is done as adjuncts to diagnosis of suspected urinary tract disease, particularly structural anomalies or mechanical-physical disturbances. They may also help validate renal function. Although there are a number of highly specialized tests, only the common recurring ones will be considered.

Intravenous pyelogram. The intravenous pyelogram (IVP) allows the radiologist to visualize the size, shape, position, and integrity of the drainage pathways of the urinary tract by tracing a radiopaque dye inserted into a vein. This is perhaps the most frequently performed test other than urinalysis and often involves nonhospitalized clients. Such clients need careful preparation for the examination.

The nurse should assess whether there is a history of allergies, especially to iodine or other radiopaque preparations. The purpose of the test should be explained, and the rationale for the preparation must be understood.

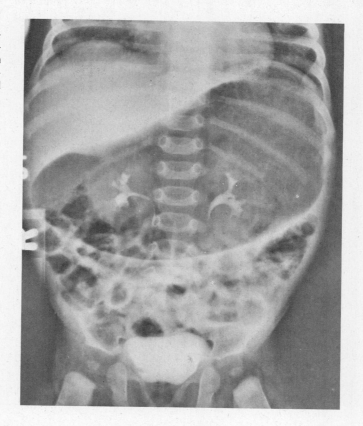

The client is dehydrated by a nothing-by-mouth regimen for approximately 6 to 8 hours because it enhances concentration of the dye, producing a clearer visualization. The colon may or may not be prepared, depending on the preferences of the radiologist. Some believe that the kidneys (which lie retroperitoneally) are likely to be obscured by shadows caused by flatus and fecal contents in the intestine. Infants may be given a formula, and small children a carbonated beverage, to distend the stomach and demonstrate the upper collecting systems to a greater advantage (Fig. 19-5). Newer contrast media do not require significant dehydration of the client. Children or adults with generalized debilitation, those who are suspected of having multiple myeloma, or those with endocrine disease should not be profoundly dehydrated.

Although rigorous bowel preparation is still required by some radiologists, it should be recalled that such a regimen exhausts clients, especially the very young child, the debilitated, or the elderly. Nurses should be cognizant of the inherent need for the individual to get up during the night to go to the bathroom if he has been given a cathartic. Assistance should be offered to prevent accidents such as a weak client's falling en route to and from the commode or incidents of incontinence in bed, which cause considerable embarrassment for him. The administration of hypnotics is of questionable value when uninterrupted sleep is probably not realistic.

A kidneys-ureter-bladder (KUB) film of the abdomen usually precedes the IVP and gives indication of the size, configuration, and position of kidneys and surrounding tissue. The dye is then injected intravenously. Clients should be

1033

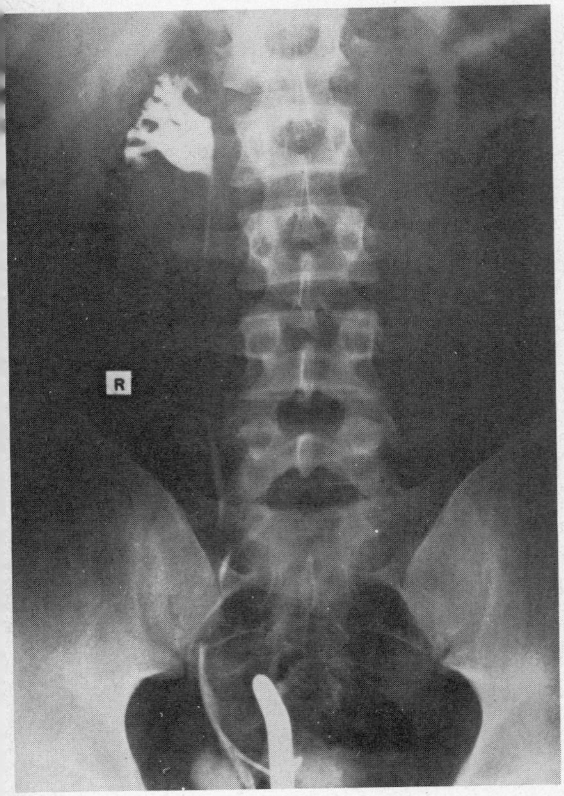

informed that they may have a salty taste in their mouth and feel flushed as the substance is introduced. The radiologist should closely observe for signs of anaphylaxis related to allergy to the dye. Emergency resuscitation equipment should be at hand. After a few minutes, films are taken to denote renal function at intervals such as 2, 5, 10, and 15 minutes after the injection of the dye. Occasionally, if an obstruction exists, an x-ray film is taken 1 or 2 hours later.

Retrograde pyelography. Retrograde pyelography is the method of choice for visualizing the upper urinary tract in many cases because (1) it enables isolated urine specimens to be obtained from the kidney and (2) renal function of the right and left kidneys can be differentiated and compared by the use of ureteral catheters and phenolsulfonphthalein.

A cystoscopy is accomplished, and ureteral catheters are threaded into the renal pelvis to obtain urine samples. Films are taken to follow the course of the ureters and to observe for obstructions or other mechanical problems. Renal function may be evaluated by introduction of a dye into the circulation and observing for its appearance in the urine flowing from each ureteral catheter. Approximately 4 to 6 minutes is the normal time for dyed urine to appear.

A dye or air can also be introduced via the cystoscope to promote visualization of the renal pelvis configuration. Later, as the ureteral catheters and the cystoscope are removed, dye is instilled to outline the ureter (Fig. 19-6).

Other tests. *Voiding cinecystourethrography* is used to demonstrate lower urinary tract abnormalities such as reflux or bladder neck obstruction. Dye is introduced into the bladder, and the structures are observed before, during, and after voiding by way of a television monitor.

Other radiological diagnostic tests used to detect disease of the urinary tract include tomographs (x-ray films that delineate tissue by levels) to study a section of kidney in detail, renal angiography, lymph angiography, retroperitoneal pneumography, cystography, urethrography, and radioisotope renograms (Fig. 19-7). The last-named test is helpful in examining renal vascularity and general ability

FIG. 19-6
Retrograde pyelography. After ureteral catheter is passed by means of cystoscopy, contrast material is injected to make right retrograde pyeloureterogram. (From Winter, Chester C., and Morel, Alice: Nursing care of patients with urologic diseases, ed. 4, St. Louis, 1977, The C.V. Mosby Co.)

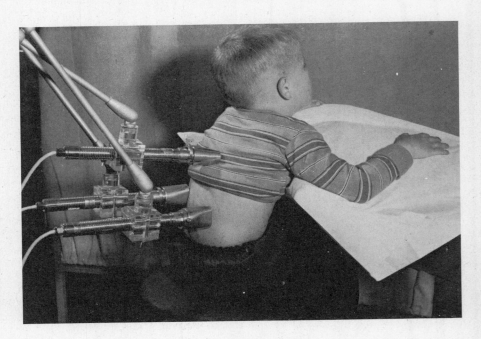

FIG. 19-7
Pediatric client having renogram made. Note probe over each kidney and additional probe over chest used to monitor blood disappearance rate of isotope-labeled test agent. (From Winter, Chester C., and Morel, Alice: Nursing care of patients with urologic diseases, ed. 4, St. Louis, 1977, The C.V. Mosby Co.)

1034

of the kidney to produce urine. It is especially useful after renal transplants to evaluate the kidney functioning and to detect early signs of homograph rejection. Isotope scanning is also used to identify nonviable kidney areas caused by tumors, infarctions, or other lesions.

Renal function tests

There are several tests designed to evaluate filtration, secretion, and resorption. Usually a battery of several tests are essential to fully assess renal function (Table 19-1).

Three common tests should be well understood by the nurse.

1. *Specific gravity of urine* indicates the percentage of solids in urine and thus the concentration capacity of the kidneys. Normal specific gravity is 1.003 to 1.030.
2. *BUN and NPN values* (blood urea nitrogen and nonprotein nitrogen) measure the efficiency of renal function to remove metabolic by-products from the blood. Normal BUN is 8 to 18 mg/100 ml, normal NPN for serum or plasma is 20 to 35 mg/100 ml, and normal NPN for whole blood is 25 to 50 mg/100 ml.
3. *Serum creatinine test* indicates glomerular functional capacity to eliminate the substances from the blood. Normal serum creatinine clearance is 0.2 to 0.6 mg/100 ml for men and 0.6 to 1.0 mg/100 ml for women.

The assessment of the urinary tract by special laboratory examinations is important when there are abdominal pains or palpable masses, fever of unknown origin, or other symptoms of urinary tract disease. Children who fail to thrive or who have repeated enuresis episodes (bedwetting beyond age 5) deserve study.

Filtration tests

The most common measurements of filtration are the urea and creatinine clearance tests. Inulin clearance may also be done. Following is the clearance formula:

$$\text{Plasma clearance (ml/min)} = \frac{\text{Urine quantity (ml/min)} \times \text{Concentration in urine}}{\text{Concentration in plasma}}$$

Urea clearance. Urea is freely filtered at the glomerulus, but approximately 40% is resorbed in the tubules by passive diffusion as water is resorbed.[3] Urea is

TABLE 19-1
Renal function tests

Test	Purpose	Nursing responsibilities
Phenolsulfonphthalein	Evaluate renal tubular excretory capacity by comparative appearance of dye in urine at timed intervals	Provide test instructions; administer 2 glasses of water before intravenous dye is injected; help client void as scheduled for 2 hours; collect and label specimens.
Urea and creatinine clearance	Measure functional efficiency of plasma filtration by the glomeruli.	Provide test instructions; administer fluid and collect specimens as indicated—both urine and blood samples for *urea clearance* test (which takes approximately 3 hours); a 24-hour urine collection and a fasting blood sample for glucose determination after the test for *creatinine clearance*.
Concentration (Fishberg)	Assess ability of kidney to concentrate urine; incorporates morning specimen collection because kidneys concentrate urine more efficiently during sleeping hours.	Provide test instructions, explaining fasting period after evening meal until midmorning the following day; urine specimens collected at hourly intervals in morning.
Dilution	Assess ability of kidney to dilute urine.	Provide test instructions: bladder is emptied and approximately 1200 ml of oral fluid is administered over 30-minute period (depending on age); specimens collected at timed intervals for 3 hours; all urine sent to laboratory.

a valid index of the glomerular filtration rate (GFR) if the urine flow rate is approximately 2 ml/min. Urea clearance is usually performed in the morning following a light breakfast in which coffee, tea, and protein foods are omitted. Water and fruit juices are given in large amounts (1000 ml in the hour before the test and 240 ml every half hour during the test).[3] At the initiation of the test the client voids and discards the specimen, but notes the exact time. One hour later the first voided specimen is saved; at the end of the next hour a second specimen is saved. At the midpoint of the examination, blood is obtained for blood urea nitrogen level.

The normal urea clearance is 75 ml/min. It is decreased in disease, which affects the GFR, and in prerenal diseases, which decrease the plasma flow rate.[3]

Creatinine clearance. Creatinine clearance is used as an index of GFR. Creatinine is an endogenous waste product, neither resorbed nor secreted by the tubules.[3] The quantity produced and excreted largely depends on muscle mass, and thus tends to remain constant in most individuals. It is a substance not influenced by protein catabolism or diet. Since creatinine is excreted primarily by glomerular filtration, the concentration rises when the GFR declines.[3]

A 24-hour urine is collected, and a blood sample for serum creatinine level is obtained. (Occasionally a 2- to 4-hour time span is used instead.) Low creatinine clearance indicates depressed renal function resulting from renal disease or circulatory impairment. Normal creatinine clearance is 110 to 150 ml/min for men, and 105 to 130 ml/min for women.

Inulin clearance. Inulin is a polysaccharide that is neither resorbed nor secreted, so it is ideal for determining plasma clearance. The test requires injection of intravenous inulin and collection of blood and urine specimens at exact times. It is, however, the most accurate measure of GFR. The normal inulin clearance rate is 124 ± 25.8 ml/min for men, and 119 ± 12.8 ml/min for women.

Tubular function tests

The PSP (phenosulphonphthalein) test is used to measure the kidney's ability to eliminate foreign substances and metabolic wastes from the blood. It is depressed in disease, which decreases the GFR.

The test requires that the client be given a light breakfast without tea or coffee. After voiding, one or two glasses of water are given before intravenous injection of the PSP dye. Urine is collected at 15, 30, and 120 minutes following injection. The percentage of dye appearing in the urine is determined colorimetrically. Normal values are 25% to 45% at 15 min, 50% to 65% at 60 min, and 60% to 80% at 120 min.

Concentration and dilution tests. These tubular function tests require ingestion by the client of a required amount of fluid and collection of serial specimens that are evaluated for quantity and quality. The value of the test is largely determined by the exactness of timing in specimen collection. The *Fishberg concentration test* mandates that the client eat a high-protein meal with limited fluids (200 ml) on the evening before the test. After this meal the individual must not eat or drink until completion of the test. On the morning of the test the first voided specimen is saved, and additional specimens are collected at the end of 1 and 2 hours. Specific gravity of each specimen is measured. It is expected that at least one sample will be 1.025. If all specific gravities are less than 1.025, depressed concentration ability of the kidney is suspected.

Dilution tests are usually performed in the morning after the client has not ingested food or fluids after the evening meal. The initial morning specimen is

collected and discarded, and the client ingests 1000 ml of water in 30 to 45 minutes. Every hour (for 4 hours), specimens are collected for specific gravity measurement. Normally one specimen will have a specific gravity below 1.003. Output is expected to be about 1200 ml in 4 hours. Low excretion quantity or a specific gravity of 1.010 or higher may indicate faulty elimination resulting from renal disease such as nephritis or the nephrotic syndrome.[3] Specific gravity is itself a measure of concentration and dilution.

Percutaneous renal biopsy

To ascertain the exact nature of glomerular structure and functioning in disease such as the nephrotic syndrome or idiopathic episodes of renal insufficiency, proteinuria, or hematuria, a direct study of nephron units extracted by needle biopsy may be desirable.

The decision to perform a renal biopsy is made only after it has been determined that the client has two functioning kidneys and that bleeding and clotting studies are within normal limits. Typing and crossmatching are completed, and at least two units of blood are immediately available for use on the day of the scheduled procedure. Baseline vital signs are also recorded.

The client is instructed that the procedure will involve his lying in a prone position (with a towel roll for abdominal support) so that the dorsal body area is maintained in straight alignment as a plane surface. Other than to lie motionless and hold a fully inspired breath on command, no other special maneuvers need be understood. Some institutions withhold the meal before the procedure, but liquids are usually permitted.

Most physicians prefer to perform a biopsy on the right kidney to avoid the area of the spleen. Since exact localization for the procedure is critical to its safety and success, it is done in the radiology department under direct radiological visualization.

The actual biopsy involves the introduction of a needle (Vim-Silverman) into the kidney cortex at a 35-degree angle using a local anesthetic. Two specimens (each containing several nephron units) are extracted for microscopic study, and a small dressing is applied over the site.

Nursing care following the biopsy is primarily directed toward preventing and detecting renal bleeding. The client is on strict bed rest until initial biopsy studies assure that no major artery has been traumatized by the procedure. Serial urine specimens are saved, and vital signs, blood studies, and other indices to detect bleeding are regularly monitored on a strict regimen. Any flank pain, fever, drop in blood pressure, or falling hematocrit level is immediately reported to the medical team. Recovery is usually accomplished in 2 to 4 days, but heavy lifting, jolting activities, and strenuous exercise should be curtailed for at least 2 weeks.

Clients who are discharged following the procedure should be instructed regarding signs and symptoms that could indicate biopsy site hemorrhage and must be certain of specific measures to take if it does occur. Printed materials are available in most institutions so that individuals may be given a copy for reference upon dismissal.

Data analysis

After collecting relevant data, the nurse organizes the data, compares them with age-appropriate norms, and identifies actual or potential nursing problems or diagnoses. Nursing diagnoses may include alterations in comfort: pain, fluid volume deficit, knowledge deficit, noncompliance, alterations in nutrition, and alterations in patterns of urinary elimination. The diagnoses can be placed in priority order for development of a nursing care plan.

Planning

PLANNING FOR HEALTH PROMOTION

Promoting urinary elimination in children

The nurse can use opportunities to instruct clients about health maintenance of the urinary system. Topics may include promoting urinary elimination, preventing urinary tract infections, and managing risks such as renal calculi or hypertension.

Toilet training. The first developmental hurdle that relates to genitourinary health is toilet training. In our society, parents are aware that this is an important achievement, and it is imperative that they have appropriate guidance during this period. The nurse should advise parents that the right time to begin toilet training is highly individualized and that it is unwise to compare their child with others of the same chronological age as an indicator of *readiness*. They should be reassured that, if their child does not achieve continence by a particular age, it does not mean they have failed or their child is slow to learn from their teachings. Furthermore, parents must understand that, if neurological structures governing voluntary voiding and continence are insufficiently developed, their best efforts will be futile. If possible, parents should establish a plan for toilet training that is mutually acceptable so that the child will face the same expectations from both parents.

The child indicates an awareness of urination by about 15 months, at which time there is an expression of discomfort at being wet. They may point at wet clothing or at a puddle on the floor. A short time later there is evidence the child knows he is wetting. Finally, at approximately 18 to 20 months, there is awareness of the fact that voiding is going to occur. This time period is when realistic toilet training can become possible unless there are concurrent stresses, such as illness, that must be coped with. Additionally, self-feeding, standing, and walking alone are normally achieved by this time. These activities are thought to be highly suggestive of psychological readiness for independent toileting.[1]

If a child is handicapped and walking is not possible, the appropriate index of *readiness* is sitting and standing balance control.

Dependable bladder reflex control is usually present when the child is 2½ to 3½ years old. At this time the bladder can contain urine for 2 hours, but this dependability is not present except during waking hours. Parents should be informed that fluid restriction before bedtime does not help gain reflex control of the bladder.

It is important that a consistent pattern of activities and rewards prevail during toilet training, even when there are the normal periods of regression to uncontrolled urination. The child should be provided with a comfortable training potty chair and training pants that reinforce the desirability and pleasure in being dry. Successes at continence and controlled voiding should be rewarded, and praise should be generously bestowed. When there is failure to perform as hoped for, the child should be reassured that parents are not angry and that there is a "next time to do better." Punishment has no place in the toilet-training regimen.

When the child reaches 3 years of age, he has usually achieved a routine pattern of voiding and exhibits responsibility for independence in this activity. However, because of distractions the toddler occasionally waits too long and has an accident. By age 4, most children are fully capable of all bathroom activity, including management of clothes, and by age 5, even nighttime control is complete.

It is crucial that nurses understand and accept that these are only average levels of developmental achievement, and that deviations in rate and rhythms might occur. However, the sequence of events tends to be highly consistent. Furthermore, readiness is as important for parents as it is for the child before embarking on the task of toilet training.

It is recommended that activities of toilet training be confined to the bathroom. The potty chair should not be placed in the bedroom or kitchen, for example, because toileting is appropriately associated only with the bathroom. When the family travels, the potty chair should be taken along so that the program of training can be continued as routinely as possible.

At the point that children are achieving independence in toileting, it is essential that their clothes are easy to manage. Slacks with elastic waistbands are more desirable, for example, than ones with belts, zippers, buckles, or buttons. Most authorities are hesitant to recommend plastic pants during training because they tend to be expressly made for containing wetness. Training pants, on the other hand, signify that remaining dry and clean is expected. They also tend to be uncomfortable when wet, and this discomfort can be a motivating influence.

The entire plan of toilet training must take into account such factors as the home's physical, social, and emotional environment, because any stresses may deter success. The reward and praise reinforcement system must fit the parents' disciplinary pattern and should be modified periodically if it fails to facilitate progress.

Games, toys, and other diversions are not appropriate while the child is toileting because it is highly desirable that all attention be focused on the task at hand. However, if there is resistance to sitting, it is not wise to force the child to sit or to have him restrained on the chair.

Children tend to void on arising, after meals, mid-morning and afternoon, and at bedtime.[1] These are good times, therefore, to take the child to the potty chair. If possible, when there is an expressed need to eliminate by the child, avoid rushing him to the bathroom because this creates tension and may make voluntary voiding less likely. At first it is important to verbally reinforce all of the steps of the progress, for example, "Let's go to the bathroom," "Now I will pull down your pants and help you sit on the potty," and so on. Consistency in language is imperative so that confusion about terms and meanings is minimized. Early in training, parents should stay with the child to be certain that the reward or reinforcement immediately follows the desired behavior.

After every training encounter, the child should be assisted in hand washing so that this behavior becomes an essential part of the entire toileting process.

The toilet training plan should be understood by babysitters and others who care for the child so that there is consistency and continuity in this developmental task achievement.

Promoting urinary elimination in adults

The nurse can instruct adult clients about promoting health habits for urination. Activity is important in keeping the tone of the overall physiological apparatus. Prolonged bed rest should be avoided whenever possible because it tends

1039

to foster fecal impactions, urinary stasis, and retention. Uncorrected gynecological conditions also may be a contributory factor. Hot baths are beneficial in reducing prolonged urinary retention, since in many persons they foster an urge to void because of stimulation of the genitalia and pelvic blood supply. Keeping the client physically active prevents apathy and promotes alertness and attention to elimination signals. Regular visits to the bathroom are desirable because they help the client associate elimination with general hygiene. Men can often void with ease while standing but cannot use a urinal in a recumbent position. Sitting on a commode in a relaxed position is helpful to others.

Incontinence is not uncommon, particularly among the elderly. As much pelvic muscular support is lost and as degeneration of the surrounding pelvic organs occurs, the normal bladder control declines. Benign prostatic hypertrophy, uterine prolapse, and cystocele are common mechanical problems that interfere with normal micturition. Infections and other inflammatory responses can also contribute to incontinence. Indwelling catheters, urinals left in place, and other similar techniques may prevent soiling of the bed or furniture, but they do little to help the client gain continence and maintain his dignity and independence. If the client is not likely to achieve continence because of his mental or physical condition, incontinence must be managed to prevent skin breakdown. General skin care and perineal care should be given scrupulous attention because urine is caustic to skin and external mucous membranes. Barrier creams can be used to protect the surrounding areas. The frequency and time of voiding should be charted to determine if there is a pattern useful in management. Restriction of fluids after 6 PM can reduce nighttime incontinence.

The elderly client may view loss of bladder control as a loss of dignity and as a reversion to the helplessness of childhood. Much of the anguish related to retention and incontinence could be avoided through a regular regimen that keeps the body in optimum shape. The fluid intake-and-output pattern of all elderly clients should be assessed on a regular basis, and potential problems that could lead to the urinary tract manifestations mentioned previously should be recognized.

Preventing infections. Young girls and women are considerably more prone to urinary tract infections than their male counterparts because their urethras are short and easily invaded by vaginal and rectal flora. It is important that they be taught to wipe or cleanse themselves from *front to back* with one stroke and discard the tissue after a single stroke. If there is vaginal or rectal drainage, it should be contained as much as possible to prevent its entering the urethra.

Soap and other strong alkaline substances should be avoided when cleansing the perineum because they tend to destroy the normal protective flora of the region that are responsible for deterring invaders from unusual sources. Effervescent bubble baths are thought to possibly transport bath water (and thus contaminants) into the urethra, especially in young girls. Some pediatricians and urologists, therefore, discourage their use.

When women become sexually active, there is yet another mechanical source of irritation to the urethra that frequently seems to be the precursor to inflammation and infection. Gentleness in coitus is essential, especially when the girl or woman is unaccustomed to the act. Some tolerance to urethral friction seems to be acquired after a period of several weeks of regular sexual activity and so eventually the potential problem is minimized. However, all women should be cautious and avoid undue mechanical trauma to the urethra by positional influence and encouraging their partners toward gentleness. Voiding before and within 15 minutes after coitus may minimize opportunities for bladder infection. Postcoital cleansing of the perineum is also desirable to minimize the activity of foreign organisms. (Men should cleanse their penis, too, for the same reason.)

Bladder stasis invites infection, and thus the bladder should be emptied regularly. Overdistension of the structures from retention is responsible for some predisposition to infection. The elderly, clients with altered neurological functioning, and others who are on prolonged bed rest are prone to the complication of stasis.

Urethral discharge and vaginal or rectal discharges deserve prompt medical intervention. Clients should understand the importance of early management of infections as a mode to discourage upper urinary tract infection. All parents and youthful or adult nursing clients should know the signs and symptoms of urinary tract dysfunction and be convinced of the need to contact a physician for assessment and intervention.

Risk management

Discouraging calculi. Clients who are known to be "stone formers" can modify their diet and increase their fluid intake and thus may be successful in preventing the development or growth of calculi, particularly in conjunction with drug therapy. Individuals who are most likely to benefit from these preventive tactics are those at risk of forming stones (for example, clients with vitamin A deficiency, those with certain endocrine disorders or long-term urinary tract infections, or those who are sedentary). Also, certain geographical localities have water supplies with a mineral content that favors urinary stones. Modifying one or more of the precursors that are linked to stone formation often is advised to discourage calculi from becoming a problem.

Preventing hypertension. Hypertension and other related cardiovascular phenomena are thought to be linked to renal damage and, ultimately, renal failure. Maintaining a standard body weight, exercising, minimizing stressors, avoiding excesses in salt, and using other recommended dietary discretions may be valuable in preventing cardiovascular disease, which leads to renal destruction.

PLANNING FOR HEALTH MAINTENANCE AND RESTORATION

Catheters

Catheters are used to (1) promote drainage or decompression of the kidney pelvis, ureters, and bladder; (2) bypass obstructions or surgical wounds; (3) splint the ureters or urethra while surgical wounds heal; (4) serve as a channel for introducing medications; (5) facilitate diagnostic tests; and (6) manage incontinence.

Urethral catheters. Although many types of catheters exist (Fig. 19-8), the three most likely to be encountered by the nurse are (1) the straight, single-lumen urethral catheter for episodic urinary drainage or urological procedures such as instillation of dyes or medications; (2) the double-lumen urethral retention catheter, usually referred to as an indwelling or Foley catheter; and (3) the triple-lumen (three-way) urethral catheter, which facilitates anchoring for prolonged drainage and irrigation (Fig. 19-9). The last two catheters are equipped with a balloon, which, after introduction, is inflated to retain it in the bladder. These catheters are usually made of latex.

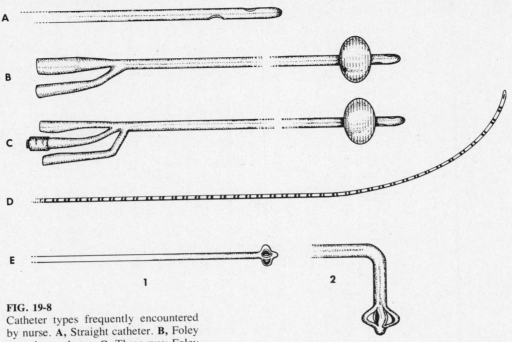

FIG. 19-8
Catheter types frequently encountered by nurse. **A,** Straight catheter. **B,** Foley retention catheter. **C,** Three-way Foley retention catheter. **D,** Ureteral catheter. **E,** 1. Malecot catheter; 2. Malecot suprapubic angle catheter.

Nephrostomy tubes and ureteral catheters. Nurses may encounter a *nephrostomy tube,* a catheter anchored in the renal pelvis through a surgical wound in the flank. It enters the pelvis by passing through the cortex and medullary substance of the kidney. A small Foley or Malecot catheter is often used. *Ureterostomy tubes* are similar to nephrostomy tubes but are inserted into the ureter through an incision above the point of pathological obstruction and passed up toward the renal pelvis. *Ureteral catheters* drain urine from one or both kidneys and are introduced via cystoscopy into the ureter. They have a tiny lumen and are long and radiopaque to facilitate x-ray study regarding their

FIG. 19-9
Three-way catheter.

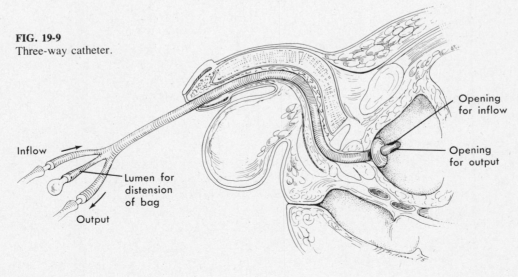

Inflow

Lumen for distension of bag

Output

Opening for inflow

Opening for output

placement. Because urine may drain from the kidney to the bladder around the catheter, a urethral catheter always accompanies ureteral catheters to prevent backflow pressure produced by improper drainage of the lower urinary tract.

Each nephrostomy, ureterostomy, and ureteral catheter is tagged to denote its placement and is attached to a unique, clearly identified drainage apparatus. Any tube that drains the kidney pelvis directly should be carefully irrigated. (It should be recalled that the renal pelvis has a capacity of 5 to 8 ml.) Always *aspirate before* adding any solutions to the renal pelvis. Only a minute amount of irrigating solution can enter, and gentle pressure and strictest aseptic technique must be used. Because the renal pelvis has a limited capacity, it is important that the catheters remain patent. They should never be clamped, and any obstruction should be managed at once. Dislodged catheters constitute an emergency because considerable renal damage can occur from excess pressure of urine in the pelvis. Although most nephrostomy and ureterostomy tubes are anchored by suturing, they can be displaced by sudden traction. Clients who have such drainage devices in place should ordinarily be placed on bed rest for their protection.

Suprapubic catheters. A cystostomy or suprapubic tube may be placed directly into the bladder through an abdominal incision. A Foley or Malecot catheter is usually used for this type of drainage. It may be used in conjunction with urethral drainage. Suprapubic drainage may be used for a long-term approach to the management of certain urinary tract dysfunctions.

Dressings are used with catheters inserted through surgical wounds, and these must be kept clean and dry to prevent excoriation of tissue, odor, and a focus for infection. The skin may be protected by using metallic paste that serves as a barrier between it and the urine-dampened dressings.

Managing clients with catheters. Catheters that enter the urinary tract are responsible for severe nosocomial infections and other complications, even when managed with scrupulous technique. Therefore many clinicians use the devices only when absolutely required—never merely to facilitate nursing care (for example, to prevent bedwetting). The risk of infection is even greater when the introduction of the catheter is complicated with trauma or if the client is being administered broad-spectrum antibiotics. The major threat of any urinary tract infection is gram-negative sepsis—a fatal condition in at least half the cases.

Catheter care begins with careful selection and preparation of equipment. A closed urinary drainage system is imperative. It should be adjusted so that the collection bag will not contact the floor even when the bed is in the lowest position. The bag should be designed so that it can be emptied without the spigot touching the floor or the collection receptacle in the process. A "sampling port" should be present, too, so that the system does not need disconnection when a sample of urine is needed. Antireflux valves have been added to most closed drainage systems to prevent any backflow of urine from the drainage tubing or bag to the bladder.

Closed urinary drainage systems are designed to discourage any disconnections that invite the introduction of microorganisms. Bladder irrigations, once considered routine for the catheterized patient, are performed only when specifically required to introduce medications, control hemorrhage, or relieve obstructions from clots or sediment. When required, a closed technique is normally used, using a three-way catheter or a method that permits the irrigation to be accomplished through the "sampling port." Whenever the port is entered to

1043

aspirate or irrigate, the site of needle entry must be prepared with alcohol or iodophor. If the tubing is disconnected for any reason, the open connection should be protected with sterile material and cleansed thoroughly again before reconnection.

Ascending infection via the outside of the catheter can be substantially reduced by meatal care. The urinary meatus should be cleansed two or three times a day with soap and water. An iodophor ointment that is bactericidal for gram-negative and gram-positive organisms should be applied. Many clients will be able to do this procedure as part of a self-care program.

The client and all nursing personnel must be aware that the drainage system must be maintained in a dependent position. Even if the device has an antireflux valve, care should be taken to always keep the drainage apparatus below the level of the bladder. (Antireflux devices do not ordinarily function properly if the bag is in a horizontal position.) Bacteria in the urine and drainage bag multiply rapidly, and any backflow of this urine into the bladder could inoculate the urinary tract with large numbers of microorganisms.

Catheters should be free-flowing. They should never be clamped except on the specific order of a physician. Residual urine in the bladder is an ideal site for the growth of organisms (Fig. 19-10).

Simple nursing measures, such as coiling and securing excess tubing on the mattress (and not permitting it to loop below the bag), instructing transportation aides regarding the proper positioning of the bag en route to x-ray or other hospital departments, and teaching the client good hygienic practices, will contribute positively to reducing the hazards of urethral catheter drainage systems.

Other considerations. The organisms that tend to create urinary tract infections are capable of easy transmission from client to client. It is known that they

FIG. 19-10
A, Urethral catheters can create pressure on blood vessels at penoscrotal angle; therefore they should *not* be taped to leg. **B,** Proper taping of male urethral catheter to abdomen. Note, there is no pressure exerted at penoscrotal angle.

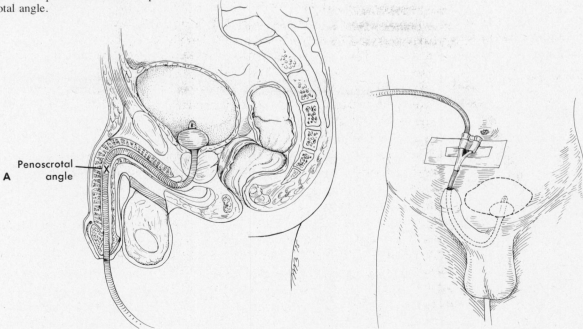

Penoscrotal
A   angle

B

tend to "jump" from one surface to another, especially when in close contact. In addition to careful hand washing among all personnel who come in contact with these clients, there are other preventive points worthy of consideration in an attempt to prevent nosocomial urinary tract infections.

It is advised to isolate any catheterized client from other clients who either have a catheter or other drainage device and/or open wounds. When drainage urine from collection bags, the nurse should not use a common container for two or more individuals. Even when there is no mechanical contact between the spigot and the device, microorganisms are transmitted by mere close association. Because clients are so vulnerable, each should have a receptacle for bag drainage that is disinfected after each use. The same principle applies to equipment used to measure specific gravity and so on.

Nurses can monitor the urinary output and order cultures on at least a weekly basis to detect the onset of bacteriuria. Institutions have various protocols for changing catheters and tubing to reduce risks to clients. Nurses who care for any catheterized client should be aware of regulations designed to minimize complications of prolonged urinary drainage. Furthermore, signs or symptoms indicative of a developing infection (fever, pain in the suprapubic or back region, foul-smelling or cloudy urine) should be promptly reported.

Elderly and confused clients may require additional precautions in catheter care management. Because the drainage tube is an abnormal appendage, it seems to serve as a source of irritation. Wrist restraints may be necessary to prevent dislodgement. The nurse will sometimes find it useful to explain to the client that the tubing is there to drain urine from the bladder and that even though he may feel pressure and bladder spasm similar to the urge to urinate or defecate, incontinence will not occur.

Exdwelling, or condom, drainage. If a male client is comatose or incontinent but retains the ability to completely empty his bladder, condom drainage may be used. There are several commercially manufactured exdwelling devices, but the nurse may need to make one, using a condom or a finger cot for a male adult and child, respectively. (The closed end of the condom or finger cot is inverted over, and attached to, drainage tubing by a small, firm ring of plastic or with a waterproof adhesive tape.) A hole for drainage is made by puncturing the condom with an object such as an applicator stick.

There are several important points to note in application of any condom drainage. Pubic hair should be shaved from the base of the penis, and the area washed and dried. Tincture of benzoin should be applied over the penis base and allowed to dry. If the foreskin is retracted, it must be eased back over the glans before the applied condom is unrolled to the base of the penis. If an erection occurs, the nurse must wait until it subsides before securing the device. Elastic tape should be applied approximately ½ inch above the condom's edge. It must not overlap the edge, and therefore any excess is cut off. The rim of the condom should be trimmed away, since it may impair circulation. Apply another piece of elastic tape to the base of the condom so that its edges come in contact with the skin and the first tape. Again, it is important that the tape ends do not overlap. Connect the device to urinary drainage. Observe the penis at 15-minute intervals during the first hour, making certain that there is no edema or discoloration of the penis and that the device is not leaking or twisted in a manner that would obstruct drainage.

Condoms should be removed and reapplied daily after skin care of the penis and perineum has been provided. Urine specimens, *except those for culture,* can be obtained from exdwelling drainage devices with dependable results.

Penile clamps (which compress the urethra) and other exdwelling apparatuses may be ordered for some incontinent clients, and each requires special nursing care considerations for safe, effective functioning. The nurse may be responsible for teaching the client and his family regarding exdwelling drainage, because incontinence is often a long-term management problem.

Urological surgery

Many surgical procedures can be performed to correct defects in the urinary tract or to remove diseased tissue or organs. Following are some common procedures:

nephrotomy Incision to remove stone.
nephrectomy Removal of kidney.
pyelotomy Incision into kidney pelvis.
ureterotomy Incision into ureter.
cystotomy Incision into bladder.
cystectomy Removal of bladder.
litholapaxy Crushing of stones by cystoscopy to facilitate removal.

Preoperative considerations include prevention and control of infections, maintenance of fluid and electrolyte balance, maintenance of excretory function, and control of pain.

The client should understand the anticipated surgical procedure regarding its objective and the postoperative regimen. In nephrectomy there should be careful explanations to assure the client that one healthy kidney can adequately handle the body's needs.

Surgical procedures involving the kidney require the same general postoperative care as for any abdominal surgery. In addition, temporary catheters may be used to drain the kidney pelvis, ureters, or bladder while healing occurs. Most clients are on a precise intake-and-output recording regimen.

Postoperatively the client should be encouraged to ambulate as soon as possible and to exercise. When confined to bed, he should rest on the operated side to promote drainage. If surgical wound drains are in place, they will be withdrawn in stages as healing takes place.

Catheters may require frequent irrigation for the first few postoperative hours. If hemorrhagic conditions result in clot obstructions, irrigations may be performed every 30 minutes. Because many older clients may be on anticoagulant therapy, this complication should be anticipated. The alert nurse will observe for bladder distension, acute retention, and signs of hemorrhage. Bowel sound return should be monitored because paralytic ileus is a frequent complication. Attention should be given to dressings. If urine appears in large quantities on any dressing, it indicates that the catheters are obstructed, preventing diversion of urine as planned.

Septicemia from gram-negative microorganisms deserves special attention because it frequently is a sequela of urological surgery or other instrumentation. Endotoxins from bacterial proliferation constrict the capillaries and pool plasma, and venous return to the heart is reduced. Profound shock, cardiac failure, and renal shutdown may result. Even with excellent therapy using steroids, antibacterial agents, and vasopressors, death ensues in half the cases. The client with

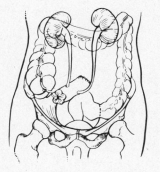

Ileal conduit and ileostomy

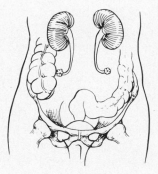

Cutaneous ureterostomy

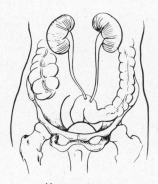

Ureterosigmoid
anastomosis

A

FIG. 19-11
A, Urinary diversions. **B,** Bedside
drainage for clients with urinary diversion and collecting appliance attached
to leg.

gram-negative septicemia is usually managed in an intensive care unit where central venous pressure and other vital signs can be monitored constantly.

This dread clinical complication can best be treated with prophylaxis, including rigorous approaches to urinary infection and avoidance of trauma that can injure the delicate structures of the tract, thus inviting inflammatory manifestations.

Urinary diversion. Surgical removal of a portion of the bladder or a total cystectomy may be performed, and a urinary diversion created (Fig. 19-11). The ureters may be attached to the sigmoid or the ileum or brought directly out to the abdominal wall. Using the bowel for diversion has some disadvantages, including hydronephrosis from slow renal draining as a result of high resistance of the bowel, infection from dilation and urinary backflow, and electrolyte disturbances from resorption of waste products.

The diversion using the ileobladder (ileal conduit) is the preferred mode because the primary problem is the client's wearing an appliance as a urinary receptacle.

Nursing considerations. Clients who have surgery that creates an alternate route for urinary elimination need personal support and instructional guidance during their adjustment period. The obvious concerns relate to the modified system for voiding and its implications in daily living patterns.

The nurse and enterostomal technician or therapist have the responsibility of introducing the client to the appliances that will serve as a receptacle for urinary voiding. A temporary appliance (a plastic pouch with an adhesive opening) will be placed over the ostomy immediately after surgery. This simple device is worn until the stoma shrinks to its nonedematous size, and then a permanent appliance is fitted. The client should understand that this will take about 4 to 6 weeks. Reassurance should include the fact that no temporary appliance will be as satisfactory as the permanent one.

At night, clients with urinary diversion have a bedside drainage system so that the urine can drain freely and sleep is not interrupted for regular emptying of the receptacle. It should be emptied about every 2 hours during the day or whenever it contains about 100 ml, if possible.

B

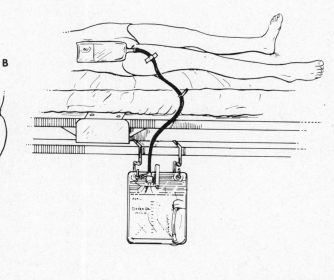

Fluids should be ingested in liberal quantities to reduce the concentration of the urine and to discourage odors created by bacteria. Other adjustments in dietary and fluid intake are probably individual, based on other preexisting considerations in health management. Some physicians, however, recommend that their clients ingest cranberry juice to ensure an acid urine to reduce the potential of infection.

Skin care is the key element to being comfortable with a system of urinary diversion. It involves a program of routines designed to reduce local irritation to the minimum.

Most stomal problems occur because of urine leaks, which irritate the stomal area, or from ripping the appliance from the skin. The appliance should always be eased from the skin with surgical adhesive remover or soap and water. Harsh solvents should be avoided. When the bag is removed, the skin should be washed with soap and water and the area patted dry. A gauze wick should be placed over the stoma at this point to prevent urine from leaking onto the prepared site. (This works only in the semirecumbent position, however.) An alternative to using a wick is for the client to bend over a basin to keep urine from draining onto the site.

In the application of the appliance, a double-faced adhesive ring is used, or a thin layer of an appropriate cement is applied over the appliance ring and allowed to become "tacky" before the ring is placed over the stoma. Care should be taken to make certain that the ring is aligned for attachment to the belt and that it is centered over the stoma. Some clients mark the area with guides before application to ensure correct positioning. The client should stand up or lie flat at the point the ring is being placed so that the skin can stretch as necessary before the cement dries.

Various powders and deodorants may be used as prescribed before the total appliance (belt and pouch) is in place because the skin under the pouch may become irritated by perspiration. Cloth pouch covers may also be used.

Although the total appliance is changed only once or twice a week, the client should follow some basic procedural guidelines to facilitate making the task as comfortable as possible.

All equipment should be gathered before beginning—the adhesive remover, cement, clean appliance and belt, gauze for wicking, powders, and soap and water. Most clients pat the skin dry with a small towel or gauze, but some prefer using dry heat from a gooseneck lamp or a hair dryer.

Unusual skin problems may be encountered by some clients, which require specialized management. There are a number of techniques and products to cope with skin irritation, many of which are available without prescription. The nurse should be familiar with products used in the local facilities for such purposes.

Stomal shrinking is not a typical problem with urinary diversion, but it may occur. The physician may order the stoma to be dilated with a sterile catheter. The nurse may be responsible for instructing the client how to correctly carry out the technique.

The client will undoubtedly have many questions regarding his personal life with urinary diversion. He should be reassured that most of his activities can continue without major adaptations. Bathing without the appliance is quite acceptable. Sexual activities may be unaltered by the surgery, and most recreational activities can be engaged in comfortably with a few modifications. Travel need not be curtailed, but clients are advised to always carry with them a complete appliance-change kit. It should carried in an attaché case or purse and not be placed in luggage that might be inaccessible to the traveler at some points.

Children as well as adults have urinary diversion. Their care involves special considerations related to developmental needs. For example, the teenager may need considerable support as he contemplates his social horizons, the future, marriage, and family life. Often, referrals to others of the same age group with a similar ostomy may be helpful in promoting full exploration of problems and anxieties.

There are over one million persons with ostomies, so that clients of every age group have peers with similar needs. In general the client cares independently for his stoma, or he has minimal help from another person (often a spouse, or a parent in the case of a young child). Nurses, however, are frequently involved in the care during a hospitalization or disability, although it may be unrelated to the ostomy, and thus should know the fundamental care routine.

Continent vesicostomy. An alternative to an ileal conduit is a vesicostomy, a procedure in which the bladder remains as internal reservoir for urine and is drained by intermittent catheterization. The bladder is closed at the urethral neck, and an external nipple valve is created from the bladder wall. The valve intussuscepts from pressure of urine in the bladder and prevents incontinence. After a 4-week healing time the client can be taught to do self-catheterization by inserting a lubricated rubber fr 12 catheter into the stoma and draining urine into the toilet. A gauze square can be placed over the stoma between drainage periods.

Implementation

COMMON HEALTH PROBLEMS OF THE NEONATE AND INFANT

Polycystic disease of the kidneys

Polycystic kidneys can occur as a congenital anomaly. If it is bilateral and involves most of the parenchymal tissue, death follows in a few days.

At birth, one or both kidneys can be affected by polycystic disease, or it may not present itself until later life. The polycystic kidney parenchyma has many blisterlike formations containing blood, mucuslike material, pus, or urine. The presence of these cysts not only interferes with normal renal function, but these cysts may rupture, creating hemorrhage and infection that affects the lower urinary tract. They tend to occur in a familial pattern, and clients who have relatives with the disorder should be viewed with this factor in mind if they have urinary symptoms indicative of the disorder. The polycystic kidney is large and creates symptomatology suggesting infection and renal degeneration. Anemia, hypertension, vomiting, and weakness are associated, particularly if the condition is bilateral.

Assessment of the potential disorder is made by excretory pyelography. Palpation should be avoided because it may cause the cysts to rupture. Medical and surgical management is limited primarily to conservation of the adequately functioning parenchyma by avoiding infection and compression damage.

Bilateral renal agenesis

Bilateral renal agenesis involves a failure of the kidneys to develop in utero and obviously leads to death shortly after birth. However, other parts of the urinary tract (such as the urethra) may not be fully developed, but the condition can be mechanically corrected by surgery if it is discovered before damage has occurred. Observation in the nursery regarding voiding is a key factor in assessment of such problems.

Exstrophy of the bladder

Exstrophy of the bladder is a congenital defect in the abdominal wall that permits the bladder to be exposed. A fissure is present where the abdomen fails to fuse and the bladder is exposed through the opening. The ureters and urethra are also exposed and continuously drain urine, causing excoriation of the surrounding tissue. Renal failure from infection or obstruction is an ultimate hazard of exstrophy of the bladder.

The cause of this defect is not known; familial tendency has not been associated with exstrophy of the bladder. The defect is three times as frequent in boys and is often associated with other defects of the genitourinary system. In boys the defect may be accompanied by undescended testes, epispadias, short penis, or inguinal hernia; in girls there may be a cleft clitoris or separated labia. The pubic bones may be separated in either sex, causing a waddling gait when the infant begins to walk.

When the client is able to tolerate surgery and abdominal size has increased (about age 2 or 3), the defect can be repaired. Several surgical procedures can be used, including ureteral sigmoid implantation, ureterostomy, and ileal conduit. Ileal conduit is the most common. An ileal bladder is formed from a section of the ileum, and the ureters are sutured to the ileal bladder. Because urine drains continuously, the client wears an ileostomy appliance over the stoma to collect urine. As the child matures, further reconstructive surgery may be necessary, particularly if other defects are present that interfere with sexual development.

The birth of a child with a congenital defect such as exstrophy of the bladder is a disturbing event for the parents and family. The nurse can facilitate bonding by accepting the client and helping the parents assume responsibility for care.

Because surgery is not performed for several years, the parents learn to bathe and diaper their infant to prevent infection and excoriation of the skin. Scrupulous cleanliness is stressed to avoid infection; petrolatum gauze may be used to lubricate the mucosa and ointments applied to protect the surrounding skin from excoriation. Other aspects of growth and development can be encouraged as the child matures.

The child may exhibit problems with self-concept and sexuality, and the nurse and parents should be sensitive to these concerns. Parent groups are often helpful in alleviating fears and providing peer support.

COMMON HEALTH PROBLEMS OF THE CHILD AND ADOLESCENT

Poststreptococcal acute glomerulonephritis

Acute glomerulonephritis (AGN) is a common parenchymal disease of childhood, believed to be caused by a nephritogenic strain of group A beta hemolytic streptococci (PS-AGN) following an upper respiratory tract infection such as tonsillitis, otitis, pharyngitis, and sinusitis, or a skin infection such as impetigo. The disease occurs predominantly in children ages 2 to 12, with the highest incidence in school-age children. Boys are affected more frequently than girls.

Pathophysiology. PS-AGN is an immune complex disease; this is supported by the findings (1) that in the latent period (about 7 days between the infection and the onset of the glomerulonephritis) an antigen common to plasma membranes of other serotypes has been demonstrated in the plasma membrane of certain streptococci, (2) that complement is utilized and hypergammaglobulinemia is evident during the active phase of the disease, and finally (3) that complement and IgG have been demonstrated on the glomerular basement membrane using immunofluorescent techniques.[4]

As cells proliferate, they occlude the lumen of capillaries, and the resultant vasospasm decreases filtration pressure. Decreased glomerular filtration leads to greater tubular reabsorption of filtered sodium and consequently contributes to edema. Vascular and tubular changes are not specific, and tubular function is usually not impaired.

Assessment. The nurse can have a significant affect on early assessment of AGN. Community health and school nurses assume responsibility for detecting carriers of beta hemolytic streptococci and obtaining cultures of skin and throat lesions. In the northern United States, upper respiratory tract infections seem to be the major precursor of AGN. However, in southern states, infected insect bites and impetigo appear to be frequently implicated in causation. Nurses should suspect any children with such conditions to be potential carriers, especially if they live in crowded housing, are poorly nourished, or are prone to illness.

Physical assessment may reveal the effects of fluid retention and edema. In early morning, edema is noticed around the eyes (periorbital edema), but as the day progresses, edema may be noticed in the abdomen and extremities. The child does not feel well and may be lethargic and irritable. There may also be headaches, dysuria, or vomiting. A significant observation is of the urine, which has a smoky brown color and is limited in volume. A thorough assessment of the cardiovascular system must be completed because tachypnea, dyspnea, dysrhythmias, gallops, venous engorgement, and cardiomegaly could signal cardiac decompensation. If complications are present, the blood pressure may be slightly elevated.

Eye grounds are to be examined for hemorrhage, exudate, and papilledema. Changes in visual acuity, seizures, headaches, or vision disturbances must also be noted because they may suggest encephalopathy.

Laboratory tests are performed to support the medical diagnosis. Urinalysis reveals hematuria, proteinuria, and increased specific gravity. The BUN and creatinine may be elevated, reflecting azotemia. Throat cultures may be positive, but many are not; the elevated antistreptolysin (ASO) titer confirms recent streptococcal infection. Other studies may include renal function studies, chest x-ray films, ECG, renal biopsy, and histology studies.

The clinical course of AGN lasts for several weeks. In the acute stage the client does not feel well, is edematous, and the urine is thick and brown. The blood pressure may be precipitously elevated. When diuresis occurs in 5 to 14 days the client feels better as weight decreases and blood pressure returns to normal.

Data analysis

Data analysis may reveal nursing diagnoses of alterations in urinary elimination, alterations in fluid volume: excess, ineffective rest and activity patterns, and alterations in nutrition. Nursing care is planned appropriately for these problems.

Planning and implementation. There is no specific medical treatment for acute glomerulonephritis, and nursing care is supportive. Only clients with oliguria or hypertension are hospitalized. Nursing goals are to (1) prevent infection, (2) reduce fluid excess, (3) maintain rest and activity patterns, and (4) provide comfort.

1051

Nursing process for common health problems

Infection. If the client has evidence of streptococcal infection, antibiotics may be administered. Some believe other family members should also receive prophylactic antibiotic therapy.

Fluid balance. During the acute stage, fluid retention may be managed by limiting sodium in the diet. If edema is mild, only added salt in the diet is restricted. However, if the edema is severe, moderate sodium restriction may be imposed. Fluids may also be limited if urinary output is below 200 to 300 ml in 24 hours. If urinary output is low, potassium may also be restricted. Protein restriction is only necessary if the client is oliguric and azotemic. Fluid balance is best evaluated by changes in weight as well as by record of intake and output, and both should be monitored daily.

Elevations in blood pressure may be associated with fluid excess. Antihypertensive drugs and diuretics may be used to lower the blood pressure.

Rest and activity. When the client is not feeling well during the acute phase, activity is usually self-limited and bed rest appropriate for recovery. Later, as the child feels better, ambulation and activity can be encouraged as the child tolerates. Bed rest also facilitates lowering of the blood pressure, which may be elevated during the acute phase.

Comfort. The nurse or parent can help the child be comfortable during the course of the illness. Daily hygiene routines and quiet play activities can be encouraged.

Complications of acute glomerulonephritis. Hypertension, cardiac decompensation, hypertensive encephalopathy, and acute renal failure are rare complications of AGN caused by hypervolemia or hypertension and require hospitalization for medical and nursing management.

Hypertension is managed with salt and water restriction and the administration of reserpine. Hydralazine may also be used. Cardiac decompensation, like hypertension, requires salt and water restriction. Furosemide (Lasix) may be given to reduce fluid overload, and digitalis may be tried to enhance cardiac efficiency. Oxygen and morphine will usually be used if pulmonary edema becomes evident. Peritoneal dialysis with hypertonic solutions is reserved primarily for children who do not respond to the other modes of management. Hypertensive encephalopathy with seizures requires emergency management to lower the blood pressure. Diazoxide (Hyperstat), diazepam (Valium), and barbiturates are drugs of choice. Renal failure requires control of fluid, protein, sodium, and potassium intake, and the correction of metabolic acidosis. Sodium-potassium exchange resins may be tried before using peritoneal or hemodialysis.

 Evaluation. Evaluation of the nursing care for a client with acute glomerulonephritis is an ongoing component of the nursing process as the client progresses from the acute phase of illness to recovery.

EXPECTED OUTCOMES

The client and/or family can:
1. Describe poststreptococcal acute glomerulonephritis.
2. Describe plans for maintaining fluid balance, including use of drugs and diets.
3. State use, dosage, time, route, and side effects of prescribed medications (antihypertensive drugs, diuretics).
4. State diet modifications (sodium restrictions, protein restrictions, fluid restrictions).

5. State plans for health maintenance, including rest and adequate fluids.
6. State plans for prevention of infection.
7. State plans for follow-up health care.

Nephrosis (nephrotic syndrome)

Nephrosis is a syndrome that may be an outcome of renal disorders (primarily glomerulonephritis) in which there are proteinuria, hypoalbuminuria, edema, and hyperlipidemia. There are three types of the syndrome. In the inherited type *(congenital nephrotic syndrome),* the clients are small for gestational age, do not respond to treatment, and usually die within 2 years. *Secondary nephrotic syndrome* occurs after known glomerular disease such as glomerulonephritis, collagen diseases, toxicity to drugs, sickle cell disease, or diabetes mellitus. However, over 80% of nephrotic syndrome in children is *idiopathic,* occuring in young children 2 to 3 years of age. This type of nephrosis is discussed here.

Pathophysiology. The major pathological changes in nephrosis occur at the basement membrane of the glomerulus. The initiating event is not known but is speculated to be an antigen-antibody reaction or biochemical change that causes increased basement membrane permeability. Increased permeability allows protein, particularly albumin, to pass through the membrane (5 to 15 g protein in 24 hours). Hypoalbuminemia decreases colloid osmotic pressure and draws fluid

FIG. 19-12
General schema for pathogenesis of nephrotic syndrome. (From James, John A.: Renal disease in childhood, ed. 3, St. Louis, 1976, The C.V. Mosby Co.)

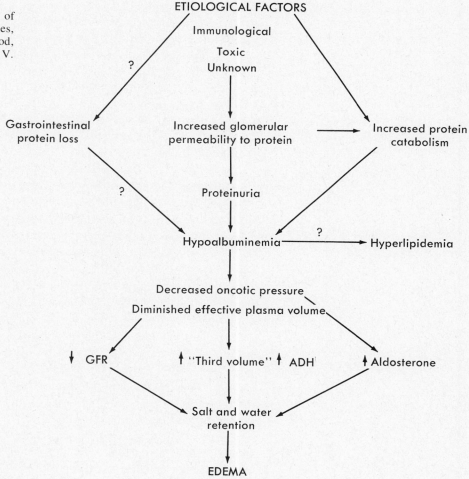

Nursing process for common health problems

out of the vascular compartments into interstitial spaces, resulting in edema. Hypovolemia also decreases renal plasma flow and glomerular filtration rate, activating the renin-angiotensin mechanism as well as volume receptors in the left atrium. The increased aldosterone and ADH responding to low volume cause salt and water retention, compounding edema. Hyperlipidemia also occurs, and serum cholesterol, triglycerides, and phospholipids may be increased as well, although the cause remains unknown (Fig. 19-12).

 Assessment. The nurse may be able to assess the changes in the young client brought about by fluid shift in the tissues. The child typically begins to gain weight over a period of several weeks. There may be puffiness around the eyes (periorbital edema), which may be noticed in the morning but disappears during the day, when edema in the abdomen and lower extremities is more evident. Pleural effusion and scrotal or labial edema are late signs. Diarrhea from intestinal mucosa edema may be noted. The skin may be susceptible to breakdown, and the client appears pale, lethargic, and irritable. The client is often malnourished, but major indications are masked by edema; subtle cues are loss of appetite and changes in the luster of the hair. Urinary output is decreased, and the urine is dark and frothy.

The diagnosis is confirmed by laboratory analysis of blood and urine. Total serum proteins are reduced, and serum cholesterol and plasma lipids are elevated. Hemoglobin and hematocrit are normal because of hemoconcentration. A low serum sodium level, proteinuria, and the presence of hyaline casts, red blood cells, and fat bodies are characteristic of the urinalysis. Renal biopsy may demonstrate glomerulosclerosis, nephritis, and membranous nephropathy.

> **Data analysis**
> *Data analysis may reveal nursing diagnoses of alterations in urinary elimination and alterations in fluid volume: excess.*

 Planning and implementation. The goal of medical therapy is to maintain a protein-free urine, prevent infection, and restore nutrition. Nursing plans are developed with the client and family to restore urinary elimination, restore fluid balance, promote nutrition, prevent infection, and provide a balance of sleep and activity. During the acute edema stage the client is hospitalized and may be subsequently treated at home.

Reducing urinary protein excretion. Steroid therapy is instituted to promote diuresis and maintain protein-free urine. Prednisone is most often used and given until the urine is free of protein for 10 to 14 days. Diuresis does not occur for several days, and it may take up to 4 weeks to be protein-free. Response to steroids often determines the course of the disease. Those who respond favorably (20% to 40%) are termed *steroid sensitive* and usually do not have recurrences; those who respond but have recurrences (60% to 80%) are termed *steroid dependent*. Five to ten percent of individuals with nephrosis are *steroid resistant* and ultimately have chronic renal failure.

Because steroids are used over a period of time, the nurse and parent must monitor side effects and the course of therapy. As the child responds to therapy with decreased proteinuria, the steroids are tapered gradually. Because the child may be cared for at home, the parents require explicit instructions for use of the drug.

Immunosuppressive drugs such as cyclophosphamide (Cytoxan) may be used with or as an alternative to steroid therapy. The nurse and parent must also monitor side effects of this drug, particularly leukopenia. If the drug is used on a long-term basis, aspermia and lack of oogenesis are risks.

Proteinuria can be evaluated by urinalysis. The nurse can monitor albuminuria and specific gravity to evaluate changes, because steroids cause diuresis and protein-free urine.

Fluid balance. Edema of nephrosis is usually resistant to diuretic therapy, but diuretics that reduce sodium retention, such as spironolactone, may be used. Salt-poor albumin may also be used for plasma-expanding properties. Low-sodium diets may be used to prevent additional fluid retention during the acute edema stage, but do not promote diuresis. Fluids may be restricted when there is massive edema. Fluid loss can be evaluated by recording intake, output, and daily weights.

Nutrition. Nutritional reserves may be slowly depleted, and attention must be directed toward restoring adequate nutritional intake. A high-protein, well-balanced diet is encouraged unless the child has azotemia and renal failure and protein is contraindicated. During the acute stage the client may be anorexic, and the nurse and parents should encourage the client as appropriate.

Infection. Because gamma globulin levels are low, the child is prone to infection. The nurse, client, and family can plan to use asepsis to prevent spread of disease. Antibiotics may be used prophylactically. Clients receiving steroids or immunosuppressant therapy are also susceptible to infection and must be observed closely.

Sleep and activity. During the acute stage the client is fatigued and is placed on bed rest. Later, as edema subsides, the child may increase activity as tolerated. During periods of bed rest the nurse and parents can turn the client, positioning his edematous body comfortably. Bone demineralization from steroid use is a hazard, and the client must not be immobile for long periods of time.

Discharge instructions. Because the cause of nephrosis may involve remissions and exacerbations, the parents can be instructed to manage care at home. Specific information should include use of drugs and diet and activity restrictions. The parents must also be encouraged to maintain health and hygiene practices favorable to preventing infections.

Evaluation. The course of nephrosis may include exacerbations and remissions, and evaluation of nursing care is appropriate at both stages. Nursing diagnoses of urinary elimination, fluid balance, and nutrition are salient.

EXPECTED OUTCOMES

The client and/or family can:
1. Describe nephrosis.
2. Recognize indications of nephrosis (weight gain, edema of eyes, abdomen, dark urine).
3. State diet modifications (sodium restrictions, high-protein diet, fluid restrictions, if necessary).
4. State use, dosage, time, route, and side effects of prescribed medications (steroids, immunosuppressants).
5. Describe activity and rest plans.
6. Monitor fluid intake and test urine for albuminuria.

7. Describe health maintenance activities for preventing infection.
8. State plans for follow-up health care.

Wilms' tumor

Wilms' tumor (nephroblastoma) is an adenosarcoma of the kidney usually occurring in children under 3 years of age. This neoplasm is a result of a defect in embryological development, which becomes manifest after birth as carcinoma. It may be unilateral or bilateral, and it affects each gender with equal incidence.

Wilms' tumor is usually discovered as a smooth, firm, tender mass in the abdomen. Low-grade fever and nausea may accompany the rapidly growing mass. Diagnosis by intravenous pyelogram and an excretory urogram must be prompt. Abdominal x-ray films or a retrograde pyelogram may also be of assistance in discovery of the mass, usually evident by a distorted kidney pelvis.

Wilms' tumor essentially constitutes an emergency, and if it is unilateral, the affected kidney should be removed without delay. Palpating the tumor and excessive handling of the client should be avoided because they favor metastasis. Prognosis is good if the tumor is discovered and treated early with surgery (nephrectomy), radiation, and chemotherapy.

COMMON HEALTH PROBLEMS OF THE ADULT

Strictures

Strictures may occur at any point along the urinary tract, resulting in an interference with the flow of urine. They may be caused by local defects in the tissue or spasmodic contractions of a neurological origin. Treatment is directed toward the cause.

Common modes of management include dilations with instruments or catheters of increasing size over a prolonged period of time, surgical incision, or plastic repair.

Renal calculi

The most common source of mechanical disturbances in the urinary tract is a result of calculi. Calculi (or stones) create obstructions to the flow of urine within the renal system. The site of the blockage and whether it is partial or complete will influence symptom development.

Urinary stasis tends to predispose to calculi formation. Certain urea-splitting organisms (*E coli, Proteus* organisms, *Staphylococcus* organisms, and *Streptococcus* organisms) tend to make the urine alkaline and thus encourage stone formation, because calcium phosphate (a constituent of calculi) is relatively insoluble in an alkaline medium. Stone formation requries that crystals must coalesce, or there must be a nidus for stone formation such as pus, blood, tumors, or a foreign body, for example, a catheter or tumor.[6]

Some urologists think that vitamin A deficiency, certain endocrine disorders, long-term recumbency, and even the mineral content of a drinking water supply can predispose to calculi.

 Assessment. Symptoms of calculi result from stone movement or its creation of an obstruction in the urinary passages.

Calculi in the calyx can interfere with renal pelvis drainage or can be large enough to create pressure, thus damaging parenchyma as well as obstructing urinary flow. Stones in the ureter can cause hydronephrosis by obstructing renal pelvis outflow (Fig. 19-13). Bladder stones can interfere with ureteral as well as urethral flow of urine in addition to creating a pressurelike sensation in the lower abdomen, especially if they are large. Calculi usually are formed elsewhere in the tract, but may become lodged in the urethra. They obstruct urinary outflow in

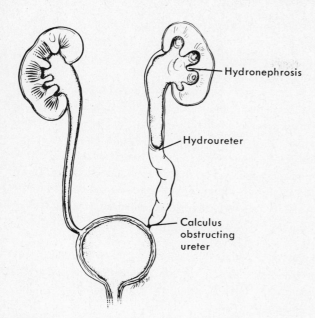

FIG. 19-13
Hydroureter and hydronephrosis as result of calculus's obstructing ureter.

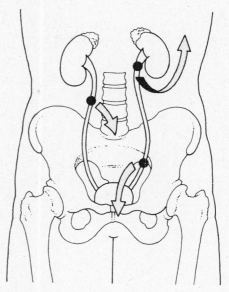

FIG. 19-14
Path of radiation of pain in renal colic is characteristic and serves to differentiate this problem from several other acute abdominal conditions. (From Budassi, Susan A., and Barber, Janet M.: Emergency nursing: principles and practice, St. Louis, 1981, The C.V. Mosby Co.)

addition to creating dysuria and pain, and require surgical removal via cystoscopy.

The client with urinary calculi will have flank or costovertebral pain that is colicky and excruciating. It may radiate to the abdomen, scrotum, or labia (Fig. 19-14). The client's face may appear ashen, and diaphoresis is pronounced. There is no comfortable position for the individual to assume. The need to void is frequently noted. Nausea, vomiting, low-grade fever, paralytic ileus, hematuria, tachycardia, and hypotension are also associated with the classic picture of renal colic.

The majority of stones are easily localized with radiological studies of the urinary tract. Small, sandylike particles that commonly suggest calculi formation may be identified by straining all urine. Hematuria, especially when accompanied by pain, may strongly indicate trauma from the movement of a calculi.

Data analysis
Data analysis may reveal nursing diagnoses of altered patterns of urinary elimination and alterations in comfort.

Planning and implementation. Calculi may be surgically removed via general surgery or cystoscopy. Large renal pelvis stones or bladder stones may require excision of the organ. Smaller stones may be crushed (via cystoscopy) and permitted to be eliminated with urinary outflow. A 10% Renacidin solution is used in some instances to decrease urine alkalinity and to dissolve calcium or phosphate deposits.[6]

Acid ash diets and high fluid intake are encouraged for many clients, because they tend to discourage calculi formation.

Individuals with colic often require hospitalization and the administration of narcotic analgesics as well as antispasmodic drugs. Agents may also be given to control the accompanying nausea and vomiting.

Clients with renal calculi are extremely prone to subsequent stone formation. They are urged to adhere to special diets and a high fluid intake for the remainder of their lives. Select individuals who are prone to calcium stones may need to curtail their dietary intake of calcium. If stones form in acid urine, an alkaline ash diet is prescribed; if they form in alkaline urine, an acid ash diet is prescribed. Drugs such as potassium acid phosphate or ascorbic acid may also be used to influence urine pH.

Clients who must remain on special dietary regimens will need support from the nurse and guidance in adhering to the prescription. Teaching must necessarily include information concerning exercise, which will minimize bone decalcification and enhance renal function.

 Evaluation. Evaluation of the nursing care plan for the client with renal calculi focuses on objectives for managing pain and promoting urinary elimination.

EXPECTED OUTCOMES

The client and/or family can:

1. Describe renal calculi.
2. State plans for promoting urinary elimination, including adequate intake of fluids (up to 4 liters per day) and frequent emptying of the bladder.
3. State diet modifications if required (acid ash, alkaline ash, calcium restrictions).
4. State use, dosage, time, route, and side effects of prescribed medications (analgesics, drugs used to alkalinize or acidify urine).
5. Describe methods for managing pain, including use of analgesics, antispasmodics, and relaxation exercises.
6. State indications for health care (pain, dysuria, hematuria).
7. State plans for follow-up health care.

Tumors   Tumors of the urinary tract may be primary or the result of metastasis. Prostatic lesions have the highest incidence of all malignancies of the genitourinary organs. Renal tumors are responsible for only 2% of cancer deaths; Wilms' tumor and hypernephroma are most commonly seen, although their incidence is low.

The onset of *renal tumors* is insidious because they grow slowly and produce few symptoms. Until the renal pelvis is eroded and hematuria ensues, no indications of disease are noticeable. Furthermore, symptoms may occur once and not return for months or even years. It is essential to emphasize that clients should be made aware of the importance of tracing the origin of all urinary tract symptoms or generalized disturbances that cannot be explained.

Bladder tumors are rare but may occur at any age. They are three times more common in men. Symptoms are hematuria, fever, cystitis, and obstruction to the flow of urine. Cystoscopy with a biopsy is the usual method of diagnosis, although a cystogram is helpful in delineating the mass. The other parts of the urinary tract are studied concurrently to determine whether the lesion may be an extension or an implant from another site of involvement.

Methods of management include surgery, irradiation, and chemotherapy by pelvic profusion, or by the local application of alkylating agents such as Thio-TEPA by catheter instillation.

COMMON HEALTH PROBLEMS OF THE OLDER ADULT

Through adult life there is little change in urinary functioning until the sixties or seventies, when blood flow to the kidneys declines and there is a decrease in the number of functional nephrons. Central nervous system degeneration may cause impairment of visceral reflexes that also help control urination. If the cerebral cortex has been affected, voiding may necessarily depend on visceral reflex. As reflex bladder emptying replaces voluntary control, the bladder loses its tone and becomes smaller. There is subsequently frequent urgency and a shortening of the warning period, which denotes the need to void. Bladder contraction occurs early in the filling stage. Retention is also common in elderly clients, especially when there are mechanical dysfunctions in the urinary tract or adjacent structures.

Stress incontinence

This condition results from relaxed pelvic musculature, causing incontinence during periods of increased cystic pressure as induced by coughing, laughing, or straining.

Frequent pregnancies or obstetrical trauma may contribute to weakening of pelvic supports, thus interfering with bladder and urethral suspension.

Surgical correction of bladder and urethral support and sphincter exercises usually will correct the problem.

Prostatic hypertrophy or neoplasm

If neoplastic growth (either benign or malignant) creates prostatic enlargement, there will be difficulty or even obstruction to voiding. Surgical removal or reduction of the prostate is required to maintain elimination efficiency and to ensure complete bladder emptying at each voiding (see Chapter 12).

COMMON HEALTH PROBLEMS THAT OCCUR ACROSS THE LIFE SPAN

Urinary tract infections

Urinary tract infections are common to individuals of all ages, but may have significant differences in cause and management in children and adults. Urinary tract infections can occur throughout the lower and upper urinary tracts. Infections of the lower urinary tract include urethritis and cystitis, whereas those of the upper urinary tract involve the kidney (pyelonephritis).

Because of the proximity of the urethra and the vaginal and rectal orifices, the incidence of infections is considerably higher in girls and women. Infants are affected more often than older children, and elderly clients are susceptible to inflammation and infection of the urinary tract.

Pathophysiology. Organisms from the bowel (*E coli, Aerobacter aerogenes, Bacillus proteus, Pseudomonas aeruginosa,* and enterococci) are responsible for most infections.

Infection may be descending or ascending (Fig. 19-15). *Descending* infections are bloodborne and occur as a result of an infectious process elsewhere in the body, especially in situations involving staphylococcal and streptococcal organisms. However, when the urinary tract is healthy, bacteria will not be filtered from the bloodstream, and urine from the kidneys, ureters, and bladder should be sterile.[5] *Ascending* infections climb to the bladder and even to the ureters and kidneys.

It is suspected that the overwhelming number of urinary tract infections in *adults* occur as a result of urethral ascent of bacteria. The male urethra is longer than the female urethra, and prostatic secretions seem to be effective against invading organisms, thus accounting for the higher incidence of infection in women. Female sexual activity also seems to contribute to inflammatory processes of the urinary tract. It is not uncommon for women to develop successive episodes of cystitis (inflammation of the bladder) with initiation of sexual intercourse, strongly suggesting that urethral ascension of organisms is partially responsible for the pathogenesis. Contamination from feces or the vaginal canal by poor perineal hygiene is responsible for many infections, especially in *children* and *older adults*.

Trauma to the external urinary meatus, especially in women, can create urethritis and ultimately cystitis from swelling and inflammation. Excessive friction to the urethra during intercourse or continued contact with undergarments or soiled sanitary napkins favors invasion of organisms.

The proximity of the female urethra and the vaginal canal can foster *cross infection,* because they are separated by only a tiny layer of tissue. Vaginal infections, especially those that cause considerable drainage, often are precursors to ascending urinary tract infections.

Instrumentation is a common cause of irritation and inflammation of the urinary tract and is usually avoidable. Catheterization and cystoscopy frequently are followed by an infection. Catheterization only for obtaining a specimen is discouraged by most authorities. Despite excellent techniques, infections seem to develop easily after *instrumentation,* which undoubtedly traumatizes the delicate mucosal lining of the urethra that ordinarily serves as a good protective barrier against bacterial invasion.

Urethrovesical reflux occurs when urine that has been forced into the urethra by a sudden increase of pressure in the bladder subsequently flows back into the bladder when the pressure returns to normal. Bacteria from the urethra are thus washed into the bladder and serve as a potential source of cystitis. This phenomenon can also occur during sexual intercourse, intermittent voiding from mechanical obstructions, or as a result of spasms at the bladder neck or in the urethra.

Bacteria in the bladder have little chance to cause infection if the urinary tract is healthy. Even when there are organisms in the cystic structure, usually they are (1) promptly destroyed by the urine properties, (2) inhibited by the antibacterial state of the bladder mucosa, (3) consumed by phagocytosis, or (4) eliminated by urination.[5]

Unfortunately, however, even the most efficient bladder-emptying leaves behind a film of urine that allows organisms to multiply rapidly before the next voiding. This problem is compounded for clients with residual urine.

Vesicoureteral reflux (urine washing from the bladder to the ureter during voiding) is a cause of ascending urinary tract infections and is responsible for creating a pool of residual urine after each voiding (Fig. 19-16). A voiding cinecystourethrogram, which permits visualization of the reflux phenomenon, confirms the pathology of reflux. Most urologists believe that all clients experience reflux to some extent but not seriously enough to promote urinary tract dysfunction. Clinical research has established that there is usually a fluid connection between the renal pelvis and the bladder, and that reverse peristalsis could transport bacteria up the ureter.

Other factors that seem to be positively related to the incidence of urinary tract infections are diabetes, the process of aging, and mechanical obstruction of the upper urinary tract. Cause-and-effect relationships are poorly understood, but research is continuing to define the etiological phenomena.

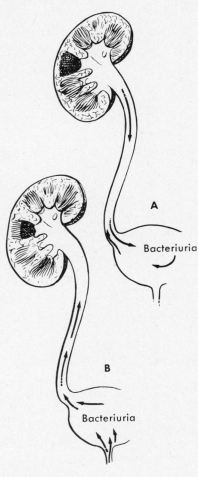

FIG. 19-15
A, Bacteriuria may be maintained by "seeding" of urine from foci of infection in kidney. **B,** Ascending route of infection. Pathogenic bacteria from external sources ascend urethra and ureters to cause bacteriuria.

Assessment. The nurse can assess the client's usual urinary habits during the nursing history.

Infants with urinary tract infections experience fever, vomiting, diarrhea, anorexia, and even jaundice. Older *children* tend to exhibit fever, chills, abdominal or flank pain, and malaise. Occasionally a urinary tract infection is asymptomatic, and the only clue that may suggest infection is failure to thrive.

If the urinary tract infection is predominantly affecting the lower urinary tract, there is frequency, dysuria, suprapubic pain, and general difficulty in voiding. The urine usually has a disagreeable odor and may contain blood or pus cells.

Indications of urinary tract infection in *adults* are similar and usually noted by frequency, dysuria, flank pain, and urinary retention. Cystitis and pyelonephritis are common.

Cystitis (inflammation of the bladder) is the most common source of urinary tract infection. The bladder becomes irritated, and frequency, urgency, dysuria, and bladder spasms occur. The bladder walls may bleed when the inflammation is severe, and gross hematuria may be present.

Pyelonephritis (inflammation of the kidney and its pelvis) may be caused by descending bloodborne organisms, but usually is linked to primary lower urinary tract infection. Flank pain, muscle spasms, chills, fever, and dysuria may be present. In severe infections, particularly those of a chronic nature, abdominal distension, vomiting, anemia, hypertension, and other signs of decreased kidney function may be apparent.

Pyelonephritis is usually unilateral and may follow manipulation, obstruction, or trauma to the urinary tract. The most frequent cause is probably obstruction, and it is removed by surgery or bypassed by perirenal drainage such as nephrostomy. Occasionally it proceeds to renal destruction or pain, and hematuria exists to the extent that a unilateral nephrectomy is performed. This infection of the kidneys is most serious, and if allowed to become chronic, it can lead to permanent renal damage from nephron loss.

Urinalysis, urine culture, and quantitative colony count are important to diagnosis. Intravenous pyelography and cystoscopic studies may also be useful adjuncts.

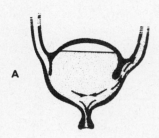
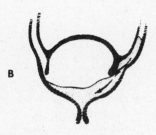

FIG. 19-16
A, Vesicoureteral reflux. During voiding, urine is forced up ureter if vesicoureteral valve is impaired and cannot shut tightly. **B,** When voiding ceases, urine refluxed into the ureter returns to bladder, and thus a pool of residual urine is produced (that is, voiding never completely empties bladder).

Data analysis
Data analysis may reveal nursing diagnoses of altered urinary elimination patterns, alterations in comfort, and noncompliance.

Planning and implementation. Sulfonamides and broad-spectrum antibiotics are drugs of choice in treating urinary tract infections while awaiting results of sensitivity studies. The elimination of bacteriuria usually requires 10 to 14 days of drug therapy. Phenazopyridine hydrochloride (Pyridium), a bladder analgesic, may be used for symptomatic relief of dysuria. Sitz baths may be used for relief of the discomforts of urethritis.

Individuals with urinary tract infections must understand the importance of following their drug therapy regimen and consuming sufficient liquids to keep micturition processes stimulated up to 4 liters per day, thus flushing out organisms that could multiply if allowed to remain for long periods of time within the bladder.

It is essential that all clients be taught signs and symptoms of developing urinary tract infections and that they seek medical attention early for definitive management. Gram-negative septicemia and renal failure are serious consequences of untreated urinary tract infections.

The nurse can instruct the client about promoting healthy urinary habits. Emphasis can be given to cleansing the perineum after defecation, voiding before and after intercourse, and avoiding bladder stasis by assuring adequate intake of fluids and voiding frequently, as often as every 2 to 3 hours while awake.

Evaluation. Evaluation of the nursing care plan is ongoing as the client recovers from the urinary tract infection.

EXPECTED OUTCOMES

The client and/or family can:
1. Describe urinary tract infection.
2. State plans for promoting urinary elimination, including adequate intake of fluids, frequent voiding, hygiene measures, and hygiene related to sexual activity.
3. State use, dosage, time, route, and side effects of prescribed medications (antibiotics, sulfonamides, urinary tract antiseptics and analgesics). State necessity for taking drug as long as prescribed.
4. State indications for health care, including pain, dysuria, hematuria, frequency, urinary retention.
5. State plans for follow-up health care.

Kidney infection

When infection invades the parenchyma of the kidney, it seems to remain confined to a wedge-shaped section unless there is extrarenal urinary tract obstruction such as a stone or tumor. In this latter case the acute infection pervades the entire kidney.[5] Urinary tract obstructions must be considered as a serious threat to the viability of a kidney. Intrarenal obstruction such as in the medullary portion of the nephron spreads quickly, and the cortex becomes involved, causing an extensive surface area to be adversely affected. (Remember that the wedge's apex is in the medulla, a small area as it relates to the surrounding cortex, Fig. 19-17.) Furthermore, the cortex is extraordinarily resistant to infection. As few as 10 bacteria can cause infection in the medulla, but up to 100,000 or more may be necessary to evoke infection in the cortex.[5]

The fate of organisms in the kidney is not well understood, and much speculation and animal experimentation revolve around the subject. There seems to be evidence of environmental phenomena that affect the viability of bacteria, and these may act on the organism itself or influence the host's defense mechanisms. Acidification of urine by ascorbic acid ingestion or certain drugs alters physiological responses to bacteria and discourages their multiplication, although these conditions do not cure the infection. Water diuresis (forcing liquids) is a fundamental part of the regimen relating to urinary tract infection. The theoretical basis has only recently been understood. It seems that extra fluids (1) change tonicity of the environment, reducing chances for bacterial survival; (2) increase blood flow and the availability of white blood cells; and (3) lower osmotic pressure and thus enhance the efficacy of the host's defense mechanisms.

The dilemma in diuresis exists because there is *not* strong clinical evidence that it is valuable consistently in infections such as pyelonephritis and that considerable diluting of antibiotics occurs, reducing their effectiveness.

1062

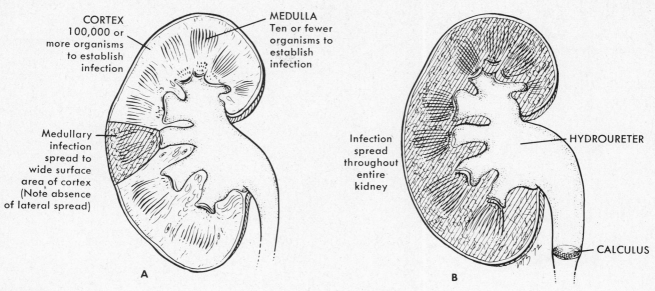

FIG. 19-17
A, Infected kidney without lateral spread of infection. Note wedge shape characteristic of medullary infection. Note also variation of vulnerability to infection of cortex and medulla. **B,** Obstruction of calculus causes infection to pervade entire renal parenchyma. Note resultant hydroureter from prolonged distension.

Neurogenic disorders affecting the urinary tract

The innervation that controls micturition is complex and is not completely understood. It is known, however, that the parasympathetic afferent fibers carry sensory impulses of the desire to void and the parasympathetic efferent fibers carry the motor impulses, making the act possible. The necessary reflex connections are thought to be in the second, third, and fourth sacral cord segments.

As the bladder fills, the sensory endings inform the client of the need to void. If it is not the proper time or place to micturate, inhibitory mechanisms from the cerebral cortex intervene, and there is voluntary control of the external sphincter. When conditions are socially correct for voiding, a series of impulses allow sphincter and perineal muscle relaxation, and thus the bladder empties. Abdominal and diaphragm muscles may assist in the act.

Children who are toilet trained feel the urge to void when their bladder contains 200 to 400 ml. The adult perceives the need for micturition at 300 to 500 ml. Since the bladder is easily distensible, adults may retain well over 1000 ml. However, such distension may cause nerve tissue trauma and result in loss of bladder tone. Clients should be instructed to empty their bladders at the first feeling of the need to void, if possible, to prevent tissue damage and bladder stasis.

There are several types of neurogenic bladders, each with its own etiology, manifestations, and appropriate intervention (Table 19-2).

Neurogenic bladder can result from congenital anomalies such as myelomeningocele, from degenerative disorders of the central and peripheral nervous systems, and from several types of cord injuries. Regardless of the cause, there is loss of continence. Voluntary control of micturition can be absent or undependable. Retention with overflow, dribbling, incomplete emptying of bladder, and precipitous or frequent voiding may occur. Bladder muscle tone is usually, but not always, impaired.

1063

TABLE 19-2

The neurogenic bladder

Type	Voluntary control	Condition of bladder; muscle tone	Bladder capacity	Micturition
Sensory atonic	Absent	Flaccid and distended; myogenic tone decreased	Considerably increased	Early stage—incomplete emptying Late stage—overflow incontinence; dribbling
Motor atonic	Absent	Flaccid and distended; myogenic tone decreased	Considerably increased	Early stage—incomplete emptying; sense of distention Late stage—overflow incontinence; dribbling
Autonomous	Absent	Myogenic tone preserved	Variable—may be increased or somewhat reduced	Early stage—inability to void; distended bladder Late stage—dribbling and straining
Reflex (automatic)	Absent	Variable—may be below normal, normal, or above normal	Variable—may be reduced or increased	Early stage—inability to void Late stage—reflex and precipitous urination
Uninhibited	Maintained by external sphincter but often insufficient to preserve continence	Normal	Decreased	Precipitous and frequent

Incontinence is of four major types: (1) *true* incontinence, where urine is not retained in the bladder and there is constant dribbling; (2) overflow incontinence, where the bladder is full, with constant dribbling; (3) *urgency* incontinence, where a small amount of urine is present in the bladder but the need to void is perceived as great; and (4) *stress* incontinence, where urine is expelled on sudden increase in the abdominal pressure (such as from laughing, coughing, or lifting). Weak supporting structures of the vesical neck, the results of surgery or obstetrical trauma, are usually among the causes.

There are several ways in which nurses can help clients achieve continence or at least improve their voiding pattern through a training program. However, before intervention and instruction can be planned, it is essential to determine the functioning of the bladder by cystometry.

Cystometric studies. Cystometric studies are designed to graphically measure the behavior of the bladder during filling and subsequent voiding. An apparatus similar to that used for continuous bladder irrigation is used. The client is asked to empty his bladder as completely as possible, and then a catheter is introduced to drain any residual urine, which is reserved for measuring. The catheter is then attached to a manometer and irrigating tubing. Sterile solution is dripped into the bladder until the first urge to void is reported. This measurement is noted as it relates to intrabladder pressure and milliliters of fluid in the bladder. The drip is continued until the urge to void is strong. This measurement is also noted, and the test continues until urgency and discomfort are experienced. When 500 to 600 ml are reached, even if no perception of the need to micturate is reported, the test is concluded so that the bladder is not injured (Fig. 19-18).

Residual urine	Infection	Etiology	Responsible conditions	Comment
Large volume	Common	Loss of sensory supply to bladder, as in lesions of posterior roots and columns	Acute (shock) stage of spinal injury; tabes dorsalis; diabetic radiculitis; subacute combined sclerosis	With the subsidence of spinal shock this type will merge into the reflex bladder unless severe myogenic disturbance has occurred through overdistention
Large volume	Common	Loss of motor supply to bladder, as in lesions of anterior horns and roots of sacral segments 3 and 4	May be part of the picture of spinal shock or occur in acute poliomyelitis	This type of bladder disturbance is also susceptible to myogenic disturbance, as above, but usually not to such severe degree
Present, usually in small or moderate amounts	Generally present	Complete interruption of reflex arc when both the sensory and motor components are destroyed	Traumatic lesions of sacral cord or conus; spina bifida manifesta; traumatic lesion of nervi erigentes	Patient may be able to express some urine by straining or manual compression
Present in variable amounts, depending on muscle tone of bladder	Often present	Complete interruption of upper motor neuron control; spinal arc present	Traumatic lesions of spinal cord above sacral level (after period of shock); spinal cord tumor; multiple sclerosis	Patient may discover "trigger areas" for induction of micturition
None	Not present	Loss of cerebral inhibitory control	Cerebral arteriosclerosis; brain tumor; brain injury; incomplete lesions of spinal cord; delayed development of cerebral inhibitory mechanism	This type shows least variance from normal bladder activity

Although the neurologist or urologist usually performs cystometric studies, the nurse may be asked to actively participate and therefore should understand the test and its implications.

Intermittent catheter drainage. The generally accepted mode of training the neurogenic bladder is by the use of intermittent catheterization. This technique has largely replaced continuous drainage or intermittent catheter clamping and drainage. The value of this newest approach is that it eliminates residual urine and avoids distension of the bladder walls, both of which invite infection. When bladder walls are stretched, the blood supply to the total surface area is reduced. This factor, in conjunction with stagnant urine, serves as an excellent medium for the rapid multiplication of bacteria.

Intermittent catheterization is usually done as a clean, not sterile, procedure, and is part of a client's self-care program. Individuals who are candidates for this instruction must be carefully evaluated to ensure their physical and psychological capabilities for dependably following the protocol. They furthermore must have the capacity to learn what is expected of them and the desire to be independent.

The procedure is treated as a sterile procedure during hospitalization to reduce the possibility of a nosocomial infection. (Certain clients may continue with a "clean" technique if they have been managed at home with it and are not too ill to continue self-care. Sterile catheters are used during hospital stays, too, unless the "clean" catheter can be stored in a closed container and isolated from sources of urinary tract organisms.)

The nurse instructs the client about the essential anatomy and the necessity for careful hand washing before catheterization. One must ensure, too, that there

1065

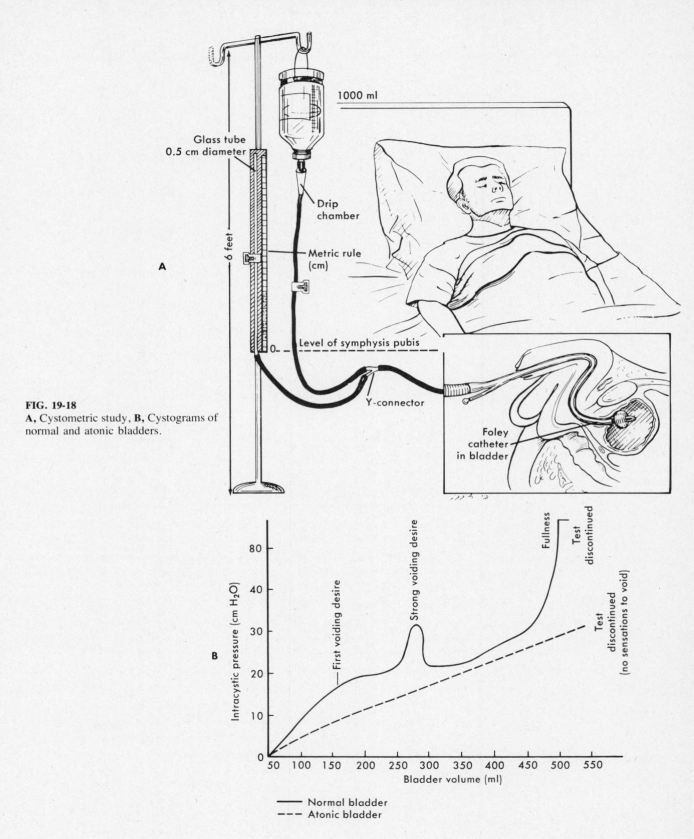

1000 ml

Glass tube
0.5 cm diameter

Drip
chamber

6 feet

Metric rule
(cm)

A

Level of symphysis pubis

0

Y-connector

Foley
catheter
in bladder

FIG. 19-18
A, Cystometric study, **B,** Cystograms of
normal and atonic bladders.

B

Intracystic pressure (cm H$_2$O)

First voiding desire

Strong voiding desire

Fullness

Test
discontinued

Test
discontinued
(no sensations to void)

Bladder volume (ml)

Normal bladder
Atonic bladder

is a good understanding about the necessity of adhering to a regular schedule for completely emptying the bladder. A typical schedule is every 3 to 4 hours during waking hours and at night on an "as needed" basis. The frequency of catheterization will depend on the amount of urine obtained at each catheterization. If high volumes are typically drained, the frequency may be increased to every other hour.

The client must have a good understanding of the signs and symptoms of urinary tract infection. The urine should be inspected as well as measured after each voiding, noting color, clarity, and odor. Most physicians will periodically request a sterile catheterized specimen for culture and sensitivity to detect any developing problems. A few prefer, in addition, to maintain the client on long-term antibiotic therapy.

The procedure is uncomplicated and can be easily learned by most individuals. Only a few steps are required:

1. Hand washing
2. Meatal cleansing with soap and water
3. Inserting the catheter and draining the bladder
4. Removing the catheter and measuring the urine
5. Washing the catheter in soap and water
6. Storing the catheter in a clean, closed container

(Catheters are reused until they become less pliable or develop defects.)

The nurse should assure the client that the procedure can be done safely in various positions. Women usually choose to sit on a commode. Men may prefer standing, however. The use of a lubricant is optional, but men may prefer one to minimize urethral irritation.

While preparing the client for self-care, the nurse must be certain to explain how to obtain supplies, offer suggestions about incorporating the procedure into daily life-style, and describe the exact steps to be taken in an emergency or problematic situation. A few clients may be instructed in the use of a sterile procedure. In such instances, more extensive follow-up on teaching is necessary to ensure compliance to sterile technique.

The use of intermittent catheter drainage is a valuable approach to neurogenic bladder dysfunction, but requires careful teaching, follow-up, and client support.

Alternatives for the client. Alternative ways of controlling voiding may need to be tried. One involves perceiving physiological responses associated with voiding other than urgency. For example, the client may perceive that he is restless, diaphoretic, and chilly, or he may note upper abdominal fullness. Responding purposefully to these clues may be useful in achieving bladder control.

If the client realizes a full bladder, trigger points may be stimulated, which cause the bladder to contract and empty. Brushing the inner aspects of the thighs or the lower abdomen, pulling pubic hair, and stimulating the anus may be useful.

Another useful technique in some cases of neurogenic bladder is the Credé method. At a determined time when voiding is likely to be occurring (calculated on the basis of fluid intake), manual compression is applied over the suprapubic area. (It is helpful to instruct female clients to bend forward at the hips to augment the effects of this maneuver.) This technique has no dangerous aspects and helps promote complete emptying of the bladder.

1067

Nursing process for common health problems

As with routine childhood toilet training, limiting fluids after the evening meal helps achieve nighttime continence. Alcohol, tea, and coffee should be avoided because they tend to act as diuretics, upsetting the micturition pattern.

Surgical correction or intervention may be required to manage some neurogenic bladders. Urinary diversion, suprapubic cystostomy, or other procedures may be tried to maintain effective drainage of the urinary tract. Ureterosigmoidostomy is not used for clients with paraplegia, however, because control of the anal sphincter has also been lost.

A relatively new concept for reflex bladder emptying consists of implanting a device in the wall of the organ, which can be triggered by an abdominal unit, with resulting micturition (Fig. 19-19).

Children with neurogenic bladders are managed similarly to the adult. However, during periods of rapid growth, relapses may occur, and this phenomenon should be discussed so that the client and his family do not feel like giving up. Persistence and patience are necessary, and mutual understanding of bladder control should be realistically based on physiological potential.

Renal insufficiency or failure

Renal insufficiency or failure can be a sudden and acute problem, or it may occur gradually over an extended period of time. End-stage renal failure is some-

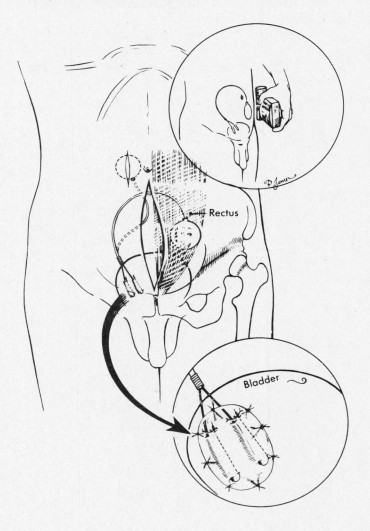

FIG. 19-19
Electronic stimulation of neurogenic bladder. (From Dodson, Austin I.: Urological surgery, ed. 4, St. Louis, 1970, The C.V. Mosby Co.)

Rectus

Bladder

times called *uremic syndrome* or *uremia*. Any degenerative condition of the renal parenchyma can result in this complication.

Pathophysiology. Renal insufficiency or failure occurs when a small number of functioning nephrons are overwhelmed by the body's demands. Renal blood flow is curbed, output is reduced, and urea, potassium, and phosphate levels rise in the blood from inadequate removal of waste products. Water excretion may be greatly reduced, and water overload and salt deficiency are the major *reversible* causes of diminishing renal function, which progresses to total renal insufficiency and eventual death.

There are agents that adversely affect renal function, creating acute or chronic renal failure. The kidney, because of its rich blood supply and involvement with metabolic activities, is especially prone to nephrotoxic substances.

The kidney concentrates and excretes many types of substances that enter the body for inhalation, ingestion, absorption, and injection. Exposure to nephrotoxins can be iatrogenic, accidental, or a suicide attempt.

Damage can be induced by direct toxicity to cells, hypersensitivity, ischemia, or mechanical obstruction.

Toxic substances such as antifreeze, solvents, insecticides, and heavy metals may create renal failure. Certain agents such as antifreeze are converted in the body from ethylene glycol to oxalic acid, which is nephrotoxic. Carbon tetrachloride is especially damaging to renal function, and damage occurs 7 to 10 days after exposure. Chlordane (an insecticide) has been implicated in anuria.

Renal failure can be caused by any condition that causes ischemia, such as anaphylaxis or shock, which produce acute tubular necrosis.

Antibiotics, antimicrobials, radiological contrast media, and certain analgesics can also create renal failure by mechanisms, including acute tubular necrosis, the nephrotic syndrome, glomerulonephritis, or interstitial nephritis.[2] The solubility of these drugs seems to be an important factor in how completely they are excreted. Crystals or sediment they leave behind can obstruct minute glomerular structures.

The nurse can help clients understand the potential hazards just described. For example, persons with diabetes, renal disease, or chronic alcoholism should not take the above-mentioned drugs without medical guidance. All persons using organic solvents should realize their potential hazard, and adequate ventilation must be assured whenever they are employed.

Assessment. Symptoms vary according to the client's age and the acute or chronic nature of the pathological processes.

Acute renal failure is said to occur when the output drops suddenly to less than 400 ml per day. There are three distinct phases in acute renal failure: (1) oliguric, (2) anuric, and (3) polyuric, or recovery. Characteristics and treatment are outlined in Table 19-3.

Azotemia is a term that describes an increase in nitrogenous wastes in the blood *without* a decreased output. Uremia is azotemia that progresses to a symptomatic state. Both azotemia and uremia can occur without oliguria. In such states fluid and electrolyte balance must be maintained solely by intake controls, so careful monitoring of blood and urine chemistries, intake and output, and central venous pressure is imperative. The nurse should understand the mechanisms of renal insufficiency and failure and be alert to signs and symptoms of its development.

1069

TABLE 19-3
Phases of acute renal failure

Phases	Characteristics	Treatment	Rationale
Oliguric	Begins shortly after insult to renal mechanisms; Oliguria with casts, hemoglobinuria, and albuminuria are likely	Sodium bicarbonate	Increases solubility of freed hemoglobin by alkalinization to minimize renal damage
		Osmotic diuresis with mannitol	Is totally filtered at the glomerulus, not reabsorbed by renal tubules; increases urine production and flushes tubules
Anuric	Nitrogenous and sulfate wastes retained with resultant acidosis and fluid overload; client may be edematous due to overhydration	Limitation of fluids to 500 to 1000 ml per day plus amount of urine output of preceding day; weighing of client at least daily	Replaces only fluid lost by insensible losses and excreted via urine; prevents overload
		Diet of high carbohydrate, moderate fat, low protein	Provides for caloric needs but prevents strain on kidneys from excreting nitrogenous wastes; prevents potassium release, which is toxic to insulted kidney
		Continuous ECG and other monitoring of potassium effects	Tissue catabolism liberates potassium; cardiac changes are evident *before* serum levels become markedly elevated
		Intravenous glucose and insulin	Causes potassium to shift to intracellular space
		Polystyrene sodium sulfonate (Kayexalate) and cathartic administration, such as sorbitol	Kayexalate is an exchange resin that binds potassium for gastrointestinal excretion; sorbitol is an osmotic, diarrhea-producing sugar, which aids excretion of resins with adequate fluid content
		Dialysis	Removes urea and other toxic substances from blood
Polyuric	Marked diuresis and electrolyte imbalances	Fluid replacement, as in phase two, with frequent determination of electrolyte values	Renal function not uniform; electrolytes haphazardly wasted

When a child is the victim, *enuresis* may be an initial manifestation. The kidney is unable to concentrate the urine, and the need to void more often is evident. Physical development may be affected because of excessive calcium losses and other changes in blood salts. Growth may be retarded, and leg aches or bone pain are not uncommon. Other symptoms characterizing uremia are to be found in all age groups and embrace not only fluid and electrolyte imbalance but also gastrointestinal, cardiovascular, and nervous system dysfunction.

Nausea and vomiting are thought to be caused by retention of acid and urea. Morning sickness similar to that associated with pregnancy can occur. As these wastes build up in the blood, the client may appear pale and is likely to complain of fatigue and other factors associated with anemia. Some adults have a foul breath and body odor resembling urine. A crystalline substance sometimes forms on the skin in late renal insufficiency and failure, which is referred to as *uremic frost*. It is usually visible on the forehead initially and may become generalized.

Cardiovascular and blood-related diseases include anemia, hypertension, and circulatory impairment. Anemia may be caused by (1) a failure of erythropoietin manufacture (produced primarily by the kidneys), needed to stimulate production of red blood cells, and (2) a reduced life span of red blood cells because of destruction resulting from an elevated BUN. The clotting mechanism is also ineffective, causing problems with easy bruising and hemorrhages throughout the gastrointestinal system. Hypertension occurs often, but complete explanation of the pathological condition is unknown. Circulatory impairment and edema may be progressive and can eventually result in pulmonary edema if they are not controlled. Pericarditis and pleuritis may also accompany renal failure.

Nervous system dysfunction may be evident. Lethargy, irritability, and even psychosis can occur. As the BUN and creatinine levels rise and the blood calcium level falls, tetany and seizures may become manifest. Clients usually progress from a clouded sensorium and drowsiness to coma, concurrent with developing acidosis.

A short, fulminating course of renal insufficiency and failure can result from several causes but is primarily caused by ischemia or the destructive activity of nephrotoxic substances. Conditions that impair normal glomerular blood flow, such as hypotension or allergic manifestations can create a clinical case of renal insufficiency. Prolonged surgical shock, severe dehydration, diabetes, and mismatched blood transfusions may be etiological factors.

The nurse may be the first to observe and interpret signs of an impending renal crisis, such as marked oliguria, edema, elevated blood pressure, and a deteriorating electrolyte status.

Close observation of certain clients should be maintained—for example, those receiving blood transfusions or victims of profound shock. Exposure to organic solvents or heavy metals should be noted. When drugs are prescribed that are known to produce papillary necrosis and scarring, the client's output should be watched, and any abnormality in quality and quantity of urine investigated.

Most persons recover from acute renal insufficiency and failure with no residual renal damage provided they receive prompt and judicious management including dialysis.

> **Data analysis**
> *Data analysis may reveal nursing diagnoses of altered patterns of urinary elimination, altered fluid volume, or knowledge deficit. The nurse and client can make appropriate plans for these problems.*

Planning and implementation. The nursing care of a client with renal insufficiency or failure is directed toward (1) correcting fluid and electrolyte imbalance and (2) removing waste products from the bloodstream by artificial means such as dialysis.

Correction of fluid and electrolyte imbalance requires constant assessment of the constituents and characteristics of blood and urine. Intake and output are recorded meticulously, often in intervals of 15, 30, or 60 minutes (Fig. 19-20). Daily weighings are routine to determine body fluid content. Dehydration can occur, which demands expansion of blood volume to keep all glomeruli working to their capacity. An adequate, but controlled, daily intake may be prescribed. Gatorade, a commercial juicelike drink, seems to produce excellent results in correcting salt, sugar, and fluid imbalances.

When oliguria or anuria is apparent, a specific water intake prescription is made, based on the client's physiological capacity as identified by weight change, urine volume, and serum sodium concentration. Water intake must be

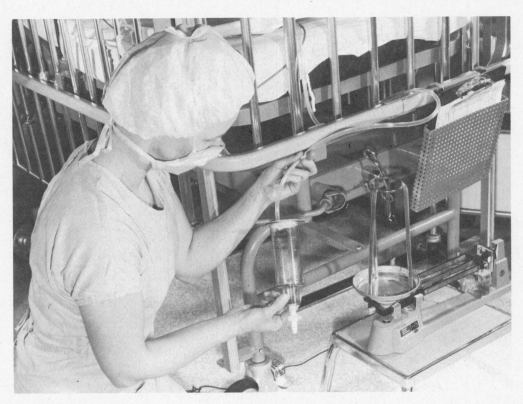

FIG. 19-20
Nurse measures hourly urine output as adjunct to fluid replacement therapy. (Courtesy Shriner's Hospital for Crippled Children, Cincinnati.)

distributed evenly throughout the day to avoid nocturnal dehydration. Orders are written in terms of specific times when fluid is to be given and of the precise amount, to maintain a satisfactory glomerular filtration rate.

Potassium imbalances are likely in acute renal failure but usually are not severe in a chronic course because of nephron compensatory devices. Prolonged anorexia and vomiting, however, can result in depletion. Exchange resins (such as Kayexalate) given orally or by nasogastric or rectal tube may be used to remove potassium from the blood.

Acidosis is an expected complication of renal failure because of loss of bicarbonates in urine and, perhaps more important, to a reduction in ammonia production and in the phosphate available for buffering action.

Maintenance of a satisfactory fluid-electrolyte and acid-base body composition is a crucial role of the physician. Oral and parenteral pharmacological agents are used to correct imbalances. Antacids are sometimes used to combat acid-base disturbances. Vitamin D may be administered to help the body absorb and use calcium for bone healing and strengthening. A low-protein diet with adequate calories and essential amino acids is likely to be prescribed. Salt is not restricted unless edema is severe.

Digitalis and antihypertensive drugs may be ordered to correct circulatory deficiencies and enhance cardiovascular activity.

The crucial part the nurse plays is monitoring intake and output and participation in the fluid-control regimen. Accuracy and punctuality are demanded in all aspects.

By explaining the regimen to the client, the nurse is more likely to enlist his cooperation. Ambulatory persons must be convinced of the critical importance of regulating intake, or they are likely to ingest fluids ad lib, because they often are thirsty and seemingly dehydrated. The dietary prescription is designed to limit the work of the kidneys as they deal with the end products of protein metabolism, but calories and essential amino acids are preserved to afford the client a sense of well-being and to maintain necessary substances for cellular nutrition. Total protein abstinence is seldom demanded now except in acute renal failure with advanced azotemia.

The client should be protected against infections, because a damaged kidney is easy prey for invading microorganisms.

Skin care should be meticulous, because the body's waste products are now largely excreted through the pores. Odor may be a problem. Bathing the client with a weak vinegar solution (1 tablespoon in 1 cup of water) may be useful in dissolving the urea crystals on the skin. The same considerations for care as employed with any gravely ill person should be followed, such as turning the client, giving frequent oral care, and promoting bowel elimination. Additional points of care may be demanded during a dialysis regimen.

Dialysis. Dialysis is indicated when the glomerular filtration rate falls below 3 ml/min, as in certain states of potassium intoxication or the uremic syndrome and in the presence of pulmonary edema induced by renal insufficiency. The purpose of dialysis is to remove waste products from the body with a dialysate solution designed to take up urea and other toxic substances that have accumulated in the blood because of renal insufficiency. Two modes of accomplishing this are peritoneal dialysis and hemodialysis. The decision to dialyze and the method selected depend on many factors. Clinicians must take into account the presence of bleeding or clotting problems, infections, hypertension, other pathological conditions of the cardiovascular system or the liver, and availability of physical, human, and economic resources.

Peritoneal dialysis. Peritoneal dialysis uses exchange catheters introduced into the abdominal cavity and permits removal and collection of certain constituents through a process of fluid exchange (Fig. 19-21). Peritoneal dialysis not only effectively corrects uremia but is also of value in removing edema fluid and exogenous intoxicants such as salicylates or barbiturates and in restoring electrolyte balance.

Peritoneal dialysis can be accomplished in several ways using the peritoneum as a dialysis membrane. Warmed dialysate is infused by gravity into the abdomen through a catheter and allowed to remain in contact with the peritoneum for approximately 30 minutes. During this time diffusion and osmosis occur. Finally the dialysate is siphoned off, and fresh dialysate is infused. This process may be repeated several times in succession before a satisfactory fluid-electrolyte acid-base balance is restored.

Newer techniques of peritoneal dialysis include the use of an automatic peritoneal dialyzing machine and the use of a long-term indwelling catheter for clients who require repeated dialysis. Home dialysis using the fixed catheter is gaining acceptance in certain locales. The continuous ambulatory peritoneal dialysis (CAPD) method permits the client to carry on routines while undergoing dialysis. Two liters of dialysate are maintained intraperitoneally and exchanged four to five times per day. This method is less complicated than the classic peri-

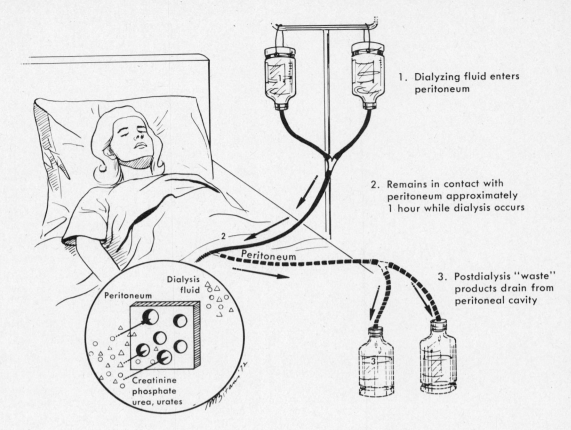

FIG. 19-21
Peritoneal dialysis.

1. Dialyzing fluid enters peritoneum

2. Remains in contact with peritoneum approximately 1 hour while dialysis occurs

3. Postdialysis "waste" products drain from peritoneal cavity

Peritoneum

Dialysis fluid

Peritoneum

Creatinine phosphate urea, urates

toneal dialysis and has several added advantages. It permits chemistry values to remain fairly constant instead of fluctuating widely from treatment to treatment. It can be accomplished without costly hospitalization and allows the client to remain mobile during treatment.

In any dialysis mode the complication of peritonitis is always a threat despite careful technique. The site of catheter insertion should be cleansed daily with povidone-iodine or another similar agent. When any tubing is connected, the junctions should be carefully cleansed. The incision site should be protected with a dry sterile dressing. Frequent cultures of the site of catheter entry and the peritoneal fluid are recommended to detect infections.

Other complications include hypotension from fluid loss, respiratory distress (from hydration imbalances that contribute to congestive heart failure and pulmonary edema), and local discomfort from intraabdominal fluid pressure. Although rare, organ perforation and hemorrhage may occur in conjunction with peritoneal dialysis, and the nurse should consider these complications if there is gross blood in the drainage or unusual pain noted by the client.

Hemodialysis. Hemodialysis involving extracorporeal circulation is five to ten times more efficient than peritoneal dialysis and has the added advantage of direct contact between the blood and the dialysate in a closed system. Furthermore, infection is less likely to develop, and it can be accomplished with considerable ease by nurses, technicians, or family members who have been trained.

Access to a major vein is essential for hemodialysis. In an emergency, the femoral vein is often used. There are several nursing responsibilities of extreme

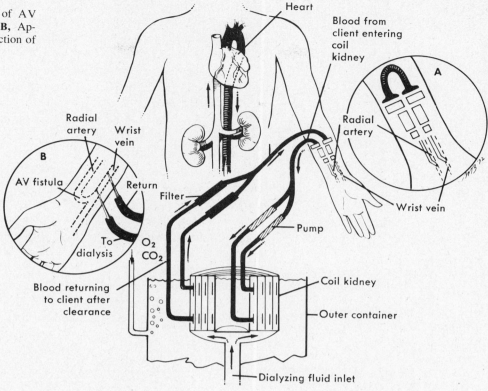

importance in the management of this cannulation. A heparin infusion must be maintained to ensure the patency of the catheter, or it will readily clot. Flushing may also be required. It is imperative that the amount of heparinized solution be judiciously controlled or a severe hemorrhagic potential could develop. Clients who have femoral vein catheters must not flex their hips or the line will be pinched off. Mobility must be reduced and all connections taped securely so that the risk of hemorrhage from accidental disconnections or dislodgements is minimized.

An arteriovenous shunt, or bypass, is implanted in the client's radial artery and forearm vein (to facilitate repeat dialysis procedures). When the two shunts are in place, they are interconnected above the skin surface to permit free circulation and prevent clotting. The bypass connection is removed when the arm is attached to dialysis and is reinserted after the dialysis. The same shunt may be acceptable for use for months, even years, with proper care.

A newer concept of dialysis incorporates a subcutaneous shunt consisting of a fistula between the radial artery and wrist vein. At each dialysis session, two venipunctures are necessary for the transport of blood to and from the hemodialysis unit (Fig. 19-22).

Care of the dialysis shunt. The dialysis shunt and the surrounding skin surface area must be protected from injury and infection. Regular site care may include a routine cleansing and the application of a dry, sterile dressing. Frequent observations should be made to ensure patency of the shunt. An audible or palpable bruit indicates the desired blood flow. The appearance of dark, separated blood in the tubing indicates clotting, and the physician must be notified at once so that steps may be taken to clear and preserve the shunt. The nurse who is not trained in hemodialysis should not attempt to clear a clotted shunt.

The shunt is usually in the forearm of clients. The nurse should take care to avoid trauma to the area. Blood pressure readings, injections, IVs, and blood sampling should be accomplished in the opposite arm.

Total blood loss can occur if the shunt is accidentally separated. Any bleeding or hematoma formation should be viewed with alarm. Direct pressure or the use of vascular clamps may be used to control bleeding until the physician is at hand to assess and manage the crisis.

Site infections are noted by the presence of inflammation, purulent drainage, and edema. Clients with Cimino-Brescia fistulas (between cephalic vein and the radial artery) or the bovine artegraft may have signs and symptoms of a *systemic* infection without any evidence of *site* infection. Fever, lethargy, or elevated leukocyte levels should be considered as indicators of serious shunt-related infection, although the site may appear normal.

Other considerations. Any client anticipating dialysis needs to understand the nature of the procedure and its implications and to be instructed regarding the apparatus and related nursing care. A family member shares such instruction if home dialysis is planned for an extended period of time. Aseptic technique, clinical recordings of intake and output and vital signs, and considerations in weighing the client should be explained thoroughly. Signs of complications, especially shock and infection, should be discussed, and intervention steps assured.

FIG. 19-23
This client relaxes during dialysis session while his wife receives instructional guidance from nurse.

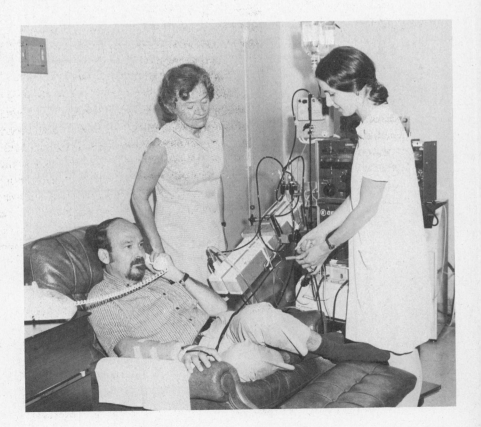

Many clients and their families are participating in a home dialysis program while awaiting a transplant opportunity (Fig. 19-23).

Newer techniques have increased the use of hemodialysis in children. Several inherent problems exist, including the small caliber of children's veins and the safety of the arteriovenous shunt, the fact that growth is halted after dialysis is begun, and the long, tedious, and frequent procedure itself. Current management of childhood renal insufficiency and failure is primarily a supportive maintenance program until adolescence is reached when adult approaches become feasible.

Complications of hemodialysis

HEPARIN REBOUND. Anticoagulation is essential for maintaining the patency of the shunt. To prevent large amounts of heparin from being taken up by the client, blood returning from the dialyzing bath is neutralized by protamine sulfate, which bonds with heparin and inactivates it. Occasionally, however, a heparin rebound is experienced several hours later when metabolic processes break down the bond between the heparin and the protamine. When this occurs, heparin is liberated in the bloodstream and clotting time increased.

HYPERTENSION. Sodium and water retention, attendant to chronic renal failure, is managed by antihypertensive drugs. These drugs, when combined with the effects of ultrafiltration inherent in dialysis, may create a hypotensive emergency. Blood pressure monitoring is a critical point in caring for a client being dialyzed so that fluid therapy is not necessary to manage a falling arterial pressure. Obviously this would place an unnecessary burden on the cardiovascular and renal systems.

HYPOTENSION. When too much extracellular fluid has been removed or if the client takes antihypertensive drugs on the day of dialysis, hypotension may occur. Careful fluid replacement with normal saline usually corrects this phenomenon.

DISEQUILIBRIUM SYNDROME. This syndrome is characterized by nausea, vomiting, headache, hypertension, seizures, and disorientation. It is thought to result from rapid removal of nitrogenous wastes, which creates an osmotic gradient between the blood and brain, thus encouraging cerebral edema formation. This unpleasant complication can be minimized, even prevented, by starting with short dialysis sessions and gradually lengthening them, giving the body a chance to build a tolerance to the effects of ultrafiltration induced by the procedure. Some clinicians use a mannitol infusion during dialysis, which replaces urea that is being removed with other osmotically active particles. This prevents the gradient effect and curtails cerebral edema formation.

Renal transplants.

Although clients with end-stage renal disease can be maintained indefinitely on a regimen of biweekly hemodialysis, renal transplant offers the only real hope of return to a normal existence. Persons are considered candidates for transplants if they have no other pathological conditions that would interfere with recovery of normal urinary function and if they indicate the desire and aptitude for cooperating in a complex program of rehabilitation. Because renal transplants are the most advanced whole organ homografts, consideration is given to both the donor and recipient.

Recipients are fully evaluated by the medical team to determine their potential for the program of renal transplant. One usual criterion is the presence of bilateral and end-stage renal failure. A series of laboratory tests and x-ray studies are performed to confirm the renal failure and to identify any other pathological condition that might contribute to further renal failure. Because a major portion of the success of an eventual transplant lies within the integrity of the family and its expressed willingness to support and participate in the management of the client, a family assessment is made by the social service worker. The final decision regarding transplant candidacy involves such factors as the age and life-style of the client, his marital and family status, and perhaps most important, his motivation and desire to receive a donated kidney. In some institutions there is a transplant committee that makes a final determination of which persons are suitable participants in the renal transplant program.

The most successful transplants involve identical twins. Others, in descending order of success, are from siblings, parents, blood relatives, nonrelated live donors, and cadavers. Since the best donors are members of the nuclear family, it is essential that everyone concerned have an opportunity to fully understand the implication of giving and receiving an organ. The decision to sacrifice a kidney is fraught with great fear for many, and therefore much support must be afforded to those involved in making such decisions. It is sometimes helpful for them to discuss their anxieties with another family who has had a successful transplant experience. Donors are not acceptable in most cases if they express any reluctance to sacrificing a kidney, have any pathological condition that might be related to renal reserve, or are women of childbearing age.

Renal transplant matches are determined by blood and tissue typing. Tissue typing is a highly sophisticated procedure and is costly. Data from potential donors and recipients are banked in computers for immediate recall, because time is of the essence, especially with cadaver donors.

Kidneys recovered from cadavers are stored in a chamber where they can be perfused with cooled, oxygenated plasma via a cannula inserted into the renal artery. Venous outflow is recirculated after being oxygenated and cooled to 8° to 10° C. Monitoring of pH and Po_2 is done at regular intervals to determine physiological viability. Even in such ideal circumstances, kidneys can remain viable for only about 2 days for transplant success. Often the kidney storage reservoir and its contents are shipped to a distant point by air for a matched recipient awaiting a donated organ.

Recipients are usually being maintained on a regular hemodialysis routine after having had a bilateral nephrectomy for control of renal hypertension. Surgical recovery from this preliminary step usually is complete in 3 weeks.

Surgical procedure. The operative procedure for removing the donated kidney is a unilateral nephrectomy in a live donor and a bilateral nephrectomy in a cadaver donor (to accommodate two recipients). Ideally the client to benefit from the transplant is prepared in an adjacent surgical suite to receive the donated organ.

The donated organ is placed in the recipient's iliac fossa on the opposite side of the body from which the organ was taken. To facilitate anastomosis of (1) the renal and hypogastric artery and (2) the renal and external iliac vein, the kidney is turned 180 degrees. Depending on its length, the ureter may be implanted into the bladder directly or anastomosed to the recipient (Fig. 19-24).

Client management after surgery involves a prolonged program of hemodialysis (until the transplanted organ assumes an efficiently functioning status) and constant observations related to immunosuppressive responses and infection.

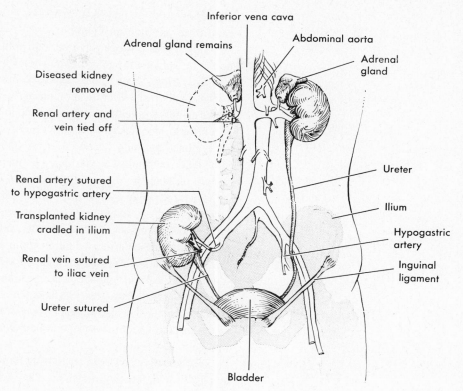

FIG. 19-24
Anatomical diagram showing position of transplanted kidney. (From Bergersen, Betty S., and others: Current concepts in clinical nursing, vol. 1, St. Louis, 1967, The C.V. Mosby Co.)

Inferior vena cava

Adrenal gland remains

Abdominal aorta

Adrenal gland

Diseased kidney removed

Renal artery and vein tied off

Renal artery sutured to hypogastric artery

Transplanted kidney cradled in ilium

Renal vein sutured to iliac vein

Ureter sutured

Ureter

Ilium

Hypogastric artery

Inguinal ligament

Bladder

Immunosuppressive responses. The greatest hazard of renal transplants is that the recipient's body will recognize the nonidentical tissue and reject it by producing antibodies that will destroy it. This potential danger exists for days, weeks, and even months after the transplant, so that the client needs unusually close observation and physiological monitoring.

Immunosuppressive agents such as steroids, antimetabolites such as azothioprine (Imuran), and serum protein substances such as antilymphocyte globulin (ALG) are used to subdue the normal immune mechanism both before and after surgery. During such therapy the client may be on reverse isolation precautions because of susceptibility to infections. Early in the postoperative period these medications are given parenterally, since the client is given nothing by mouth. Dosages are adjusted according to kidney function and white blood cell count.

Strict isolation is usually maintained until the wound has healed. Catheter care, dressing changes, and other procedures must be performed with impeccable technique. Gowns, masks, and gloves are employed, and care taken to ensure that anyone who enters the room is free of infections.

The research and clinical experience in renal transplants indicates that all clients encounter a rejection crisis, and thus both the recipient and his family should be prepared for this event. Signs and symptoms of rejection that the nurse must be able to note are hypertension, malaise, fever, oliguria, anorexia, headache, edema, and tenderness over the transplanted site. Because steroids mask signs of inflammation, fever may not be evident. When a rejection is suspected, alterations in hydration, diet, and medications are made because the body is unable to cope normally with fluids and rid itself of metabolic wastes. Some nephrologists think that local irritation of the transplant site is an important indicator in recognition of rejection.

During the postoperative period, both the transplant recipient and his live donor are anxious to see positive results of the surgical experience. Urine output may be varied. Some clients have anuria or oliguria, whereas other experience a massive diuresis. Careful monitoring of fluids and electrolytes must be maintained to serve as indices of renal function, a guide for fluid replacement, and as a criterion for further necessity of dialysis. Urine and blood analyses are routinely done, and intake and output are scrutinized. Weights are ordered to determine fluid status and are considered by many clinicians to be the best indicator of body fluid content.

Client teaching is essential in the postoperative period for both the donor and recipient. Urinary hygiene is vital content. Clues that indicate inflammation or mechanical disturbances of the bladder, ureters, or kidneys must be well known so that any further urinary complications can be avoided. It should be recalled that both clients are reliant on a single kidney for survival.

Despite careful management, the transplanted kidney may fail to function, and removal is necessitated. Some nephrologists will attempt a second transplant on the opposite side. However, if there are three or four successive failures, further transplants seem unwise, and hemodialysis may be continued for an indefinite period of time.

Fortunately, however, increasing numbers of recipients are able to return to active life with few modifications. They have achieved their ultimate goal—staying alive without hemodialysis. There is little modification in their life-style, but caution must be exercised in relation to contact sports, and childbearing is usually forbidden because the transplanted kidney is situated in the abdomen with little protection from trauma.

Although care of the renal transplant client is a relatively new phenomenon in nursing, more nurses will have the opportunity to participate in this exciting innovation in organ transplant science. Most nurses who work in a special program such as the renal transplant one are highly skilled in the specialty and are an integral part of the health team. They must be equipped to be especially cognizant of the many needs of family members and appreciate their potential contributions to the client's management.

 Evaluation. Plans for the client in renal failure may involve correction of fluid and electrolyte imbalance or removing waste products from the blood by use of peritoneal dialysis or hemodialysis. If renal failure is chronic, dialysis may be used or the client may have a kidney transplant. Evaluation of nursing care, therefore, depends on goals for care, and evaluations are made continuously as objectives are modified.

EXPECTED OUTCOMES
The client and/or family can:
1. Describe renal failure.
2. Describe use of therapeutic modalities such as dialysis or renal transplant.
3. Manage dialysis if done at home, or shunt care if done at a dialysis center.
4. Maintain adequate urinary output.
5. State diet and fluid modifications.
6. State use, dosage, time, route, and side effects of prescribed medications.

7. Describe plans for health maintenance (rest, activity, prevention of infection).
8. State indications for health care.
9. State plans for follow-up health care and use of community resources.

Trauma

Trauma to the urinary tract is most serious when it affects the kidney itself. Crushing blows or penetrating wounds can cause parenchymal hemorrhage or even displacement of the organ. Contusion usually creates hematuria and infection, requiring bed rest and pharmacological therapy. Laceration may occur, and a medical emergency is thus created, since one fifth of the total cardiac output is received in the renal area. Nephrectomy may be necessitated in severe cases. It is not uncommon for traumatized kidneys to develop degenerative disease.

Bladder injuries may result from fracture in the pelvic regions or severe blows to the abdomen. If the bladder ruptures, urine flows into the retropubic space in the peritoneum, and there is pain, shock, and inability to void. As soon as the diagnosis is made, surgical repair should be performed.

Children are especially prone to renal trauma, since only 2 to 3 cm of tissue is in the space between the skin surface and the kidney itself. Falls from bicycles, being struck by a car, and other blow-type injuries result in such trauma, but they are frequently overlooked because other injuries may appear more serious.

Hemorrhage and shock are the primary problems in renal trauma.

Evaluation

Nursing care for the client with a health problem of the urinary system is evaluated continuously as plans are developed for the client for health promotion maintenance or restoration. Common nursing diagnoses may include altered urinary elimination, alterations in comfort: pain, knowledge deficit, alterations in nutrition, noncompliance, or fluid volume deficit, and plans are made accordingly. Evaluation determines effectiveness of plans, and the client and nurse may decide the problem is resolved or that the plan should be modified or continued. When the client has reached his highest level of wellness, the nurse-client relationship is terminated and the client assumes responsibility for his health care.

EXPECTED OUTCOMES

The client and/or family can:
1. Describe the health problem.
2. State plans for promoting urinary elimination, including assuring adequate fluid intake and avoiding urinary stasis.
3. Discuss plans for preventing urinary tract infections, including hygiene measures and assuring adequate fluid intake.
4. State use of therapies, including diet, medications, dialysis, and surgical interventions.
5. State indications for health care, including pain, dysuria, frequency, oliguria, hematuria, pyuria, fever, urinary retention.
6. State plans for follow-up health care.

Nursing process for common health problems

Summary

The nursing process helps the nurse and client plan comprehensive nursing care for the client with common health problems of the urinary system. The nurse and client identify actual or potential nursing problems and plan for health promotion, maintenance, or restoration.

During the assessment stage the nurse collects data about the client's patterns of urinary elimination across the life span and relates the information to data collected from developmental, social, and psychological histories, and data obtained from physical assessment. Data analysis may reveal nursing diagnoses of altered patterns of urinary elimination, actual or potential fluid volume excess or deficit, pain, or noncompliance.

The nurse and client can plan for health promotion, maintenance, or restoration. Goals for health promotion may include promoting urinary elimination habits, preventing infections, and risk management. Plans for health maintenance and restoration are developed for clients with altered elimination who may have urinary tract surgery.

Health problems of the urinary system occur across the life span. Congenital anomalies such as polycystic kidney or exstrophy of the bladder are noted in the neonate and infant, whereas poststreptococcal acute glomerulonephritis and nephrosis are health problems of the child. Strictures, renal calculi, tumors, and incontinence are typical of adult health problems; urinary tract infections, neurogenic disorders, and renal failure occur across the life span. Plans are implemented for each of these problems as appropriate for the client's age and stage of development.

Evaluation is an integral part of the nursing process that allows the nurse and client to determine the outcome of plans according to established criteria. Ultimate expected outcomes are for the client to achieve his own optimal health.

References

1. Brandt, Patricia A., Chinn, Peggy L., and Smith, Mary Ellen: Current practice in pediatric nursing, St. Louis, 1976, The C.V. Mosby Co.
2. Brundage, Dorothy: Nursing management of renal problems, ed. 2, St. Louis, 1980, The C.V. Mosby Co.
3. Harrington, Joan DeLong, and Brener, Etta Rae: Patient care in renal failure, Philadelphia, 1973, W.B. Saunders Co.
4. Hughes, James E.: Synopsis of pediatrics, ed. 5, St. Louis, 1980, The C.V. Mosby Co.
5. Lilly Research Laboratories: Kidney and urinary tract infections, Indianapolis, 1971, Eli Lilly and Co.
6. Winter, Chester C., and Morel, Alice: Nursing care of patients with urologic diseases, ed. 4, St. Louis, 1977, The C.V. Mosby Co.

Suggested readings

Barrett, Nancy: Continent vesicostomy: the dry urinary diversion, Am. J. Nurs. **79**(3):462-464, 1979.

Beber, Charles: Freedom for the incontinent, Am. J. Nurs. **80**(3):482-484, 1980.

Cianci, Judith, and others: Renal transplantation, Am. J. Nurs. **81**(2):354-355, 1981.

Davis, Virginia, and Lavandero, Ramon: Caring for the catheter carefully . . . before, during, and after peritoneal dialysis, Pt. 2, Nursing 80 **12**(10):67-71, 1980.

Denniston, Donna, and Burn, Kathryn: Home peritoneal dialysis, Am. J. Nurs. **80**(11):2022-2026, 1980.

Ellis, P.D., editor: Renal failure, Crit. Care Q. **1**(2):1-91, 1978.

Gross, Susan, and Algrim, Corrine: Teaching young patients and their families about home peritoneal dialysis, Nursing 80 **10**(12):72-73, 1980.

Hetrick, Anne, and others: Nutrition in renal disease: when the patient is a child, Am. J. Nurs. **79**(12):2152-2154, 1979.

Irwin, Betty: Hemodialysis means vascular access and the right kind of nursing care, Nursing 79 **9**(10):49-53, 1979.

Juliani, Louise: When infection leads to acute glomerulonephritis, here's what to do, Nursing 79 **9**(10):40-45, 1979.

Lavandero, Ramon, and Davis, Virginia: Caring for the catheter carefully . . . before, during and after dialysis. Pt. 1, Nursing 80 **10**(11):73-79, 1980.

Luke, Barbara: Nutrition in renal disease: the adult on dialysis, Am. J. Nurs. **79**(12):2155-2157, 1979.

Oestreich, Sandy J.: Rational nursing care in chronic renal disease, Am. J. Nurs. **79**(6):1096-1099.

Sorrels, Alice J.: Continuous ambulatory peritoneal dialysis, Am. J. Nurs. **79**(8):1400-1401, 1979.

Stark, June: BUN/creatinine, Nursing 80 **10**(5):33-38, 1980.

NURSING PROCESS

for clients with common health problems of the

20 Cardiovascular system

Assessment

Data analysis

Planning

Implementation

Evaluation

Health problems of the cardiovascular system remain the primary cause of death in the United States and represent significant losses from illness and disability. Common health problems occur across the life span, but may be unique to certain age groups. Congenital heart disease and inherited disorders such as hemophilia or sickle cell disease, for example, have peak incidence in infancy, whereas rheumatic fever occurs during childhood, and rheumatic heart disease and Hodgkin's disease are common to young adults. Ischemic heart disease (angina pectoris and myocardial infarction) and hypertension are notable diseases of adulthood; others include peripheral vascular disease and atherosclerosis. Anemia and leukemia are universal to all ages. The purpose of this chapter is to help the nurse develop skills necessary to assess clients with common health problems of the cardiovascular system; to plan nursing care for health promotion, maintenance, and restoration; to implement plans; and to evaluate expected outcomes.

Overview of the cardiovascular system

The cardiovascular system consists of three interdependent parts: the heart (pumping mechanisms), blood vessels (flow-regulating mechanisms), and blood (delivery and regulatory mechanisms). The interaction of these components maintains a dynamic state of optimum oxygen delivery to the cells.

THE HEART

The heart is the organ that circulates oxygenated blood to the body and returns deoxygenated blood to the lungs for exchange of gases. Separate chambers within the heart prevent mixing of oxygenated and deoxygenated blood, and valves assure forward flow of the blood. The right atrium receives deoxygenated blood from the superior and inferior venae cavae and coronary system. This blood passes through the tricuspid valve to the right ventricle to be pumped to the lungs via the pulmonary artery. Oxygenated blood returns from the lungs through the pulmonary veins to the left atrium. The blood in the left atrium flows through the mitral valve to the left ventricle and is pumped through the aortic valve to the aorta for systemic and coronary circulation. Disruption of the flow in the heart chambers can result in inadequate oxygenation, mixing of arterial and venous blood, and reduced cellular perfusion. Examples of such problems to be considered later are congenital heart defects and valvular weakness or stenosis.

Myocardial blood supply

The myocardium receives its source of blood supply during diastole from the coronary arteries originating in the sinus of Valsalva. The left coronary artery branches into two arteries: (1) the anterior descending artery to supply the anterior two thirds of the septum and right bundle branch, and (2) the circumflex artery to supply the left atrium and ventricle. The right coronary artery (posterior descending) supplies the sinoatrial (SA) node, atrioventricular (AV) junction, posterior bundle branch, posterior one third of the septum, right ventricle, and diaphragmatic surface of the left ventricle. Coronary veins return blood to a sinus that empties into the right atrium for direct circulation into the lungs.

The concept of myocardial blood flow is important to the understanding of ischemic heart disease, a syndrome characterized by myocardial ischemia or anoxia. Significantly, coronary artery disease is the major type of heart disease in middle adulthood. Later discussions focus on the preventive aspects and therapeutic interventions used to maintain oxygen supply in the myocardium.

Conduction system

Rhythmic contraction of the heart depends on orderly transmission of electrical impulses from the base to the apex of the heart. The transmission of impulses is believed to occur by the spread of a local current from cell to cell through low-resistance pathways rather than through a syncytium, or interconnected network of cells, as once thought. The passage of ions from cell to cell thereby couples the cells electrically.

Each cardiac fiber has the unique property of being able to initiate contractions, but an organized pattern is established by the "pacemaker," the SA node in the right atrium. Impulses from the SA node travel to the left atrium via Bachmann's bundle and down internodal pathways to the AV junction (AV node and His area) where a slight delay occurs until atrial contraction is complete. The impulses continue from the AV junction to the bundle of His via atrionodal, nodal, and nodal His pathways, and on to the Purkinje fibers, resulting in ventricular contraction. It should be recalled that the conduction system is also dependent on the movement of the electrolytes sodium and potassium, which, as they exchange places across the cell membrane, cause depolarization and repolarization.

Irregularities in conduction impose serious hazards to pumping mechanism. Dysrhythmias may cause either extremely rapid or extremely slow heart rates, both of which can result in insufficient pumping of oxygen. Pump failure (congestive heart failure and cardiogenic shock) and cardiac standstill are examples of serious outcomes of dysrhythmias.

Nervous system control

The rate of impulse formation, conduction, and strength of contraction is regulated by the autonomic nervous system through the right and left vagus nerves of the parasympathetic nervous system and the sympathetic nervous system. The autonomic nervous system is mediated by neurotransmitters contained in the postganglionic nerve fibers and, when released, bind to specific receptors on the surface of myocardial cells. Acetylcholine regulates the vagus nerve; norepinephrine, the sympathetic nerves.

The vagus and sympathetic nerves have opposite effects on the events in the cardiac cycle. The vagus nerve decreases the role of impulse formation in the SA node, slows the speed of conduction through the AV node, and reduces the force of atrial and probably ventricular contraction. The sympathetic nerves, on the other hand, increase the rate of impulse formation, conduction, and force of contraction.

The autonomic nerves are further influenced by reflex changes in pressoreceptors in the aortic arch and carotid arteries. Pressoreceptor response to increases in internal or external pressure stimulate the cardioinhibitory center, which inhibits the accelerator center and slows heart rate. Conversely, decreases in pressure in these areas ultimately increase heart rate.

Finally, the heart rate is controlled by oxygen and carbon dioxide levels, blood pH, electrolytes, and certain drugs.

The pumping action of the heart is governed by laws of *automaticity* (initiation of impulses), *conductivity* (transmission of impulses), *excitability* (response stimuli), *refractoriness* (delay in response to stimuli), and *rhythmicity* (regular formation and conduction of impulses). These laws facilitate adaptation of the changing needs for oxygen from moment to moment and throughout the life span.

Adaptation to the need for oxygen is influenced by *intrinsic* as well as *extrinsic* factors. When there is need for increased oxygen delivery, such as during exercise, obesity, digestion, emotional stress, metabolic disease, hemorrhage, anemia, and use of certain drugs, cardiac output increases. In instances when there is less demand for oxygen, such as resting states, hypervolemia, or increased blood viscosity, the heart responds accordingly. This reciprocal relationship between the pumping mechanisms and oxygen requirements assures a dynamic equilibrium in meeting the need for oxygen.

Cardiac output

Cardiac performance is determined by the chamber size and amount of blood returned to and pumped from the heart and is influenced by blood viscosity and total peripheral resistance (TPR). Stroke volume and cardiac output are two parameters of cardiac performance with which the nurse should be familiar. *Stroke volume* is defined as the amount of blood pumped from the ventricles during each contraction of the heart (about 70 ml of blood in an adult) and depends on the blood available from venous return for ejection, the size of the chamber, and the force of the myocardial contraction. *Cardiac output* is the amount of ventricular outflow and is calculated by multiplying the stroke volume by the heart rate. Because the heart rate depends on many factors, the cardiac output varies according to the need for oxygen. Cardiac output is influenced by preload and afterload. *Preload* refers to the resting force of the myocardium and depends on the stretching potential of the left ventricle (left ventricular end diastolic pressure) and the volume of blood remaining in the left ventricle after diastole. *Afterload* refers to the resistance to ventricular ejection offered by the peripheral blood vessels (TPR). These concepts are useful to the understanding of hemodynamic monitoring and pharmacological therapy used to increase or reduce cardiac output.

BLOOD VESSELS

The blood vessels provide transportation for the blood pumped from the heart to the cells. Variances in structure of the arteries, capillaries, and veins assure flow in the vascular circuit.

Arteries

Arteries, composed of several cell layers, are elastic to accommodate the pressure as blood is pumped from the left ventricle. The lining of the artery (intima) is smooth to propel blood, but, unfortunately, it has an affinity for certain lipids and tends to acquire plaques during aging. Known as *atherosclerosis,* this plaque formation gradually impedes arterial flow and is believed to be the basis of many ischemic processes. The middle layer of the artery, the media, is elastic to accommodate pulsatile forces. This media, too, is affected by aging, and calcium deposits in later life limit its elasticity, a state known as *arteriosclerosis*. The outer arterial layer, the adventitia, supports the artery as it courses through tissue systems. Hypertension, aneurysms, obstructions, and inflammations are common interferences with cellular oxygenation from arterial causes.

Microcirculation

Smaller arteries (arterioles) distribute oxygen, but the actual exchange of oxygen and carbon dioxide occurs in the capillaries. These one-celled vessels branch into all tissues and adjust locally to the demands for oxygen by increasing the microcirculation in areas of high nutrient exchange. Venules, emptying into veins, provide return deoxygenated blood for reoxygenation in the lungs.

Veins

The veins are less elastic and depend largely on muscular action to provide forward flow of circulating blood. Valves, which are especially prevalent in the lower extremities, prevent back flow. The veins are called capacitance vessels because they can distend and accommodate 75% of the blood volume. Venous stasis and weakened valves contribute to varicosities (varicose veins), a common problem of venous return to be discussed later.

Flow regulation

Laws of physical science govern flow-regulating mechanisms. The concept of *pressure gradient* is useful in understanding that blood will flow from an area of greater pressure (the heart) to an area of lesser pressure (the blood vessels). The concept of flow *resistance* explains that resistance is offered by the size of the tube (vessel diameter) and the viscosity of the fluid (blood). Arterial blood pressure then is a reflection of the cardiac output and the resistance. Changes in pressure or resistance will alter flow regulation.

Intrinsic and extrinsic factors alter and adjust the flow rate to meet the need for oxygen. The contractility of the vascular smooth muscle is regulated by hormones (primarily epinephrine) and the sympathetic nervous system, both of which produce vasoconstriction. The action of hormones on adrenoreceptors of the cell membrane causes vasoconstriction or vasodilation. Norepinephrine binds with alpha receptors, whereas epinephrine binds with either alpha or beta receptors. Activation of alpha receptors causes vasoconstriction; beta receptors cause vasodilation. Although adaptive in most instances, vasoconstriction can have deleterious effects when the peripheral vasculature is already obstructed. Peripheral vascular disease and hypertension are thought to result from this action. Cellular oxygen needs also stimulate flow-regulatory mechanisms. Factors such as altitude, disease (anemia), and certain drugs influence and maintain vascular dynamics.

BLOOD AND LYMPHATICS

The blood is the transport medium for oxygen, carbon dioxide, and metabolites. Furthermore, the blood mediates internal regulation of acid-base balance, thermal controls, and hormonal regulation. The blood contains formed elements responsible for delivery of oxygen to the cells, phagocytosis, hemostasis, and fibrinolysis. Fifty-five percent of the blood is plasma; the remaining formed elements are the red blood cells (erythrocytes), white blood cells (leukocytes), and platelets (thrombocytes).

The red blood cells, numbering 4.5 to 5.0 million per cubic millimeter of blood are conveyors for the respiratory pigment hemoglobin. Hemoglobin carries the oxygen to the cells. The role of the red blood cells in transporting hemoglobin is vital, and therefore a balance of production and destruction of the cells is necessary to assure adequate oxygen delivery. It should be recalled that iron and vitamin B_{12} are necessary nutrients in the maintenance of red blood cell production; without these elements a state of nutritional anemia will occur.

The white blood cells (5000 to 10,000 per cubic millimeter of blood) are components of the body's protective system and are involved primarily in phagocytizing harmful substances. Types of white blood cells and precursors are varied, and exact roles are now being identified. There are two types of leukocytes, granular and nongranular. Granular leukocytes (granulocytes) include polymorphonuclear neutrophils, polymorphonuclear eosinophils, and polymorphonuclear basophils. Nongranular leukocytes include lymphocytes and monocytes. Lymphocytes originate from lymphocytic stem cells in the bone marrow, but are processed in the thymus gland before they become functional and are known as T cells or T lymphocytes; they provide cellular immunity. Other cells are differentiated in unknown lymphoid structures and are referred to as B cells or B lymphocytes; these are responsible for antibody production. Monocytes, on the other hand, are produced in the bone marrow from monoblast cells. Leukemia, involving any variety of these cells, is a tumor process that disrupts oxygen delivery mechanisms by crowding out other formed elements.

Hemostasis is assured by the platelets, the third major formed element in the blood. There are approximately 250,000 to 500,000 platelets per cubic millimeter of blood. Platelets are instrumental in initiating the clotting process, a complex mechanism whereby the conversion of fibrinogen to a fibrin clot prevents hemorrhage. Hemorrhagic states are rare and often caused by a defect in one of the clotting factors. Hemophilia is a well-known example.

A balance between clotting and bleeding is maintained by the fibrinolytic system, which controls and regulates the enzymatic breakdown of both fibrinogen and fibrin.

The delivery and regulatory roles of the blood respond to oxygen saturation and the need for greater or lesser delivery. Bleeding, clotting, or changes in blood volume may act to affect delivery mechanisms.

The *lymphatic circulation* can be considered an adjunct to the delivery and regulatory roles of the cardiovascular system, although its prime function is production of immune antibodies. The lymph phagocytizes bacteria and disposes of chemical wastes from the cells, both of which are transported in lymphatic channels. The lymphatic channels follow venous channels and, like the veins, depend on valves and muscular action to assure forward flow. Regional lymph nodes collect and redistribute the fluid between venous and lymphatic systems as needed. Enlarged lymph nodes are a visible result of an infectious process in the body. Lymph tumors, such as Hodgkin's disease, are discussed later because they present a threat to lymph flow.

Assessment

NURSING HISTORY

The nurse has a significant role in assessing the client's cardiovascular system. Assessment is done across the life span and may include neonatal appraisal, well-child examinations, or health appraisals of adolescents and adults. In critical care settings, information must be gathered rapidly, and the nurse sets priorities for the information needed to plan care. The nurse uses the data to formulate nursing diagnoses and integrates the findings from the physical, diagnostic, and hemodynamic assessment with information gathered in the nursing history.

Health history

The health history is used to collect data about the client's usual health habits that reflect circulation and exchange of oxygen. The history should be obtained during the initial contact with the client to obtain baseline information.

The nurse should determine if the client is having pain. The pain should be described as to location, duration, precipitation of onset, and what has been done to relieve it. Chest pain is of particular significance, and the location and radiation patterns should be carefully described. Pain in the calves of the legs may be related to oxygen deprivation, and the nurse should determine if the pain is continuous or intermittent, and how much exercise the client can tolerate. This type of pain is usually associated with arterial insufficiency. Pain caused by venous insufficiency is intensified by prolonged sitting or standing. The nurse should also determine neurovascular integrity and ascertain if the client experiences burning, numbness, or tingling.

The nurse should also assess the client's respiratory status. Does the client have difficulty breathing? Shortness of breath? Orthopnea (sitting upright to breathe)? Paroxysmal nocturnal dyspnea? What is the effect of exercise on breathing?

The effects of circulatory effectiveness can be determined by weight gain. Has the client gained weight? Is there edema? If edema is present, when does it occur? What relieves it?

The nurse can inquire if the client has any problems with bleeding. Does he notice unusual bruising? Is there prolonged bleeding?

Finally, the nurse should determine exercise tolerance. Is the client easily fatigued? Does the child, adolescent, or adult have decreased exercise tolerance? Does the client assume unusual postures such as squatting or the knee-chest position (infants) to relieve stress of exercise?

The health history can also be used to determine past health problems, medications used, and the potential for inherited diseases. The nurse can inquire about previous illnesses and ask specifically if the client has relatives who have

Nursing process for common health problems

hemophilia, sickle cell anemia, leukemia, rheumatic fever, congenital heart disease, diabetes mellitus, hypertension, or ischemic heart disease.

Information from the diet history can be related to the client's cardiovascular status. The nurse should note diets that contain excess calories, fat, cholesterol, and sodium.

The health history can also be used to determine risk for cardiovascular disease. Cardiovascular disease is the most common cause of death in adults, and risks associated with this health problem have been identified. Information about the client's usual habits such as diet, exercise, smoking, and drinking, as well as usual blood pressure levels, can be obtained in the health hazard appraisal to identify the individual's potential risk.

Developmental history

The structures of the cardiovascular system change markedly as the individual ages. The nurse must be cognizant of the effects of physical development on the heart rates, production of formed elements in the blood, and blood pressure to interpret these parameters as they relate to the client's age (Table 20-1).

Neonate. During the first period of reactivity, a major change in the cardiovascular status occurs. Fetal circulation converts to independent circulation of life. This change is thought to be initiated as the lungs inflate with extrauterine oxygen. Lowered pulmonary vascular resistance allows four times more blood from the right heart to enter the lungs. The pressure of blood coming to the left heart then causes closure of the foramen ovale, and the ductus arteriosus is no longer functional. The heart rate during the first period of reactivity is rapid, 130 to 150 beats per minute. The rhythm continues to be irregular through the second period of reactivity and stabilizes about the sixth hour after birth. Since the heart rate is rapid, assessments of rate and rhythm must be made with a stethoscope.

The heart rate of the newborn can be scored on the *Apgar* scale (see Chapter 2). This rating gives the physician an indication of the newborn's ability to meet the need for oxygen. A heart rate over 100 beats per minute is given the highest rating of 2; rates below 100 are scored as 1. Absence of a heart rate is scored as 0 and indicates the need for resuscitation.

During the neonatal period the blood pressure is at its lowest because the left ventricle is not pumping a full load of blood. The systolic blood pressure of the newborn ranges from 40 to 70 mm Hg and rises to 80 mm Hg within a month. The blood pressure of the newborn can be obtained by milking the blood of a

TABLE 20-1
Age-related vital signs

Age group	Heart rate (per minute)	Respiratory rate (per minute)	Blood pressure (mm Hg)	
Neonate	130-150	36-60	Systolic	20-60
Infant	125-135	40-46	Systolic	70-80
Toddler–school age	65-105	20-24	Systolic	90-100
			Diastolic	60-64
Adolescent	65-100	16-22	Systolic	100-120
			Diastolic	70-80
Adult	60-100	12-20	Systolic	100-120
			Diastolic	70-80
Older adult	60-100	12-18	Systolic	130-140
			Diastolic	90-95

limb toward the heart and securing a small blood pressure cuff to retain the blood ("flush technique"). The sphygmomanometer is deflated slowly, and the pressure is read when color returns to the limb. Blood pressure assessments of the newborn are not done routinely, because they are difficult to obtain and may vary with each reading.

The source of formed elements in the blood also changes at birth. The erythrocytes, leukocytes, and thrombocytes (which were formed by the spleen, liver, and lymph during fetal life) are now formed in the bone marrow. At the time of birth the supply of erythrocytes increases to provide for oxygen needs during and immediately after delivery. Destruction of the erythrocytes is accomplished by the liver, and physiological jaundice (icterus) may be apparent for several days until liver function matures and is able to accommodate destruction of additional erythrocytes. The clotting process is unstable during the neonatal stage, owing to decreased prothrombin stores. Vitamin K may be given soon after birth to stimulate prothrombin production.

Infant. The need for oxygen during infancy is met by a normally rapid heart rate of about 130 beats per minute. The rhythm, however, is irregular until puberty. The heart rate may increase when the infant cries, nurses, or defecates and should not be taken immediately after these activities.

Toddler, preschooler, and school-age child. The heart rate slowly stabilizes to meet the need for oxygen during periods of growth. The pulse rate, easily obtained by compressing a peripheral artery, ranges from 85 to 105 beats per minute during the preschool years to 65 to 80 during the school-age years. The blood pressure can be obtained by conventional methods, but the cuff should be selected to fit the youngster's arm. The cuff should be 1.2 times the diameter of the arm. Normal blood pressure ranges from 90/60 to 100/64.

Adolescent. During puberty the heart increases to its adult size. Until this time heart murmurs or irregularities of rhythm may be benign. During adolescence the heart rate stabilizes and assumes a regular rhythm. There is a slight sex difference established at this time, with a normal heart rate of 65 for men and slightly higher for women. The blood pressure is about 100/70. The heart rate of the young adult is more similar to that of the adolescent than to that of the mature adult.

Adult. The physiological effects of aging are observed markedly in the cardiovascular system. Influenced by environment and heredity, these changes are manifested in early adult years. Blood vessels become less elastic and may be obstructed by deposits of calcium and fatty acids (cholesterol and triglycerides). Cardiac reserve diminishes as does exercise tolerance. Hypertension, ischemic heart disease, and peripheral vascular ischemia are common in this age group.

Older adult. In the older adult, the cardiac reserve, stroke volume, and cardiac output are diminished by as much as 30% to 40%. The heart rate at rest remains unchanged but takes longer to return to normal ranges after stress. Furthermore, the heart does not respond to stress with marked increases in rate, and for this reason pulse determinations in older people are less reliable assessments. Decreased elasticity as well as calcification and fibrosis of the arteries impedes arterial flow. These factors, coupled with increased peripheral resistance, cause diminished supplies of oxygen to vital organs such as the heart, brain, liver, and kidneys. Clinical evidence of decreased oxygen supplies is evident in older individuals and accounts for the most common cause of death in this age group.

Nursing process for common health problems

Social history

The nurse can obtain data about the client's life-style and recognize the effects of educational background, economic resources, religious affiliation, and ethnic and cultural heritage on the client's cardiovascular health.

Educational level. Nursing care for the client with health problems of the cardiovascular system includes health teaching for promotion, maintenance, and rehabilitation. The nurse should identify the client's and family's educational background to plan appropriate teaching programs. Many clients have sophisticated knowledge about their health and body function; others have little understanding of their health needs or problems. Because the nurse must be able to adapt teaching to all educational levels, it is important to determine the client's present level of understanding.

Economic factors. Cardiovascular disease is the number one disease affecting persons in the United States. Economic losses arising out of disruption of lifestyles from cardiovascular disease represent personal as well as societal losses. Time lost from work, hospitalization expenses, and potential changes in occupation are serious economic burdens for the involved individuals.

Psychological history

Information about the client's psychological status is necessary to develop a comprehensive care plan. The nurse can gather this information by helping the client identify stresses in his life and the resources he has available to cope with stress, illness, and change.

Stress. Stress of daily living is not unusual, and the amount tolerated varies among individuals and for each individual at any one time. Because stress is related to health and illness, it is important for the client and nurse to be aware of stress impinging on the client. Common stressors are environment, work, family relationships, diet, financial responsibilities, and change, and the nurse can identify to what extent these may be stressors for each client.

Coping resources. The nurse and client can also identify usual *coping mechanisms,* because these will be used to deal with the stress of illness. Psychological coping mechanisms may include anger, denial, or intellectualization. Other coping resources are the client's family and support group and economic and educational resources. Some clients may use biofeedback, relaxation exercises, or drugs to manage stress. Clients can be described as active copers or passive copers, depending on their role in problem solving. The nurse must therefore be aware of the client's coping style as well as his coping mechanisms and coping resources when planning nursing care.

Physical assessment

Physical assessment of the cardiovascular system involves an orderly examination of the heart and blood vessels. Skills of *inspection, palpation, percussion,* and *auscultation* are used to collect these data.[22]

Heart

Inspection. The forcefulness of pulsations of the heart can be observed by watching cardiac movement on the chest. Inspection is performed with the client supine and the chest exposed. Cardiac movement is observed at the point of maximum impulse (PMI), which is usually located at the mid-clavicular line at the fifth intercostal space (Fig. 20-1). Increased work of the heart at the right ventricle may cause a lift (heave) that can be observed with each palpation.

Palpation. The PMI can be palpated to identify heart size and rate of pulsation. The normal PMI is about the size of a nickel; enlargements may indicate left ventricular hypertrophy. The PMI is palpated for *thrills,* vibrations that occur as the blood flows through narrow or damaged valves.

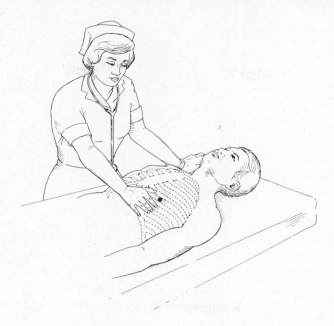

Percussion. Percussion of the heart is done to determine size and location of borders and involves percussing the borders from the lateral chest wall to the midline. The point of change from resonant to dull indicates the cardiac border. This information is likely to be difficult to obtain in clients with emphysema or obesity, and a chest x-ray film provides more reliable information about heart size and location.

Auscultation. The heart's pumping can be listened to with a stethoscope to determine heart rate and rhythm and to identify heart sounds, murmurs, or rubs. A good-quality stethoscope (with a bell and diaphragm) and a quiet environment are essential to cardiac auscultation. The client should be in a supine position with the head slightly elevated; infants and young children may be more likely to be quiet if held by the parent.

Rate and rhythm. The nurse can listen to the heart to determine the rate and rhythm. The stethoscope can be placed over the apex (mitral area) to hear the heart beat, which is counted for 1 minute. The nurse can palpate the carotid or radial arteries while listening to the heart beat to detect pulse deficits. The heart rate and rhythm vary with age (Table 20-1).

Heart sounds. Heart sounds reflect the opening and closing of the valves and are heard at specific points on the chest wall where the sounds are best transmitted at the aortic, pulmonic, mitral, or tricuspid areas (Fig. 20-2). Each site should be auscultated with the bell and diaphragm of the stethoscope, allowing adequate time for auscultation.

The *first heart sound* (S_1) is produced by asynchronous closure of the mitral and tricuspid valves and is heard loudest at the apex or mitral area. The first heart sound actually has two components (the mitral closing [M_1] and the tricuspid closing [T_1]), but because the valve closings normally occur so close together, only one sound is heard. If the two heart sounds are distinct, or split, when auscultated at the mitral area, there may be late closure of the valves, a pathological condition of a bundle branch block.

FIG. 20-2
Anatomic areas used to locate heart sounds.

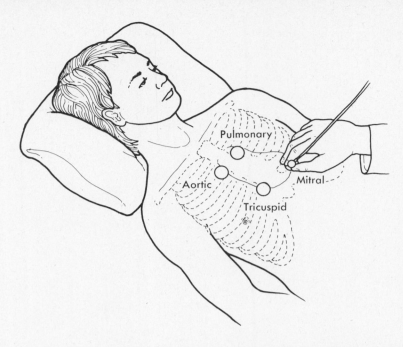

The *second heart sound* (S_2) is caused by the asynchronous closure of the pulmonic and aortic valves. The aortic valve (A_2) closes slightly before the pulmonic valve (P_2), but these sounds are heard as one sound, loudest at the base or aortic area. The second heart sound may be auscultated to hear a physiological split sound of the slight delay in closure of the pulmonic valve on inspiration. This is because of a decrease in intrathoracic pressure that ultimately increases the flow to the right atrium, increases right ventricular filling, increases right ventricular stroke volume, and consequently prolongs right ventricular ejection. This split can be heard at the pulmonic area. Splitting on expiration is usually abnormal and may indicate an atrial septal defect or pulmonic stenosis.

The *third heart sound* (S_3) is a low-pitched sound heard best with the bell of the stethoscope at the mitral area, and reflects ventricular vibrations produced by rapid filling of the ventricles during diastole. S_3 occurs just following S_2 and resembles the pronunciation of the word "Ken$_{S_1}$-tuc$_{S_2}$-ky$_{S_3}$. This sound is normal in children and young adults (physiological S_3), but is abnormal in adults and may indicate heart failure, postmyocardial infarction damage, mitral or tricuspid incompetence, or other cardiac pathological conditions.

The *fourth heart sound* (S_4) is a low-pitched sound heard over the mitral area. This sound is caused by resistance to ventricular filling in late diastole because of increased ventricular diastolic pressure or impairment of ventricular distensibility and, because of the ventricular resistance, the atrium contracts more forcefully and produces the fourth heart sound. The sound, if present, occurs just before S_1 and resembles pronunciation of the word "Ten$_{S_4}$-ne$_{S_1}$-see$_{S_2}$. The sound may be normal in children and young adults but in adults is associated with systemic and pulmonary hypertension, aortic and pulmonic stenosis, myocardial infarction, and other cardiac disease.

Murmurs. Murmurs are sounds produced by vibrations within the heart and great vessels caused by increased turbulence of flow. The flow through the heart and vessels can be changed by constriction or dilation of a valve or vessel, stenosis, or increase in flow rate. The murmurs are heard over the area in which the murmur occurs. Murmurs are described by their location, timing, intensity, pitch, and quality.

LOCATION. The location of the murmur is described as the location where the sound is loudest. Anatomical landmarks are used for descriptive purposes. Additionally, the nurse can note whether the murmur is confined to the area (fixed) or radiates to other locations on the chest wall.

TIMING. Murmurs can be described by the time they occur in the cardiac cycle. Murmurs occur during systole (systolic murmurs) or diastole (diastolic murmurs). Murmurs can be further described as to the extent of time during systole or diastole. Pansystolic murmurs, for instance, occur through entire systole from S_1 to S_2.

INTENSITY. The sound of the murmur can be graded by its intensity:

Grade 1 = Very faint
Grade 2 = Faint
Grade 3 = Moderately loud
Grade 4 = Loud
Grade 5 = Very loud
Grade 6 = Loudest possible

PITCH. The velocity of blood flow through the valves determines the pitch of the murmur. Murmurs may be described as low, medium, or high pitched. Low-pitched murmurs have a flowing quality; high-pitched murmurs, a whistling quality.

QUALITY. The quality of the murmur aids description and refers to the character of the sound and its onset and progression. Murmurs can be flowing, harsh, whistling, musical, rumbling, or raspy. Crescendo murmurs increase in intensity after onset; decrescendo murmurs decrease in intensity after onset; crescendo-decrescendo murmurs increase and decrease in intensity.

Rubs. The sound produced by the interfacing of the parietal and visceral surfaces of the pericardium caused by inflammation of the pericardial sac is referred to as a *pericardial friction rub*. The sound is a scratchy, grating sound that can vary in intensity, duration, and location depending on the position of the client, phase of respiratory cycle, or length of time the surfaces are in contact. Pericardial friction rubs are heard with pericarditis or after myocardial infarction.

Blood vessels. The blood vessels (the veins and arteries) can be inspected, palpated, and auscultated to determine adequacy of venous and arterial circulation. A systematic approach to each limb and the vessel facilitates examination.

Inspection. Observing the color, size, shape, and symmetry of the limbs and digits provides significant information about peripheral vascular circulation. The skin should be observed for color. Inadequate circulation may produce pallor, rubor, or cyanosis.

Pallor can reflect decreased oxyhemoglobin levels caused by reduction of hemoglobin, loss of blood flow (shock), or edema. Pallor is observed on the skin surfaces around the face, nail beds, mucous membranes, or the conjunctiva. Pallor in dark-skinned individuals is best observed in mucous membranes. Rubor, or reddish hue to the skin, is caused by increased blood flow in the skin surfaces. This may be caused by fever or exposure to cold.

Cyanosis gives special information about oxygen delivery to the cells and

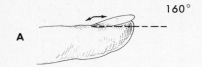

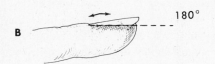

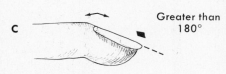

FIG. 20-3
Clubbing. **A,** Normal angle of nail. **B,** Slight clubbing. **C,** Severe clubbing. (From Abels, Linda Feiwell: Mosby's manual of critical care, St. Louis, 1979, The C.V. Mosby Co.)

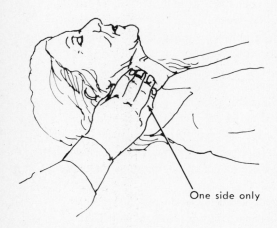

FIG. 20-4
Palpating carotid pulse. (From Wasserberger, Jonathan, and Eubanks, David H.: Practical paramedic procedures, ed. 2, St. Louis, 1981, The C.V. Mosby Co.)

reflects deoxygenation of the blood. When deoxygenation reaches levels of 3 to 4 g/100 ml of blood, mild cyanosis appears, whereas overt cyanosis appears at 5 g/100 ml of blood. Cyanosis can be differentiated as peripheral and central. Peripheral cyanosis occurs in states of low cardiac output such as found in pump failure. Central cyanosis is caused by circulatory inadequacies of oxygenation, usually from pulmonary disease, obstructions, or congenital or acquired heart defects in which there is mixing of deoxygenated and oxygenated blood. Clinically, peripheral and central cyanosis cannot be distinguished, but assessments of cyanosis are essential for planning nursing interventions. Cyanosis is best visualized with good lighting. Vascular areas such as the tongue, lips, earlobes, and nailbeds offer best visualization. Cyanosis in dark-skinned individuals can be detected by inspecting mucous membranes of the mouth.

Circulation in the extremities is noted by inspecting the fingers and toes for hair growth, the nailbeds for presence of clubbing, and the digits for capillary refill. Absent or inadequate circulation to the extremities may be reflected by absence of hair growth, and the nurse can look at each digit to determine the presence of hair. *Clubbing* (Fig. 20-3) is believed to be a response to chronic hypoxia in which the vascular bed at the end of the digits increases and the angle of the nail is decreased. *Capillary refill* can be tested by pressing the tip of the nail to produce blanching and observing return of color. Prolonged filling time is indicative of inadequate circulation.

The veins in the extremities can be observed for distension, occlusion, or dilation. Veins of the lower extremities should be observed for presence of erythema, distension, or swelling indicative of thrombosis, thrombophlebitis, or varicosities. *Homan's* test can be done to determine pain of thrombophlebitis. The client dorsiflexes his foot; if pain occurs, the test is positive, indicating pain from phlebitis, not pain from muscle spasm.

The veins of the neck should be observed for distension and pulsation. Venous pressure can be estimated by observing the jugular vein. The nurse can slightly occlude the vein and allow it to fill. Venous distension, which is visible in the supine position, will disappear as the head of the bed is elevated. If venous pressure is elevated, distension is visible with the bed elevated at 45 degrees, and the veins are engorged when the bed is at a 90-degree angle. Venous distension can be more accurately described from a reference point such as the suprasternal angle. Venous distension greater than 2 cm from this point when the bed is elevated at a 45-degree angle is abnormal.

Hepatojugular reflux can be observed if venous pressure is elevated, as in right heart failure or hypovolemic (cardiogenic) shock. To determine elevation of venous pressure, the nurse applies pressure over the right upper quadrant of the abdomen for 30 to 45 seconds. The blood returns to the right heart and produces engorgement of the neck veins if the heart is not able to accommodate the additional fluid load.

Palpation. The extremities can be palpated to note temperature, edema, and pulsation. All extremities should be felt for warmth. It is important to note the point where the temperature changes occur and differences in the opposite limb.

Edema can be assessed over a bony prominence such as the medial malleolus, anterior tibia, and sacrum. The nurse can press the area for 5 seconds and measure the pitting on a scale of +1 to +4:

+1 = Slight indentation that disappears rapidly

+2 = Indentation that disappears in 10 to 15 seconds
+3 = Deep indentation that disappears in 1 to 2 minutes
+4 = Marked indentation that disappears in 5 or more minutes

The carotid and peripheral pulses should be palpated and counted for 1 minute. The carotid pulse is located by sliding the finger tips laterally across the thyroid cartilage and moving them into the groove between the trachea and sternocleidomastoid muscle (Fig. 20-4). The carotid artery should be palpated lightly to avoid stimulating the carotid sinus, which could induce a bradycardia. The femoral pulses are found in the groin below the inguinal ligaments. Firmer pressure may be required to locate these pulses. The popliteal arteries are more easily found with the knee flexed and using both hands if necessary (Fig. 20-5, *A*). The dorsalis pedis (Fig. 20-5, *B*) and posterior tibial (Fig. 20-5, *C*) pulses can be felt using lighter pressure and, if faint, can be marked with ink for future identification. If the nurse is not able to palpate the pulse, a Doppler unit may be used to enhance identification of the pulse. Pulses are graded according to palpable blood flow:

0 = Absent, not palpable
+1 = Barely palpable, thready and weak
+2 = Slightly reduced
+3 = Normal volume, easily palpable
+4 = Bounding, abnormally forceful

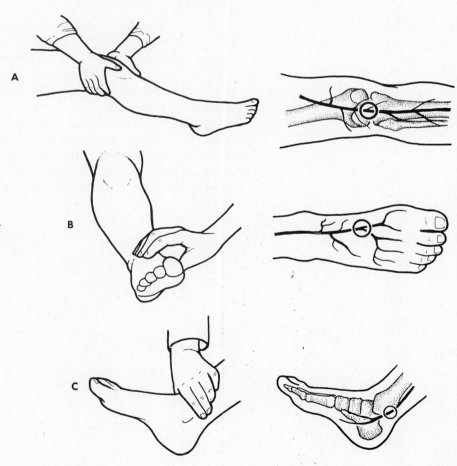

FIG. 20-5
Location and palpation of arteries of lower extremity. **A,** Popliteal. **B,** Dorsalis pedis. **C,** Posterior tibial.

Nursing process for common health problems

Auscultation. The arteries can be auscultated using the bell of the stethoscope over the artery. Normal arteries do not produce sounds, but in the presence of obstruction, such as in arteriosclerosis, a blowing sound, or *bruit,* can be heard. The carotid arteries, abdominal aorta, and femoral arteries can be auscultated to verify adequacy of blood flow.

HEMODYNAMIC ASSESSMENT

In addition to data from the nursing history and physical assessment, the nurse may gather and/or interpret data from hemodynamic monitoring. The data obtained from monitoring are useful for establishing nursing diagnoses and priorities of problems, as well as providing ongoing information and patterns of incipient changes during critical illness.

There are various types of monitoring equipment, and the nurse should be familiar with the equipment used in a particular setting and be able to explain its use to the client and family. It cannot be emphasized too strongly that monitoring does not take the place of reasoned clinical assessment or negate the involvement of the nurse in the client's plan of care.

Electrocardiogram

The electrocardiogram (ECG) is a graphic record of the electrical conduction pattern that represents myocardial depolarization and repolarization. The electrical currents can be detected on the skin by use of electrodes placed on opposite poles of the electrical field. The current changes are amplified and recorded on graph paper or reflected on an oscilloscope.

The electrodes, or leads, are placed on the limbs (or shoulders) and various points of the precordium. Suction cups, disks, or needles may be used to secure the leads. Most monitoring is done using the three standard limb leads placed on the right arm (shoulder), left arm (shoulder) and left leg, or a point below the rib cage (Fig. 20-6). The axis of lead I is from the negative electrode on the right arm to the positive electrode on the left arm; the axis of lead II is from the negative electrode on the right arm to the positive electrode on the left leg. The axis of lead III is from the negative electrode on the left arm to the positive electrode on the left leg. More complete electrocardiographic data (12-lead ECG) can be obtained by adding electrodes to points around the precordium.

Before placement of the electrode, the skin should be cleansed with alcohol and, if necessary, shaved. Depending on the type of electrode used, an elec-

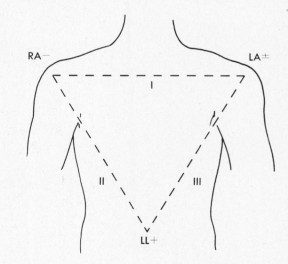

FIG. 20-6
Standard limb leads.

trode paste may be applied to the skin to facilitate conduction. Topical leads should be changed every 8 to 24 hours to prevent skin irritation. Disposable, prelubricated disks generally are changed every 3 to 4 days unless the client complains of skin irritation, in which case the disks are changed daily and the sites rotated. Electrodes should not be placed over bony areas, skin folds, or areas needed for defibrillation.

To obtain a bipolar lead, it is necessary to use positive, negative, and ground electrodes. Placement of electrodes determines the leads, and the lead that gives the best display of QRS-complex and P-wave activity is used. The electrodes should be placed in areas where muscle activity will offer minimal interference. Chest leads are most suited to long-term monitoring. Fig. 20-6 shows lead placement for standard chest lead II, which is most frequently used for monitoring, because it gives the best visualization of P-wave activity.

The ECG is recorded on graph paper on which the horizontal lines indicate voltage and the vertical lines indicate time. Letters are used to designate the positive and negative deflections from the isoelectric line caused by depolarization and repolarization of the heart (Fig. 20-7).

BASIC ECG COMPLEXES

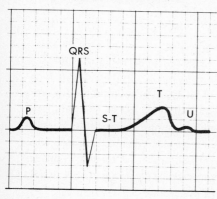

FIG. 20-7
Normal ECG. (From Goldberger, Ary L., and Goldberger, Emanuel: Clinical electrocardiography: a simplified approach, ed. 2, St. Louis, 1981, The C. V. Mosby Co.)

P wave   = Depolarization of atria
QRS complex = Depolarization of bundle of HIS and Purkinje fibers, and ventricle
PR interval   = Time of conduction from atria to ventricles
ST segment   = Recovery or repolarization of ventricles
T wave   = Recovery after contraction of ventricles
U wave   = May represent hypokalemia; often insignificant

A normal ECG is influenced by the age, sex, and size of the client. In addition, if the client has been taking digitalis or quinidine preparations or other drugs, the rate and rhythm may be altered.

The client should receive an explanation of this procedure so that he will be relaxed and a basal heart rate obtained. The equipment is grounded, with no chance of electrical damage to the client, and the procedure is painless. Knowing this may relieve some clients' fears.

ECG interpretation. Interpretation of the ECG is complex and not within the scope of this text. Nurses, however, should be familiar with a basic approach to ECG interpretation and be able to recognize common dysrhythmias.

A systematic approach to reading an ECG is helpful. Analysis of cardiac rhythms can be made and compared with normal cycles by looking at a 6-second record of the ECG.[1,10,28]

1. *Rate*. First determine atrial and ventricular rates. Several methods can be used.
   a. Quick estimate: In a 6-second strip, count number of cycles of P to P intervals (atrial rate) and R to R intervals (ventricular rate) and multiply by 10 (6 seconds × 10 = rate per minute). N = 60 to 100 (adults).
   b. More accurate estimate: Count "large boxes" between cycles (P to P atrial rate; R to R ventricular rate) and divide into 300 (300 large boxes in 1-minute strip); or count number of "small boxes" between consecutive R or P waves and divide into 1500 (1500 small boxes in a 1-minute strip). This method is helpful for calculating rapid rates.

c. Estimates of irregular rhythms: Count several P to P or R to R cycles and the number of 0.04-second (small) boxes between them. The former figure divided by the latter and multiplied by 1500 gives rate per minute.

2. *Rhythm.* To determine the rhythm, it is helpful to have calipers or a ruler and paper. The points of the calipers are placed on a P to P or R to R cycle and compared with subsequent cycles in the strip. The rhythm should be noted as regular or irregular.

3. *Configuration.* Identify the presence, shape, and duration of each component of the cycle.

   a. P wave. Present or absent? Direction of inflection? Precedes QRS?

   b. PR interval. Duration (number of small boxes × 0.04)? N = 0.12 to 0.20 second.

   c. QRS complex. Shape? Duration (number of small boxes × 0.04)? N = <0.10 second.

   d. ST segment: Elevated or depressed?

   e. T wave. Direction? Height?

   f. U wave. Present or absent?

Artifacts may confuse the interpretation of ECGs. Two common ones are a wandering baseline (Fig. 20-8) and somatic tremor (Fig. 20-9). A tremulous, uneven baseline may be caused by muscle tremors, as might occur if the client is tense, coughs, turns, or shivers. Placing the electrodes outside a muscle mass may prevent this phenomenon. A wandering baseline can be caused by inadequate grounding or improper placement or connection of electrodes. This artifact can be remedied by securing the placement of electrodes.

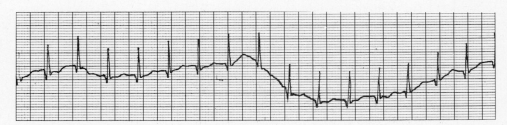

FIG. 20-8
Wandering baseline. (From Conover, Mary B.: Understanding electrocardiography: physiological and interpretive concepts, ed. 3, St. Louis, 1980, The C.V. Mosby Co.)

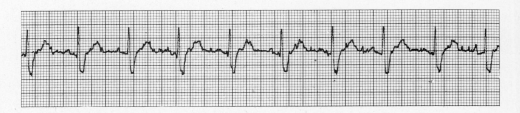

FIG. 20-9
Somatic tremor. (From Conover, Mary B.: Understanding electrocardiography: physiological and interpretive concepts, ed. 3, St. Louis, 1980, The C.V. Mosby Co.)

Finer discriminations of the heart's electrical activity may be determined by the *electrogram,* or intracardiac ECG. Electrode-tipped catheters are placed in the right atrium (atrial electrogram), in the septal leaflet of the tricuspid valve (bundle of His electrogram), or over the entire surface of the heart (surface mapping) to detect focal points of irregular cardiac conduction.

Use of ECG. The ECG can be used in a variety of settings. It is useful in physical examination and mass-screening programs to determine cardiac pathological conditions, often before such conditions are manifested clinically. The record of the ECG is usually retained for comparisons with changes at a later date.

Dynamic electrocardiography allows the collection of ECG data while the client pursues usual activities. A compact recording device such as a Holter monitor can be worn by the client. Chest leads are used to obtain the ECG, which can be stored and recorded for a 24-hour period. The client keeps a record of his activities for the specified time period, and the record can then be correlated with events recorded by the ECG.

The ECG can also be used when the heart rate must be monitored on a continuous basis, such as in emergency departments, mobile intensive care units, surgery or cardiac catheterization, or in coronary care units when the client is critically ill. At this time the tracing is shown on an oscilloscope, which gives immediate visualization of the electrical pattern of the heartbeat. Newer forms of communication make it possible to transmit ECGs over telephone wires so that the client may receive the services of a specialist at a distant medical center. The ECGs may be sent from emergency vehicles, clients' homes, or small hospitals that do not have the services of a cardiologist. The equipment for obtaining ECGs has been compacted so that it is easily portable and can be used outside a

FIG. 20-10
Nurse interprets ECG transmitted by telemetry.

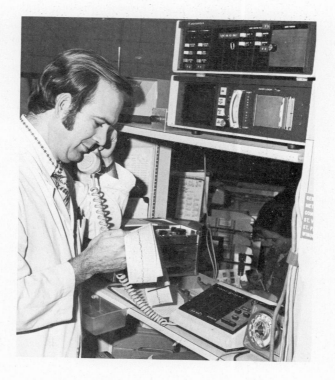

health care facility. Computer analysis of ECG tracings is also used in clinical settings. The computer monitors rate and analyzes changes in rate and QRS morphology. This capability for displaying, analyzing, and storing aids immensely in rapid, accurate diagnosis of dysrhythmias.

Telemetry

To provide mobility for clients who must be monitored, information about cardiac conduction can be transmitted via electrodes attached to a portable transmitter and displayed at a central monitoring station (Fig. 20-10). Usually the client wears the battery-operated transmitter pinned to his gown or in a pocket and is instructed to remain within the area of the receiving station. The system can also be adapted to transmit over telephone lines.

Vectorcardiogram

Whereas electrocardiography measures only the magnitude and direction of the electrical changes within the heart, a vectorcardiogram can be used to record changes in spatial orientation, magnitude, and force of myocardial conduction. Leads applied to the chest transmit data on a graph or oscilloscope in the forms of vector planes or loops. The P loop represents atrial activity; the QRS complex, ventricular depolarization; and the T loop, ventricular repolarization.

Venous pressure

Venous pressure reflects the pressure of the blood against the veins. It changes with differences in the heart rate, vessel size, and blood volume. Increases in venous pressure can be observed in distended jugular veins. A rise in venous pressure can also be detected when the client raises his hands above his heart. Normally the veins collapse as the hands are raised, but if the veins remain full of blood, the venous pressure is elevated.

Central venous pressure

Central venous pressure (CVP) reflects the pressure of the blood in the right atrium and therefore is a measurement of cardiac efficiency, blood volume, peripheral resistance, and right ventricular pressure. CVP provides useful information in instances of increasing blood volume, as in pump failure (cardiac decompensation, right heart failure) and states of vasoconstriction or decreased blood volume (in states of shock, septic shock, hypovolemia, vasodilation, and burns). CVP is also useful in detecting hemodilution before changes in the hematocrit are noticed. A 3- to 5-cm drop in CVP can reflect a loss of 10% of the blood volume.

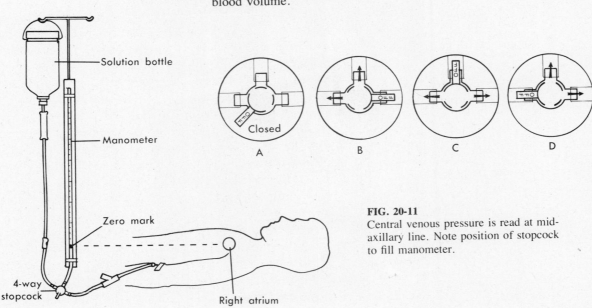

FIG. 20-11
Central venous pressure is read at midaxillary line. Note position of stopcock to fill manometer.

NORMAL HEMODYNAMIC PRESSURE RANGES

Right atrium
A wave	<8 mm Hg
V wave	<8 mm Hg
Mean	2-6 mm Hg

Right ventricle
Systolic	20-30 mm Hg
Diastolic	0-5 mm Hg
End-diastolic	2-6 mm Hg

Pulmonary artery
Systolic	20-30 mm Hg
Diastolic	10-20 mm Hg
Mean	10-15 mm Hg

Pulmonary artery wedge
A wave	12-15 mm Hg
V wave	12-15 mm Hg
Mean	4-12 mm Hg

Left atrium
A wave	12-15 mm Hg
V wave	12-15 mm Hg
Mean	4-12 mm Hg

Left ventricle
Systolic	100-140 mm Hg
Diastolic	0-5 mm Hg
End-diastolic	5-12 mm Hg

Pulmonary artery catheterization

To obtain a measurement of CVP, it is necessary to insert a catheter into the superior vena cava or right atrium (Fig. 20-11). After scrupulous skin preparation, the catheter is passed from a cutdown or puncture site in the antecubital, subclavian, jugular, or basilic vein to the right atrium. At this point the catheter can be attached to a precalibrated manometer or a strain-gauge transducer and a flush solution. To use a precalibrated monitor to determine CVP readings, the intravenous infusion is discontinued and the fluid is permitted to run into the manometer. The manometer must be placed at a point level with the right atrium, usually at the midaxillary line. The manometer is read when the fluid levels off in the manometer. Respirations may cause a certain amount of fluctuation in the fluid level, and the reading should be obtained at the highest point of fluctuation. If the client is using a ventilator, its use should be discontinued if possible during the reading of CVP.

To use the transducer, the transducer is attached and calibrated according to the manufacturer's directions. The CVP is read with the transducer at the midaxillary line and the client in a supine position or a predetermined position used for each reading. When the stopcock at the transducer is turned off to the intravenous fluid, the wave form is visible on the oscilloscope. The reading should be obtained at the highest point of fluctuation.

Aseptic technique is observed to prevent entry of microorganisms and phlebitis. An antibacterial ointment should be applied to the insertion site as the dressing is changed and the line changed every 24 to 48 hours. Solutions with a pH of 7 may also help prevent phlebitis. Medications, especially vasopressors or antidysrhythmic drugs, should not be given through the CVP line because they will distort interpretation. Normal CVP is 6 to 12 cm of water when the catheter is in the superior vena cava, and 0 to 12 cm water when in the right atrium.

Cardiac hemodynamics may be measured more accurately by the use of a special flow-directed catheter (Swan-Ganz catheter) placed in the pulmonary artery. Pressure changes here reflect variances in left heart activity and help identify incipient pulmonary edema or the reduced cardiac output concomitant with dysrhythmias or a failing infarcted heart, shown in the material at left. Effects of fluid and pharmacological therapy may be monitored, but the real value lies in the ability for early detection of pressure changes that can occur many hours before a change in CVP or other clinical evidence is present. The use of the catheter is extended by the capability of withdrawing blood samples for blood gas analysis, pulmonary angiography, measurement of cardiac output by thermal dilution, pacing, or recording of His bundle activity.

The catheter (Fig. 20-12) is inserted through a peripheral vein (usually median basilic) into the subclavian vein where pressures can be obtained in the right atrium and right ventricle. The catheter is then advanced through the pulmonic valve into the pulmonary artery (Fig. 20-12). At this point the pulmonary artery pressure (PAP) is recorded and reflected by means of a transducer to a monitor, which displays the pressures in wave form. PAP is usually recorded every hour for critically ill clients.

Additional information can be obtained by advancing the catheter into the pulmonary artery wedge position (PAWP), pulmonary artery occluded position (PAO), or pulmonary capillary wedge pressure (PCWP). The balloon is inflated to obtain pressure readings but must not remain inflated at the risk of pulmonary infarction. (A normal A wave reading is 12 to 15 mm Hg.) Changes in wave form

FIG. 20-12
Flow-directed, balloon-tipped catheter showing inflation of balloon in right atrium and consequent "floating" of catheter through right ventricle and out to distal PA branch. Balloon is deflated, advanced slightly, and reinflated slightly to obtain PAW pressure. (From Daily, Elaine K., and Schroeder, John S.: Bedside hemodynamic monitoring, ed. 2, St. Louis, 1981, The C.V. Mosby Co.)

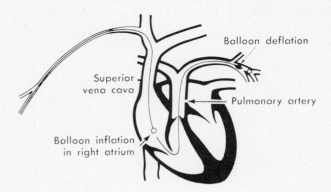

indicate that the wedge position has been obtained. Balloon inflation should never exceed the manufacturer's recommendation, and the balloon should be deflated once the wedge pressure is recorded. Clients who are using respirators should be temporarily disconnected, if possible, from ventilatory assistance to obtain accurate PAWP readings. These data are usually recorded every 4 hours.

The insertion site should be observed frequently and dressings changed according to agency policy. The line should be continuously flushed with a heparinized saline solution. Medications should not be infused through this line.

Left ventricular end diastolic pressure (LVEDP) is another parameter of cardiac function that may be used to monitor vital changes in critically ill persons. LVEDP correlates with pulmonary artery end diastolic pressure and thus reflects left ventricular function. A normal reading is 5 to 12 mm Hg.

Cardiac output

Exact measurements of cardiac output are valuable in monitoring cardiac performance of critically ill persons.[13] Precise information about the pumping efficiency and circulating blood volume is useful in assessment and intervention of clients with pump failure, myocardial infarction, congenital heart defects, and after open-heart surgery. Cardiac output increases in diseases such as anemia, thyrotoxicosis, and conditions of increased metabolism. Decreases in cardiac output are usually caused by inadequate venous return, bradycardia, and hypovolemic states (hemorrhage and shock).

Determinations of cardiac output are based on the Fick principle, which states that the rate a substance delivered in a fluid is distributed in a moving fluid is equal to the product of the flow rate and the difference between concentration at sites proximal and distal to the area. Dye indicators and thermal indicators are the most common methods used to determine cardiac output. Both methods are highly sophisticated measurements of cardiac function and are usually done in medical facilities with specialized support services.

In the dye-dilution method a dye is inserted in the venous circulation, and the amount of circulated dye in an artery is measured. Established dye-dilution curves are used as a basis to calculate the cardiac output. This method is not usually feasible to obtain serial measurements.

Bedside monitoring of the cardiac output can be done more easily by the thermal indicator technique. In this method a four-lumen flow-directed catheter is used. One lumen is placed in the superior vena cava or right atrium, and a thermistor in the pulmonary artery. When a substance (usually 5% dextrose) of a known temperature is instilled in the atrial catheter, the temperature is measured by the thermistor in the pulmonary artery. Temperature-dilution curves are

FIG. 20-13
Arterial line used to monitor intraarterial blood pressure. Note flush system and monitor.

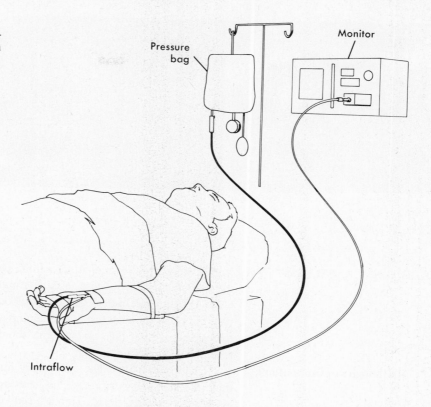

Pressure bag

Monitor

Intraflow

calculated by the computer and displayed on the monitor. Changes in cardiac output over a period of time are more significant than one-time assessments, and this method permits serial monitoring without discomfort to the client once the catheter is inserted (N = 4 to 8 L/min).

Intraarterial blood pressure

Accurate measurements of the blood pressure of critically ill clients in states of shock and those with dysrhythmias, accelerated hypertension, or valvular obstruction may be obtained by using an intraarterial catheter (arterial line) to determine systolic, diastolic, and mean blood pressures (Fig. 20-13). A catheter flushed with heparinized saline is inserted into an artery, usually the radial artery.

If the radial artery is used, it is necessary to verify the presence of ulnar artery flow. This is known as the *Allen test* and is performed by occluding the ulnar and radial arteries with the examiner's fingers. The client's hand should be elevated in this position for 5 minutes to drain circulation. When the ulnar artery is released, the blood flow should return to the hand, indicating adequate circulation in the ulnar artery.

A transducer attached to the catheter converts pressure to voltage that can be read on a monitor. A transfer blood pack unit or other pressure device around the heparinized saline is inflated above the point of systolic blood pressure to maintain the catheter in the artery.

The insertion site should be inspected frequently for thrombus formation and inflammation. The line should be flushed continuously with heparinized solution and after drawing blood gases to prevent formation of microemboli. A continuous flush intraflow system (Fig. 20-14) can be used for this purpose. At least every 8 hours the system should be calibrated with the monitor according to the instructions with the equipment.

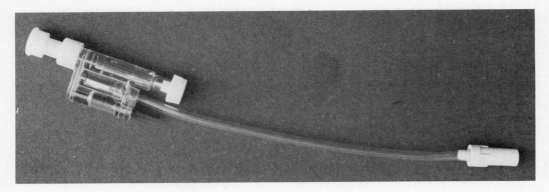

FIG. 20-14
Intraflow flush system.

DIAGNOSTIC ASSESSMENT

Various diagnostic examinations can be performed to assess interferences with the need for oxygen. These tests determine cardiac efficiency, patency of the blood vessels, and indices of various blood components. The nurse should prepare the client for each test by explaining what will be done and what he can do to cooperate. After the test the nurse should assess the client for any untoward reactions to the examination.

Radiological examinations

Chest x-ray film. The chest x-ray film is a simple measure used to determine the size and position of the heart and great vessels. Calcification of the vessels may also be noted. This test can be used in mass-screening programs to detect gross cardiac pathological conditions.

Angiocardiogram. To obtain an angiocardiogram, a dye is inserted into the heart through a catheter in the antecubital vein. Roentgenograms are taken as the dye fills the chambers of the heart. Valvular defects can be noticed as the dye outlines the structures. The client should not have anything by mouth for 6 to 8 hours before this test, and a sedative may be given for apprehension. After the test the nurse should observe the insertion site for bleeding or thrombosis.

Cardiac catheterization. Cardiac catheterization is a more complex procedure in which a catheter is inserted in the peripheral veins or arteries and is threaded through the chambers of the heart.[7,20] Dye may be inserted to visualize cardiac structures or blood samples obtained and analyzed for physiological data about blood flow, oxygen and carbon dioxide content, and pressure variances within the four chambers of the heart and the aorta as well as structural abnormalities.

Before the examination the physician explains the purpose of the catheterization and procedures to be used. The procedure is not without risk of dysrhythmias, perforation, pericardial tamponade, thrombus, cardiac arrest, electrolyte imbalances, or allergic reactions caused by contrast media, and the client should be informed by the physician of these potential complications and should sign a permit. The nurse can offer additional information as required by the client. Booklets, instruction sheets, and media aids may be used to enhance explanations.

Before the procedure the client receives nothing by mouth. Infants may be given a solution of dextrose and water 2 to 3 hours before the catheterization to prevent dehydration and hypoglycemia. A sedative is given immediately before

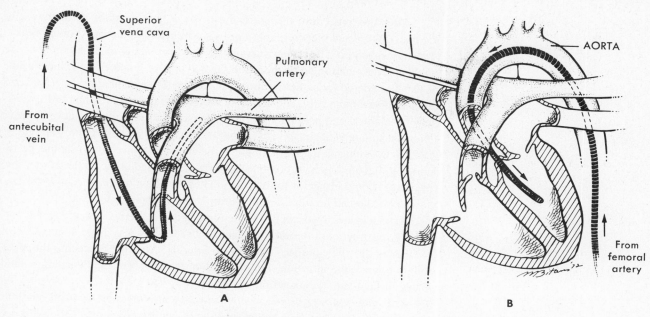

FIG. 20-15
Cardiac catheterization. **A,** Right heart. **B,** One approach to left heart.

the catheterization; infants and children may be given a general anesthetic to prevent crying and restlessness during this procedure, which can take several hours.

Examination of the right heart is accomplished by threading the catheter from a cutdown site in a peripheral vein to the right atrium, right ventricle, and pulmonary artery (Fig. 20-15, *A*). The left side of the heart may be approached in several ways. The catheter may be inserted in a retrograde manner through the aorta to the left atrium and left ventricle (Fig. 20-15, *B*). The catheter can also be guided into the coronary arteries and dye injected to visualize the arteries. In another approach the catheter is inserted with a bronchoscope by a stab wound through the main bronchus to the left atrium or left ventricle.

While the catheter passes through the chambers of the heart, the physician observes its progress with fluoroscopy and may use cineradiography to obtain moving pictures. Pressure readings and blood samples may be obtained from the heart chambers and blood vessels. The client's heart is continuously monitored by an electrocardiogram during the catheterization. Nitroglycerin may be given to dilate the coronary arteries for improved visualization or to treat angina. Atropine may be given intravenously for bradydysrhythmias.

Most clients are awake during the procedure and may be aware of the movement of the catheter and the insertion of the dye. They may notice extra heart beats while the catheter is threaded through the chambers of the heart. Some individuals experience a feeling of warmth when the dye is inserted. Numbness and tingling may be felt at the point of catheter insertion from temporary circulatory obstruction. These feelings are normal, and the client should be prepared for them.

Nursing process for common health problems

After this procedure the nurse must assess the client for disturbances of cardiac rhythm and bleeding, thrombosis, or infection at the site of and distal to catheter insertion. The client is usually on bed rest for 4 to 24 hours after the procedure, depending on the insertion site and type of procedure; the longer time is usually ordered for catheterizations done using the femoral arteries. Vital signs are monitored frequently, and the nurse should note the rate, rhythm, and character of the apical and peripheral pulses. The pulses distal to the point of catheter insertion should be taken to verify adequate circulation. The extremity should be felt for warmth; numbness or tingling and blanching or cooling should be reported to the physician. A compression dressing is used at the cutdown site, and the nurse should inspect it for bleeding. Thrombophlebitis may occur at the cutdown site and can be treated with warm, sterile compresses.

Arteriogram. Dye can be inserted into specific arteries to demonstrate narrowing, obstructions, thrombi, or aneurysms. Clients may have a sensation of warmth as the dye circulates through the arteries. After the procedure the nurse should observe the insertion site for bleeding or thrombosis and encourage fluid intake to facilitate dye excretion.

In *coronary artery arteriography* (selective arteriograms) contrast media is injected into the coronary arteries for the specific purposes of locating arteries and determining patency and flow rates. These studies may also be done at the time of cardiac catheterization. A catheter is inserted through the ascending arch of the aorta to the aortic valve where it enters the right and left coronary arteries. Dye is then instilled through the catheter to visualize the patency of the arteries.

Radionuclide studies. Radioactive drugs can be administered to obtain noninvasive radiographic images of the heart and vessels. Two methods are radionuclide angiography and myocardial imaging.

Radionuclide angiography is obtained by injection of a radioactive substance such as pertechnetate ^{99m}Tc into the venous system. Visualization of the heart, great vessels, and lungs is obtained with a high-speed scintillation camera.

Myocardial imaging is performed with the use of radioisotopes, such as ^{43}K, that concentrate in a normal, well-perfused myocardium. The drug is injected intravenously and detected by scanning techniques. Underperfused areas indicate myocardial ischemia or infarct. Other isotopes, such as technetium, accumulate in areas of the myocardium that are underperfused and are used to estimate blood flow and areas of cell damage.

Venogram. Dye may also be inserted into veins for the purpose of outlining obstruction or lesions. The nurse should observe bleeding at the site of dye insertion.

Lymphography. Radiopaque dye can be inserted in lymphatic channels (lymphangiogram) or lymph glands (lymphadenogram) to detect obstruction or hyperplasia. The procedure is lengthy, often taking up to 8 hours. Children may be restrained and sedated to ensure cooperation. In a lymphangiogram the lymphatic channels are located in a web of the extremities, and then dye is inserted slowly at the rate of 7 ml/hr. Periodic x-ray films are taken as the dye is absorbed into the lymphatic circulation. The obstruction is indicated when the dye is unable to pass. The blue dye discolors the skin at the insertion site and may be present for 1 to 2 weeks. Excretion of the dye will be noticed until the dye is absorbed. The dye is usually retained in lymph nodes for as long as a year, making follow-up x-ray films easier to obtain.

After the procedure the client should rest and may appreciate a back massage. A mild analgesic may be ordered for discomfort. A dressing is applied to the insertion site and should be observed for bleeding or drainage. Complications of this procedure are rare, but the nurse should observe the client for pulmonary emboli (from dye absorbed in venous circulation) or thrombophlebitis.

Hematological studies

Blood specimens can be obtained to measure various indices of blood components. When a blood specimen is drawn, the nurse should observe the site for bleeding and, if necessary, apply pressure to the puncture site for several minutes. Often specimens must be obtained daily for purposes of comparison, and the sites should be varied so that the client does not become bruised or sore in any one area.

Complete blood count. The complete blood count gives an indication of the type and number of formed elements in the blood. The counts are compared with normal values for age and are used to determine interferences with the oxygen supply.

Hematocrit value. The hematocrit value expresses the relationship of the formed elements in the blood to the total blood volume. The hematocrit value is lowered when the blood volume increases, as in congestive heart failure. The hematocrit value rises when blood volume is lost, as with bleeding, shock, and burns. Normal ranges for hematocrit are 45 to 50 vol/100 ml in men and 40 to 45 vol/100 ml in women.

Coagulation time. The time for the clotting mechanism to become active is expressed as the coagulation time. See Table 20-2 for coagulation factors. This test is useful when clients are receiving heparin, a drug that prolongs coagulation time. Normal coagulation time is 9 to 12 minutes. The Lee-White coagulation time is about 7 to 15 minutes.

Prothrombin time. A prothrombin time test measures how long it takes for prothrombin to become active in the clotting process. This test is used for clients who are receiving coumarin derivatives that lengthen the prothrombin time. Normal prothrombin time is 11 to 18 seconds.

Partial thromboplastin time (PTT). PTT is a blood study that determines deficiencies in all coagulation factors except factor VII. This test is used for clients who are receiving anticoagulants to detect changes in the coagulation process. The normal time is 39 to 59 seconds.

Activated partial thromboplastin time (APTT). APTT detects deficiencies in thromboplastin formation and is used to evaluate effectiveness of anticoagulants.

Erythrocyte sedimentation rate (ESR). The ESR indicates the extent to which red blood cells settle to the bottom of a test tube containing a sample of blood. The sedimentation rate rises during inflammatory processes such as rheumatic fever and myocardial infarction. Normal ESR is 0 to 20 mm/hr.

Serum cholesterol. The amount of cholesterol in a sample of blood is determined to indicate the likelihood of obstruction of blood vessels by atherosclerotic processes. The normal level is 150 to 280 mg/100 ml of blood.

Serum triglyceride. Triglycerides are simple lipids that may contribute to atherosclerosis. Normal range is 140 to 200 mg/ml of blood.

Serum enzymes. When tissue has been damaged, certain enzymes are released. These enzymes are released during tissue damage, but forms of the

TABLE 20-2

Coagulation factors

Factor	Name
I	Fibrinogen
II	Prothrombin
III	Tissue thromboplastin
IV	Calcium
V	Proaccelerin (accelerator globulin)
VI	Previously called accelerin (no longer in use)
VII	Proconvertin
VIII	Antihemophilic factor (AHF)
	Antihemophilic globulin (AHG)
IX	Plasma thromboplastin component (PTC) (Christmas factor)
X	Stuart-Prower factor
XI	Plasma thromboplastin antecedent (PTA)
	Antihemophilic factor C
XII	Hageman factor

enzymes (isoenzymes) specific to myocardial tissue injury provide more accurate data about myocardial tissue injury. (See discussion later in this chapter.)

SGOT = Serum glutamic-oxaloacetic transaminase; 15 to 45 units/ml is normal.

SGPT = Serum glutamic-pyruvic transaminase; 5 to 36 units/ml is normal.

LDH = Lactic dehydrogenase; 60 to 1000 units/ml is normal.

CPK = Creatine phosphokinase; 0 to 20 IU/L is normal.

Other studies

Phonocardiogram. A phonocardiogram is a visual record of heart sounds. The record is useful in analyzing heart sounds, particularly in children whose heart rate is rapid. In some instances the use of the phonocardiogram may eliminate the need to perform a cardiac catheterization or angiography.

Echocardiogram. An echocardiogram is a record of ultrasonic waves that bounce an echo off varied structures of the heart. An ultrasonoscope (probe) is used to send the impulses to the heart wall so that heart movement, the amount of blood, and the thickness of the heart wall can be determined and recorded on an oscilloscope or graph paper. This test is particularly useful to detect valve functioning, left ventricular activity, presence of tumors, congenital heart disease, or pericardial effusion.

No special preparation is required before the test because it is not invasive. The test is usually done in a laboratory, but may be done at the bedside if the client is too ill to be transported. The client is positioned lying turned slightly to his left side; the head may be elevated 15 degrees.

Ultrasound. The size, position, and movement of the heart can be determined by the use of high-frequency waves passing through matter and reflected as a visual record. No special preparations are required for this noninvasive procedure.

Venography. Venography is used to detect the presence of thrombus formation in the veins. A radioactive substance such as radioactive urokinase or fibrinogen that will be incorporated in the thrombus is given intravenously and the area scanned. Areas of increased uptake demonstrate the presence and location of the thrombus.

Plethysmography. This test measures variations in electrical resistance associated with changes in blood volume. Electrodes are applied to the extremity and the data recorded on graph paper. The venous flow is occluded with a cuff and changes recorded as blood pools in the extremity.

Bone marrow aspiration. A specimen from the bone marrow may be obtained to ascertain the type and amount of elements formed there. An easily accessible bone such as the sternum, iliac crest, or tibia is used. Generally the tibia is used with infants. The site is antiseptically cleansed and anesthetized with a local anesthetic, and a short needle is inserted to aspirate the bone marrow. The specimen is put on a slide that is stored in a preservative and later examined microscopically.

If the client is upset, a sedative may be given before the procedure. Young children may be held or restrained to prevent movement during aspiration. The client may feel sensation of pressure as the specimen is aspirated, but the procedure is not unduly painful. A bandage is put over the site, and unusual bleeding should be reported to the physician.

Measurement of capillary fragility. Interferences with clotting can be determined by measuring capillary fragility (Rumpel-Leede test). A blood pressure cuff is placed on the client's limb and inflated to a pressure midway between those used to measure systolic and diastolic blood pressure. The cuff remains in place for 5 to 15 minutes. Normally a few capillaries will break, causing small hemorrhages known as petechiae. When the platelet count is low and the clotting mechanism is impaired, the number of petechiae will increase.

Vanillylmandelic acid test (VMA). Vanillylmandelic acid is a metabolic breakdown product of catecholamines. Detecting increased catecholamine production as occurs in tumors of the adrenal medulla (pheochromocytoma) is useful in diagnosing the presence of this tumor.

For this study a 24-hour urine sample is obtained. The specimen should be refrigerated during collection and stored in a container with a preservative of 6 N hydrochloric acid. False-positive results can be obtained if the client has included in his diet chocolate, coffee, tea, vanilla, or fruits of any kind. For this reason the client should abstain from these foods for 3 days before the test.

Renin test. Renin is an enzyme that stimulates the release of angiotensin II. Angiotensin II raises systemic blood pressure by a vasoconstricting action and by stimulation of the release of aldosterone from the adrenal gland. In the presence of kidney disease or decreased blood flow to the kidneys, renin is released and may be identified as a possible contributing factor in the diagnosis of hypertension.

Renin levels may be determined by radioimmunoassay or by collection of renal vein samples by catheterization of the inferior vena cava. Because renin is stimulated by sodium intake and an upright position, the client may be asked to follow a special diet and ambulate for 4 to 6 hours before obtaining blood samples. In one procedure the client follows a 9 g sodium diet for 3 days before the test. A fasting blood sample is drawn from the client, who is recumbent after 6 hours of sleep. The client then walks or stands for 4 hours, and another blood sample is drawn, iced, and sent to the laboratory for radioimmunoassay.

Schilling's test. Schilling's test is used to measure the presence of vitamin B_{12} in the body. In pernicious anemia this vitamin is not present. Radioactive vitamin B_{12} is given orally, and its excretion is measured in the urine. The client receives nothing by mouth after midnight and is given an oral dose of radioactive vitamin B_{12} in the morning. The client may also be given a loading dose of intramuscular vitamin B_{12} to assure sufficient vitamin B_{12} in the body so that the diagnostic dose is not used. The urine is saved for 24 hours, and the excreted vitamin B_{12} is measured. If the body has adequate reserves of B_{12}, only 10% to 20% of the vitamin should be excreted. Less than 10% excretion is indicative of pernicious anemia.

Stress tests (exercise tolerance tests, treadmill tests). The myocardial oxygen requirements during exercise can be determined when the client exercises while his heart rate and rhythm are monitored. This test can be done to estimate the extent of coronary artery disease, evaluate the effectiveness of cardiac surgery or drug therapy, and measure capacity for exercise.

The test is performed as the client exercises, either by walking up and down steps (Master's two-step exercise test) or, more commonly, as the client walks forward on a backward-moving treatmill set at various speeds. Stress testing can also be done with the client riding a stationary bicycle or with the use of a pace-maker or drugs to increase heart rate. The client is monitored by an electrocardiogram as he attempts to achieve his maximal heart rate according to standards for age and weight. The submaximal heart rate is the rate at which ischemic changes will occur in the presence of coronary artery disease.

Before the test the nurse and physician should explain the test and elicit the client's cooperation. The client can be instructed to wear loose-fitting clothing and shoes with rubber soles. He should eat a light meal before the test and abstain from drinking coffee or alcohol. The client should also be instructed to report fatigue or chest pain, because the test will be stopped on a signal from the client.

The client is monitored during the test and the test is stopped if the client's blood pressure decreases, if he is short of breath, or has chest pain or dysrhythmias (PVCs 8 to 10 per minute or ventricular tachycardia). Facilities for defibrillation and resuscitation must be easily accessible.

Data analysis

When the nurse has gathered necessary and appropriate data from the nursing history, hemodynamic monitoring, or diagnostic studies, the data are compared with norms to detect deviations and formulate a list of nursing problems or diagnoses. Problems or diagnoses may be of an immediate or long-term nature, actual or potential. Common nursing diagnoses may include ineffective airway clearance, alterations in cardiac output, alterations in comfort, ineffective coping, fluid volume deficit, impaired gas exchange, knowledge deficit, noncompliance, alterations in self-concept, or alterations in tissue perfusion.

Planning
PLANNING FOR HEALTH PROMOTION

To ensure adequate oxygen to the client's cells, the nurse can help the client develop health habits that will promote the exchange of vital gases. The nurse may conduct programs planned to identify client risks for cardiovascular disease and instruct about risk prevention or management. The nurse may also participate in health teaching, which directs the client toward promoting circulation, preventing infection, and obtaining genetic counseling. Instruction about adequate nutrition is also essential in encouraging a diet sufficient for preventing nutritional anemias, and the nurse may help the client select appropriate meals and nutritious diets.

Risk factors and risk management

A variety of factors have been identified as being associated with cardiovascular diseases, particularly atherosclerotic heart disease (coronary artery disease), and hypertension.[33,43,57] The factors have been identified from retrospective and prospective studies. One of the earliest studies to identify the relationship of certain factors and the likelihood of heart disease was the Framingham Heart Study.[5,57] Subsequent studies using a variety of populations have confirmed the original findings. Risks include nonmodifiable factors such as age, gender, race, and family history, and modifiable factors of hypertension, smoking, hypercholesterolemia, obesity, glucose intolerance, sedentary life-style, stress, alcohol abuse, and environmental contaminants. Major risks are hypertension, smoking, and hypercholesterolemia; others are considered contributory.

There are a variety of tools available to assess risk factors and predict the possibility of death from cardiovascular disease. One method is the health hazard appraisal in which data are collected about the client's family background, current health status, and health habits, and compared with norms for age, sex, and race. Other tools include nursing histories and health habit analysis formats.

Once the risk is identified, the nurse can help the client plan risk management strategies. Risk management may include prevention of the risk, eliminating the risk that is present, or managing the risk after cardiovascular disease has been diagnosed. Many risk management strategies involve behavior modification, and instruction may take place in individual counseling settings or in group or community education programs.

Awareness of risk for cardiovascular disease has contributed to decline in atherosclerotic heart disease, and some believe atherosclerosis is indeed preventable.[38] Since the mid-1960s the death rate from atherosclerotic heart disease has decreased 15% to 25%. Although the decrease is not related to elimination of any one risk factor, it is believed that a change in several health habits has decreased death rates.[56] The role of the nurse in health instruction can therefore be vital to health promotion and prevention of atherosclerotic heart disease.

Nonmodifiable risk factors. The nurse can help the client recognize factors that contribute to risk for heart disease. Although age, sex, race, and genetic or family history cannot be altered, they contribute to risk of disease and are particularly significant in the presence of other risk factors.

Age. Atherosclerosis is a disease of middle age. Although predeterminants of atherosclerosis may be evident in childhood, clinical manifestations are usually not evident until the client is age 40 or 50. The incidence of disease increases markedly after this period.

Gender. The incidence of cardiovascular disease is greater in men until age 65, when the incidence equalizes. Various theories are offered to explain the sex-related difference. Some attribute it to the higher estrogen levels of premenopausal women because there may be a relationship of estrogen to high-density lipoproteins, which are inversely related to atherosclerosis and ischemic heart disease.

Race. The incidence of ischemic heart disease is higher in whites. The incidence of hypertension, however, is two times greater in blacks. These differences have been related to genetic background, environment, and life-style, although causal relationships have not been established.

Genetic history. Family history appears to be a significant risk factor for predisposition to heart disease. Diabetes mellitus and hypertension are two inherited risks for heart disease, and it is believed that family history may be more related to these specific risks than heart disease per se.

Modifiable risk factors. Major modifiable risk factors are hypertension, smoking, and hypercholesterolemia. Less significant although contributory, are obesity, glucose intolerance, sedentary life-style, stress, alcohol abuse, and caffeine abuse. Because these factors are amenable to prevention or change, the nurse and client can plan to alter one or more of these factors.

Hypertension. Hypertension is known to be a precursor of atherosclerosis and is associated with risk for ischemic heart disease. Mechanisms of atherogenesis are not clear, but it is believed that the injury to the intima caused by increased ranges of blood pressure may precipitate plaque formation. Others have identified an increased infiltration of lipids into blood vessels during states of elevated blood pressure.[38] The risk for heart disease increases with increases in systolic and diastolic pressure. Risk can be four times greater if the diastolic blood pressure is higher than 105 mm Hg.

Prevention. Because hypertension is believed to be caused by increased sodium in the diet and obesity, prevention is directed toward controlling sodium and calorie intake. Health instruction about nutrition begins during the prenatal period and is implemented in the diet of the neonate. Salt should not be added to the diet, and calories can be planned to accommodate the needs of the growing child.

Risk management. Control of hypertension may be the most significant factor in reducing the incidence of ischemic heart disease.[43] Once diagnosed, hypertension is treated with a sodium-restricted, calorie-controlled diet, diuretics, and, if necessary, antihypertensive drugs. The nurse can help the client comply with his therapeutic regimen. Therapy must be continued for a lifetime, and compliance with this program is imperative. Continued interest and follow-up by the nurse have been demonstrated to improve compliance.[50]

Hypercholesterolemia. Retrospective and prospective studies have identified the relationship of high fat and high cholesterol diet intake and high serum cholesterol levels with increased incidence of ischemic heart disease.[5,43] Cholesterol is transported in the bloodstream by lipoproteins that have varying amounts of cholesterol, protein, triglycerides, and phospholipids. Lipoprotein complexes can be classified as to the density and amount of cholesterol carried as chylomicrons, very-low-density lipoproteins (VLDL), intermediate-density lipoproteins (IDL), and high-density lipoproteins (HDL). Sixty to seventy-five percent of cholesterol is carried on the low-density lipoproteins, and these are therefore more closely associated with hypercholesterolemia. High-density lipoproteins, however, have an inverse relationship with the incidence of ischemic heart disease. Most researchers prefer to examine total cholesterol, and the risk for heart disease is increased threefold when total cholesterol levels are elevated.[38]

Triglycerides are carried primarily by chylomicrons, very-low-density lipoproteins, or intermediate-density lipoproteins. Elevation of serum triglycerides is also associated with heart disease.

The role of diet and hypercholesterolemia has been controversial, although most researchers agree that diets high in total fat and cholesterol contribute to increased serum cholesterol levels. Countries such as Japan, for example (where the total fat in the diet is less than 10% and the fat intake is from unsaturated fats), have a significantly lower rate of heart disease.

Prevention. The role of cholesterol, lipids, and carbohydrates in producing atherosclerosis is a subject of current research. Saturated fats appear to contribute to atherosclerotic formations, and many suggest a lifetime diet that is low in saturated fats, with emphasis in early years. Triglycerides, the simple lipids contained in lard, butterfat, olive oil, coconut oil, and soybean oil, have been suggested as a cause of atherosclerosis and should be restricted in the diet. Other diets in which carbohydrates are restricted are being used in an attempt to lower serum triglyceride levels by reducing serum pre-beta-lipoproteins, a combination of lipid and protein that is produced from carbohydrates and that can be influenced by dietary modification.

FAT-CONTROLLED DIET

Purpose:	Reduce fatty acids and prevent atherosclerosis.
Meats and eggs	Trim fat from meat; broil or boil meat; limit eggs to three a week.
Milk	Skim milk, buttermilk.
Fruits and vegetables	All allowed except avocado.
Breads and cereals	All allowed except biscuits.
Foods to avoid	Whole milk, cream, butter, ice cream, mayonnaise, sour cream, cheese, cakes (except angel food), cookies, duck, goose, fried foods, pork, meats canned in oil, nuts, peanut butter, creamed foods, chocolate.
Suggestions	1. Select meat with minimal marbling of fat. Trim excess fat from meat. Baste meat with unsaturated oil and seasonings. Broil or bake meat to permit drippings to drain off.
	2. Use unsaturated oil to make salad dressings and to bake.

In spite of controversy, most authorities agree that hypercholesterolemia can be prevented by reducing the intake of fats, particularly saturated fats.[38,43] As with any diet instruction, nutrition for health begins before birth and continues during the lifespan. Diets low in cholesterol and saturated fat are advised to maintain a serum cholesterol below 140 mg/100 ml (see fat-controlled diet, above).

Risk management. Clients with elevated serum cholesterol levels can dramatically reduce them by following a low-cholesterol diet.[38] Antilipidemic drugs may be used along with controlling the fat in the diet. These drugs appear to lower the level of circulating blood lipids and may prevent further atheromatous formations. Clofibrate (Atromid-S) and cholestyramine resin (Cuemid) are two such drugs.

Smoking. The hazards of tobacco smoking are produced by the inhalation of nicotine and carbon monoxide. The nicotine is a vasoconstrictor that compromises arteries already narrowed by atherosclerosis. Carbon monoxide reduces the oxygen-carrying capacity of the blood and puts added workload on the heart. Some believe smoking also contributes to atherogenesis because increased plaque formation has been found on autopsies of smokers.[43] The incidence of cigarette smoking has not dropped dramaticallly for all ages and sexes in spite of warnings by the Surgeon General and media campaigns of various health agencies. The incidence has decreased for men but not women, and many predict an increased incidence of ischemic heart disease in women. The incidence of smoking has also increased among adolescents.[43]

Prevention. Tobacco smoking may be considered as a drug addiction and, consequently, the most appropriate prevention is to not acquire the habit. Health instruction can be designed for target populations of school-age children and adolescents. Because smoking is often associated with stress, appropriate stress management strategies can also be emphasized.

Risk management. Once the habit has been acquired, it may be difficult for the client to quit smoking. The nurse can help the client identify resources and approaches to quitting smoking once the client has expressed the desire to do so. Often hospitalization for ischemic heart disease and enforced abstinence provides a stimulus for quitting. Many hospitals, health care centers, or community agencies sponsor smoking cessation clinics, and the nurse may refer the client to these.

Sedentary life-style. Controversy exists as to the exact relationship of activity to the development of heart disease. Generally it is believed that there is little difference between the moderately active person and one who has active exercise, but there is a positive relationship for those who have very sedentary life-styles and development of heart disease. Inactivity may contribute to peripheral pooling and stress the cardiovascular system. Prolonged inactivity of sitting or lying in one position particularly contribute to venous stasis and problems of venous circulation such as varicosities and thrombophlebitis. Prolonged bed rest presents potential problems of cardiac as well as extracardiac hazards of immobility. The risk factor for inactivity is also related to obesity and hypertension. The potential for glucose intolerance and hypertriglyceridemia may also be related to sedentary activity because, once the individual increases his activity, serum glucose and triglyceride levels are lowered.

Prevention. Although changing an inactive life-style may not prevent ischemic heart disease, the benefits of activity warrant an exercise program incorporated into daily activity. Exercise can be included in programs for school-age children and adolescents learning about health and hygiene. Training in individual, noncompetitive sports such as swimming is one positive approach to developing life-long habits of recreational enjoyment of exercise.

Risk management. Exercise programs of regular sustained activity have been developed for individuals with sedentary life-styles who are at risk for cardiovascular disease or have had ischemic heart disease (angina pectoris, myocardial infarction) or peripheral vascular disease. An exercise program should be planned with a health professional and individualized for age, sex, and present health status as well as preferences for activity. Many communities have resources for individual or group exercise programs. Participation in these programs often sustains motivation for continuing exercise. Clients with known heart disease may be included in special programs that provide medical supervision and monitoring of heart rate and rhythm by ECG while the client exercises.

The exercise program contains three components: warmup, workout, and cooldown.[15] The *warmup* phase is used to increase cardiovascular and musculoskeletal efficiency and limber up muscles. This phase lasts 5 to 10 minutes, but can increase in cold weather or during prolonged absence from exercise. Walking or limbering exercises are done at this time. The *workout* phase should improve cardiac condition and, in planned programs, may be designed to reach a specified target heart rate. The duration and intensity of this phase depends on the individual's health and objectives for exercise and can be met by walking, jogging, or swimming. The *cooldown* phase allows slowing of the cardiovascular system, dissipation of heat, and removal of lactic acid. Cooldown may be accomplished by walking at a slow rate for 5 to 10 minutes.

The benefits of exercise can be obtained in three to five exercise periods of 20 to 40 minutes each week. The program can begin slowly and increase as the client tolerates. The client should be instructed about the benefits of a regular program as opposed to erratic periods of exercise, about appropriate dress for the weather, and about exercising at least 1 hour after a meal. Clients with heart disease should report chest pain or undue fatigue precipitated by exercise.

Obesity. Obesity is defined as 20% over ideal weight. Although not an independent risk factor, obesity adds to the cardiac workload and is a known risk for hypertension and hyperlipidemia, and should be prevented or eliminated.

Prevention. Dietary and exercise habits to prevent obesity begin during prenatal development and infancy when adipocytes are developed. Instruction about diets restricted in sodium, sugar, and calories is essential for rearing healthy children of normal weight.

Risk management. Weight-reduction programs can be instituted for clients who are overweight and most particularly for clients with hypertension. The nurse can counsel the client about meal planning for weight reduction or refer the client to programs of behavior modification. Significant and permanent weight loss requires motivation and compliance with dietary prescription, and the nurse can help the client obtain reward for change in behavior.

Stress. Several researchers have identified a positive relationship between psychological stress and cardiovascular disease.[25] A behavior composite has been identified and labeled as a type A coronary-prone personality. Individuals demonstrating this behavior are intense, competitive individuals who are conscientious and wish to be respected for their accomplishments. They anticipate and react to events before their occurrence and often do several jobs at one time. Interpersonal relationships tend to be egocentric, and these persons are easily angered and frustrated and may have repressed hostility. These individuals, in contrast to type B personalities who approach life situations in a less intense manner, are at a greater risk for heart disease.

Stress and change as identified on critical life event scales may also contribute to cardiovascular disease. Several studies have demonstrated sudden cardiac deaths after traumatic life events.[25] Stress may also accumulate over time and contribute to maintaining elevated blood pressure, thus increasing the risk of heart disease and other diseases associated with hypertension.

Prevention. The first step to preventing stress is for the client to identify stressors in his life and the coping resources he has to deal with them. Stress prevention is planned to balance stressors with coping resources. Clients identified as type A personalities can often learn to modify their reaction to stressful events or to eliminate unnecessary stresses from their lives.

Risk management. Stress management skills can be used for clients whose stress levels represent potential or actual risk for cardiovascular disease. Stress management may be learned in individual counseling or group settings. Many use behavior modification techniques, relaxation exercises, or biofeedback. Other approaches may include the temporary use of sedatives or tranquilizers.

Glucose intolerance. Glucose intolerance has been identified as a contributory risk to ischemic heart disease. Individuals with serum glucose levels greater than 120 mg/100 ml are at twice the risk for heart disease, and diabetes mellitus has been demonstrated to be a precursor of coronary heart disease.

Prevention. Some forms of glucose intolerance (diabetes mellitus type II) may be related to obesity, and prevention of glucose intolerance may be managed by maintaining weight at normal levels. Others relate glucose intolerance to lack of exercise, a risk that reverses by increasing exercise.

Risk management. Clients with glucose intolerance caused by diabetes mellitus and not managed by weight control and exercise must be encouraged to follow a therapeutic plan for preventing hyperglycemia and glucosuria. The plan may include the use of pharmacological agents such as insulin to lower serum glucose levels.

Alcohol abuse. The effects of alcohol on the cardiovascular system appear to be related to the amount of alcohol used. Moderate use of small amounts of alcohol have relaxing social benefits as well as positive effects as a vasodilator. Alcohol has also been linked to enhancing high-density lipoproteins that are inversely related to ischemic heart disease.

Continuous consumption of large amounts of alcohol, however, has recently been associated with cardiac toxicity.[32] Alcoholic cardiomyopathy may decrease myocardial function and precipitate heart failure or dysrhythmias. The uptake of triglycerides may be increased with alcohol use.[2] Prolonged alcohol use causes structural changes in the myocardium and myocardial capillaries, and sclerosis and fibrosis in the small arteries may lead to microinfarcts.[2]

Prevention. As with other addictions, prevention may be facilitated by instruction about the dangers of alcohol abuse. Health information should be directed toward warning about the adverse effects of alcohol abuse on the cardiovascular system as well as other hazards.

Risk management. Clients identified as alcohol abusers can be referred to individual or group counseling or to community withdrawal programs.

Caffeine. Excessive amounts of caffeine are known to cause cardiac dysrhythmias, tachycardia, and extrasystoles. Individuals can therefore be instructed to limit intake of caffeine in products such as coffee, tea, some soft drinks, or chocolate.

Environmental risks. Contaminants in foods, air, water, and drugs have been linked to cardiovascular disease. Although no one factor is causal, environmental pollutants may contribute to total risk.

The minerals in the client's water supply may contribute to heart disease. Areas with high-sodium-content water may be associated with hypertension, and clients in these areas may be advised to use distilled or purified water.

Sidestream smoke from cigarette smoking, driving in traffic with carbon monoxide wastes, or working in tunnels in which carbon monoxide buildup is evident may contribute to risk of cardiovascular disease or compromise already involved cardiovascular system. Clients with coronary artery disease, for example, can develop chest pain in smoke-filled rooms. It is believed that the increased carboxyhemoglobin levels cause hypoxia and increase myocardial oxygen demand.

The use of oral contraceptives has been linked to cardiovascular disease, particularly thrombus formation and hypertension. Women already at risk for these diseases must be informed of the additional risk of using oral contraceptives.

Other risks. Recent evidence has linked *vital capacity* of the lungs to heart disease. Individuals with decreased vital capacity have a higher incidence of heart disease. This is believed to result from changes in oxygenation that increase cardiac workload. *Gout* is also known to correlate positively with heart disease. Individuals diagnosed as having gout are at twice the risk for ischemic heart disease.

Promotion of circulation

Circulation is promoted when free flow of the blood through the vessels is permitted. Constricting clothing can impede arterial circulation and should not be worn. Round garters, girdles, panty girdles, and belts are common sources of constriction. Sitting with the legs crossed at the knees obstructs circulation in the popliteal area, and sitting with the thighs flexed can constrict femoral circulation. It is desirable to vary body position and avoid long periods of pressure on the blood vessels. Turning during sleep is a natural movement that promotes circulation, but if the person is unable to turn himself, the nurse or family should do it for him.

Venous circulation is promoted by competent valves and muscle movement against the veins. Standing for long periods of time may produce a strain on the valves as they attempt to overcome gravity. If the person finds it necessary to stand, he can be encouraged to wear support stockings. These hose compress the muscles of the legs and help overcome gravity. The hose should be put on before the person gets out of bed and pulled on evenly from the toes to below the knee or to the groin. Walking also promotes venous return by the pressure of the muscles on the veins. Persons who must be on their feet can be encouraged to flex their legs and walk as much as possible.

Circulation is also promoted by warmth, which causes vasodilation. The body should be kept warm with clothing suitable for the weather. Extra clothing should be worn when the person is outside in cool air. Socks can be worn in bed if circulation to the extremities is poor. The inside environment should be warm, and blankets should be used as needed at night to keep the person warm. Alcoholic beverages produce peripheral vasodilation and may be ordered to promote circulation. Nicotine in tobacco, however, constricts vessels, and smoking is not advisable.

Prevention of infection
Certain microorganisms can cause cardiac infections that may impair delivery of oxygen to the cells. Syphilis is one disease that can cause permanent damage to the myocardium or cardiac valves. Early diagnosis and treatment of syphilis are imperative to prevent this residual damage. *Staphylococcus* and *Streptococcus* organisms can enter the body through the oral route, often during dental procedures. Prophylactic antibiotics may be given to individuals at risk for heart disease to prevent infections from these organisms. Streptococcal throat infections are thought to precede rheumatic fever. All persons with throat infections should be evaluated by a physician and treated before further systemic damage results. German measles (rubella) may cause fetal damage during the first trimester of pregnancy when cardiac structures are developing. Women should have adequate prenatal care and immunization against rubella to prevent congenital heart defects that can result when the fetus is exposed to rubella.

Genetic counseling
Interferences with oxygen to the cells that are genetically determined can be avoided through genetic counseling by a physician or geneticist. Hemophilia and sickle cell anemia are two such diseases. The couple may be given information about the chances of their offspring's being born with an inherited disease and options for conception considered.

Role of nutrition
Adequate nutrition is essential in promoting oxygen to the cells. The diet should be well balanced and contain sufficient calories to meet the metabolic needs of the individual, but it should not cause the client to become overweight. Large meals increase cardiac demands; small, frequent meals are preferable.

The diet should also contain sufficient vitamins and iron to prevent anemia. Iron supplements are usually used in the diet of infants. When food from all four food groups is obtained daily, the diet should be adequate to prevent nutritional anemias.

PLANNING FOR HEALTH MAINTENANCE AND RESTORATION

Planning for clients with common health problems of the cardiovascular systems requires plans that are developed to give the client access to health care facilities as well as plans for managing cardiac emergencies in specific health care settings. Plans and protocols may be developed for each, and the nurse should be familiar with emergency protocols in the community as well as those used in the hospitals or other health care facilities.

Planning in the community

Because cardiovascular disease is the most common health problem and deaths attributed to atherosclerotic heart disease often occur outside the hospital, the community can develop a coordinated plan by which emergency health care facilities are available to the citizens. The development of community-based plans has been facilitated by the Emergency Medical Systems Service Act of 1973 (PL 154) in which funds were designated to develop or upgrade facilities for life support.

The emergency medical system (EMS) may provide care at three levels: bystander response, basic life support, and advanced life support.[19] The first level includes citizens trained in lifesaving skills such as cardiopulmonary resuscitation; the second level includes firemen, police officers, and emergency medical technicians (EMTs) trained in life support measures and the facilities for transporting victims to health care facilities. At the third level the plan includes professionals trained in advanced life support activities that can be delivered in a mobile intensive care vehicle or in emergency departments or critical care units of the hospital. All individuals should know how to contact the emergency medical system, and many (one in five) should know how to provide basic life support with mouth-to-mouth ventilation and external cardiac compression.

Planning for basic life support: cardiopulmonary resuscitation (CPR)

In situations of respiratory or cardiac arrest, ventilation and circulation can be restored by emergency procedures of mouth-to-mouth ventilation and/or external cardiac compression (ECC). These procedures can be used by citizens and ancillary or professional health team members trained in resuscitation procedures. The American Heart Association and American National Red Cross have developed standards and training programs for certifying personnel in rescue procedures.[58] The Joint Commission for Accreditation of Hospitals (JCAH) lends further support to training of personnel in these techniques by requiring personnel in member institutions to provide training and review annually for employees.

Cardiopulmonary resuscitation procedures of basic life support can be administered by one or two rescuers and involves procedures of mouth-to-mouth ventilation and external cardiac compression that may be used singly or together (cardiopulmonary resuscitation, CPR).[19,58] The sequence of the procedures involves: (1) establishing unresponsiveness, (2) establishing breathlessness, and (3) establishing pulselessness. The procedures are similar for victims of all ages, but must be modified for the size of the victim as well as age-related rates for respiration and heart beat.

Unresponsiveness. Unresponsiveness can be established by shaking the victim and providing verbal stimuli such as calling the victim's name. Time should not be wasted in determining pupil response or other procedures to establish levels of consciousness.

Breathlessness and ventilation. After establishing unresponsiveness, the rescuer can hyperextend the victim's neck and look, listen, and feel for spontaneous respirations. If none are present, the rescuer should give four quick breaths to inflate the client's lungs.

Mouth-to-mouth ventilation. Mouth-to-mouth ventilation is the most effective way to restore oxygen to the cells when supplemental oxygen and assistive devices are not available. The exhaled air from the rescuer is used to inflate the victim's lungs. The rescuer can double his tidal volume by taking deep breaths, which provide 18% oxygen, 2% carbon dioxide, and an arterial oxygen tension (PaO_2) of 50 to 60 mm Hg.

The procedure for adults and children follows:

1. Position victim on his back and open airway by hyperextending airway using (unless contraindicated by spinal cord injury) head tilt/neck lift (Fig. 20-16) or head tilt/chin lift (Fig. 20-17).
2. Establish breathlessness by looking, listening, and feeling for respirations.
3. Pinch nostrils.
4. Make seal over mouth of victim.
5. Exhale, noting lung compliance of victim and observing rise and fall of chest to gauge effectiveness of ventilation.
6. Ventilations are delivered at rate of 12 per minute for adults, 15 per minute for children.

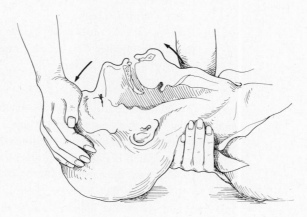

FIG. 20-16
Head tilt/neck lift maneuver. (From Ellis, Patricia Diane, and Billings, Diane M.: Cardiopulmonary resuscitation: procedures for basic and advanced life support, St. Louis, 1980, The C.V. Mosby Co.)

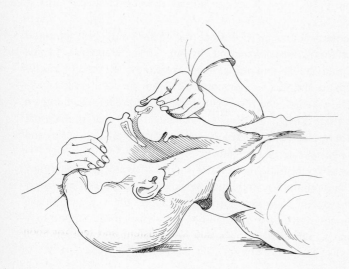

FIG. 20-17
Head tilt/chin lift maneuver. (From Ellis, Patricia Diane, and Billings, Diane M.: Cardiopulmonary resuscitation: procedures for basic and advanced life support, St. Louis, 1980, The C.V. Mosby Co.)

Nursing process for common health problems

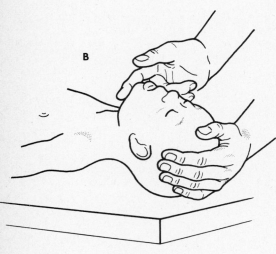

FIG. 20-18
Head tilt maneuver for infant. **A,** Head tilt/neck lift. **B,** Head tilt augmented by chin lift.

The procedure for infants and neonates follows:

1. Position infant on his back. Because neck and trachea are more pliable and neck muscles not developed, head and neck must be supported and extreme hyperextension is not required. Airway may be opened by head tilt/neck lift (Fig. 20-18, *A*) or head tilt augmented by chin lift (Fig. 20-18, *B*).
2. Establish breathlessness by looking, listening, and feeling for respirations.
3. Make seal over victim's nose *and* mouth.
4. Deliver gentle breaths to inflate lungs, observing rise and fall of chest for effectiveness of ventilation.
5. Ventilations are delivered at rate of 20 per minute.

Mouth-to-nose ventilation. Mouth-to-nose ventilation can be accomplished by breathing into the victim's nose if there is an obstruction in the mouth, if there is a mouth injury, or if a seal cannot be maintained with the mouth. The following procedures are used:

1. Position victim on his back and hyperextend airway with head tilt/chin lift maneuver.
2. Close victim's mouth.
3. Breathe into victim's nose: adults, 15 times per minute; children, 20 times per minute. The rescuer must remove his mouth from victims' nose to allow exhalation.

Mouth-to-stoma ventilation. Mouth-to-stoma ventilation is similar to mouth-to-mouth ventilation. It is not necessary to tilt the head; the rescuer should make a seal over the stoma and ventilate.

Pulselessness and external cardiac compression. After ventilating the victim with four quick breaths, the rescuer can determine presence of a pulse. In adults and children, the carotid pulse on the side of the rescuer is easily palpated for 5 to 10 seconds. The brachial pulse is more easily identified in infants and neonates and should be palpated for 5 to 10 seconds to identify presence or absence. If there is no pulse, the rescuer can initiate external cardiac compressions (ECCs).

In hospital or emergency vehicle settings the victim may be monitored with facilities for determinations of rate and rhythm (ECG, telemetry). In this instance, changes of rate and rhythm and cardiac arrest may be noted instantly. If the client is monitored and the rescuer notes a rhythm of ventricular tachycardia or ventricular fibrillation, the rescuer may deliver a precordial thump, a blow to the sternum (Fig. 20-19), to create a mechanical low-energy electrical stimulus to the heart that may result in depolarization of the cells, asystole, and (ideally) return of a normal rate and rhythm.

Once pulselessness is verified, the rescuer should activate the emergency medical system. In the community this may be done by sending someone to dial 911 or otherwise obtain transportation and advanced life support. In the hospital or other agencies, assistance and facilities for advanced life support may be obtained by paging a code such as "Code 1" that summons members of a resuscitation team.

FIG. 20-19
Precordial thump. (From Abels, L.:
Mosby's manual of critical care, St.
Louis, 1979, The C.V. Mosby Co.)

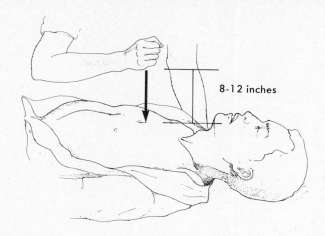

8-12 inches

External cardiac compression (ECC). ECC is used to stimulate circulation. The heart is compressed between the sternum and spine by using manual pressure while the victim is positioned on a firm surface. The rhythmic compressions force oxygenated blood through the blood vessels to maintain a systolic blood pressure of 100 mm Hg. The procedure is not without hazards, and if it is done improperly, there is a danger of fracturing the sternum or ribs and lacerating the liver or spleen.

The procedure for adults follows:

1. Position victim on hard surface such as floor. If victim is in bed, a bed board, tray, or cardiac arrest board must be positioned under the victim's back.
2. Expose victim's chest and identify landmark for hand position on lower one third of sternum. This can be done by palpating rib cage to xiphisternal junction (Fig. 20-20) and placing two or three fingers on notch.

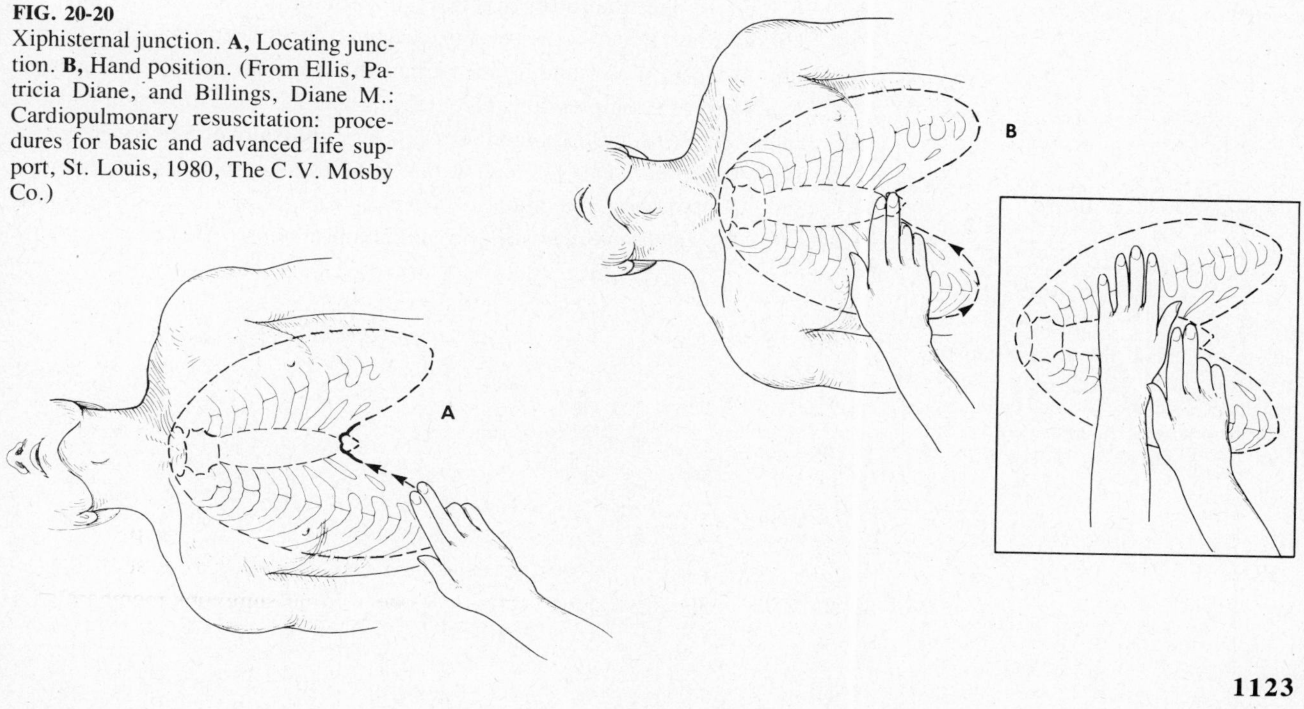

FIG. 20-20
Xiphisternal junction. **A,** Locating junction. **B,** Hand position. (From Ellis, Patricia Diane, and Billings, Diane M.: Cardiopulmonary resuscitation: procedures for basic and advanced life support, St. Louis, 1980, The C.V. Mosby Co.)

FIG. 20-21
Rescuer's position for external cardiac compression. Note fingers interlocked to prevent pressure on rib cage. (From Ellis, Patricia Diane, and Billings, Diane M.: Cardiopulmonary resuscitation: procedures for basic and advanced life support, St. Louis, 1980, The C.V. Mosby Co.)

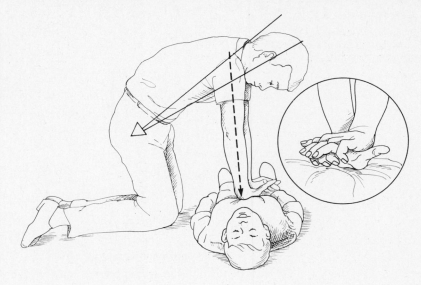

Heel of other hand is placed proximal to fingers for appropriate compression point. Rescuer then can place other hand on top of hand on sternum, and with arms extended and using weight of body for compression (Fig. 20-21), compresses sternum 1½ to 2 inches. Compressions should be given rhythmically without bouncing or releasing contact with chest. Fingers may be interlocked to keep them off chest (Fig. 20-21).

3. Compressions are given at a rate of 80 to 100 per minute.

The procedure for children follows:

1. Position victim on hard surface.
2. Expose chest and identify landmark for compression. In children over 5 years of age, the lower one third of sternum is used as for adults. In children less than 5 years of age, the liver and spleen lie higher in abdominal cavity and middle of sternum is therefore a more appropriate landmark for compression. Heel of one hand is used for compression in children (Fig. 20-22). Compression for children over 5 years of age is done at depth of 1 to 1½ inch at rate of 60 to 80 compressions per minute. Compression for children under 5 years of age is done at depth of ½ to 1 inch and rate of 80 to 100 compressions per minute.

FIG. 20-22
Heel of one hand placed mid-sternum provides adequate compression for children under 5 years. (From Dison, N.: Clinical nursing techniques, ed. 4, St. Louis, 1979, The C.V. Mosby Co.)

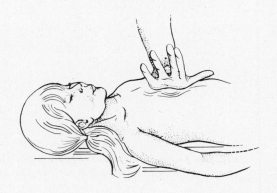

FIG. 20-23
External cardiac compression for infants. Note rescuer uses two fingers mid-sternum for compression.

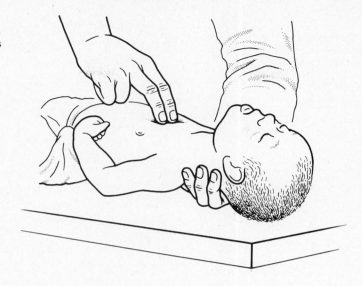

The procedure for infants and neonates follows:

1. Position victim on hard surface with rescuer's hand supporting victim's neck (Fig. 20-23).
2. Expose chest and identify landmark for compression. Heart of infant or neonate is higher in chest, and midsternum is used as compression point. This can be identified at nipple line. Two or three fingers are used to compress sternum ½ to 1 inch (Fig. 20-23) at rate of 100 compressions per minute.

Cardiopulmonary resuscitation (CPR). CPR is the combination of efforts of mouth-to-mouth ventilation and external cardiac compression used by a single

---

PROTOCOL FOR CARDIOPULMONARY RESUSCITATION

1. Establish unresponsiveness.
2. Call for help.
3. Position victim on back.
4. Hyperextend neck and establish breathlessness.
5. If no response, deliver four quick ventilations.
6. Verify pulselessness, activate emergency medical system.
7. Begin external cardiac compressions at age-appropriate depth and rate; alternate with ventilations.
   a. Adults: 15 compressions 1½ to 2 inches, followed by two breaths for rate of 60 compressions and eight ventilations per minute.
   b. Children: 80 compressions per minute at depth of 1 to 1½ inches interspersed with one ventilation every fifth compression.
   c. Neonates and infants: 100 compressions per minute at depth of ½ to 1 inch with one ventilation every fifth compression for ventilatory rate of 20.
8. Evaluate effectiveness of resuscitation efforts every 1 to 3 minutes.
9. Establish entry into health care system for definitive therapy.

Adapted from Performance tests for one rescuer CPR and infant resuscitation, American Heart Association.

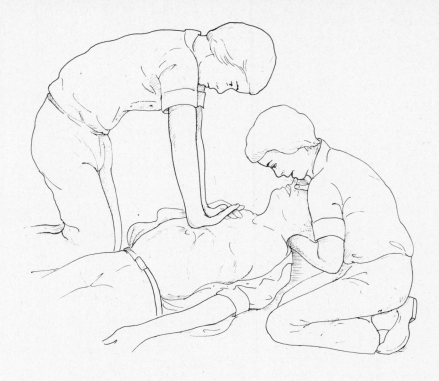

FIG. 20-24
Two-person rescue. Note position of rescuers on opposite sides of victim. (From Ellis, Patricia Diane, and Billings, Diane M.: Cardiopulmonary resuscitation: procedures for basic and advanced life support, St. Louis, 1980, The C.V. Mosby Co.)

rescuer or preferably two rescuers during situations of respiratory and cardiac arrest. If only one rescuer is available he can alternate ventilations and compressions (see protocol on p. 1125). If a second rescuer is available, one rescuer can perform ventilations while the other delivers external cardiac compressions. The rescuers should position themselves on opposite sides of the victim, if possible (Fig. 20-24). When one rescuer becomes exhausted, it is advisable to switch positions. The compression rate can be slowed during two-rescuer CPR and mnemonics used for counting out loud (''one one thousand, two one thousand'') to ''five one thousand'' to keep a regular rate and signal the rescuer doing ventilations to breathe on every fifth count.

Once CPR is initiated, the rescuers should obtain advanced life support. The victim can be transferred to an emergency vehicle (mobile intensive care unit) or, if hospitalized, to an intensive care unit where equipment and personnel are available for definitive therapy.

Planning for advanced life support

Advanced life support refers to the adjunct equipment and drugs used to reverse cardiac death and may be administered in a mobile intensive care unit (MICU), an emergency department, or in the hospital. Plans and protocols can be developed for specific situations but generally involve establishing an intravenous route for administration of drugs, using ECG monitoring equipment, using oxygen therapy devices for establishing and maintaining an airway and delivering oxygen, administering intravenous fluids, and assessing, planning, and evaluating care. These procedures are discussed where appropriate throughout the text.

Implementation

COMMON HEALTH PROBLEMS OF THE NEONATE AND INFANT

Congenital heart disease

Abnormalities of the development of the heart and great vessels during uterine life are manifested at birth or several years thereafter as defects of cardiac output or circulation of oxygenated blood.[51] The defects are described as *acyanotic* or *cyanotic,* depending on circulation of the blood through the heart. In acyanotic defects there is no mixing of unoxygenated blood in the systemic circulation, and these defects may not be evident clinically until later in life. Patent ductus arteriosus, coarctation of the aorta, aortic stenosis, pulmonic stenosis, ventricular septal defects, and atrial septal defects are examples of acyanotic defects. With cyanotic defects, on the other hand, there is mixing of pulmonic and systemic circulation that is ultimately incompatible with life. Cyanotic defects may be present even though clinical cyanosis is not. Tetralogy of Fallot, transposition of great vessels, tricuspid atresia, and truncus arteriosus are examples of cyanotic heart defects.

Pathophysiology. The cause of congenital heart disease is related to defects of embryonic development during the fifth to eighth week of gestation when the heart and great vessels are forming. Disruption of development may be precipitated by prenatal factors such as maternal infection during the first trimester. Rubella, influenza, or chickenpox are common causative agents. Genetic factors may also contribute to congenital heart defects. There is an increased incidence of congenital heart disease in families where a parent or sibling has a congenital heart defect. The incidence of cardiac defects is also increased in individuals who have other chromosome defects such as Down's syndrome. Finally, environmental factors may contribute to faulty embryonic development. These may include radiation, poor maternal nutrition, or maternal use of drugs such as alcohol or LSD.

Congenital heart disease occurs in 8 to 10 of 1000 live births. Clients at risk are those with parents or siblings with congenital heart disease.

Assessment. The nurse can assess the neonate's or infant's cardiovascular status immediately after birth and during subsequent health appraisals. At this time a nursing history and physical assessment are done to determine effectiveness of cardiac output and identify potential or actual health problems attributed to congenital heart disease. The congenital defects may be described as acyanotic or cyanotic.

Acyanotic heart defects. Acyanotic heart defects (Fig. 20-25) are not immediately incompatible with life. Oxygenated blood is supplied to the cells, but as the child's needs for oxygen increase, there is added strain on the defective heart and there is potential for the defect to become cyanotic. The child becomes fatigued, irritable, and dyspneic and may faint. Often the defect is not observed until the child participates in screening examinations where murmurs are detected or has a complete physical examination, including an ECG. Noninvasive studies of the heart as well as cardiac catheterization may be used to diagnose the exact defect.

Patent ductus arteriosus. A patent ductus arteriosus occurs when this fetal structure does not close, and there is a communication between the pulmonary artery and the aorta. The ductus arteriosus is a normal structure in fetal circulation, but if it does not close at birth, the duct continues to shunt circulating blood. Fortunately the increased pressure of the blood at the aorta forces oxygenated

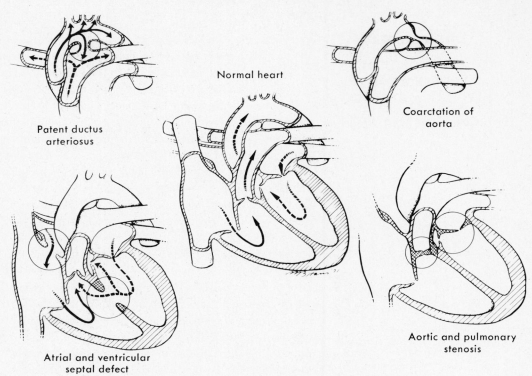

FIG. 20-25
Acyanotic heart defects.

Normal heart

Patent ductus
arteriosus

Coarctation of
aorta

Atrial and ventricular
septal defect

Aortic and pulmonary
stenosis

blood into the pulmonary artery through the patent ductus, thereby increasing the amount of blood circulating through the lungs.

The duct that remains open in about 15% of preterm births causes the neonate to have signs of respiratory distress such as grunting, tachypnea, and retractions.[55] Because these neonates are unable to tolerate surgery, they may be treated palliatively with aspirin or indomethacin (Indocin) or with prostaglandin synthesis inhibitors, which cause constriction of the smooth muscle in the ductus arteriosus.

As the child grows, he may become dyspneic and have an enlarged heart, left ventricular hypertrophy, or a characteristic "machinery type" heart murmur. The diastolic blood pressure may be low. The systolic blood pressure increases because of the left ventricular hypertrophy, and the increased stroke volume causes increased aortic pressure. This defect is diagnosed by the physical findings and confirmed by ECG, cardiac catheterization, and echocardiogram.

The defect may be closed by a surgical approach. When the child is between 1 and 5 years of age and able to withstand thoracic surgery, the patent duct may be ligated or divided to produce closure. The prognosis for this surgery is good, and no limits are placed on the child's activity after recovery.

Coarctation of the aorta. In coarctation of the aorta, the aorta is constricted at some point. The constriction may be proximal or distal to the ductus arteriosus. The defect is usually not immediately noted unless the constriction is severe. It is important, therefore, to screen children during health appraisals, particularly if they are to be involved in athletic activities.

Characteristically there is an increased blood pressure proximal to the defect with a decrease distally. The blood pressure is higher in the arms than in the legs.

The pulses in the arm are strong, but the femoral and popliteal pulses are weak. Occasionally the child has a soft, high-frequency heart murmur. The diagnosis is confirmed by aortography.

The defect can be corrected by removing the constricted portion of the aorta and anastomosing the ends or inserting a graft. The surgery is usually not done until the child is at least 3 to 5 years old and involves a thoracic approach to surgery that is not as involved as open-heart surgery.

Aortic stenosis. In this defect a stricture may occur above or below the aortic valve, or the valve itself may be incompetent and may restrict, or completely obstruct, blood flow. The child becomes fatigued and dizzy when the cardiac output is reduced. These signs are most evident as the increasing demands of oxygen for growth are not met. A serious outcome may be sudden death after exertion. There is also a characteristic systolic murmur heard at left sternal border. Diagnosis is based on an ECG, which shows left ventricular hypertrophy, and on cardiac catheterization by which the stricture is visually indicated.

The stenosis is relieved by an incision into the valve and is done when the child is able to withstand surgery.

Pulmonic stenosis. In pulmonic stenosis there is a stricture of the pulmonic valve. Depending on the severity of stenosis, the child experiences dyspnea, fatigue, syncope, and ultimately congestive heart failure. This stenosis is diagnosed by systolic heart murmurs, ECG, echocardiogram, and cardiac catheterization. The stenosis is corrected by incision into the valve, valvulotomy, and is done when the child is 2 to 3 years old. The prognosis is favorable.

Ventricular septal defect (VSD). An opening in the ventricular septum is another area where congenital defects cause interference with oxygen supply. If the opening in the ventricle is small and low, the child is asymptomatic because circulation through the heart is not interrupted. About 50% of small defects close spontaneously before the child is 3 years old. If the defect is larger and higher in the septum, an increased volume of blood is pumped to the pulmonary circulation through the defect, and there may be a strain on the right side of the heart. The child experiences dyspnea and fatigue. He may have heart failure, and upper respiratory tract infections are common. The diagnosis is based on a loud parasystolic murmur heard at left lower sternal border and confirmed by cardiac catheterization and echocardiography.

The defect can be closed by suturing the defect or, if it is large, by inserting a patch graft of plastic sponge. If a patch graft is used, the fibrous tissue of the heart invades the graft and secures its position in the heart. These surgeries are done by the open-heart method. The prognosis is very good. Some physicians recommend that young children with large defects who cannot tolerate surgery undergo palliative banding procedures to decrease pulmonary blood flow and peripheral resistance until corrective surgery is done at a later date. Operative risk makes the procedure controversial.

Atrial septal defects (ASD). Atrial septal defects result from an open foramen ovale or openings in the atrial septum. Pressure on the left side of the heart is increased, and blood circulates from the left atrium to the right atrium, causing left-to-right shunting and providing increased flow of oxygenated blood to the right side of the heart. The child may be subject to fatigue and frequent respiratory tract infections. A heart murmur may be noticed. The heart appears enlarged on chest x-ray films, and the diagnosis is confirmed by cardiac catheterization.

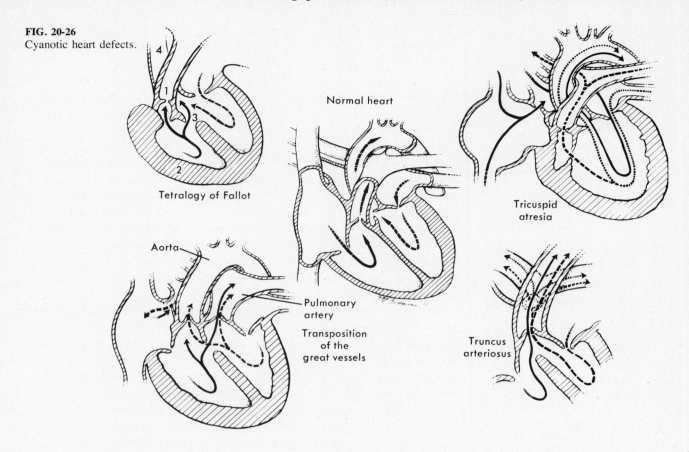

FIG. 20-26
Cyanotic heart defects.

Tetralogy of Fallot

Normal heart

Tricuspid atresia

Aorta

Pulmonary artery

Transposition of the great vessels

Truncus arteriosus

The defect can be closed by suturing or inserting a graft, requiring open-heart surgery. The prognosis is good.

Cyanotic heart defects. Cyanotic heart defects (Fig. 20-26) are potentially dangerous to life. There is mixing of pulmonic blood into the systemic circulation, and the need for oxygen to the cells is not met. Indications of inadequate oxygenation are evident at birth, and the nurse should be alert to identifying the cues of inadequate oxygenation. The most noticeable sign is difficulty in breathing. Dyspnea is particularly marked during feeding or defecation. At these times the accessory muscles are used, and there is rib retraction and flaring of the nares. Infants may breathe better in the knee-chest position, which increases venous return by occluding the femoral vein. The entrapment of venous circulation increases oxygen saturation and decreases the workload of the right ventricle. Some infants may assume this position spontaneously. Cyanosis, visible in highly vascular areas, is a valuable indicator of congenital heart defects. The nurse should note where it occurs, how long it lasts, and if it is more evident during activity. The neonate may also be observed to be extremely restless or lethargic and to have poor muscle tone. There may be metabolic acidosis from an increase of lactic acid released during aerobic metabolism.

Difficulty in feeding, especially coordinating sucking, swallowing, and breathing, may be reported by the mother. Tachycardia, enlarged liver, and overt heart murmurs are other signs to be observed in the neonate.

1130

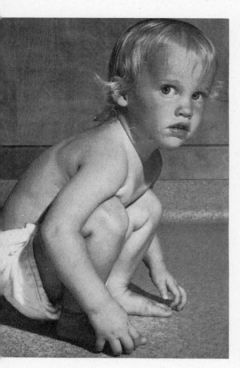

FIG. 20-27
Child with cyanotic heart defect squats to increase cardiac flow. (From Ingalls, Joy A., and Salerno, M. Constance: Maternal and child health nursing, ed. 4, St. Louis, 1979, The C.V. Mosby Co.)

As the child develops, he will gain weight slowly, because of the calorie expenditure in the exertion of feeding. He may squat frequently, a position that relieves dyspnea and increases venous blood return to the heart by occluding the femoral vein (Fig. 20-27).

To compensate for the inadequate oxygen supply to the cells, there is an increase in the number of erythrocytes. This polycythemia causes distension of peripheral capillaries and gives a "clubbed" appearance to the fingers and toes (Fig. 20-3). Clubbing is generally noticed in the thumbs first and may be preceded by a shininess and loss of wrinkles in the extremities. Polycythemia may predispose to thrombosis formation or thrombophlebitis from the increased viscosity of the blood. Other compensatory mechanisms include increased heart rate and increased contractile force of the heart. Because cyanotic defects are not compatible with life, surgical correction is required soon after birth. Palliative procedures may be attempted until the child is old enough to tolerate more lengthy corrective surgery.

Tetralogy of Fallot. The tetralogy of Fallot is the most common cyanotic heart disease in children and is composed of four heart defects: (1) pulmonary stenosis, which produces (2) right ventricular hypertrophy, (3) a ventricular septal defect (VSD), and (4) an overriding aorta that receives blood from both ventricles and right-to-left shunting through the VSD. The newborn with tetralogy of Fallot is extremely cyanotic, lethargic, and limp. There is dyspnea and later clubbing of the fingers. The infant is small and does not gain weight. As he becomes older, he is observed to squat frequently to relieve dyspnea. He is prone to respiratory tract infections. The diagnosis is based on clinical symptoms, murmurs, ECG, x-ray films, phonocardiogram, and cardiac catheterization.

Palliative surgery is attempted during early childhood to meet increasing demands for oxygen during periods of growth. Subsequent surgery during the school years is necessary to achieve permanent correction. Two common approaches to palliative surgery are the Blalock-Taussig and the Waterson procedures. The Blalock-Taussig procedure involves an end-to-side anastomosis of the right subclavian or carotid artery to the right pulmonary artery. The Waterson procedure involves a side-to-side anastomosis of the ascending aorta to the right pulmonary artery. These procedures increase the oxygenated blood and relieve the symptoms of cyanotic heart disease.

Corrective surgery is done when the child is in good health and able to tolerate lengthy surgery. The heart defects are corrected by relieving the pulmonary stenosis and closing the ventricular septal defect and correcting the overriding aorta. This requires open-heart surgery when the child is 3 to 4 years old. Some surgeons prefer to do the corrective surgery at one time to avoid the risks of two major surgeries.

Transposition of the great vessels. When the great vessels are transposed, the aorta and pulmonary artery are anatomically reversed. Unless there is a patent ductus arteriosus or atrial or ventricular septal defect to provide mixing of arterial and venous blood, the newborn will not live.

Transposition of the vessels is noted, depending on the presence of concomitant defects by severe cyanosis. Cyanosis is less severe if there is a PDA or ASD or VSD, but heart failure is soon evident. The diagnosis is based on cardiac catheterization, echocardiography, and x-ray film.

Palliative surgery may be performed to create defects to allow mixing of blood. In one procedure, *balloon septostomy,* a balloon-tipped catheter is inserted during cardiac catheterization to create or enlarge an intraatrial septal defect. In the *Blalock-Hanlen* procedure an atrial septal defect is created. In the *Edwards* procedure the right pulmonary veins are repositioned so that oxygenated blood flows into the right atrium. The *Mustard* procedure is used for permanent correction. The atrial septum is excised, and an intraatrial baffle is created so that oxygenated blood from the pulmonary veins returns to the right ventricle for circulation to the body and deoxygenated blood returns from the venae cavae to the left ventricle and pulmonary artery for circulation to the lung. Mortality with this defect has been greatly improved with initial palliative and corrective procedures accomplished with open-heart surgery techniques.

Tricuspid atresia. The tricuspid valve is closed in tricuspid atresia, and no opening exists from the right atrium to the right ventricle. There must be an opening in the atrial septum and a patent ductus arteriosus to sustain the life of the newborn so that unoxygenated blood can be shunted to the pulmonary circulation. The infant is cyanotic, dyspneic, and easily fatigued. The ECG demonstrates left ventricular hypertrophy from added demands on the heart. A shunting procedure (pulmonary-to-artery anastomosis) may be attempted as a palliative measure to increase blood to the lungs, and later corrective surgery is done to repair the defect.

Truncus arteriosus. In truncus arteriosus only one vessel, the aorta, receives blood from the ventricles. The defect occurs as a result of failure of division of the bulbar trunk into the pulmonary artery and aorta. Consequently this structure overrides both ventricles and results in pulmonary and systemic circulations. There are several types of this defect. In one type the right and left pulmonary arteries arise from the posterior wall of the truncus. In another type, the right and left pulmonary arteries arise from the posterior wall of the truncus. In another type the right and left pulmonary arteries originate from the lateral walls of the truncus. In still another form the pulmonary arteries are absent, and the arterial supply to the lung is through the bronchial arteries. There is usually a harsh systolic heart murmur apparent within the first week of life.

Truncus arteriosus is repaired surgically. Palliative surgery is accomplished by banding the pulmonary arteries to increase the blood flow to the lungs. When the child is older, corrective surgery is performed to close the VSD so that the truncus arteriosus arises from the left ventricle. The pulmonary artery is excised from the aorta and attached to the right ventricle, and a prosthetic valve conduit is inserted. The prognosis depends on the severity of the defect.

Data analysis
Data analysis is concluded after obtaining the nursing history. Although congenital defects may vary, common nursing diagnoses may include alterations in cardiac output, ineffective family coping, impaired gas exchange, fluid imbalance, self-care deficit, knowledge deficit, or alterations in tissue perfusion.

Planning and implementation. Correction of congenital heart defects may require expensive surgery, lengthy hospitalization, and care at home for the infant before and after surgery. Families and the client must draw on many coping resources to manage the change in family life-style when a child has a congenital heart disease. The nurse helps the family plan to manage the care of their child and, during acute crisis of surgery, initiates and directs nursing care.

Cardiac surgery. Improved techniques of cardiac surgery have made possible earlier and more complete correction of congenital heart defects. Although much cardiac surgery is done for children, adults may also require surgical correction of weak or stenosed valves, revascularization procedures for obstructed coronary arteries, or heart transplants.

There are two basic approaches to cardiac surgery. *Open-heart surgery* involves opening the heart to correct various defects. This surgery is made possible by equipment for cardiopulmonary bypass that provides extracorporeal circulation while surgery is performed on the heart. Open-heart surgery is used to correct congenital defects, insert prosthetic valves, revascularize coronary arterial supply, repair thoracic aortic aneurysms, and perform heart transplants. In *closed-heart surgery* the myocardium is not invaded, and cardiac circulation is not interrupted. A valvulotomy or mitral commissurotomy may be done by this approach.

Open-heart surgery is performed with the use of a cardiopulmonary bypass machine that permits extracorporeal oxygenation during surgery. A cannula is inserted into the superior and inferior venae cavae, and the deoxygenated blood is diverted to the cardiopulmonary bypass machine where carbon dioxide and oxygen are exchanged in the oxygenator. The oxygenated blood is returned to the systemic circulation through a cannula in the ascending aorta. Myocardial circulation is maintained by cannulas in the coronary arteries.

Hypothermia is used as an adjunct to open-heart surgery. This slow cooling of the body reduces metabolism and needs for oxygen, particularly to vital tissues such as the kidneys and brain. When the surgery is completed, the client is slowly returned to normal body temperature so that shivering does not increase metabolism and the need for oxygen. The heart is defibrillated and the use of a bypass machine discontinued.

During surgery, vital signs are monitored continuously. An ECG is used to detect irregularities of rate or rhythm of the heart. An EEG is used to determine cerebral activity and the effect of hypoxia on the brain. The temperature and blood pressure are also monitored continuously.

Nursing care of the client having open-heart surgery. Nursing care of the client having open-heart surgery occurs in four phases: (1) maintenance of optimum health before surgery, (2) preoperative nursing care, (3) postoperative nursing care, and (4) rehabilitation. The client may be in contact with four different groups of nurses, and a continuous care plan is imperative as the client moves from home or a hospital unit to a cardiac surgery unit, rehabilitation unit, and home again. Although principles of nursing care for clients of all ages are similar in each phase, the nurse must adapt the care plan to the age and developmental stage of the client and his family.[61]

Health maintenance before surgery. Maintaining health before surgery depends on the client's age and current health status.[27] Infants with congenital defects, for example, may be cared for at home until they are able to tolerate surgery. Adults, on the other hand, may be severely restricted in activity because of chest pain or heart failure before revascularization procedures, or valve replacement.

Nursing process for common health problems

INFANTS AND CHILDREN. Because most congenital heart defects are not repaired immediately, the nurse and the family must cope with the infant's special needs. The infant is usually managed at home, and it may be helpful to the family to have a community health nurse visit in the home to make suggestions for care.

Nursing care for the newborn with a heart defect is directed toward providing oxygen to the cells, and efforts are made to lessen the activity of the infant. The baby may breathe more easily in Fowler's position or in the knee-chest position. The newborn should be fed regularly so that he does not have to cry to obtain a feeding. Less energy is used in nursing if the holes in the nipple of the bottle are enlarged. If possible, the mother should be encouraged to feed her baby, either by breast or bottle. Supplemental oxygen can be given by mask if needed. The use of gavage feedings should be avoided when possible, because the insertion of the feeding tube is stressful and only serves to increase oxygen demands.

Dietary and pharmacological therapy may be used to reduce fluid retention, which can put a strain on the heart. Low-sodium formula may be used initially, and later as the infant's diet is expanded, the parents can be instructed in foods that are low in sodium. Cardiotonic glycosides may be used if evidence of cardiac decompensation appears. If these drugs are given at home, the parents should be instructed how to give the medication and recognize signs of toxicity to report to the physician.

As the infant grows, he should be permitted to mature naturally. Developmental tasks such as weaning and toilet training can be pursued at a normal pace. The toddler is naturally more active and can participate in activities as his strength allows. The toddler with a congenital heart defect tires easily and will usually limit his play of his own accord. A sensible balance of rest and activity, however, should be followed.

Parents of children with congenital heart defects are naturally concerned with the growth and behavior of their child. Often, parents tend to be overprotective, perhaps from fear or guilt. The nurse can give explicit guidelines for activity during this precorrective phase so that the parents feel more comfortable with the child. Family discipline and values should be maintained. This is often difficult because the child with a heart defect may become cyanotic when upset, which may frighten his parents and make them hesitate to enforce discipline. However, even with his special needs, the child with a congenital defect should fit within the family structure.

ADULTS. Adults who are facing open-heart surgery may have severe chest pain or dyspnea that limits activity. Fatigue is common, and frequent rest periods are required to conserve energy. The client may have heart failure and can be managed with digitalis, diuretics, and a sodium-restricted diet. The nurse can help the client and family follow the medical plan until surgery can be performed.

The client should be at his maximum level of health before admission. He should be in nutritional health and free of infections. The client should also visit his dentist to verify that tooth decay is not a site of bacterial growth.

Preoperative nursing care. Principles of preparing a client of any age for cardiac surgery are basically similar for clients of all ages. The equipment used for children is smaller, however, and instructions must be appropriate to developmental needs and maturational levels of children or adults.

INFANTS AND CHILDREN. When preparing infants and children and their parents for cardiac surgery, the nurse should assess the age, the child's understanding of the surgery, and the relationship the child has with his parents. Simple explanations of what will happen and who will be with him should be given to the child before the procedure is done. If possible, the parents should be present to reassure the child. Above all, information should be honest.

Approaches using play therapy may be useful in preparing the child for cardiac surgery. Role playing with dolls or puppets can help the child work through feelings of fear and hostility. The nurse can also demonstrate the use of equipment and procedures by role playing. Storytelling is another approach in preparing the child for surgery and hospitalization. Some hospitals have written stories about the surgery that parents can read to the child at home before he comes to the hospital.

OLDER CHILDREN, ADOLESCENTS, AND ADULTS. Older children, adolescents, and adults usually respond to preoperative explanations that are given directly and honestly. The client will be better able to cooperate after surgery if he knows what to expect. Some adults benefit from group discussions about impending surgery or from discussing the surgery with a client who is recovering from a similar operation. Many hospitals have highly developed teaching programs that may include written surgery guides, visual media, and tours of the postoperative nursing unit.

Family support is vital during the preoperative period, and attempts should be made to preserve family integrity. If rooming-in is available, one of the parents may stay with the child to give him a sense of security during these procedures. More liberal visiting hours should be available for adults who face cardiac surgery so that family members can stay as they are needed.

Religious support is important to many clients, and they may wish to have visits from a religious counselor. Most hospitals have a chaplain who may visit if the client indicates a desire.

Diagnostic tests and laboratory examinations will be performed before surgery to assess organ function and obtain baseline data. The client will also be typed and cross-matched for blood.

Physical preparation for the client having cardiac surgery is similar to that for the client having chest surgery because a thoroctomy or sternotomy incision is used. The client may be instructed to bathe or take showers with an antiseptic soap for several days before surgery. All diuretics, cardiac glycosides, antidysrhythmics, and anticoagulants should be discontinued for 3 to 5 days before surgery. Immediately before surgery the nurse should use a checklist to be sure that all preoperative procedures have been completed and preoperative medication given if ordered.

Postoperative nursing care. Postoperative nursing care is given in a specialized nursing unit where medical and nursing personnel are constantly available. The goals of nursing care for the client who has had cardiac surgery are to (1) maintain a supply of oxygen to the cells, (2) maintain cardiac output, (3) maintain warmth, (4) maintain fluid and electrolyte balance, (5) provide a balance of rest and activity, and (6) provide physical and psychological comfort.

Nursing process for common health problems

MAINTAINING OXYGEN TO THE CELLS. When the client returns from surgery, the nurse must maintain an open airway. An endotracheal tube is used at least until the client has recovered from anesthesia. Pressure-controlled or volume-controlled ventilators may be used for the first 24 hours after surgery to increase pulmonary reserve and prevent atelectasis. Some physicians prefer using a tracheotomy and assisted oxygen ventilation from a respirator; other clients may receive oxygen by a nasal cannula or a humidity tent. Regardless of the type of ventilatory support, the airway should be suctioned as necessary to prevent obstruction.

As ventilation improves, the ventilatory devices are removed, and 40% oxygen is administered per T-pieces on the endotracheal tube. The nurse should evaluate the client's response to this change by listening to breath sounds to detect rales or rhonchi and observe the client for indications of respiratory distress such as rapid pulse, dyspnea, wheezing, or cyanosis. If there is respiratory obstruction from secretions, the nurse should suction the client frequently. Suctioning stimulates the cough reflex, and trapped mucus can be raised. The client is encouraged to take deep breaths and cough every hour to prevent respiratory tract obstruction and pneumonia. Percussion and postural drainage is given every 1 to 2 hours to stimulate drainage and expectoration of mucus. *Postperfusion lung syndrome* (atelectasis and pulmonary edema) may occur 6 to 24 hours after surgery. There may be cyanosis, increased heart rate, lowered blood pressure, and hemorrhage, all of which contribute to hypoxemia. Nursing care is directed to prevent this syndrome.

Chest tubes are used to promote reexpansion of the lungs (see Chapter 21). Serous drainage and air are removed from the intrapleural cavity, anterior mediastinum, and occasionally the pericardial space via the tubes placed in underwater seal drainage. The tubes should be stripped, or milked, frequently to prevent obstruction from blood clots. The nurse should observe and record the amount of drainage hourly. During the first hours after surgery as much as 100 ml per hour may be drained (adults), but the amount decreases gradually as lungs reexpand. An increase in bleeding indicates hemorrhage, and the surgeon should be called immediately. The nurse should also observe the client for pneumothorax and mediastinal shift. The chest tubes are removed in 24 to 48 hours when the lungs have reexpanded.

The nurse should evaluate oxygenation in peripheral circulation by feeling the extremities for warmth, checking the pedal and radial pulses, and observing the color of the skin. Peripheral circulation and oxygen to the cells are promoted by active and passive exercises of the extremities. The client should turn or be turned every 2 hours to ensure adequate circulation. The nurse may also exercise the limbs during the bath; this is particularly important for the client who has undergone myocardial revascularization procedures in which segments of the saphenous vein have been removed for grafting.

Children are naturally more active, but adults may need to be encouraged to move. Elastic stockings may be ordered by the physician to promote venous return and prevent thromboembolism. Anticoagulants such as aspirin or low-dose heparin may also be used to prevent thrombus or embolus formation.

MAINTAINING CARDIAC OUTPUT. During the first several days after surgery, it is imperative that cardiac function and circulation of fluids be optimal. The nurse monitors vital signs and urinary output to identify potential problems of altered cardiac output, such as hypotension, oliguria, dysrhythmias, or changes in level of consciousness, and plans to prevent these problems with appropriate nursing actions.

Vital signs are evaluated continuously and recorded at least every 15 minutes until stable during the immediate postoperative period. A cardiac monitor and an indwelling thermometer are used to give instant information. An indwelling arterial line is used to monitor the blood pressure, which should be maintained at 110 to 150 mm Hg systolic. Drugs, such as nitroprusside (Nipride) or dopamine, or blood or plasma may be used to maintain blood pressure. Hypertension is common immediately after surgery because of peripheral vasoconstriction and hypothermia, but should return to normal ranges in a few hours.

Frequent determinations are also made of pulmonary artery pressure, CVP, electrolytes, and arterial blood gases. The client may feel overwhelmed by this equipment, and as often as possible, the personnel who are interpreting the data should offer an explanation of the equipment, and the nurse and surgeon should give reassurances of his progress.

In addition to assessing the vital signs, the nurse should observe all dressings for bleeding. If anticoagulants are being used, there may be bleeding from the dressing or in the chest tube drainage, or there may be hematuria. Internal bleeding may be manifested by shock, and changes in the vital signs should be reported to the surgeon immediately.

Cardiac rhythm is observed on the ECG. Dysrhythmias, such as atrial fibrillation, premature ventricular contractions, or heart blocks, can be detected and drugs or pacemakers used to correct them. Most surgeons suture temporary pacemaker wires in the atria and ventricles in anticipation of dysrhythmias. The apical-radial pulse should be taken frequently to determine pulse deficits. Dysrhythmias, myocardial infarction, hemorrhage, sepsis, emboli, and cardiac arrest are not uncommon complications of cardiac surgery in adults.

Neurological signs and the level of consciousness should also be determined frequently because these are reflective of cerebral perfusion and therefore adequate cardiac output. As the client warms up from hypothermia, his pupillary response, handgrip, and level of consciousness should improve rapidly. Any untoward signs should be reported to the surgeon.

Urinary output as a parameter of renal perfusion is a critical indicator of cardiac output sufficient for fluid transport and elimination. Low doses of dopamine may be used to assure renal artery vasodilation and urinary output.

MAINTAINING WARMTH. As the client returns from surgery, he must be kept warm. Hypothermia from surgery may last several hours, and a blanket, warmer, or radiant warmer for infants should be used to prevent heat loss and shivering.

MAINTAINING FLUID AND ELECTROLYTE BALANCE. Fluid balance is critical after open-heart surgery, particularly in children and older adults. Fluid restriction is usually imposed, owing to the retention of fluid in interstitial spaces caused by priming solutions used with the pump oxygenator and sodium retention stimulated by elevated aldosterone and ADH levels responding to stress. Diuretics may be used to promote the shift of fluids from intravascular to extracellular compartments.

Fluid needs, balanced by determinations of weight, left atrial and ventricular pressures, and urinary output, are met by intravenous infusions during the first 24 to 48 hours. The infusions must be regulated carefully to prevent circulatory overload and resultant pulmonary edema or heart failure, or, conversely, low cardiac output syndrome.

Blood loss alters fluid balance and must be replaced on a per volume basis. Some institutions use computer systems to monitor this loss. Whole blood, packed blood cells, or plasma expanders may be used as needed. Red blood cells are often destroyed because of hemolysis occurring during the use of cardiopulmonary bypass. Iron and folic acid preparations therefore are used for 1 to 2 months after surgery to stimulate production of red blood cells. There may be a platelet deficiency from sequestration of platelets in the extracorporeal system and dilution of blood from priming solutions. Platelet-rich blood may be infused to compensate for the loss. Decreased thrombin and prothrombin cause clotting defects, and the nurse should be alert to unusual bleeding.

To ensure a balance of fluids, the urine output must approximate fluid intake, and the hourly urine output determination should be recorded. During the first hour after surgery the urine output may be increased from the hemodilution from the pump oxygenator. A Foley catheter or pediatric urine collector may be used to collect urine for measurement. The specific gravity of the urine is also determined. Because cardiopulmonary bypass equipment causes hemolysis of red blood cells, the urine may be blood-tinged for the first 3 to 4 hours after surgery. Persistent hematuria may indicate a sludging process in which the hemolyzed red blood cells accumulate and cause acute tubular necrosis. Prerenal failure is manifested by decreased cardiac output and gradually decreasing urinary output and should be reported.

Electrolyte status is monitored frequently and replacements given as needed. The nurse should be alert to changes in the client's condition that indicate electrolyte imbalance. Potassium levels should be monitored, particularly as deficits or excesses produce dysrhythmias and acid-base changes. Potassium loss can occur from ADH secretion; excesses are caused by potassium released into the bloodstream as a result of red blood cell hemolysis.

A nasogastric tube may be inserted to prevent distension or nausea and vomiting. The tube should be irrigated as ordered and accurate record of intake and output kept. The nurse can listen for bowel sounds, which should return to 4 to 6 hours after surgery. Absence of bowel sounds and abdominal distension should be reported to the surgeon.

The client is usually permitted a clear liquid diet when gastrointestinal function returns. The diet may be limited in sodium to prevent fluid retention. All oral intake must be recorded accurately and added to the total of intravenous fluids to determine the daily fluid intake.

PROVIDING BALANCE OF REST AND ACTIVITY. Providing a balance of rest and activity is difficult during the first few days after surgery. The client is constantly interrupted for determinations of vital signs, collection of blood specimens, respiratory therapy, and other procedures, and he is unable to sleep. Sleep deprivation may become acute on the third or fourth day after surgery, and many clients become disoriented and depressed. Sleep needs are met by a secure, quiet environment, and the nurse should plan care to provide such a setting.

Many clients experience a transient psychosis in settings of sensory deprivation. Clients may have illusions, delusions, or even hallucinations. This is particularly true of individuals who are accustomed to being independent and in control of their activities. The nurse can use several strategies to create an envi-

1138

ronment that maintains a semblance of reality. Visits from the family, toys for children, early ambulation, and private rooms with windows, clocks, calendars, and familiar clothes all help orient the critically ill individual.

Activity is limited by the use of monitoring equipment and intravenous tubing, but the client should be encouraged to move. The joints may become stiff with disuse, particularly the left shoulder, which may be painful to move because of thoracotomy incision. Diversional activity is usually not necessary at this time, but quiet music may be relaxing for adults. Children may have a favorite soft toy in bed with them.

By the second or third postoperative day the chest tubes and ventilating assist equipment are removed, and the client is encouraged to sit on the side of the bed and progress to sitting in a chair. Ambulation is allowed as the client tolerates and is facilitated when the monitoring lines are discontinued.

PROVIDING PHYSICAL AND PSYCHOLOGICAL COMFORT. Often the need for physical and psychological comfort assumes less priority when lifesaving needs are critical. The nurse, however, should be alert to simple measures that will make the client more comfortable.

During the first few days the client will need a sponge bath and a back massage. Diaphoresis is not unusual after surgery, and the nurse should change linens and bathe the client as needed. A change of position is often all that is needed to relieve a backache or a pressure point. Pain medication is usually given in small doses to prevent central nervous system depression, but it should be offered as needed. Oxycodone (Percodan), administered orally, is often sufficient to manage postoperative pain in adults.

The support of the family during this period is important to the psychological well-being of each client. The family is encouraged to visit as often as possible. Young children are not accustomed to being separated from their parents and

	Complication	Prevention	Management
TABLE 20-3 Common complications of open-heart surgery	Cardiogenic shock (low cardiac output syndrome)	Prevent by maintaining fluid volume and pumping status	Manage with fluid volume, afterload reduction with sodium nitroprusside, balloon pump; inotropic support such as isorpoterenol
	Dysrhythmias	Prevent with hydration, oxygenation, electrolyte balance, pain relief	Manage with antidysrhythmic drugs, pacing, cardioversion/defibrillation, CPR
	Thrombosis and pulmonary embolism	Prevent with low-dose heparin, exercise, antiembolism stockings	Manage with heparin to increase clotting time to twice normal; ligate vena cava
	Bleeding	Prevent with infusion of platelets	Manage with blood replacement, surgery
	Wound infection	Prevent with asepsis	Manage with antibiotics, debridement
	Renal failure	Prevent with hydration	Manage with sodium and water restriction, dialysis
	Electrolyte imbalance	Prevent by maintaining balance of potassium, calcium, magnesium, sodium, and chloride	Manage with replacement as necessary
	Postoperative psychosis	Prevent by orienting client to person, time, place; provide periods for sleep	Manage by orientation, transfer out of intensive care unit, promoting sleep, and rest

need physical contact with their parents to maintain security. The nurse can encourage the parent to hold the child's hand and cuddle him when visiting. Adolescents and adults also derive support from family interest and should be permitted frequent visits with their family.

The nurse should understand the concern of the family while they await word of their family member's progress. The nurse can facilitate conferences with the surgeon so that the family is told of the progress. Family members have needs, too, and the nurse should understand that their demanding or hostile behavior may be a reflection of their anxiety.

Several coping mechanisms may be used to handle the stress of cardiac surgery, and the nurse should be able to recognize these behaviors. Regression and depression are coping mechanisms that the client who has undergone cardiac surgery may use. Regressing to a more comfortable mode of behavior is particularly noted in children. The nurse and parents should not scold the child who wets the bed or asks to be fed. Adults often return to dependency states, and these needs must be met before independent forms of behavior are evident.

COMPLICATIONS. Complications of open-heart surgery are minimized by advances in surgical procedures and constant nursing care in specialized settings. Several complications, however, may occur and require appropriate intervention.[24] Complications are listed in Table 20-3 and discussed where appropriate in the text.

REHABILITATION AND DISCHARGE INSTRUCTIONS. After the critical 2 to 7 days have passed, the client is usually transferred to a progressive care or regular nursing unit for recovery. Activity is increased gradually in preparation for return to the client's normal life-style.

The client, nurse, and family should anticipate behavior and activity changes that may occur as a result of improved health after surgery. Parents of infants or young children can prepare to facilitate activities that promote growth and development. Family dynamics may be altered by increased energy and relief of pain in adolescents and adults, and it is useful for the family to prepare for possible role changes as activity tolerance increases. Before discharge the surgeon should indicate how much activity is permitted.

At home the client continues to increase activity gradually, and schedules depend on the age of the client and postoperative recovery. Children usually return to school in 4 to 6 weeks, and adults gradually resume usual activities in 6 weeks to 6 months.

Exercise rehabilitation programs are particularly useful to adults who have had valve repair or revascularization procedures. The client may be referred to a rehabilitation program or instructed in individualized exercise.

After discharge the client must continue to maintain health habits to prevent complications or further cardiovascular health problems. The nurse can provide information about health promotion and risk prevention or management. If the client is to follow a special diet or use medications, these also must be discussed.

Evaluation. Evaluation of nursing care for the client with congenital heart disease occurs during each stage of the nursing care plan and focuses on the expected outcomes set forth in the planning stage of the nursing process.

EXPECTED OUTCOMES BEFORE SURGERY

The client and/or family can:
1. Describe the health problem.

2. Describe the therapeutic plan to maintain health before surgery.
   a. Diet (sodium restrictions, fat restrictions, calorie restrictions).
   b. Medications (use, time, dosage, route, side effects).
   c. Activity (limitations, if any).
3. Demonstrate physical and psychological readiness for surgery.

EXPECTED OUTCOMES AFTER SURGERY

The client and/or family can:
1. Describe the progression and resumption of usual activities.
2. State use, time, dosage, route, side effects of prescribed medications.
3. List foods on special diet (sodium restrictions, fat restrictions, calorie restrictions).
4. State signs of complications to report to physician (chest pain, incisional pain, dyspnea, weight gain, cyanosis, fatigue).
5. Describe plans for health maintenance.
   a. Normal growth and development.
   b. Risk prevention and/or management.
6. Recognize resources for continuity of health care: physician, nurse, community health agencies.

Sickle cell disease   Sickle cell disease is an inherited defect of the oxygen-carrying component of the red blood cell, hemoglobin.[17,41] The disease is carried as *sickle cell trait* by as many as 10% of the involved population, but is not clinically significant until the defect is present as *sickle cell anemia.*

Pathophysiology. Sickle cell disease is an autosomal recessive genetic defect. Valine, an amino acid, is substituted genetically for glutamic acid in the beta-hemoglobin chain, forming hemoglobin S instead of hemoglobin A. During periods of oxygen deficiency the hemoglobin S (HGS) assumes a sickle shape. The sickled red blood cells clump together and obstruct blood flow in the capillaries, producing ischemia and its clinical manifestations.

Sickle cell disease is found primarily in blacks; 1 in 10 carry the trait while as many as 1 in 500 may have the disease. These individuals are usually asymptomatic because only 25% to 45% of the hemoglobin is abnormal (HGS), but they may become symptomatic under stress of oxygen deprivation or demand such as anemia, exercise, infection, pregnancy, surgery, or high altitudes. When they marry a person who is also a carrier of the trait, there is a chance that one in four of their offspring will have sickle cell anemia. One half of the other offspring will be carriers of the trait.

Identification of persons who carry the trait is urged so that the couples who wish to have a family can be aware of the risk of having a child with sickle cell anemia. Many communities offer screening programs in which a simple screening test, *Sickledex,* can be used to identify carriers. Prenatal diagnosis can be made by amniocentesis, because adult hemoglobin is present in the fetus after 20 weeks' gestation. Parents can then make decisions about abortion.

Assessment. The nurse can assess infants and children during health appraisals to determine alterations of cardiac output. Clinical manifestations of sickle cell disease appear in individuals with sickle cell anemia, but are usually not noticed until the infant is 3 to 4 months old because fetal hemoglobin, which lasts up to 6 months, inhibits sickling. The onset may be gradual or sudden and is characterized by remissions and exacerbations. There may be slow weight gain, and the child is usually small for his age. The child is usually pale, weak, anorexic, irritable, and susceptible to infection.

Nursing process for common health problems

Exacerbations known as *sickle cell crisis* are precipitated by situations of decreased oxygen such as stress, coldness, and dehydration. The hemoglobin S crystallizes, causing obstruction and ischemia. The onset of the crisis may be recognized by anorexia, fever, irritability, and pain. Pathological changes that occur are a result of red blood cell destruction as well as the increased viscosity of the blood, causing sluggish circulation in the capillaries. End organ necrosis follows. All organs may be affected, and there may be swelling, pain, congestive heart failure, renal failure, enlarged spleen, leg ulcers, nausea, vomiting, headaches, drowsiness, and cerebral vascular accidents. Dactylitis, ischemic necrosis of the small bones of the hands or feet, results in swelling of the soft tissues and warmth and tenderness of the extremities. Priapism in men occurs from stasis and occlusion of venous blood flow.

There are four main types of sickle cell crises. The most common and most painful is the *vasoocclusive* crisis. The small blood vessels become occluded, and the blood supply to the vital organs is diminished. In the *sequestration* type of crisis, sickled red blood cells collect in the spleen. The client becomes pale and lethargic, and the spleen is enlarged. Hypovolemic shock may occur and can lead to death. In an *aplastic* crisis the production of red blood cells in the bone marrow is decreased. The client is pale, lethargic, and dyspneic because of a lack of circulating oxygen. In a *hyperhemolytic* crisis there is increased destruction of red blood cells. This type of crisis is recognized by jaundice and low back pain. The diagnosis is based on identification of the hemoglobin S.

> **Data analysis**
> *Data analysis may reveal nursing diagnoses of alterations in cardiac output, alterations in comfort, impaired gas exchange, ineffective family coping, alterations in tissue perfusion, fluid imbalance, and knowledge deficit.*

Planning and implementation. The nurse plans with the client, family, and health team to manage the child during crisis and provide instructions for preventing future episodes. Therapeutic intervention is directed toward increasing the blood volume so that the sickled cells can circulate freely and providing supportive care for pain and tenderness. Alkaline fluids can be offered to modify the acid pH, which seems to promote sickling. Some recommend the use of sodium citrate or sodium bicarbonate to create an alkaline blood pH. Urea therapy may be used to prevent formation of hydrophobic bonds between the HGS molecules. Side effects of this therapy are diuresis, drowsiness, and coma, and the nurse should monitor the client receiving urea.

Analgesics can be given to allay pain. A restful environment should be established so that the need for oxygen is not increased, and the client should be kept warm. Transfusions with whole blood or packed cells may be of some benefit. Transfusions may be of particular use during pregnancy to prevent abortions, stillbirths, and maternal deaths, which are frequent outcomes of pregnancy in women with sickle cell anemia.

Nursing care is supportive. The client can be positioned comfortably, and when he is turned, the nurse should support the painful joints. The family should be included in the nursing care, and, if possible, one of the parents should room-in and care for the client.

When the crisis is resolved, the child returns home. Attempts should be made to maintain a normal life-style and encourage normal development. Maintenance of health is particularly important for this child. The parents should provide a well-balanced diet, keep the child warm, prevent infections, and promote free circulation to avert precipitation of crisis. Some communities have a parents' club where parents of children with sickle cell anemia can discuss mutual problems and provide support for each other.

 Evaluation. Evaluation is an ongoing component of the nursing process.

EXPECTED OUTCOMES

The client and/or family can:
1. Describe sickle cell disease.
2. Recognize indications of impending sickle cell crisis.
3. Use health maintenance strategies to prevent sickle cell crisis.
   a. Maintain warmth.
   b. Prevent physiological and psychological stress.
   c. Maintain adequate fluid intake.
4. State use, time, dosage, route, and side effects of prescribed medications.
5. Describe normal patterns of growth and development.
6. State indications for need for follow-up health care and where to obtain it.
7. Describe available community resources.

Hemophilia

Hemophilia is a defect in the clotting process that causes bleeding episodes. This disease can be classified as mild, moderate, or severe, depending on the amount of defective clotting factor.

Pathophysiology. Several clotting factors are necessary to prevent bleeding, and a defect in any one of them may be inherited. The most common, however, is hemophilia A, a sex-linked recessive disorder in which there is a deficiency of factor VIII, antihemophilia factor (AHF). The disease is passed to boys through the mothers. Other forms of hemophilia, however, may be passed to both sons and daughters. Those at risk are those from families in which the trait has been identified.

 Assessment. Unless the disease is severe and bleeding occurs during circumcision or minor injury in the newborn nursery, hemophilia is usually not detected until the toddler stage when the young boy is physically active. The parent notices that the child bruises easily and bleeds for long periods of time if cut. Internal bleeding, which may be manifested by pallor and tachycardia, may occur. If there is bleeding into the joints (hemarthrosis), these areas become swollen, painful, and ankylosed. The diagnosis is confirmed by blood analysis identifying the clotting factor deficiencies and disorders of clotting function. Bleeding time, however, is normal.

Data analysis
Data analysis may reveal nursing diagnoses of alterations in cardiac output, alterations in comfort, ineffective coping, and potential for injury.

 Planning and implementation. Nursing care is planned to minimize and control bleeding episodes and instruct families in providing safe environments for the child. No cure for hemophilia exists, but bleeding can be prevented and controlled with a concentrated antihemophilic factor, *cryoprecipitate*. This costly substance can be given when bleeding is anticipated, such as before dental or surgical procedures. It is most useful, however, during bleeding episodes. Often the client or members of the family are instructed how to give cryoprecipitate, thus avoiding trips to the emergency unit. Adverse reactions to cryoprecipitate are similar to a transfusion reaction, and the family and client should be alerted to recognize this potential occurrence.

Initial bleeding can be controlled by putting direct pressure at the site of bleeding for 10 to 15 minutes and elevating the involved part. Applications of ice may also be used. Fibrin foam is available to use in preventing blood loss during injury. Topical epinephrine (Adrenalin) may be used to induce vasoconstriction. If blood loss is severe, it may be necessary to provide transfusions with whole blood or packed red blood cells. Persons with hemophilia should carry a card identifying their disease so that they can obtain prompt treatment if they are injured. Family members should also know how to cope with a bleeding episode so that blood loss can be prevented. Furthermore, the client should not use aspirin because its anticoagulant properties can prolong bleeding.

Bleeding into the joints may require immobilization until swelling subsides. Casts or braces may be used for this purpose and the client encouraged to maintain range of motion of uninvolved limbs. When hemostasis is assured, the involved limb can be exercised.

Providing normal maturational experiences for the child with hemophilia is a difficult task for the family. The parents may wish their child to participate in all activities, yet are aware of the consequences of a slight injury. The nurse can help the parents find a suitable balance that permits independence and safety for the growing child.

The environment during the toddler period should be as safe as possible, because falling and bumping into furniture can cause bleeding. The child can wear protective padding and a helmet when learning to walk. Stuffed furniture is safer in the child's surroundings. In the hospital the side rails of the crib should be padded so that the child does not hurt himself by rolling into them.

The school-age child should be directed toward quiet activities, and sports that involve body contact are to be avoided. Swimming and bowling are examples of sports that offer exercise but are not injurious to the body. As the child learns self-care activities, he should be taught to use sharp objects cautiously. Nail files, pins, and jewelry can cause a bleeding episode. A soft toothbrush should be used, because slight pressure on the gums can cause bleeding. In the hospital, utmost care should be used when inserting intravenous or intramuscular needles. Small-gauge needles are preferable, and the nurse should be sure there is no bleeding after withdrawal of the needle.

Adolescence presents new problems. The adolescent may become obese from lack of exercise and compensatory eating. The adolescent is encouraged to develop interest in areas of a less active nature; swimming is one such sport. It is also important to plan realistic career goals that will not require dangerous physical activity. Girls with hemophilia may experience menstrual periods that are prolonged or irregular.

Several community resources may be available to families of individuals with hemophilia. The National Hemophilia Association has local chapters that meet to discuss mutual problems. Suggestions for home care may be made by the community health nurse who visits in the home. Sheltered workshops and financial aid may be available for clients who have need of these services.

 Evaluation. Evaluation of the nursing care plan is an ongoing component of the nursing process.

EXPECTED OUTCOMES

The client and/or family can:
1. Describe hemophilia.
2. Recognize impending bleeding episodes.
3. Minimize bleeding episodes by providing a safe environment, avoidance of use of aspirin.
4. Control bleeding episodes with direct pressure, elevation of affected part, fibrin foam, ice, or use of cryoprecipitate.
5. State limitations of activity appropriate for growth and development.
6. Describe therapeutic plans for immobilization of involved limbs.
7. State indications for health care services and availability of community resources for families with members who have hemophilia.

COMMON HEALTH PROBLEMS OF THE SCHOOL-AGE CHILD

Rheumatic fever

Rheumatic fever is an inflammatory process involving the mesenchymal supporting tissues of the body, particularly the joints, heart, and blood vessels. It is discussed here because of the changes that occur in the heart, although many classify it as a collagen disease.

Pathophysiology. Rheumatic fever is believed to be an autoimmune or hypersensitivity reaction to group A beta hemolytic *Streptococcus* organisms that produce connective tissue damage. The streptococcal infection, which may have had earlier systemic evidence as a sore throat, causes inflammation and scar tissue formation in the heart valve, particularly the mitral valve. The characteristic *Aschoff bodies,* which are composed of reticuloendothelial cells, plasma cells, and lymphocytes around a necrotic center, cover the valves. Scar tissue, which forms during healing, leaves the valves stenosed. The inflammation can also involve the endocardium, myocardium, and pericardium.

More than 100,000 new cases of rheumatic fever are diagnosed yearly. School-age children 6 to 15 years are most often affected. The disease tends to occur in cold, humid climates and in environments where living conditions, hygiene, and nutrition are substandard. There also appears to be a familial tendency. Rheumatic fever is potentially preventable by early identification and treatment of streptococcal sore throats. Screening programs in which throat cultures are periodically obtained from the individuals at risk may be of value in identifying and treating the streptococcal infection and thereby preventing rheumatic fever.

 Assessment. Nurses, particularly those in school health settings, may be involved in health appraisal of school-age children and have an opportunity to assess their cardiovascular and respiratory health status to identify children with rheumatic fever. This is particularly significant because rheumatic fever is potentially preventable. The onset of the disease occurs as an upper respiratory tract infection with chills, fever, and tonsillitis. The client recovers, but the symptoms recur in 2 to 5 weeks. The symptoms are variable and may include major or minor symptoms. According to Jones' diagnostic criteria, two major or one major and two minor symptoms preceded by beta hemolytic streptococcal infection are diagnostic for rheumatic fever. The five major symptoms are *polyarthri-*

1145

tis (warm, reddened, swollen joints), *carditis* (involving early valvular incompetency and stenosis of mitral and aortic valves, increased pulse at rest, or while sleeping), *chorea* (neurological involvement from perivascular changes in the central nervous system), *subcutaneous nodules* (noted on extensor surfaces of joints), and *erythema marginatum* (characteristic rash over trunk and inner aspects of arms). Minor symptoms include history of rheumatic fever, arthralgia, fever, and laboratory data such as electrocardiographic changes (prolonged PR and QT intervals), elevated erythrocyte sedimentation rate, presence of C-reactive protein, an elevated antistreptolysin O, anemia, and leukocytosis.

When these symptoms subside, there may be little, if any, residual damage. The likelihood of recurrence of the infection is high, and pathological changes that cause heart damage are evident at this time.

> **Data analysis**
> *Data analysis may reveal nursing diagnoses of alterations in cardiac output, alterations in comfort, disturbances in sleep pattern, or alterations in tissue perfusion.*

Planning and implementation. Nursing care is planned to relieve the symptoms and prevent recurrence of the inflammation. Aspirin is given for analgesic and antiinflammatory effects. Because large doses of aspirin are used, antacids should be used and salicylate levels obtained periodically. Cortisone may be used if joint involvement is severe. Antibiotics such as penicillin are given to prevent or reduce infection.

Bed rest is also part of the therapeutic plan until the inflammation subsides, although the value of strictness and length of the rest is debatable. Because the child will most likely be cared for at home, the nurse helps the family make plans for taking care of the child at home. The home should be arranged to make nursing care simple for the family. A high hospital bed may be easier for the person giving care. These may be rented or borrowed from a "community loan closet." Back rests, foot cradles, and bed trays can be made from large cardboard boxes. The child's room should be quiet but accessible to the one giving care. It may be easier to have the bedroom area on the same floor as the kitchen and bathroom to avoid needless steps. The community health nurse can demonstrate a bed bath and the use of a bedpan or improvised commode if complete bed rest has been prescribed for the child.

During the acute phase of the illness the child does not feel well. Nursing care given by the nurse or parent should be done slowly and gently. A bed bath can be soothing, and at this time the parent should pay particular attention to proper body alignment and position to prevent deformities of the inflamed joints. Range-of-motion exercises can be done to prevent contractures. Pain medication may be given as ordered to relieve joint pain. Skin care is important, and even though children are more likely to move and reposition themselves, it is necessary to observe the skin for breakdown. The child who has been in bed all day may find it difficult to sleep at night, and a sponge bath and back rub before the child goes to sleep will help him relax.

Nutrition and elimination needs are important to the bedfast child. If the child is not hungry, he does not need to be forced to eat. Attractive meals suitable for his age and taste may stimulate his appetite. Because the child is on bed rest, the need for calories is reduced. An increased protein and carbohydrate diet is necessary for healing, and fluids should be forced to prevent dehydration and ensure adequate urinary output. It is also important to encourage fluids when the temperature is elevated. The child should avoid becoming constipated, and the parent should offer the use of the bedpan or commode on a regular basis.

As the child feels better, his activity may be increased. He will undoubtedly feel like playing, and parents should devise games and toys that may be used in bed. Often a game bag can be made so that the toys can be kept orderly near the bed. Later the child may have visitors and perhaps do some schoolwork. If possible, a visiting teacher or a telephone hookup to the classroom can be arranged.

As the child recovers, his activities are resumed slowly. The parents may need to guide the child in good health habits and help him maintain a balance of activity and rest. The American Heart Association has a program to help parents cope with the child with rheumatic fever and may work with state and local agencies in offering financial assistance to the family.

The client who has had rheumatic fever must use extreme caution to prevent streptococcal infections. Some recommend prophylactic use of antibiotics on a continuous basis. Benzathine penicillin, 1.2 million units IM monthly, may be used, or oral prophylaxis with 200,000 units of penicillin twice a day, or 1 g sulfadiazine once daily. Prophylaxis duration is not certain but may be discontinued in the adult years because the incidence of streptococcal infections decreases with age and in those without cardiac involvement. Prophylaxis is particularly important before surgery, oral surgery, or invasive dental procedures such as teeth cleaning, and should be instituted as a lifelong health practice. Protocols may include a combination of intramuscular and oral routes or be administered only by the oral route. In the former plan, 1 million units (30,000 units/kg pediatric dose) of aqueous penicillin G mixed with 600,000 units of procaine penicillin G is given intramuscularly 30 minutes to 1 hour before the procedure and followed with 500 mg (250 mg pediatric doses for clients under 60 lb) phenoxymethyl penicillin orally every 6 hours for eight doses. The oral regimen includes an initial dose of 2 g (1 g pediatric dose) phenoxymethyl penicillin followed by 500 mg (250 mg pediatric dose) every 6 hours for eight doses.

With earlier diagnosis and treatment of rheumatic fever, fewer residual effects will be noted. Scarring of the mitral and aortic valves, however, predisposes to mitral or aortic stenosis later in life. These may be treated surgically to release the stenosis or replace the valve.

 Evaluation. The nurse and client/family evaluate the nursing care plan at appropriate points of care.

EXPECTED OUTCOMES
The client and/or family can:
1. Describe rheumatic fever.
2. Describe therapeutic management.
    a. Medications: use, time, dosage, route, and side effects of prescribed medications.
    b. Diet: maintenance of nutrition appropriate to age of client.
    c. Activity: limitations and use of bed rest.
3. State need to prevent recurrence of beta hemolytic streptococcal infection by use of prophylactic antibiotics, particularly before surgery or invasive dental procedures.
4. State indications for continued health care services and use of community resources.

**COMMON HEALTH
PROBLEMS OF THE
YOUNG ADULT**

Hodgkin's disease

Hodgkin's disease is a malignant tumor process of the lymphatic circulation. The cause of the tumor formation is not known, but is suspected to be of viral origin, because clustering of individuals attending the same schools or living in the same community has been reported.

Pathophysiology. The disease is believed to originate in the thymus gland or thymus-dependent areas of lymph nodes and may be a T cell disease.[29] There are several histological patterns of the disease: increased lymphocytes, decreased lymphocytes, nodular sclerosis, or mixed cell types. The prognosis varies with the type of involvement.

Hodgkin's disease is a disease of young adults ages 15 to 35, although there may be a second peak of incidence at ages 55 to 75. Approximately 7000 individuals are diagnosed with Hodgkin's disease each year.

 Assessment. Hodgkin's disease is noted by presence of nodes in the lymph circulation, which gradually increase in size. Cervical lymph nodes are often the first to be detected. The obstruction to lymphatic circulation causes pain, impaired circulation, and edema. There may be fever, weight loss, malaise, night sweats, or pruritus. The nodes soon obstruct vital organs or may metastasize to the heart, lungs, or liver. The diagnosis is based on physical findings, biopsy, lymphangiogram, and the identification of *Sternberg-Reed* cells in the biopsy. Some encourage performing an exploratory laparotomy to identify the presence and extent of nodular involvement.

Data analysis
Data analysis may reveal nursing diagnoses of alterations in cardiac output, alterations in comfort, fear, and alterations in tissue perfusion.

 Planning and implementation. For the purposes of diagnosis and treatment, the tumors are classified histologically and staged clinically as to extent of involvement (see material on p. 1149). Treatment protocols can be developed for intervention for each stage, keeping deleterious effects of therapy to a minimum. Radiation therapy and chemotherapy, singly or in combination, are the two most common approaches used to induce remissions and, in some instances, cure.

High-power radiation using the linear accelerator has proved tumoricidal in many individuals with Hodgkin's disease. Radiation therapy is generally effective in stages I and II; when tumors are identified and staged, therapy can be more specific. Radiation therapy should be used with caution in children and adolescents because retarded growth and skeletal deformities have occurred because of radiation therapy.

Current approaches to chemotherapy suggest that the use of several drugs in a cyclical fashion is more effective than the single use of any one drug and does not cause additional toxicity. In one protocol nitrogen mustard, vincristine sulfate (Oncovin), prednisone, and procarbazine hydrochloride (MOPP) are used. These drugs may produce mild to serious side effects. Nausea and vomiting are not uncommon for most of these drugs. Use of prednisone may result in metabolic and electrolyte changes. Antineoplastic drugs often cause uric acid crystal formation, and allopurinol (Zyloprim) may be given to prevent this complication.

ANATOMICAL STAGING OF HODGKIN'S DISEASE

Stage I: Involvement of a single lymph node region (I) or of a single extralymphatic organ or site (L_E).

Stage II: Involvement of two or more lymph node regions on the same side of the diaphragm (II), or localized involvement of extralymphatic organ or site and of one or more lymph node regions on the same side of the diaphragm (II_E).

Stage III: Involvement of lymph node regions on both sides of the diaphragm (III), which may also be accompanied by localized involvement of extralymphatic organ or site (III_E) or by involvement of the spleen (III_S) or both (III_{SE}).

Stage IV: Diffuse or disseminated involvement of one or more extralymphatic organs or tissues with or without associated lymph node enlargement. The involved extralymphatic site should be identified by symbols used for pathological staging:

H+ for liver	P+ for pleura
L+ for lung	O+ for bone (osseous)
M+ for marrow	D+ for skin

Symptoms A or B: Each stage is subdivided into A and B categories: B for those with certain general symptoms and A for those without. B symptoms are as follows:
1. Unexplained weight loss of more than 10% of body weight in the 6 months before admission.
2. Unexplained fever with temperatures above 38° C.

NOTE: Pruritus alone will no longer qualify for B classification.

Nursing intervention during therapy is supportive. The nurse should be alert to the client's emotional state and offer opportunities for the client to express his feelings in a therapeutic environment. The nurse should also plan to alleviate the discomforts that may arise from radiation therapy or chemotherapy. Comfort measures, use of antiemetics to manage nausea, and maintenance of fluid and electrolyte balance are all appropriate strategies.

Although previously considered to have a less than favorable prognosis, Hodgkin's disease now holds a brighter future. Early diagnosis and staging procedures as well as recent advances in radiation and chemotherapy have improved response rates and, in some instances, induced total remission, particularly for histological type of lymphocyte predominance.

☞ **Evaluation.** The nursing care plan for the client with Hodgkin's disease may occur over a period of time, during diagnosis, remission, and exacerbation, and the nurse-client relationship may be supportive or facilitative.

EXPECTED OUTCOMES

The client and/or family can:
1. Describe Hodgkin's disease.
2. Describe the therapeutic plan.
   a. Chemotherapy.
   b. Radiation therapy.
3. Maintain health status while receiving therapy.
   a. Fluids and nutrition.
   b. Activity and rest.
   c. Urinary and bowel elimination.
4. Use coping resources to maintain physical and psychological health.
5. Identify community resources for physical and psychosocial support for clients with Hodgkin's disease.

Infectious mononucleosis

Infectious mononucleosis is an acute inflammation of the lymph tissue of young adults 15 to 25 years of age. Infection is caused by the Epstein-Barr virus, which can be transmitted by oral contact such as occurs during kissing. The incubation period is 2 to 6 weeks. During the prodromal period of 3 to 5 days the client has nonspecific symptoms of fatigue, anorexia, or malaise. The acute stage lasts 7 to 20 days, and the client experiences a sore throat, headache, fever, chills, nausea, diaphoresis and malaise. During the convalescent period of 2 to 6 weeks the client may continue to be weak and tired.

The disease is acute in onset and self-limiting. During the infection the lymph nodes and spleen produce excess lymphocytes, and the liver is affected by the lymphatic proliferation.

The treatment for infectious mononucleosis is symptomatic. The client is confined to bed rest during the acute illness. Isolation procedures are not required, although the client may be communicable through the convalescent period. Analgesia, antipyretics, and antibiotics are used to manage symptoms.

Pericarditis

Pericarditis is an inflammation of the pericardium and may occur in acute or chronic forms. The inflammation may be caused by a variety of viral or bacterial infections, neoplastic disease, surgical trauma, or myocardial infarction. The acute inflammation rests in the pericardium and may cause fluid accumulation in the pericardial sac (pericardial effusion). As the inflammation becomes *chronic,* the pericardial membrane becomes thickened, scarred, and restricts movement during systole and diastole (constrictive pericarditis).

Pericarditis is a disease of young adults. Individuals at risk are those with lowered resistance to infection or previous history of infection elsewhere in the body.

The symptoms of the disease are related to the constriction of the pericardial sac. In acute pericarditis a pericardial friction rub can be heard. There may be chest pain and dysrhythmias. If the pericardial sac fills with fluid, there is pressure on the heart (cardiac tamponade), producing tachycardia, hypotension, decreased cardiac output, and shock. If the pericardial sac is restricted by scar tissue, there may be signs of heart failure. Diagnosis is difficult because the symptoms are similar to other cardiac disease. Chest x-ray films reveal an enlarged heart.

The objectives of therapy are to treat the inflammation and relieve the fluid or constriction of the pericardium. Antibiotics and steroids are used for the infectious/inflammatory process, and a pericardial tap (pericardiocentesis) to remove fluid or a pericardectomy to remove scar tissue may be performed. Digitalis may be used for dysrhythmias and other specific therapies used if the client is in heart failure.

Myocarditis

Myocarditis is an inflammation of the myocardium that can result from viral or bacterial infections, hypersensitivity reactions, or may occur with endocarditis or pericarditis.

The symptoms of the disease are nonspecific, and the client may have chills, fever, anorexia, chest pain, dyspnea, and dysrhythmias. The danger of pericardial tamponade (compression) exists if there is pericardial effusion resulting from pericarditis.

Therapeutic management involves the use of antibiotics and bed rest. Steroids may be used for acute inflammations and digitalis for dysrhythmias or prevention of heart failure.

Bacterial endocarditis

Bacterial endocarditis is an inflammation of the endocardium. The disease is classified by severity and cause as *acute bacterial endocarditis* (ABE) or *sub-*

1150

acute bacterial endocarditis (SBE). Acute bacterial infections are caused by *Staphylococcus aureus,* whereas the subacute form of the disease is usually caused by *Streptococcus viridans* or, rarely, *Staphylococcus aureus.* Both diseases can be preceded by rheumatic fever or syphilis as well as congenital valve disease. Portals of entry are commonly from oral surgery, dental procedures, genitourinary surgery, or use of contaminated needles. The inflammatory process produces calcification and scarring of the valves and endocardium and may result in valvular insufficiency or stenosis.

Bacterial endocarditis is a disease of young adults. Risk is increased with exposure to infection, particularly through dental and surgical procedures. Prophylactic use of antibiotics (penicillin) before these procedures is therefore recommended. Risk also increases if the client has had rheumatic fever because the scar tissue provides crevices in which bacteria lodge and cause recurrence of the infection.

The onset of *acute* bacterial endocarditis is sudden and characterized by a high fever, chills, diaphoresis, leukocytosis, and heart murmurs. Emboli may be released if the fragments of infection on the valves become dislodged. Heart failure may occur in several days if there are incompetent valves. The onset of *subacute* bacterial endocarditis is less sudden, and the client has malaise, chills, fever, perspiration, joint pain, and petechiae. The diagnosis is confirmed by blood culture.

Antibiotics are used to treat the infection. The client is usually hospitalized and bed rest must be prescribed for 2 to 6 weeks until the infection subsides. Antipyretics may be used to reduce the fever. If heart failure or valve damage is present, these must be treated as well.

Convalescence may seem lengthy to the young adult who is involved in developing a career and planning for his family. The nurse can suggest suitable diversional activities while the client must be inactive. Nutrition is provided with well-balanced diets, and energy expenditure is balanced with periods of rest.

COMMON HEALTH PROBLEMS OF THE ADULT

Atherosclerosis

Atherosclerosis is a multifaceted process in which there is a thickening and hardening of the medium and large muscular arteries, notably the coronary, carotid, basilar, abdominal aorta, and iliac arteries. Ultimately the lesions in the arteries obstruct blood flow to tissue and major organs, manifested as coronary artery disease, myocardial infarction, peripheral vascular disease, aneurysms, and cerebrovascular accidents (stroke).

Pathophysiology. The underlying pathophysiological mechanism of artery obstruction is *plaque* development, which many researchers believe starts in early childhood. In early stages the plaques contain smooth muscle cells and cholesterol; later, plaque formation is complicated by deposition of fibrous proteins, complex carbohydrate products, and calcium. The lipid streaks attract molecules of low-density type proteins, which cause smooth muscle cells to enter the intima and attach. The smooth muscle cells produce collagen and, with the muscle cells and lipids, form plaques. Small blood vessels grow into the plaque, and as they rupture and bleed, increase the size of the plaque and initiate scar tissue formation and fibrosis, two processes that further enlarge the plaque.

Clinical manifestations of plaque formation in the coronary arteries may be caused by obstruction and stenosis of the artery or thrombogenic factors, causing rupture of the plaque and ulceration. In the aorta, thinning of the media beneath the plaque causes weakening, aneurysm formation, and rupture of the artery.

Several theories are offered to explain plaque formation. The theories focus on the role of smooth muscle cells in plaque development, the role of cholesterol in plaque development, disintegration of platelets, and arterial endothelial damage.[5] Other researchers have focused on the relationship of aging, metabolic events of lipid metabolism, hypoxia, environmental stress, or the process of atherogenesis. Risk factors associated with atherogenesis are discussed elsewhere in this chapter.

Ischemic heart disease

Ischemic heart disease (atherosclerotic heart disease) is a specific manifestation of atherosclerosis in the coronary arteries. Plaque formation occurs at bifurcation points in the arteries, particularly of the left anterior descending (LAD) coronary artery, the right coronary artery (RCA), and, rarely, the circumflex artery. Obstruction is a slow process, resulting from plaque accumulation or rupture and clot formation, causing a temporary or permanent obstruction of blood flow distally. Collateral circulation develops around the site of atheromatous obstruction, ensuring exchange of gases and nutrients to the myocardium. Failure of collateral circulation to provide adequate oxygen supply to the cells results in coronary artery disease, the temporary obstruction of blood flow (angina pectoris, preinfarction angina), or permanent obstruction and tissue death (myocardial infarction).

Ischemic heart disease (coronary artery disease, myocardial infarction) is the most common health problem and the primary cause of death in the United States.[33] Although epidemiological data reveal changes in death rate and risk, this disease continues to challenge health professionals to direct efforts toward prevention and management of the disease.[33,56,58] Ischemic heart disease currently affects individuals between 40 and 70 years of age, and more than 4 million Americans have a history of ischemic heart disease.[33] Although the death rate from myocardial infarction is decreasing, the event is the most common cardiac emergency, and the mortality rate is as high as 20% after the first attack.

Risk factors associated with heart disease include smoking, hypercholesterolemia, hypertension, elevated serum glucose, gender (men more than women), age (increases with age), genetic background, and the effects of sedentary life-style and stress. These are discussed earlier in this chapter.

Pathophysiology. Coronary artery disease and myocardial infarction are ischemic response of the myocardium caused by a temporary or permanent narrowing of the coronary arteries. Oxygen is needed in the myocardial cells for the process of aerobic metabolism in which adenosine triphosphate (ATP) is released for energy. Unlike other organs that have fewer oxygen needs, the heart extracts about 70% oxygen in the resting state. The amount of oxygen needed to perform the work of the heart is expressed as myocardial oxygen consumption (MVO_2) and is determined by the heart rate, myocardial contractility, and wall tension (tension in the chamber dependent on the chamber size and pressure exerted by blood volume in the chamber).

The normal heart can adjust easily to increased demands for oxygen by increasing rate, force of contraction, or volume of blood through the chambers. In hearts in which there is obstruction to myocardial blood flow, the supply of oxygen becomes insufficient to meet current demands. Instances of temporary or total obstruction cause a state of anoxia and an environment in which aerobic glycolysis meets energy needs. Accumulation of lactic acid and loss of intracellular potassium are results of aerobic glycolysis and predispose to dysrhythmias and heart failure.

Hypoxemia and lactic acidosis impair left ventricular function. The strength of contraction is reduced, and wall motion of the ischemic segment may be hypokinetic. Ultimate left ventricular failure results in reduced stroke volume, decreased cardiac output, increased left ventricular end-diastolic pressure and pulmonary artery wedge pressure, and clinical states of heart failure.

The extent of ischemia depends on the nature of the coronary artery obstruction (temporary or permanent) as well as the location and size of the obstruction. Three clinical manifestations of myocardial ischemia include angina pectoris, the temporary narrowing of the coronary artery, preinfarction angina in which angina is refractory and infarction imminent, and myocardial infarction or permanent obstruction of the artery.

Angina pectoris

Angina pectoris is the temporary occlusion of the coronary arteries attributed primarily to atherosclerosis, infrequently to aortic stenosis, pulmonary embolism, or anemia. The temporary occlusion is brought about by the difference in oxygen supply and oxygen demand, and factors of either origin can precipitate angina pectoris. Inadequate oxygen supply may occur as a result of hypotension, hypovolemia, anemia, vessel spasm, or drugs that cause vasoconstriction. Angina also occurs because the coronary arteries are unable to dilate to accommodate the increased oxygen demand required during activity such as exercise, REM sleep, emotional stress, eating heavy meals, or sexual intercourse.

Assessment. The most common manifestation of inadequate oxygen supply is *chest pain,* and the nurse should note time, location, duration, and precipitating factors. When the coronary arteries are narrowed, the client experiences chest pain, because the heart is unable to supply the myocardium with needed oxygen. The chest pain is believed to occur when the arteries are at least 75% occluded. The cause of the pain is not known, but may be a result of chemical irritation to the nerve fibers or a manifestation of the stretching of coronary blood vessels that stimulate nerve endings in the vessel.

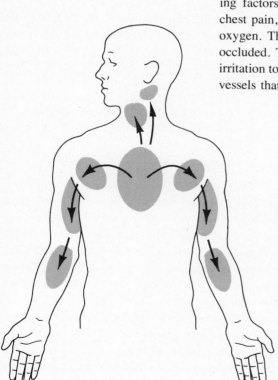

FIG. 20-28
Radiation pattern of chest pain from myocardial ischemia.

The pain is typically described as crushing substernal pain that radiates by way of afferent sympathetic fibers to ganglia at the base of the neck to the left arm, lower jaw, interscapular area, and even to the epigastrium (Fig. 20-28). The right arm may also be involved. The client may experience a sensation of tightness in his chest and a choking feeling as he gasps for breath. This pain, unlike the pain of preinfarction angina or myocardial infarction, lasts only 3 to 5 minutes and is relieved by rapid-acting coronary artery vasodilators such as nitroglycerin. Because the pain is transient, it may be confused with gastrointestinal symptoms or pulmonary disease.

The pain of angina may be described further by specific features. *Nocturnal angina* awakens the client during sleep. It is believed that the increase in metabolic activity of REM sleep causes the pain. *Variant angina* (Prinzmetal's angina) is not related to exertion and probably reflects intermittent coronary artery spasm. The episodes of pain are cyclical and tend to occur at one time of day. The pain of variant angina is usually longer and more severe. The dangers of this angina are lethal dysrhythmias and sudden death. *Angina decubitus* occurs when the client is recumbent and is relieved by sitting or standing. It is possible that left ventricular failure, brought about by increased intrathoracic blood volume while recumbent, may initiate the chest pain.

The client with angina, in addition to chest pain, may experience *dyspnea*. Left ventricular compliance and increases in left atrial and pulmonary pressures cause interstitial pulmonary edema and dyspnea. The client may have orthopnea (sitting up to breathe), dyspnea on exertion, or paroxysmal nocturnal dyspnea.

Physical assessment may reveal the presence of third and fourth heart sounds or a split-second heart sound. Tachycardia, elevated blood pressure, and premature beats or ectopic rhythms are not unusual.

The diagnosis of angina is made primarily on symptoms. The ECG may be normal; stress testing is advised to demonstrate the effect of exercise on myocardial activity.

Data analysis
Data analysis may reveal nursing diagnoses of alterations in comfort, fear, alterations in cardiac output, lack of knowledge, and noncompliance.

Planning and implementation. Nursing goals are planned with the client and may include (1) increasing the supply of oxygen to the myocardium, (2) reducing the demand for oxygen, and (3) helping the client prevent further episodes of angina. Initially the client may be hospitalized for diagnosis and therapeutic management, but later he may be able to manage future episodes of chest pain at home.

Increasing oxygen to the myocardium. Nitrates and beta adrenergic blocking agents are used to relieve coronary spasm and decrease oxygen demand. When oxygen is restored, the pain subsides.

Nitrates are used to relax smooth muscle and thereby decrease arterial systolic pressure and myocardial oxygen demand. Nitrates may be rapid acting or long acting. Nitroglycerin tablets, which are administered sublingually, may be taken at the onset of the angina attack. Occasionally the client learns which situations might produce angina, and nitroglycerin can be taken prophylactically. Nitroglycerin acts within 2 to 5 minutes, and, if the pain is not relieved, the dosage may be repeated two or three times at intervals of 5 minutes. If relief is not obtained, then the client must seek further medical help, because there may be permanent obstruction of the coronary arteries. Nitroglycerin is not habit forming and can be used repeatedly. It should be stored in a dark, airtight container, because it is sensitive to light and decomposes rapidly. The supply of the drugs should be refrigerated and only a few tablets carried with the client. A stabilized form of nitroglycerin, Nitrostat, has been developed. This drug has uniform potency and can be carried without fear of decomposition. These drugs may cause flushing and dizziness, and the client should be alert for feelings of faintness.

Amyl nitrate, another rapid-acting vasodilator, is prepared in perles that must be crushed to release vapors that are then inhaled. Some clients may prefer carrying this medication with them for use during angina attacks. This drug also causes flushing and dizziness.

Long-acting vasodilators may be prescribed to prevent narrowing of the coronary arteries. These drugs are taken on a routine basis, and the client should be instructed when to take them. Pentaerythritol tetranitrate (Peritrate) and isosorbide dinitrate (Isordil) are commonly used for this purpose. Side effects of these drugs include flushing and headache.

Nitrol ointment provides vasodilation up to 3 to 6 hours and is particularly useful for management of nocturnal angina if applied before sleep. The ointment is applied to the skin in a ¼- to 1-inch ribbon that is measured with paper accompanying the product. Although the ointment is absorbed from any surface, the chest is convenient and has psychological benefits of being near the heart.[31] The ointment is spread over a 6- × 6-inch area (not rubbed in) and covered with plastic wrap taped to the skin. The excess is removed and the skin cleansed before the next application.

Beta-adrenergic blocking agents such as propranolol (Inderal) may be used if nitrates are not effective in managing pain. These drugs act to decrease oxygen requirements by decreasing the heart rate and redistributing blood flow to nonischemic portions of the heart.[47] Side effects such as nausea, vomiting, and diarrhea are minor; extreme fatigue, bronchoconstriction, sexual difficulties, heart failure, bradydysrhythmias, heart block, and hypoglycemia represent more serious side effects and should be brought to the attention of the physician. The client should be cautioned not to discontinue the drug, since abrupt withdrawal may cause dysrhythmias, angina, or myocardial infarction from sudden increased responsiveness to sympathetic stimuli.

Reducing demand for oxygen. Limiting activity enables the heart to meet minimum demands. The client should stop his activity at once and rest. If the client is at work, he should notify health personnel; if at home, he should call the physician and emergency medical system. Some clients are reluctant to acknowledge the chest pain or dismiss it as indigestion. Proceeding with activity only puts additional strain on the heart, and it is imperative that the client rest immediately.

When the diagnosis of angina has been confirmed, the client must learn to adjust his activity so that he does not place undue strain on his heart. A moderate amount of exercise may be encouraged to increase myocardial strength, but exertion, mental stress, or overactivity may be harmful at this time.

Eliminating precipitating factors. The nurse plans with the client to identify precipitating factors and develops a plan for modification of risk factors and precipitating events as well as a program of medication and exercise. Because myocardial ischemia can be precipitated by heavy meals, smoking, cold weather, or emotional stress, the client must learn to adjust his life to prevent events that could produce angina. The nurse must understand the client's life-style, his reaction to his illness, and his family patterns when helping him plan to eliminate factors that produce angina.

Many persons with angina are overweight, and the client is usually put on a reducing diet. In addition to being limited in calories, the diet may be also limited in saturated fats (see fat-controlled diet on p. 1115). Saturated fats contribute to atherosclerosis, and when the diet is followed, saturated fats and animal fats are eliminated and polyunsaturated fats used instead.

Eating, especially heavy meals, increases the demand for oxygen and puts a strain on the heart. The client may find it less tiring and more satisfying to eat five or six small meals instead of three main meals.

Nicotine in tobacco produces vasoconstriction and limits the oxygen supply to the myocardium. The client should be aware that all forms of tobacco are hazardous to his health, and if he uses tobacco, he should be encouraged to stop. It is difficult to break the smoking habit, particularly at a time when the client must give up certain foods and activities. The nurse should be understanding of the client's feelings when helping him give up his habit. Community resources such as smoking clinics may be helpful to the person who is trying to quit smoking.

A cold environment can also produce vasoconstriction and a strain on the heart. In an attempt to generate warmth, the metabolism rises when the person is cold, and the demand for oxygen rises accordingly. The client with angina should dress appropriately for cold weather and should avoid strenuous exercise such as walking uphill or shoveling snow when it is cold.

Many clients worry that sexual intercourse may precipitate an attack of angina. The client can be instructed to use nitroglycerin before intercourse and follow suggestions about sexual activity that are given to clients who have had myocardial infarctions.

Emotional stress increases the production of epinephrine, which has a vasoconstricting effect on the coronary arteries. The client should be aware of situations in his life that cause emotional stress and plan to avoid them or cope with them in a less stressful manner.

Exercise programs for cardiac conditioning are valuable to increase collateral coronary circulation, prevent further angina, and contribute to general wellness. The programs are planned for the individual and depend on his cardiac capacity and interests in exercise. The objective of the program is to increase resting heart rate to 85% of maximal heart rate.[15] Stress testing with ECG is done to obtain baseline information, and a specific plan is developed for the client. The exercise can be obtained by walking, jogging, bicycling, or swimming with gradual and regular increases until the target heart rate is reached. Many communities have cardiac rehabilitation centers or programs that are associated with health care agencies or community service agencies, and the nurse can facilitate the client's attendance at one of these programs.

Preinfarction angina is characterized by the onset of severe, abrupt chest pain that is longer (greater than 15 minutes) than the pain experienced by individuals with angina. Furthermore, the pain may be brought on by episodes of minimal stress, hence incapacitating the client from performing many activities of daily living. The pain is resistant to nitrate therapy but is often relieved by narcotics. The client may have severe dyspnea and is likely to develop heart failure if not treated immediately. Coronary artery angiography reveals obstruction in coronary blood flow, and the ECG findings are indicative of myocardial insufficiency.

Therapeutic intervention is aimed at preventing infarction and restoring the client to a functional life-style. Objectives of therapy are similar to those for individuals with angina, but approaches are rigorous. The client is usually hospitalized in a coronary care unit where he can be monitored continuously.

Bed rest in a quiet environment is prescribed. The client should be positioned with the head of the bed elevated 60 to 90 degrees to enhance venous pooling, reduce venous return, and thereby decrease ventricular load and relieve dyspnea. Oxygen may be administered to reduce myocardial ischemia and lower the heart rate, thereby increasing time for diastolic filling and increasing cardiac output.

Pharmacological intervention includes the use of beta adrenergic blocking agents, propranolol (Inderal), and, if there is left ventricular failure and hypervolemia, digitalis and diuretics may be used. Vasodilators such as nitroprusside (Nipride) are used to lower the left ventricular end-diastolic pressure, decreasing peripheral resistance and ultimately decreasing myocardial oxygen demand. Inotropic support is provided, if needed, with dopamine.

More definitive intervention such as surgical approaches may be attempted to assure oxygen supply to the myocardium. These approaches are used particularly if the client has repeated episodes of angina and coronary vessel obstruction is progressing. Such intervention has inherent risks, and candidates are selected carefully from those who are not improving with medical therapies and who have three-vessel involvement with adequate left ventricular function and an ejection fraction greater than 50%.

1. An *endarterectomy,* the removal of atheromatous plaques that line the coronary arteries, may be attempted. These plaques can be scraped out or forced out with gas under pressure, thus enabling a free flow of blood to the myocardium. This approach is rarely used, however.
2. *Ligating the internal mammary artery* has proved to increase coronary blood flow by increasing the amount of blood diverted to the coronary artery. This approach may be successful in selected individuals.
3. *Blood vessel transplants* have been used to bypass occluded coronary arteries. A vein segment, usually from the saphenous vein, is ligated and removed for transplantation to the coronary arteries or used to bypass obstructions by anastomosis from the ascending aorta to the coronary artery (usually the left anterior descending, right coronary, or circumflex artery) (Fig. 20-29). This is an open-heart surgical approach, and nursing care is described elsewhere in this chapter. Following the surgery, radiographic studies are done to determine patency and flow rates. Long-term results of this surgery are not known, but current evidence indi-

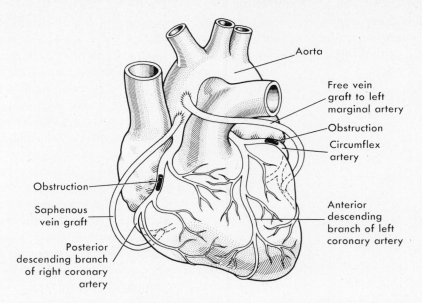

FIG. 20-29
Coronary artery bypass grafts.

cates 60% to 80% patency after 5 years. Results seem to improve if two or three arteries are grafted during the procedure. The value of this surgery for the client is not only the freedom from pain and increased exercise tolerance but also the improved quality of life.

4. *Angioplasty*. Newer approaches to plaque removal include percutaneous transluminal coronary angioplasty (PTCA). The procedure is similar to a cardiac catheterization, and a vinyl balloon is inflated to exert pressure, forcing exudation of fluid and dilation of obstructed arteries.[49] The mass is compressed, compacted, and remodeled, thereby increasing the diameter of the artery. Nursing care is similar to that following cardiac catheterization.

Myocardial infarction

A myocardial infarction (MI, coronary occlusion, coronary thrombosis, or heart attack) is the total occlusion of a coronary artery, which may be small and focal or large and diffuse. The cause of the obstruction is not known, although hemorrhage beneath an atherosclerotic plaque and thrombus formation are presumed to be precipitating factors. Recent research indicates that thrombus formation may be secondary to infarction, since edema associated with infarction impairs blood flow in the coronary artery, causing stasis and thrombus formation.[13]

Pathophysiology. Within 30 seconds following the occlusion, metabolic changes occur as a result of ischemia. Anaerobic glycolysis is initiated to provide energy sources, resulting in lactate production. Additionally, there are changes in membrane electropotential owing to loss of sodium pump activity and changes in the transmembrane potassium gradient.

After about 20 minutes, cellular changes, including rupture of lysozymes and structural defects of the sarcolemma, become irreversible in the center of the infarcted zone. There is, however, an ischemic zone surrounding the infarct, which is composed of normal or near normal cells (Fig. 20-30). This area of ischemia is potentially viable if adequate circulation is reestablished. The objective of therapy, therefore, is to preserve this area and prevent extension of the central zone of necrosis.

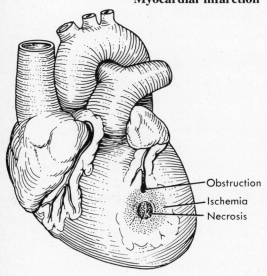

FIG. 20-30
Myocardial infarction, zones of necrosis, and ischemia.

1158

Myocardial infarction impairs ventricular function and predisposes to hemodynamic changes. These may include reduced contractility, reduced stroke volume, abnormal wall motion, decreased ejection fraction, increased left ventricular end-systolic and end-diastolic volumes, and increased ventricular end-diastolic pressures. Compensatory mechanisms postpone deterioration of cardiac output and perfusion. These may include reflex sympathetic stimulation to increase heart rate, vasoconstriction, ventricular hypertrophy, and sodium and water retention. These compensatory mechanisms, however, increase myocardial oxygen demand, and therpeutic intervention is planned to optimize oxygen delivery and reduce demand.

Healing of the infarcted myocardium occurs over a period of several weeks. Within 24 hours there is cellular edema and leukocytic infiltration. Cardiac enzymes are released from the cells at this time. Tissue degradation and removal of necrosis occurs on the second or third day. Scar tissue formation begins in the third week as fibrous connective tissue replaces necrotic tissue. A stable scar is established within 6 weeks to 3 months.

Myocardial infarction most often occurs in the left ventricle and can be described by the area involved. A *transmural* infarction involves the entire myocardial wall; a *subendocardial infarction* is limited to the inner portion of the myocardium.

Assessment. The client who has a myocardial infarction notices a sudden, sharp, viselike, crushing substernal pain that may radiate to his left arm, both arms, or jaws. The pain may last for as long as 30 minutes and is not relieved by nitroglycerin or rest. The pain may be confused with indigestion or gallbladder pain and may be initially dismissed by the client. Oxygen deprivation to the myocardium weakens the force of contraction of the heart, and circulation may be slowed. The individual becomes restless and may even pace and open windows for fresh air. Later he becomes diaphoretic, ashen, and dyspneic. Sympathetic nervous system stimulation causes tachycardia and a rise in blood pressure, but vagal stimulation may also occur, causing a slower heart rate and a drop in blood pressure. Most clients have premonitory symptoms such as increased angina, fatigue, or indigestion. The client is usually anxious, a condition that tends to intensify the pain and dyspnea.

Physical assessment reveals a pale, diaphoretic client in severe pain. Nausea and vomiting may occur from vagal stimulation. Third and fourth heart sounds may be heard on auscultation as well as murmurs or a pericardial friction rub. The ECG may reveal findings typical of myocardial infarction—pronounced Q waves, T wave inversion, and ST segment elevation—and the client should be monitored continuously for dysrhythmias, such as premature ventricular contractions, which are not uncommon immediately following the infarction.

Laboratory studies support the evidence of an infarction. The sedimentation rate and white blood cell count rise in response to the tissue death. The body temperature is usually elevated to 101° F (38.3° C) for the first few days. Enzymes such as SGOT, LDH, and CPK, which are released at the time of tissue necrosis, are observed within 24 hours. CPK is the earliest and most specific of the enzymes to be detected. (Blood for enzyme studies should be obtained immediately, because enzymes from muscle injury from injections can distort values.) The nurse should be aware of variations of enzyme levels during the course of myocardial infarction (Table 20-4). Isoenzymes (molecular forms of enzymes

TABLE 20-4

Serum enzyme changes in myocardial infarction

Enzyme	Normal value (per ml serum)	Onset	Peak	Duration
CPK (creatine phosphokinase)	6 to 30	2 to 5 hours	24 to 48 hours	2 to 5 days
CPK-MB			18 hours	24 to 36 hours
SHBD (serum alpha-hydroxybutyrate dehydrogenase)	50 to 250	6 to 12 hours	48 to 72 hours	1 to 3 weeks
SGOT (serum glutamic-oxaloacetic transaminase)	12 to 40	6 to 10 hours	24 to 48 hours	3 to 5 days
SGPT (serum glutamic-pyruvic transaminase)	6 to 53	6 to 10 hours	24 to 48 hours	5 days
LDH (lactic dehydrogenase) (total) increases slowly	150 to 300	6 to 12 hours	48 to 72 hours	10 or more days
LDH$_1$	Isoenzymes change before total LDH levels increase. LDH$_1$ increases 4 hours earlier than			
LDH$_2$	LDH$_2$ but after 24 hours there is a significant reversal of LDH$_1$ and LDH$_2$ ratio			

with different physical and chemical properties) are used to aid diagnosis. Isoenzymes are site specific and help determine the tissue involved and differentiate from other injury. CPK-MB and LDH are specific for myocardial tissue injury, and characteristic patterns of onset, peak, and duration can be used to support medical diagnosis and monitor progress.

Radiographic studies may show an enlarged heart, and specific areas of necrosis can be noted by myocardial imaging techniques. Echocardiographic findings can be used to estimate hemodynamic function and may reveal areas of asynergy or dysynergy.

Hemodynamic data obtained by monitoring catheters and cardiac output studies provide specific information about myocardial function. Left ventricular stroke volume and cardiac output may be diminished, whereas the left ventricular end-diastolic and end-systolic volumes may be increased.

Data analysis

Data analysis may reveal nursing diagnoses of alterations in cardiac output, alterations in comfort: pain, fear, alterations in tissue perfusion, fluid imbalance, knowledge deficit, noncompliance, or ineffective coping.

Planning and implementation. The nursing care plan must be developed immediately, because approximately 60% of deaths from myocardial infarction occur within the first 2 hours after the onset of chest pain.[58] During the initial phase of nursing care, emergency plans or protocols may be instituted to obtain health care assistance for the client. Health care services may be provided in the community, in an emergency vehicle, at an emergency department, or in the hospital. During the recovery phase the client is in a coronary care or intensive care unit, and the nursing care plan is developed with the client to prevent further myocardial damage. During the rehabilitation phase of care the client assumes increasing responsibility for his care and plans for return to his community.

Emergency care. Emergency care for the client having a myocardial infarction is directed toward providing rest and comfort and identifying potential complications of dysrhythmias or cardiac arrest. The first responder can loosen the client's collar and position him so that he can breathe easily. He should be supported in whatever position is comfortable for him, usually Fowler's position so that he does not have to exert himself to be comfortable. While medical help is being obtained, someone should remain with the client and calm him with verbal support. A heart attack is a frightening experience for the victim and his family, and the atmosphere should be quiet and supportive.

Medical assistance should be obtained as soon as possible and facilities for basic and advanced life support obtained. At this time priorities are established and protocols instituted.

Oxygen is given immediately to relieve dyspnea and assure cellular oxygenation during the first critical 20 minutes of ischemia. Oxygen should be given as soon as facilities are available in the industrial clinic, ambulance, emergency unit, or coronary care unit. Nasal oxygen with a cannula extending 1 cm into the nares is usually used, because the setup is comfortable for the client and supplies sufficient supplemental oxygen. Others prefer a mask because the percentage of oxygen administered can be regulated. Oxygen is also needed when narcotics are used for pain relief, because the respiratory center may be inhibited.

An intravenous infusion of D_5W or lactated Ringer's solution is started to provide access for administration of drugs. An ECG recording is obtained and interpreted for dysrhythmias. Morphine may be given for chest pain. If dysrhythmias are present, they are treated immediately. Atropine is used for bradydysrhythmias and lidocaine for premature ventricular contractions (PVCs) or ventricular tachycardia.

Recovery. When emergency care has been given, the client is transported to a coronary care unit for continuous observation and therapeutic intervention. At this time the nurse evaluates response to previous interventions and obtains essential data for a nursing history. A care plan is developed for the individual and may include goals to (1) relieve pain, (2) relieve dyspnea, (3) prevent dysrhythmias, (4) decrease myocardial oxygen demand, (5) reduce cell injury, (6) prevent complications, and (7) help the client integrate the experience of a myocardial infarction.

The family should not be neglected when the client is admitted to the coronary care unit. The physician usually informs the family of the client's diagnosis as soon as possible. The nurse can accompany the physician to facilitate answers to the family's questions at a later time. The nurse should also explain visiting policies in the unit and indicate waiting room facilities. If possible, the nurse should plan to consult with the family during the client's stay in the coronary care unit to inform them of his progress and give them opportunities to assist in planning nursing care.

Pain relief. Chest pain is acute when the client has a myocardial infarction. The pain compounds the anxiety and dyspnea, and relief should be offered immediately. Narcotics such as meperidine (Demerol) hydrochloride or morphine are used. They may be given intravenously if the client is in shock, because there is diminished absorption from intramuscular sites.

The nurse should observe the client for the effect of the narcotic. If pain relief is not obtained in 15 to 20 minutes, the physician should be notified because the infarction may have extended. Some clients are hesitant to ask for pain medication, and the nurse should be alert to nonverbal cues that indicate pain. The nurse should also observe the client for respiratory rate depression when narcotics are used. Pain unrelieved by narcotics and rest may be treated with propranolol (Inderal), nitroprusside (Nipride), or intravenous nitroglycerin. These drugs reduce the oxygen demand, the blood pressure, or reduce afterload (nitroglycerin) and relieve pain by reducing cardiac distension of nerve fibers.

Relief of dyspnea. Oxygen is used to increase arterial oxygen and thereby reduce difficulty of breathing. The client may be more comfortable in a semi-Fowler's position to increase lung expansion and diaphragm movement as well as relieve pooling in pulmonary vessels. Dyspnea is also relieved as left ventricular function improves and pulmonary congestion is lessened.

Preventing dysrhythmias. Dysrhythmias, particularly atrioventricular heart block and ventricular fibrillation are the greatest threat to life immediately after a myocardial infarction and 90% of clients have dysrhythmias within 72 hours after infarction. The nurse gathers data from the ECG, electrolyte levels, and the client's vital signs to identify potential or incipient dysrhythmias. Because hypoxemia increases myocardial ischemia, oxygen is used to decrease myocardial oxygen demand and the likelihood for dysrhythmias. Antidysrhythmic drugs may be used to treat or prevent dysrhythmias. Continuous infusions of lidocaine (Xylocaine) are often used during the first 48 to 72 hours to prevent premature ventricular contractions (PVCs), the precursors of ventricular tachycardia and ventricular fibrillation. Clients with heart block (first-, second-, or third-degree AV block) may be treated with adrenergic agents such as atropine sulfate or temporary cardiac pacing.

Decreasing myocardial oxygen demand. Myocardial oxygen demand is determined by heart rate, afterload, preload, and myocardial contractility. A balance of oxygen supply and demand can therefore be achieved by pharmacological therapy to support the ischemic myocardium. Myocardial oxygen demand can be reduced with the use of nitrates to dilate coronary arteries and peripheral venous circulation. Rapid-acting intravenous nitroglycerin may be used in a continuous drip to improve coronary blood flow and cause preload and afterload reduction by venous dilation. Longer-acting nitrates such as Isordil may be used subsequently. Propranolol (Inderal) may also be used to decrease myocardial oxygen demand by decreasing the heart rate and contractility.[47]

Physical and psychological rest are significant to recovery from a myocardial infarction. The weakened heart is unable to meet more than basal needs, and the client must avoid superfluous activity while collateral circulation develops. Most physicians limit the client's activity and plan care to prevent increasing metabolism from eating, straining to defecate, or emotionally exciting situations.

Initially the client may be on bed rest. This may mean the client does not bathe, feed, or turn himself. These activities are done by the nurse. Many clients resist forced dependency, and the nurse should use approaches that help the client obtain needed rest and yet preserve his dignity. The nurse can allow the client choices as appropriate to give him a feeling that he is still in control of the situation. The nurse should anticipate the needs of the client so that he does not have to turn himself or reach for a glass of water, for example.

Activity programs can begin in the coronary care unit to include passive range-of-motion exercises and later increasing to active exercises as the client tolerates. Progression of activity depends on the extent of infarction, presence of dysrhythmias, presence of complications and age, sex, and general health of the client.[64]

Bed rest presents cardiac as well as extracardiac hazards of immobility.

Individuals who must rest in bed have an increased cardiac workload, diminished cardiac reserve, orthostatic hypotension, and greater risk for thrombus formation. Furthermore, there is a reduction in maximal oxygen uptake (O_2 max), decreased circulating blood volume, reduced plasma volume, and increased viscosity of the blood. Extracardiac hazards of bed rest also include diminished vital capacity of the lungs, decreased muscle strength, urinary stasis, and psychological stress.

To prevent these hazards, many advocate early, progressive activity programs to minimize cardiac deconditioning and promote psychological well-being that often results from activity. Anticoagulants (heparin followed by warfarin [Coumadin]) are used to prevent thromboembolic effects of bed rest. Antiembolic hose may also be used.

Dietary restrictions may be imposed to assure metabolic rest. Intravenous fluids and clear liquids are offered for the first few days to simplify digestion and reduce cardiac workload. Coffee, tea, and some colas containing caffeine, a cardiac stimulant, may be removed from the diet. Some maintain that oral fluids should be served at room temperature, since hot fluids can cause abdominal distension and cold fluids can produce vasoconstriction and vagal stimulation, which could cause a serious bradycardia. Other evidence suggests, however, that ice water does not produce deleterious effects, and since it is refreshing to clients, it can be offered.[34] Later the diet is advanced to several small meals a day. The diet may be restricted in sodium (see low-sodium diet p. 1172), fat (see fat-controlled diet, p. 1115), or calories as the situation warrants. Others advocate the use of a skim-milk diet consisting of frequent feedings of skim milk to meet basal metabolic needs during the first 4 to 5 days. It is felt that this diet aids in prevention of postinfarction gastric ulcer formation.

The client should avoid becoming constipated. Straining to defecate increases the cardiac workload and may produce Valsalva's maneuver (expiration against a closed glottis). This maneuver produces reduced venous return, lowering of the blood pressure, bradycardia, and possible syncope. Constipation is not uncommon, because the client is on bed rest, has a limited diet, and may be receiving opiates. Stool softeners are usually ordered to prevent this problem, and most physicians permit the use of a bedside commode. This offers a more natural position for defecation, and there is less strain on the heart when the client can use the commode.

Psychological rest is promoted by eliminating sources of stress. In the coronary care unit the environment should be quiet and relaxing. Outside stimulation from television, newspapers, radio, or visitors is usually limited. The family can help plan for psychological rest by eliminating known sources of stress and avoiding subjects that upset the client. Often the client is concerned about his family or business, and the nurse and family can determine how best to reassure him.

Sleep needs are important during this period of healing. The nurse should plan vital sign assessments and treatments so the client can have several uninterrupted periods for sleeping through a complete 90-minute cycle.

Reducing cell injury. Recent data about the nature of the ischemic zone surrounding the infarct have directed researchers to attempt immediate interventions that may reduce myocardial cell injury in this area. These may include the use of calcium antagonists such as verapamil, administration of glucose-insulin-potassium infusions, use of hydrogen receptors or steroids, infusion of streptokinase in the blocked coronary artery to dissolve a clot, or infusion of nitroglycerin to reduce coronary artery spasm. Many of these approaches are in research trial stage and the nurse may participate in documentation of use of these drugs.

Preventing complications. Complications of a myocardial infarction are a result of deficits of myocardial perfusion and may involve problems associated with myocardial contractility or conduction. Complications are usually evident within the first few hours, and with use of monitoring equipment and nursing assessment can be detected in incipient stages. The location and extent of necrosis determines the likelihood of serious complications. Common complications are dysrhythmias, pump failure (cardiogenic shock or congestive heart failure), and pulmonary edema; myocardial rupture and pericarditis (postmyocardial infarction syndrome, PMIS) are less common. The nurse should be alert to the possibilities of these complications and report ominous signs.

Fatal *dysrhythmias* may develop when necrotic tissue is present along conduction pathways and occur in about 40% of persons with myocardial infarction. With the use of continuous monitoring equipment, many of these rate and rhythm irregularities can be detected before they cause ventricular fibrillation or cardiac arrest. When dysrhythmias do occur, they may be treated with antidysrhythmic drugs (such as intravenous lidocaine hydrochloride), cardiac pacing, cardioversion, or cardiopulmonary resuscitation.

Pump failure (congestive heart failure and cardiogenic shock) occurs in about 25% of persons with myocardial infarction. *Pulmonary edema* is the result of left heart failure and must be treated immediately. *Myocardial rupture,* although rare, occurs 4 to 10 days after the infarction and is associated with massive infarction. *Pericarditis* occurs in less than 10% of clients after a myocardial infarction, but the nurse can assess the client for pericardial friction rub, chest pain that increases on inspiration, and fever. Pericarditis occurs 1 to 14 days after the myocardial infarction and may be caused by a virus or autoimmune disorder. Analgesics and rest are used for treatment. *Thromboembolism,* particularly pulmonary embolism, are not infrequent causes of death following myocardial infarction. Low-dose heparin therapy may be used to prevent thromboembolism in high-risk clients.

Integrating the experience. The client's reaction to the myocardial infarction is the sum of his personality, socioeconomic status, family role, age, previous hospitalizations, and the value he places on health. The reactions to this illness take on many forms as the client attempts to integrate this critical experience within the framework of his personality.[11,25] The nurse must be alert to the meaning of behavior and assist the client as he attempts to cope.

This assisting relationship pervades the entire hospitalization but is probably most intense when the critical days are past, and the client has time to ponder what has happened to him. He may deny the experience or pass it off as a bad case of indigestion. He may feel euphoric at having lived through the heart attack and claim to feel better than he ever has. He may also be angry and wonder why this has happened to him. The anger is often displaced onto family members or the nurse. The experience may be totally intellectualized, and the client may become knowledgeable about monitors, ECGs, and his drugs. Regression or depression may also be reactions to this illness. Aggressive sexual behavior is not uncommon in middle-aged men. These coping mechanisms appear to be necessary in the recovery process, and the nurse should be supportive as the client attempts to resolve his feelings about his illness.

Rehabilitation. The client's return to his former state of health should begin soon after the critical period is over. The physician gives realistic guidelines for activity, and the nurse can help the client anticipate how he will live within this framework.[64]

When the critical first 3 to 7 days are over, the client is transferred to another nursing care unit for several weeks of recovery. In some hospitals the client is transferred to a progressive care unit. This intermediate care unit has facilities for telemetry, enabling the client freedom of movement and yet security of monitoring.

The transfer from the coronary care unit should be accomplished smoothly. The nurse from the nursing unit should meet the client before he arrives and help him plan for his care there. Conferences with the nursing team in the coronary care unit and written care plans are helpful in providing continuity of care.

The client may view the transfer with relief or apprehension. Some see the transfer as a sign of progress and welcome the change. Others may fear losing the security of the intensive nursing care and the relationship with the nurses in that unit. Transfer is best done during the day when personnel are sufficient to meet the client's needs. The client may feel more secure in a two-bed room. Often it is helpful for the nurse to be available after the transfer to answer questions and dispel fears.

When the client has adjusted to the progressive care nursing unit, the nurse, client, and family may begin discussing plans for rehabilitation. Many hospitals have formal education programs for individuals or groups; at other institutions the nurse or physical therapist initiate instructions with the client. Regardless of facilities, personnel, or teaching strategies, the client ultimately assumes responsibility for understanding information about his physical activity, drug therapy, diet modifications, and risk reduction.

Activity. Transfer from a coronary care unit does not indicate freedom for activity. It is helpful to be able to instruct the client as to the amount of activity in which he can participate. A useful tool is metabolic equivalents (METS); METS represent the energy used per kilogram of body weight per minute (approximately 3.5 cc of oxygen) and serve as guidelines for the client's activity (Table 20-5). The physician prescribes activity levels, allowing for increases for one MET during the acute phase to nine METS during recovery. Instructions such as these are more easily followed if examples and choices are given.

When the client has regained strength, he may be sent home to rest for several more weeks. Household and career responsibilities are resumed gradually, often on a part-time basis at first. The client may participate in a cardiac rehabilitation program.

Many clients are concerned about resuming sexual activity.[8,46,52] The nurse can create an atmosphere in which questions can be asked and information freely given. Most physicians agree that sexual intercourse can be resumed if the client can walk up stairs without anginal pain. Cardiac stress during intercourse can be minimized if the client initiates intercourse when he is rested and in a comfortable environment. Intercourse should be avoided if the client is fatigued or cold and after heavy eating or drinking. Although choice of positions for inter-

TABLE 20-5

Metabolic equivalents for 70 kg person

Activity	Calories per minute	METS	Activity	Calories per minute	METS
Housework			**Self-care**		
Hand sewing	1.4	1	Rest, supine	1.0	1
Sweeping floor	1.7	1.5	Sitting	1.2	1
Machine sewing	1.8	1.5	Standing, relaxed	1.4	1
Polishing furniture	2.4	2	Eating	1.4	1
Peeling potatoes	2.9	2.5	Conversation	1.4	1
Scrubbing, standing	2.9	2.5	Dressing, undressing	2.3	2
Washing small clothes	3.0	2.5	Washing hands, face	2.5	2
Kneading dough	3.3	2.5	Bedside commode	3.6	3
Scrubbing floors	3.6	3	Walking, 2.5 mph	3.6	3
Cleaning windows	3.7	3	Showering	4.2	3.5
Making beds	3.9	3	Using bedpan	4.7	4
Ironing, standing	4.2	3.5	Walking downstairs	5.2	4.5
Mopping	4.2	3.5	Walking, 3.5 mph	5.6	5.5
Wringing by hand	4.4	3.5	Propulsion, wheelchair	2.4	2
Hanging wash	4.5	3.5	Ambulation, braces and crutches	8.0	6.5
Beating carpets	4.9	4			
			Recreational		
Industrial			Painting, sitting	2.0	1.5
Watch repairing	1.6	1.5	Playing piano	2.5	2
Armature winding	2.2	2.0	Driving car	2.8	2
Radio assembly	2.7	2.5	Canoeing, 2.5 mph	3.0	2.5
Sewing at machine	2.9	2.5	Horseback riding, slow	3.0	2.5
Bricklaying	4.0	3.5	Volleyball	3.0	2.5
Plastering	4.1	3.5	Bowling	4.4	3.5
Tractor ploughing	4.2	3.5	Cycling, 5.5 mph	4.5	3.5
Wheeling barrow 115 pounds, 2.5 mph	5.0	4.0	Golfing	5.0	4
			Swimming, 20 yards per minute	5.0	4
Horse ploughing	5.9	5.0	Dancing	5.5	4.5
Carpentry	6.8	5.5	Gardening	5.6	4.5
Mowing lawn by hand	7.7	6.5	Tennis	7.1	6
Felling tree	8.0	6.5	Trotting horse	8.0	7
Shoveling	8.5	7.0	Spading	8.6	7
Ascending stairs	9.0	7.5	Skiing	9.9	8
17 pound load, 27 feet per minute			Squash	10.2	8.5
Planing	9.1	7.5	Cycling, 13 mph	11.0	9
Tending furnace	10.2	8.5			
Ascending stairs	16.2	13.5			
22 pound load, 54 feet per minute					

Adapted from Exercise equivalents, Colorado Heart Association. Metabolic equivalent equals approximate resting energy expenditure.

course is a personal matter, there may be less stress with the client in a side-lying or supine position. The client is the best judge of the stress of intercourse and should report palpitations that persist 15 minutes after intercourse, anginal pain, or feelings of fatigue the following day.

Drug therapy. The client can begin to assume responsibility for medications that he will be taking when he is discharged. Formal or informal teaching programs can be used to instruct the client about the use, dosage, and untoward effects of each drug. In some settings the client may administer his own medications so he becomes familiar with the drugs while under health care supervision.

Diet. The client may follow a calorie-restricted, low-fat and/or sodium-restricted diet. The nurse and dietitian can plan with the client and his family to provide instruction about these diets. A diet history of the client's usual eating patterns can be used as a basis for modifications required by restrictive diets.

Risk factor modification. Health instruction about risk factor modification continues throughout the rehabilitation process. The client and family become increasingly aware of specific risks that can be modified and can begin implementing plans for change during this time.

Evaluation. Evaluation of client expected outcomes for the client with ischemic heart disease occurs at each stage of the nursing care plan, after emergency care and stabilization, following recovery, and during rehabilitation. Evaluation of outcomes during one stage provides data for planning during the next, thus assuring continuity of care.

EXPECTED OUTCOMES
The client and/or family can:
1. Define ischemic heart disease.
2. Accept health problem and use appropriate coping resources.
3. State how to manage chest pain and obtain emergency medical services.
4. Identify risk factors and state plans for risk prevention and risk management.
5. Identify precipitating factors of chest pain and state how to prevent or manage.
6. Describe therapeutic plan for the following:
   a. Activity: exercise rehabilitation, limits on activity during rehabilitation.
   b. Medication: use, dosage, time, and side effects of prescribed medication.
   c. Diet: sodium-restricted, fat-restricted, calorie-restricted.
7. State indications for follow-up health care and availability of community resources for health maintenance and rehabilitation and emergency medical services.

Heart failure

Heart failure (pump failure, congestive heart failure) is a condition in which the cardiac output is insufficient for metabolic demands of the body.

Pathophysiology. Under normal conditions the heart responds to changing metabolic demands with a variety of compensatory mechanisms to maintain cardiac output. These may include (1) sympathetic nervous system response to baroreceptors or chemoreceptors, (2) stretching of cardiac muscle and dilation to accommodate increases in volume, (3) renal artery vasoconstriction and activation of the renin-angiotensin system, and (4) responses of serum sodium and ADH regulation of fluid reabsorption. Failure of these compensatory mechanisms may be precipitated by increases in circulatory blood volume pumped against an increased vascular resistance by a heart stretched to its physiological limit. Rapid heart rates shorten filling time in the ventricles and coronary arteries, reducing cardiac output and permitting inadequate oxygenation to the myocardium. Increased wall tension from dilation increases oxygen demand and the heart enlarges (hypertrophy). Ultimately, and particularly in an already damaged or ischemic heart, mechanical pumping efficiency fails.

Heart failure may be described as life-sided heart failure or right-sided heart failure, depending on the primary source of failure. Failure of one side of the heart is subsequent to failure of the other, and clinical manifestations often reflect total pump failure. *Left heart failure* exists when cardiac output from the left ventricle is less than the volume received from the right side of the heart. Increases in left atrial pressure followed by increases in pulmonary filling pressure cause transudation of fluid into the interstitial tissues of the lung and result in pulmonary congestion and, ultimately, pulmonary edema. *Right heart failure,* which follows, occurs when the output of the right ventricle is less than the blood volume received from the systemic circulation.

Heart failure can also be described as acute or chronic. *Acute failure* is usually precipitated by stress that exceeds compensatory mechanisms and may result in cardiogenic shock. *Chronic heart failure,* often referred to as congestive heart failure, develops over a period of time and is usually the end result of increasing inability of physiological mechanisms to compensate.

Heart failure is a sequel to several forms of heart disease and therefore may involve clients of all ages. Neonates with congenital heart disease, for example, or adults with atherosclerotic heart disease or hypertension are likely to have concomitant heart failure. Middle-aged and older adults, however, are more often involved.

Following are common precipitating causes of heart failure:

1. *Causes attributed to the heart*
   Myocardial infarction
   Myocardial ischemia
   Angina pectoris
   Dysrhythmias
   Pericarditis, myocarditis, endocarditis
   Valvular disease
   Congenital heart defects (patent ductus arteriosus)
   Constrictive heart disease (constrictive pericarditis, tamponade)
2. *Causes attributed to the blood vessels*
   Hypertension
3. *Causes attributed to the oxygen-carrying capacity of the blood*
   Anemia
   Hemorrhage
4. *Other causes*
   Hyperthyroidism
   Obesity
   Pregnancy
   Stress
   Infection
   Hypervolemia

 Assessment. Physical examination of the client in acute heart failure reveals a client with clinical evidences of inadequate circulation and fluid accumulation. As the left ventricle becomes ineffective in propelling oxygenated blood from the pulmonic circulation, the fluid accumulates in the lungs. Slight exertion may produce dyspnea (dyspnea on exertion). The client may have a cough that occurs with effort or even during sleep. The client may expectorate mucus and be easily fatigued. Rales and rhonchi may be heard in the lung. Fatigue during feeding is most evident in newborns.

As fluid continues to accumulate in the lungs, the client has *orthopnea* (must assume an upright position to facilitate breathing) and *paroxysmal nocturnal dyspnea* (awakens in the night with an attack of extreme difficulty in breathing). Sitting facilitates respirations by causing venous pooling, thereby decreasing venous pressure. Orthopnea can be recognized in newborns who can sleep only in an upright position on the nurse's or parent's shoulder. Rales and hemoptysis may be evident. There may be a frothy cough caused by the increasing accumulation of fluid in the interstitial cells and alveoli of the lungs.

Hypoxia occurs as cardiac output and oxygen saturation of the blood decrease. The client is fatigued, and as cerebral oxygenation diminishes, he may become dizzy, confused, drowsy, or even unconscious. Lethargy may be observed in infants and children.

Pulmonary edema is a serious result of left-sided failure. Fluid accumulates rapidly in the lungs, and the client may have Cheyne-Stokes respirations and may become cyanotic. The client is extremely anxious. The heart rate is rapid, CVP increases, and urinary output drops. The client may expectorate frothy, pink-tinged mucus. Auscultation of the lungs reveals rales. The third heart sound is present, and a gallop rhythm from the rapid heart rate can be heard. Pulmonary edema requires immediate intervention to restore oxygen to the cells.

Right-sided heart failure usually develops shortly after left-heart decompensation. Systemic circulation is slowed, blood returning to the vena cava eventually backs up, and increased hydrostatic pressure causes fluid to accumulate in the peripheral tissues. Fluid shifts from intercellular compartments to interstitial and intracellular areas. Renal flow is decreased because these fluid shifts set up compensatory mechanisms of aldosterone release and sodium retention, which further aggravate the cycle of fluid retention.

The accumulation of fluid in the tissues (edema) soon becomes evident. In neonates and infants it is likely to appear around the eyes and as hepatomegaly. Adults may first note fullness in constricted areas such as fingers with rings. Weight gain, however, is the most reliable indicator of fluid retention, since 5 to 10 pounds can be gained before clinical evidence appears.

Edema may be described as *pitting edema,* because when tissues are pressed, the indentation remains. Edema also tends to be *dependent* (below the level of the heart), because gravity influences fluid collection. The nurse should therefore assess edema in dependent areas such as the feet or in the sacral area if the client is supine. The sinusoids of the liver and spleen collect excess fluid, causing enlargement and tenderness of these organs. The fluid may accumulate in the abdominal cavity from increased intravascular pressure, forcing serous fluid out of the portal circulation. This state is known as *ascites.* If tissues become too engorged, the skin may crack and fluid escape. Gastrointestinal symptoms such as nausea, vomiting, or anorexia result from the presence of ascites. Decreased urine output and distended jugular veins are other indications of right-sided heart failure.

Monitoring and frequent assessments are significant to the early recognition of incipient heart failure or pulmonary edema. The CVP is elevated, and peripheral veins may be distended as well. Heart failure may be diagnosed by the clinical symptoms, ECG, chest x-ray films, increased circulation time, a rise in the CVP and pulmonary artery pressures, and arterial blood gas analysis, which reveals hypoxemia.

Data analysis
Data analysis may reveal nursing diagnoses of alterations in cardiac output, fluid imbalance, disturbances in tissue perfusion, knowledge deficit, and noncompliance.

Planning and implementation. The nurse plans care that will stabilize oxygen needs and demand. In acute heart failure the client may be critically ill and may be in an intensive care unit for continuous observation. As the failing heart is supported, the client may be transferred to a progressive care unit where he can assume responsibility for managing his own care.

Goals of care are to (1) improve cardiac output, (2) restore oxygen to the cells, and (3) reduce fluid accumulation. Nursing care is given to support these goals and is planned for the individual client, his needs, and his age.

Improving cardiac output. Cardiac output must be maintained or restored to provide oxygen to the cells. This may be accomplished by afterload reduction and use of positive inotropic agents. If the blood pressure is low, dopamine may be used to maintain perfusion pressure.

Cardiac glycosides are used to improve myocardial strength. They act by increasing cardiac output, prolonging conduction time, and increasing the refractory period. Initially these drugs are given in a *digitalizing* dose to obtain maximum cardiac efficiency. When the greatest effectiveness of the drug is obtained, a lower *maintenance* dose may be used. Serum digitalis levels should be monitored when the client is first receiving these drugs to detect toxic doses. (Therapeutic serum digitalis levels are digoxin, 0.9 to 2.0 ng/ml, and digitoxin, 14 to 24 ng/ml.)

Nausea and vomiting may be side effects of cardiac glycosides, but when they are accompanied by anorexia, bradycardia, premature ventricular contractions, mental confusion, blurred vision, and dizziness, the client may be experiencing *digitalis toxicity*. Digitalis intoxication can occur from rapid digitalization; presence of renal disease, vomiting, or diarrhea; and concurrent use of diuretics, which cause potassium depletion. Increasing potassium reserves may reverse the symptoms of toxicity. Potassium supplements such as Kaon, Kaochlor, Kay Ciel, or potassium chloride may be used. Foods high in potassium, such as bananas and orange juice, can also be used to prevent potassium depletion.

The nurse should be thoroughly familiar with the use of cardiac glycosides and count the pulse of each client for 1 full minute before giving these medications. Irregularities and bradycardia should be reported to the physician. Generally, if the pulse rate is lower than 60 beats per minute in adults or 90 to 110 beats per minute in infants and children, the physician should be notified before the drug is given. The nurse should also be alert to dosage changes and know the difference between maintenance and digitalizing doses. Dosages for infants are small, and an overdose could be a serious error. It may be helpful to prepare intramuscular doses in a tuberculin syringe, which is calibrated in 0.1 ml units. Doses for the elderly should be monitored carefully because the drug is more slowly metabolized. Risk of toxicity also increases with renal failure, hypoxia, hypokalemia, or clients who have had cardiac surgery.

Maintenance doses of cardiac glycosides may be continued on an indefinite basis at the home. The client should be taught the importance of taking the exact prescribed dose each day. He may also be instructed to report irregularities of his pulse or signs of digitalis toxicity. If the medication is given to infants or children, the nurse can instruct the parents in approaches in giving the medication. If the physician wants the pulse to be counted, the nurse can instruct the parents in this technique.

1170

Vasodilators may also be used to increase cardiac output by decreasing arterial resistance. These drugs include nitroprusside (Nipride), hydralazine (Apresoline), and prazosin (Minipress).

The client should be positioned to avoid needless energy expenditure. If the client has orthopnea, he should be supported in high Fowler's position. Pillows on an overbed table may be used to support the client's arms. Neonates should be placed in an Isolette with the head elevated 20 to 30 degrees. The client should be turned frequently to promote circulation and to prevent tissue breakdown caused by pressure from edema. When bathing the client, the nurse should use lotion to soften the skin and prevent irritation and breakdown.

Mental rest is as important as physical rest. Sedatives may be used to promote rest. The nurse may identify sources of anxiety and plan with the client, family, and nursing team to eliminate them.

Providing oxygen to cells. Supplemental oxygen may be used to assure adequate oxygen to the cells. Nasal or mask oxygen is usually used for adults, and an incubator or humidity tent is used for infants and children. When the client has acute pulmonary edema, the oxygen may be given under pressure. The nurse should evaluate the client's response to oxygen therapy and observe his color, respirations, and vital signs.

Morphine may be given to improve respiratory efficiency. When it is used in small doses, respirations are not dangerously depressed. Morphine has the added benefit of increasing venous capacitance.

Reducing blood volume. When the heart is decompensated, it has difficulty circulating the blood, and fluid accumulates in the tissues. The blood volume can be reduced by the use of diuretics, sodium-restricted diet, and rotating tourniquets. If necessary, a paracentesis can be done to remove excess fluid in the abdominal cavity. Changes in daily weight, CVP, and pulmonary artery pressure are good indices of progress in reducing the blood volume. As blood volume is reduced, cardiac strength should improve and oxygen is restored to the cells.

Diuretic therapy. Diuretics are used to promote rapid elimination of fluids. Mercurial and thiazide diuretics are often used, and as much as 500 to 2000 ml fluids can be eliminated in a day.

When the client is receiving diuretics, the nurse should offer assistance for voiding. The client may be weak or hesitant to ask for the bedpan or to go to the bathroom, and the nurse should anticipate these needs. Diapers on infants should be changed frequently. Intake and output should be recorded carefully.

The nurse should observe the client for electrolyte loss when diuretics are used. Electrolyte loss can be especially critical in infants and older persons and may appear rapidly. The client may also be receiving cardiac glycosides and following a low-sodium diet, and electrolyte loss can be further potentiated. Abdominal cramps, weakness, lethargy, or muscle spasm should be noted.

The effectiveness of the diuretic can be evaluated by changes in daily weight. When the client is weighed, he should be weighed at the same time each day with the same clothes and on the same scales. If the client is unable to stand on the scales, the stretcher-bed scales should be used.

Sodium-restricted diet. Restricting sodium intake is another way in which the blood volume can be reduced. Sodium causes water retention, and eliminating dietary sources of sodium may prevent and control fluid retention. The client in heart failure requires a 2 g or less sodium diet.

Nursing process for common health problems

The diet is based on known sodium content in food and table salt (see below). Table salt contains 40% sodium; 1 teaspoon of salt contains 2400 mg of sodium; and a normal diet averages 5 to 8 g of sodium per day. By the elimination of table salt in seasoning foods, the diet can be maintained at approximately 3 g sodium per day. A *mild sodium-restricted diet* can be observed if the client avoids salt in seasoning and cooking. A *moderate sodium-restricted diet* (1 g/day) can be observed by eliminating salt as well as foods with known sodium content. A *strict low-sodium diet* (500 mg/day) is followed by eliminating all salt in cooking and seasoning and all foods with natural sodium content. To follow a very low sodium-restricted diet (250 mg/day), it is also necessary to use specially prepared low-sodium foods such as low-sodium bread and milk.

Persons on strict low-sodium diets may need to purchase special sodium-restricted foods. Lonalac is a milk formula that can be purchased at most food markets. Sodium-free baking soda and baking powder are sold at drugstores and can be used in home cooking. In some areas the sodium content of drinking water may be high, and the client should check with local authorities for content. Home water softeners can also be a source of sodium in the water. In these instances distilled water can be used for drinking purposes.

The American Heart Association has several booklets that may be helpful to persons following this diet.

Persons who are following sodium-restricted diets should be alert to indications of sodium depletion. Vomiting, diarrhea, and excessive perspiration can potentiate sodium loss, as can diuretics. Lethargy and abdominal cramps should be reported to the physician immediately.

SODIUM-RESTRICTED DIET

Purpose	1. Prevent or control fluid retention in cardiovascular disease such as coronary artery disease, congestive heart failure, hypertension. 2. Prevent electrolyte imbalance in metabolic diseases. 3. Prevent fluid retention in renal disease such as nephritis and nephrosis. 4. Control ascites in liver disease.
Meats	All; but avoid pork, lunch meats, seafood, canned meat.
Milk	Low-sodium milk for very low sodium-restricted diet.
Fruits and vegetables	Most fresh fruits and vegetables.
Breads and cereals	Puffed rice, puffed wheat, shredded wheat, farina, oatmeal, rice, potatoes, unsalted breads, unsalted melba toast, noodles.
Foods to avoid	Foods prepared with seasonings and leavenings: monosodium glutamate, salt, onion salt, baking soda, baking powder; salted foods: nuts, popcorn, pretzels, crackers, bouillion; foods preserved in salt; canned foods, some frozen foods, sauerkraut, pickles; dairy products: cheese, ice cream, sherbet, malted milk; green vegetables: celery, spinach, turnips, greens; beets; carrots; carbonated beverages; maraschino cherries; medicines with a sodium base; toothpaste; tomato juice.
Suggestions	1. Use salt substitute in seasoning if permitted by physician. 2. Season foods with lemon, parsley, and so forth. Marinate meat before cooking. 3. Use low-sodium baking powder and potassium baking soda. 4. Read labels carefully—sodium is added as seasoning or preservative in many foods. Look for words: salt, soda, leavening, sodium.

Rotating tourniquets. Applying tourniquets to the limbs to decrease venous return is another method used to reduce circulating blood volume. The venous circulation in the limb is restricted, and the workload of the heart is lessened. Tourniquets are usually used during severe decompensation and pulmonary edema and only until cardiac strength is improved. Some researchers advise against the use of tourniquets, because trapped blood may cause increased central venous pooling, and they suggest allowing blood to pool in the lower extremities in a dependent position. Tourniquets are rarely used in children, although blood may be trapped by having the legs lowered 20 to 30 degrees. Use of hemodynamic monitoring to assess heart failure in incipient stages has reduced the need for these measures.

Tourniquets are applied initially to two legs and one arm to reduce the greatest circulatory load, and are rotated so that each limb is occluded for 45 minutes and free for 15 minutes. The tourniquets are applied midway on the upper arms and thighs. Rubber tourniquets, blood pressure cuffs, or automatic rotating tourniquets are removed and reapplied in a systematic fashion. If manual tourniquets are used, it is helpful to have a graph to indicate the rotation pattern and the time to change each tourniquet (Fig. 20-31). Automatic rotating tourniquets inflate mechanically, and the dial may be set to determine how often each cuff is inflated and deflated (Fig. 20-32). These tourniquets are convenient and save disturbing the client for each rotation.

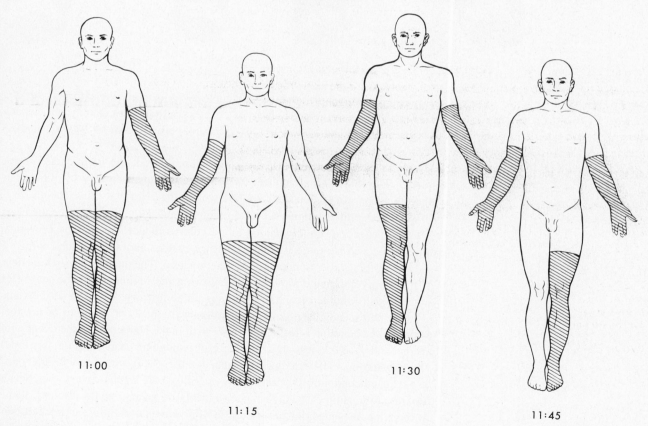

11:00

11:15

11:30

11:45

FIG. 20-31
Rotating tourniquets. Tourniquets are applied to three limbs and rotated every 15 minutes.

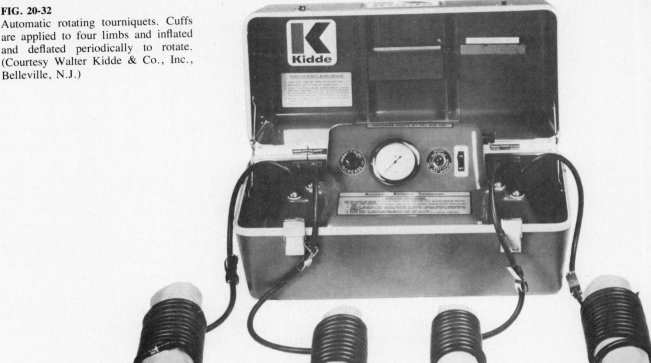

When tourniquets are in use, the nurse should observe the extremity for circulation. The tourniquet should not constrict arterial circulation, but venous circulation should be occluded. The peripheral pulses should be present, and the limb warm and of normal color.

When circulating blood volume has been reduced, the tourniquets are removed. They should be removed one at a time in sequence every 15 minutes so that the added circulation does not overwhelm the heart and cause shock.

Discharge instructions. Cardiac function is usually restored when the heart is strengthened and the circulating blood volume reduced. It may be necessary for the client to continue to take cardiac glycosides and diuretics and follow a sodium-restricted diet to maintain cardiac function. The nurse can help the client or his family anticipate problems in following the regimen at home and offer suggestions for home care. The client should be instructed to report indications of heart failure such as weight gain, dyspnea, fatigue, or swelling of the feet or hands. A community health nurse may visit in the home or help the client with his diet and should assess any indications of impending heart failure at this time.

Evaluation. The nursing care plan for the client with heart failure must be evaluated continuously, particularly in critical care settings where the client's response to nursing care may change suddenly, requiring modification of plans. At this time, expected outcomes include hemodynamic stability, absence of pulmonary or systemic congestion, electrophysiological stability, and absence of complications.

EXPECTED OUTCOMES

The client and/or family can:
1. Describe heart failure.
2. Describe the therapeutic plan:
   a. Medications (digitalis, diuretics, potassium, propranolol): state use, time, route, dosage, side effects.
   b. Diet: sodium-restricted.
   c. Activity: limitations, if any.
3. State indications of problems requiring health care (weight gain, dyspnea, edema, fatigue.)
4. State plans for follow-up care and use of community resources.

Cardiogenic shock

Cardiogenic shock (low output syndrome) occurs when the heart is damaged and cardiac output is greatly reduced. This syndrome is often related to pump failure, although the two, in fact, may be separate entities. The pathophysiological changes are a result of the decreased cardiac output, and severity is related to decreased stroke volume. The arterial blood pressure falls, and perfusion of tissue is inadequate. Vital organs such as the brain, heart, lungs, and kidneys are immediately affected by lack of oxygenation.

Pathophysiology. The diseased heart is unable to contract synchronously or forcefully, and blood flow to the aorta is diverted. The left ventricular end-diastolic pressure (LVED) and left atrial pressures (LAP) increase from inefficient systolic outflow. Ultimately, pulmonary artery pressures increase, and fluid shifts into pulmonary interstitial space and alveoli, reducing surface area for gas exchange. In the face of inadequate oxygenation, anaerobic metabolism ensues with resultant lactic acid accumulation and metabolic acidosis.

The cause of cardiogenic shock is generally attributed to the left ventricle, which has become weakened from a myocardial infarct and is unable to supply stroke volume to meet the cellular oxygen needs. Damage of 40% of the heart from myocardial infarction precipitates shock. Other causes of shock may be dysrhythmic conduction, valvular defects, or complications of open-heart surgery. The ineffective ventricular contraction also lowers coronary artery perfusion, further compounding pump failure. Although similarities of shock states are apparent, the unique facets of cardiogenic shock are discussed here.

Assessment. The nurse must make continuous assessments of clients with compromised cardiac activity to detect changes indicative of cardiogenic shock in incipient stages. Even with early diagnosis, the mortality rate is approximately 80%.[9] The nurse analyzes data from the nursing history and uses physical assessment skills and data from hemodynamic monitoring to determine inadequate cardiac output.

In the initial stages of cardiogenic shock, hypoxemia is manifested by diminished blood supply to vital organs. Cerebral hypoxemia is noted by restlessness, confusion, and agitation. The client will have central cyanosis as determined by observation of the vascular bed of the tongue. The skin is cool and moist from decreased peripheral circulation. Urinary output will be diminished (less than 20 ml/hr) as a result of inadequate renal perfusion. Vital signs reflect a hypoxic state. The systolic blood pressure drops below 100 mm Hg (usually the systolic blood pressure drops before the diastolic blood pressure), and the nurse should be alert to this narrowing pulse pressure. The pulse increases, and dysrhythmias may result from an irritable myocardium. CVP increases along with pulmonary artery pressure, and end-diastolic pressure as intravascular vol-

1175

ume increases. The cardiac output is less than 2.2 L/min. The blood gases confirm an elevated PCO_2 and decreased PO_2.

To adjust to the loss of arterial pressure, the adrenal glands release epinephrine and cortisol in attempts at vasoconstriction to augment perfusion of vital organs. If therapeutic intervention is not instituted, prolonged hypoxemia causes lactic acidosis, loss of myocardial contractility, vascular tone, and, ultimately death.

> **Data analysis**
> *Data analysis may reveal nursing diagnoses of alterations in cardiac output, alterations in tissue perfusion, and fluid imbalance.*

Planning and implementation. The nursing care plan is developed immediately to restore circulation. The client may be in an intensive care setting where goals for nursing care include (1) restoring blood volume, (2) improving myocardial contractility, and (3) increasing oxygen to the cells.

Restoring blood volume. Intravenous fluids and plasma expanders, such as dextran, albumin, or hespan, are given immediately to restore blood volume and correct electrolyte and acid-base balance. Blood volume is circulated more efficiently if the client is in a supine position, and unless there is evidence of pulmonary edema, the client should be placed comfortably in this position. Elastic hose may be used to facilitate venous return. Nursing evaluations must be made frequently to note intravenous flow rate, CVP, LAP, PAP, PAWP, arterial blood pressure, urine output, neurological signs, and skin temperature as evidence of improving cellular perfusion.

Improving myocardial contractility. Pharmacological agents are used to stimulate myocardial contraction and increase vascular resistance. The drugs used are determined by the client's response to therapy and are individualized to his needs. Some agents act synergistically, and doses must be regulated accordingly; others have multiple effects on the cardiovascular system, and benefits are weighed against side effects. Commonly used drugs are positive inotropic agents to increase myocardial contractility and cardiac output (digitalis drugs) and catecholamines to increase blood pressure and heart rate; examples are dopamine (Intropin), isoproterenol (Isuprel), norepinephrine (Levophed), and epinephrine (Adrenalin). Vasodilator agents such as nitroprusside (Nipride), nitroglycerin, and phentolamine (Regitine) are used to reduce afterload and preload. Dopamine and nitroprusside may be used together for their combined effects of afterload and preload reduction and increasing myocardial contractility.

If pharmacological intervention is not successful, mechanical devices such as the intraaortic balloon pump or external counter-pulsation devices may be used. These devices are used primarily in research centers where highly skilled personnel and equipment are available.

The *intraaortic balloon pump* is used in instances of left ventricular failure as might occur in pump failure or in function failure following cardiopulmonary bypass surgery.[3,13,16,18] In this procedure a balloon-tipped catheter with connections to a mechanical pump is inserted through the femoral artery to the

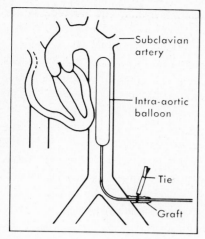

FIG. 20-33
Placement of intraaortic balloon. Insertion is made through side arm graft via cutdown on common femoral artery. Balloon position is just distal to left subclavian artery. Ties around graft secure catheter in place without jeopardizing perfusion to leg distal to insertion site. (From Daily, Elaine K., and Schroeder, John S.: Techniques in bedside hemodynamic monitoring, ed. 2, St. Louis, 1981, The C.V. Mosby Co.)

descending thoracic aorta (Fig. 20-33). The balloon is then inflated with helium or carbon dioxide. Once connected to the mechanical pump, the balloon is programmed to inflate during diastole, thereby augmenting contractions of the left ventricle during diastole and lowering intraaortic pressure during systole. The mechanical pump can be set to inflate during diastole on a ratio, for instance, of 1:2, 1:4, and 1:8 beats. As the client's status improves, he is gradually weaned from the pump. In addition to monitoring parameters of cardiac function for the client by the use of the balloon pump, the nurse should inspect the insertion site and assess all pulses distal to insertion for adequate circulation. The client should remain in a semi-Fowler's position during use of the balloon pump to prevent advancement of the balloon in the thoracic aorta. Foot drop can become a complication of use of the balloon pump, and the nurse should position the client and institute range-of-motion exercises to prevent this phenomenon.

The *external counterpulsation device* is being used in some areas to prevent consequences of cardiogenic shock by increasing diastolic pressure and lowering systolic pressure to rest the failing heart. This externally applied device consists of water-filled bags that fit with an airtight seal from the ankles to the waist. The pressure in the device is synchronized with the ECG to exert a counterpressure to the normal cardiac cycle, that is, to increase pressure during diastole, causing improved myocardial and coronary flow, and to lower pressure during systole by exerting a negative pressure, resulting in increased stroke volume and systemic blood flow.

Within the 3-hour average treatment time, marked changes in shock reversal have been observed. The diastolic blood pressure rises, and mean and peak systolic pressures increase; urinary output improves, as does the client's mental response. The nurse should offer emotional support while the device is in use and make continuous assessments of changes in the client's hemodynamic status.

Increasing oxygen to cells. Supplemental oxygen is given by mask or ventilator, and the nurse should determine response to this intervention. Vasodilators may be used to increase perfusion of vital organs. If lactic acidosis occurs, sodium bicarbonate may be given to correct the results of anaerobic metabolism.

 Evaluation. As circulating volume is restored and cardiac function stabilized, the nurse continues to evaluate response to the therapeutic plan and reassesses data to identify the potential for other problems. The client may be transferred to a progressive care unit where supportive therapy and instruction may be included in the care plan.

EXPECTED OUTCOMES

The client will:
1. Maintain adequate blood volume for hemodynamic stability.
2. Maintain adequate myocardial contractility.
3. Maintain adequate tissue perfusion.
4. Be free of complications.

Dysrhythmias

A dysrhythmia is an irregularity of the heart rate or rhythm. Dysrhythmias are caused by disturbances of mechanisms of impulse formation or conduction. These may include nervous system disturbances, metabolic changes such as acidosis, electrolyte imbalances (particularly hypokalemia, hyperkalemia, and hypocalcemia), hypoxia, trauma, electrical shock, and, most commonly, myocardial infarction. Changes in rate or rhythm are potentially life threatening because cardiac output and myocardial contractility are compromised.

     Assessment. The nurse has frequent opportunities to assess heart rate and rhythm during health appraisals or while taking vital signs for clients in health care facilities. Clients with actual or potential disturbances of cardiac rate or rhythm may be monitored on an ECG, telemetry, or Holter monitor, and the nurse can use these data to identify incipient dysrhythmias. Dysrhythmias can be classified by their threat to life or by anatomical site of origin (Table 20-6). Common dysrhythmias are discussed in this text by site of origin (Table 20-7), and the reader is referred to additional texts for advanced concepts of dysrhythmia interpretation.[1,10,28]

Sinus dysrhythmias. Deviations from normal sinus rhythm may be a response to respiration, exercise, rest, medications, or disease. The dysrhythmias are usually not serious, because the origin of the heartbeat remains in the pacemaker and the rhythm is normal. In many instances the client may not be aware that these dysrhythmias are present. Two such dysrhythmias are sinus bradycardia and sinus tachycardia.

TABLE 20-6
Classification of dysrhythmias

Site of origin	Prognosis
Sinoatrial (SA) node Sinus tachycardia Sinus bradycardia Sinus arrhythmia Sinoatrial (SA) arrest or block	**Minor dysrhythmias** Sinus tachycardia Sinus bradycardia Sinus arrhythmia Premature atrial contractions (less than 6/min) Premature ventricular contractions (less than 6/min) Premature AV nodal contractions (less than 6/min) Wandering pacemaker
Atria Premature atrial contractions (PAC) Atrial tachycardia Atrial flutter Atrial fibrillation Atrial standstill	**Major dysrhythmias** Premature atrial contractions (more than 6/min) Atrial tachycardia Atrial flutter Atrial fibrillation Premature ventricular contractions (more than 6/min) Ventricular tachycardia Premature AV nodal contractions (more than 6/min) AV nodal rhythm Sinotrial (SA) arrest or block Delayed AV conduction (first-degree heart block) Second-degree AV heart block (2:1 or 3:1 block) Complete AV heart block (third-degree block) Bundle branch block
Atrial ventricular (AV junction) Premature AV nodal contractions (PNC) AV Nodal tachycardia AV Nodal rhythm Delayed AV conduction (first-degree heart block) Second-degree AV heart block (2:1 or 3:1 block) Complete AV heart block (third-degree block)	
Ventricles Premature ventricular contractions (PVC) Ventricular tachycardia Bundle branch block Ventricular fibrillation Ventricular standstill	**Death-producing dysrhythmias** Ventricular fibrillations Ventricular standstill (asystole) Electromechanical dissociation Slow idioventricular rhythm

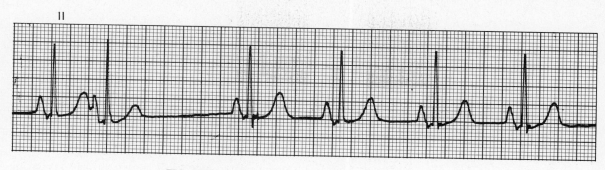

FIG. 20-36

Premature atrial contraction. (From Conover, Mary H.: Cardiac arrhythmias: exercises in pattern interpretation, ed. 2, St. Louis, 1978, The C.V. Mosby Co.)

Atrial flutter. Atrial flutter (Fig. 20-37) is a serious dysrhythmia in which an irritable focus stimulates rapid (300 to 350 per minute) atrial contractions. The ventricles respond to some of the atrial stimuli, and consequently the ventricular rate is also rapid. Angina or congestive heart failure may result. Antidysrhythmic drugs may restore normal rhythm; cardioversion may be necessary in some instances.

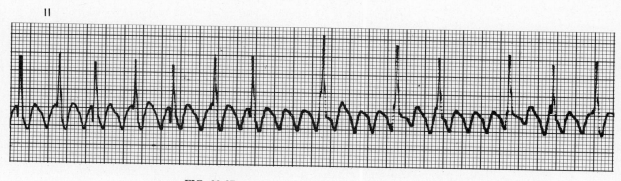

FIG. 20-37

Atrial flutter. (From Conover, Mary H.: Cardiac arrhythmias: exercises in pattern interpretation, ed. 2, St. Louis, 1978, The C.V. Mosby Co.)

Atrial fibrillation. Atrial fibrillation (Fig. 20-38) is an unorganized contractility of atrial myocardium. There may be as many as 400 beats per minute. The ventricles do not respond to all stimuli, and the ventricular rate is usually 150 to 180 beats per minute and irregular. The pulse deficit may be detected by counting the apical-radial pulse. This dysrhythmia is common and associated with mitral stenosis and regurgitation, heart failure, open-heart surgery for mitral valve replacement, and congenital heart defects. Release of emboli is a hazard of the rapid rate and incomplete atrial emptying. Heart failure is likely if the dysrhythmia is not treated. Antidysrhythmic drugs and cardioversion are used to reverse the dysrhythmia. Anticoagulants may be used for chronic atrial fibrillation, to prevent emboli formation.

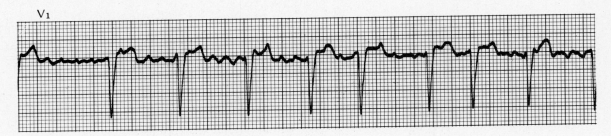

FIG. 20-38
Atrial fibrillation. (From Conover, Mary H.: Cardiac arrhythmias: exercises in pattern interpretation, ed. 2, St. Louis, 1978, The C.V. Mosby Co.)

Heart blocks. These dysrhythmias result in the blocking of impulses in the AV node, in the bundle of His, and at bundle branch origins. The heart block exists when impulses from the atria are not conducted to the ventricles. The heart block may be first degree (prolonged conduction time from the atria to the ventricles), second degree (occasional stimulation of the ventricles), or third degree (in which the ventricles do not receive any atrial stimulation.) Heart block may be a temporary complication of an acute heart disease or may exist as a chronic problem.

First-degree heart block. First-degree heart block (Fig. 20-39) is a delayed conduction between the atria and ventricles, measured on the ECG as being longer than 0.20 seconds. This heart block may be caused by digitalis toxicity, myocardial infarction, or coronary artery disease. Clinical evidence of first-degree heart block is not evident. If the problem is drug related, the dose may be modified.

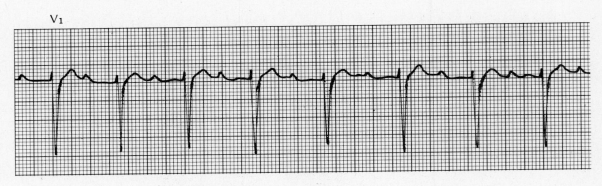

FIG. 20-39
First-degree heart block. (From Conover, Mary H.: Cardiac arrhythmias: exercises in pattern interpretation, ed. 2, St. Louis, 1978, The C.V. Mosby Co.)

Second-degree heart block. Second-degree heart block (Fig. 20-40) is characterized by prolonged conduction and occasional dropped beats. There are two forms of this heart block, Mobitz type I (Wenchebach) and Mobitz type II, differentiated by the increased conduction time and dropped beats. Second-degree heart block is a serious dysrhythmia that has the potential for becoming a third-degree (complete) block or inciting premature ventricular contractions. The pulse rate becomes slower, and if this block persists, the client may have effects of decreased cardiac output and heart failure. Pharmacological agents to stimulate the heart (atropine, isoproterenol [Isuprel]) or a pacemaker may be used to treat the block and prevent heart failure.

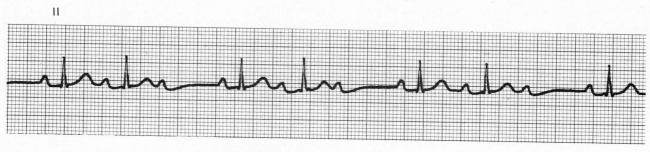

FIG. 20-40
Second-degree heart block, type I (Wenchebach). (From Conover, Mary H.: Cardiac arrhythmias: exercises in pattern interpretation, ed, 2. St. Louis, 1978, The C.V. Mosby Co.)

Third-degree heart block. In third-degree heart block (complete heart block) (Fig. 20-41), no stimuli from the atria pass to the ventricles to stimulate ventricular contraction. Ventricular pacemakers initiate occasional contractions at the inherent rate of 20 to 40, but these are inadequate to maintain cardiac output. Third-degree heart block can be associated with congenital heart defects, but more often with myocardial infarction or as a complication of open-heart surgery. Third-degree heart block is an emergency situation treated with resuscitation procedures, isoproterenol, or temporary cardiac pacing.

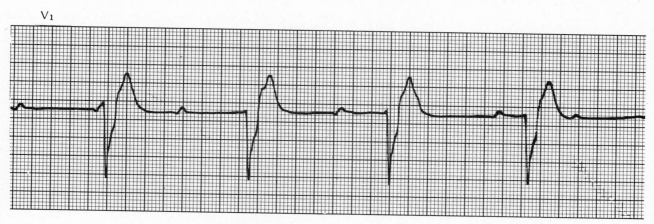

FIG. 20-41
Third-degree (complete) heart block. (From Conover, Mary H.: Cardiac arrhythmias: exercises in pattern interpretation, ed. 2, St. Louis, 1978, The C.V. Mosby Co.)

Stokes-Adams syndrome is a particular form of complete heart block characterized by angina, dizziness, confusion, and syncope. A permanent pacemaker is inserted to provide ventricular stimulation.

Nursing process for common health problems

Ventricular dysrhythmias. In these dysrhythmias the ectopic focus is in the His-Purkinje system. Ventricular dysrhythmias warrant special observation, since most of these have the potential for being lethal.

Premature ventricular contractions. Premature ventricular contractions (PVCs) (Fig. 20-42) are ventricular beats that occur before the next expected heart beat. PVCs, although not unusual in infants and older individuals, are often indicators of ventricular irritability and may be precursors of ventricular tachycardia or ventricular fibrillation. PVCs are serious when they occur more than two in a row, six per minute, or if the R wave comes near or on the T wave, or if they are multifocal, that is, originate from different sites in the ventricle. PVCs are commonly associated with myocardial infarction, cardiac infections, heart failure, or hypokalemia.

The onset of frequent PVCs is treated with a bolus of lidocaine (Xylocaine) followed with a continuous infusion of the drug. Many prefer using a lidocaine infusion to prevent PVCs in high-risk clients, such as those with myocardial infarction.

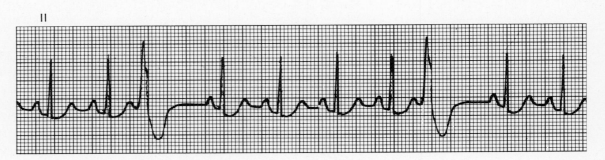

FIG. 20-42
Premature ventricular contraction. (From Conover, Mary H.: Cardiac arrhythmias: exercises in pattern interpretation, ed. 2, St. Louis, 1978, The C.V. Mosby Co.)

Ventricular tachycardia. In ventricular tachycardia (Fig. 20-43) the ventricular rate is 150 to 250 beats per minute. This is a potentially serious dysrhythmia that may result in shock or congestive heart failure and is often a precursor to ventricular fibrillation. Antidysrhythmic drugs such as lidocaine or bretylium (Bretylol) are administered rapidly. Cardioversion may also be employed.

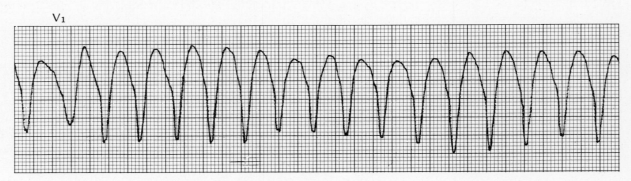

FIG. 20-43
Ventricular tachycardia. (From Conover, Mary H.: Cardiac arrhythmias: exercises in pattern interpretation, ed. 2, St. Louis, 1978, The C.V. Mosby Co.)

Ventricular fibrillation. Ventricular fibrillation (Fig. 20-44), the rapid, disorganized beating of the ventricles, is incompatible with life. Ventricular contraction is ineffective, and the client exhibits the clinical evidence of cardiac arrest. Resuscitation procedures and defibrillation must be instituted at once.

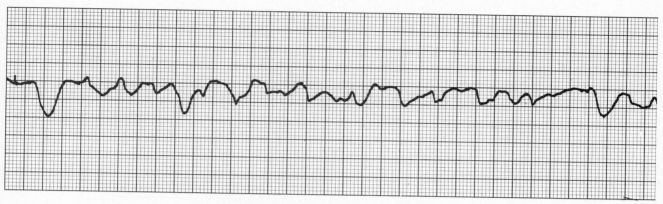

FIG. 20-44
Ventricular fibrillation. (From Conover, Mary H.: Cardiac arrhythmias: exercises in pattern interpretation, ed. 2, St. Louis, 1978, The C.V. Mosby Co.)

Cardiac arrest. Cardiac arrest is the cessation of impulse formation or conduction. Respiratory arrest often precedes (particularly in neonates, infants, and children) or immediately follows cardiac arrest, and a more accurate term may be cardiopulmonary arrest. Cardiac arrest may be caused by disruption of impulse formation or conduction or cardiac contraction. Dysrhythmias of cardiac arrest are ventricular fibrillation, asystole, electromechanical dissociation (EMD), or slow idioventricular rhythm.

Asystole. Asystole (cardiac standstill) is an absence of impulse formation or conduction. There is no mechanical activity, and the client has clinical signs of cardiac arrest (unresponsiveness, breathlessness, pulselessness). The ECG reveals absence of any electrical activity (Fig. 20-45).

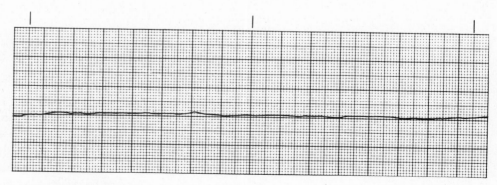

FIG. 20-45
Asystole. (From Wasserberger, J., and Eubanks, David: Practical paramedic procedures, ed. 2, St. Louis, 1981, The C.V. Mosby Co.)

Nursing process for common health problems

Electromechanical dissociation. Electromechanical dissociation (EMD) refers to presence of electrical activity but absence of mechanical contraction of the heart. The ECG may reveal rhythms such as normal sinus rhythm or heart block, but the client does not have a pulse or blood pressure (Fig. 20-46). EMD is usually caused by severe heart damage in which the hypokinetic myocardium is unable to contract effectively, or occasionally by cardiac tamponade.

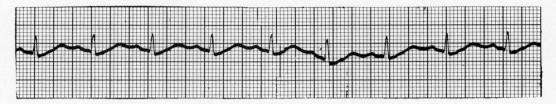

FIG. 20-46
Sinus rhythm with electromechanical dissociation. (From Goldberger, Ary, and Goldberger, Emanuel: Clinical electrocardiography: a simplified approach, ed. 2, St. Louis, 1981, The C.V. Mosby Co.)

Slow idioventricular rhythm. A slow idioventricular rhythm is produced by erratic impulse formation and conduction. The ECG reveals wide QRS complexes indicative of impulse formation in the ventricles (Fig. 20-47). Conduction and contraction are not adequate, however, to support circulation, and the client rapidly becomes unresponsive and may not have a palpable pulse.

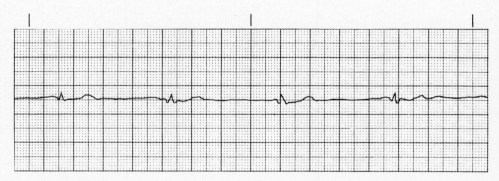

FIG. 20-47
Slow idioventricular rhythm. (From Wasserberger, J., and Eubanks, D.H.: Practical paramedic procedures, ed. 2, St. Louis, 1981, The C.V. Mosby Co.)

Cardiopulmonary arrest can be recognized by the absence of ventilatory efforts and impulse formation or conduction. Cerebral hypoxia occurs rapidly, and the client loses consciousness. Breathing is absent, and there is no pulse. The client will be pale, cool, and, as hypoxemia persists, pupils are dilated. Life-threatening dysrhythmias that warn of cardiac arrest are third-degree heart block, PVCs, and ventricular tachycardia, whereas ventricular fibrillation, EMD, and asystole are observed on the monitor with the clinical evidence of cardiopulmonary arrest.

Vital organs cannot tolerate the absence of circulating oxygen longer than 3 to 5 minutes in adults and 5 to 8 minutes in infants and children. *Clinical death* occurs at the time of cardiac or respiratory arrest. *Biological death* occurs when there is cellular anoxia, usually 3 to 8 minutes after clinical death. Resuscitation measures must therefore be instituted at the time of clinical death to prevent irreversible biological death.

> **Data analysis**
> *Data analysis includes interpretation of rate and rhythm changes as well as clinical evidence of the effects of the dysrhythmia. Nursing diagnosis may include alterations in cardiac output, alterations in tissue perfusion, and fear.*

Planning and implementation. Immediate action is required to manage dysrhythmias. The nurse may continue to assess the client with minor dysrhythmias but must determine the potential for change to a major dysrhythmia and be prepared to implement plans or protocols. Clients with major dysrhythmias may be treated to prevent the outcomes of prolonged disturbances in impulse formation and conduction such as heart failure or lethal dysrhythmias. Pharmacological agents, cardioversion or defibrillation, or external or internal pacing may be used. Cardiopulmonary resuscitation and advanced cardiac life support measures are instituted for the client demonstrating death-producing dysrhythmias. The nurse must anticipate the plans likely to be used to manage a variety of dysrhythmias and be prepared to intervene instantly.

Pharmacological management of dysrhythmias. Antidysrhythmic drugs can be used to control dysrhythmias of myocardial ischemia or irritability or to treat longstanding disturbances of impulse conduction. The drugs may be administered orally or intramuscularly, but in life-threatening situations are administered intravenously as a bolus or a continuous infusion. Some drugs may be administered directly into the heart. Specific drugs are listed in Table 20-8.

Cardioversion and defibrillation. *Cardioversion* is the delivery of a low voltage electrical stimulus (3 to 5 watts/sec/kg body weight) to the heart. The stimulus is synchronized with the ECG to interrupt the dysrhythmia at the peak of the R wave (ventricular depolarization) so that normal impulse formation and conduction can be reestablished. *Defibrillation* is the delivery of an unsynchronized low-voltage-to-high-voltage electrical stimulus to the heart to disrupt fibrillation by creating a momentary asystole so that normal rate and rhythm can be established. Cardioversion may be an elective procedure when pharmacological therapy is ineffective in controlling dysrhythmias. Defibrillation is most often an emergency procedure used in ventricular tachycardia (client unresponsive) or ventricular fibrillation.

To deliver the voltage for cardioversion or defibrillation, for adults, large electrodes (paddles) are applied to the apex of the heart and at the second intercostal space below the right clavicle at the base of the heart at the left of the lower sternum at the midclavicular line (Fig. 20-48). Electrode paste or saline sponges are used so the skin is not burned. If time permits, the procedure can be explained to the client and a sedative given. At the time electrical current is

TABLE 20-8
Common pharmacological agents used to manage dysrhythmias

Drug	Antidysrhythmic action	Use	Dose
Atropine	↑ Heart rate	Sinus bradycardia AV block Reverse drug-induced bradycardia	IV: 0.5 mg q.5 min
Bretylium (Bretylol)	↑ Threshold for ventricular fibrillation ↑ Contractility ↑ Automaticity	Ventricular tachycardia Ventricular fibrillation	Bolus: 5-10 mg/kg Infusion: 1-2 mg/min
Digitalis	↑ Contractility ↓ Heart rate ↑ AV refractoriness ↑ Ventricular automaticity	Atrial fibrillation Atrial flutter Paroxysmal atrial tachycardia	Digitalizing: 0.75-1.5 mg in 24 hrs Maintenance: 0.125-0.5 mg q.day
Phenytoin (Dilantin)	↓ Automaticity ↑ AV conduction	Paroxysmal atrial tachycardia Ventricular ectopy	IV: 50-100 mg q 5 min to 1 g Oral loading: 1 g in 24 hrs Maintenance: 300 to 500 mg/day
Propranolol (Inderal)	↓ Heart rate ↓ Contractility ↓ Automaticity ↓ Conductivity ↑ AV node refractoriness	Sinus tachycardia Atrial dysrhythmias Ventricular ectopy Ventricular dysrhythmias	IV: 1 mg/min Oral: 10-200 mg q.i.d.
Lidocaine (Xylocaine)	↓ Automaticity ↓ Conductivity ↑ Fibrillation threshold	Premature ventricular contractions Ventricular tachycardia	Bolus: 50-100 mg Infusion: 1-4 mg/min
Disophyramide (Norpace)	↓ Contractility ↓ Excitability ↓ Automaticity ↓ Conductivity ↑ AV node conduction	Ventricular ectopy Ventricular tachycardia	Oral loading: 200-300 mg Maintenance 100-200 mg q.6 hr
Procainamide (Pronestyl)	↓ Automaticity ↓ Excitability ↓ Conductivity ↓ Contractility	Ventricular ectopy Supraventricular tachycardia	IV bolus: 50-100 mg q 5 min up to 1 g Infusion: 1-4 mg/min Oral loading: 1 g Maintenance: 250-500 mg q.3-4 hr
Quinidine sulfate	↑ AV node conduction ↓ Excitability ↓ Conductivity ↓ Contractility ↑ Automaticity	Atrial dysrhythmias Ventricular ectopy Ventricular tachycardia	Oral: 200-400 mg q.4-6 hr

discharged, all personnel must stand clear of the bed so that voltage is not conducted to them. Defibrillation may be repeated at higher voltages if initial attempts are not successful. The procedure is evaluated by the return of a normal or life-sustaining rhythm, but the nurse should continue to assess the client for changes in heart rate and rhythm.

Cardiac pacemakers. Cardiac pacemakers are used to provide electrical stimulation to the myocardium to depolarize the atria and/or ventricles.[23,30,39] A battery provides the source for the electrical stimulation, and an electrode catheter implanted in the epicardium conducts the electrical charge.

Pacing may be temporary or permanent. A temporary pacemaker may be used during emergency situations, such as atrioventricular blocks, PVCs, ventricular tachycardia, or asystole, as the electrical stimulus overrides the dys-

FIG. 20-48
Paddle placement for defibrillation.

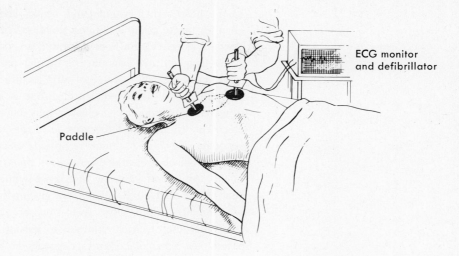

rhythmic conduction. Temporary pacemakers may also be used after open-heart surgery in anticipation of treatment of potential dysrhythmias. *Permanent* pacemakers are used for chronic conduction defects such as sinus bradycardia, sick sinus syndrome, chronic heart block, or chronic myocardial damage.

Pacing may be obtained from external or internal sources. An *external pulse generator* is usually used for temporary pacing, and the source for pulse generation is obtained from a monitoring console or a battery suspended on an IV pole or carried in a cloth pouch pinned to the client's gown. The pacing catheter is placed in the heart, usually in the right ventricle. An *internal pacemaker* is usually used when permanent pacing is required. The pulse generator is compact and can be implanted in the pectoral muscle or in the subcutaneous tissue of the abdomen, and the electrodes are inserted in the myocardium. Overgrowth of the endothelial cells secures the electrodes in place (Fig. 20-49).

The pacemaker can be inserted by several approaches. In the *transthoracic (percutaneous) approach* the electrodes are inserted in the ventricles by means of a needle placed directly through the chest wall. This method is usually used for temporary emergency pacing. The *transvenous approach* can be used for temporary or permanent pacing. In this instance the electrode is positioned with the aid of fluoroscopy by threading the pacing catheter through the jugular, basilic, or cephalic vein to the endocardial surface of the right ventricle. After open-heart surgery the pacing electrodes are placed via the *thoracotomy* or *mediastinal incision*. If pacing will be permanent, the battery is implanted in the subcutaneous tissue of the chest. In instances of permanent pacing, a thoracotomy incision may be used to secure the electrodes to the epicardium *(epicardial approach)*. The pulse generator is then sutured in the pectoral muscle or in surrounding subcutaneous tissue. The electrodes may be inserted into the epicardium or endocardium. Temporary pacing usually involves an epicardial approach, whereas permanent pacing electrodes are secured in the endocardium with a transvenous approach.

There are several *modes* of pacing that can be used for individual client needs. These include the continuously discharging mode with fixed or adjustable rates, synchronous, demand, and sequential modes. *Continuously discharging* (asynchronous) pacemakers provide stimuli to the atria or ventricles, regardless

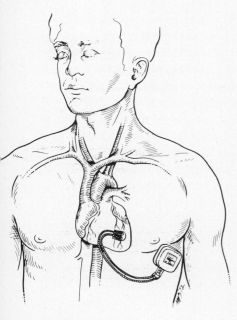

FIG. 20-49
Implanted pacemaker.

1189

Nursing process for common health problems

of the heart's own spontaneous beats. The rate can be fixed or adjusted to changes in the client's clinical situation. In *synchronous* pacing the electrical stimulus is provided at a preset rate if a spontaneous heart beat does not occur. Atrial-triggered synchronous ventricular pacemakers have an electrode in the atria that senses the voltage of atrial contraction and, if inadequate, stimulates ventricular contraction via an electrode in the ventricle. A ventricular QRS-triggered synchronous pacemaker may be placed in the ventricle to provide electrical stimulation if the voltage of the heart's ventricular contraction is inadequate. *Demand* pacemakers provide electrical stimulus at a preset rate if a spontaneous heart beat does not occur. *Sequential* pacemakers have an electrode in the atrium and ventricle that sense within the ventricle the last ventricular beat to the next atrial beat. *Atrial* pacing occurs when there is no atrial beat or if the atrial rate is slow, as in sinus bradycardia.

When the electrical stimulus to the atria or ventricle is stimulated by the pacemaker, a pacemaker artifact appears on the ECG (Fig. 20-50). The nurse can note frequency of paced beats and evaluate pacemaker effectiveness with the clinical state of the client.

When pacemakers are used, the nurse should observe the insertion site and note the heart rate. The dressing at the insertion site for temporary pacing may be changed frequently, and antibiotic cream may be ordered. If a femoral vein is used as the insertion site, the client should be instructed not to sit in high Fowler's position. Temporary pacemakers are liable to electrical interference, and the wires on older models should be insulated (a rubber glove can be used) and all equipment grounded. The effectiveness of the temporary pacemaker can be evaluated by observing the client for adequacy of heart rate and cardiac output (pulse, color, level of consciousness). If the client is ambulatory, the battery pack may be worn in a carrier around the waist.

When the pacemaker is implanted, there may be initial swelling and bruising at the site of implantation. The client may be advised to rest in bed for the first 48 hours after implantation so that epithelialization can occur around the implanted electrodes. After this time the client should be encouraged to do range-of-motion exercises, particularly if the pacemaker is implanted in the pectoral muscle. These exercises stimulate circulation and promote absorption of edematous fluid. Analgesia may be used for the first few days if the client is uncomfortable. The pulse rate should be counted frequently for the first few days, and if the client is monitored, the nurse should observe the rate and rhythm.

The nurse can instruct the client with a permanent pacemaker how to make

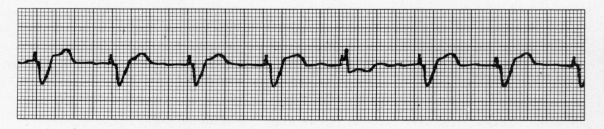

FIG. 20-50
Pacemaker artifacts. (From Conover, Mary H.: Cardiac arrhythmias: exercises in pattern interpretation, ed. 2, St. Louis, 1978, The C.V. Mosby Co.)

observations about the functioning of the pacemaker. The instructions should be given in a way that will make the client feel confident about having a pacemaker, because many clients fear dependency on a battery to sustain their life. Although each type of pacemaker is unique and requires special care, the client should know how to count his pulse. A decrease in heart rate of 5 to 10 beats in a minute is indicative of battery power loss. The client should also be instructed to report episodes of dizziness or fainting, which could indicate dislodging of the catheter.

The electrical stimulation of some pacemakers may be interrupted by high-frequency electrical equipment. In the hospital, ultrasonic oxygen and diathermy may interfere with the pacemaker. At home the client should avoid close proximity to automobile engines, spark plugs of lawn mowers and snowmobiles, microwave ovens, and dentist drills. The client should also know that the pacemaker may set off the alarm system of the airport weapons detection devices. The client should carry a card with him to indicate that he has an implanted pacemaker and give information about the model number, serial number, and pacing rate.

The batteries of the pacemaker need to be changed on a periodic basis. Newer batteries have been developed that last up to 10 years, but some clients still must come to the hospital every 2 years to change the batteries. The batteries are changed in a simple surgical procedure. The client is usually hospitalized while the battery is changed with the client under local anesthesia, and the rhythm is observed for several days. Some batteries can be charged at home with a recharging unit that is worn in a vest. The procedure takes about 1 hour and can be performed while the client reads or watches television.

The client or his family must learn to recognize indications of battery power loss and, in addition to counting his pulse, may use facilities for pacemaker

TABLE 20-9
Essential drugs used for cardiopulmonary resuscitation

Drug	Use	Dosage	
		Adult	Infant/child
Atropine	Sinus bradycardia	0.5 mg q.5 min	0.005-0.03 mg/kg
Bretylium tosylate (Bretylol)	Ventricular tachycardia; ventricular fibrillation	Bolus: 5 mg/kg Infusion: 1-2 mg/min	
Calcium chloride	Electromechanical dissociation; ventricular standstill	250-500 mg/kg q.10 min	25 mg/kg
Dopamine hydrochloride	Cardiac output; peripheral vasoconstriction	2-20 μg/kg/min; effects depend on dose	2-10 μg/kg/min
Epinephrine (Adrenalin)	Cardiac arrest; perfusion pressure	0.5-1.0 mg q.5 min	0.1 ml/kg of 1: 10,000 solution
Isoproterenol hydrochloride (Isuprel)	Bradycardia	2-20 μg/min	0.1 μg/kg/min
Lidocaine (Xylocaine)	Ventricular ectopy	Bolus: 1 mg/kg Infusion: 1-4 mg/min	0.5 mg/kg
Procainamide (Pronestyl)	Ventricular ectopy	Bolus: 100 mg (20 mg/ min) q.5 min Infusion: 1-4 mg/min	
Sodium bicarbonate	Maintain arterial pH; prevent metabolic acidosis	1 mEq/kg initially followed by 0.5 mEq./kg q.10 min	1 mEq/kg diluted 1:1 with sterile water

1191

Nursing process for common health problems

battery checks. These may include periodic attendance at special clinics for clients with pacemakers where equipment is available to check the battery, or telephone hookups with the clinic in which the battery can be checked over the telephone wires. The client can also set his radio at 550 kw, and the pacemaker next to the radio will produce a click before each heart beat (pulsation) if the battery is functioning properly.

When the client goes home, it may be helpful to have a community health nurse visit in the home. Many clients are elderly and fearful of being active or of dislodging the pacemaker. Actually the client can resume all activities except body contact sports. The client should also be instructed to avoid the Valsalva maneuver, which may slow the heart rate. The nurse can follow through on instructions given in the hospital and assess the vital signs to determine pacemaker effectiveness.

Cardiopulmonary resuscitation and advanced cardiac life support. When cardiopulmonary arrest is noted, the nurse must institute resuscitation procedures. Basic life support measures of mouth-to-mouth ventilation and external cardiac compression can be instituted until equipment and personnel for advanced life support are summoned according to plans. At that time, determined by the specific dysrhythmia of cardiac arrest, intravenous lines are established,

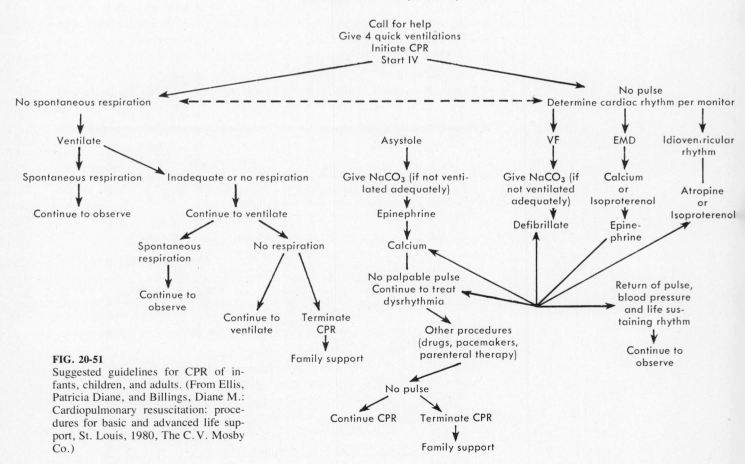

FIG. 20-51
Suggested guidelines for CPR of infants, children, and adults. (From Ellis, Patricia Diane, and Billings, Diane M.: Cardiopulmonary resuscitation: procedures for basic and advanced life support, St. Louis, 1980, The C. V. Mosby Co.)

1192

defibrillation instituted, pharmacological agents administered (Table 20-9), and airway support systems (oxygen administration, endotracheal infiltration, masks, or ventilators) used as needed (Fig. 20-51).

Termination of resuscitation should be considered if there is no improvement of the client's status after 30 minutes of ineffective support or the rescuer is exhausted.[19,58] Others consider failure after repeated attempts to defibrillate. Termination of rescue efforts represents a difficult decision and an intense feeling of frustration for those involved.

Recovery from a cardiac or respiratory arrest, on the other hand, may have a profound psychological effect on the client and his family.[35] Recent evidence indicates that some individuals who experienced clinical death have reported witnessing the resuscitation efforts as if they were hovering over the rescue attempt. The client may wish to relive the experience by verbalizing his feelings and fears, and the nurse should be available to support the client as he recovers from this crisis.

 Evaluation. The nursing care plan for the client with a dysrhythmia is developed with objectives of restoring normal heart rate and rhythm. Pharmacological agents, cardioversion and defibrillation, temporary or permanent pacemakers, or cardiopulmonary resuscitation may be used to achieve these objectives, and evaluation of plans is done continuously as the client responds to implementation of the plans.

EXPECTED OUTCOMES

The client can:
1. Describe the dysrhythmia.
2. Maintain or obtain normal heart rate and rhythm.
3. State plans for complying with therapeutic interventions:
   a. State use, dosage, route, time, and side effects of prescribed medications.
   b. State use and care of pacemaker (if used).
   c. Take his own pulse.
4. State indications of health problems requiring health care services, including slow or irregular pulse.
5. State plans for follow-up health care and use of community resources.

Hypertension

Hypertension is an elevation of blood pressure above age-related standards. Normal blood pressure is a reflection of cardiac output (heart rate and stroke volume) and peripheral resistance. Alterations in any one of these factors, heart rate, stroke volume, or peripheral resistance, will therefore produce a change in the systemic arterial blood pressure.

Hypertension can be defined by type (see material on p. 1194) or by progression of the disease (Table 20-10). *Essential* or *primary* hypertension is the most common type and involves 85% to 95% of the individuals with the disease. There is no identifiable cause of this type of hypertension, and the onset is insidious with a slow, progressive increase in the blood pressure over a period of years. *Secondary* hypertension accounts for 5% to 15% of the population with hypertension. Secondary hypertension is attributed to an underlying pathological condition that, when treated, will cause the blood pressure to return to normal. *Benign* hypertension refers to insidious onset, whereas *malignant* hypertension refers to rapidly progressing hypertension.

Pathophysiology. The cause of primary hypertension is not known, although many etiologies have been identified. The disease is probably multifac-

Primary (essential) hypertension
No known cause

Secondary hypertension
Coarctation of the aorta
Pheochromocytoma
Primary aldosteronism
Renovascular disease
Cushing's syndrome
Pituitary tumors
Toxemia of pregnancy
Long-term stress
Head injury
Brain tumors
Long-term use of drugs: amphetamines and
oral contraceptives

toral and involves dynamic interactions of sodium regulation by the kidneys, aldosterone metabolism, norepinephrine metabolism, and environmental and genetic factors.[40]

Sodium regulation may be one of the major contributing causes of essential hypertension. Increased sodium retention causes water retention and hypertension. The kidney excretes sodium and water to return blood pressure to normal, but in essential hypertension this mechanism does not occur and the blood pressure remains elevated, because of the increased fluid volume and cardiac output. Genetic influences and high-sodium diets may be underlying causes of the altered sodium excretion in the kidneys.

Increased peripheral resistance may be caused by sympathetic nervous system stimulation by norepinephrine. Inappropriate secretion of renin also increases peripheral resistance. It is theorized that renal artery ischemia causes the release of renin, the precursor of angiotensin II, a pressor that constricts arterioles and increases the blood pressure. Prolonged constriction of the blood vessels contributes to vascular sclerosis and vessel damage. There is intraarteriolar thickening and replacement of the smooth muscle and elastic tissue lining with fibrotic tissue. Hemorrhage and necrosis further damage the vessels and perpetuate increased vascular resistance.

Regardless of the cause of primary hypertension, the ultimate consequence of the increased cardiac output and increased peripheral resistance is damage to target organs supplied by the blood vessels. In the heart, increased resistance is compensated by increased force of myocardial contraction, and over time the left ventricle hypertrophies to accommodate the increased workload. Increased blood volume after each systole increases pressure in the chambers of the heart until blood flow backs up in the pulmonary veins and capillaries of the lungs. Additionally there may be angina, myocardial infarction, or heart failure.

TABLE 20-10
Phases of primary hypertension

Phase	Blood pressure range	Comments
Prehypertensive	$\frac{<160}{90\text{-}95}$ mm Hg	Blood pressure elevated intermittently; as children may have had elevated blood pressure
Benign hypertension		
Mild (stratum I)	90-104 mm Hg	Occurs in older adults; limited retinopathy
Moderate (stratum II)	105-114 mm Hg	
Severe (stratum III)	>115 mm Hg	
Malignant hypertension	>130 mm Hg	Occurs in young adults; characterized by sudden rise in blood pressure and rapid decline of renal function; physical findings of papilledema and protein casts in urine
Acute hypertension	>140 mm Hg	Physical findings of encephalopathy: confusion, headache, coma, seizures, papilledema

TABLE 20-11

Risk factors of primary hypertension

Factor	Comments
Age	Highest incidence age 30 to 40
Race	Incidence twice as great in blacks; incidence three times greater for black men; incidence five times greater for black women
Gender	Complications of hypertension increase in men
Family history	Seventy five percent of clients with hypertension have family history of hypertension
Obesity	Increased weight in childhood or middle age increases risk of hypertension
Serum lipids	Increased triglycerides or cholesterol increase risk of hypertension
Diet	Increased risk with high-sodium diets; increased risk in industrialized societies with high-fat, high-caloric diets
Smoking	Risk related to amount smoked and number of years

Hypertension is a disease of middle adulthood involving over 35 million individuals.[33] It has been estimated that one in six individuals have high blood pressure. Hypertension is rare in children and is usually the secondary type of hypertension, although it is necessary to identify children and adolescents who may be at risk for primary hypertension as adults.[48]

Individuals at risk for hypertension can be identified (Table 20-11). The nurse can help identify these clients during health hazard appraisals, screening programs, and when obtaining a nursing history.

 Assessment. Because it is estimated that one half of individuals with hypertension are not diagnosed, the nurse has a significant role in assessing clients with hypertension.[40] The most easily detected indication of hypertension is an elevated blood pressure for the client's age (Fig. 20-52). Although these figures are arbitrary, they provide guidelines for diagnosis and treatment. The blood pressure should be taken using an appropriate size cuff with functioning equipment in a quiet environment. A Doppler probe may be used to listen to faint pressure sounds, particularly those of infants and young children. The pressure should be measured in each arm with the client standing, sitting, or lying down. Two readings should be obtained 1 to 2 minutes apart to identify the systolic pressure and diastolic pressures of fourth and fifth sounds. Both diastolic pressures should be recorded; the fourth sound is diagnostic in children, the fifth in adults. To confirm the diagnosis the blood pressure must be elevated at three successive readings on separate days.

Early in the course of the disease (mild hypertension) the client may have *headaches* from vasoconstriction or *epistaxis* from nasal capillary hemorrhage. As the vascular damage progresses, the client has *blurred vision,* or even blindness, and *shortness of breath.* There may be dizziness, syncope, or angina. Headache may become more severe as spasms and occlusive disease of the cerebral vessels increase. In malignant stages the arterioles are fibrotic, and there may be end organ disease such as renal failure, retinopathy, cerebrovascular occlusion, myocardial infarction, or heart failure.

Physical examination findings may include retinal changes observed on ophthalmoscopic examination, an enlarged heart, and possibly the presence of a fourth heart sound. Neurological changes related to cerebral artery damage may be noted. The client may be overweight.

Laboratory studies may be done to differentiate essential from secondary hypertension. An intravenous pyelogram, renal function studies, renin and

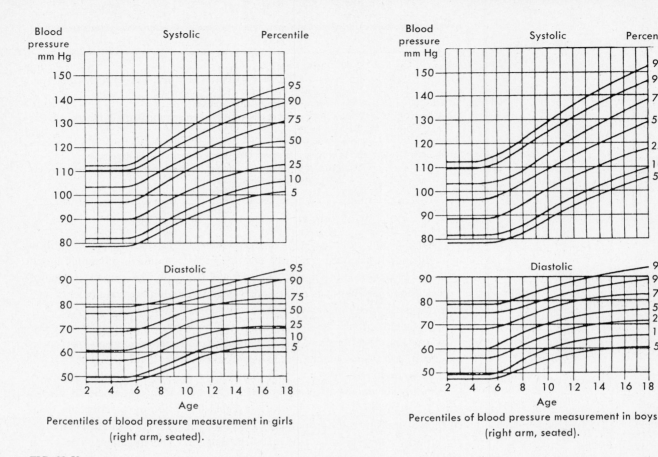

FIG. 20-52
Age-related diagnostic standards for hypertension (above 95th percentile). (From American Heart Association: Standards and report of the task force on blood pressure control in children.)

vanillylmandelic acid determinations may be obtained to rule out these causes. A chest x-ray film and ECG are obtained to determine cardiac status. Other tests include blood studies for glucose, cholesterol, triglycerides, calcium, potassium, and BUN.

> **Data analysis**
> *Data analysis may reveal nursing diagnoses of alterations in cardiac output, alteration in tissue perfusion, fluid imbalance, knowledge deficit, and noncompliance.*

Planning and implementation. The objective of the nursing care plan is to reduce the blood pressure and maintain pressures at normal levels. This may involve a program of health maintenance and, depending on the severity of the hypertension, may require diet restriction and pharmacological intervention with diuretics or antihypertensive drugs. Clients with diastolic pressure less than 105 mm Hg (mild hypertension) may be managed with a program that includes dietary control of sodium and calories and a reduction of risk factors. If the diastolic blood pressure is greater than 105 mm Hg (moderate hypertension), diuretics may be prescribed. If the blood pressure is not maintained with this regimen, antihypertensive drugs are added. Accelerated hypertension is treated with potent, rapid-acting antihypertensive agents, such as nitroprusside or minoxidil.

The nurse helps the client assume responsibility for his individual plan to reduce blood pressure. Goals for lowering the blood pressure may include (1) obtaining physical and mental rest, (2) reducing the circulatory load, (3) blood pressure reduction with pharmacological agents, and (4) assuming responsibility for the therapeutic plan. Most clients are treated on an outpatient basis, but may be hospitalized to obtain rest, initiate drug therapy, or manage a hypertensive crisis.

Balancing activity and rest. The client with hypertension must learn to modify his life-style so that he obtains emotional and physical rest. Occasionally he may be hospitalized so that stresses of his life may be limited. Mild sedatives or tranquilizers may be used to ensure rest. At this time the nurse can help the client plan to modify his activities so that those requiring exertion or involving competition might be restricted. Stress management is useful to minimize sympathetic nervous system stimulation. Some suggest biofeedback mechanisms and relaxation exercises to accomplish this.

Reducing circulatory load. Limiting the dietary intake of sodium can control sodium retention and the increased blood volume that may contribute to hypertension. The diet may limit only the salt used in cooking or in seasoning foods, or it may be more severely restricted to foods with a high natural sodium content (see low-sodium diet earlier in this chapter). The diet may also be reduced in calories to prevent or control obesity. The nurse and dietitian can make suggestions for following these diets and making them more palatable.

Thiazide diuretics such as chlorothiazide (Diuril) may also be used to reduce circulating blood volume. These drugs are known to have antihypertensive effects and are often used as an adjunct to other forms of pharmacological therapy. The nurse should observe the client for signs of sodium and potassium depletion when he is using these drugs and following a sodium-restricted diet.

Reducing blood pressure with pharmacological agents. Several types of antihypertensive drugs are used to lower the blood pressure. They act at various sites to lower blood pressure by several physiological mechanisms, and the nurse should be familiar with actions and side effects of each. The drugs can be used singly or in combination to control the blood pressure at a normal level. Commonly used drugs are sympathetic nervous system depressants such as reserpine; selective sympathetic nervous system depressants such as guanethidine (Ismelin) sulfate, methyldopa (Aldomet), or hydralazine hydrochloride (Apresoline); ganglionic blocking agents such as pentolinium (Ansolysen) tartrate; and amine-oxidase inhibitors such as parglyline hydrochloride (Eutonyl). Beta adrenergic blocking agents such as propranolol (Inderal) or metoprolol (Lopressor) can be used to decrease the heart rate and reduce cardiac output. Clonidine (Catapres) stimulates alpha receptors in the brain to inhibit the sympathetic vasomotor center and sympathetic outflow. Prazosin (Minipres) blocks peripheral sympathetic nerve activity at alpha receptors to cause peripheral vascular dilation. Clients resistant to other drugs may receive minoxidil (Loniten), a potent vasodilator.

These drugs produce a rapid lowering of the blood pressure, and the client should be aware of some of the side effects and the precautions he should observe. Lowered blood pressure can cause the client to become dizzy. He should rise slowly from a lying or sitting position to prevent fainting from orthostatic hypotension. He should also avoid standing for long periods of time, because the blood may tend to pool in the peripheral vessels when antihypertensive drugs are used. Rest produces vasodilation, which, when combined, with antihypertensive drugs may cause the client to faint. The client should not take hot baths or become overheated during the summer. Many of these drugs are potentiated by alcohol, tranquilizers, and other drugs, and the client should inform his physician if he uses these drugs. If the client becomes dizzy or has blurred vision, he should not drive or operate heavy machinery. Some drugs, particularly guanethidine, cause premature ejaculations and impotence. The client should be informed of these possibilities so that his cooperation in following prescribed therapies can be enlisted. The client should carry an identification card to indicate that he is taking antihypertensive drugs.

In states of accelerating hypertension or hypertensive crisis, potent antihypertensive drugs are used to lower rapidly rising blood pressures. Diazoxide (Hyperstat) and sodium nitroprusside (Nipride) are two such drugs. They are administered intravenously with utmost caution to slowly lower the diastolic blood pressure. They act to produce peripheral vasodilation. Side effects such as diaphoresis, headache, dizziness, and nausea and vomiting may be evident and can be reduced by slowing the infusion. These effects disappear when use of the drug is discontinued.

Diazoxide and nitroprusside are rapid acting and must be administered in a setting such as an ICU where the client can be monitored with an intraarterial line and side effects can be observed immediately. The drugs are infused via an infusion pump so the flow rate can be regulated.

Hyperglycemia occurs in the majority of individuals who receive diazoxide, and the nurse should monitor glucose levels, particularly in persons with diabetes mellitus. Hyperglycemic effects disappear when the drug is discontinued. Sodium retention has been noted with use of this drug, and the nurse must observe the client for fluid retention or impending pump failure. Diazoxide should be administered in a peripheral vein and caution used to prevent extravasation. The drug is given undiluted by the rapid intravenous push method. The client should be recumbent when receiving this medication, and frequent assessments of blood pressure changes noted.

Nitroprusside is mixed in 500 to 1000 ml of solution. The solution may have a brownish tint when mixed, and since nitroprusside is unstable when exposed to light, the solution should be covered with aluminum foil to prevent decomposition. Great caution should be used when administering this drug to older adults, because they are more sensitive. Use with children has not been established.

Assuming responsibility for the plan. Compliance with the therapeutic plan is the crucial factor in blood pressure control, and the client should be involved in formulating a plan of care and should understand the importance of the therapeutic regimen.[36,44,63] Compliance increases as the client participates in decision making.[14] Teaching groups are helpful in which clients with similar problems can share their experiences. If the client is to take his own blood pressure at home, the nurse should instruct him in the appropriate technique. The diet and pharmacological therapy should be reviewed and the client given an opportunity to demonstrate his understanding of the therapeutic plan. Most forms of hypertension can be controlled. Moderation in activity, limitation of sodium intake, and pharmacological therapy enhance oxygen delivery to the cells and prevent serious oxygen impairment in vital organs.

Other problems. The client with hypertension may have other problems that persist until the blood pressure approaches normal ranges. The nurse can help the client cope with these by offering instruction and supportive care. Headaches are treated with analgesia and usually disappear as the blood pressure is reduced. Nosebleeds may be packed to control bleeding. Clients with visual problems can be referred to an ophthalmologist.

Complications. Complications of hypertension may include cerebral infarction, renal failure, ischemic heart disease, or hypertensive encephalopathy, often referred to as end organ disease. These are discussed where appropriate in the text.

 Evaluation. Evaluation is an ongoing component of the nursing process and helps the nurse and client with hypertension judge the effectiveness of individual goals.

EXPECTED OUTCOMES

The client and/or family can:
1. Define hypertension.
2. Maintain blood pressure in normal range by:
    a. Obtaining mental and physical rest.
    b. Following diet plans (sodium-restricted, calorie-restricted).
    c. Following prescriptions for medications (diuretics, antihypertensive agents).
3. Identify risk factors for hypertension and state plans to prevent or manage modifiable risks.
4. State indications requiring health care.
5. Describe plans for follow-up health care and can state available community resources for health care.

Peripheral arteriovascular disease

Peripheral vascular disease of the arteries is one aspect of an arterioatherosclerotic process. Blood flow is slowed by narrowing and obstruction of the arteries in the extremities. Atherosclerosis begins as accumulation of fatty streaks and plaques in the intimal layer of the artery. Narrowing and arterial obstruction is potentially aggravated by high-cholesterol diets, obesity, hypertension, smoking, heredity, or other risk factors. Ultimately, arteriosclerosis, calcification, and impaired elasticity of the medial layer of the artery are evident, contributing to health problems such as arteriosclerosis obliterans, Raynaud's disease, Buerger's disease, or aneurysm formation.

Arteriosclerosis obliterans. This form of peripheral arterial disease is an obstructive, degenerative process of the medial and intimal layers of peripheral arteries. It is an end-stage result of atherosclerosis in which the artery (usually the femoral or carotid) loses elasticity and is obstructed by plaque formation.

Arteriosclerosis obliterans is a disease of middle-aged individuals, particularly men. Those with risk factors of hypertension, obesity, smoking, and diabetes mellitus are candidates for peripheral arterial disease.

The nurse can use the health history to elicit information about risk factors, health habits, and life-style. A physical examination of the extremities reveals evidence of disrupted oxygenation. There is coldness of the extremities, decreased peripheral pulses, pallor, bruits, tingling, and muscle cramps at night.

1199

Because the femoral artery is usually the first to become obstructed, claudication and numbness and tingling in the legs are noted. Decreased blood supply to the hypogastric artery may cause impotence. The reduced oxygen supply predisposes the client to skin ulcers and infections of the extremities. Serum cholesterol and triglyceride levels may be elevated. Angiography may be done to demonstrate location and extent of obstruction.

Therapeutic intervention is directed toward promoting arterial circulation and preventing infection. Symptomatic relief may be obtained when the client is conscientious in observing principles of good health, but pharmacological intervention and surgical approaches are often required.

Arterial circulation is promoted when the client is warm. The nurse can instruct the client to avoid chilling and cold environments and dress appropriately for cold weather. Direct applications of heat are usually not used because heat increases the metabolism and the need for oxygen.

Circulation is also promoted by body position and exercise. The client should not cross his legs or flex his knees or hips for prolonged periods of time. The client may elevate the head of his bed on blocks to increase arterial circulation to the extremities at night. Walking stimulates circulation, and the client should have planned periods of moderate exercise. He should not smoke.

Because oxygen supply is limited in the extremities, the client is sensitive to infections. He must observe daily hygiene habits of cleanliness and safety of the involved parts. Even the slightest indication of an inflammation should be reported to the physician.

Vasodilation may be achieved by pharmacological therapy or surgery. Vasodilators such as isoxsuprine hydrochloride (Vasodilan) may be used. Papaverine relaxes smooth muscles of the blood vessels and is used to prevent spasm. Tolazoline hydrochloride (Priscoline) is an adrenergic blocking agent used for vasodilating effects at the arterioles.

The client should follow a fat-controlled diet, and if overweight, should also restrict calorie intake. If hypertension or diabetes mellitus is diagnosed, the therapeutic plan for these diseases should be followed carefully.

Antilipemic agents may be used to decrease serum lipid levels. Some are clofibrate (Atromid-S) and cholestyramine (Questran) and are used depending on type of hyperlipidemia.

Surgical approaches such as aortoiliac (Fig. 20-53, A) and femoropopliteal bypasses (Fig. 20-53, B) may be performed to reestablish circulation. A segment of the saphenous vein or a synthetic graft may be inserted to provide continuity for distal circulation. Nursing care is similar to that for the client having aneurysm repair. Other surgical approaches include *endarterectomy* (reaming out plaques from the intima and media using balloon catheters or instruments) or *patch grafting* of the involved portion of the artery, or total grafting with end-to-end anastomosis. Severing the sympathetic nerves prevents vasoconstriction, and a sympathectomy may be performed for selected individuals.

Raynaud's disease. Raynaud's disease is produced by a spasm of the arteries, which causes blanching of the fingers and toes. There may be numbness and tingling in the extremities and atrophy of the nails. This disease occurs most often in young women and may have a genetic origin. These clients are susceptible to infection, and gangrene may occur rapidly. The diagnosis is based on clinical symptoms.

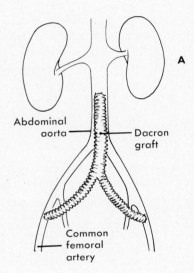

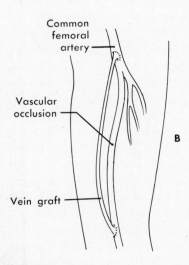

FIG. 20-53
Bypass graft. **A,** Aortoiliac. **B,** Femoropopliteal.

Raynaud's disease is a chronic condition and is managed by observing health habits to promote circulation. It is important for the client to maintain arterial circulation by exercise. Vasodilating drugs can be prescribed, and a sympathectomy can be done to provide vasodilation.

Buerger's disease. In Buerger's disease (thromboangitis obliterans), an inflammation of the arteries and veins, ultimately causes ischemia. Eventually there is thrombus formation, which may produce scarring when the inflammation subsides. Young men are most often affected by Buerger's disease. The client notices coldness in the extremities and numbness and tingling in the feet and hands, and redness may be observed along the lines of the veins and arteries. Peripheral pulses may be weak or absent, and the muscle cramps that occur after exercise may be relieved by rest. This phenomenon is known as *intermittent claudication,* which is the time from the onset of pain upon exercise to the time the pain is relieved by rest. The pain is related to the impaired oxygen supply to the muscle.

It is important to reestablish circulation and prevent complications of ischemia. If the client uses tobacco, he must stop. The client should observe health habits that promote circulation; that is, he should keep warm and avoid sitting or standing in one position. Skin care is vital to prevent infections that may result from tissue ischemia in the extremities. Care of the feet is described in Chapter 9. Vasodilators may also be used to prevent further vessel narrowing, and a sympathectomy may be done to promote vasodilation.

Buerger-Allen exercises may be prescribed to promote circulation and establish collateral circulation. In the starting position for these exercises, the client lies supine in bed. He first raises his legs for 2 to 3 minutes until they blanch. If the client is unable to hold his legs in this position, he can rest them on a box or an inverted chair back that has been padded and placed on the bed. Next, the client lowers his legs to the floor for 5 to 10 minutes and then returns to the starting position for 5 to 10 minutes. These exercises should be done five to ten times, three times a day.

An oscillating, or rocking, bed may be used to accomplish the same purpose of promoting circulation. The client remains in a bed that slowly elevates and lowers his body continuously.

Aneurysm. An aneurysm is an enlargement of an artery. The enlargement can occur from congenital weakness, infections, trauma, or arteriosclerosis and atherosclerosis.

Pathophysiology. Arteriosclerosis is the most frequent cause of aneurysms and usually occurs in older persons, men ages 60 to 70. The aneurysm is described by the shape of the enlargement (Fig. 20-54). A *saccular* aneurysm is an outpouching of a portion of the artery, whereas a *fusiform* aneurysm involves the total circumference of an area of the artery and has a spindle shape. When the media and intima separate, the aneurysm is referred to as a *dissecting* aneurysm.

Assessment. The enlargement of the artery may be noticed by an increase in blood pressure, pain at the site, dyspnea, or visible pulsation of the artery. *Dissecting aneurysms* of the abdominal aorta (AAA) are sudden in onset and represent a life-threatening emergency. Pain is severe and may be located in the abdomen or radiate substernally to the back, shoulders, or legs. The client may have nausea and vomiting, and the client may appear to be in shock even though the blood pressure is elevated. The blood pressure may be 10 mm Hg higher in the

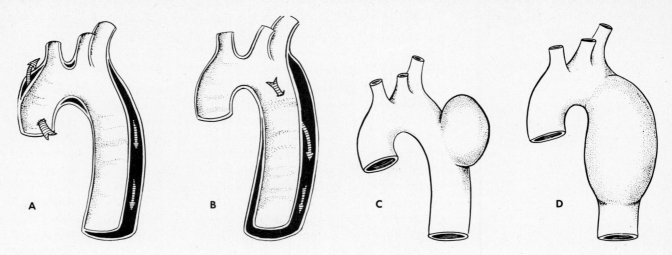

FIG. 20-54
Types of aneurysms. **A** and **B,** Dissecting. **C,** Saccular. **D,** Fusiform.

thighs than in the arms. There may be hemorrhage if the aneurysm ruptures. The enlarged artery may press on other structures or produce venous distension. The diagnosis is confirmed by arteriography.

> ***Data analysis***
> *Data analysis may reveal nursing diagnoses of alterations in cardiac output, alterations in comfort: pain, fluid imbalance, or alteration in tissue perfusion.*

Planning and implementation. The nursing care plan for a client with an aneurysm is developed to meet the needs of the individual client. Attempts are made to remove or repair the aneurysm before it ruptures and, if possible, to lower the blood pressure before surgery. If the anuerysm is small, the artery may be resected and anastomosed. Larger aneurysms are usually resected, and a graft is used to establish arterial continuity. If the aneurysm is on the thoracic aorta, it is necessary to perform open-heart surgery. Because larger aneurysms and dissecting aneurysms of the abdominal aorta are potentially life threatening, the client may be admitted to a surgical unit or an intensive care ward.

Nursing care of the client having peripheral vascular surgery: abdominal aortic aneurysm repair. Nursing care is planned for preoperative, postoperative, and rehabilitation phases of surgery. Clients with small aneurysms may have been prepared for surgery before being admitted to the hospital, whereas clients with acute dissecting aneurysms may have been admitted directly to an ICU without any preparation. The care plan must therefore be developed for the needs of each client.

Preoperative nursing care. Goals for preoperative care are to (1) lower the blood pressure and prevent rupture of the aneurysm, (2) manage pain, and (3) provide preoperative instructions.

REDUCING BLOOD PRESSURE. Blood pressure can be lowered by use of drugs and decreasing circulating blood volume. Potent antihypertensive drugs such as nitroprusside (Nipride) are used to lower the blood pressure to a systolic pressure of 100 to 120 mm Hg.[4] The client must be monitored continuously when these drugs are used. Propranolol (Inderal) may also be used to reduce the force of cardiac output to prevent vessel rupture. If necessary, diuretics are used to decrease blood volume.

PAIN. Analgesia may be used to manage pain. The nurse can use measures to make the client comfortable and therapeutic communication skills to allay anxiety that compounds pain.

PREOPERATIVE INSTRUCTIONS. The nurse can instruct the client and family about surgical approaches and what to anticipate after surgery. The client and family should be informed of procedures and nursing care he can expect.

Postoperative nursing care. After surgery, goals for nursing care may include (1) maintaining circulation, (2) maintaining ventilation, (3) maintaining fluid and nutrition balance, and (4) providing comfort. The client may be in an intensive care setting for several days after surgery for monitoring of vital signs and fluid status, and the nurse and client plan for increasing independence as the client progresses.

MAINTAINING CIRCULATION. Arterial circulation is promoted by warmth and gravity. The client should be kept warm and free from chilling. The head of the bed may be elevated slightly to increase circulation in the extremities. The nurse should avoid gatching the bed or having the client in a high Fowler's position, because this pressure may obstruct arterial flow.

Effectiveness of circulation can be evaluated by inspecting the extremities and counting the distal pulses. The legs and feet should be warm, normal in color, and have rapid capillary refill. Numbness, tingling, coldness, and pallor are ominous signs. The nurse should locate the femoral, popliteal, dorsalis pedis, and posterior tibial pulses and count the pulse at each location. A Doppler probe can be used if the pulses are not easily palpated. Absence of pulses should be reported to the physician.

Blood volume and blood pressure may be regulated to maintain circulation and prevent rupture of the incision or graft. Fluids may be restricted for several days and diuretics administered as needed. Potent antihypertensive drugs may be used to maintain the blood pressure in normal ranges. The nurse can evaluate fluid status by weighing the client daily and observing CVP and PAP pressures. An arterial line is used for continuous evaluation of the blood pressure.

Antiembolism stockings may be used because clients are at high risk for thrombophlebitis. Ambulation is encouraged soon after surgery, but the client should dorsiflex his feet periodically while in bed.

Perfusion to the kidneys is important, particularly if surgery was performed on the abdominal aorta in proximity to the renal arteries. The nurse must monitor urine output and report decreases in output, oliguria, or changes in specific gravity to the surgeon.

MAINTAINING VENTILATION. Immediately after surgery it is imperative to maintain a patent airway. An endotracheal tube may be used with a ventilator or supplemental oxygen. The nurse must suction the client's trachea frequently and evaluate breath sounds for presence of rales. Arterial blood gas values may be used to evaluate oxygen exchange. The nurse should observe the client for "wet lung syndrome,'' which can occur after surgery. This is believed to be caused by an inflammatory response to massive resections, especially if the thoracic aorta is removed, or from increased fluid in retroperitoneal space that moves into interstitial spaces of the lungs. Frequent turning, percussion, and postural drainage help avert this pulmonary complication.

MAINTAINING FLUID AND NUTRITION BALANCE. For several days after surgery the client receives nothing by mouth. It is of utmost importance to prevent gastric distension and stress on the suture line of the grafted vessel. For this reason a nasogastric tube or a gastrostomy tube is used to assure outlet for fluids and gas. A suction source is usually used until peristalsis returns. At this time the client may be given sips of water, and if the water is tolerated, the gastric decompression may be discontinued. Nausea and vomiting that stress the incision are also to be avoided, and antiemetics must be given at early indications of nausea. Nutrition is provided by intravenous fluids until diet progression is ordered, about 3 to 7 days after surgery.

Fluids are used to maintain hydration without overloading the circulation. The nurse can evaluate fluid status using intake and output records, monitoring the CVP, and clinical evaluation of the client's skin turgor and body temperature.

PROVIDING COMFORT. The nurse should plan care for the comfort of the client. Pain medication may be given as needed. An abdominal binder can be used to make turning, coughing, and deep breathing easier.

The nurse can help the client turn from side to side, but the client should avoid flexing the knees or hips. The client is usually allowed to ambulate in several days, and pain medication may be used before ambulation to encourage this activity.

Discharge instructions. During the rehabilitation phase the client increases ambulation and prepares to return to his previous life-style. The nurse can help the client and family learn health habits that promote circulation and to modify risk factors that contribute to aneurysm development.

 Evaluation. Expected client outcomes are evaluated continuously during the course of the client's hospitalization for abdominal aneurysm repair. Outcomes from the preoperative nursing care plan may provide data for planning postoperative care.

EXPECTED OUTCOMES

The client will:
1. Describe aneurysm and aneurysm repair.
2. Maintain hemodynamic stability.
3. Maintain circulation through grafted vessel.
4. Be free of complications.
5. Describe plans for health maintenance:
   a. State restrictions on activity.
   b. State use, dosage, time, route, and side effects of prescribed medications.
   c. Identify risk factors and state plans for prevention and management of modifiable risks.
6. State plans for follow-up health care.

Thrombophlebitis (venous thromboembolic disease)

Thrombophlebitis is an inflammation of a vein. The term *venous thrombosis* more accurately defines the condition of a blood clot that has formed inside a blood vessel, whereas *thrombophlebitis* refers to the inflammation that initiated the clot formation. *Phlebothrombosis* refers to the thrombus as the initiating factor of the inflammation. The clinical course of the disease is similar regardless of the sequence of events, but concern is directed particularly to deep vein thrombosis (DVT), which has a 50% chance of dislodging and forming an embolus.

Pathophysiology. Thrombus formation occurs as a result of venous stasis, enhanced coagulability of the blood, or endothelial or vessel damage. These can be precipitated by a variety of factors.

Venous stasis is common in individuals who are immobile or otherwise confined to bed from the ineffectiveness of the soleus muscles in propelling venous blood flow. Those who stand for long periods of time, sit with knees and thighs bent, who wear constricting clothing such as girdles or elastic hose, or who have increased abdominal pressure from obesity, tumors, or pregnancy are also victims of venous stasis. Although venous stasis per se does not cause thrombus formation, it accelerates the process once initiated.

Hypercoagulability of the blood as noted by increased prothrombin time and increased number of platelets can occur following trauma, childbirth, and myocardial infarction and can incite thrombosis. Interestingly, this phenomenon occurs 7 to 10 days after injury.

Thrombus formation can also be caused by endothelial damage. This is likely to occur as a result of intravenous infusions and cannulation. Diseases in which there is endothelial damage may also contribute to thrombosis. Buerger's disease is one example.

Individuals at risk for thromboembolic disease are obese, those prone to venous stasis, and women who use oral contraceptives. Surgery and trauma carry the highest risk for precipitating thromboembolic disease, and the risk increases with age.[21] The onset is believed to occur intraoperatively. In addition to the stasis of recumbency, cardiac output is decreased and circulation slowed. Thirty percent of individuals having surgery have deep vein thrombosis.[6] Orthopedic surgery of the hips and lower extremities presents a high risk, as does surgery involving a retropubic approach to prostatectomy. The presence of cancer at the time of surgery may also increase the risk of thrombosis formation. Venous thrombosis is also associated with myocardial infarction, and the incidence is two to three times greater if complicated by heart failure.

Nursing care for clients with thromboembolic disease must be directed toward preventing venous stasis by instructing clients in health maintenance strategies, discouraging the hazards of immobility, and using caution with intravenous infusions and sticks. These aspects of nursing care can be included in care plans for any client who has had surgery or who has real or potential problems of immobility.

Assessment. The nurse can anticipate potential problems of venous stasis in clients who have had surgery or are immobile. The signs and symptoms of thrombophlebitis depend on the location of the involved vein. Thrombophlebitis of superficial veins is noticed by redness, warmth, tenderness, and palpation of a hardened vein. There is usually fever as a result of the inflammation. Thrombophlebitis in deeper veins of the legs (deep vein thrombosis), on the other hand, is evidenced by edema, swelling, pain, redness, and warmth. The swelling can be noted by measuring the circumference of the calf. Pain is aggravated by movement, and *Homan's sign* (pain on dorsiflexion of the foot) can be elicited to differentiate muscle spasm from thrombophlebitis. Some clients with deep vein thrombosis do not demonstrate symptoms, making diagnosis difficult. The medical diagnosis is based on clinical evidence, venography, ultrasound, Doppler flow studies, or impedance plethysmography.

> ### Data analysis
> *Data analysis may reveal nursing diagnoses of alterations in cardiac output, alterations in comfort: pain, fluid imbalance, and alteration in tissue perfusion.*

Planning and implementation. The nursing care plan is developed initially to prevent thrombus formation. The nurse and client may plan before surgery or anticipated immobility to initiate actions that avert hazards of stasis and immobility. These may include active and passive exercises, use of antiembolism stockings, early ambulation, if possible, and avoiding knee gatching.

Thrombus formation may be prevented by low-dose heparin, 5000 units intravenously every 8 hours for 7 days.[6] This dose of heparin is lower than that which causes bleeding and is believed to neutralize activated clotting factor X before clot development. Because bleeding is not a side effect of this dosage of heparin, frequent monitoring of coagulation time is not necessary. Low-dose heparin therapy is contraindicated after hip or bone surgery, abdominal prostatectomy, or brain surgery.

Heparin is administered subcutaneously into the fat tissue of the lower abdominal wall or above the iliac crest (Fig. 20-55, *A*). The skin can be gently wiped with alcohol and rolled to lift the subcutaneous fatty tissue. The heparin should be deposited at a 90-degree angle (Fig. 20-55, *B*). It is recommended that the nurse not aspirate when giving heparin to prevent hematoma formation. The

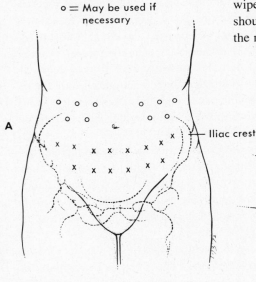

x = Preferred sites
o = May be used if necessary

Iliac crest

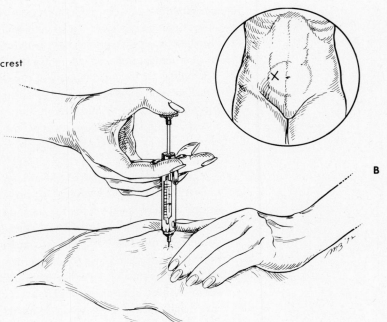

FIG. 20-55
Injection technique for giving heparin subcutaneously. **A,** Sites. **B,** Skin is rolled and syringe held at a 90-degree angle. (Courtesy Wyeth Laboratories, Philadelphia.)

1206

site should not be massaged after withdrawing the needle, but the alcohol sponge may be pressed gently on the site. The site must be rotated for each injection. If heparin therapy is to be continued for a period of time, a long-dwelling catheter needle with a catheter plug, also known as a heparin lock or heparin well, may be inserted in the vein for ease of administration. When heparin is given by this route, the infusion site should be observed for inflammation. A return blood flow should be ascertained and aseptic technique used. The first dose should contain 0.2 ml more than prescribed to fill the tubing.[26] Subsequent doses keep the medicine flushed through the tubing.

If thrombosis does occur, the nursing care plan is developed to (1) reduce the inflammation, (2) prevent embolism, and (3) relieve pain.

Reducing inflammation. Inflammation can be relieved by warm, moist soaks. A heating unit with low heat may be used to keep the soaks continuously warm. The warmth dilates the vein and contributes to the development of collateral circulation. This approach is particularly useful for thrombophlebitis of superficial veins caused by intravenous infusions. Some physicians believe, however, that using heat to dilate blood vessels may precipitate embolism and order applications of ice.

Preventing embolism. An inflammation of the vein predisposes to the danger of embolus formation, particularly pulmonary or coronary emboli.[12] To prevent this danger, bed rest is prescribed for the client. The physician may order the affected part to be elevated to prevent venous congestion. The client should rest quietly in bed and avoid activities that cause sudden increase in venous return such as coughing or straining. Performance of these activities affects the Valsalva maneuver (expiration against a closed glottis). The intrathoracic pressure increases, causing decreased venous return. With straining, the cardiac output is reduced and the diameter of the femoral vein enlarges. When the glottis is opened and the intrathoracic pressure drops, venous return is suddenly increased and the increased flow through the enlarged femoral vein may release the thrombus. The client should therefore be instructed to breathe through his mouth to avoid closing the glottis.

Elastic stockings or bandages may be used to promote venous return. Elastic stockings should be ordered to fit the individual client and may extend from the toes to below the knee or to the groin. At no time should the stockings or bandages constrict the popliteal area. The stockings or bandages can be removed for bathing the leg, and the nurse should inspect the skin for signs of breakdown. The client may be instructed to wear elastic stockings or bandages at home to prevent further thrombophlebitis. The nurse should instruct the client to put on the stockings or bandages before getting out of bed so that venous blood does not pool in the feet.

Anticoagulants may be used to prevent extension of the clot. Heparin or warfarin (Coumadin) may be given in prophylactic or therapeutic doses. Heparin is a rapid-acting anticoagulant that acts primarily as an antagonist to the thrombin formation. Heparin may be given intravenously, intramuscularly, or subcutaneously.

Bleeding is a dangerous side effect of the therapeutic doses of heparin, and the nurse should observe the client for early signs of bleeding, such as hematuria and bruising. The client should not use a straight razor or a hard-bristle toothbrush when taking anticoagulants, because slight injury can cause bleeding. Clotting times should be checked frequently so that the dose of heparin can be appropriately adjusted. Protamine sulfate is an antidote for heparin.

Coumarin derivatives such as dicumarol, warfarin (Coumadin), and phenindione (Hedulin) are longer-acting anticoagulants that interfere with prothrombin formation. These drugs may take up to 3 days to become effective and are often started with a rapid-acting anticoagulant for peak effectiveness when heparin is to be discontinued. Many drugs, such as aspirin, phenothiazines, and antihistamines, interact with coumarin drugs, and the client should have the anticoagulant dose adjusted to these drugs. The client should be aware that he will bleed easily while taking these drugs and should take care not to injure himself. Menstrual flow in women increases, and there might be a slight hematuria. If the client is taking the drug on an indefinite basis, he should carry a card that indicates he is using this drug. Prothrombin times should be determined frequently for regulation of an effective anticoagulant dose. Vitamin K (Mephyton) is an antidote for coumarin anticoagulants.

Vasodilating drugs may be used to reduce vessel spasm at the site of thrombus formation. These drugs improve circulation and thereby increase the rate of thrombus absorption.

In some instances, activators of the naturally occurring fibrinolytic enzyme system, streptokinase and urokinase, may be infused intravenously. These drugs prevent damage of DVT by lysis of the thrombus and perhaps by reducing plasma viscosity and decreased tendency for aggregation of red blood cells. Early lysis may reduce the edema and tenderness in the involved extremity. The major complication of therapy is bleeding, and these drugs are therefore not advised for clients who have had recent surgery or to dissolve myocardial or cerebral thrombi.

If conservative therapy does not resolve the thromboembolic disease, or if embolism appears, imminent surgical approaches may be attempted. The involved vein or the vena cava may be ligated to prevent the circulation of the embolus. In other approaches, intracaval devices such as grids or umbrellas can be inserted in the vena cava to impede embolus circulation yet allow free circulation of the venous blood. These may be inserted with the client under local anesthesia (see Chapter 21).

Relieving pain. Pain is managed with analgesics. Aspirin or drugs containing aspirin are usually not given, since aspirin interferes with platelet aggregation and alters dosage requirements of heparin. Enforced bed rest also limits pain, but the nurse can help the client change positions and provide comfort measures as needed.

Discharge instructions. When the client has recovered, he should be instructed to avoid situations of decreased mobility, constriction of circulation, and injury. The physician may prescribe oral anticoagulants such as warfarin, and the nurse should instruct the client on the use of these drugs.

Evaluation. Evaluation of the nursing care plan for the client with venous thromboembolic disease is a continuous component of the nursing process.

EXPECTED OUTCOMES

The client and/or family can:
1. Define venous thromboembolic disease.
2. Describe health maintenance plans for:
   a. Activity: exercise; avoid standing or flexing legs while sitting.

gery, compression dressings are applied to the incisions, and elastic bandages are used to secure them.

Immediately after surgery the nurse can assess the client for bleeding. Any bleeding on the bandages should be marked with a pen so that an increase can be noted. At no time should the elastic bandages be removed, since they provide compression to control bleeding. The nurse should also palpate and count the popliteal and pedal pulses to evaluate peripheral circulation.

Promoting circulation is important after surgery, and as soon as the client has recovered from anesthesia, he is encouraged to walk to stimulate development of collateral circulation. The nurse should accompany the client for the first few times, because he may be unsteady on his feet. Walking is usually painful for several days, and a narcotic may be ordered for pain. The pain medication may be given before the client gets out of bed, but the nurse should observe him for dizziness and support him as he ambulates.

When the client is in bed, he should be positioned to aid venous return. The foot of the bed may be elevated, and at no time should the knee be gatched or the head of the bed raised in high Fowler's position. The client should be discouraged from sitting on the side of the bed, because this obstructs circulation in the femoral veins and arteries.

The client is usually discharged in 2 to 3 days but is instructed to rest at home. He should avoid periods of standing, but walking is helpful in promoting venous return. The client should also be instructed in health habits that will prevent recurrences of his varicosities.

Varicose ulcers

Varicose ulcers may develop on the skin surrounding deep varicosities from venous stasis and lack of oxygen to the cells. The ulcer may be treated by frequent cleansing, wet-to-dry soaks, karaya dressings, or enzymatic debridement with streptokinase-streptodornase (Varidase) or fibrinolysin-desoxyribonuclease (Elase). Larger ulcers may be treated with pressure bandages or protective medicated paste boots such as Unna's boot. Finally, skin grafting may be attempted if conservative measures do not cause healing.

Valvular heart disease

Valvular heart disease is a result of stenosis or insufficiency of the valves of the heart. *Stenosis* occurs when the cusps of the valve become fibrotic, calcified, and may even fuse. The pressure in the involved chamber increases because of the resistance of the stenotic valve. As pressure increases, the workload of the myocardium increases and there may be dysrhythmias, heart failure, or cardiogenic shock. Valvular *insufficiency* occurs when the valves retract and no longer close completely. There is leaking and regurgitation during systole. The cardiac workload increases because of incomplete emptying and increasing demand for tissue oxygenation.

Valvular heart disease is usually the result of a previous cardiac infection, such as rheumatic fever or cardiac syphilis, but also may be congenital. This obstructive process is usually slow in onset and affects older persons who may have had a cardiac infection during childhood. The diagnosis is based on the client's history, phonocardiography, electrocardiogram, echocardiography, and cardiac catheterization.

Aortic stenosis may be the result of scarring, thickening, or fusion of the cusps of the aortic valve. The client complains of fatigue and anginal pain because blood flow to the coronary artery is decreased by the lower pressures in the aorta. Syncope may occur as a result of inadequate blood supply through the aortic valve. Characteristic heart murmurs may be heard, and there is an elevation of left ventricular pressure. Congestive heart failure is the ultimate outcome of aortic stenosis. When the client has become incapacitated, the physician may consider performing surgery to insert a prosthetic valve.

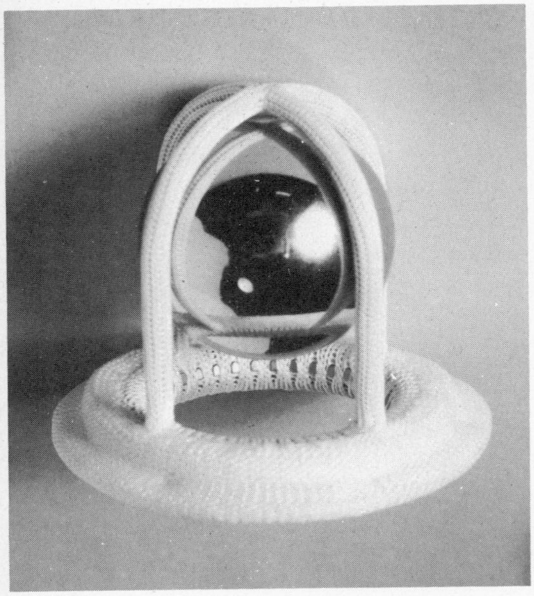

Aortic insufficiency involves the failure of the leaflets of the aortic valve to close completely. This is usually a residual damage from rheumatic fever or cardiac syphilis. The heart increases in size as it attempts to compensate for the inefficient valve. The client becomes fatigued and is eventually unable to cope with daily activities. The valve can be replaced during open-heart procedures.

Mitral stenosis is the most common complication of rheumatic fever. The mitral valve becomes inflamed, scarred, and eventually stenosed. Pressure in the left atrium increases, and pulmonary stasis can lead to pulmonary edema. The client complains of fatigue and dyspnea on exertion. There is usually a diastolic murmur present. If the stenosis is not complete, the client may be treated conservatively with rest, sodium-restricted diet, and cardiac glycosides. If the client is a good operative risk, several surgical approaches may be used. A mitral commissurotomy involves dilating the stenotic valve with the physician's finger or a dilator through a closed-heart surgical technique. Later, if the commissurotomy is not successful, a prosthetic or Porcine valve may be inserted (Fig. 20-57). These are inserted with open-heart surgical techniques. Long-term anticoagulant therapy is necessary if a prosthetic valve is used, whereas short-term (several months) therapy is used for Porcine valves.

Mitral insufficiency involves the failure of the leaflets of the mitral valve to close. Blood regurgitates to the left atrium, and the volume overload eventually causes the client to become fatigued and have dyspnea on exertion. There is a systolic murmur present. Open-heart surgery may be attempted to replace the valve with a prosthesis.

Cardiac syphilis

Cardiac syphilis is a manifestation of the tertiary stage of syphilis. This stage usually occurs 15 to 30 years after the initial infection. The aorta and aortic valves are most often affected by the scarring and plaque formation. The aorta may become inflamed, producing an aortitis, and if the media is involved, there may be an aortic aneurysm. When the aortic valves are scarred, aortic insufficiency may result. These complications can be prevented by early case finding and treatment of syphilis in the primary stage. Ultimate treatment involves surgical repair of the damaged valves or aneurysm.

COMMON HEALTH PROBLEMS THAT OCCUR ACROSS THE LIFE SPAN

Anemia

Anemia is an imbalance of the rate of formation and destruction of the red blood cells. The imbalance may be caused by (1) decreased production of red blood cells, (2) disorders of maturation and erythropoiesis, and (3) blood cell breakdown (hemolysis) or loss. Anemia can also be described by morphological characteristics (size, shape, color) of the red blood cell.

Anemia is a disease that involves individuals of all ages. It can be evident at birth as hemolytic anemia of the newborn, as a genetic defect such as sickle cell anemia, in nutritional disorders such as iron deficiency anemia or folic acid deficiency anemia, or in states of insidious or frank blood loss.

Assessment. Regardless of the cause of anemia, the effects on oxygen-carrying capacity are similar, and the nurse has a significant role in assessing these. Using the nursing history, the nurse can ascertain information about the cardiovascular system as well as include a dietary history, history of previous

FIG. 20-57
Mitral prosthesis. (Courtesy Edwards Laboratories, Santa Ana, Calif. From Duffy, Margery, and others, editors: Current concepts in clinical nursing, vol. 3, St. Louis, 1971, The C.V. Mosby Co.)

health problems, and genetic history. Significant information to obtain includes adequacy of nutrients during growth (infancy, childhood, adolescence, and pregnancy) and dietary sources of nutrients necessary to erythrocyte formation—iron, folic acid, and vitamin C. A financial history is useful to determine if poverty is a basis for poor diet. Other data from the history include presence of other diseases that interfere with red blood cell formation or destruction such as malnutrition, malabsorption syndromes, diseases of the stomach or small intestine, gastric disorders, cancer, or bleeding states. Neonates should be observed for presence of hemolytic disease and a genetic history elicited from blacks at risk for sickle cell disease.

A physical examination shows the client to be pale, weak, and fatigued. There may be anorexia, malaise, coldness of the extremities, and bleeding from superficial tissues as the anemia progresses. The heart responds to the lack of circulating red blood cells with increased rate and hypertrophy. Dyspnea and increased respirations also occur in an attempt to correct cellular hypoxia. The anemia may be insidious in onset or appear suddenly, and the severity of the symptoms corresponds to the onset. Bone marrow aspiration and CBC are used to confirm the diagnosis.

Data analysis
Data analysis may reveal nursing diagnoses of alterations in cardiac output, impaired gas exchange, knowledge deficit, alterations in nutrition, and sleep pattern disturbances.

Planning and implementation
Iron deficiency anemia. Iron deficiency anemia is the most common anemia and occurs in 20% of women and in one half of women who are pregnant. Less than 3% of men have iron deficiency anemia.

Iron deficiency anemia is caused by inadequate dietary intake of iron or faulty use in the bone marrow from blockage of its release in the reticuloendothelial cells. Iron is particularly required during periods of growth (infancy, pregnancy), and dietary deficiencies are most apparent at these times. Blood loss from menstruation, hemorrhage, or malabsorption syndromes also precipitate iron deficiency anemia. Red blood cells become smaller, and the proportionate hemoglobin is reduced, producing a microcytic, hypochromic type of anemia.

A balance of dietary intake, use, and excretion of iron must be maintained. Diets that contain 12 to 15 mg of iron should be provided each day, because only 5% to 10% of the iron is absorbed. Of this iron, two thirds is used for hemoglobin formation, and one third is stored in the liver, spleen, and bone marrow. During stress states, the reserves are depleted first, and the gastrointestinal absorption increases to maintain current hemoglobin use. Iron loss is especially critical in infants because erythropoiesis in the bone marrow does not occur until the child is 2 months old and red blood cell destruction is greater than red blood cell production.

Therapeutic intervention centers around improving dietary patterns, and the nurse plays an instrumental role in client instruction. Foods that contain sources of iron, such as eggs, enriched breads, spinach, liver, meats, and molasses, should be offered daily. The diet should also contain a source of vitamin C (such as orange juice, strawberries, cantaloupe, and tomato juice), which is needed for the absorption of the iron. The nurse may suggest resources for food planning and procurement of nutritious food.

Iron preparations may also be used to supplement dietary sources of iron. Iron drops are commonly used for infants until their diet contains sufficient meats to provide a natural source of iron. Other oral preparations of iron may be given to children and adults. These are usually best given between meals because they are absorbed more efficiently in an acid environment. Giving the medications with orange juice is helpful because the vitamin C contained in the juice promotes absorption of iron. If the oral preparations are in a liquid form, they should be given with a straw to avoid staining the teeth. The iron tends to cause the stool to become dark, and the client should be prepared to observe this change.

If the anemia is severe, iron-dextran (Imferon), the parenteral preparation of iron, may be given intramuscularly. The Z-track technique (Fig. 20-58) should be used for injection to assure deposition of the medication in the muscle and prevent staining the tissues. The medication is drawn into a syringe with a 2-inch needle, and 0.5 cc of air is drawn into the syringe. The needle should be changed before the medication is injected into the muscle; a site is selected in the upper outer quadrant of the buttock; and the skin is pulled laterally. The medication is injected at a 90-degree angle, with 0.5 cc of air to seal the medication in the muscle; 10 seconds later the skin is released and the needle withdrawn. Walking promotes the absorption of the iron, but tight clothing such as girdles should not be worn because they could force the medication out of the muscle.

The individual with iron-deficiency anemia may feel constantly fatigued after doing simple tasks. The child with anemia is pale and does not have energy to play. Nursing care is directed toward providing rest for the client, even to the point of assisting with bathing and eating, which may be too tiring. The environment should be warm and blankets available for use on the bed. Nightgowns with a drawstring bottom or feet may be used for infants who kick off their covers. The client's appetite may be poor, and nursing measures to stimulate the appetite, such as mouth care and appetizing food, should be used. Mouth care should be given gently because the gums may bleed easily.

When anemia is corrected, the oxygen-carrying capacity improves, and color and energy to meet daily needs are restored. The client should be aware of the role of iron in maintaining his health and should be instructed in the principles of a well-balanced diet.

Aplastic anemia. Aplastic anemia involves depression or inactivity in bone marrow, resulting in inadequate production of white cells and platelets as well as red blood cells. It may be caused by certain drugs and chemicals, especially chloramphenicol, sulfonamides, antineoplastic agents (especially the alkylating agents and vinca alkaloid), insecticides, and benzene preparations. Aplastic anemia may be treated by removing the causative agent, administering steroids, and administering blood transfusions. The prognosis is generally favorable, and nursing management is similar to that for the client with leukemia, because bruising, hemorrhage, and overwhelming infections are likely complications.

Maturational anemias. *Pernicious anemia* is caused by the absence of the intrinsic factor, a blood factor that is necessary to use vitamin B_{12} in the formation of red blood cells. The intrinsic factor is formed in the lining of the stomach,

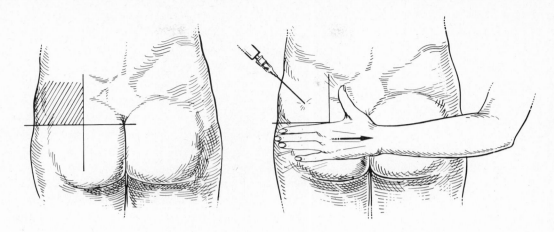

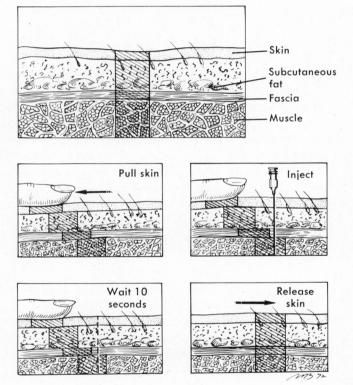

FIG. 20-58
Z-track technique for intramuscular injection of Imferon. Skin in upper outer quadrant of buttock is pulled laterally and medication injected; after 10 seconds; needle is withdrawn and skin released. (Reprinted with permission of Merrell Dow Pharmaceuticals Inc., subsidiary of The Dow Chemical Co., Cincinnati, Ohio 45215.)

but it may be absent because of a hereditary defect. The intrinsic factor is also missing when the client has a malignancy in the stomach or has had a gastrectomy. The size of the red blood cell enlarges, as does the hemoglobin value, producing a macrocytic, hyperchromic anemia, although the total number of erythrocytes decreases and they assume an abnormal shape. Middle-aged persons are most often affected by pernicious anemia. In addition to the symptoms of anemia (weakness, fatigue, and pallor), the client may have a sore, burning mouth and a smooth, red tongue. The nervous system is also involved, and the client may notice numbness, tingling, loss of touch, and lack of sense of position, and may even have a reversible psychosis. The diagnosis is confirmed by a gastric analysis, or Diagnex Blue test, which reveals absence of free hydrochloric acid, and by Schilling's test.

This chronic anemia is treated with intramuscular injections of cyanocobalamin (vitamin B_{12}). Because vitamin B_{12} is not used from oral or dietary sources, it must be given intramuscularly in monthly doses. The client may learn to give his own injection or have a family member assist him.

Folic acid deficiency anemia is another disorder of erythrocyte maturation that may be caused by inadequate dietary sources (particularly in malnutrition or infants receiving only a milk diet) when there is an increase in demand for folic acid (stress, growth, pregnancy) or interference with folate metabolism, particularly by alcohol ingestion. This is a macrocytic anemia. The symptoms are similar to those of pernicious anemia and are reversed with a normal diet of foods rich in folic acid or supplemented with 0.25 to 1 mg folic acid orally daily for 1 to 2 weeks.

Hemolytic anemia. Destruction of red blood cells may be caused by toxins, infections, blood incompatibility, and certain medications. The hemolytic process is more rapid than replacement in the bone marrow, and anemia results.

Hemolytic disease of the newborn (erythroblastosis fetalis) is a form of hemolytic anemia that occurs when there is an incompatibility (isoimmunization) of the fetal and maternal bloods. Although incompatibility between A, B, and O blood types is possible, the major incompatibility occurs when the mother has Rh-negative blood, the father has Rh-positive blood, and the fetus is Rh-positive. Fetal red blood cells may cross the placental barrier, causing the mother to form anti-Rh antibodies. These enter fetal circulation and cause destruction of fetal red blood cells. More antibodies are formed with each subsequent pregnancy, and although the first newborn may not have hemolytic disease, subsequent children undoubtedly will.

The newborn with hemolytic disease is anemic and has an enlarged liver and spleen from the body's attempts to create new red blood cells to replace those that were destroyed. The newborn is also jaundiced, because the immature liver is unable to excrete the excessive bilirubin that is released as a product of red blood cell hemolysis. Jaundice of the skin and sclera occurs within the first 36 hours, and if the serum bilirubin level rises above 20 mg/100 ml of blood, kernicterus, or brain damage from the excessive bilirubin, may follow.

The possibility of erythroblastosis fetalis can be detected by parental blood studies, which are usually a part of the prenatal examination. If there is a possibility of a blood incompatibility, samples of the amniotic fluid may be obtained by amniocentesis during the prenatal course to detect the presence of rising bilirubin levels and an increase in the number of immature red blood cells. The amniotic fluid is usually a deep yellow if the fetus has an isoimmunization problem.

If the fetus appears to be in danger from rising bilirubin levels, an intrauterine exchange transfusion can be performed. A special needle is inserted through the mother's abdomen to the uterus and the abdomen of the fetus. Rh-negative blood is transfused to the fetal peritoneal cavity, where it is absorbed into the peripheral circulation. This procedure is not without risk of maternal or fetal infection, fetal injury, or premature labor.

An anti-Rh gamma globulin (RhoGAM) has been developed, which can be given to the mother within 72 hours after the birth of each Rh-positive baby to prevent antibody formation. RhoGAM can also be used after spontaneous or therapeutic abortion. When known clients with isoimmunization problems are admitted for delivery, a blood sample should be sent to the laboratory for antibody screening and cross-matching with Rh-immune globulin. After delivery, a sample of cord blood is also analyzed for Rh determination. RhoGAM is then administered intramuscularly to the postpartum or postabortal client within 72 hours of delivery. The use of this drug should drastically reduce the number of neonates with this hemolytic disease.

If the bilirubin level is elevated at birth, the neonate can be treated with phototherapy or an exchange transfusion to reduce rising bilirubin levels. *Phototherapy* is based on the principle that exposure to light reduces the serum bilirubin level by photooxidation.[37] This approach is preferred if the hemolytic disease is mild or in instances of hyperbilirubinemia of prematurity. The newborn is placed in a crib or incubator with a canopy of fluorescent lights. His eyes are closed and covered to prevent light damage. The shields should be removed periodically, however, so that the eyes can be inspected and visual stimulation provided. As much skin surface as possible should be exposed. A diaper can be placed under the client to prevent soiling the crib. Male newborns should be diapered to prevent priapism (continuous erection) caused by stimulation from the light. Turning the client every 4 hours exposes all skin surfaces adequately. The therapy may be continued as long as a week until the bilirubin levels return to normal. The neonate should be observed for a greenish, loose stool or rash, which is a common side effect of phototherapy. Anemia may recur in 1 to 8 weeks; therefore it is important to continue frequent assessments of hemoglobin levels. Using phototherapy is simple and less costly than an exchange transfusion and presents fewer risks.

If the bilirubin levels rise above 10 mg/100 ml of blood, an *exchange transfusion* may be done immediately after birth to replace the newborn's blood with compatible donor blood. If the transfusion is to be done, the umbilical cord should be kept moist for this procedure. A catheter is inserted in the umbilical vein, the neonate's blood is withdrawn, and donor blood is inserted (about 20 ml at a time) until approximately 500 ml is exchanged, usually twice the amount of donor blood as infant's blood volume.

After the transfusion, the newborn is placed in an incubator with high humidity and oxygen. The nurse should observe vital signs and assess the utilization of oxygen in the cells. Complications that could result from the transfusion include heart failure from circulatory overload, air embolism, bacterial infection, or cardiac arrest, and the nurse should monitor cardiovascular functions frequently to detect untoward changes. The newborn is usually fed within 24 hours, and if he is bottle-fed, the holes in the nipples should be enlarged to prevent fatigue during feeding.

Anemia from blood loss. Anemia can also result from a slow loss of blood or a rapid hemorrhage. Persons with bleeding ulcers, ulcerative colitis, and certain malignancies may have slow blood losses that may result in anemia. Blood loss may also occur during or after surgery or following traumatic injury.

Therapeutic intervention is directed toward replacing the lost blood.[53] Whole blood, plasma, or packed cells may be used (see Chapter 8).

Evaluation. The nurse and client can evaluate outcomes of nursing care on an ongoing basis.

EXPECTED OUTCOMES

The client and/or family can:

1. Describe anemia.
2. State plans for therapeutic management:
   a. State use, time, dosage, route, and side effects of medication (iron, vitamin B$_{12}$, folic acid).
   b. State diet prescription (iron rich, folic acid rich).
3. Describe plans for health maintenance:
   a. Rest and exercise.
   b. Warmth.
   c. Adequate fluids and nutrition.
   d. Promotion of activities for growth and development.
4. State plans for follow-up health care and indicate community resources for clients with anemia.

Leukemia

Leukemia is the proliferation of immature white blood cells and their precursors. The white blood cells are produced in such numbers that they accumulate, infiltrate, and eventually decrease the production of other blood constituents, notably the red blood cells, platelets, and polymorphonuclear leukocytes.

The cause of leukemia is not known, but it is considered to be a neoplastic process. Some theories favor a viral cause, others a genetic basis that causes increased susceptibility to leukemia. There also seems to be a familial basis; and environmental effects of ionizing radiation, as noticed during atomic bombings, have been known to increase the number of persons with leukemia.

Pathophysiology. The mechanism by which the proliferated cells prevent normal hematopoiesis is not known, although disruption can occur at any stage of cell differentiation (stem cells or blast cells). One theory supports the overcrowding of the immature cells in the bone marrow spaces; others attribute the disruption to substances released by the immature cells that inhibit hematopoiesis.

Leukemias are described by the course of the disease as acute or chronic and by the type of cell involved as lymphocytic or myelogenous. Individuals of all ages may have leukemia, although the type and onset appear to be age specific.

Acute lymphocytic leukemia (ALL) is the most common form of leukemia and affects children 2 to 5 years of age. It is the most common childhood cancer and second leading cause of nonaccidental death in children. The cell involved is the lymphoblast, an immature form of the lymphocyte that invades the bone marrow, bloodstream, and lymph nodes. The onset is abrupt, and death ensues in 4 months if no treatment is instituted. The use of chemotherapy produces remissions in 90% of individuals, and 5 years after treatment many (30% to 40%) are in remission and some cured.

Acute myelogenous leukemia (AML) refers to a leukemia involving the granulocytes. This is a disease of all ages, although it is more common in adults. Survival time of untreated AML is predicted to be 3 to 4 months; with chemotherapy, survival times of 2 years have been reported.

Chronic lymphocytic leukemia (CLL) is a defect of the B-lymphocyte that occurs after stem cell differentiation. The cells invade the bone marrow, bloodstream, and lymph nodes and produce involvement of the liver and spleen. This is a disease of adults over age 35. The onset is insidious, and mean survival rates are longer (3 to 4 years) than for the acute form of the disease. Treatment is not instituted, however, until the symptoms are similar to those in the acute form.

Chronic myelogenous leukemia (CML) involves primarily granulocytes, and the origin of the carcinogenesis is believed to be in the stem cell. Furthermore, a unique chromosome, known as the *Philadelphia chromosome,* can be detected in the blood of individuals before the development of CML. The chromosome is undoubtedly involved in the development of CML.

There are two phases of cell proliferation, a chronic phase and a blastic phase. The chronic phase, in which an increase in proliferation of granulocytes crowding out the erythrocytes, lasts for several years. The blastic phase or blast crisis has an abrupt onset of increased myeloblast proliferation. This is a disease of middle adulthood and increases in frequency with age. The onset is insidious and, as the disease progresses, resembles acute myelogenous leukemia. A survival time of about 3 years is enhanced by chemotherapy.

 Assessment. The client with leukemia exhibits the affects of anemia and reduced platelet count. He is fatigued, weak, pale, and dyspneic, and the temperature, pulse, and respirations are elevated. There is a tendency for easy bleeding, particularly in the gums and mucous membranes of the mouth. Petechiae may appear on all parts of the body. The client may be anorexic and have bone pain. The lymph glands, liver, and spleen enlarge, and the client is susceptible to infection. The rampant production of cells eventually involves the central nervous system, causing headache, nausea and vomiting, papillary edema, and generalized effects of increased intracranial pressure.

The diagnosis of leukemia is confirmed by blood analysis and bone marrow aspiration. Tissue cultures and special staining techniques aid in identifying the type of cell involved. Diagnosis of the involved cells aids therapy, because some approaches are more effective for various types of cells and untoward effects of therapy can be minimized.

Data analysis
Data analysis may reveal nursing diagnoses of alterations in cardiac output, alterations in comfort, fear, ineffective coping, knowledge deficit, disturbances in self-concept, and alterations in tissue perfusion.

Planning and implementation. There is currently no cure for leukemia, but long-term remissions can be induced by various chemotherapeutic agents, radiation therapy, or bone marrow transplants and leukophoresis. The type of intervention depends on the cell type involved and the age and health of the client.

Chemotherapy. The goal of chemotherapy is to induce remission, which is defined as normal bone marrow with less than 5% blast cells and absence of clinical symptoms. Purine antagonists such as mercaptopurine, folic acid antagonists such as methotrexate (Amethopterin), antimetabolites such as cytosine araboside (Cytosar), alkylating agents such as vincristine sulfate (Oncovin), and cyclophosphamide (Cytoxan) may be used. Antibiotics such as daunorubicin appear to be effective in remitting the disease. Corticosteroids such as prednisone are also useful. These drugs are more effective in producing a remission when used in combination. Prednisone and vincristine, for example, have been observed to cause 90% remissions. The use of antineoplastic drugs in a cyclical fashion has also been found to prolong remission and reduce side effects of multiple agent therapy.

Nursing process for common health problems

Before administration of chemotherapeutic agents, the client should be evaluated for extent of disease, bone marrow status, and complete blood count. Packed cells, platelets, and antibiotics may be given before the initiation of chemotherapy to prevent hematological complications.

Response to chemotherapy differs between children and adults; better responses are achieved in children. Adults generally do not respond well to steroid therapy, and remission is brief. Purine antagonists, however, are useful in many instances of adult therapy.

The nurse should be aware of the side effects of these drugs and know that the client may feel uncomfortable while under treatment. Alopecia is a common side effect, and when the drugs are given intravenously, a tight rubber band on the scalp or a scalp cap can be inflated to constrict cerebral blood vessels to prevent infusion of the drug at the hairline. If hair loss is severe, wigs may be worn until the hair begins to grow, about 3 months after therapy. The client usually has nausea and vomiting when receiving these chemotherapeutic agents, and the nurse can give mouth care and incorporate appropriate comfort measures in the nursing care plan. The client should not receive immunizations or vaccinations if he is taking immunosuppressive drugs and should report exposure to communicable diseases to the physician. The client should also be instructed not to take vitamins with folic acid while receiving folic acid antagonists, such as methotrexate, because these drugs negate the effectiveness of the chemotherapeutic agent. Aspirin should not be used during chemotherapy, because platelet depression and bleeding are enhanced by its use.

The central nervous system is resistant to chemotherapeutic intervention because those agents do not cross the blood-brain barrier. To prevent central nervous system damage, most treatment plans include prophylactic treatment with radiation therapy and intrathecal methotrexate. Success of therapy is monitored by frequent assays of cerebrospinal fluid obtained by lumbar puncture. Others advocate the use of an Ommaya reservoir, a silicone tube inserted into the ventricles through which chemotherapeutic agents can be inserted under strict aseptic conditions.

Radiation therapy. In some instances radiation therapy may be used as an adjunct to chemotherapy. Long-term side effects of radiation therapy, such as interference with bone growth and sterility, are dangerous in children, and, consequently, use of radiation therapy must be judicious in the young.

Bone marrow transplant. Bone marrow transplants have been attempted to induce remissions, particularly for clients with chronic myelocytic leukemia, ALL, or AML, who have responded poorly to chemotherapy.[59,62,65] Before transplant the client receives total body radiation to destroy bone marrow function, and donor bone marrow is transfused at 10 ml/kg body weight.[54] The nurse should observe the client for signs of rejection such as rash or liver disease.

Leukopheresis. Leukopheresis therapy involves removing the blood to separate out the leukocytes and replacing the remaining blood. This may be done in clients with chronic lymphocytic leukemia to reduce the number of circulating white blood cells.[50,60]

Nursing care for the client with leukemia is planned for individual needs of the client and family. The care plan may be developed for clients during acute stages of illness when nursing care is supportive, during remission when nursing care is facilitative, or in terminal stages of the disease when the family, client,

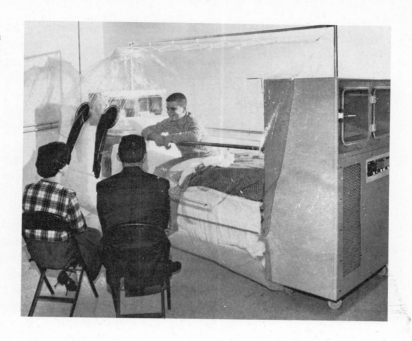

and health team face the client's imminent death. Goals may include (1) preventing infection, (2) managing bleeding, (3) maintaining fluid and nutrition balance, (4) providing comfort measures, and (5) maintaining client and family support systems.

Preventing infection. The client is prone to infection when a proliferation of immature white blood cells and leukopenia occur as a result of drug therapy. The infection may be bacterial, viral, or fungal in origin, and nursing care is planned to reduce the risk of infection by use of aseptic technique and avoiding creating ports of entry for microorganisms. The client may be placed on reverse isolation. Some institutions use a life island, an enclosed plastic tent that protects the client from environmental hazards during states of severe leukopenia (Fig. 20-59). The client can see and communicate with family and nursing staff but remains protected. Nursing care is given through gloved ports. Others, however, feel that isolation is disruptive to psychosocial development at a time when the client most needs human support systems. In these instances the client may be in a private room and protected by clean technique in nursing care procedures. Antibiotics may be given prophylactically. Infection is the most common cause of death in the client with leukemia, and scrupulous care should be provided for prevention.

Managing bleeding. Bleeding is a problem of clients with leukemia during the acute stages of the disease because of the crowding and reduction of platelets and during chemotherapy and radiation therapy if thrombocytopenia is a consequence of therapy. The nurse should be gentle in giving care. A soft toothbrush should be used if the gums are bleeding, and small needles should be used for injections. Aspirin should not be used, because it interferes with platelet production and may prolong bleeding time.

Maintaining fluid and nutrition balance. The client with leukemia who is receiving chemotherapy must be encouraged to obtain adequate fluids and nutrition. For the anorexic client, easily digested and well-balanced meals should be

1221

offered. If the client has sore gums or bleeding in the mouth, a bland diet can be used. Fluids should be encouraged when antimetabolite drugs are used, because the formation of uric acid crystals increases as neoplastic cells are destroyed. Allopurinol (Zyloprim) may be used to prevent uric acid crystal formation, and sodium bicarbonate may be given to alkalinize the urine, because uric acid is more soluble in an alkaline urine. Intravenous fluids may be used to ensure adequate urinary output. Total parenteral nutrition may be used to support nutrition as necessary.

Providing comfort measures. During exacerbation of the disease the client may be uncomfortable or in pain. Infiltration of vital organs by white blood cells may cause infarction and pain. Analgesics and narcotics may be used as needed. Comfort measures such as bathing, turning, and frequent hygiene can be offered regularly to clients who are confined to bed.

Maintaining client/family support systems. The diagnosis of a fatal illness is a devastating experience for the client, family, and the health team. The nurse should assess the client's and family's knowledge of the diagnosis and acceptance of the disease to make a care plan. There may be many reactions to the diagnosis of leukemia, and the nurse offers support and understanding as the client and family deal with this crisis. Support from a religious counselor may be invaluable at this time.

The family should be part of the care plan. If the client is a child, one of the parents may wish to stay in the room and take part in his care. Adults may wish their family to be with them as often as possible, and the nurse can be flexible with visiting hours.

In the terminal stages of leukemia the client is weak, irritable, and easily fatigued. There may be bleeding from the mouth and general malaise. Many clients fear being alone during this phase of their illness. Attentive nursing care that demonstrates concern for the client and his family provides fundamental support during the time of his death.

Families of children who die from leukemia often have difficult adjustments to the loss of the child. There may be guilt, anger, and blaming. As many as 50% of these marriages end in divorce.[45] The nurse may have an important role in encouraging families to return to the hospital for counseling or referring them to appropriate community resources.

Evaluation. The nursing care plan for the client with leukemia is developed according to individual needs during diagnosis, exacerbation, remission, or terminal illness, and evaluation is appropriate during each of these stages.

EXPECTED OUTCOMES

The client and/or family can:
1. Describe leukemia.
2. Use appropriate individual and family coping resources.
3. Demonstrate sensitivity to changes in self-concept.
4. State plans for health maintenance:
   a. Prevention of infection.
   b. Adequate fluids and nutrition.
   c. Adequate urinary and bowel elimination.
5. State use, dosage, time, route, and side effects of prescribed antineoplastic medications. Manage side effects (nausea, vomiting, bleeding, alopecia, anorexia, uric acid formation).

6. State indications for health care services (bleeding, pain, petechiae, infection, fever, decreased urine output).
7. Describe plans for follow-up care.
8. Describe community resources available to clients and families with leukemia.

Disseminated intravascular coagulation

Disseminated intravascular coagulation (DIC) is not a disease entity as such, but a phenomenon that is a result of various stress states and toxic conditions, causing a syndrome of concomitant activation of the blood-clotting (release of thrombin) and fibrinolytic systems. Hypercoagulability and decreased clotting responses primarily in the arterioles, venules, and capillaries follow. Depletion of the clotting factors and platelets results in hemorrhage and stagnation of the blood flow in the circulation.

DIC may be recognized by various cues, mainly those arising from the hemorrhagic state: petechiae, ecchymosis, hematuria, hematemesis, epistaxis, and oozing from infusion sites or infection sites. Blood studies reveal a thrombocytopenia, prolonged prothrombin time, increased partial thromboplastin time, and reduced fibrinogen levels.

The nurse should be alert to the possibility of DIC on the basis of the above cues and suspect its presence at times when there has been tissue or endothelial cell injury or red blood cell, white blood cell, or platelet damage. States such as hypotension, septicemia, hypoxemia, cancer chemotherapy, obstetrical emergencies (such as placenta abruptio, sepsis, or fetal death), burns, toxin ingestion, and tumor processes have been known to precipitate DIC.

Intervention is directed toward halting bleeding mechanisms. Heparin is given as an antagonist to thrombin to inhibit intravascular clotting, and whole blood or platelets may be used to supply clotting factors. The preexisting stress state must also be managed to remove precipitating factors.

Nursing care during episodes of DIC should be supportive. If the client is bleeding, provisions for rest, fluids, and nutrition should be made. A safe environment is necessary for the client receiving heparin. Oxygen therapy may be used as needed. Observations of urinary output are critical because fibrin deposits may be excreted. The client will appreciate comfort and hygiene measures that are supportive during the course of an episode of DIC.

Evaluation

During the evaluation stage of the nursing process the nurse and client make judgments about outcomes of care planned for health promotion, maintenance, and restoration for common problems of the cardiovascular system. Nursing diagnoses may include alterations in cardiac output, alterations in tissue perfusion, knowledge deficit, noncompliance, alterations in comfort: pain, ineffective airway clearance, ineffective coping, fluid volume deficit, impaired gas exchange, and alterations in self-concept.

EXPECTED OUTCOMES

The client and/or family can:
1. Describe the health problem.
2. State plans for health promotion of the cardiovascular system, including risk factor identification and management, promotion of circulation, prevention of infection, and provision for appropriate nutrition.

3. State use of therapies, including surgery, pharmacological agents, and special diets.
4. State indications for health care, including pain, weight gain, changes in vital signs, difficulty in breathing, and changes in color of skin and nailbeds.
5. State plans for follow-up health care and use of community resources.

While evaluating client outcomes, the nurse and client may decide that the problem is resolved or that the plan should be continued or modified to attain problem resolution. The nurse-client relationship is terminated as problems are resolved and the client assumes responsibility for his optimal level of wellness.

Summary   The nursing process is a method for identifying nursing problems, planning, implementing, and evaluating nursing care for clients with common health problems of the cardiovascular system across the life span. The role of the nurse may be dominant in life-threatening situations of cardiovascular crisis, or facilitative and supportive as the client assumes responsibility for his own health care.

During the assessment stage of the nursing process the nurse collects and analyzes data pertinent to the client's cardiovascular health status. Significant data include the client's health history; developmental, social, and psychological histories; and physical assessment. Data obtained from hemodynamic monitoring is also used to formulate nursing problems or diagnoses.

The nurse and client plan for health promotion, maintenance, and restoration. Health promotion involves preventing and managing modifiable risk factors associated with health problems of the cardiovascular system and instructing clients about promoting circulation, preventing infection, planning adequate nutrition, and, in some instances, genetic counseling. Because sudden death from cardiovascular health problems can occur in the community or health care facilities, clients, families, and nurses must be able to plan for emergency care and cardiopulmonary resuscitation.

Common health problems of the cardiovascular system occur throughout the life span. Problems of the neonate or infant include congenital heart disease, sickle cell anemia, and hemophilia. Rheumatic fever and cardiac infections are associated with school-age children and young adults. The majority of health problems of the cardiovascular system, however, occur in adulthood and are the primary cause of death in the United States. Atherosclerosis, ischemic heart disease, hypertension, heart failure, cardiogenic shock, peripheral vascular arterial and venous diseases are salient. Anemia and leukemia occur in all age groups and represent significant health problems. The nurse and client implement plans to restore the client to his highest level of wellness associated with these problems.

The nurse and client evaluate objectives specified in the planning stage of the nursing process. Client expected outcomes are unique to each client and appropriate to his growth and development across the life span. Evaluation determines if objectives for promotion, maintenance, and restoration of health for problems of the cardiovascular system have been achieved and that the client has indeed obtained his optimal level of wellness.

References

1. Andreoli, Kathleen, and others: Comprehensive cardiac care, ed. 4, St. Louis, 1979, The C.V. Mosby Co.
2. Barboriak, Joseph, and Menahan, Lawrence: Alcohol, lipoproteins, and coronary heart disease, Heart Lung **8**(4):736, 1979.
3. Begley, Linda: External counter-pulsation for cardiogenic shock, Am. J. Nurs. **75**(6):967-970, 1975.
4. Bramoweth, Ellen: Acute aortic dissection, Am. J. Nurs. **80**(11):2010-2012, 1980.
5. Braunwald, Eugene, editor: Heart disease, a textbook of cardiovascular medicine, vol. 2, Philadelphia, 1980, W.B. Saunders Co.
6. Chamberlain, Susan: Low-dose heparin therapy, Am. J. Nurs. **80**(6):1115-1117, 1980.
7. Cogen, Roberta: Preventing complications during cardiac catheterization, Am. J. Nurs. **76**(3):401-405, 1976.
8. Cole, Collier, and others: Brief sexual counseling during cardiac rehabilitation, Heart Lung **8**(1):124-129, 1979.
9. Collier, Sue: Cardiogenic shock: principles of management. In Current practice in critical care, vol. 1, St. Louis, 1979, The C.V. Mosby Co.
10. Conover, Mary H.: Cardiac arrhythmias, ed. 2, St. Louis, 1978, The C.V. Mosby Co.
11. Cook, Rosa Lee: Psychosocial responses to myocardial infarction, Heart Lung **8**(1):130-135, 1979.
12. Cudkowicz, Leon, and Sherry, Sol: The venous system and the lung, Heart Lung **7**(1):91-96, 1978.
13. Dailey, E., and Schroeder, J.: Techniques in bedside hemodynamic monitoring, ed. 2, St. Louis, 1981, The C.V. Mosby Co.
14. Daniels, Linda, and Kochar, Mahendar: Monitoring and facilitating adherence to hypertension therapeutic regimens, Cardiovasc. Nurs. **16**(2):7-12, 1980.
15. Dehn, Michael: Rehabilitation of the cardiac patient, the effects of exercise, Am. J. Nurs. **80**(3):435, 1980.
16. Dorr, Kathleen: The intra-aortic balloon pump, Am. J. Nurs. **75**(1):52-55, 1975.
17. Doswell, Willa: Sickle cell anemia, you can do something to help, Nursing 78 **8**(4):65-70, 1978.
18. Eckhardt, Erica: Intraaortic balloon counterpulsation in cardiogenic shock, Heart Lung **6**(1):93-98, 1977.
19. Ellis, P.D., and Billings, D.M.: Cardiopulmonary resuscitation, procedures for basic and advanced life support, St. Louis, 1980, The C.V. Mosby Co.
20. Finesilver, Cynthia: Reducing stress in patients having cardiac catheterization, Am. J. Nurs. **80**(10):1805, 1980.
21. Fitzmaurice, Joan: Venous thromboembolic disease: current thoughts, Cardiovasc. Nurs. **14**(1):1-4, 1978.
22. Fowkes, William C., and Hunn, Virginia K.: Clinical assessment for the nurse practitioner, St. Louis, 1973, The C.V. Mosby Co.
23. Furman, Seymour: Recent developments in cardiac pacing, Heart Lung **7**(5):813-826, 1978.
24. Futral, Joel: Postoperative management and complications of coronary artery bypass surgery, Heart Lung **6**(3):477-485, 1977.
25. Gentry, W. Doyle, and Williams, Redford: Psychological aspects of myocardial infarction and coronary care, ed. 2, St. Louis, 1979, The C.V. Mosby Co.
26. Geolot, Denise, and McKinney, Nancy: Administering parenteral drugs, Am. J. Nurs. **75**(5):788-793, 1975.
27. Glancy, D. Lulce: Medical management of adults and older children undergoing cardiac operations, Heart Lung **9**(2):277, 1980.
28. Goldberger, Emanuel: Treatment of cardiac emergencies, ed. 2, St. Louis, 1979, The C.V. Mosby Co.
29. Groër, Maureen, and Shekleton, Maureen: Basic pathophysiology, a conceptual approach, St. Louis, 1979, The C.V. Mosby Co.
30. Hammond, Cecile: Protecting patients with temporary transvenous pacemakers, Nursing 78 **8**(11):82-86, 1978.
31. Hansen, Mary, and Woods, Susan: Nitroglycerin ointment—where and how to apply it, Am. J. Nurs. **80**(6):1122-1124, 1980.
32. Haughey, Cynthia: Alcoholic cardiomyopathy, Nursing 80 **8**(10):54, 1980.
33. Heart facts 1981: Dallas, Texas, 1980, American Heart Association.
34. Houser, Doris: Ice water for MI patients? Why not? Am. J. Nurs. **76**(3):432-434, 1976.
35. Lee, Anthony, editor: The Lazarus syndrome: caring for patients who've returned from the dead, RN **41**(6):53-64, 1978.

36. Long, Madeleine, and others: Hypertension: what patients need to know, Am. J. Nurs. **76**(5): 765-770, 1976.

37. Lucey, Jerold F.: Neonatal jaundice and phototherapy, Pediatr. Clin. North Am. **19**(4):827-839, 1972.

38. Mallison, Mary: Updating the cholesterol controversy: verdict—diet does count, Am. J. Nurs. **78**(10):1681, 1978.

39. Manwaring, Mary: What patients need to know about pacemakers, Am. J. Nurs. **77**(5):825-830, 1977.

40. Marcinek, Margaret: Hypertension, what it does to the body, Am. J. Nurs. **80**(5):928-932, 1980.

41. McFarlane, Judith: Sickle cell disorders, Am. J. Nurs. **77**(12):1948-1954, 1977.

42. McFarland, Mary: Fat embolism syndrome, Am. J. Nurs. **76**(12):1942-1944, 1976.

43. McIntosh, H., and others: Introduction to risk factors in coronary artery disease, **7**(1):126-149, 1978.

44. Mitchell, Ellen: Protocol for teaching hypertensive patients, Am. J. Nurs. **77**(5):808-809, 1977.

45. Morse, Margaret Lawley: Acute lymphocytic leukemia of childhood, care of the child and family. In Peterson, Barbara, and Kellogg, C.J., editors: Current practice in oncologic nursing, St. Louis, 1976, The C.V. Mosby Co.

46. Puksta, Nancy: All about sex after a coronary, Am. J. Nurs. **77**(4):602-605, 1977.

47. Ram, C. Venkata: Clinical applications of beta adrenergic blocking drugs: a growing spectrum, Heart Lung **8**(1):116-123, 1979.

48. Report of task force on blood pressure control in children. Pt. 2, Pediatrics **59**(5):Suppl., 1977.

49. Ring, Ernest, and others: Early experience with percutaneous transluminal angioplasty using a vinyl balloon catheter, Ann. Surg. **191**(4):438-442, 1980.

50. Rossman, Maureen, and others: Pheresis therapy: patient care, Am. J. Nurs. **77**(7):1135-1141, 1977.

51. Sacksteder, Sara, and others: Common congenital cardiac defects, Am. J. Nurs. **78**(2):266-272, 1978.

52. Scalzi, Cynthia, and Dracup, Kathy: Sexual counseling of coronary patients, Heart Lung, **7**(5): 840-845, 1978.

53. Scarlato, Michael: Blood transfusions today, what you should know and do, Nursing 78 **8**(2):68-72, 1978.

54. Schwitter, Georgeann, and Beach, Judith: Bone marrow transplantation in children, Nurs. Clin. North Am. **11**:49-57, 1976.

55. Smith, Mary Ellen: Nonsurgical closure of patent ductus arteriosus in preterm infants, Heart Lung **8**(2):308-310, 1979.

56. Stallones, Reuel: The rise and fall of ischemic heart disease, Sci. Am. **243**(5):53-59, 1980.

57. Stamler, Jeremiah, and others: Coronary proneness and approaches to preventing heart attacks, Am. J. Nurs. **66**(8):1788-1793, 1966.

58. Standards and guidelines for cardiopulmonary resuscitation and emergency cardiac care, J.A.M.A. **244**(5):453-509, 1980.

59. Stream, Patricia: Bone marrow transplantation: an option for children with acute leukemia, Ca. Nurs. **3**(3):195-199, 1980.

60. Tenczynski, Janie: Leukopheresis: the process, Am. J. Nurs. **77**(7):1133-1134, 1977.

61. Thorpe, Constance: A nursing care plan—the adult cardiac surgery patient, Heart Lung **8**(4): 690, 1979.

62. Walker, Patricia: Bone marrow transplant: a second chance for life, Nursing 77 **7**(1):24-25, 1977.

63. Ward, Graham, and others: Treating and counseling the hypertensive patient, Am. J. Nurs. **78**(5):824-828, 1978.

64. Winslow, Elizabeth Hahn, and Weber, Terese: Rehabilitation of the cardiac patient, progressive exercise to combat the hazards of bed rest, Am. J. Nurs. **80**(3):440, 1980.

65. Zimmerman, Susan, and others: Bone marrow transplantation, Am. J. Nurs. **77**(8):1311-1315, 1977.

Additional readings

Abels, Linda: Mosby's manual of critical care, St. Louis, 1979, The C.V. Mosby Co.

Abramson, Harold, editor: Resuscitation of the newborn infant, St. Louis, 1973, The C.V. Mosby Co.

American Heart Association: Heartbook, a guide to prevention and treatment of cardiovascular diseases, New York, 1980, E.P. Dulton.

Arbeit, Sidney, and others: Recognizing digitalis toxicity, Am. J. Nurs. **77**(12):1936-1945, 1977.

August-Miller, Susan: Dealing with sudden death: the survivors, Crit. Care Q. **1**(1):71-77, 1978.

Aure, Beverly: Intrauterine transfusions, the nurse's role with expectant parents, Nurs. Clin. North Am. **7**(4):817-826, 1972.

Bivalec, Lorraine, and Berkman, Joanne: Care by parent, Nurs. Clin. North Am. **11**:109-113, 1976.

Buickus, Barbara: Administering blood components, Am. J. Nurs. **79**(5):937-941, 1979.

Cain, Rebecca, and others: Variant angina: a nursing approach, Heart Lung **8**(6):1122-1125, 1979.

Clapp, Mary Jo: Psychosocial reactions of children with cancer, Nurs. Clin. North Am. **11**:73-82, 1976.

Cullins, Laura: Preventing and treating transfusion reactions, Am. J. Nurs. **79**(5):935-936, 1979.

Daly, Catherine R., and Kelly, Elizabeth: Prevention of pulmonary embolism: intracaval devices, Am. J. Nurs. **72**(11):2004-2006, 1972.

Davis, Julian, and others: Current treatment of sickle cell disease, Curr. Prob. Pediatr. **10**(12):1980.

DeHoff, Janet L.: What you should know about interpreting cardiac enzyme studies, Nursing 76 **6**(9):69-70, 1976.

Desotell, Susan: A brighter future for leukemia patients, Nursing 77 **7**(1):19-24, 1977.

Dracup, Kathleen, and others: The physiologic bases for combined nitroprusside-dopamine therapy in postmyocardial infarction heart failure, Heart Lung **10**(1):114-120, 1981.

Fagan-Dubin, Linda: Atherosclerosis: a major cause of peripheral vascular disease, Nurs. Clin. North Am. **12**(1):101-108, 1977.

Fenn, John: Reconstructive arterial surgery, Nurs. Clin. North Am. **12**(1):129-142, 1977.

Fergusson, Jean: Late psychologic effects of a serious illness in childhood, Nurs. Clin. North Am. **11**:83-93, 1976.

Foley, Genevieve, and McCarthy, Ann Marie: The child with leukemia: in a special hematology clinic, Am. J. Nurs. **76**(7):115-119, 1976.

Franciosa, Joseph: Nitroglycerin and nitrates in congestive heart failure, Heart Lung **9**(5):873, 1980.

Frantz, Angelina: Keeping up with automatic rotating tourniquets, Nursing 78 **8**(4):31-35, 1978.

Fuller, Ellen: The effect of antianginal drugs on myocardial oxygen consumption, Am. J. Nurs. **80**(2):250, 1980.

Gildea, Joan, and others: Congenital cardiac defects, pre- and postoperative nursing care, Am. J. Nurs. **78**(2):273-278, 1978.

Greene, Trish: Current therapy for acute leukemia in childhood, Nurs. Clin. North Am. **11**(1):3-19, 1976.

Greenfield, Diane, and others: Children can have high blood pressure, too, Am. J. Nurs. **76**:770-772, 1976.

Gyuldy, Jo-Eileen: Care of the dying child, Nurs. Clin. North Am. **11**:95-107, 1976.

Haughey, Brenda: CVP lines: monitoring and maintaining, Am. J. Nurs. **78**(4):635-638, 1978.

Hill, Martha: Helping the hypertensive patient control sodium intake, Am. J. Nurs. **79**(5):906-909, 1979.

Hirsch, Ann: Postmyocardial infarction syndrome, Am. J. Nurs. **79**(7):1240-1241, 1979.

Houser, Doris: What to do first when a patient complains of chest pain, Nursing 76 **6**(11):54-56, 1976.

Hultgren, Herbert N., and others: Clinical evaluation of a new computerized arrhythmia monitoring system, Heart Lung **4**(2):241-251, 1975.

Kapoor, Amar, and Dang, N.S.: Reliance on physical signs in acute myocardial infarction and its complications, Heart Lung, **7**(6):1020-1025, 1978.

Keaveny, Mary Ellen, and Wiley, Loy: Hodgkin's disease: the curable cancer, Nursing 75 **5**(3):48-54, 1975.

Koch, Janice: Code pink: a system for neonatal resuscitation, J. Obstet. Gynecol. Neonatal Nurs. **7** (5):49-53, 1978.

Lancour, Jane: How to avoid pitfalls in measuring blood pressure, Am. J. Nurs. **76**:773-775, 1976.

Lavin, Mary Ann: Bed exercises for acute cardiac patients, Am. J. Nurs. **73**(7):1226-1227, 1973.

LeBlanc, Dona: People with hodgkin's disease: the nursing challenge, Nurs. Clin. North Am. **13**(2):281-300, 1978.

Lieberman, Ellen: Blood pressure and primary hypertension in childhood and adolescence, Curr. Prob. Pediatr. **10**(4):1980.

Long, Gail: Managing the patient with abdominal aortic aneurysm, Nursing 78 **8**(8):21-27, 1978.

Martinson, Ida: The child with leukemia: parents help each other, Am. J. Nurs. **76**(7):1120-1122, 1976.

Mattea, Judith, and Mattea, Edward: Lidocaine and procainamide toxicity during treatment of ventricular arrhythmias, Am. J. Nurs. **76**(9):1429-1430, 1976.

Mechner, Francis: Patient assessment: examination of the heart and great vessels, Pt. I. Am. J. Nurs. **76**(11):1, 24, 1976.

Melker, Richard: CPR in neonates, infants and children, Crit. Care Q. **1**:49-65, 1978.

Miller, Karen: Assessing peripheral perfusion, Am. J. Nurs. **78**(10):1673, Oct. 1978.

Miller, William: Minimizing the risks of adult heart disease, Pediatr. Nurs. **5**(1):B-D, 1979.

Moore, Karen, and Maschak, Barbara: How patient education can reduce the risks of anticoagulation, Nursing 77 **7**(9):24-29, 1977.

Moore, Susan: Pericarditis after acute myocardial infarction: manifestations and nursing implications, Heart Lung **8**(3):551-558, 1979.

Moser, Marvin: Hypertension, how therapy works, Am. J. Nurs. **80**(5):937-941, 1980.

Murray, Jay, and others: CVP monitoring, side-stepping potential perils, Nursing 79 **7**(1):43-47, 1977.

Nauright, Lynda: Identifying hypertensive adolescents, Pediatr. Nurs. **5**(2):34, 1979.

O'Brian, Bonnie, and Woods, Susan: The paradox of DIC, Am. J. Nurs. **78**(11):1878, 1978.

Peoples-Verga, Carolyn: Get into hypertension to improve patient compliance, Nursing 76 **6**(10):32-35, 1976.

Pochedly, Carl: Acute lymphoid leukemia in children, Am. J. Nurs. **78**(10):1714, 1978.

Sexton, Dorothy: The patient with peripheral arterial occlusive disease, Nurs. Clin. North Am. **12**(1):89-99, 1977.

Shearer, JoAnne, and Caldwell, Mary: Use of sodium nitroprusside and dopamine hydrochloride in the postoperative cardiac patient, Heart Lung **8**(2):302-309, 1979.

Shor, Vivian: Congenital cardiac defects, assessment and case finding, Am. J. Nurs. **78**(2):256-261, 1978.

Sivarajan, Erika, and Halpenny, C. Jean: Exercise testing, Am. J. Nurs. **79**(12):2162-2170, 1979.

Smith, Raw: Invasive pressure monitoring, Am. J. Nurs. **78**(9):1514-1521, 1978.

Stephenson, Hugh E., editor: Immediate care of the acutely ill and injured, St. Louis, 1974, The C.V. Mosby Co.

Strong, Arlene: Caring for cardiac catheterization patients, Nursing 77 **7**(11):60-64, 1977.

Stuart, Eileen, and others: Nursing rounds: care of the patient with a mitral commissurotomy, Am. J. Nurs. **80**(9):1611, 1980.

Tanner, Gloria: Heart failure in the MI patient, Am. J. Nurs. **77**(2):230-234, 1977.

Webb, Watts, and Brunswick, Richard: Management of acute dissections of the aorta, Heart Lung **9**(2):284, 1979.

Wollnik, Lorraine: Management of the child with cancer on an outpatient basis, Nurs. Clin. North Am. **11**:35-48, 1976.

Woske, Martha, and Kratzer, Joan: Cardiac teaching: Preparing the patient for a different life, Nursing 77 **7**(5):25-26, 1977.

Ziesche, Susan, and Franciosa, Joseph: Clinical applications of sodium nitroprusside, Heart Lung **6**(1):99-103, 1977.

NURSING PROCESS

for clients with common health problems of the

21 Respiratory system

Assessment

Data analysis

Planning

Implementation

Evaluation

Common health problems affecting the respiratory system are common across the life span. Although infections account for many of the health problems, other factors such as trauma and environment may also be responsible. Regardless of the source, each may have an effect on the ability of the client to meet oxygen needs, the degree of which depends on the extent of the involvement. This chapter presents information about some of the common health problems affecting the respiratory system in children and adults. Information is presented about assessment and about strategies that can be used for planning and implementing care. Such strategies are useful in helping the client promote, maintain, and restore health. Information related to evaluating a care plan for common respiratory problems is also presented.

Overview of the respiratory system

All cells of the body require an adequate and continuous supply of oxygen. For the body to receive adequate and continuous oxygen, certain factors are necessary:

1. The respiratory center in the brain must be active and responsive to blood-gas concentrations.
2. The nerve pathways must be intact so that stimuli may be transmitted from the brain to the respiratory muscles.
3. The respiratory muscles must function properly.
4. The airway must be patent so that oxygen can be delivered to the cells and carbon dioxide can be removed.
5. The alveoli must be able to expand.
6. The capillary bed must be adequate to enhance diffusion.
7. There must be an adequate supply of oxygen within the atmosphere.
8. The hemoglobin must be adequate to carry oxygen to the cells.
9. The cardiovascular system must be intact so that blood can be circulated to all tissues of the body.

Respiration is the process by which the cells receive the oxygen supply for cellular metabolism and remove carbon dioxide, a metabolic waste. The process includes *ventilation,* the delivery of atmospheric air (inspiration) to the alveoli, and the removal of gas (expiration) after it has given up oxygen and received carbon dioxide; *diffusion,* the movement of oxygen across the alveolar membrane and capillary wall into the blood, and diffusion of carbon dioxide in the opposite direction; and *circulation;* the transport of oxygen and carbon dioxide in the blood and body fluids to the body cells, where oxygen is taken up and carbon dioxide given off.

The continuous process of respiration is accomplished through the integrated function of the upper and lower respiratory tracts, which begin at the nose and ends at the alveolar surface. The upper tract (which comprises the nose, pharynx, larynx, and upper part of the trachea) helps filter, warm, and humidify the air before it reaches the alveoli (gas-exchanging units) within the lung. For example, air is filtered of dust, bacteria, and other tiny particles as it passes through the nasal and oral cavities, pharynx, and larynx to the tracheobronchial tree. The bony structures and the rich blood supply of these passages condition the air to body temperature as it passes through.

The lower tract begins at the lower end of the trachea (carina) and extends to the alveoli, thus consisting of the lower end of the trachea, bronchi, bronchioles, and the alveoli in the lungs. As air passes through these structures, various protective defenses are mobilized. The tracheobronchial tree contains numerous goblet cells and cilia. The mucinous secretions from these cells moisten the inspired air and prevent drying of the delicate structures. The cilia, by their wavelike motions, facilitate removal of the foreign particles by propelling these particles and mucus upward into the bronchioles and trachea, where they are expelled by the action of the cough reflex. The lymphocytes and macrophage cells are essential for cleansing the deeper surfaces of foreign particles. These cells accomplish this function by moving particles to the upper passages or into the lymph nodes of the lung, where filtering takes place.

CONTROL AND REGULATION OF RESPIRATION

The respiratory center is composed of neurons that are located in the cerebral cortex, pons, medulla, and hypothalamus. The cerebral cortex is responsible for voluntary breathing acts, whereas the pons and medulla are responsible for involuntary breathing. The pons and medulla are composed of neurons that induce inspiration and expiration. All respiratory center activity is transmitted to the medulla; therefore, it is classified as the primary respiratory center. The higher centers (cerebral cortex and hypothalamus) modify the discharge of the medullary neurons. The peripheral and central chemoreceptors and afferent impulses from the lungs also modify the medullary neurons. The medullary center affects the muscles of respiration by means of the phrenic and thoracic nerves, which innervate these muscles. This complex series of events controls the rate and depth of breathing and, as a result, influences overall alveolar ventilation.

Peripheral and *central chemoreceptors* are collections of specialized cells located at the bifurcation of the common carotid artery (carotid body) and near the arch of the aorta (aortic body). The most potent stimulus for peripheral chemoreceptors is hypercapnia with hypoxemia. A Pa_{CO_2} above 40 mm Hg and Pa_{O_2} below 60 mm Hg will stimulate them. When the chemoreceptors are stimulated, respirations increase in rate and depth, which results in an increase in alveolar gas exchange. Factors such as acidosis, hyperglycemia, decreased cardiac output, and increased body temperature influence these receptors, but to a lesser degree. Central chemoreceptors are more sensitive to Pa_{CO_2} than are peripheral receptors.[24]

The *pneumotaxic* center is located in the pons and is responsible, along with the medulla, for giving rhythmic quality to respirations.

The *Hering-Breuer* reflex is a pulmonary reflex that helps control respiration by affecting the depth of breathing. The receptors involved are probably located in the bronchi and bronchioles. On inspiration, the lungs inflate and the reflex is stimulated, which in turn activates the inspiratory center and inhibits the lung from expanding further.

Assessment

NURSING HISTORY

Health history

The nursing history should include information about the client's health, development, social and psychological states.

The health history is particularly important. If the client has a specific problem, the following questions may be asked.

When did the problem develop? How did the problem start? Did it develop suddenly or over a long period of time? What has been done to obtain relief? What medications have been taken? Are nose drops frequently used? (Gives information about aspiration potential.)

Did other symptoms accompany the problem? For example, vomiting? Did the client have loss of appetite? Has the client been easily fatigued? Has there been weight loss? Fever? Chills? Sweating? Night sweats? Shortness of breath?

Has anyone in the family recently had an upper respiratory tract infection? Has there been exposure to tuberculosis? How many respiratory tract infections (colds, flu) are experienced per year? Are there any known allergies? Is there a family history of cancer or chronic lung disease? When was the last tuberculin test? What was the reaction?

Nursing process for common health problems

A number of symptoms may be experienced in relation to a problem affecting the respiratory system. The nurse should make specific assessments in relation to these in an effort to formulate a plan of care. Some of these symptoms include dyspnea, chest pain, cyanosis, voice quality, stridor, cough, and the presence of secretions. Data obtained about each of these can be enhanced by keen observation and listening.

Dyspnea. Dyspnea, a subjective symptom in which breathing requires excessive effort, is often experienced. It is indicative of a discrepancy between the need for ventilation and the ability to meet that need.[32] Descriptions that may be given by the client to describe dyspnea are "shortness of breath," "tightness," and "can't get my breath." Assessment gives information about the extent and severity of the difficulty. Specific assessments that should be made in relation to the dyspnea include: activity, time of day, duration, posture and onset.

> *Activity:* It is necessary to assess whether it occurs more often at rest or during or after activity. If the dyspnea occurs during activity, the type of activity should be noted. For example, does it occur while the client is engaging in activities of daily living (dressing, bathing, or eating)? Specifically how does it affect activities of daily living? Does it occur while walking on level ground or while climbing stairs? How many steps? Does the child experience dyspnea during vigorous play?
>
> *Time of day:* Is it nocturnal, or does the client have paroxysmal nocturnal dyspnea?
>
> *Duration:* Does it tend to persist, or is it short term?
>
> *Posture:* What position does the client assume? Is the client orthopneic? Children with severe orthopnea and dyspnea tend to sit cross-legged leaning forward over a couple of pillows or bed tables.
>
> *Onset:* Did it occur suddenly, or over a period of time?

The nurse should also assess for other symptoms and behaviors. Does a cough or diaphoresis accompany the dyspnea? Is there a change in the color of the skin? What are the pulse and respiratory rates? What behaviors are exhibited during or after an attack? Is the client anxious, restless, fidgety, or confused? These may indicate a reduction in oxygenation to the brain. Is there nasal flaring? Nasal flaring is an indication of air hunger. What measures does the client employ to obtain relief?

Chest pain. When the nurse collects data regarding chest pain, information should be obtained about the following:

> *Onset, location, and radiation:* Did it occur suddenly? Is it generalized or localized? Does it radiate?
>
> *Duration and character, or quality:* Is the pain scratchy, or is it dull, sharp, or stabbing? In what phase of ventilation is the pain felt, inspiration or expiration? Is it worse on inspiration or expiration?
>
> *Frequency:* How often is the pain felt?
>
> *Factors that precipitate or relieve the pain:* Is it worse on coughing? Is the pain relieved when a certain position is maintained?
>
> *Effects of the pain on activity:* What is the relationship of the pain to eating, swallowing, exertion, rest?

Cyanosis. Cyanosis, a bluish discoloration of the skin and mucus membranes, occurs when a reduced level of hemoglobin is present in the blood. Because the hemoglobin must be reduced in excess of 5 g/100 ml,[44] it is not a reliable sign of the state of oxygenation. Second, it is a subjective assessment that depends on factors such as thickness of skin, lighting, pigmentation and the observer's perception,[32] and activity. An awareness of these guidelines is essential as cyanosis is assessed. It indicates a disturbance in gas exchange between alveolar air and pulmonary capillary blood.

In making assessments of cyanosis, the nurse should observe skin areas that are thin, unpigmented, and where capillaries are superficial and numerous: for example, the tip of the tongue, buccal mucosa, cutaneous surfaces of the lips, tips of fingers and toes, nail beds, earlobes, and tip of nose. The skin of the newborn is thin; therefore cyanosis may occur readily, particularly in areas that are highly vascular, such as the heels. *Peripheral cyanosis,* or cyanosis of the tip of the nose or ears, is normal in the newborn. In adults it might be evident when there is diminished blood flow to these parts, as when they are cold. To adequately evaluate cyanosis, consideration should be given to factors such as lighting, activity, condition of the environment, duration, and distribution. Adequate lighting should be available as this assessment is made. Natural light is best. The use of fluorescent light may make "normal colored" skin appear cyanotic.

Activity and environment: Infants should be inspected when they are quiet or sleeping in a warm environment. Determine whether or not emotional or physical factors precipitate cyanosis. Does the color become worse when coughing or crying? Does cyanosis occur when the client assumes a certain position? Does it occur after activity?

Duration: Is it transient or does it persist?

Distribution: Is there discoloration of the conjunctiva or mucous membranes of the mouth, or is it limited to the extremities? The former is indicative of a central type of cyanosis, whereas the latter is a peripheral type that results from blood stasis.

Voice quality: Does the client speak in short, jerky sentences? Is vocalization limited? Are sounds weak? Does the speech have a nasal quality? Is hoarseness present?

Stridor. Stridor, a harsh, high-pitched sound, is associated with an obstruction about the larynx.

General assessment: When was the noisy breathing first heard? Assessments should be made in regard to the timing of the stridor. Does it occur during inspiration, expiration, or both? Is the stridor accompanied by a normal voice quality? Is the stridor high pitched or low pitched? Does dyspnea or coughing accompany it? Does posture affect the sound? If so, does it affect the sound more or less?

Pediatric assessment: Assessments should be made as to what the child was doing before the sound was first heard. Was he playing with a small object? Was he playing with a toy? If so, is the toy missing any parts? Was he eating?

These assessments are valuable in helping the physician establish a diagnosis.

Nursing process for common health problems

Cough. A cough is a reflex mechanism that facilitates the removal of foreign material from the bronchi and secretions from the lungs. The physiological mechanism responsible for a cough is a deep inspiration followed by momentary closure of the glottis and a sudden explosive expiration. The mechanism is aided by maximal contraction of the muscles of expiration. The purpose of this is to produce high-velocity air flow through the airways to propel mucus or foreign material out of the system. Coughing is relatively rare in the newborn. The character and severity of the cough depend on a number of factors: the disease process; the amount of mucus, fluid, or foreign material; and the part of the respiratory system involved.

In assessing this symptom, the nurse should determine the frequency, duration, type, and circumstances related to the cough.

Frequency and duration: Is there persistent throat clearing? Is the cough paroxysmal or persistent? Is it exhausting?

Type: Is it productive or nonproductive? Is it a hacking, dry, or bubbly cough? The latter type of cough is indicative of stimulation from the lower respiratory tract. Is it throaty, barking, or hoarse? A cough of this nature indicates involvement of the larynx and pharynx. Is it voluntarily induced?

Circumstances and activities: Is the cough worse after eating, walking, or being treated? What about the occurrence of the cough? Does it occur most often on rising, during the day, or at night? Is it associated with fear or discomfort? Does it occur when the client assumes a certain position?

Secretions. Other pertinent assessments that require observation include whether the client breathes through his mouth or nose or the presence or absence of secretions. If present, the nurse should determine the type, color, consistency or viscosity, amount and odor.

Type: Is it purulent or mucoid? Purulent secretions indicate some type of infection. Mucoid secretion is caused by oversecretion of bronchial mucus, as may occur in asthma and bronchitis.

Color: Is it blood tinged *(hemoptysis)?* Certain medications (such as those containing catecholamines) produce pink secretions that resembles blood-tinged secretions of pulmonary edema. The nurse should therefore validate whether the client has taken medications that may have altered the color of the secretions. If hemoptysis is present, is the secretion streaked with blood, or is it grossly bloody? Is it bright red or dark? Does it accompany coughing? How long has the client experienced the symptom?

Consistency or *viscosity:* Is it thin, tenacious, stringy, or frothy?

Amount: Is the amount small, moderate, or copious? Does it separate into layers after standing? As closely as possible, estimation of the amount should be given in milliliters.

Odor: Is there an odor present? If so, is it fruity or foul?

Developmental history

Neonate. The respiratory system in the neonate is immature. This particularly accounts for the rapid, shallow breathing. In a resting state the normal respirations are synchronous and range from 35 to 60 per minute, with a slight irregular rhythm or pattern that is largely diaphragmatic. The infant breathes through his nose and tolerates mouth breathing very poorly.

The dimensions of the respiratory structures and three of the four sinuses (ethmoid, sphenoid, and maxillary) are small and gradually increase throughout the stages of development. The number of alveoli in proportion to body size is approximately one tenth of the alveoli in the adult. The neonate has an excessive amount of hemoglobin to allow more oxygen to be carried per unit of blood, and a greater uptake of oxygen from the lungs.

Infant. The respiratory center of the infant is more developed, and as a result the respirations become more regular and are nondiaphragmatic. This pattern continues until the early school-age period. The respiratory rate decreases to about 44 breaths per minute. It is not uncommon to hear a young infant grunt during breathing, especially while asleep. Such pattern is thought to be caused by vibrations of air passing over the soft palate while breathing. This grunting should not be confused with grunting experienced in respiratory distress syn-

TABLE 21-1

Anatomical and physiological considerations of the pediatric respiratory system

Anatomy and physiology	Significance	Age anatomy matures
Immature thermostatic control Large body surface	↓ Ability to adjust to temperature changes	6 Months to 1 year
Decreased subcutaneous fat	↓Ability to maintain temperature T↓ 36.5 C causing ↑ metabolic rate, ↑ oxygen consumption and metabolic acidosis	
Low cardiac stroke volume High cardiac rate	↑Rate doubles cardiac output (twice that of an adult) to meet needs for ↑ metabolic rate	After 6-8 years
Small length and diameter of airway	Predisposition to obstruction, infection, and atelectasis	Resolves with age and growth
Large head, short neck, soft larynx and weak shoulder girdle	Predisposition to upper airway obstruction by position alone Rationale for neutral head position with roll under shoulders for maintaining airway patency during CPR	2 Years
Narrow nasal bridge, obligate nasal breathers	Predisposition to nasal obstruction by foreign body, trauma, or surgery with significant airway compromise	6 Months
Large tongue	↑Likelihood of airway occlusion	2 Years
Large, U-shaped epiglottis	↑Sensitivity to edema, trauma, and infection ↑End expiratory pressure during respiratory failure	2 Years
Cricoid cartilage most narrow aspect of trachea causing funnel shape	↑Susceptibility to trauma, edema, and infection 1 mm of edema can compromise airway 75%*	Varies with age and growth
Active lymph tissue	Infection and edema can cause occlusion of upper airway	Active—6 year atrophy after 12 years
Diaphragm, primary muscle in respiration	Resulting large negative pressure Abdominal contents can compromise diaphragmatic movement	4 to 5 Years
Immature development of intercostal and abdominal muscles	These muscles cannot be relied upon for respiratory effort Infant compensates with ↑ in respiratory rate	Transition from abdominal to costal breathing at 2 to 3 years; completed by 7 years
Right and left mainstem bronchi at 55-degree angles	Intubation of either mainstem bronchus equally possible High risk of bilateral aspiration	1 to 2 Years
Immature bronchial muscle	↓Potential for bronchospasm	2 to 3 Years
Bronchioles large in diameter and length	Bronchioles constrict and shorten on expiration, collect mucus	Matures with age and growth
Immature alveolar system causing ↓ number of alveoli and ↓ surface area	↓Diffusion ↑Shunting	8 Years
Lung compliance relative to body weight	Pressure requirements for ventilation equal adult requirements	

From Crowley, Constance M., and Morrow, Alice I.: A comprehensive approach to the child in respiratory failure, Crit. Care Q. **3:**27-43, June 1980.
*Mellins, R., Chernick, V., Doershuk, C., and others: Respiratory care in infants and children. New York, American Lung Association, 1971, p. 3.

drome, which occurs when the child expires against a closed glottis. Breath sounds in the infant are loud and harsh because the sounds of the tracheobronchial tree are transmitted through less tissue. As the infant grows, the number and size of the alveoli continue to increase.

Child. The respiratory center continually matures. By the time the child is 5 years of age, the rate becomes approximately 20 to 25 respirations per minute. It remains relatively stable until the early adolescent period. Respirations are characteristically costal. About 8 years of age, the number of alveoli present equals that of the adult. The frontal sinuses are developed about this age period because the skull has grown large enough to allow space for them (Table 21-1).

Adolescent. The respiratory rate decreases to a normal standard of 17 to 22 breaths per minute between the ages of 10 to 14 and to 15 to 20 around the fifteenth year of life, at which age it remains stable. Metabolism increases because of the growth spurt during this period, and therefore more oxygen is needed to meet the energy needs of the body. The sphenoid sinus fully develops after this age period.

Adult. A rate of 15 to 20 respirations per minute is established during early adulthood. All the respiratory structures reach their adult size.

Older adult. During later maturity, characteristic changes are noted in the character of the thorax and other respiratory structures. The thorax becomes stiffer, and the lungs become less elastic; thus expansion of the rib cage is limited, and the lungs are poorly aerated. Metabolism also decreases. As a result, the residual volume increases, and the vital capacity decreases, resulting in an alteration in the diffusion mechanism of the lungs.

Social history

When information about the social history is obtained, it is essential to obtain data about smoking, occupation, and environmental factors, because each may have an effect on the client's health.

Smoking data. Whether the client smokes or has stopped smoking, data should be obtained about the type, duration, frequency, amount, and whether or not client inhaled the smoke (Table 21-2). Because of the effect of sidestream smoke on the nonsmoker, the nurse should inquire whether there is close proximity or frequent contact with smokers in closed or poorly ventilated rooms. Sidestream smoke has been documented to be hazardous to health (see Chapter 4).

TABLE 21-2
Smoking data

	Presently smokes	Previously smoked
Type	What does client smoke? Cigarette? Cigar? Pipe?	What did client smoke? Cigarette? Cigar? Pipe?
Duration	How long has client smoked? At what age did client start smoking? Has client ever stopped smoking? For what period of time? When did client stop? Why did client stop? If smoking has been resumed, why?	How long has it been since client smoked? How long did client smoke: Months? Years? Why did client stop?
Amount	How many cigarettes does client smoke per day?	How many cigarettes per day did client smoke?
Frequency	Is client a chain smoker?	Was client a chain smoker?
Inhalation	Does client inhale?	Did client inhale?

Occupational data. In obtaining data about the occupation, questions such as type of occupation and whether there is or has been exposure to irritating substances on the job, such as dust, fumes, chemicals, vapor, and if so, the duration of exposure. Information about exposure to radiation, cotton, coal, and asbestos is also helpful.

Environmental data. Inquire whether the client lives in a highly polluted area. Ask if there is adequate humidification in the home.

Psychological history

The psychological history should include information about (1) the client's attitude toward his illness, (2) the effect the illness has on the life-style (for example, has it been necessary to make changes in the life-style?), (3) feelings about the illness and therapy, and (4) attitudes of family toward the illness and therapy. Such information can be useful as the nursing care plan is developed.

Physical assessment

Physical assessments of the chest give the nurse an opportunity to establish baseline information as well as provide a framework for detecting any changes that might occur in a client's condition. These parameters include *inspection, palpation, percussion,* and *auscultation.*

Inspection. Inspection, or visual observation, is the first step in performing respiratory assessment. (Palpation during inspection is common.)

The nurse should first assess the shape of the client's chest, observing its anteroposterior diameter. A comparison should be made of findings against the *normal* appearance of the chest (Fig. 21-1, *A* and *B*). The observation may reveal a *pigeon chest, barrel chest,* or *funnel chest* (Fig. 21-1, *C, D,* and *E*). Other changes (deformities) may also be evident; for example, kyphosis, scoliosis, and scars may be present and indicative of previous surgery.

Observing the lungs for *expansion* and *symmetry* is also essential. These assessments can best be made if the nurse places the palms of the hands against the client's chest at the area of the seventh rib. The thumbs should touch or nearly touch, and the fingers should be spread apart (Fig. 21-2). As the client inhales deeply, the chest will expand and the fingers will spread farther apart. As the assessment is made, compare movement of both sides. Do both sides expand at the same time? Do they expand equally? Both the anterior and pos-

FIG. 21-1
Normal and abnormal chest shapes. **A,** Normal infant. **B,** Normal adult. **C,** Barrel chest. **D,** Funnel chest (pectus excavatum). **E,** Pigeon chest (pectus carinatum).

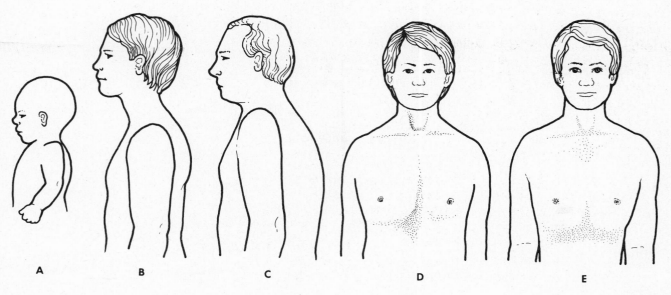

A   B   C   D   E

Nursing process for common health problems

terior chest should be observed. Pain and discomfort may be responsible for producing asymmetric movements.

Other assessments that can be made include the position of the trachea. Is it in the midline (which is normal), or is it deviated to one side or the other?

Assessing for *retractions* is also important. Retractions are seen most prominently in the lateral chest. They are indicative of abnormally labored breathing. If retractions are present, the nurse should note the type. Are they infraclavicular, supraclavicular, suprasternal, or intrasternal retractions? Fig. 21-3 presents a guide for observing retractions.

The rate, depth, rhythm, and character, or quality, of *respirations* must be assessed. All assessments must be made for at least 1 full minute. In assessing the *rate* of respirations, the nurse should observe whether the rate is normal (eupnea), realizing that the rate varies with age (Table 21-3 and Fig. 21-4), or if there are variations from normal: slow (bradypnea), rapid (tachypnea) (Fig. 21-5), or periods of cessation (apnea). Bradypnea exists when the rate per minute falls below 30 in infants, 20 in children, and 10 in adults; whereas tachypnea occurs when the rate per minute is over 50 in infants, 30 in children, and 20

FIG. 21-2
Position of hands for palpation of thoracic excursion.

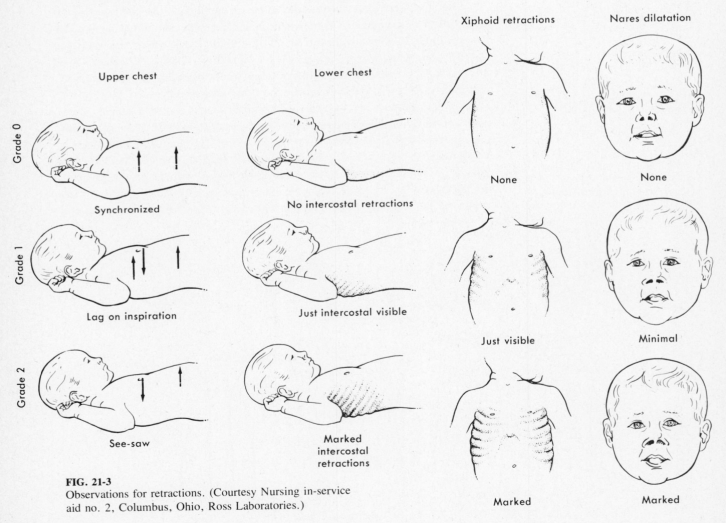

FIG. 21-3
Observations for retractions. (Courtesy Nursing in-service aid no. 2, Columbus, Ohio, Ross Laboratories.)

1238

TABLE 21-3
Respiratory rates at varied age
levels

Age	Average respiratory rate (per min)
Neonate	30-50
Infant (6 mo)	20-30
Early childhood (2 yr)	20-30
Later childhood (9-10 yr)	16-24
Adolescent	12-16
Adult	14-18

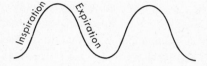

FIG. 21-4
Spirogram of normal respiration. (From
Glover, Dennis W., and Glover, Margaret McCarthy: Respiratory therapy:
basics for nursing and the allied health
professions, St. Louis, 1978, The C.V.
Mosby Co.)

in adults.[30] If apnea is present, it is important to assess whether the episodes are intermittent. Intermittent apnea is common in premature infants with central nervous system immaturity. Short periods of apnea are also considered normal in the neonatal period.

In inspecting the *depth,* the nurse should note whether the client's breathing is normal, deep, or shallow. Deep, gasping-type breathing is *hyperpnea* (hy-perventilation). Slow shallow breathing (hypoventilation) is diminished in depth (Fig. 21-6). It may be observed in clients with severe pain, those with broken ribs, those who are heavily sedated, and those who have copious secretions.

Assessments of the *rhythm* should include observation of the intervals of respirations. Are the respirations equally spaced or irregular? What is the ratio of inspiration to expiration? Normally, expiration is longer than inspiration. For example, the ratio is normally 1:2 or 1.5:2.[30] The neonate has a tendency to breathe irregularly. As a result, the nurse should note the persistence of the change in rhythm because this gives a better indication of respiratory difficulty. Patterns indicative of deviation from the normal breathing cycle (often a serious one) are *Biot's respirations* —irregular periods of apnea that are followed by several breaths that are even in rate and depth; *Cheyne-Stokes respirations,* which are characterized by periods of hyperpnea alternating with periods of apnea; and *Kussmaul* respirations—an increased depth of breathing (Fig. 21-7). It is necessary to observe the client over several minutes in order to make ac-curate assessments.

As assessments are made of the client's respirations, assessments must also be made of the *pulse rate* (rapid or slow) and of its *rhythm* (regular or irregu-

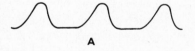

A   B

FIG. 21-5
Spirograms of **A,** bradypnea, and **B,** tachypnea. (From Glover, Dennis W., and Glover, Margaret McCarthy: Respiratory therapy:
basics for nursing and the allied health professions, St. Louis, 1978, The C.V. Mosby Co.)

FIG. 21-6
Spirograms of **A,** hyperventilation, and
B, hypoventilation. (From Glover, Dennis W., and Glover, Margaret McCarthy: Respiratory therapy: basics for
nursing and the allied health professions, St. Louis, 1978, The C.V.
Mosby Co.)

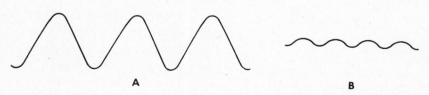

A   B

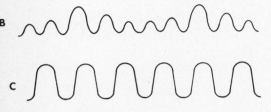

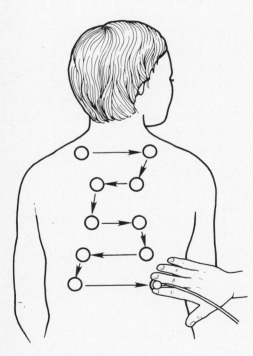

FIG. 21-7
Spirograms of abnormal breathing patterns. **A,** Biot's respirations. **B,** Cheyne-Stokes respirations. **C,** Kussmaul's respirations. (From Glover, Dennis W., and Glover, Margaret McCarthy: Respiratory therapy: basics for nursing and the allied health professions, St. Louis, 1978, The C.V. Mosby Co.)

FIG. 21-8
Sequence for auscultation of posterior thorax with a stethoscope (note technique for holding the stethoscope).

Nursing process for common health problems

lar) and *volume* (weak or strong). Normally the ratio of respiratory rate and pulse rate is 1:4. The pulse rate is an objective way of monitoring airway patency as well as determining the degree of hypoxia. An increase in pulse rate is one indication of the body's attempt to compensate for hypoxia.

The *character* or *quality* of respiratory and abdominal movements must be observed. Are the movements abdominal or diaphragmatic, costal or thoracic? Respiratory movements are more diaphragmatic in neonates and men and more costal in women. The diaphragmatic breathing in the neonate is largely the result of the weak intercostal muscles. Abdominal movements predominate in infancy, and the transition to costal respirations is gradual until about age 7. Costal breathing movements predominate in adults. The nurse must also assess whether accessory *muscles* such as the sternocleidomastoid and platysma muscles are being used during respiration.

Types of breathing patterns

abdominal, or diaphragmatic, breathing Occurs when the abdomen protrudes on inspiration, and movement of the chest wall is insignificant. (This type breathing is often seen in clients with pleurisy and upper thoracic injuries.)

thoracic, or costal, breathing Occurs when movement of the chest dominates. (It is commonly seen in clients with gastric distension, abdominal pain, and paralysis.)

paradoxic breathing Occurs when the chest wall on one side moves in the opposite direction. (This type breathing is common in clients with flail chest injuries.)

Palpation. Palpation is the next step in respiratory assessment. It delineates pain, masses, pulsations, or thrills of the thorax. To delineate pain, it is always best to start away from the area where the client states the pain is felt and palpate toward the area. In this way the specific pain area can be more accurately pinpointed. Such information is helpful for documentation in the record and for reporting to the physician.

Since *vibrations* of sounds are transmitted to the wall of the chest, they can be palpated. Such transmission is referred to as *vocal fremitus*. To palpate vocal fremitus, the examiner, in sequence, places the palmar surface of the fingers over specific areas of the chest the same manner as for assessing expansion. The nurse starts at the top of the chest slowly, moves downward and instructs the client to repeat "99" or some other phrase. A comparison is made of the findings on either side. In men, vocal fremitus is more palpable because male voices have a lower pitch than female voices. It is also palpated more easily in thin persons. Decreased vocal fremitus is indicative of total airway obstruction and the presence of fluid or air in the pleural space. Secretions in the lungs and any conditions that increase the density of the lungs (such as atelectasis, pneumonia) increase the fremitus.

Although assessments may be made with the client in the supine position, it is better to have the client maintain a sitting position. The hands should be warm.

Percussion. Percussion is the tapping of the surface of the chest wall to produce sound. *Resonance* is a normal "hollow" sound in lung percussion. Characteristically, it is low pitched and nonmusical in quality. The *tympanitic* sound is usually loud, musical, and long. This sound is the result of air in an enclosed area. *Dullness* occurs in areas of high density, as in lung consolida-

FIG. 21-9
Relationship of the lobes of the lungs to
the thorax: *1*, upper lobe; *2*, middle
lobe; *3*, lower lobe.

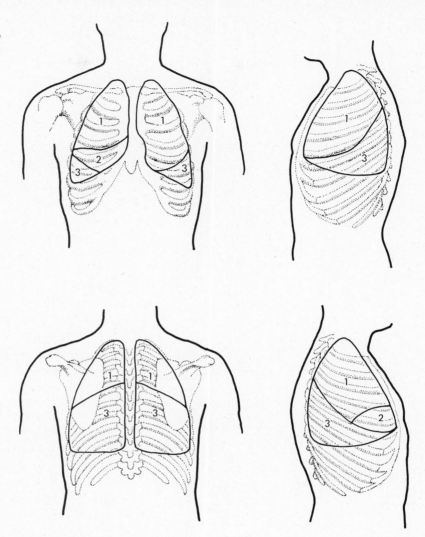

tion or pneumonia. *Flatness* is a short, nonmusical sound of high frequency
that is usually heard over solid organs and fluid, as in pleural effusion.

Auscultation. Auscultation involves listening to sounds within the chest.
With the diaphragm of the stethoscope pressed firmly (to decrease sound by skin
or hair rubbing against the diaphragm) against the chest wall, breath, voice,
and abnormal sounds can be heard on auscultation. The head of the stethoscope
should be warm. The client should be instructed to breathe slightly more deeply
than normal. The posterior chest should be examined first. It is best to use a
systematic approach beginning at the right scapular area and comparing the
sounds heard on this area with those of the left scapular area. All areas of the
lungs should be covered (Figs. 21-8 and 21-9). On completion of the examination of the posterior chest, auscultation should be repeated on the anterior
chest (Fig. 21-10). The environment should be quiet, and the client should assume an upright position, if possible. Rest periods should be provided as often
as necessary.

Assessment of breath sounds. Breath sounds are produced as air moves in
and out of the lungs. These are *normal* sounds and can be heard through the

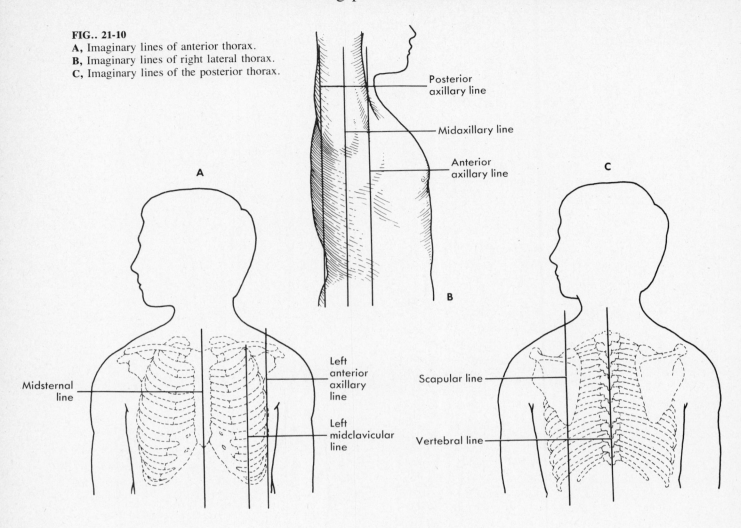

FIG.. 21-10
A, Imaginary lines of anterior thorax.
B, Imaginary lines of right lateral thorax.
C, Imaginary lines of the posterior thorax.

lung. There are three types of breath sounds: vesicular, bronchial, and broncho-vesicular. They should be evaluated as to pitch, intensity, quality, and duration. *Vesicular* breath sounds, heard over most of the lungs, are characteristically soft and low pitched (because of the increased distance from the main airway) and are heard *longer* during the inspiratory phase than the expiratory phase. The sound during expiration is nearly inaudible. In contrast, *bronchial* breath sounds are louder (high pitched) and have a coarser sound, that is, longer during expiration. There is a pause between inspiration and expiration. These sounds can be heard by placing the stethoscope over the trachea close to the suprasternal notch (Fig. 21-11, *A*). They are not heard over the normal lung. *Bronchovesicular* sounds are nearly equal in duration on inspiration and expiration. These sounds are best heard where bifurcations of the large airways occur (manubrium sterni and intrascapular regions) (Fig. 21-11, *B*). If bronchovesicular sounds are heard in other areas of the lung, they represent an abnormality. Fig. 21-12 shows diagrams of breath sounds.

Assessment of voice sounds. Following assessment of breath sounds, an assessment of voice sounds should be made. When voice sounds are auscultated,

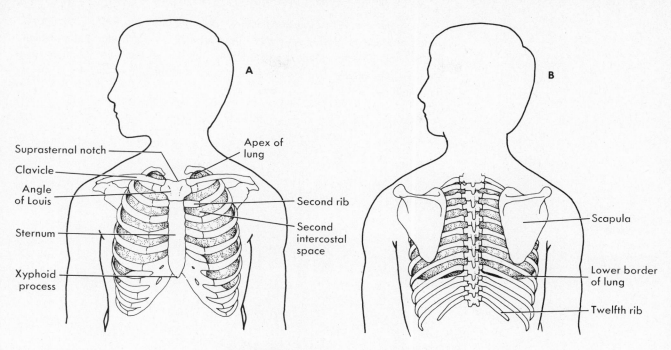

FIG. 21-11
Anatomical landmarks: **A,** anterior chest; **B,** posterior chest.

the client is asked to repeat "99" as the examiner listens to the chest. The intensity of the sounds will either increase or decrease depending on the nature of the chest. For example, the presence of fluid or air in the pleural space decreases the intensity, whereas consolidation in the tracheobronchial tree increases the voice sounds because sound transmission is improved. Terms used to describe voice sounds are *bronchophony* (clear and distinct sounds associated with consolidation), *pectoriloquy* (hearing syllables of whispered words), and *egophony* (hearing loud "eee" to "aaa" sounds with a nasal quality.) In the latter the client repeats "e," but the examiner hears an "a" sound during auscultation. Each of these is heard when the lung tissue is compressed or consolidated (such as over pleural effusion).

Assessment of adventitious sounds. Adventitious sounds are abnormal lung sounds that are superimposed on normal breath sounds. These sounds are produced as a result of secretions, exudates, or obstructions in the alveoli and tracheobronchial tree. Rales, rhonchi, and wheezes are common examples.

Rales, distinct, crackling or gurgling sounds, are most often heard during inspiration. Characteristically, they are disconnected sounds or vibrations that result from the bubbling of air through fluid. *Rhonchi* are musical sounds or vibrations that are heard continuously and are usually longer. *Wheezes* are continuous sounds that are usually heard during expiration but may be heard during any phase of respiration. The nurse should evaluate wheezing in relation to variables such as position and coughing. To help the nurse evaluate these variables, a number of questions may be raised. Does the wheeze occur when the client lies on one side but not the other? Does coughing accompany wheezing? (Wheezing that does not subside with coughing is suggestive of obstruction.)

Nursing process for common health problems

Another sound that can be heard on auscultation is the *pleural friction rub,* which produces a grating sound or vibration as the visceral and parietal pleura rub together. These sounds are heard when the two surfaces are inflamed, as in pleurisy. The pleural friction rub is associated with breathing and is not affected by coughing.

FIG. 21-12
Location, **A,** and characteristics, **B,** of breath sounds. (**B** from Malasanos, Lois, and others: Health assessment, ed. 2, St. Louis, 1981, The C.V. Mosby Co.)

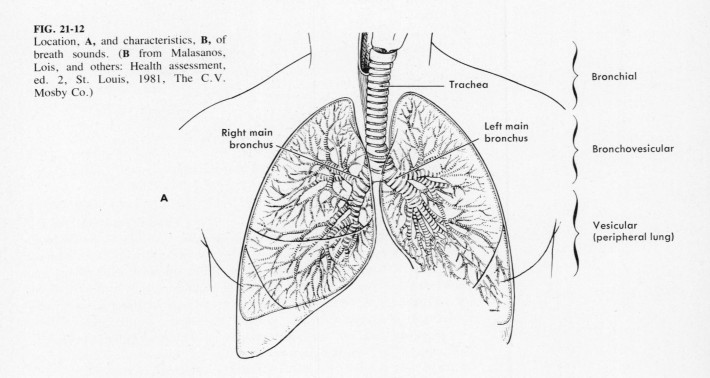

Sound	Duration of inspiration and expiration	Diagram of sound	Pitch	Intensity	Normal location	Abnormal location
Vesicular	Inspiration > expiration 5:2		Low	Soft	Peripheral lung	Not applicable
Broncho-vesicular	Inspiration = expiration 1:1		Moderate	Moderate	First and second intercostal spaces at the sternal border over major bronchi	Peripheral lung
Bronchial (tubular)	Inspiration < expiration		High	Loud	Over trachea	Lung area

DIAGNOSTIC ASSESSMENT

Diagnostic studies used to detect pulmonary diseases may include radiographic tests, direct visualization, biopsies, and laboratory studies (hematological, cytological, and bacteriological). Skin tests, pulmonary function studies, and bronchospirometry are also useful diagnostic tests.

The nurse has a major responsibility in preparing the client for the specific test. Inherent within this responsibility is knowing the purposes and procedural aspects of the tests. Before the examination, the nurse should explain the test to the client and inform him of his responsibilities during the test. Afterward, the client should be made as comfortable as possible and observed for reactions and possible complications.

Radiographic evaluations

Radiological studies are perhaps more common than other diagnostic tests. These are widely used for screening and diagnostic purposes and give evidence of lesions within the respiratory passages that cannot be detected on direct examination. Radiographic methods commonly used to detect respiratory diseases include chest x-ray films, tomography, fluoroscopy, angiography, bronchography, and sinus x-rays.

Routine chest x-ray films. Several views may be taken for routine examination of the chest: posteroanterior (PA), lateral, oblique, and lateral decubitus. In either view, the x-ray is taken following a deep inspiration and breath holding to prevent movement of the diaphragm. The *posteroanterior* and *lateral* views are commonly used to reveal information about the thoracic cavity. The lateral view is considered to be extremely important because it provides information about areas that are not evident on the PA view. If the client is ambulatory, he stands and leans his chest against the x-ray plate while the film is taken. Films may also be taken with the client in a sitting or lying position. The *oblique* view facilitates localizing a lesion and projecting it free from overlying bony structures or the heart. It may be made in either the right or left anterior or posterior position. Right or left *lateral decubitus* roentgenograms are obtained to demonstrate the fluid level in the chest, as in pleural effusion.

Often the hospitalized client is too ill to go to the radiology department for x-ray examination. In such instances, a portable x-ray unit is moved to the client's bedside. The plate is placed under his back, or in the desired position, and the film is taken.

Tomography. Tomography (planigraphy, laminography, or sectional radiography) is a technique used to demonstrate intrathoracic lesions (such as cavities, cysts, or calcifications) that are obscured by overlying structures. It demonstrates lesions that are poorly seen on routine chest x-ray films.

Fluoroscopy. Fluoroscopy is a radiological technique used to observe the motion of pulmonary and cardiac structures. Information can be obtained as to how the zones of the lungs behave during the respiratory cycle.

Pulmonary angiography. Pulmonary angiography involves the rapid injection of a radiopaque dye into the pulmonary circulation. It provides information about pulmonary vascular anatomy and is useful in determining the site of pulmonary embolism. One of two approaches may be used. More commonly, a catheter is inserted, with the use of a fluoroscope, through the venous system, through the chambers of the heart, and into the pulmonary artery via the right brachial vein. With the other approach, a catheter is inserted through the femoral venous system and the inferior vena cava into the pulmonary artery. A specified amount of radiopaque contrast medium is injected. The physician observes for two defects: a filling defect and a cut-off defect. The latter is an abrupt cessation of the radiopaque flow at the site of obstruction, whereas the former is the negative image made by the embolus in the stream of radiopaque material. Because most emboli are not totally occlusive, some radiopaque material passes around them and flows distally. Hence, the filling defects are more common. Cardiac dysrhythmias may occur as the catheter passes through the chambers of the heart.

Bronchography (bronchogram). Bronchography is a roentgenographic visualization of the size, shape, patency, and number of bronchi. An iodized liquid (such as Dionosil), which is opaque to x-rays, is used because the similarity in density of the bronchi and lung tissue prohibit visualization of the bronchial tree on routine chest x-ray films. Visualization may be limited to a part of a lung *(selective bronchography),* an entire lung, or both lungs.

The iodized liquid is instilled into the bronchial tubes and their branches by way of a catheter that has been passed through the nose into the bronchi. A laryngoscope is passed through the pharynx, larynx, and trachea by way of the mouth. During the examination, the client assumes various positions to facilitate passage of the liquid into the bronchi. X-ray films are taken as the client assumes the varied positions.

Bronchography can be performed under either general or topical anesthesia. In children, it is usually done under general anesthesia. Preparation for bronchography includes withholding foods and fluids for 6 to 8 hours before the examination. For children, water may be withheld only 4 hours before the procedure to avoid dehydration. Premedication with a sedative and atropine are usually prescribed to relax the client and dry up secretions, respectively.

Oral hygiene should be provided and dentures should be removed. Coughing and deep breathing should also be encouraged.

To prevent coughing and gagging during passage of the tube, a local anesthetic is sprayed into the pharynx, larynx, and trachea. The client's color, pulse, and respirations should be monitored closely. After the examination the client should be given nothing by mouth until the gag reflex returns. Percussion and postural drainage are usually employed to facilitate evacuation of dye from the respiratory passages. A chest x-ray film may be obtained 24 hours after bronchography to help evaluate how well the contrast medium has cleared the bronchial passages.

Lung scan (pulmonary scintiphotography). Pulmonary scanning procedures involve the use of a scanning device that records an outline of pulmonary radioactivity following injection or inhalation of radioactive particles.

Perfusion scanning. When perfusion scanning is done, macroaggregates of albumin tagged with radioactive particles (such as ^{131}I) are injected intravenously. Because of the small particle size, they pass readily through the venous system and right side of the heart, into the lung, and become lodged in the capillary bed. These particles are most often injected with the client lying in a supine position because this position affords uniform concentration of the particles throughout the lung. If they are injected with the client in the upright position, the particles concentrate more at the base rather than throughout the lung. Several films (scintiscans) are taken to give a pictorial representation of the distribution of the radioactive particles in various regions of the lung. Usually four views (anterior, posterior, left lateral, and right lateral) are taken, because lesions may show up on only one of the four views. When a disease process impairs the blood flow, the radioactive particles become temporarily trapped. As a result, a blank area shows up on the film. This gives an outline of the pulmonary lesion.

As the particles decrease in size, they are flushed from the lungs by the bloodstream and eventually reach the liver, where they are removed primarily by Kupffer's cells. There the particles are phagocytized and rapidly metabolized. The iodine is excreted in the urine.

Another method of pulmonary scanning is *ventilation scan*. The client is instructed to breathe a tracer amount of a radioactive gas (^{133}Xe) and oxygen from a spirometer.

After a single inhalation of the gas, the client holds his breath, and the total lung capacity, or the distribution of the ^{133}Xe throughout the bronchi and alveoli, is recorded with a scintillation camera. Under aeration, the occurrence of pneumoconstriction in embolized lung regions has been documented. To minimize this effect, the client is instructed to take several deep breaths before the initial inhalation of ^{133}Xe. This facilitates normal ventilation to these areas. The client may maintain a supine or erect position, and the procedure usually takes 5 to 10 minutes.

An alternative method of ventilation scanning is the *radioaerosol inhalation scan*. The client inhales an aerosol mist of ^{131}I or ^{99}Tc tagged in serum albumin. It is considered useful in detecting regional airway obstructions.

Sinus x-ray films. Sinus x-ray films are taken to obtain information about the size and position of the sinus, as well as to detect lesions within the cavities. Several sinus views may be taken. If information is needed about all sinuses, the *nose-chin* position is used. The film is taken with the client's mouth open and with the nose and chin on contact with the film. The posteroanterior (PA) view is useful in revealing information about the frontal sinus. The client sits with his head in an upright position, and his nose and forehead placed against the film. For both of these, the rays are projected through the occiput. A lateral view gives information about the sphenoid, ethmoid, and frontal sinuses. To obtain additional information on the sphenoid sinus, a projection may be made through the floor of the mouth.

Examination by direct visualization

One group of examinations can be made with the use of an instrument that views the part in question through a lighted tube. For example, rhinoscopy (interior of nasal cavities), laryngoscopy (interior of the larynx), bronchoscopy (interior of the bronchial tree), mediastinoscopy (interior of the mediastinum), and view of the sinus cavities by transillumination.

Rhinoscopy. Rhinoscopy is the examination of the interior of the nasal cavities. When nasal examinations are to be performed, the nurse should have in readiness ample lighting, preferably a head lamp and head mirror. In addition, the instruments specified for nasal examinations should be on hand. These may come prepackaged or separate. Probably the most widely used nasal instrument is the nasal speculum. A pharyngoscope may be used to examine the posterior nose and nasopharynx.

Before the test, a vasoconstrictor drug such as epinephrine (Adrenalin) may be applied to shrink the nasal mucosa. This practice permits better exposure. Occasionally an anesthetic may be applied to the nasal mucosa to decrease discomfort from the passage of the tube.

Nursing process for common health problems

The procedure should be explained to the client. The age of the client will determine how the client is handled during the procedure. It may be necessary to place the infant or young child on the knee and tilt the head backward with one hand while the other hand is used to restrain the legs. Older children or adults may be instructed to sit in front of the examiner with the head slightly elevated.

Laryngoscopy. An examination of the larynx may be performed either indirectly or directly. When the *indirect method* is used, the client sits all the way back in the chair with his head and shoulders brought forward. The client is instructed to stick out his tongue, or the physician may grasp it. A warmed mirror is used to visualize the back of the throat. The larynx is examined while the client phonates sounds as *ah* or *e-e-e-e*.

The *direct method* is used to examine lesions of the larynx and to remove tissue for examination. Preparation for the direct laryngoscopic examination is similar to that for a bronchoscopic examination. A sedative is administered an hour before the examination. It is usually carried out with the client under local anesthesia, although it may be done with a general anesthetic.

Bronchoscopy. A bronchoscopy is a procedure performed to visualize larger branches of the tracheobronchial tree. In addition, it may be performed for diagnostic purposes (to view a diseased area, or to obtain tissue for biopsy to ascertain the cause of a cough, hemoptysis, or a bronchial obstruction) or for therapeutic purposes (to aspirate secretions, and to remove a foreign body). The procedure and preparation are similar to those for a bronchogram (see discussion earlier in this chapter).

Foods and fluids are withheld for 6 to 8 hours before the test to prevent aspiration of particles during and after the test; dentures are removed; and oral hygiene should be administered. In an effort to allay apprehension, the client is usually sedated before the examination.

Because of the nature of the examination, the client is likely to be apprehensive after he is informed about the test. The nurse should provide as much support as is needed. Questions are often raised about whether breathing will be impaired and the extent of the pain. The client should be informed that he will be able to breathe, although fullness in the pharynx may be felt. Pain is nil. He should be informed of the importance of following instructions given by the physician. The nurse can promote relaxation by instructing the client to breathe through his nose while keeping his mouth opened. This should be practiced during the preexamination period.

A bronchoscope is inserted through the mouth, pharynx, larynx, and trachea into the bronchi after these have been anesthetized with a local anesthetic. A general anesthetic may be used for a child. The examination is carried out in a dark room to facilitate visualization. During the examination, the client's color, pulse, and respirations should be carefully monitored. Hypoxemia may occur, especially in the presence of pulmonary disease. Dysrhythmias have also been reported.

The position the client is allowed to assume after the examination depends on his state of awareness. If a general anesthetic has been administered, he is placed in a lateral Sims' position until he recovers from anesthesia. This position facilitates drainage of mucus and saliva from the oropharynx, which might irritate the lung tissue. Suction may be required. When the client regains consciousness, he may be placed in an upright position and encouraged to breathe deeply. Fluids and foods should be withheld until the cough, swallowing, and gag reflexes return. The nurse should check for the return of the latter by touching the back of the client's throat with a tongue blade or wisp of cotton and noting whether the client gags. If a gag occurs, fluids are permitted.

Since talking causes added strain to the muscles of the vocal cords, it should be discouraged. Provisions should be made for communication. The call light should be within easy reach, and a pad and pencil should be left at the bedside to be used as necessary.

Laryngeal edema and hemorrhage are major complications that may occur after bronchoscopic examination. Hemorrhage is more likely to occur if a biopsy was taken during the examination. A pneumothorax may also occur as a result of a ruptured bronchus.

Following the procedure, the nurse should monitor vital signs and other signs indicative of hemorrhage and respiratory obstruction. Significant changes should be reported to the physician. A sputum specimen may be collected for 24 hours after bronchoscopy. Some form of humidification may be prescribed to lessen the chances of laryngeal edema developing.

Flexible fiberoptic bronchoscopy (FFB). The fiberoptic bronchoscope (fiberscope) is a flexible tube that transmits light and a clear image around corners. Because of its flexibility and smaller diameter, it causes less trauma than the conventional rigid bronchoscope. It has also been considered valuable because it can pass constricted or distorted areas of the bronchus[66] and allows for subsegmental visualization. Fiberoptic bronchoscopy is often performed at the bedside. The client may maintain a sitting or recumbent position.

Other measures similar to those discussed under bronchoscopy are performed. For example, the client is premedicated with atropine sulfate and meperidine (Demerol) hydrochloride or diazepam (Valium). Nothing is permitted by mouth for at least 4 to 6 hours before the examination to minimize the risk of regurgitation and aspiration.

The nose, oropharynx, and hypopharynx are sprayed with 1% lidocaine. After lubricating the fiberscope (with surgical jelly or lidocaine ointment), the physician passes the tube transnasally to a point behind the epiglottis, where additional anesthetic is dropped through the biopsy channel onto the vocal cords. The fiberscope is then carefully advanced through the vocal cords, and more lidocaine is instilled down the mainstream bronchus. This application may be sufficient to complete the procedure, although others may require more anesthetic. During each instillation the client is instructed to take a deep breath and hold it for a brief period. If the client coughs, this facilitates movement of the anesthetic over the cords and thus helps maintain laryngeal anesthesia. Once the fiberscope is in place, a systematic inspection is made of the bronchial segments. Biopsy specimens (brush or forceps) may be taken of the lesions that are apparent. A suction tube such as a Lukens tube may be used to collect a specimen for cytology or culture. Normal saline washings may be employed to facilitate visibility after manipulation.

Whenever either of these procedures (conventional or FFB) is performed, complete monitoring and resuscitative equipment should be on hand. Oxygen is administered during the procedure.

Mediastinoscopy. For the mediastinoscopic examination, a small incision is made in the suprasternal notch, and an instrument (mediastinoscope) is inserted through the incision into the mediastinum. Once the instrument is in position, the mediastinal structures are inspected and a biopsy specimen is taken. A mediastinostomy is usually performed with the client under general anesthesia.

Transillumination. Transillumination is a method of examining the frontal and maxillary sinuses by directing a beam of light against them. The procedure is done in a dark room. If the light does not penetrate the sinuses, a pathological condition is suspected. The detection of fluid in the sinus indicates an obstruction to drainage. No special preparation is necessary.

Lung biopsy

A lung biopsy involves the aspiration of secretions with a needle. Two approaches can be used: the *transtracheobronchial* (TTB) and the *transthoracic*. The latter includes the percutaneous needle lung biopsy (NLB), or aspiration, and the open thoracotomy technique (open lung biopsy). The *aspiration* technique (NLB) provides material for cytology and culture; whereas the *cutting* technique (open thoracotomy) involves obtaining small specimens of lung tissue for analysis.

The transtracheobronchial biopsy is performed during bronchoscopy with the aid of a fluoroscope. One example of this approach is *bronchial brushing,* which can also be obtained through a bronchoscope. With the bronchial brush method, a flexible catheter under fluoroscopic control is passed through the nasopharynx and vocal cords into the bronchial tree. When the tip of the catheter has been guided into the proper place, a flexible brush is passed through the catheter in the area of the lesion. Once in place, the brush is manipulated (pulled back and forth) into the lesion, withdrawn, and smeared onto glass slides for staining. The smear specimen is then inoculated into various culture media and slides for mycobacteria and fungi or for routine bacterial and viral studies.

Premedication is generally not necessary. A local anesthetic, such as topical viscous lidocaine (Xylocaine) hydrochloride, is injected into the nasopharynx, and a 2% lidocaine solution may be injected via the cricothyroid membrane.

Pleural biopsy

A specimen for a pleural biopsy may be obtained via a percutaneous needle biopsy. Before the biopsy, pleural fluid is aspirated to ascertain the position of the needle in the pleural space, and subsequently prevent puncturing the lung. Following the procedure a chest radiograph is taken to assess the status of the lung. Complications following a pleural biopsy include pneumothorax and hemorrhage.

Laboratory studies

Laboratory studies are performed on the blood or secretions of respiratory passages. These include hematological, cytological, and bacteriological studies.

Hematological studies. Hematological studies are used to give estimations of total and differential leukocyte counts. These examinations are valuable in distinguishing between pyogenic infections and tuberculosis. In addition to the leukocyte count, a complete blood count and sedimentation rate may be determined to help diagnose respiratory disorders.

Cytological studies. Cytological studies may be performed on sputum, tracheobronchial secretions, and pleural fluid to detect the presence of carcinoma cells. The Papanicolaou technique is used for this purpose.

Bacteriological studies. Bacteriological studies may be made of secretions from the nasopharynx, chest, and pleural cavities. *Smears* and *cultures* of secretions from these areas are helpful in determining specific disease-producing organisms in a number of respiratory disorders. *Blood cultures* may also be taken to identify the specific organisms responsible for producing severe infections of the lungs. Cultures and smears of sputum may also be indicated.

Sputum studies. Sputum studies are generally part of the routine examination of clients with respiratory disease.

Microscopic and bacteriological studies may be made of the sputum to diagnose respiratory diseases. Microscopic studies may reveal the causative organism in many infections, for example, bacterial pneumonias and tuberculosis. Exfoliative cell studies may be useful in the diagnosis of bronchogenic cancer.

A morning specimen, obtained immediately on arising in the morning is most desirable, because abnormal bronchial secretions tend to accumulate during sleep. However, the specimen may be collected throughout the day, provided material is raised from deep within the bronchial tree. Instructions should be given regarding the difference between sputum and saliva. The client should be instructed to cough and breathe deeply and to collect secretions that come from deep within the chest. Saliva and secretions from the nose and pharynx should not be collected.

Methods of collection. There are a number of procedures for collecting sputum specimens. In some institutions the client may be sent directly to the laboratory to submit a fresh specimen for immediate processing. In others, sputum specimens are collected on the nursing unit in a small sputum container for a varied number of hours. The latter, we believe, is more commonly the procedure of choice.

Sputum specimens may be collected during and after postural drainage. Special inhalation treatments may be prescribed for clients who are unable to raise sputum. With this method, heated saline in propylene glycol or distilled water is placed in a nebulizer. The nebulizer is attached to compressed air. A fine mist is produced that, when inhaled, travels to the lower respiratory tract and stimulates mucus secretion. The client coughs up the sputum, which is collected in the usual manner. Warm drinks (such as tea, bouillon, or hot lemonade) may also be administered to help stimulate the flow of mucus.

Tracheal aspirations may be used to obtain sputum from weak or unconscious clients. Commercial containers are available that permit the nurse to collect sputum directly from within the respiratory tract. The apparatus is attached to the suction catheter. As secretions are aspirated, they flow from the respiratory passages into the container. Chances of contamination are decreased with this method.

Another method that may be used in collecting sputum specimens is gastric lavage. The test is carried out before breakfast, and the gastric contents are examined for swallowed sputum. See Chapter 17 for discussion of passage of a gastric tube. After the tube is in place, gastric secretions (approximately 50 ml) are aspirated, placed in a sterile container, and sent to the laboratory for examination.

Regardless of the procedure, the nurse should be familiar with factors that may alter the results of the test. The nurse must know whether a sterile container or one with a fixative (such as ether, acetone, or alcohol) is to be used. Fixatives are valuable in that they facilitate prompt fixation of cells and cessation of autolytic changes. Because cells are either partially or completely separated from the blood supply long before they are expectorated, some autolytic changes have already taken place. Therefore, rapid fixation is essential. The practice of having the client expectorate into a fixative solution at the bedside decreases autolytic changes that may occur when there is a delay in taking the specimen to the laboratory. Any time lapse between specimen collection and fixation results in a decrease in quality of cellular detail and subsequently invalid results. Hence, specimens should be taken to the laboratory immediately after they are obtained. In instances where there is a delay in delivering a culture specimen to the laboratory, it should be refrigerated to prevent growth of bacteria.

Skin tests for tuberculosis

The tuberculin test is used as an aid in the diagnosis of tuberculosis and for purposes of screening in high-risk populations. The basis for such a test is the fact that infection with *Mycobacterium tuberculosis* produces sensitivity to certain products of the organism. It has been recommended that the test be performed routinely at the end of the first year of life.

Two preparations of tuberculin antigen are available for diagnostic testing: *purified protein derivative* (PPD) and *old tuberculin* (OT). Purified protein derivative is more accurate and is used more often than old tuberculin. Several strengths of PPD are available: first, intermediate, and second. Most commonly skin testing is performed with intermediate strength PPD. However, first strength is generally used for those individuals who are thought to be highly sensitized. Second strength may be used for individuals who do not react to the intermediate strength, those suspected of being positive reactors, or for individuals who may have depressed immune systems, but never as the first test. The intracutaneous (intradermal) techniques for administering the tuberculin are the Mantoux test, jet injection, and multiple puncture. Of these, the Mantoux test is most commonly used and preferred.

Mantoux test. With the Mantoux method, a measured amount of tuberculin solution of known concentration, usually 0.1 ml containing 5 tuberculin units (TU), is injected intracutaneously with a tuberculin syringe. The production of a distinct wheal about 6 to 10 mm in diameter is an indication that the tuberculin was injected accurately. Within 48 to 72 hours after the injection, a reading is taken to determine the presence or absence of induration. Readings should be made in the presence of adequate lighting and with the forearm slightly flexed at the elbow. The area should be inspected by direct light from a side view against the light and palpated by gentle stroking with the fingers. Measurement of the area should be made transversely to the long axis of the forearm, and the findings recorded in millimeters. It is helpful to use a caliper for measuring.

The Mantoux test is frequently performed by the nurse. It is very important for the nurse to be aware of factors that affect the results, some of which are discussed here. Tuberculin is more sensitive to effects of light than heat, which is one reason for storing it in the refrigerator; the light goes out when the door is closed. Since dilute solutions of tuberculin deteriorate with age, tuberculin should be refrigerated, and once it has been opened, it should be discarded after a few weeks. Also, there is an increased chance of contamination and growth of microorganisms within the solution when tuberculin is allowed to stand at room temperature. When diluted in a buffered diluent, the tuberculin protein is absorbed in various amounts by glass and plastics. Although a small amount of stabilizer is added to the diluent by the manufacturer to reduce absorption, the nurse should follow guidelines that will minimize reduction in potency by absorption.

The tuberculin should never be transferred from one container to another, and once the syringe is filled, the skin test should be performed immediately. Instructions given by the manufacturer should be closely adhered to so as to assure that the prescribed amount is administered. Failure to adhere to these guidelines will result in false positive readings.

Tuberculin *anergy,* or failure to have a positive test in the presence of tuberculosis, may occur in various acute fulminating infections such as miliary tuberculosis and measles, during corticosteroid or immunosuppressive therapy, and in elderly and debilitated individuals.

Jet injection. With the jet injection method, a jet gun is used to administer, under high pressure, the prescribed dose of tuberculin intracutaneously.

With the standard test dose, the intracutaneous Mantoux and jet injection tests are interpreted as follows:

0 mm to 4 mm of induration = Negative reaction
5 mm to 9 mm of induration = Doubtful reaction
10 mm or more of induration = Positive reaction

A positive reaction (10 mm or more) represents specific sensitivity with *M tuberculosis,* whereas a doubtful reaction indicates sensitivity that may be the result of either atypical mycobacteria or *M tuberculosis.* When a doubtful reaction occurs, it is recommended that the test be repeated at a different skin site. A negative reaction indicates either a lack of tuberculin sensitivity or a low-grade sensitivity.[2] Repeat tests are usually not necessary unless there is clinical evidence that the individual has tuberculosis.

Various sites may be used for intradermally injecting tuberculin. The volar or dorsal surface of the forearm is the preferred site and is, therefore, most frequently used. Other sites may be used, particularly when clients are apprehensive about the injection. For example, the posterior thorax may be used for children to prevent their seeing the injection process.)

Multiple puncture tests. Another method sometimes used in tuberculin tests is puncturing through a film of liquid tuberculin. The Heaf, tine, Sterneedle, and Mono-vac tuberculin tests are examples. They contain prongs that are pressed downward for 1 or 2 seconds to a predetermined depth (1 to 2 mm) on the volar surface of the forearm after it has been cleansed with alcohol or acetone. As with the Mantoux test, readings are taken within 48 to 72 hours. The test results are interpreted as follows: positive if fesiculation is present, doubtful if the induration around one or more of the puncture sites is 2 mm or more in diameter, and negative if the induration around the puncture sites is less than 2 mm in diameter. If the reaction is doubtful, the physician usually orders a Mantoux test. In measuring, the diameter of the largest induration (papule) should be recorded.

The multiple puncture method, commonly used for screening purposes, is particularly advantageous for testing children because only one person is needed to administer the test. Children also are thought to show less fear and feel less pain when this method is used.

Assessment of pulmonary function

Pulmonary function tests are performed to evaluate respiratory function of a client with known lung disease, progression of disease (in clients with chronic lung disease), and response to therapy. They are useful in preoperative evaluation of clients for resectional surgery. These tests are usually limited to children 6 years old and older who can follow instructions.[57] Young children's and adolescent's performances may be variable.[64] Generally no special preparation is required. However, the client should be informed that during the test, the physician or technician will provide instruction about breathing at various times.

Spirometry. Spirometry is the means by which key lung capacities, volumes, and flow rates are measured. The measurements vary according to the age, gender, height, and weight of the client. These measurements follow:

Lung capacity measurements

total lung capacity (TLC) Amount of air contained in the lung after a maximal inspiration (IC + FRC).

vital capacity (VC) Maximum amount of air that can be expired after the deepest inspiration possible.

inspiration capacity (IC) Maximal amount of air a person can breathe after a normal expiration.

functional residual capacity (FRC) Amount of gas remaining in the lungs after a normal expiration.

Lung volume measurements

tidal volume (TV) Volume of air inspired or expired during each respiratory cycle, including both dead space and alveolar volume.

inspiratory reserve volume (IRV) Maximal volume of air that can be inspired after normal inspiration.

expiratory reserve volume (ERV) Maximal volume of air that can be expired after a normal expiration.

residual volume (RV) Volume of air retained in the lungs after a maximal expiration.

minute volume (MV) Volume of air inspired per minute.

Flow rate measurements

forced expiratory volume (FEV, FEV_1, FEV_2, FEV_3) Measures the volume of air forcibly exhaled after a maximal inspiration in 1-, 2-, and 3-second intervals.

maximal expiratory flow rate (MEFR) The total amount of air expired per minute, breathing as rapidly as possible.

maximal inspiratory flow rate (MIFR) Measures the amount of air inspired per minute breathing as rapidly as possible.

peak expiratory flow rate (PEFR) Measures the highest rate of flow, sustained for 10 seconds or more, at which air can be expelled from the lungs.

Blood gas analysis   Blood gas analysis is a measurement of the partial pressure of oxygen and carbon dioxide in the blood. These measurements are analyzed to assess the client's oxygenation status and the acid-base status. Measurements are made of *actual oxygen tension* (Pa_{O_2}), the measurement of the partial pressure exerted by oxygen in arterial blood; *arterial carbon dioxide tension* (Pa_{CO_2}), measurement of the partial pressure exerted by carbon dioxide in arterial blood; *arterial oxyhemoglobin saturation* (Sa_{O_2}) measurement of the percentage of oxygen combined with hemoglobin; arterial pH; and bicarbonate (HCO_3). Bicarbonates differentiate respiratory from metabolic causes. It should be noted that only Pa_{O_2}, Pa_{CO_2}, and Sa_{O_2} give blood gas measurements. However, all parameters (including pH and HCO_3) are included for all blood gas analyses. The Pa_{O_2} and Pa_{CO_2} are expressed in mm Hg, whereas the Sa_{O_2} is expressed in percentage.

Arterial blood is desirable for two reasons: (1) it more likely represents a mixture of blood that comes from various parts of the body, and (2) it gives information about the ability of the lungs to oxygenate the blood. Venous specimens, drawn through a central venous catheter, may be used, although they do not afford the most accurate reading. Unclotted blood is used to determine blood gas values. Therefore, to prevent clotting, blood is withdrawn with a heparinized glass syringe. The syringe is iced until blood gas determination can be made. The ice lowers the temperature and subsequently reduces metabolism, causing less alteration in the Pa_{O_2}, Pa_{CO_2}, and pH values.

Specimens for arterial blood gas determinations are usually drawn anaerobically from the radial, brachial, or femoral arteries. During the early neonatal period, arterial blood may be obtained from an umbilical artery catheter that has been passed above the bifurcation of the aorta. The temporal artery may also be used. This site is considered ideal for infants, because the oxygen tension in other arteries may be lower because of fetal shunting involving flow through the ductus arteriosus. A stab wound may be made in the infant's heel, finger, or earlobe to obtain an arterialized capillary blood sample. With the latter approach, the first drop of blood is discarded, and the subsequent blood is collected in a heparinized capillary tube. Once the blood sample has been obtained, constant pressure must be applied to the site of the arterial puncture for at least 5 minutes. If the client is receiving anticoagulant therapy or has a blood dyscrasia, pressure should be applied for a longer period of time. The puncture site should be checked again within 5 minutes after pressure is released to assess whether or not a hematoma has formed. Severe pain may be indicative of hematoma formation.

When blood gas determinations are made, notation should be made as to whether the client was breathing room air. If not, the concentration, number of liters, and method of administration of oxygen should be indicated. Notations should also be made of vital signs, level of consciousness, and amount of activity at the time the sample was taken. It might also be helpful to record the withdrawal site. Such information is helpful in analyzing the results. For example, saturation values may differ depending on whether the sample was obtained above (temporal artery, earlobes) or below (umbilical artery) the ductus. Samples taken above the ductus may be slightly higher.[61] Normal blood gas values are given in Table 21-4. One variable that may affect these norms is age. The Pa_{O_2} and Sa_{O_2} in older persons tend to be near the lower part of the normal range, whereas younger individuals tend to have high normal values.

The nurse should also be knowledgeable about the following terms. *Hypercapnia (hypercarbia)* is increased arterial carbon dioxide tension. It usually results from hypoventilation and is often accompanied by hypoxia. *Hypocapnia (hypocarbia)* is reduced arterial carbon dioxide tension. It results from hyperventilation. *Hypoxemia* is a deficiency of oxygen in arterial blood. As a result, the oxygen content is insufficient to meet tissue needs. Numerically, hypoxemia is considered to be present when the Pa_{O_2} drops below 50 mg Hg, with a corresponding 16 ml/100 ml, provided the concentration of hemoglobin is normal.[47]

TABLE 21-4

Normal blood gas determinations

Blood gas	Adult		Neonate (arterial blood)
	Arterial blood	**Venous blood**	
pH	7.35 to 7.45	7.31 to 7.41	7.30 to 7.39
Pa_{O_2}	85 to 100 mm Hg	35 to 40 mm Hg	63 to 87 mm Hg
Pa_{CO_2}	38 to 42 mm Hg	41 to 51 mm Hg	31 to 35 mm Hg
Sa_{O_2}	96% to 98%	70% to 75%	94%
Actual bicarbonate (HCO_3)	23 to 25 mEq/L	23 to 25 mEq/L	19 to 20 mEq/L
Base excess	−2 to +2	−2 to +2	—

Data analysis

After the nurse collects the necessary data about the client, the data are compared with norms appropriate to the age, gender, and development of the client. Consideration is also given to the family and social background. Potential or actual diagnoses that may be established include ineffective airway clearance, ineffective breathing patterns, impaired gas exchange, grieving, ineffective coping, alterations in cardiac output, fear, and alterations in comfort.

Planning

PLANNING FOR HEALTH PROMOTION

As the nurse develops a plan of care for clients with problems involving the respiratory system, consideration should be given to health promotion strategies, as well as objectives specific to restoration and maintenance. Inherent within the latter are varied therapies that are used in the care of these clients. These therapies must also be considered as the care plan is developed. Any condition that interferes with the delivery of an adequate supply of oxygen to cells threatens the survival of the cells. The nurse can therefore be most effective through teaching good health practices in an effort to help prevent conditions that interfere with maintenance of adequate oxygen.

Adequate ventilation must be provided within the environment if adequate oxygen is to be maintained. Individuals should be encouraged not to sleep or work in stuffy or smoke-filled environments. Smoking should be discouraged.

When individuals work in dusty environments, they should be encouraged to wear a mask or some other protective device to prevent inhalation of irritating dust and fumes. When nasal congestion occurs, individuals usually attempt to obtain some relief. Nose drops, sprays, and inhalers can easily be purchased over the counter and are thought to give prompt relief. Overuse of any of these should be discouraged, because the use of local medications for as long as 3 days, even if prescribed, may lead to chronic congestion or damage to the mucous membranes. When antibiotic instillations, drops, or sprays are used, sensitization may be produced, and damage to the olfactory function may occur.

Proper clothing should be worn to coincide with environmental temperatures to reduce conditions that might lead to congestion.

Clients should be educated about ways in which they can prevent inhaling foreign objects. Food should be chewed thoroughly, and care must be maintained not to eat small bones or hard particles that could easily be aspirated. The purchase of toys with small parts that can be easily pulled off should be discouraged.

PLANNING FOR HEALTH RESTORATION AND MAINTENANCE

Maintaining airway patency

In caring for clients with problems that interfere with the delivery of oxygen to the cells, the nurse must develop a plan to meet the following objectives: (1) maintain a patent airway; (2) restore or maintain adequate gaseous exchange; (3) reduce metabolic demands; and (4) prevent and control infection.

One way in which the respiratory passages respond to irritation or infection is by increasing the amount of secretions. Viscosity of the secretions is also increased. It is important that these secretions be removed from the respiratory passages to keep the airway open. The client should be adequately hydrated to keep the secretions thin so that they can be easily expectorated. Various forms of nebulization therapy and drugs may be prescribed to help thin respiratory tract secretions. See discussion of nebulization later in this chapter.

Once these secretions are thinned, they must be removed from the respiratory tract. Clients who find expectoration offensive may limit removal of the sputum. The nurse must help the client understand the importance of raising the secretions and expectorating rather than swallowing them. Ample containers and tissue must be provided, and the nurse must observe the amount, color, and character of the sputum.

If the cilia are unable to propel secretions upward to where they can be expectorated, the client must be encouraged to cough. Coughing is an effective means of clearing secretions from the lower respiratory tract and, as a result, facilitates maintenance of airway patency. If the client is able to cough, the nurse must instruct him to cough effectively so that these secretions may be raised. If secretions are allowed to remain within the tracheobronchial tree, they become a primary source for bacterial growth and for the formation of mucus plugs that may obstruct the air passages.

Several approaches have been suggested to facilitate effective coughing. Each of these recognizes the importance of proper positioning before the exercise is carried out. Before the coughing procedure is actually carried out, the client's position may be changed from side to side to help loosen secretions while at the same time increasing coughing effectiveness. To help the conscious client cough effectively, the nurse *assists him to a sitting position*. This position facilitates maximal chest expansion. Before the cough, he should be instructed to *breathe deeply* so that a large volume of air can enter the lung, thus dilating the deeper air passages. As a result, air is forced behind the mucus to facilitate its removal. The client is then instructed to exhale forcibly until the cough reflex is stimulated. The continuous flow of air through the trachea and the buildup of carbon dioxide trigger the cough reflex. Coughing exercises should be performed at least five times every 1 to 2 hours.

When the client is too weak to cough or coughs ineffectively, endotracheal stimulation with a catheter may be performed. The value of this procedure is that it stimulates the cough reflex, thus producing violent coughing. Adequate suctioning equipment should be in readiness in case the client is unable to expectorate the secretions independently.

Nasal hygiene is also a very important aspect of care. Any added mucus accumulation will irritate the tissue about the nostril, and if not removed, the mucus may interfere with the entrance of air. The client should be encouraged to blow his nose periodically during the day to help remove secretions. The nostrils should be cleansed several times a day with moistened applicators to relieve dryness and irritation. Petrolatum or some form of lubricant may be applied to relieve dried membranes.

Relieving apprehension and fear. Because life depends on breathing, the client who is dyspneic is naturally anxious and apprehensive. Any difficulty in breathing tends to make death seem more imminent. To alleviate the apprehension and fear associated with dyspnea, the nurse must direct efforts toward calming the client. Comfort measures must be provided. Oxygen should be administered to relieve dyspnea. It may be necessary to elevate the head of the bed. In this position the abdominal organs do not press against the diaphragm, there is more room for lung expansion, and as a result, breathing is made easier. However, if the client is more comfortable in another position, the nurse should permit him to assume the position. Whatever position the client assumes, he must be well supported to prevent added strain on the respiratory muscles.

1257

Often, the client is so severely dyspneic that he fears his next breath will be the last. In these cases, the nurse should remain as close by the client as possible or allow a family member or friend to stay with him. It may be necessary to hold the young infant or child for short periods. He should be assured that his signal for attention will be heeded. As necessary and if the client desires, the nurse should consult the chaplain to visit him. This practice is also thought to lessen apprehension.

For information concerning the importance of alleviating emotional outbursts, see Table 21-5.

Restoring or maintaining adequate gas exchange

Inhalation therapy is prescribed to restore pathophysiological alterations of gas exchange toward the normal level. It aims at adequate oxygenation and proper elimination of carbon dioxide. This is accomplished through administration of therapeutic gases (oxygen and carbon dioxide mixtures). Pressure breathing devices, resuscitators, and respirators are means by which therapy is accomplished. Inhalation therapy is usually used for the hospitalized client, although it may be used in the home under adequate supervision.

Reducing metabolic demands

Stress of any nature, whether physical or emotional, has an effect on the respiratory status. If the temperature is elevated, metabolism increases. As a result, greater demands are placed on pulmonary ventilation. If the client has dyspnea, he tires easily and uses a great deal of energy for breathing. If he becomes upset, his respirations become deeper and faster. The nurse must therefore intervene by helping the client decrease the metabolic demands of the body. As the metabolic demands are decreased, oxygen requirements are also decreased. The nurse should plan to reduce metabolic demands by maintaining rest and activity, reducing the efforts of breathing, and maintaining nutrition, hydration, and elimination.

Maintaining rest and activity. If bed rest is prescribed, the nurse should inform the client of the importance of bed rest and what it entails. If he understands the rationale for reduced activity, he is more likely to cooperate.

Activities should be planned so that the client will have an opportunity to rest between activities. In this way, the client has an opportunity to restore himself. Any factor within the environment that reduces the client's ability to rest should be eliminated. The environment should be free of loud noises. Visitors should be limited. He should be assisted with activities of daily living. When it is necessary to administer physical care to the client, it should be carried out in a calm and unhurried manner. All treatments and procedures should be explained to the client in terms that are easily understood by him.

If the client is unable to sleep, nursing measures such as a backrub at bedtime or warm fluids may promote relaxation and subsequently enhance sleep. Often it may be necessary to communicate this problem to the physician so that medication can be prescribed. When drugs are prescribed, they should be used cautiously, especially if they have the potential of depressing the central nervous system, which would affect respiratory efficiency. When coughing interferes with the client's ability to rest, medications should be prescribed to relieve the cough.

When bed rest has been prescribed for the client, range-of-motion exercises must be carried out two or three times each day to maintain muscle tone and joint mobility. These exercises should be carried out slowly, and the client should be allowed frequent periods of rest to prevent overtaxing his respiratory reserve.

When activity is increased, the client must be assessed for his tolerance to increased activity. The vital signs should be assessed before, during, and after the activity, and a comparison made of the three. The nurse should also assess (1) whether the coughing episodes increase with activity, (2) whether breathing becomes more difficult, and (3) how much fatigue has been caused. Each of these observations should form a basis for later activities.

As often as necessary, diversional activities must be planned to help relieve anxiety. Whatever is planned should be based on the client's interest and needs. The planned activities should not be physically overtaxing. Soft, cuddly toy animals for infants, dolls or plastic cars for toddlers, and crayons and coloring books for preschoolers are useful diversional toys that could be brought to the hospital. Puzzles also provide diversion for children of school age. If the client has a small, portable hobby, he should be permitted to bring it to the hospital. None of these requires expenditure of lots of energy. If the client is ambulatory, he may provide his own activity by visiting other clients. When possible, he should be allowed to spend time in the lounge or visit the gift shop within the hospital. The client who moves around by wheelchair must also be permitted these activities. Television, radio, magazines, and newspapers are means of diversion that are health oriented and can be used for both the ambulatory and bedridden client. These do not require exertion that would tax the client physically. They are also a means of keeping him oriented to the time and happenings outside the hospital environment. Other resources such as the occupational therapist may be consulted to help the client plan activities.

If the client has an emotional outburst of crying, sobbing, or anger, the nurse must direct efforts toward finding the cause and trying to alleviate it as soon as possible, because each of these emotions has an effect on metabolic activity. The nurse must be aware of covert manifestations that indicate anxiety and stress. Being uncooperative, indifferent, or demanding indicates some form of stress.

The nurse must develop and maintain a therapeutic relationship with the client and should listen and communicate with him. Both verbal and nonverbal communications must be used. Ample time is needed for the nurse to assess, validate, and develop a plan with the client. If the client is afraid, just spending extra time with him, using nonverbal forms of communication such as a touch or a smile, may be all that is necessary to reassure him. The young child may be held. If the client has questions about his illness, his questions should be answered. The nurse should first assess what the client already knows, then give explanations accordingly.

Decreasing effort of breathing. To decrease the effort of breathing, adequate room ventilation must be provided. Cool, fresh air should be circulated within the environment. Any client who has difficulty breathing should not be made to feel closed in. Curtains should not be drawn around the client, because this act only serves to make him feel more closed in. Clothing should be light, but warm. Large meals and gas-forming foods should be avoided because they produce pressure on the diaphragm and, as a result, interfere with thoracic expansion. The client should be encouraged to maintain a position that facilitates easier breathing. A semi-Fowler's position is usually maintained.

Maintaining nutrition and hydration. Clients who have respiratory problems may have difficulty maintaining adequate nutrition and hydration. The sources of the problem are many. The nurse has a responsibility of finding out the source and implementing a plan accordingly. Often, the client lacks the strength to chew because so much energy is used in trying to breathe. A chronic cough may be exhausting and may be responsible for anorexia. A diminished or lost sense of taste may cause the client not to have an appetite. Eating often brings on attacks of coughing and dyspnea. Therefore, in an effort to prevent these attacks, the client may not eat. Some have irritated throats, which often present a problem, and may affect the client's ability to take in adequate foods and fluids.

It is a nursing function to help the client maintain adequate nutritional and fluid intake. When coughing is severe, medications must be prescribed to help relieve the cough. The nurse must encourage and help the client to select foods that are easy to chew and swallow if dyspnea is a problem. Frequent small meals should be provided rather than large meals. Gas-forming foods should also be discouraged. Meals should be attractively prepared. Odors within the environment must be eliminated. Sputum should be expectorated in a proper container and disposed of as often as necessary.

Provisions should be made for oral hygiene every 2 or 3 hours throughout the day and before meals. Such measures help improve the client's appetite, provide moisture for the mouth, and prevent infection. An infection in the mouth only compounds the problem. Hard candies are refreshing and help keep the mouth moist. Chewing gum may be offered unless it impairs the ability to breathe or causes abdominal distension that would impair lung expansion. The lips should be lubricated several times a day to prevent dryness.

The nurse should also assess the status of the client's hydration. Some are mouth-breathers and thereby lose large amounts of fluids by the oral route. Ample fluids should be provided. Cool fluids are soothing. It is a common practice for clients to drink through a straw. However, such practice requires more effort, especially for the weak, dyspneic client. Therefore fluids permitted should be offered directly from a glass to lessen energy requirements, prevent swallowing of air and the resultant abdominal distension, and possibly promote increased fluid intake. The condition of the client's skin and mucous membranes should be observed daily. Before the nurse develops a plan, information should be obtained about the client's normal intake-and-output pattern, because this information should provide a basis for the plan. The client should also be weighed daily.

Maintaining elimination. The sources of bowel problems for the client with respiratory problems are often related to inactivity and physical status. Many of these clients are weak, and they tend to tire easily. Any activity often precipitates attacks of coughing and dyspnea. They therefore tend to limit any activity that will produce added stress. Tracheostomized clients cannot strain unless the tracheostomy opening is closed off, because of the loss of Valsalva's maneuver. The abdominal muscles may be weak.

Constipation is not only uncomfortable, but it also limits breathing effectiveness. The overfilled bowel produces added pressure against the diaphragm, which results in limiting the space for adequate lung expansion and resultant ineffective breathing. The nurse must therefore plan measures that will prevent bowel problems. The plan should be based on the client's elimination schedule. The client must be helped to select adequate roughage in the diet. If certain foods are known to have a laxative effect on the client, these should be supplied. Fruit juices and fluids should be encouraged to stimulate peristaltic activity and supply enough water for the feces. The client should be instructed to engage in physical

TABLE 21-5

Common problems: possible strategies of care for clients with respiratory interferences

Problem	Possible effect	Possible source	Actions, assessments, or implications	Rationale	Expected outcome
Apprehension and anxiety	Increased demand for energy	Stress (such as illness, feeling of helplessness, lack of control, insecurity, or fear) Breathlessness	Once cause is determined, use measures to relieve apprehension or anxiety 1. Create environment conducive to ventilation of fears and concerns 2. Spend time with client; be a good listener 3. Provide for anticipatory guidance (for example, let client know what to expect, what is expected of him); permit client to make some decisions about aspects of care (for example, in which arm would client prefer to have the intravenous infusion started? Would client prefer to be bathed before or after breakfast or later during the day?) 4. Encourage family support and participation in care 5. Plan for consistency of care as much as possible 6. Supply oxygen 7. Keep call light within easy reach 8. Check positioning	Facilitates expression of fears and concerns, thus helping alleviate or reduce apprehension Permits client to exert some control and to predict what will happen	Decreased apprehension and anxiety
Cough	Increased demand for energy	Irritation from external stimuli (smoke, smog, dust, or gas) or internal stimuli (inflammatory process or allergic response)	Make pertinent assessments Eliminate external stimuli if possible Instruct client to obtain medical consultation rather than employ self-treatment with nonprescription medicine	Prevent hypersensitization to medicines	Decreased episodes of coughing
		Position	Help client maintain a position that relieves the cough	Irritating and nonproductive coughs often interfere with activity and rest	
Dyspnea	Increased demand for energy	Emotional reaction (tension or anxiety); illness	Make detailed assessments about the nature of dyspnea Give instructions on a breathing pattern, especially in severe states, that promotes complete exhalation and improves gas exchange 1. Begin instructions when client is not experiencing dyspnea or when dyspnea is minimal 2. Plan for practice sessions Lessen emotional reaction, such as fear, panic, and helplessness (see Apprehension)	When dyspnea is minimal, client is more likely to note reduction in stress state (such as air hunger), thus may be more motivated to continue practicing	Dyspnea will be lessened
		Position	Position client in position that tends to relieve dyspnea (usually semiupright position is desirable) Provide balance between activity and rest Provide oxygen when indicated Instruct client to avoid gas-producing foods	Facilitates greater lung expansion	

Continued.

TABLE 21-5, cont'd

Common problems: possible strategies of care for clients with respiratory interferences

Problem	Possible effect	Possible source	Actions, assessments, or implications	Rationale	Expected outcome
Increased volume of secretions	Dilution of irritant, thus facilitating removal from body (protective)	Inflammatory process	Make assessments Increase fluid intake to as much as 3 to 4 liters per day, if not contraindicated Encourage ambulation if not contraindicated Instruct client on deep breathing Change positions frequently Give frequent mouth care	Facilitates thinning of secretions Facilitates mobilization of secretions, thus preventing pooling Promotes comfort and prevents infection	Thinner secretions, which are easily expectorated
Thick secretions	Increased difficulty in removal, thus becoming ideal medium for infection				
Pain	May interfere with ventilation, produce shallow breathing, and as a result decrease alveolar aeration	Inflammation or trauma	Make pertinent assessments Administer analgesics as prescribed, but cautiously Assess respiratory rate and client's behavior (restlessness or confusion) before administration of medications	Certain analgesics (such as morphine) depress respiratory and cough reflexes Cerebral hypoxemia may occur	Feels less pain

exercises. He should be encouraged to heed the defecation impulse. As much as possible, the client should be allowed to use the sitting position during the act of defecation. If these measures are not adequate, it may be necessary to consult the physician so that medications (such as stool softeners) or other measures may be prescribed to prevent constipation.

Nursing intervention must also be planned so that any problem that will cause a further alteration to the ability to meet oxygen needs will be eliminated (Table 21-5).

Preventing and controlling infection

The client should be protected from any source of infection. Any person who has a respiratory tract infection should not be permitted to care for or visit the client. Any additional infection only serves to increase the need for oxygen. The client who has a respiratory tract infection should be isolated from other clients. The environment must be clean. The nurse should educate the client and his family in regard to preventive measures and therapy. Principles of medical asepsis should be taught. Such pointers as proper handwashing, proper disposal of sputum, and covering the cough and sneeze should be included in the instructional plan.

The client's temperature should be assessed frequently. If the client is a mouth-breather or if he has frequent coughing spells, the temperature should be taken rectally to ensure a more accurate reading.

The client's resistance must be built up with an adequate supply of nutrients and fluids. Vitamins may be prescribed as necessary. Whatever guidance and teaching are done should take the client's culture and religion into consideration.

Oxygen therapy

Oxygen therapy is a means of maintaining the physiological need for oxygen. It is generally prescribed when the amount of oxygen in the blood and tissues is insufficient to meet the body's needs. When this occurs, hypoxia, which may be related to several mechanisms, may exist. Several types of hypoxia have been identified.[30] These include the following.

1. *Hypoxic hypoxia* occurs when there is decreased diffusion of oxygen from the lung into arterial blood. It therefore may occur in lung problems such as atelectasis, pneumonia, and pulmonary edema.
2. *Anemic hypoxia* occurs in the presence of insufficient hemoglobin, as may occur in anemic problems.
3. *Ischemic hypoxia* occurs when tissue perfusion is decreased. Situations in which there is an obstruction of blood flow to tissues or a low blood volume or pressure may produce ischemic hypoxia.
4. *Histotoxic hypoxia* occurs when the tissues are poisoned, as may occur from substances such as sodium cyanide.

Assessment of the need for oxygen. The nurse must continually assess the client for signs of hypoxia. Such signs as increased pulse rate, dyspnea, rapid shallow breathing, cardiac dysrhythmias, drowsiness, headache, disorientation, excitement, apprehension, flaring nostrils, yawning, restlessness, cyanosis, and intercostal and substernal retractions are indications of hypoxia.

In the neonate, however, cyanosis and pallor are most unreliable. Even with the presence of adequate oxygenation, cyanosis or pallor may be evident because of superficial vasoconstriction from lowered body temperature. Because cyanosis may not be evident until the Pa_{O_2} is below 50 mm Hg even in the adult, it should not be used as a lone determinant of oxygen need. An increase in pulse rate is an objective indicator of the need for oxygen because it indicates the body's attempt to compensate for a decreased amount of oxygen to tissue.

Failure to recognize hypoxia will result in deterioration of cerebral, adrenal, cardiac, renal, and hepatic functions.

Planning for oxygen therapy. When oxygen therapy is prescribed, the nurse should direct a plan of care toward promoting comfort, promoting safety, and maintaining an adequate oxygen supply.

Promoting psychological and physical comfort. Whenever oxygen is prescribed, the client should be informed of the purpose and principles of therapy. Such explanations are essential in allaying fear and anxiety. Similar explanations should also be given to the family, because many people have misconceptions about the use of oxygen therapy. Explanations should also be given if the client is a young child. If the child is frightened, allowing him to have a favorite toy may be instrumental in calming him. If the client is frightened as therapy commences, the nurse should remain with him until he becomes calm. As therapy continues, the nurse must continually provide reassurance by attending to the client's needs. Comfort measures such as hygienic care and skin care must be provided. The client should be repositioned at least every 2 hours to maintain the integrity of the skin. Because oxygen has a drying effect on the mucous membranes, oral and nasal hygiene should be administered every 2 hours, and the intake of fluids should be encouraged.

Promoting safety. In promoting safety, the nurse must have an understanding of the following properties of oxygen so that precautionary measures can be taken before therapy is actually started:

1. *Oxygen is odorless, colorless, tasteless, and heavier than air.* Therefore

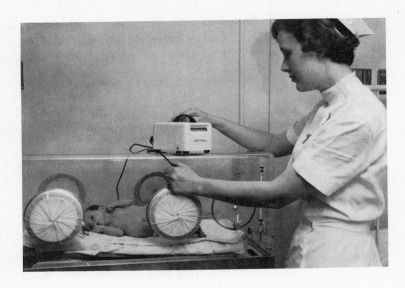

FIG. 21-13
Nurse analyzes oxygen concentration of the incubator. First, the accuracy of the analyzer must be assessed. Then air is drawn into the bulb by squeezing it a desired number of times (five to ten). The button on the analyzer is pressed, and the oxygen concentration is recorded on the dial. (From Smith, Robert M.: Anesthesia for infants and children, ed. 4, St. Louis, 1979, The C.V. Mosby Co.)

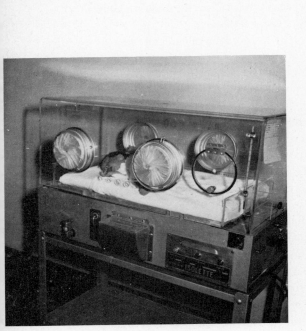

FIG. 21-14
Incubator supplies oxygen, humidity, and warmth. (From Smith, Robert M.: Anesthesia for infants and children, ed. 4, St. Louis, 1979, The C.V. Mosby Co.)

it may escape into the environment without being noticed. To maintain an adequate oxygen supply when a tent is used, the canopy (tent) must be securely tucked under the mattress with cotton blankets.

2. *Oxygen supports combustion.* Therefore no-smoking rules must be enforced. Matches and cigarettes should be removed from the room, and the client, as well as visitors, should be instructed not to smoke. "No Smoking" signs should be displayed where they can be easily seen. Electrical equipment such as call bells, heating pads, or electric razors should not be allowed in the proximity of oxygen. A hand bell should be used instead of an electric one. If it is necessary to suction a client who is using oxygen it may be necessary to discontinue the oxygen while the suctioning procedure is being carried out. Mechanical toys also should not be allowed near oxygen. Oil, grease, alcohol, and wool have a low combustion point and may ignite spontaneously in the presence of oxygen. They therefore should not be used. A cotton blanket rather than a wool one should be used to provide warmth for the client in an oxygen tent.

3. *Oxygen has a drying effect on the mucous membranes and may cause varying degrees of irritation.* Therefore, regardless of the method of oxygen administration (cannula, catheter, or mask) some form of humidification is necessary. Usually oxygen is bubbled through a bottle of distilled water. These bottles (or humidifiers) should be maintained at the desired level to assure maximum efficiency. When the reservoir is filled at near capacity, oxygen has to travel through more water. Consequently the client will receive more relative humidity because the oxygen is in contact with the water for a longer period of time. Conversely a decrease in the water level decreases the efficiency of the humidifier.[30]

When a catheter or cannula is used for the confused or disoriented client, it may be necessary to apply soft restraints to prevent unnecessary pull on the tubes.

Maintaining an adequate oxygen supply. Regardless of the route used to administer oxygen, it must be remembered that oxygen is a drug. It is therefore essential that the concentration be strictly controlled, and assessments be made to determine the effectiveness of the therapy. Maintenance of the flow rate (such as liters per minute) is essential in controlling the concentration. Therefore, when oxygen is administered, the nurse must make frequent assessments of the oxygen concentration to determine its adequacy. The analysis of oxygen concentration can be made with the use of an oxygen analyzer (Fig. 21-13). Arterial blood gas determinations are also essential in making decisions about the needed oxygen concentration.

The frequency of making determinations will depend on the state of the client. In some instances it may be necessary to make assessments at half-hour or hour intervals, whereas with others a much longer interval may be acceptable. The nurse should evaluate information from the client's record and use it as a basis for determining frequency of oxygen analysis.

One of the assessments that must be made while oxygen is maintained is the client's response to therapy. These assessments should include vital signs, color, degree of respiratory distress, behavior, and level of consciousness.

Oxygen toxicity may occur when there is prolonged exposure of the lung tissue to high oxygen concentrations. Changes may occur in the lung, including alveolar edema, pulmonary congestion, intraalveolar hemorrhage, and hyaline membrane formation. The client may complain of substernal pain, sore throat, and cough within 8 to 10 hours of receiving high concentrations of oxygen.

Methods of administering oxygen therapy. Oxygen may be administered by several methods. The method selected will depend on the client's age, ventilatory status, and condition. The selected method will be one that will deliver the adequate oxygen concentration. Although the administration of oxygen has become a function of the respiratory therapist, the nurse must be aware of the aspects of oxygen therapy and plan so that desired oxygen concentration, temperature, and humidity are maintained.

The *incubator* is frequently used for the premature or small infant to provide oxygen, humidity, and warmth similar to the intrauterine environment (Fig. 21-14). The physician prescribes the temperature and humidity in the incubator according to the infant's needs.

The infant's temperature should be assessed every hour until it becomes stabilized, after which the intervals between assessment may be increased. Nursing care is administered through portholes. When the nurse feeds the infant, he is raised to a semi-Fowler's position. He should be bubbled and allowed to remain slightly elevated for a short while after feeding. Various types of incubators are available. A detailed discussion of the varied types is beyond the scope of this book.

The *humidity tent,* such as the *CAM* or *Mistogen tent* (which is often used for infants and young children), provides a mist at a particle size that adequately assists in the transport of oxygen into the terminal alveoli. Small moisture particles that vary in size from 1 μ to 5 μ are desirable. The smaller the size of the particles, the deeper the penetration of the tracheobronchial tree. The small child can be enclosed in the tent completely (Fig. 21-15), whereas only the head and upper torso of the older child are enclosed. Before the child is placed in the tent, it should be flooded with oxygen. Because the fine mists aid in hydration, it is essential that accurate records be kept of intake and output.

The *oxygen tent* is suitable for administering a moderately high concentration of oxygen, as well as providing a means of humidification. It also has a cool-

FIG. 21-15
CAM tent is cooled and ventilated electrically. Note that the child has adequate room for play. (From Ingalls, A. Joy, and Salerno, M. Constance: Maternal and child health nursing, ed. 4, St. Louis, 1979, The C.V. Mosby Co.)

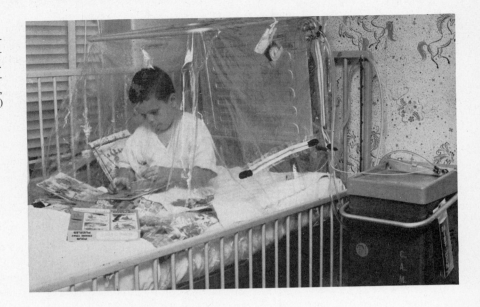

ing effect by convection. The *hood* or *face* tent fits under the chin, around the client's face, and provides oxygen therapy as well as a high-humidity environment. These are used primarily for children.[23]

Oxygen can be administered nasally by catheter or by cannula. Although *catheters* are infrequently used, two techniques may be used for delivering oxygen by this method. With the oropharyngeal technique (deep technique), oxygen is delivered directly into the oropharynx. As much as 30% oxygen concentration may be delivered with a flow rate of 4 to 5 L/min, and 40% concentration at 6 to 7 L/min. With the second technique (shallow technique), the catheter tip is placed only in the nasopharynx.

When oxygen is delivered by nasal catheter, the nurse should choose a catheter that is comfortable to the client's nose. Generally a French catheter, size 8 to 10, is recommended for children, size 10 to 12 for women, and size 12 to 14 for men. The flow rate should be started at 3 to 4 L/min before the catheter is inserted. A water-soluble lubricant should be used to lubricate the tip. The catheter should be checked for patency. One method for checking patency is to dip the tip of the catheter in water and observe for bubbling.

When the oropharyngeal technique is used, the desired depth of insertion is determined by measuring the distance from the ear lobe to the external nares. After insertion, the catheter should be observed approximately opposite the uvula. If the catheter is inserted too far, gastric distension may result. If the client appears to be swallowing air, the catheter should be withdrawn slowly until swallowing ceases. For the nasopharynx technique the catheter is inserted until the tip touches the back of the nasopharynx. It is then withdrawn about ½ inch. Once the catheter is in the desired position, it should be taped to the tip of the nose.

Even when oxygen is administered by catheter, movement should not be hampered. Tubing should be pinned to the bedding or clothing, with enough slack to facilitate movement. The catheter should be changed at least every 8 hours, or whenever it becomes obstructed, and a clean catheter inserted into the opposite nostril. The nares should be cleansed of secretions frequently to ensure a patent airway and to reduce irritation that may be caused by oxygen. Frequent oral hygiene is also important to alleviate dryness, remove secretions, and prevent infection.

The nasal *cannula* is commonly used. With this method the concentration of oxygen is controlled by adjusting the oxygen flow 2 to 8 L/min to deliver a concentration of 30% to 40%. Two small soft plastic prongs are placed in the external nares. The prongs are held in place by a headband that fits over the ears. These should be adjusted to the client's comfort. Mouth breathing should be discouraged, because it causes the concentration of oxygen to be diluted. Similar care is administered to the client with a cannula as with a catheter. Both methods are advantageous in that they do not interfere with eating or talking or hamper movement.

When a client is not able to tolerate a nasal catheter or cannula, because of excessive drainage or nasal obstruction, a *face mask* may be prescribed. The mask fits around the nose and mouth and is capable of delivering concentrations of oxygen from 40% to 80%. When oxygen is started by mask, the flow should be started at an excessive rate (8 to 10 L/min) and gradually decreased to 4 to 6 L/min, or as prescribed, when breathing approaches normal. If the client is anxious, the nurse may find it helpful to allow him to place the mask around his face before the headband is applied. This lessens the closed-in feeling. Once the client accepts the mask, the headband should be adjusted so it fits snugly but not too tight. Oxygen should not be permitted to escape from the top of the mask and blow into the client's eyes. To prevent skin irritation, the mask should be removed at least every 2 hours, and the face washed and dried. Powder may be applied to the face to keep it dry. The position of the mask, the presence of leaks and kinks, and the water supply in the humidifier should be assessed hourly.

Various types of masks are used. The *Venturi mask,* which is based on the Venturi principle, delivers precise fixed concentrations of 24%, 28%, 35%, and 40% oxygen. A prescribed gas flow is used for each type. For example, 40% require 8 L/min, and 24% require 4 L/min. An aerosol humidity source is not required for Venturi masks that deliver 30% concentration and below. However, the higher (that is, 35%, 40%) should have a humidity source.[30] In fact, these (above 30%) are humidified by an adjunctive aerosol therapy that is generated by compressed air. These masks are commonly used to begin oxygen therapy in clients with chronic obstructive pulmonary disease because high concentrations of oxygen might depress ventilation. It prevents abrupt changes in Pa_{O_2} and Pa_{CO_2}[23] and is therefore an effective method of controlling inspired oxygen. Although expensive, the Venturi mask is beneficial for home use, especially by clients who tend not to keep the liter flow low. *Nonbreathing masks,* which do not permit carbon dioxide to accumulate, and *partial rebreathing masks* are used to increase the $F_{I_{O_2}}$. A tight fit and gas flow affect proper functioning of the bag. Flow rates should be adequate to prevent the bag from collapsing on inspiration.[50] These masks are often used for the client who hyperventilates.

Oxygen may also be administered through a *tracheostomy* either by a special tracheal mask or catheter. These methods are particularly useful when the client has a cuffed tracheostomy. Portable oxygen is also available for the ambulatory client. Such units may be prescribed for home use.

Special rooms have been designed in some facilities to deliver oxygen. Oxygen is piped into the room, and the client can be cared for as he would be in an ordinary room.

Hyperbaric oxygenation is a means of delivering large concentrations of oxygen to the cells over a brief period of time. Oxygen is administered in a pressure chamber, which delivers oxygen at three times the pressure that is ordinarily breathed. Hyperbaric oxygenation has proved to be most effective as therapy for anaerobic infections (such as tetanus and gas gangrene) and carbon monoxide poisoning; as cancer therapy when combined with radiation; in cardiovascular surgery; and in the relief of arterial insufficiency of the extremities. Numerous articles are available on the uses of hyperbaric oxygenation. The reader should refer to them for details regarding compression and decompression, complications that can arise, and overall hazards of oxygen administered at such high concentrations.

Terminating oxygen therapy. Analysis of oxygen concentration and blood gas determinations are particularly necessary when preparation is being made for terminating oxygen therapy. The physician may order a gradual lowering of the oxygen concentration. Analysis must be made with each decrease in flow rate. If, during this approach, the client needs more oxygen, analysis should be made of the concentration before it is increased. Any possible factor associated with the need for an increase should be evaluated. For example, did the client appear to need more oxygen after engaging in an activity, such as eating a meal?

Besides a reduction in flow rate, an approach that may be employed is to discontinue therapy for a brief period on a trial basis. When either approach is used, the nurse should frequently assess the client's physiological and emotional response to a decrease in therapy. The observations should be reported to the physician. The presence of an increased pulse rate, respiratory distress, and other signs of hypoxia warrant continuing oxygen therapy.

Intermittent positive pressure breathing

Intermittent positive pressure breathing (IPPB) is pressure greater than atmospheric pressure at the airway opening during inspiration (Fig. 21-16). As a result, a greater amount of air enters the lungs with or without increased FI_{O_2}. Such therapy may be provided to improve delivery of medication (in clients unable to coordinate their breathing pattern), to improve coughing and expectoration (by delivering aerosolized medication), to lower a rising Pa_{CO_2},[3] to facilitate lung expansion, and to promote adequate ventilation without increased effort by the client. For example, the postoperative client has a tendency to hypoventilate because of pain, tight bandages, and sedation. Clients who remain in bed or who are seriously ill also tend to breathe ineffectively. Although proper nursing care (including coughing and deep breathing exercises) is considered more effective, IPPB therapy may be prescribed to facilitate adequate ventilation, thus preventing pulmonary complications. The nurse should be aware of precisely what the IPPB treatment is to accomplish. If removal of secretions is the primary concern, then coughing should be encouraged following therapy. See discussion of effective coughing methods earlier in this chapter.

The device may be adjusted to cycle automatically (pressure assisted) or may be triggered by the client's own inspiratory effort (client controlled). The later approach is used more often.

The physician prescribes the amount of pressure, oxygen concentration, medication, and length and frequency of therapy. It is usually prescribed three to

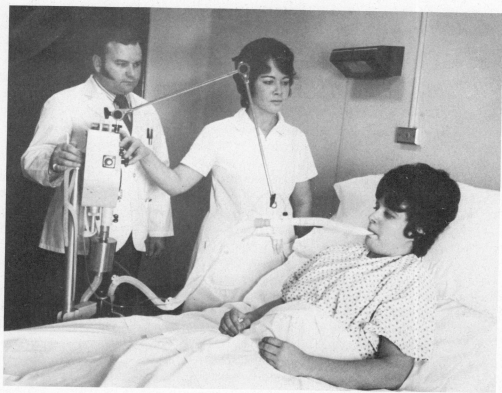

FIG. 21-16
Respiratory therapists administer inspiratory positive pressure breathing to client. (Courtesy St. Francis Hospital Center, Beech Grove, Ind.)

four times a day for 10 to 15 minutes for children and 15 to 20 minutes for adults. If the client is having severe respiratory distress, treatments may be prescribed at more frequent intervals. The respiratory therapist administers therapy. However, in the absence of a therapist, the nurse must observe the client to evaluate the ventilatory pattern, response to therapy, and whether the therapeutic objectives are being obtained without complications.[3] The need for necessary changes should be communicated with the physician. As therapy is begun, the client should be instructed to sit up straight, relax, and breathe deeply on inspiration. He should be permitted to stop during the treatment to cough and expectorate secretions. The client should be observed for signs of hyperventilation. When the client hyperventilates, carbon dioxide is rapidly eliminated, and an intracellular alkalosis may result. Such complaints as head and chest pain, numbness and tingling of the fingers and toes, vertigo, syncope, and in extreme states, carpopedal spasms may occur. These symptoms warrant discontinuation of therapy and notification of the physician or respiratory therapist.

If the client receives sympathomimetic drugs such as isoproterenol (Isuprel) hydrochloride, he should be observed for symptoms of palpitation, rapid increase in pulse rate, tremors, nervousness, dizziness, and headache. If they occur, therapy should be discontinued. Other medications that are commonly prescribed include isoetharine hydrochloride (Bronkosol), acetylcysteine (Mucomyst), and pancreatic dornase (Dornavac).

Parameters that may be used to determine the therapeutic benefit of IPPB therapy include pulmonary function, blood gas analysis, sputum production, or evidence of improved expectoration, or decreased respiratory symptoms.[3]

1269

Incentive spirometry

Incentive spirometry, frequently prescribed for clients postoperatively, encourages a voluntary maximal sustained inspiration as the client inhales through a spirometer.[23] The goal is to provide an incentive for maximal inspiratory effort. The spirometer contains a signal that goes on when the preset inspiratory volume is inhaled and remains on until inspiratory flow ceases. The inspiratory volume is preset and is increased by increments.

Aerosol therapy

Aerosol therapy is commonly administered to clients with infections and obstructive pulmonary diseases. When administered for these purposes, it acts as a vehicle for administering drugs in the form of a mist to the lower respiratory passages.

Aerosols of distilled water or normal saline are used to liquefy secretions and improve mucociliary transport. Detergents such as propylene glycol or glycerine decrease viscosity of secretions by reducing surface tension.[46] Mucolytic agents (for example, acetylcysteine) change the physical characteristics of bronchial secretions and increase mobilization. Other medications that may be administered are antibiotics, steroids, vasoconstrictors, and bronchodilators. Such therapy may be administered intermittently (four to six times per day) or continuously. When used continuously, aerosols are usually used along with assisted ventilation.

Devices used to generate aerosols are *nebulizers* and *humidifiers*. The former forms a cloud or mist, whereas the latter increases the water vapor content. A number of nebulizers in clinical use deliver varied particle size. For example, an ultrasonic nebulizer produces particle sizes over a small range of 0.5μ to 3μ, a jet nebulizer produces particle sizes between 0.5μ to 15μ, and a hand bulb nebulizer reduces a solution to a mist of fine particles 3μ to 5μ in diameter. When aerosol therapy (for example, ultrasonic nebulizer) is prescribed in conjunction with IPPB, the client should be instructed to exhale as much as possible, gently bite down on the mouthpiece and seal the lips around it so that air does not escape. He should then inspire deeply (to increase tidal volume), hold the breath 1 to 2 seconds (to facilitate the particles being deposited deeply and uniformly), and exhale completely. Following the therapy, the client should be encouraged to cough forcefully.

Most nebulizers distribute large quantities of water over short periods of time. As a result, alterations in fluid balance (such as overhydration) may occur. Therefore accurate records must be kept of intake and output whenever any form of aerosol therapy is prescribed. The appearance of dyspnea either during or following therapy may be an indication of an excessive deposit of moisture in the airway resulting in increased airway resistance.[30] The physician should be notified if dyspnea occurs.

Ventilation therapy

Ventilation therapy (mechanical ventilation) is a means of augmenting respiratory gas exchange by the use of a mechanical device (such as a ventilator).

Indications for ventilation therapy
1. To relieve respiratory insufficiency without increasing the work of breathing, by increasing tidal volume, actively inflating the lungs, and providing a means for more adequate ventilation.
2. To administer aerosol therapy deeply into the poorly ventilated lungs.
3. To improve alveolar gas exchange by effecting more uniform aeration.
4. To promote better bronchial drainage.

5. To establish a more effective cough by ventilating beyond retained secretions.

6. To eliminate buildup of carbon dioxide in the blood, thereby preventing acidosis.

7. To provide deep breathing exercises, thereby improving the tone of the respiratory muscles and improving pulmonary circulation.

Types of ventilation. There are many types of ventilators available. Basically, these can be divided into two main classifications: pressure cycled and volume cycled.

Pressure-cycled ventilators permit air to flow into the client's lung until a predetermined pressure is reached. When the pressure is reached, a valve closes, the inspiratory phase ceases, and expiration begins. The cycle then is repeated. The pressure is preset, hence the name pressure-cycled. The Bird and Bennett PR-1 and PR-2 are examples of pressure-cycled ventilators.

Any form of obstruction, as from excessive mucus, will alter the cycle. Inspiration is shortened; therefore the rate of cycling increases. If any leakage occurs in the system, the inspiratory phase is prolonged because it takes longer for the pressure to build up, resulting in prolonged inspiration. The nurse should therefore listen for changes in rhythm of the cycle and plan some form of implementation. For example, suctioning the client often relieves the obstruction that is responsible for the change. If this measure does not relieve it, the physician and possibly the respiratory therapist should be notified immediately. If the inspiratory cycle is prolonged, the system should be checked for leaks. Pressure-cycled ventilators, because of imprecise ventilation, have just about disappeared from routine use.

The *volume-cycled ventilator* delivers a predetermined volume of gas into the client's lung with each breath. The volume may range up to 2000 cc or more.[30] When the volume is delivered, the inflation cycle stops, and the lungs are permitted to deflate, which is followed by a repetition of the cycle. Again, any form of obstruction or leakage alters the cycle. Volume ventilators have a safety feature or control that limits the system's pressure, which functions to prevent delivery of high pressures. For example, when the pressure limit is reached, an alarm (visual or audible) is activated, and some of the volume is not delivered. Examples of volume-cycled ventilators for the infant are Babybird, Bourns, Bio-med MVP-10, and Amsterdam; for the adult, the Engstrom, Bennett MA-1, and Emerson and Ohio Critical Care ventilators.

These ventilators have certain controls (sighs, sensitivity disconnect alarms) and accessory attachments (humidifiers, spirometers, intermittent mandatory ventilation (IMV), CPAP, PEEP). Discussion of the latter two follow.

Continuous positive airway pressure (CPAP or CPPB) is a *nonmechanical* means of ventilation. (CPAP differs from PEEP in that the client on CPAP is breathing spontaneously, and may not be on a ventilator; whereas the client is controlled by a ventilator on PEEP).[30] It provides continuous positive airway pressure by maintaining pressures above zero at the end of the expiratory phase. As a result, collapse of the alveoli is prevented because air within these structures is forced to be retained. An endotracheal tube or face mask may be used to deliver measured concentrations of oxygen. The use of an aneroid manometer facilitates constant monitoring of the pressure. Weaning, by lowering expiratory pressure, takes place gradually over a period of several days. This procedure has primarily been used as therapy for neonatal respiratory distress syndrome. Adequate skin care around the face is essential.

Positive end expiratory pressure (PEEP) refers to a ventilatory pattern in which a positive airway pressure is applied with inspiration and expiration. Such pressure does not fall to zero at the end of expiration. Hence, it is very useful in a number of diseases where arterial hypoxemia is manifest. It may be used with mechanical ventilation whether the client has an endotracheal tube or tracheostomy.

Levels commonly used for PEEP are 5, 10, and 15 cm. On expiration, the desired PEEP level should be reached but should begin rising on the next inspiration to the desired peak inspiratory pressure. PEEP is effective in that it causes the alveoli and smaller airways to be opened for a longer period of time in addition to increasing the lung volume, thus enhancing the distribution of oxygen throughout the lungs.

When PEEP is used, the client's cardiovascular status (heart rate, blood pressure) should be monitored closely. The urine output and arterial blood gases are also frequently monitored. It is also important that close checks be made of the ventilator, because any minor change may alter the PEEP reading.

Client assessments during ventilation therapy. When ventilatory therapy is employed, assessments of the client's oxygen status, blood gas determinations, and analyses of the oxygen concentration are frequently made. Any marked changes in these must be reported to the physician.

Frequent assessments must also be made of the client's vital signs, increasing rate and character of pulse and respirations, blood pressure, skin color, level of consciousness, secretions, urinary output, degree of chest expansion, breath sounds, and other physical assessments as previously mentioned. When medications are used for nebulization, the nurse must be aware of signs of drug overdosage and report the appearance of these to the physician. Signs indicative of water intoxication (weight gain and behavior changes such as confusion, inattentiveness, weakness, and edema) should be observed. This is particularly important for the child.

Oxygen toxicity is a potential hazard, especially when the concentration of oxygen is greater than 40%. Substernal chest pain is a common sign of oxygen toxicity.

Because the incidence of stress ulcers tends to increase with the length of time a client is on a ventilator, the nurse should anticipate this and observe the client for gastrointestinal bleeding. The nasogastric drainage and stools should be tested for guaiac and observed for the overt appearance of blood.

The nurse must also observe the machine to ensure proper functioning. The pressure, oxygen concentration, set respiratory rate, set volume, water level on humidifier, and position of artificial airway should all be observed at regularly scheduled intervals.

Implementing care during ventilation therapy. Regardless of the form of therapy, the nurse must help the client maintain the integrity of all systems. Clients receiving ventilatory therapy require constant attention. Measures must be carried out to prevent skin breakdown and muscle contractures. The client's position should be changed frequently. He must be positioned to facilitate effective breathing (that is, in a semi-Fowler's position) unless contraindicated. Adequate humidification must be employed. Adequate fluids and nutrition must be provided. Frequent oral and nasal hygiene must be given. Patency of the airway must be maintained. This can be accomplished by suctioning as frequently as necessary. Measures must be employed to maintain adequate elimination.

Emotional support must be provided to the client and the family. Care should be provided in a confident, assured manner. Such action will undoubtedly facilitate a calming feeling in the client and minimize feelings of helplessness. When family members are present, some time should be spent with the family answering the questions, informing them of the indications and rationale for therapeutic routines.

Artificial airways

Artificial airways are used to ensure an opened airway, facilitate administration of a high oxygen concentration and humidification, and facilitate mechanical ventilation. These are accomplished through the use of an oropharyngeal airway, nasopharyngeal airway (Fig. 21-17), endotracheal tube, or tracheostomy.

Oropharyngeal airway. An oropharyngeal airway is generally placed in the oral cavity and provides an airway down to the pharynx. In addition, in the unconscious client it helps maintain the tongue in a normal position, thus preventing the tongue from falling back and blocking the airway. Its use also enhances pharyngeal suctioning. These airways come in various sizes (Fig. 21-18). Whenever they are used, the client should always maintain a lateral position, to prevent the device from being aspirated.

Endotracheal intubation. Endotracheal intubation is often employed when airway assistance is needed for 1 or 2 days and when anesthesia is administered. Endotracheal tubes may be inserted through the mouth (*orotracheal*) by the physician via a laryngoscope (Fig. 21-19, *A*). The orotracheal tube extends from the mouth to just above the bifurcation of the trachea (Fig. 21-19, *B*). After orotracheal intubation, an oropharyngeal airway is usually inserted to prevent the

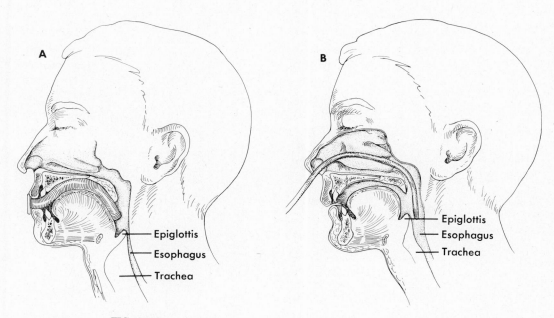

FIG. 21-17
A, Oropharyngeal airway. **B,** Nasopharyngeal airway.

1273

FIG. 21-18
Various sizes of oropharyngeal airways. (From Smith, Robert M.: Anesthesia for infants and children, ed. 4, St. Louis, 1979, The C. V. Mosby Co.

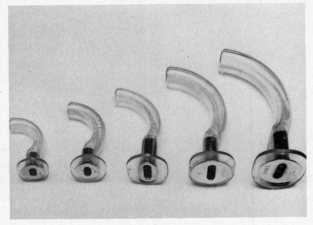

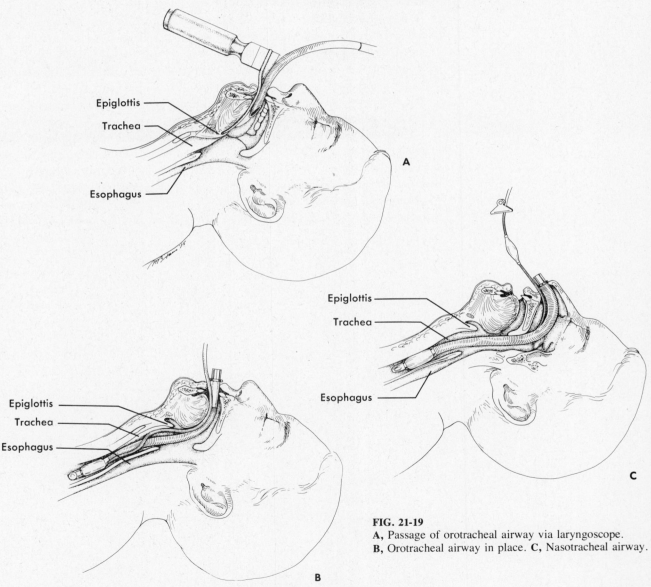

Epiglottis

Trachea

Esophagus

A

Epiglottis

Trachea

Esophagus

C

Epiglottis

Trachea

Esophagus

B

FIG. 21-19
A, Passage of orotracheal airway via laryngoscope.
B, Orotracheal airway in place. **C,** Nasotracheal airway.

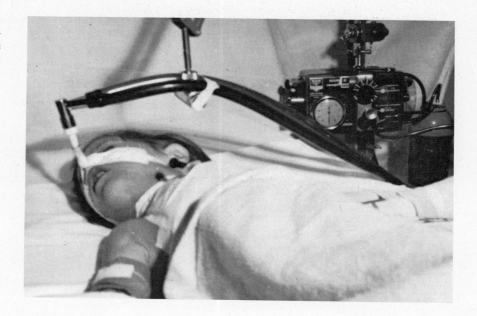

client from occluding the tube by biting. The tube may also be inserted through the nares (*nasotracheal,* Figs. 21-19, *C,* and 21-20). This route facilitates better tolerance and subsequently the tube can be continued for a longer period of time.[12]

Endotracheal tubes have an inflatable cuff, except those used for infants and small children. The narrow cricoid ring in infants and small children ensures an adequate tracheal seal, thus making the use of a cuffed tube unnecessary. However, in adolescents the trachea grows larger than the larynx. Hence a cuff is needed to seal off the tube. When cuffed tubes are used, precautions similar to those with a cuffed tracheostomy tube must be taken (Table 21-6).

Endotracheal tubes are made of hard rubber or plastic and are very uncomfortable; therefore, they are tolerated better by the unconscious person. If the client requires a tracheal airway beyond 2 days, a tracheostomy is generally performed. Usually the maximum time an endotracheal tube is left in place is 5 days. Table 21-7 shows selection of sizes of endotracheal tubes.

Whenever endotracheal tubes are used, the nurse must develop a plan that will enhance maintenance of the airway. Especially with infants, the tube must be maintained in proper position because even the slightest movement may result in displacement of the tube into the right main bronchus and occlude the left one by bypassing it.[4]

Secretions must be removed from the oropharynx as often as necessary by suctioning. If secretions accumulate around the base of the tube, the secretions must be suctioned through the tube. See discussion of principles of suctioning later in this chapter. Frequent assessments should be made of the client's vital signs, respiratory status, and emotional state. It is particularly important to bilaterally auscultate the lungs to determine if both lungs are being ventilated. Occasionally endotracheal tubes are placed beyond the bifurcation of the bronchus, resulting in only one lung being aerated.

Tracheostomy. A tracheostomy is the creation of an artificial opening into the trachea through which breathing occurs. The incision is made on the anterior

TABLE 21-6

Endotracheal intubation: nursing assessment and implementation

Stage of intubation	Rationale
Preintubation	
1. Explain procedure to client and family.	Explanation regarding what to expect is essential in lessening anxiety.
2. Inform client and family of the inability to speak while tube is in place, but once the tube is removed, the client will be able to speak.	With the tube in place, air does not pass over the vocal cords; therefore, sounds are not produced.
3. Establish a method of communication: writing or nonverbal.	Provides a means of maintaining contact with the environment.
4. Assess for loose, chipped, or capped teeth.	
5. Removal dental prosthesis, or any foreign object or secretion.	Protects client from possible dislodgement during intubation.
6. Obtain necessary equipment (laryngoscope with straight and curved blades, Magill forceps and a swirl adapter, tracheal tube, oropharyngeal airway or bite block, tape, inflating syringe, phenylephrine hydrochloride, lidocaine hydrochloride, Ambu bag, suctioning equipment, oxygen, guide wire, and water soluble lubricant).	Enhances successful intubation. The laryngoscope facilitates passage of the ET tube. The airway or bit block prevents damage or occlusion of the tube if the client bites down. The lubricant facilitates passage and prevents trauma.
7. Check function of equipment (such as cuffs for leaks, or laryngoscope for batteries and bulbs.)	Ensures proper functioning of equipment before actually starting procedure.
Intubation	
1. Provide psychological support during the process of intubation (such as explaining what is occurring).	Explanation and reassurance help lessen anxiety.
2. Properly position client at midchest height of physician, in a sniffing position, with the head anteriorly displaced and hyperextended.	Reduces need for physician to bend. The sniffing position creates a relatively straight line through the oropharyngeal and tracheal passageways.
3. Flood with oxygen immediately before and after intubation.	Ensures adequate oxygenation. Client is deprived of oxygen during procedure.
4. Secure tube to face and bite block.	Prevents accidental extubation or dislodgement of the tube into the right main bronchus. Bite block is used to prevent client from biting down, thus preventing obstruction of the tube.
5. Observe for signs indicating developing complications: cessation of breathing, crowing respiratory sounds, wheezes.	Apnea, aspiration, laryngospasm, bronchospasms, and tube displacement are immediate complications of intubation.
6. Assess blood pressure and heart rate at frequent intervals.	
7. Auscultate the chest bilaterally immediately after intubation and at least at hourly intervals thereafter.	To evaluate airway patency, distribution of air, and abnormal breath sounds. Decreased breath sounds on either side indicate inadequate ventilation of the respective lung.
8. Assess symmetry of chest.	To evaluate distribution of air.
9. Secure order for chest x-ray films.	Confirms placement of tube.
10. Suction secretions as often as necessary.	Secretions increase because of irritation caused by the tube. Remove secretions and prevent aspiration.
a. Auscultate following suctioning.	Auscultate to evaluate effectiveness of suctioning. Suctioning can stimulate vagus nerve and produce dysrhythmias.
b. Assess apical pulse rate and quality.	
11. Maintain high humidity and oxygen concentration as prescribed.	Prevents drying of secretions. Excessive dryness could result in destruction of the alveolar-capillary membrane. Oxygen is given to facilitate adequate oxygenation. With humidification, water is absorbed and can thus alter fluid volume.
12. Maintain strict intake and output.	
13. Reassure client through verbal communications, as well as by such actions as calmness and an air of confidence.	
14. Follow up on established means of communication.	
15. Turn side to side hourly and perform active and passive exercises.	Facilitates movement of secretions. Stimulates circulation.
16. Provide frequent oral hygiene.	
17. Restrain the restless, agitated client.	Prevents dislodging the tube.
Preparation for extubation	
1. Suction secretions from airway through the tube before it is removed.	Prevents aspiration of secretions during process of removal.
2. Adequately oxygenate the client before removal.	Maintains adequate oxygen supply to cells.
Postextubation	
1. Observe for signs of complications: stridor, dyspnea, cyanosis, or crowing respiratory sounds.	Laryngeal edema may develop 1 to 3 hours after intubation. Laryngeal spasms and subglottic edema may also occur. Hoarseness is commonly experienced.
2. Monitor vital signs, respiratory status closely for: quality and rate of respiration, chest sounds, symmetry of chest, and color. Evaluate blood gases.	
3. Assess degree of mental alertness and client's behavior.	
4. Instruct client regarding frequent turning, coughing, and deep breathing.	Stimulates circulation, facilitates movements of secretions, and prevents alveolar collapse.

neck below the second and third tracheal cartilages, and the tracheostomy is maintained by an outer and inner cannula (Fig. 21-21). The outer cannula fits directly into the tracheal opening. The inner cannula fits into the outer cannula. A third part, the obturator, is used at the time of insertion to prevent trauma.

Cuffed tracheostomy tube. The cuffed tracheostomy tube has the advantage of providing a closed system, thus preventing air from entering or escaping the upper respiratory passages. As a result, better ventilation is maintained, because it is usually used in conjunction with positive-pressure ventilators. It also reduces the possibility of aspiration of secretions when the laryngeal and pharyngeal reflexes are absent.

To seal the encircling balloon around the trachea, it is inflated *slowly* with the least amount of air necessary. Usually from 1 to 3 cc of air may be needed to provide an adequate seal. A slight air leak should always be left to decrease pressure in the trachea and prevent ischemic necrosis, thus decreasing chances of a tracheal esophageal fistula developing. (If the cuff pressure is allowed to exceed systemic circulation pressure in the tissue [around 25 mm Hg], a reduction in blood circulation occurs.[24]) Signs that may be used to determine the *least* adequate amount of air are (1) aphonia in the conscious client, because sound is absent when air flows over the vocal cords and (2) absence of an audible escapage of air from the nose, mouth, and tracheostomy tube when the tube is briefly occluded.

Distal to the inflating balloon is a small test balloon that is used as a guide in determining when the cuff balloon is inflated. When the distal balloon becomes inflated, this indicates that the cuff balloon is also inflated. The test balloon remains inflated as long as the cuffed balloon is.

A syringe that has been filled with the desired amount of air and a hemostat with padded rubber tubing are needed to inflate the cuff. The rubber tubing prevents damage to the small-bore tubing. The hemostat is clamped over the tubing after the balloon is inflated to prevent air from escaping from the tubing. The nurse should record that amount of air needed to inflate the tubing so that one is readily aware if a significant increase in the amount of air is needed for inflation. If the amount increases significantly, the physician should be notified, because it might be an indication of tracheal dilation. If the cuff has been in place

TABLE 21-7

Selection of sizes of endotracheal tubes

Age (yr)	Weight (lb)	Anatomical distance (cm)			Endotracheal catheter size			Length of catheter (cm)	Tidal volume (cc)
		Teeth to carina	Teeth to cords	Length of trachea	French*	Portex Magill*	Outside diameter (mm)	Orotracheal*	
6-7	44-55	15.5	9.5	6	25, 26, 27	3, *4*, 5	8.3-9	*15*, 16, 17	250-350
7-8	44-55	15.5	9.5	6	25, 26, 27	3, *4*, 5	8.3-9	*15*, 16, 17	275-375
8-9	55-70	15.5-17	9.5-10	6.3	26, *27*, 28	4, *5*, 6	8.7-9.3	15, *16*, 17	275-375
9-10	55-70	15.5-17	9.5-10	6.3	26, *27*, 28	4, *5*, 6	8.7-9.3	15, *16*, 17	350-400
10-12	70-85	16.3-18.5	10.0-11	6.3	28, *29*, 30	5, *6*, 7	9.3-10	16, *17*, 18	400-500
12-16	85-130	17.5-25	11.0-15	6.5-7	31-32	6, *7*, 8	10.0-11.3	17, *22.5*, 24	400-500
Adult	130-200	28.0-32	12.0-15	10.0-14	34-36	7, 8, *9*, 10	10.7-13.3	*23*, 26	450-550

From Smith, Betty J.: Fundamentals of anesthesia care, St. Louis, 1972, The C.V. Mosby Co.
*The numbers in italics indicate the average size for the particular age group.

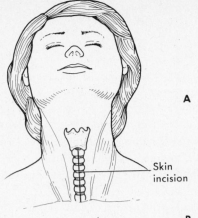

Skin incision

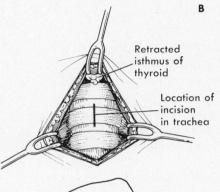

Retracted isthmus of thyroid

Location of incision in trachea

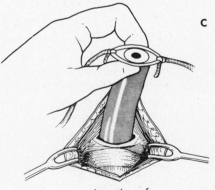

Insertion of tracheostomy tube

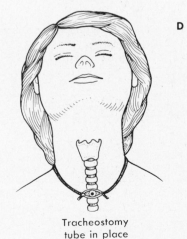

Tracheostomy tube in place

FIG. 21-21
Creation of a tracheostomy. **A,** Skin incision (note position of head). **B,** Location of incision in trachea. **C,** Insertion of tracheostomy tube. **D,** Tracheostomy tube in place.

for some time, a small additional amount of air may be needed because of some tracheal dilation. The physician should be consulted whenever difficulty is experienced in inflating the cuff. The nurse should be aware of signs that indicate leakage or rupture of the cuff. Deflation of the test balloon while the tubing is clamped is one sign of leakage. Signs of rupture are an increase in the amount of air needed to inflate the balloon, absence of resistance to the increased volume, withdrawal of more air than was injected, and absence of aphonia.

At one time, routines were established for deflating the cuff to eliminate the possibility of tracheal ischemia and necrosis. However, the use of low-pressure cuffs (such as the Lenz tube) and minimal leak technique have eliminated the need for periodic deflation of the tube.

Need for tracheostomy. Tracheostomies are performed for a number of reasons. In contrast to practices of years past, they are performed not only to maintain a patent airway in a respiratory emergency (such as from respiratory tract obstruction) but also for preventive reasons. When a tracheostomy is performed for preventive reasons, it is done to (1) improve and maintain ventilation, (2) prevent or relieve hypoxia that may be caused by accumulation of secretions in the pulmonary tree, and (3) reduce the work of breathing for a weak or critically ill client.

The nurse should be aware of signs that indicate respiratory distress. Signs such as gasping respiration, sternal retraction, labored breathing, tachycardia, and cyanosis are significant and should be reported to the physician immediately.

On recognizing the need for a tracheostomy, the nurse prepares the necessary equipment, including a tracheostomy tray, sterile gloves, an antiseptic, and an anesthetic. The client should be instructed about the procedure. A small pillow or blanket may be placed under the client's shoulders to hyperextend the neck, thus bringing the larynx and trachea closer to the surface. A small towel may be used for the child. The nurse selects the appropriate tube size for the client (Table 21-8).

In an emergency situation, there will be little or no time for preparation and explanations about the experience. However, when the procedure is planned, adequate explanations should be given to the client. Explanations of the meaning, effect, and outcome of the tracheostomy should be a part of the information. The client should be given a description of the tracheostomy tube and be told its purpose and how it works when in place. He should be permitted to examine the equipment. He should be told what to expect and what is expected of him. The routines of tracheostomy care should be explained. Important during this period is assuring the client that someone will be in constant attendance with him during the early posttracheostomy period. Instructions about coughing and deep breathing should be given.

Means of communication should be discussed. The client should be informed that when a tracheostomy is performed, the expired air passes out below the level of the cords rather than over the vocal cords. As a result, sounds are

TABLE 21-8

Suggested tracheostomy tube sizes for various age levels

Age	Size
Newborn	00 to 0
1 month to 1 year	1
1 to 3 years	2
3 to 6 years	3
6 to 12 years	4
12 years and over	5

not possible. Therefore some method of communication should be established. A pen or pencil and pad or a magic slate are common methods to use. If necessary, the use of the magic slate should be demonstrated. If the client is unable to write, a simple system of communication should be established. If the tracheostomy is to be temporary and if the larynx is intact, the client should be told that covering the tracheostomy opening for very brief intervals will allow sounds to be produced as the cover permits air to flow over the vocal cords. The nurse might cover the opening for the client if he is unable to do so himself.

Because the infant cannot communicate by speaking or writing, it is difficult for the nurse to develop a system for nonverbal communications. Therefore the nurse will have to anticipate his needs. Strategies such as pointing to pictures or using lip reading may prove valuable for the older child.

The nurse should discuss other limitations with the client. He will not be able to strain because elimination of the glottis from the air route decreases his ability to perform activities associated with Valsalva's maneuver (forcibly pressing against a closed glottis). While eating, the client should be instructed to tilt the head forward (anteflexion) to prevent aspiration. When the head is anteflexed, the esophagus opens wide and the epiglottis closes completely. Hyperextension favors aspiration because in this position the esophagus narrows, and a direct route is opened into the trachea. As a result, foods and fluids may flow easily into the trachea.

Complications that may occur following a tracheostomy include dislodgement, obstruction of the tube by secretions, bleeding, and subcutaneous emphysema. These are more likely to occur during the first week. Between the second and third week, complications are thought to be related to excessive cuff compression of endotracheal mucosa (tracheal stenosis). The nurse's awareness of these will guide assessments of symptoms that might be indicative.

Tracheostomy care. When a tracheostomy has been performed, the client has a tendency to be frightened. The nurse should relate a feeling of confidence by being calm. A frightened client produces an increased amount of mucus, causing more distress and further endangering the patency of the airway. For the child, the nurse should use a gentle touch and a confident expression as methods to calm him.

The client should be observed frequently. This is particularly important for infants; because of the small size of the tube, it can easily become obstructed. The nurse must not forget that the tracheostomized client cannot call for help. The call light must therefore be kept within easy reach. Paper and pencil should be provided for the older client.

Three main principles should serve as a guide in caring for clients with tracheostomies: a patent airway must be maintained, cleanliness must be promoted, and drying and crusting of the mucosa must be prevented.

1. Maintain a patent airway.
   a. Observe the tube for accumulation of excessive secretions, and suction as often as needed. The tracheostomy tube acts as a foreign body to the respiratory passage, and the response is an increase in the amount of secretion. The trachea might have to be suctioned as often as every 10 to 15 minutes during the first 24 hours. The frequency of suctioning decreases after the first couple of days.

b. Observe for signs of airway occlusion.
(1) Changes in vital signs—increased pulse rate, increased shallow respirations, decreased blood pressure, and low-grade fever.
(2) Changes in mental attitude—restlessness and anxiety.
(3) Changes in respiratory status—wheezing, whistling, bubbling, gurgling, rattling, and dyspnea.
c. Observe for air leaks around the trachea. To detect air leaks, the nurse palpates the exposed skin near the wound and listens for crackling sounds.
d. Observe the position of the client. The client should be elevated to a semi-Fowler's position. This position facilitates more effective breathing and coughing. It also promotes drainage of accumulating fluid, as well as prevents fluid from pressing on the airway. Positioning a smaller infant and young child is perhaps more challenging. The infant's neck must be constantly observed. A desirable position for the infant is one in which he is flat. A small pillow may be placed under his neck and shoulders. Arm splints may have to be used to prevent the young child from pulling out the tube. See Chapter 8 for discussion of restraints.
e. Observe the position of the tracheostomy tube.
2. Promote cleanliness. The nurse should remove the inner cannula and cleanse it as often as necessary.
3. Prevent drying and crusting of the mucosa.
a. Remove secretions as they accumulate.
b. Provide some form of moisture or humidification. Often, the physician may order 2 to 3 ml of sterile saline to be instilled directly into the tube before suctioning to aid in loosening secretions and to provide a stimulus for the cough reflex.
c. Provide adequate hydration.

Maintaining a patent airway: suctioning. Suctioning is performed to remove accumulated secretions from the respiratory tract and is an absolute necessity. The client is not able to produce an effective cough, and the secretions are usually excessive in the initial period because the tracheostomy tube stimulates secretions. Explosive coughing is not possible because pressure cannot be built up against the closed glottis. Suctioning should therefore be performed as often as necessary. During the first 24 hours this might be as often as every 10 to 15 minutes. The intervals between aspirations lengthen as the quantity of secretions decreases. With a reduction in the amount secreted, the aspiration span may lengthen to 1- or 4-hour intervals. Retained secretions are an excellent medium for bacteria, and the removal of these by suctioning reduces the possibility of an infection.

Before suctioning is started, the nurse must obtain the client's cooperation and relieve his apprehension. The technique therefore should be explained to the client, and the nurse's hands should be washed.

TRACHEOBRONCHIAL SUCTIONING WITH CATHETER. If suctioning is to be effective, consideration must be given to the type, size, and diameter of the catheter. A whistle-tip catheter is most desirable because its smooth, rounded end permits mucus to be removed more effectively. The diameter of the catheter

TABLE 21-9

Catheter sizes for various age groups

Age group	Size (French scale)
Infants	5 and 8
Children	10
Adults	14 and 18

From Aspiration techniques, The H-Line **2:**8-9, Fall/Winter 1968.

TABLE 21-10

Force of suction for various ages

	Inches (Hg)	mm (Hg)
Infants	3 to 5	60 to 100
Children	5 to 8	100 to 110
Adults	8 to 15	110 to 140

From Aspiration techniques, The H-Line **2:**8-9, Fall/Winter 1968.

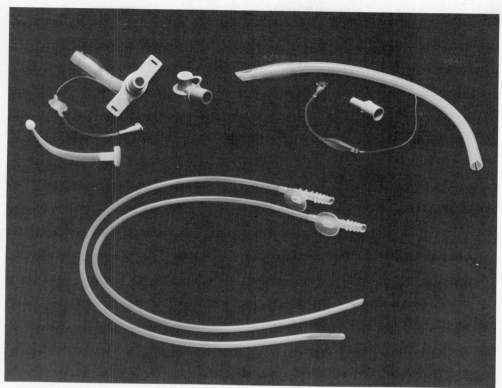

FIG. 21-22
Vent on aspiration catheter permits intermittent aspiration. Note cuffed tracheostomy and endotracheal tubes. (Courtesy Protex Division, Smith Industries, Inc., Woburn, Mass.)

should be large enough to remove the mucus but not so large that it obstructs the airway. A catheter that is not more than two thirds of the size of the opening of the tracheostomy tube meets this criterion. Suggested catheter sizes have been established, and they should be adhered to as closely as possible (Table 21-9).

A Y or T valve attachment should be attached to the suctioning catheter. Commercial catheters with vents are also available (Fig. 21-22). Such attachment provides a vent that permits the nurse to intermittently control the suctioning by covering and uncovering the vent. As a result, pressure does not build up within the catheter, and damage to the tracheobronchial membrane is lessened.

PROCEDURE. The force of suctioning must be maintained, but strong suction should be avoided. Ranges in suction force for mucus aspiration have been suggested (Table 21-10).

The suctioning process removes not only secretions but air as well. As a result, the client experiences a feeling of suffocation and tends to become apprehensive during suctioning. The nurse therefore must be concerned with timing as a factor in effective suctioning. Suctioning should be intermittent. Intermittent suctioning not only relieves feelings of suffocation, but prevents damage to the tracheal membrane. A single suctioning for an adult should not extend over 10 to 15 seconds during a 3-minute period. Excessive suctioning can block a segment of the lung, causing the segment to collapse. Though rare, cardiac arrest resulting from reflex vagal stimulation in the presence of extreme hypoxia may also occur. After each 10-second suctioning, the vent should be opened, and the catheter removed. The client should be permitted to rest for 3 minutes before the procedure is repeated. Oxygen may also be administered during the rest period. The

1281

10-second suctioning and 3-minute rest periods should be continued until no secretions are obtained. However, judgment must be used in deciding whether to strictly adhere to the suctioning-rest interval. If secretions are thick and copious and if they interfere with the client's breathing, the nurse must alter the intervals and must suction the client until the secretions are adequately removed and breathing is well established. In many institutions, it is a common practice to increase the concentration of oxygen to 100% for 1 minute before and after suctioning.

Sterile technique is the usual practice for tracheostomy care. This practice employs the use of sterile gloves and a sterile catheter at each suctioning.

Before suctioning, the catheter should be moistened with normal saline to prevent trauma to the mucous membrane as the catheter is inserted. If secretions are to be adequately removed, the catheter must be inserted far enough to obtain secretions.

In deciding the length to insert the catheter, the nurse must be familiar with the policy of the employing institution. Some physicians recommend the catheter be inserted not more than 5 inches (12 cm) without specific orders. However, it may often be necessary to enter the bronchi in order to remove secretions. For deeper suctioning, the nurse must instruct the client to assume various positions, depending on which bronchus is to be suctioned. To suction the left bronchus, the client should be instructed to turn slightly onto his left side, with his head turned to the far right. To suction the right bronchus, the client turns his body to the right and his head to the far left. These positions make the bronchus that is to be suctioned more readily accessible. The catheter should be directed toward the direction of the bronchus to be suctioned. To prevent laryngeal spasms, the client should be instructed to inhale as the catheter passes the larynx.

As the catheter is advanced, the vent should be opened. Once the catheter is in the desired position, the vent should be closed off with the finger or thumb, and suctioning started. As the catheter is withdrawn, the catheter should be gently rotated 360 degrees between the thumb and forefinger. The same measure (opening the vent) should be practiced if the catheter adheres to the mucosal lining. If the client coughs during suctioning, the catheter should be removed to prevent buildup of pressure. Coughing also facilitates removal of secretions, thereby performing the work of suction. After the procedure, the catheter should be cleansed by drawing saline through it to remove retained secretions.

During suctioning, the nurse should note the amount, color, odor, character, and consistency of the secretions, the rate and character of the client's respirations, and the reaction of the client to the procedure.

When the client is monitored (for example, by telemetry) observation for the development of dysrhythmias should be made. In addition to these assessments, breath sounds and chest assessments should be made following suctioning.

It is often necessary to suction the nasopharynx as well as the tracheostomy. When this is the case, two catheters should be used, and care must be maintained to prevent cross contamination of the nose and throat and the tracheostomy; for example, by proper labeling when indicated.

SUCTIONING BY OTHER ROUTES. When the nurse suctions a client through other routes, the same principles discussed under tracheobronchial suctioning must be applied. It should be performed as gently and quickly as possible. A Y-connecting catheter must be used. The catheter should be large enough to remove secretions, and most of all, the client must be prepared for the procedure.

1. *Oropharyngeal suctioning.* The nurse depresses the client's tongue with a tongue blade, places the top of the catheter into the pharynx, and aspirates secretions.

2. *Nasopharyngeal suctioning.* The nurse inserts the catheter tip into one nostril and advances it along the floor of the nasal cavity. Suction is applied, and the client is aspirated as the catheter is withdrawn. Secretions from the other nostril can be aspirated in the same manner.

3. *Endotracheal suctioning.* Endotracheal suctioning is often carried out by the physician, although the nurse with adequate preparation may also perform endotracheal suctioning. With the client in a sitting position, this provides an effective way of inducing coughing as well as removing secretions. He is instructed to hyperextend his neck, and extend his tongue. These practices permit the glottis to come in line with the trachea, thereby facilitating passage of the catheter into the pharynx and trachea rather than into the esophagus. He is also instructed to inhale as the catheter tip is advanced to prevent spasms of the larynx. The catheter is not attached to suction while it is being passed. The client will cough as the catheter tip enters the trachea. If the catheter is in the trachea, air exchange will be noted at the end of the catheter, and the client will not be able to produce sounds. Once the position of the catheter is ascertained, tracheal suctioning is applied as the catheter is withdrawn.

Promoting cleanliness. The inner tube of the tracheostomy should be removed and cleansed frequently. Various methods may be employed for cleansing. One method is to scrub the inside of the inner tube with a soft brush or pipe cleaner while running cold water through the tube. Cold water prevents mucus from coagulating. If mucous material has become encrusted, the inner tube may be soaked in a basin of a specially prepared solution for several minutes. While the inner tube is soaking, the outer tube should be suctioned to remove accumulated secretions. After the inner cannula has been soaked, it should be rinsed well with water. Shaking the tube is all that is required to remove excess water. Before reinsertion, a careful inspection should be made to see that bristles or lint have not adhered to the tube, because they may be aspirated into the respiratory passages. Holding the tube toward the light is an excellent way of checking for the presence of a foreign object.

To remove the inner cannula, the locking device should first be turned at the center of the flange. This allows the inner tube to be released. (To remove the inner laryngectomy tube, the locking device should be turned counterclockwise to release.) Then the outer tube is held steady, and the inner tube is gently pulled out with a curving motion toward the client's chest. The airway should be checked for patency. Suction if needed.

To reinsert the inner cannula, first the outer cannula is supported by placing the finger and thumb against the flange. The inner cannula is inserted with a curving motion upward toward the client's chin. Then the tracheostomy tube is locked in place by turning the lock. (To lock a laryngectomy tube, the inner tube is turned clockwise.)

The outer cannula is usually removed by the physician. It may be changed as often as every fourth day. Changing the cannula sooner may be hazardous because the trachea may seal when it is removed, thus causing the airway to become occluded.

The dressing under the cannula should be changed as often as needed. By keeping the dressing clean, irritation and maceration of the skin are prevented. Gauze tracheostomy dressings should be used because they do not have loose strings that can be aspirated.

Each time the dressing is changed, the area around the tracheostomy tube should be cleansed with soap and water and observed for signs of inflammation and edema.

Tapes hold the outer tubing in place and should be tied securely. The nurse must remember that if the tapes are too loosely tied, there is a possibility that the tubes will become displaced. If they are tied too tightly, the client suffers much discomfort. The correct tension of the tapes can be obtained by securing the knot when the client's head is slightly flexed. The tapes should be tied at the side of the neck. These should be changed as needed. It is good practice to have two people available when tapes are changed. One to hold the tube in place and the other person to replace the tapes. If the client is not critically ill, he may be asked to assist.

As soon as possible, the client should be taught how to care for the tracheostomy himself.

Preventing dryness

HUMIDIFICATION. Air that enters through the tracheostomy is not properly conditioned (warmed, moistened) and is irritating. This happens because the tissue that normally helps moisten inspired air is bypassed. Therefore humidification must be provided to protect the mucosa from drying and crusting. Humidification also prevents the secretions from becoming thick and viscous, thus preventing an obstruction and infection.

Humidification might be delivered by several means. Nebulizers and humidifiers are generally used for this purpose. Portable nebulizers can be used in conjunction with a tracheostomy collar to provide humidification (Fig. 21-23). Ultrasonic nebulizers may also be used. The incubator or mist tent may be used for the infant. These may be used with a respirator or mask. These are generally used with caution, because alterations may occur in fluid balance (water intoxica-

FIG. 21-23
Tracheostomy collar for humidification. Collar normally fits directly over tracheostomy. (From DeWeese, David D., and Saunders, William H.: Textbook of otolaryngology, ed. 6, St. Louis, 1982, The C.V. Mosby Co.)

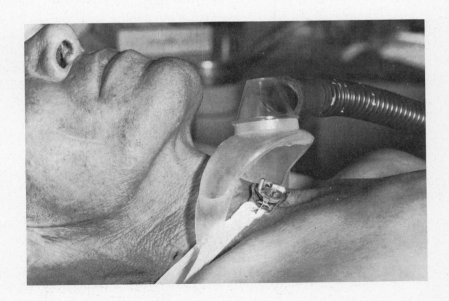

tion). Usually the therapist keeps accurate records of the amount of solution used for nebulization in an effort to prevent alterations in fluid balance.

Humidifiers are usually used when the client is being maintained on a respirator.

A wet gauze may be placed over the opening. This practice not only moisturizes but also filters out foreign objects such as dust particles.

T TUBE. A T piece is a plastic tube in the shape of a T that is used to deliver humidity with oxygen. It is frequently used in conjunction with a tracheostomy or endotracheal tube. The perpendicular portion fits over the tracheostomy or endotracheal tube. Oxygen is given in one end of the vertical, or cross, portion, and expired air exits through the other end of the vertical portion.

Nursing implementation during an emergency. If the tube accidentally becomes dislodged, as from violent coughing, the nurse should *immediately* spread the trachea vertically with an unclamped hemostat or tracheal dilator (Fig. 21-24). The nurse must signal for help and remain with the client until the physician arrives. If a physician is not available or cannot be reached, the nurse should insert a duplicate outer cannula, using the obturator to prevent trauma, provided it can be done without force. The obturator is removed, inner cannula reinserted, and tapes tied. To care for such an emergency the following equipment should always be at the bedside: two sterile curved hemostats or a tracheal dilator and a complete duplicate sterile tracheostomy (or laryngectomy) set.

Removal of the tracheostomy. The nurse must assess the client's ability to bring up secretions on his own and whether or not deep aspiration is needed. These factors help the physician decide when to discontinue the tracheostomy. Varied ways may be used for discontinuing a tracheostomy. One simple method is to simply remove the tube and place several strips of tape over the opening after the skin has been pulled together. The edges adhere within a few days after removal. The process of *decannulation* is also used. With this process, closure of the tracheostomy opening is a gradual process. The process is started by partially closing off part of the tracheostomy opening with a cork and gradually increasing it to complete closure or the size of the cannula may be reduced daily.

FIG. 21-24
Nurse should dilate the trachea with a tracheal dilator if the tracheostomy tube becomes dislodged accidentally.

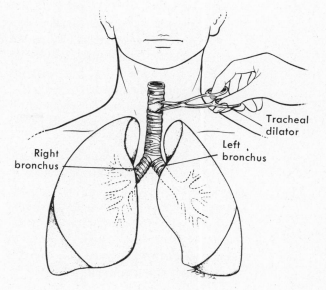

Tracheal dilator

Left bronchus

Right bronchus

When a tube size becomes two or more sizes smaller, it can be removed.

During the process, the nurse should assess the client's tolerance to the occlusion by observing his respiratory status and vital signs. When the client can tolerate complete closure, the tracheostomy tube is removed, and the opening permitted to heal. A tracheal button is sometimes used to temporarily close the tracheostomy opening. An emergency tracheostomy set should be left close at hand in case the client develops subsequent respiratory difficulty.

Discharge instructions for client with tracheostomy. Because of the nature of some respiratory conditions, the client may be discharged from the hospital with the tracheostomy tube in place. In these instances, the nurse must teach the family, particularly if the client is a child, how to care for the tracheostomy. The principles of care, specific observation, and signs and symptoms to report should comprise the instructions. Instructions should be given as to where equipment may be purchased. In caring for children particularly, parents should be told the importance of not allowing water to enter the tube as might happen during the bath. Referral should also be made to the community health nurse for follow-up care.

Thoracentesis
The aspiration of fluid from the pleural cavity is accomplished by a procedure known as thoracentesis. This procedure may be performed for diagnostic or therapeutic purposes. When performed for diagnostic reasons, the aspirated fluid is cultured for bacteria or examined for the presence or absence of abnormal cells. When performed for therapeutic reasons, ample fluid is removed to facilitate comfort and easier breathing.

A thoracentesis is performed by the physician under sterile conditions. The skin is cleansed with an antiseptic at the site of entry. The area is anesthetized, and a long aspiration needle is inserted through the anesthetized skin and chest wall into the pleural cavity, and fluid is withdrawn. The amount withdrawn depends on whether the test is performed for diagnostic or therapeutic purposes. If the procedure is performed for diagnostic purposes, 20 to 30 ml of fluid is aspirated. Larger amounts are withdrawn for therapeutic purposes.

Usually the physician informs the client about the purpose of the procedure and how it will be performed. However, the nurse should reinforce the physician's explanations. The client should be instructed about his responsibilities during the test. Instruction should be given as to the position he is to assume during the procedure. Positions are maintained that increase the intercostal spaces, thereby lessening trauma during the procedure. Infants are placed with their chest across a pillow. Children and adults sit in bed and lean over an overbed table or sit on the edge of the bed and lean over an overbed table with the feet supported on a stool or chair. In instances in which the client is too ill to assume either position, a lateral position with the affected side uppermost is used.

In an effort to decrease secretions and prevent laryngospasms, atropine may be administered during the procedure. To prevent trauma, the client is discouraged from coughing or moving after the needle is inserted.

Before the test, vital signs and state of the client should be assessed to establish a baseline for later evaluation. During the procedure the nurse supports the client in the desired position. Frequent observations should be made of the rate and character of pulse and respirations, color, and general appearance. At the completion of the procedure the specimen should be sent to the laboratory and frequent assessments made for untoward effects such as persistent cough and hemoptysis, which may indicate damage to the lung. Significant changes in the vital signs may indicate hemorrhage and impending shock because of a shift of fluid from the vascular spaces into the pleural cavity.

Chest surgery

Preoperative care. Before chest surgery, a number of diagnostic tests are performed (such as chest x-ray studies, sputum analysis, skin test, pulmonary function tests, bronchoscopy, and electrocardiogram). These may be done before or after the client is admitted. The nurse should explain each test to the client. When a decision is made to perform surgery, the nurse reinforces the physician's explanation. (Postoperative expectations are also discussed.) Explanations should be made in terms that are easily understood by the client.

Adequate nutrition must be provided in the preoperative period. A diet high in protein, with supplemental vitamins, may be ordered to help promote postoperative healing.

Chest physiotherapy should be discussed and demonstrated, and ample time must be allowed for the client to practice deep breathing and effective coughing methods as well as practice splinting the operative site and coordinating the actual pressure that is applied while splinting and coughing. The nurse should work closely with the respiratory therapist. The client must be told that turning, coughing, and deep breathing will be done every 2 hours. Instructions should be given as to the proper way to perform these exercises. Instructions to breathe deeply may be understood by the adult but not by a young child. In dealing with young children, the nurse must be especially imaginative. For the child, play therapy is instrumental in explaining procedures. A 2-year-old child knows how to blow out his breath. Blowing games may be used to make the child breathe deeply. The nurse instructs the child to blow, with the understanding that the longer he blows, the greater the inspiration he will have to make. This method accomplishes the same goal as more direct methods accomplish with adults.

Similar imaginary games may be practiced to accomplish other objectives. Special incentive spirometers are available for children. These have bright lights and play music if inspiratory volume is maintained. Arm and leg exercises should be taught and their importance stressed.

The client should be told that he will receive oxygen and that chest tubes will be attached to chest drainage during the postoperative period. Pain medications will be available, and intravenous therapy will be administered. The nurse must assure the client that each of these are normal and not related to a precarious state.

Ample time should be allowed for the client to express his fears and anxieties about the surgery. Regardless of the source of fear, the nurse should provide support. If the client has misconceptions about the surgery, the nurse should correct these. All the client's questions should be answered, and any special problem brought to the attention of the appropriate person (physician, social worker, or chaplain).

On the evening before surgery, the operative area is shaved, and the client is given a sedative. An enema may also be prescribed. The morning of surgery, medications will be administered to allay apprehension, reduce secretions, and prevent laryngospasm. Endotracheal anesthesia is used to keep the lungs expanded during surgery.

1287

Nursing process for common health problems

Postoperative care. In the postoperative period, the nurse assesses the client for signs of complications and plans care for maintaining airway patency and lung expansion, promoting comfort, and maintaining nutrition, hydration, and activity.

Postoperative assessments. The nurse observes the client for signs of blood loss. The vital signs should be assessed as often as every 15 minutes in the immediate postoperative period. Close attention is paid to the character of the pulse and respiration. The frequency of assessing vital signs decreases as they become stabilized. The dressing should be checked for excessive drainage. Since fluids flow downhill, the nurse should check for drainage on the back where the drainage has run to a lower level. Changes in color should be assessed by checking the lips, ear lobes, nail beds, and mucous membranes. The level of consciousness should also be assessed. Observations are made for the presence of a pneumothorax. Dyspnea, cyanosis, and acute chest pain are signs of pneumothorax and should be reported to the physician immediately.

Frequent assessment should be made of chest sounds. The lungs should be auscultated to detect alteration in normal breath sounds, which, if present, suggest fluid overload.

Maintaining patent airway and promoting comfort. When the client returns from surgery, he is placed in a supine position with his head turned to the side until he reacts from anesthesia. After he reacts, he is placed in a semi-Fowler's position, provided his vital signs are stable. In this position, pressure on the diaphragm is decreased, and aeration, breathing, drainage, and lung expansion are facilitated. The water seal drainage system is checked for proper functioning.

As soon as the client completely reacts, the nurse is able to evaluate the effectiveness of preoperative teaching. Turning and coughing should be started and continued at least every 2 hours. Deep breathing should be encouraged more frequently—five to six times per hour.

Tight and binding dressings, especially on the abdomen and chest, often inhibit ventilation because the thorax is unable to expand to its fullest on inspiration. This is an added reason to encourage turning, coughing, and deep breathing exercises.

Pain medications should be given as frequently as necessary. Pain inhibits coughing, because when pain is felt, the client tends to splint the chest and as a result breathe shallowly in order to decrease the pain. This interferes with adequate ventilation and results in retained secretions, which may block the small airways. Because little oxygen reaches the alveolar capillaries and little carbon dioxide is removed, hypoxia and hypercapnia may result. The nurse must therefore help the client cough in a way that causes the least amount of pain. A sitting position must be maintained, and the client's chest should be supported. The nurse's hands should be placed over the incision while the client breathes deeply and coughs (Fig. 21-25). A pillow may also be used for splinting. As soon as his condition indicates, he is encouraged to perform these without assistance. It may be necessary to administer these before coughing and deep breathing exercises. When depressant drugs such as morphine and meperidine (Demerol) hydrochloride are prescribed, the nurse must carefully observe the client for signs of respiratory depression after they are administered. A respiratory rate of less than 12/min warrants consulting the physician before the medication is administered.

Excessive secretions in the tracheobronchial tree interfere with blood gas

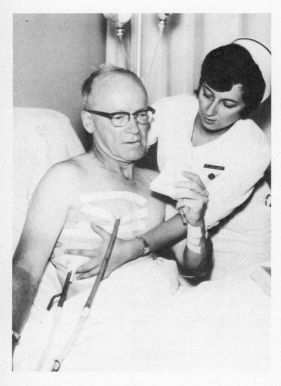

FIG. 21-25
Nurse splints the client's incision during coughing exercises. The sitting position facilitates a more effective cough. (Courtesy Marie E. Collart, Columbus, Ohio.)

exchange, and may lead to postoperative atelectasis and pneumonia. Coughing, suctioning, and other measures that promote removal of secretions should be employed as frequently as necessary.

Various forms of respiratory therapy may be prescribed to facilitate lung expansion and loosen secretions. Aerosol and IPPB therapy with isoproterenol (Isuprel) hydrochloride are commonly prescribed. IPPB is cheaper and effective. Expectorant drugs may also be prescribed to decrease the thickness of the mucus and facilitate its removal.

Maintaining hydration and nutrition. If the client receives intravenous fluids, frequent assessments must be made of the rate of infusion and the state of hydration because of the danger of pulmonary edema. The nurse must be aware of the symptoms of pulmonary edema so that their appearance can be reported to the physician immediately. These symptoms include cyanosis, dyspnea, blood-tinged frothy sputum, moist respirations, and distended neck veins.

As soon as the nausea ceases, clear fluids may be given. Solid foods are advanced to the client's tolerance. Energy foods in the form of carbohydrates should be encouraged to coincide with increased activity.

Maintaining activity. The muscles of the thorax aid respiration and assist with movement of the shoulder girdle. Muscles of the shoulder girdle are attached over a large area of the thorax. When chest surgery (such as a thoractomy) is performed, the motor nerve supply to part of the muscle is divided, and the muscles that affect movement of the head, trunk, upper extremity, and rib cage are cut. Therefore, any movement of the arm will be painful, and some limitation may be noted in the function of the affected parts. However, the nurse must assist the client with range-of-motion exercises, beginning on the evening of surgery, to prevent stiffness of the arm and development of a frozen shoulder. In the days following, these exercises should be performed two or three times a day. For a complete discussion of principles of range of motion see Chapter 10.

Leg exercises should also be encouraged, to improve muscle tone and thus facilitate adequate blood flow and discourage clot formation. The client may be instructed to mimic bicycle riding and actively move the calf muscles by dorsiflexing each foot. The latter may be encouraged every 5 minutes during the waking hours.

As soon as the client's condition permits, he is allowed out of bed. Ambulation, with assistance, is usually encouraged within 24 hours. Such activity may be brief and limited to sitting in a chair at the bedside. Nonetheless, it is essential in preventing muscle spasms, improving comfort, actively reducing postoperative weakness, and decreasing the risk of phlebitis and pulmonary embolism. If drainage tubes are in place, the nurse must be cautious not to dislodge the chest tubes when activities are increased.

Discharge instructions. In preparing the client for discharge, the nurse works closely with the client, his family, and physician. The nurse instructs the client to maintain good oral hygiene, continue exercises at home, obtain adequate rest, maintain good nutrition, avoid upper respiratory tract infections, and seek medical help at the onset of a respiratory tract infection.

Chest drainage. When a pneumothorax occurs or when chest surgery is performed or if the chest is punctured by a weapon, air enters the pleural cavity and causes a disruption in the negative intrapleural pressure.

A small amount of air entering the chest will cause partial collapse of the lung. As the entrance of air increases, the lungs will continue to collapse because the air within the lung will exit through the bronchus.[35] As the amount of air continues to increase in the pleural cavity, the lung will collapse completely, particularly if the air cannot leave the chest. Blood may also ooze from the chest wall or from a small vessel and accumulate in the pleural space. Both the air (and fluid) must be removed. If measures are not taken to reestablish negative pressure (for example, by removing air and fluid within the space), the following pathological conditions may result: (1) the lung on the opposite side will collapse; (2) the trachea and mediastinum will become compressed toward the unoperated side; (3) the compressed lung will lose its function; and (4) the space between lung and chest wall will become vulnerable to infection, and empyema may result. To prevent these problems, a chest drainage system (water seal, airtight system) is used.

Types of chest drainage systems. One, two, or three bottles, attached to the closed system, may be used. A single tube or two tubes may be placed in the chest wall to remove air and fluid. When two tubes are used, one is placed anteriorly through the second intercostal space to provide an avenue for the rising air, and the second is placed posteriorly between the eighth or ninth intercostal space to drain the fluid.

Regardless of the number of bottles used, the principle of the system is the same: *to evacuate air and fluid from the chest cavity* and, simultaneously, *to act as a one-way valve preventing a back-flow of air and fluid into the chest.* Consequently the lungs reexpand.

One-bottle system. When the one-bottle drainage system is used, the bottle is attached to a catheter that extends from the client's chest. Two rods are placed through a tightly sealed cap—one long and one short. To prevent the entrance of air, the long rod extends not more than 2.5 cm below the surface of the fluid to provide the seal. As a result, air does not reenter the client's chest. This distance is important because the positive pleural pressure has to replace the fluid volume before air can escape. The short tube is open to the air. As the client breathes, water fluctuates (rises on inspiration and falls on expiration) in the water-seal rods. On expiration, air from the pleural space bubbles through the rod into the water. Drainage fluid also passes into the bottle on expiration. The one-bottle system is mainly used after a pneumonectomy and to drain transudate (exudate) from the chest. Gravity drainage is all that is necessary to remove fluid from the chest (Fig. 21-26, *A*).

Two-bottle system. When a two-bottle system is used, the first bottle (the trap bottle, or collection bottle, so named because it collects chest fluid drainage) is placed between the client and the water-seal bottle (second bottle). (The use of this bottle eliminates the need to constantly adjust the depth of the water-seal rod as fluid drains from the pleural space, because the rod in this bottle is above fluid level.) The principle of this system remains the same. As air and fluid flow from the chest they enter the trap bottle, and the air is forced out of the bottle through the rod that goes into the water-seal bottle, where it bubbles out under water and exits through the exit tubing (Fig. 21-26, *B*).

Three-bottle system. This system is indicated when air leaks are excessive. In the three-bottle system, the *first* bottle (trap bottle) is attached to the catheter that extends from the client's chest. A *second* bottle is attached to the trap bottle and provides the *water seal.* This is accomplished by enclosing the water-seal

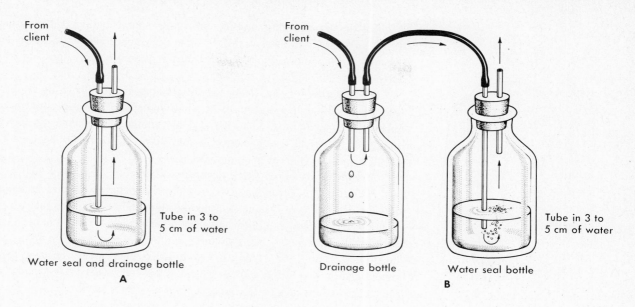

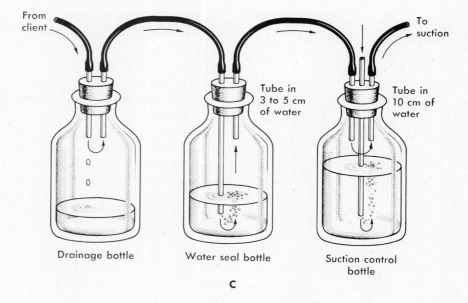

FIG. 21-26
A, One-bottle drainage system. **B,** Two-bottle drainage system. **C,** Three-bottle drainage system.

From client

Tube in 3 to 5 cm of water

Water seal and drainage bottle

A

From client

Drainage bottle

Water seal bottle

Tube in 3 to 5 cm of water

B

From client

To suction

Drainage bottle

Water seal bottle

Tube in 3 to 5 cm of water

Suction control bottle

Tube in 10 cm of water

C

drainage tube to run through a tightly sealed cap and through a second tube, which forms a connection to the *third* bottle—the pressure-regulating bottle (suction control bottle). The suction control bottle, which is placed between the water seal and suction source, is valuable in that it prevents excessive pressure from being exerted within the client's chest. Pressure regulation is accomplished by submerging the long tube through the center of the cap to a depth ranging from 10 to 20 cm (the normal negative pressure in the chest). It serves to regulate the amount of suction applied to the client's pleural cavity. Therefore, regardless of the source of negative pressure from the suction outlet, the suction reaching the chest will be no more than the length of the submerged rod. For example, when the suction is turned on, the pressure above the water level in the third bottle will be the negative pressure that is transmitted to the pleural cavity.[35] If the suction exceeds the desired centimeters of water pressure, air will enter the third tubing from the outside, go through the water, into the space above the water, and out through the suction machine. As a result the desired negative pressure is maintained (Fig. 21-26, *C*).

Modification for age. When the chest drainage system is set up for the infant and young child, the bottle must be small enough to permit accurate measurement of the small losses, and the drainage tubing should be light enough not to impede the infant's movements. A small bottle (230 ml) may be used. For the child, a special 1000-ml flask may be used.

Modifications of the bottle drainage system

Heimlich chest drainage valve. A flutter valve that can be attached to a chest catheter and drainage system has been developed. The setup has the same effect as the water seal and the following added advantages: (1) the client can be ambulatory while the chest is being drained, and the drainage bag can be held at any level (Figs. 21-27 and 21-28); (2) clamping is unnecessary because the valve functions in any position; (3) the danger of air entering the chest is nil because the valve remains intact and connected to the catheter even if the valve casing is broken; and (4) it is small and can be discarded after use.

Another advantage is that suction is not necessary for thoracic drainage with the use of the flutter valve. According to Heimlich, the few cases where suction is indicated are continuing massive pneumothorax and mediastinal drainage, because it is the expansion of the lung in the pleural cavity that enables the valve to function. When suction is indicated, further security can be gained by placing the valve between the chest tube and the suction drainage apparatus. Even if the bottle is damaged the valve prevents air and fluid from refluxing into the chest.

Pleur-Evac. The Pleur-Evac is a plastic disposable unit that incorporates the three-bottle setup into one unit. The unit is compartmentalized and has a chamber for drainage collection, water seal, and pressure regulation. The same number of milliliters of water is added to the water-seal and pressure-regulating chambers that would be used if bottles were employed. Each chamber is calibrated so that the amount of drainage and water levels can be easily determined. The unit is readily attached to the bed and provides an outlet for the removal of drainage.

Argyle double-seal. The Argyle double-seal chest drainage unit (Fig. 21-29) is a compact, four-chambered unit. Except for the extra chamber, it is similar to the three-bottle system. For example, fluid and air drain from the client into a collection chamber. (This three-column chamber has an overflow pattern.) The first chamber is graduated in 5-ml increments up to 200 ml to facilitate pediatric use.[11] Air passes from the client into the underwater seal chamber. The second chamber is the water seal. The third chamber regulates the amount of negative pressure applied to the client, and the fourth chamber, found left of the collection chambers, is an underwater seal and manometer. The manometer gives an actual measure of the amount of negative pressure that is being applied to the client. The black ball, found at the water level, enhances instant visual assessment of the amount of pressure reaching the client. This fourth chamber is considered an added safety feature that functions to relieve pressure buildup with the system.

Emerson postoperative pump. When suction is needed, a suction source such as the Emerson postoperative pump, an electrical pump, is attached to the

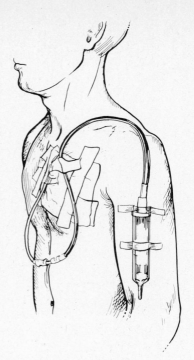

FIG. 21-27
Valve can be attached to arm to facilitate mobility. (Courtesy Dr. Henry J. Heimlich, Cincinnati, Ohio.)

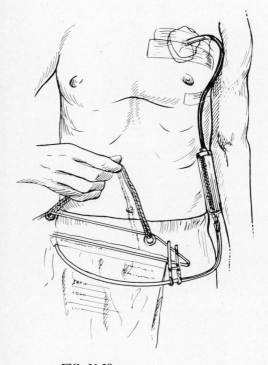

FIG. 21-28
Valve chest drainage permits early ambulation. Drainage bag can be carried at any level because the valve prevents a backflow of drainage. (Courtesy Dr. Henry J. Heimlich, Cincinnati, Ohio.)

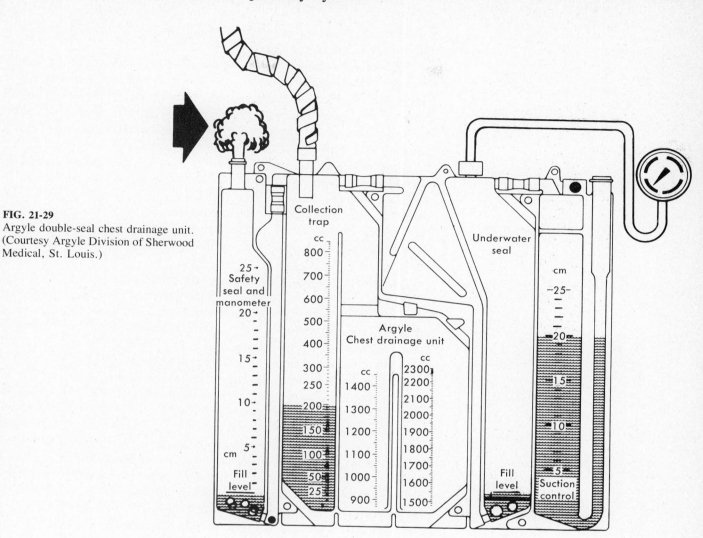

FIG. 21-29
Argyle double-seal chest drainage unit.
(Courtesy Argyle Division of Sherwood
Medical, St. Louis.)

system. A negative pressure of 10 to 15 cm is applied. The amount of pressure can be changed as indicated.

Planning and implementing care for the client with a chest drainage system. Nursing care should be directed toward promoting safety, maintaining patency of the drainage tube, making assessments, and preventing complications.

Promoting safety. Several precautions must be taken. First, all equipment (bottles, solution, and tubing) must be sterile. Next, the system must be airtight, and the tube in the water-seal bottle must be below water level to form the seal. The nurse secures all connections with adhesive tape to safeguard them from being pulled apart. Pins should not be used to secure the tubing because they may puncture the tube, thereby producing an air leak. Finally bottles must be kept below the level of the chest to prevent backflow of fluid and air within the chest. Placing the bottles at a distance of 18 inches (45.72 cm) below the chest level is often recommended. Electrical beds should be locked in place to prevent them from being accidentally lowered. Housekeeping and ancillary personnel, family members, and friends should be instructed not to lower the bed for cleaning or other reasons.

Care must be taken to see that bottles are not kicked over or accidentally broken. The bottles may be taped to the floor with large strips of adhesive, or they may be placed in a specially designed rack. Aseptic technique must be used when the bottles are changed. Because clients with chest tubes can so easily develop tension pneumothorax, chest tubes should *never* be clamped. This is especially true if an air leak, even if minimal, is present.[83]

Often, it may be necessary to transport a client with chest tubes to the radiology department or some other special area within the hospital. When this is necessary, the tubing should not be clamped during the transfer. The drainage receptacles, however, must be placed below the level of the client's chest at all times. Whenever possible, procedures should be done at the bedside to eliminate hazards inherent to transfer, such as displacement of tubes or backflow of drainage.

Maintaining patency of the drainage tube. The nurse plans care to facilitate reexpansion of the lungs. The patency of the tube must be continually checked. Small clots may lodge in the tubing and prevent proper drainage; therefore, if prescribed, the tubing should periodically be milked, or stripped, with a downward motion away from the client's chest.

Tension in the tube must be prevented. The client should be instructed to avoid letting his body weight compress the tubing. A trough can be made by bringing the ends of linen together around the tubing and pinning the ends with safety pins. Pillows or adhesive tape can be used for this purpose. A rubber band can be looped around the tubing and pinned to the bed to facilitate movement.

Making assessments. The nurse must continually observe the amount, color, and consistency of drainage. Increments of fluid drainage should be assessed at regularly scheduled intervals, and a notation made of the date and time of the reading. As much as 200 to 500 ml of bloody drainage may be lost within the first 24 hours. An amount over 500 ml in 24 hours is considered excessive. If more than 100 ml appears in 1 hour, the physician should be notified. Within 36 hours after surgery the drainage decreases in amount and becomes serous. Accurate intake and output records must be kept.

The nurse must *observe for fluctuations* (such as rising and falling of the column of water) in the water-seal bottle. The water rises with increased negative pressure during inspiration and falls during expiration. In the Pleur-Evac system, the liquid rises on the right side of the chamber and falls on the left side. Fluctuations indicate that a constant negative intrapleural pressure is being maintained and that the lung is not adhering to the chest wall. Fluctuations usually occur for at least 36 to 72 hours after surgery. After this period, the lungs have usually reexpanded; therefore fluctuation will not be noted. If fluctuations cease before this period, the nurse should check the patency of the tube, because blood clots or kinks may have occluded the tubing. The chest should be auscultated at frequent intervals.

In the early chest drainage period, bubbling may appear in the water-seal bottle. Bubbling may appear intermittently with coughing, expiration, or movement. *Bubbling should not occur during inspiration.* It represents expulsion of air from the chest and displacement of air from the tubing by fluid draining from the chest. Persistent bubbling indicates the presence of small leaks from the surface of the lung, which usually diminish over a 24- to 48-hour period. However, mechanical causes may also be responsible for persistent bubbling. For example, there may be a leak in the tubing, or air may be sucked into the chest around the tubing. The nurse should also check the pressure gauge when suction is used.

Preventing complications. The client should be placed in a semi-Fowler's position. Controversy seems to exist among physicians regarding position changes. Some advocate turning the client from side to side every 2 hours. Others prefer the client to lie on the affected side. Those who prefer the latter position believe that it decreases pain, facilitates drainage, and prevents spread of infection to the unaffected side. Regardless of the restrictions placed on position, the nurse should encourage the client to cough and breathe deeply and engage in other activities that are directed toward preventing complications. Measures should be taken to lessen pain from these activities.

Removing tubes. Chest x-ray films are usually taken daily to ascertain the rate and amount of lung reexpansion and the presence of atelectasis, infection, or mediastinal shift. When the lungs become fully expanded and there is no evidence of air or fluid within the pleural cavity, the drainage system is discontinued. In a client with a spontaneous pneumothorax, the appearance of a small amount of serosanguineous fluid, in the tubing or bottle that has previously been clear, is an indication for removal.[83] The pink drainage is the result of complete reexpansion of the lung, forcing out residual air pockets and subsequent layering over of surfaces and drainage of any pleural fluid.

Before the physician removes the tubes, the client is instructed to take a deep breath and to exhale (Valsalva's maneuver) as the tubing is swiftly withdrawn. This maneuver prevents air from entering the chest and facilitates removal of residual fluid. The area is then covered with a Vaseline or petroleum gauze and a dry dressing and secured with tape. Following removal, the nurse must make frequent observations for signs of air leakage and for symptoms of respiratory distress. It is not uncommon for fluid to drain from the small opening as during coughing or straining. Such drainage, which is darker and more serous than fresh blood, comes from the diaphragmatic sulcus, and it is desirable that it be removed.[83] Since the dressing serves as a one-way valve, it is common practice that the dressing not be removed but reinforced for the first 48 hours. Following this period, the dressing is usually removed.

Planning for emergencies: accidental removal of chest tube. If a chest tube accidentally becomes dislodged, measures should be taken to prevent air from entering the chest (such as covering the opening to prevent the entrance of atmospheric air). The physician should be notified and preparation made for reinsertion. Solution for cleansing the area (such as Betadine) and necessary tubing should be readied. Immediate reinsertion is important because edema of the tissue causes the opening to close rapidly.[83]

Implementation

COMMON PROBLEMS OF THE NEONATE

Congenital laryngeal stridor

Congenital laryngeal stridor is a noisy (crowing) sound produced on inspiration. The noisy breathing may occur shortly after birth and persist until the second year of life. Crying and excitement generally make the stridor worse and produce cyanosis. Sleep and rest tend to cause the sound to diminish.

The basic factor responsible for producing the stridor is immaturity of the larynx. By age 2, the flabby structures have matured enough to permit normal breathing. For this reason, usually no treatment is indicated. However, if the stridor is severe and if the neonate is not able to maintain adequate oxygenation, a tracheostomy may be performed.

Choanal atresia

Choanal atresia is a congenital defect in which one or both of the posterior nares fail to canalize. The obstruction is usually caused by a membrane, although it may also be caused by cartilage or a bony growth.

Assessment. It is usually unilateral. When the obstruction is bilateral, the infant breathes through his mouth. Feeding is impossible because he cannot breathe and suck at the same time. Varying degrees of cyanosis may be experienced. An infant with a unilateral obstruction may have no symptoms unless he develops an infection in the opposite upper respiratory passage. The diagnosis is made shortly after birth. Inability to pass a small catheter or probe through the nose into the pharynx confirms the diagnosis.

Planning and implementation. The objective of therapy is to remove the obstruction in an effort to provide a patent airway. If the obstruction is bilateral, a surgical emergency exists because the infant may suffocate unless an airway is established. Emergency treatment consists of piercing the membrane and establishing a communication between the anterior and the posterior nares. Probes are often used to perforate the membranous obstruction. Periodic dilation of the nasal passages may be necessary to keep them patent. If the obstruction is unilateral, surgery may be delayed until the child is several years old. Radical surgery may be performed when the obstruction is the result of a bony growth.

The objectives of nursing care should be to (1) help the infant maintain oxygenation as nearly adequate as possible and (2) maintain nutritional intake. Strategies related to the former objective include keeping the nasal passages clean and protecting the infant from respiratory tract infections. Because breathing is difficult when the neonate attempts to eat, feeding often presents a problem. He should be fed slowly, and the nipple should be large enough to permit adequate fluid to pass but not so large that excessive amounts of milk enter the mouth. Frequent rest periods should be provided during feedings. To prevent aspiration of fluids, the infant should be held while feedings are administered. The neonate's tolerance to feedings should be closely assessed. If excessive respiratory difficulty is noted, it may be necessary to maintain nutritional intake by other means, such as by giving an intravenous feeding.

Idiopathic respiratory distress syndrome of the neonate (IRDS)

Previously termed *hyaline membrane disease,* respiratory distress syndrome (RDS) is a disease that primarily affects premature infants. The exact cause of the syndrome is unknown, but an absence, inactivation, alteration, or deficiency of surfactant has been documented.[25] Surfactant, a lipoprotein material that is thought to be secreted by the alveolar membrane, lines the alveoli and is responsible for lowering the alveolar surface tension, thus decreasing the tendency of the alveoli to collapse. An impairment in surfactant results in a collapse of the alveoli at the end of expiration, and the alveoli must reexpand completely with each inspiration.

The fetal lung begins synthesizing surfactant during the second trimester, but not until the thirty-fourth or thirty-fifth week are significant amounts produced. Through examination of the amniotic fluids, determinations can be made of the production of fetal surfactant. Low concentrations of surfactant in the fluid are predictive of IRDS, whereas adequate concentrations are indicative of normal pulmonary function.[40]

Factors such as maternal diabetes mellitus, toxemia, placenta previa, abruptio placenta, anemia, and cesarean delivery predispose the newborn to IRDS.[75] Maternal bleeding and decreased birth weight also tend to increase the incidence. Infants who weigh between 1000 to 1500 g are most commonly affected. With cesarean births, the incidence increases with decreasing gestational age. Whether a cesarean section or the indications for this type of delivery increase the susceptibility is controversial. However, reports have shown that IRDS is less frequent in full-term infants, whether delivered vaginally or by cesarean section. The disorder is more common among male infants, and the incidence tends to increase in infants of diabetic mothers.

Pathophysiology. IRDS is characterized by destruction of the alveolar capillary membranes, increased permeability of the pulmonary capillaries, and interstitial edema.[47] As a result of alveolar damage, surfactant is depleted and subsequently the lungs become airless, and fibrin collects on the epithelial wall. The fibrin formation is thought to resemble hyaline material, hence its original name. Because of the damaged lungs, there is poor gaseous exchange; as a result a number of symptoms are experienced by the infant.

Assessment. IRDS becomes apparent as early as 1 to 6 hours after birth. Signs, any two of which are thought to be significant, indicative of RDS are tachypnea (as many as 65, or even higher, respirations per minute), cyanosis, expiratory grunt, and labored breathing (as evidenced by nasal flaring during inspiration and retractions of the sternum and lower costal margin[40,61]). Cyanosis is caused by intrapulmonary shunting through atelectatic areas, and by extrapulmonary shunting through persistent fetal channels.[75] Grunting (expiratory in nature and having been described as a whimper, whine, or cry) is thought to represent an attempt to overcome expiratory atelectasis. Each time the infant grunts, expiration is prolonged. As a result, the pressure within the alveoli is maintained, preventing alveolar collapse.

As the condition worsens, short periods of apnea may be noted. These episodes may be relieved by tactile stimulation. Retractions may also become more pronounced, the respiratory rate decreases, and periods of apnea become more frequent. Blood gas analysis reveals decreased oxygen concentration, increased carbon dioxide content, increased acidity, and decreased concentration of buffer base. Clinically, metabolic and respiratory acidosis is manifest.

Data analysis
Data analysis may reveal nursing diagnoses of ineffective breathing patterns, alteration in tissue perfusion, alteration in cardiac output, and impaired gas exchange.

Planning and implementation. The nurse in the nursery should closely observe all infants, particularly premature infants, infants of diabetic mothers, and those delivered by cesarean section for signs of IRDS. The nurse must have a thorough knowledge of the characteristic patterns of the newborn's respiratory rate and skin color. Any change in either of these warrants consultation with the physician.

Various forms of therapy have been used. Infants with RDS are preferably treated in neonatal intensive care units. Because lack of oxygenation and increased acid content are basic manifestations of the syndrome, therapy is directed toward improving tissue oxygenation and correcting acid-base imbalance. Tissue oxygenation is accomplished with the use of oxygen and ventilatory therapy, whereas intravenous therapy and alkali and temperature regulation are employed to correct acidosis.

Maintaining tissue oxygenation. Oxygen therapy is administered via an incubator, a mask, head hood, or endotracheal tubes, and is carefully regulated. Some institutions use oxygen liberally, whereas others use it more sparingly. Because it may be necessary to administer greater than a 40% concentration of oxygen, the infant should be observed closely for signs of retrolental fibroplasia (see Chapter 13) or oxygen toxicity (see discussion earlier in this chapter).

The administration of oxygen therapy requires a thorough understanding of the purpose, its use and care. See a complete discussion of oxygen therapy earlier in this chapter.

Ventilatory therapy methods are used when there is an inability to maintain arterial oxygen tension at desired levels and when acidosis increases even with fluid and base therapy. The *hypoxic test* has been reported to be an objective method for determining the need for ventilatory assistance. The infant breathes 100% oxygen for 20 minutes. If, at the end of this time period, the arterial Pa_{O_2} is less than 50 mm Hg, ventilatory assistance is indicated.[40] Either manually or mechanically assisted ventilation may be used. CPAP is used to prevent expiratory alveolar collapse. PEEP or CDP (continuous distending pressure) may also be used. (See discussions of these earlier in this chapter.)

Maintaining proper environmental temperature. The nurse must maintain the infant's body temperature as close to normal as possible. Any increase or decrease in body temperature brings the homeodynamic mechanisms into action. In an attempt to return the temperature to a normal range, tissue metabolism increases and results in both an increased use of oxygen and production of lactic acid, causing further production of acidosis. Because of the effect of a raised temperature, the thermal environment must be maintained at a level that will produce the least metabolism. Temperatures (such as rectal, skin, and incubator) should be monitored carefully and frequently, and adjustments made accordingly.

Assessment of the environmental temperature is accomplished by suspending an air thermometer probe tip from the top of the incubator. A telethermometer is used with a probe to monitor the skin temperature. The probe is taped to an exposed part of the infant. In addition to monitoring the temperature, the nurse should closely monitor the pulse and respiration.

Correcting acidosis. To reduce acidosis, intravenous fluids containing 10% glucose (to provide calories) and a buffer base such as sodium bicarbonate may be prescribed. Blood gas analyses are made periodically during the day, and adjustments in the amount of buffer are made on the basis of these results.

Since glucose in the urine produces a diuretic effect, the urine should be monitored frequently for the presence of glucose. Glycosuria is an indication to gradually decrease the concentration of glucose until the urine becomes free of glucose. Such a measure is important because if the increased excretion of water and electrolytes continues, the purpose of fluid therapy would be defeated.

Evaluation. The infant with IRDS has problems with ineffective breathing, alterations in cardiac output, impaired gas exchange, and alterations in tissue perfusion. The nursing care plan must focus on objectives for improving the breathing status.

EXPECTED OUTCOMES

The family can:
1. Describe idiopathic respiratory distress syndrome.
2. State plans for follow-up health care and use of community resources.

Sudden infant death syndrome (SIDS)

Sudden infant death, commonly referred to as crib death or cot death, is the sudden and unexpected death of an infant who was either well or almost well before death and whose death remains unexplained after the performance of an autopsy. It is a leading cause of death during the first year of life, occurring most frequently between the second and fourth months of life. It is thought to affect 2 to 3 of every 1000 live births. Infants considered at greatest risk for SIDS are those of adolescent mothers, especially premature babies, or infants of low birth weight, and those of black or Indian ancestry.

The mechanism of sudden infant death is not known. Several earlier theories have been disproved including accidental suffocation by bed clothing, regurgitation, and hypersensitivity to cow's milk. Other mechanisms, including immunological, biochemical, respiratory, have been suggested, but are unconclusive.

It occurs most frequently during sleep, usually between the hours of midnight and 9:00 AM.[19] Most deaths occur unobserved, silently, and without struggle.

Data analysis
Data analysis may reveal nursing diagnoses of ineffective family coping, grieving, knowledge deficit, and fear.

 Planning and implementation. Nursing care should be directed toward providing support to the family. When the death occurs, the initial reaction of family members is likely to be shock and disbelief, which may persist for several weeks. Following this period, guilt feelings may be experienced. The nurse can provide added support by supplying family members with explanations about SIDS, answering their questions, and creating an environment in which family members can readily express their feelings. A community health nurse referral should also be made so that continuity of care can be provided, especially because family members may not have assimilated all the information during the immediate days following the death.

 Evaluation. The nursing care plan for parents who have had an experience with SIDS is based on diagnoses such as ineffective family coping, grieving, knowledge deficit, and fear. The plan is evaluated on an ongoing basis.

EXPECTED OUTCOMES

The family can:
1. Discuss SIDS, including theories related to possible causes and risk factors.
2. Verbalize feelings and concerns about the death.
3. State plans for follow-up expression of concerns.

COMMON PROBLEMS OF THE INFANT AND CHILD

Croup

Croup is a syndrome characterized by a barking cough or brassy, hoarseness, suprasternal and intercostal retractions,[29] inspiratory stridor, and restlessness, all of which are caused by laryngeal obstruction. It may be severe enough to produce cyanosis. Attacks of croup are usually acute but brief and generally occur at night. A number of variables have been related to croup: age, gender, time of year. Two types of croup are discussed: viral and bacterial.

Viral croup. Croup with a viral origin is most commonly caused by one of the adenoviruses; parainfluenza types 1, 2, 3; influenza type A virus; or the respiratory syncytial virus (RS). An upper respiratory tract infection precedes the onset by as much as a week or more.

Laryngotracheobronchitis. Laryngotracheobronchitis is an acute infection of the larynx, trachea, and bronchi. The infection is usually viral in origin.[80] Parainfluenza types 1, 2, and 3 are commonly responsible, type 1 being the usual cause. Adenoviruses, respiratory syncytial viruses, influenza viruses, and rhinoviruses have also been implicated. Boys between the ages of 3 months to 3 years are most often affected, and it is most common during the winter months. The more frequent occurrence in boys is not understood. However, the higher incidence during colder weather has been related to the frequent incidence of respiratory tract infections during the winter.

Pathophysiology. Mechanisms that have been documented to produce the obstruction include edema and inflammation (of the larynx, trachea, and bronchi) and muscle spasms.

 Assessment. The infection may come on abruptly or follow an acute respiratory tract infection. It is accompanied by a high fever, as high as 105° F (40.5° C), hoarseness, and a croupy cough. As the condition continues, tachypnea, restlessness, dyspnea, and signs of laryngeal obstruction are noted. Seizures may occur as a result of the temperature elevation. Death may occur from occlusion of the bronchial tree by viscid mucus or from obstruction of the larynx by edema. The condition is serious and demands prompt therapy.

 Planning and implementation. Therapeutic care is planned to maintain a patent airway and to prevent infection and promote rest and comfort.

To facilitate a patent airway, the child is placed in a cool, high-humidity atmosphere (for example, a mist tent). A croupette, croup room, or mask may also be used.[29] Such therapy reduces the viscosity of the mucus and soothes the lining of the tracheobronchial passages. A cool environment is preferred because the coolness counteracts the inflammatory conditions of the larynx. Oxygen is administered in combination with mist therapy, but *not* alone, because it dries the mucosa and further thickens the viscid mucus. The oxygen, by relieving hypoxia, will help alleviate anxiety, apprehension, and increased respiratory efforts. A tracheostomy may be performed if the obstruction is severe.

Mucus secretions are increased in the anxious child. Such response only endangers the patency of the airway. Therefore adequate emotional support should be provided. The nurse should spend time with the child, and parents should also be allowed to spend extra time with the child.

The child must be adequately hydrated. Adequate fluids not only meet the fluid requirement but also increase the moisture of the mucous membrane of the respiratory passages. Oral fluids should be at room temperature rather than cold. Continuous intravenous therapy may be prescribed.

Accurate records should be kept of intake, and antibiotic therapy may be prescribed if a secondary bacterial infection has developed. Sedatives are contraindicated because of their depressant effect on the respiratory center. Output, in addition to the specific gravity of urine, should be monitored at frequent intervals.

Often during the early stage the less acutely ill client is treated in the home. At home treatment usually include the use of a vaporizer, increased fluid intake, and bedrest. Prevention of the disease is essential. The nurse must instruct parents to limit the child's exposure to upper respiratory tract infections. If the child gets a cold, he must be protected from further infection. The importance of reporting signs of infection to the physician should be emphasized so that severe attacks can be prevented. Antibiotic therapy may be prescribed when an infection develops.

Acute spasmodic croup. Spasmodic croup, usually viral in origin, is characterized by airway obstruction. In addition, in some cases, laryngeal irritation, and immaturity of the larynx have been attributed as causes.

Assessment. The onset is sudden, dramatic, and alarming. Characteristically the attack occurs at night with a barking cough and stridor and tends to progress rapidly. Cyanosis may also occur. Usually the child is frightened, which increases the severity of the symptoms. The attack gradually subsides within 1 to 3 hours. The morning following the attack, a periodic croup cough may be noted. Subsequent nocturnal attacks may occur.

Planning and implementation. Nursing care should be planned to lessen respiratory distress. Care must be implemented in a calm, efficient manner. Such an approach can be instrumental in reassuring the child and the family, and subsequently enhance their calmness. All activity should be minimized so that adequate rest can be obtained. It is essential that accurate documentation of the child's behavior and symptoms be made (for example, restlessness, apprehension, respiratory and pulse rate, breathing pattern, general appearance).

Once the child is calm and has been made comfortable, the nurse must spend time with the parents. Their questions should be answered. Explanations of the use and function of all forms of therapy should be provided. Often, therapy is continued at home. Therefore explanations not only serve to lessen anxiety, but are useful in facilitating home care.

Other forms of therapy include humidification and use of medication. Drugs such as diphenhydramine elixir, syrup of ipecac, and corticosteroids are used. When syrup of ipecac is used, subemetic doses are prescribed. Following the administration of ipecac, the nurse should assess and document the effect of the drug.

Methods of humidification. Humidification may be provided by either a croup tent, croupette, or mist tent. The croup tent is one method of providing a humid environment. Oxygen can also be provided via the tent. A croupette is used to provide cool humidification (or mist) with oxygen administration. It is used for infants, and children up to around 10 years of age, and is useful in reducing hypoxia, reducing and liquefying secretions, and in reducing mucosal edema. It also provides a cool environment. Mist tents provide a high humidity environment (Fig. 21-30).

Croupettes and tents heighten barriers to communication. They also require the nurse to make frequent assessments of the respiratory status and of possible

FIG. 20-30
Ultrasonic mist has gained favor because the small mist particles penetrate the respiratory passages better than former misting techniques. The equipment is compact and relatively easy to handle. In real therapeutic situations, the mist may be so dense that the child is obscured. Side rail is down for picture only. (Courtesy Children's Health Center, San Diego, Calif.)

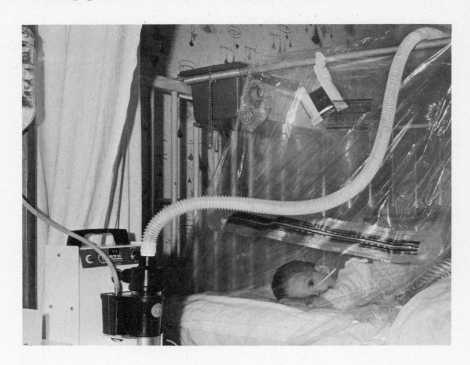

impending laryngeal obstruction. Chilling should be prevented by frequently changing clothing and bed linen.

The nurse should also provide emotional support for the child. The child should not be alarmed by the tent. Any type of fear only serves to cause further respiratory distress. Therefore, it is important to explain to the child what is happening. He should not be left alone until he is calm, and care should be taken so that he can see. A favorite toy should be allowed in the tent, but consideration given to the type of toy when oxygen is being used.

Home modifications. In the home, the bathroom may provide a high-humidity environment. The door is closed, and hot water is allowed to flow in the bathtub or shower. Water must be allowed to constantly drain from the tub; and the mother should stay with the child. Sheets may be draped around a table, and a commercial vaporizer used to provide steam. (Commercial *cool* vaporizers are also available.) If a vaporizer is not available, a kettle may be improvised for a vaporizer. It should be refilled frequently. When improvisions are made, care must be taken to make the tent as stable as possible. Parents should also be informed of the hazards of burns from such treatment; they should be instructed on all safety precautions.

Bacterial croup. *Acute epiglottitis* is a bacterial infection of the epiglottis, aryepiglottic folds, and supraglottic area that causes obstruction of the airway.[72] The infection is caused by *Haemophilus influenzae* type B. It is more commonly seen in children (usually boys) between the ages of 2 and 5 years, but may occur in any age group. There is no seasonal incidence; however, it develops more rapidly than viral croup.[2]

Assessment. Signs of marked respiratory distress (stridor and retractions), anxiety, restlessness, and temperature elevation develop rapidly. Tachycardia and tachypnea also develop. Hoarseness generally does not occur, because the larynx is usually not involved; the voice sounds are muffled. The older child is likely to complain of a sore throat and dysphagia. Pooling of secretions may be noted as a result of difficulty swallowing. The child tends to mouth breathe, and insists on sitting up learning forward with the neck hyperextended.

The diagnosis is established on physical examination on the basis of symptoms and from direct visualization of the epiglottis. (A cherry red, edematous epiglottis is a characteristic finding.) This examination should be done with extreme caution and skill. (When visualization is done, the nurse must have oxygen, suction, self-inflating bag, laryngoscope, and nasotracheal tubes available.[72] A tracheostomy setup should also be on hand. Although useful in establishing a diagnosis, throat cultures should not be done because of the possibility of producing sudden obstruction. Leukocyte counts may also be obtained, and lateral airway radiographs taken.[39]

 Planning and implementation. Immediate hospitalization, usually in an intensive care facility, is essential. Emergency creation of an artificial airway (tracheostomy or nasotracheal intubation) may be necessary.[5] Before an artificial airway is established, the child should be maintained in an upright position to prevent airway obstruction. Some form of humidification (to loosen the crust) and oxygen may be prescribed. The child is extubated when the epiglottis appears normal, usually 2 to 3 days after antibiotic therapy is started.

Antibiotic therapy, usually ampicillin, is prescribed. This medication may be prescribed for intravenous administration in divided doses during the acute phase. Afterward oral antibiotics are prescribed. Although controversial, corticosteroids may be given for their antiinflammatory effect. Adequate hydration should be maintained throughout the course of therapy.

The child and his family must receive adequate emotional support. The calm manner in which care is administered, and being attentive to the client's concerns will enhance such support.

Evaluation. The client with croup may have problems with ineffective breathing and impaired gas exchanges. The nurse and the client's family evaluate plans developed to enhance breathing.

EXPECTED OUTCOMES
The client and/or family can:
1. Describe croup.
2. Describe plans for home management including preparation and use of humidification methods.
3. Discuss safety factors in relation to home management.
4. State plans for follow-up health care.

Bronchiolitis

Bronchiolitis is an acute viral infection of the bronchioles. It is commonly seen in infants less than 2 years of age and most frequently around 6 months. Boys are more commonly affected, and its occurrence is during the winter and spring.

The respiratory syncytial influenza B virus is most frequently responsible for causing bronchiolitis. Usually the infant is exposed to a respiratory tract infection by a family member.

Pathophysiology. In bronchiolitis, viral organisms colonize the mucosa of the bronchiole and result in necrosis. The triad—cellular debris, edema, and mucus—obstructs the airway, and atelectasis subsequently results. Although the child may be able to get air into the lungs, he has difficulty expelling it because of it being trapped distal to the obstruction.[73] The obstruction interferes with normal gas exchange, and as a result the child becomes hypoxic and develops respiratory acidosis.

Assessment. The progression of the disease varies from mild to alarming severity. It usually begins as an upper respiratory tract infection. A cough, low-grade temperature, and nasal discharge are usually present at onset. Within 2 days, tachypnea (as high as 80), with nasal flaring retractions and, in severe cases, cyanosis may occur. These signs and symptoms occur as a result of partial obstruction of the bronchiolar lumen by exudate and edema.[77] Crying, feeding, and activity tend to make the symptoms worse. An expiratory wheeze may occur with activity. The infection usually lasts about 7 to 10 days.

Planning and implementation. Therapy is planned to maintain oxygenation, to maintain hydration, and to promote rest.

Maintaining oxygenation. Oxygen therapy is administered to correct hypoxemia, which occurs as a result of poor ventilation and perfusion. It also allows restlessness and anxiety. Other strategies that facilitate oxygenation are used, such as placing the child in a semi-Fowler's position. This position makes breathing easier because the abdominal organs do not press against the diaphragm. Consequently there is more room for lung expansion. The child is usually placed in a high-humidity environment. This liquefies secretions and makes coughing up of the mucus easier. If the child is not able to bring up secretions, suctioning should be used.

Maintaining hydration. Infants tend to be dehydrated because of poor fluid intake and increased insensible losses from tachypnea. The poor intake of oral fluids is usually a result of severe respiratory distress. Therefore intravenous therapy with electrolytes is prescribed for replacement therapy. Care must be taken not to overhydrate the child. Intake and output must be carefully monitored. The specific gravity must be checked each time the child voids to establish some guide to the hydration status. Usually a specific gravity reading between 1.008 and 1.015 is consistent with adequate hydration. A specific gravity reading below 1.008 may indicate overhydration, whereas a reading above 1.015 is indicative of dehydration. The nurse must carefully assess for signs indicating overhydration (for example, breathing difficulty, moist rales, tachycardia) and dehydration (for example, thick secretions and poor skin turgor).

Promoting rest. The nurse must provide emotional support to the child and his family by carefully attending to his needs, explaining aspects of care, and answering questions. Because the virus is transmitted by droplets, respiratory isolation is maintained.

Tonsillitis

The lymphoid tissues of the oropharynx and nasopharynx consists of the adenoids, lateral hands, fascial tonsils, and lingual tonsils, which are referred to as *Waldeyer's ring*. This tissue is present throughout childhood (from around 3 years of age to the adolescent period). After this period most of the ring atrophies. The exception is the lingual ring, which may appear larger.

Enlargement of the tissue often occurs during periods when there is an infection, for example, tonsillitis and adenoiditis.

Tonsillitis is an infection that often complicates an upper respiratory tract infection, usually pharyngitis. The *Streptococcus* organism, most often the beta-hemolytic type, is the most frequent offender in acute tonsillitis. Various fungi and other bacteria have also produced attacks of tonsillitis.

 Assessment. Sore throat, difficulty in swallowing, fever, and general malaise are common symptoms. Headache, muscle pain, and otalgia may also occur. During the inflammation, the mucous membrane around the throat is inflamed and studded with white or yellow patches. The temperature may be elevated as high as 102° to 103° F (38.8° to 39.4° C). Throat cultures are usually taken to detect the causative organism.

> **Data analysis**
> *Data analysis may reveal nursing diagnosis such as alterations in comfort or alterations in nutrition.*

 Planning and implementation. Therapy is directed toward relieving pain and preventing infection. Throat irrigations and analgesics such as codeine are helpful in relieving pain. Antibiotic therapy (for example, penicillin) is given for 10 days to combat the infection. Bed rest should be enforced. Compliance is often a problem. Therefore adequate information should be given to the parents so that compliance is enhanced. To help the client maintain nutritional intake, a light diet and adequate fluids are encouraged. Both of these measures help the client maintain resistance to infection.

Adenoiditis   Adenoiditis, an infection of the adenoids, usually accompanies acute tonsillitis. In older children and adults it may occur alone. When an infection occurs, the adenoids tend to enlarge and may obstruct the airway and eustachean tubes.

 Assessment. Symptoms indicate nasal obstruction (for example, mouth breathing, noisy breathing, especially when awake, and snoring during sleep). More specifically, these are caused by blockage of the posterior nasal channel by the adenoids. Headache, nasal and postnasal discharge, fever, malaise, drooling, and changes in the voice are also evident.

> **Data analysis**
> *Data analysis may reveal nursing diagnoses of ineffective breathing patterns and sleep pattern disturbance.*

 Planning and implementation
Tonsillectomy and adenoidectomy (T and A). A tonsillectomy is indicated when attacks of tonsillitis occur repeatedly. Adenoidectomy is especially indicated for persistent infection. However, surgery usually is not performed during an acute attack or for 2 to 3 weeks after any infection. Certain blood dyscrasias, such as aplastic anemia, hemophilia, or leukemia, contraindicate surgery.

Tonsillectomies may be performed at any age, although not before 3 to 4 years of age. They are more commonly performed in preschool and school-age children. In the child, a tonsillectomy and adenoidectomy are usually performed at the same time. The adenoidectomy is particularly a more useful operation for the child than the adult because children often have large, obstructive adenoids.

Nursing process for common health problems

Preoperative preparation. Once the decision is made to perform both a tonsillectomy and an adenoidectomy, the client should be adequately prepared for the experience. If the client is a child, surgery should be explained in terms that can be understood. The child should be informed about the surgery, the necessity for it, how surgery will affect him, and the limitations that will be experienced in the early postoperative period. Parents can be instrumental in preparing their child for surgery, although the nurse should assist the parents in preparation as much as necessary. Comic books and coloring books on the subject are available and are excellent resources for hospital and surgical preparation. These books discuss the entire hospital experience. The discussions are presented in language that can be easily understood by the child. The preschool child should have the material read to him by the parents or nurse. Doll play therapy is also helpful.

The child may be admitted to the hospital the morning of surgery, provided all preparation is done ahead of time. However, the child is usually admitted to the hospital the evening before surgery. When he is admitted, the nurse should familiarize him with the hospital environment. The nursing history should include questions regarding a recent infection or recent exposure to a contagious disease. (He should also be observed for any signs of infection.) The nurse should examine the school-age child for loose teeth. The presence of these should be reported to the physician before the anesthetic is given. Data should be obtained for vital signs and bleeding tendencies. Any abnormalities in vital signs should be reported. Bleeding and clotting times are usually obtained on admission. The results should be reviewed and evaluated, and any abnormal values should be reported to the physician. (Any tendency to hemorrhage is treated with vitamin K.)

Several hours before surgery, fluids and foods are withheld to prevent aspiration after the anesthetic is given. Preoperative medications (such as barbiturate and atropine) are given before surgery.

Intraoperative care. General anesthesia is usually used for the child, whereas local anesthesia is commonly used for adults. During surgery the child is placed in a supine position with the head hyperextended. The position prevents blood from flowing into the lower part of the throat. The mouth is opened with a mouth gag, and the tonsils and adenoids are removed with the use of snares. Aspiration of secretions is performed continuously during the procedure to remove the excess blood and lessen the chance of pulmonary complications.

Postoperative care. After surgery the client is placed in a prone position. A pillow is placed under the chest and abdomen to prevent aspiration of vomitus and to promote drainage of secretions from the mouth. Frequent assessments for signs of hemorrhage should be made. Postoperative bleeding is most likely to occur within the first hour following surgery. Indications of hemorrhage are frequent swallowing, changes in vital signs, tachycardia, restlessness, drop in blood pressure, and vomiting of bright red blood. Emergency equipment (epinephrine, gauze sponges, and suctioning equipment) should be available.

An ice collar may be ordered to relieve pain. If so, it must be kept cold. Ice chips, cold bland fluids, and foods may be given after the nausea has subsided. Milk, carbonated beverages, and synthetic juices may also be given. The natural acid juices (tomato and orange) are usually not given because they tend to irritate the throat. Spices, rough foods (such as popcorn), and extremely hot liquids are also avoided. Aspirin may be ordered to promote comfort.

Rest periods should be encouraged the day after surgery and periodically during the days following. Generally the child is discharged on the first postoperative day.

In preparing the child for discharge, the parents should be given a list of diet instructions. This practice is customary but not a necessity because the child generally limits the diet to foods that do not hurt.

Delayed hemorrhage is likely to occur around the fifth to seventh postoperative day. It is during this period that the tonsillar fossae and adenoid space separate. Therefore parents should be told to observe for signs of bleeding such as nosebleed, hemoptysis, frequent swallowing, and vomiting of blood. If these signs occur, the parents should be instructed to take the child to the emergency unit or the physician's office. Failure to relieve delayed bleeding may result in major blood loss. Instructions should also be given regarding medications and activity for the child. The child can usually return to normal activity within 1 to 2 weeks.

Cystic fibrosis

Cystic fibrosis is an inherited disease involving the exocrine glands.[48] It is inherited as an autosomal recessive trait.

Cystic fibrosis is considered a major cause of chronic pulmonary disease in the infant, child, and young adult. It occurs most commonly in whites and has been documented to occur in approximately 1 in 1500 to 1 in 2500 per live birth.[14] At this time, individuals with cystic fibrosis live 25 years or more.

Pathophysiology. Cystic fibrosis affects many organ systems.[74] A basic defect that has been observed in cystic fibrosis is obstruction of exocrine gland ducts or the passageways into which exocrine secretions are discharged, namely, the bronchioles, bronchi, paranasal sinuses, salivary ducts, small intestine, pancreatic ducts, bile ducts, uterine cervix.[48] The obstruction results from highly viscous abnormal mucous secretions; consequently the secretions (for example, pancreatic enzymes) do not enter the duodenum. Subsequently, foods are poorly absorbed, especially fats and proteins because these substances normally are broken down by these enzymes. The fat-soluble vitamins (A, D, E, K) are also poorly absorbed. Malfunctioning of the mucociliary transport and increased secretions obstruct the lungs[11] and lead to air trapping and atelectasis. Fibrotic changes also occur in the lungs and pancreas (for example, replacement of the pancreatic acini by fibrotic tissue).[74]

The pulmonary secretions of clients with cystic fibrosis provide an excellent medium for bacterial growth. As a result, pulmonary infections are frequent and present a serious threat to life. The prim   ʾfecting organism is *Pseudomonas aeruginosa* or *Staphylococcus aureus;* ι. ʌever, *Diplococcus pneumoniae, Haemophilus influenzae, Klebsiella pneumoniae, Escherichia coli, Proteus vulgaris, Candida albicans,* and *Aspergillus fumigatus* may also produce an infection.[48] Respiratory complications of cystic fibrosis include bronchiectasis, pneumothorax, and cor pulmonale.

Assessment. In cystic fibrosis, signs indicative of both pulmonary and gastrointestinal involvement are present. The pulmonary signs include tachypnea, a chronic, unproductive cough, shortness of breath (especially with activity), barrel chest, clubbed fingers, and cyanosis.[42]

Gastrointestinal involvement is manifested by frequent, bulky, foul-smelling, greasy, or frothy stools. Flatus is excessive. The smell is offensive because of the presence of a large amount of malabsorbed fats and proteins; it is

1307

frothy because of the sugar ferment. The stools may also be clay-colored. The child may have a voracious appetite but fail to gain weight. Abdominal distension is also present, and there is slow muscular development.

Bowel obstruction from thick, mucoid secretions (referred to as *meconium ileus* in the infant and *meconium ileus equivalent* in the older child and adult) may also develop.[42] Prolapsed rectum may develop in these children.

The diagnosis is made by clinical observation, chest x-ray study, a positive sweat test (sweat chloride above 60 mEq/L), an absent or low pancreatic iso-amylase concentration in serum, and measurement of duodenal trypsin, which is decreased or absent.

Data analysis
Data analysis may reveal nursing diagnoses of alteration in nutrition, ineffective airway clearance, alteration in bowel elimination, ineffective family coping, grieving, impaired home maintenance management, and knowledge deficit.

Planning and implementation. The therapeutic plan is designed to provide adequate nutrition and promote respiratory function. Diet modification (for example, low fat, high protein, high calorie) are instituted to compensate for faulty pancreatic function. The fat content of the diet is reduced and the amount of protein increased. Protein can be added to the diet with powdered milk. Total calories must be doubled because one half of the nutritional value is lost in the stool. Calories can be added by increasing the carbohydrate in the formula or by adding more fruits and meats during meals. In addition, fat-soluble vitamins A, D, E, and K and sodium chloride are added to compensate for losses in the frequent stools. Pancreatic enzymes are given with each feeding or meal to aid digestion. When new foods are added to the infant's diet, the mother is instructed to observe the color of the stools as an indication of how well the food is being tolerated. The diet may be difficult to follow, and the mother may appreciate suggestions from the nurse or dietitian.

Maintenance of free respiratory passage is necessary to support life. Most deaths from cystic fibrosis result from pulmonary complications. As a result, a program of nebulization therapy and exercises to promote drainage of accumulating mucus in the lungs should be begun immediately. Nebulization is used to deposit water and medication in the bronchial tree where mucus obstructs exchange of vital gases. Mist tents, ultrasonic nebulizers, aerosol treatments, or intermittent positive pressure breathing treatments may be used to loosen secretions. The nurse or physical therapist should teach the parents how to do clapping, cupping, and vibrating exercises to help dislodge mucous plugs. These treatments should be done before meals so that the client will be able to obtain nutrition without choking. Lung lavage with isotonic saline solution is being used experimentally to remove mucus from deep in the lung. Copious amounts of the solution are given through a catheter that is inserted through the bronchi to the base of the lungs. The fluid is drained out, and with it, the mucus.

During acute states, nursing care should be supportive. If the client has diarrhea, his buttocks should be cleansed carefully, and an ointment may be applied around the rectum if it becomes excoriated. The odor from the stool is foul, and a deodorant may be used in the room and around the bed. Lowered resistance may cause slow healing, and the skin may be easily broken down. The nurse should observe the client's skin and protect it from irritation by turning the client frequently and using lotion on areas of friction.

With early diagnosis and treatment many clients live to adulthood. The diet and respiratory therapy that is started in the hospital is continued at home. A community health nurse can be helpful in assisting the parents to make adaptations to home life. Most children use mist tents to sleep in, and some form of nebulization may be required. These can be an expense to most families, and community resources may be mobilized to defray the cost. Some communities have a Cystic Fibrosis Association, which can be instrumental in helping parents and supplying needed equipment to care for their children at home.

As the child matures, the parents must help him find a balance of independence and security within his capabilities. Some communities have special schools for children with health problems where therapy can be carried out during the school hours. Other areas have summer camps so that the children can enjoy recreation away from home, yet be in a safe environment.

Clients who reach adulthood will need to plan realistic goals for career and marriage. The client who is considering marriage should understand the risk of passing the disease to his or her offspring and should obtain genetic counseling. Male clients with cystic fibrosis are usually sterile.

Evaluation. The nursing care plan for the client with cystic fibrosis is based on diagnoses such as alteration in nutrition, ineffective airway clearance, ineffective family coping, grieving, and knowledge deficit. The plan is evaluated on an ongoing basis.

EXPECTED OUTCOMES

The client and/or family can:
1. Explain cystic fibrosis, including the cause, genetic relationship, and organ systems involved.
2. State plans for maintaining nutritional status.
3. Demonstrate performance of home care techniques such as chest physiotherapy.
4. Describe signs indicative of early lung infection.
5. State plans for health maintenance.
6. State plans for follow-up health care.

Miliary tuberculosis

Miliary tuberculosis is a generalized hematogenous disease with multiple tubercle formation. It may occur following primary infection or by reactivation of a dormant focus years later.[58] Because the body's defenses are overwhelmed, lesions are not only found in organs with an elevated Pa_{O_2}, but in others as well (for example, liver, spleen, bone marrow, meninges). It is a frequent occurrence in infants and young children.

Pathophysiology. The tubercles, which gain entry through the lymphatics, result from the lodgement of the tubercle bacilli in small capillaries. The miliary lesion may be confined to the lungs or affect distant organs. For example, erosion of the bacilli into the pulmonary artery results in limitation of the lesion to the *lung* because the organisms, which are filtered out by the alveolar capillary bed, become trapped in the alveolar circulation and hence do not reach arterial systemic circulation. However, massive invasion of the organisms into the pulmonary arteries results in their gaining entry through the alveolar capillaries and into systemic circulation, thus affecting varied organs. Erosion of a caseous focus into a pulmonary vein may have the same effect. Sites most commonly affected by miliary tuberculosis are the liver, spleen, lymph nodes, kidneys, adrenal glands, prostate gland, seminal vesicles, fallopian tubes, endometrium, meninges, bone marrow, and retina.[58]

 Assessment. Symptoms depend on the organs affected. The onset is usually acute and accompanied by fever, dyspnea, cough, cyanosis, and prostration; or symptoms are indicative of chronic illness (fatigue, weakness, and weight loss). Splenomegaly and anemia are common.

Because varied organs may be affected, diagnostic assessments may include chest roentgenogram; funduscopic examination of the eyes; and aspiration biopsies of the liver, lymph node, and bone marrow to detect caseating granulomas and tubercle bacilli. Therapy is basically the same as for pulmonary tuberculosis.

COMMON HEALTH PROBLEMS OF THE ADOLESCENT

Fractures of the nose

Fractures of the nose are not uncommon, possibly because the nose is exposed and unprotected. Children frequently sustain nasal fractures from falls, but often these are not evident until adolescence when a deformity is noted. Adolescents who engage in active sports also frequently sustain nasal fractures. Both nasal obstruction and external deformity may result.

Whenever a child falls and hits his nose or whenever the older individual sustains a blow on the nose, he should be seen by a physician. X-ray films may be taken to ascertain whether a displacement is present. Immediate care is usually planned to control bleeding and prevent swelling by application of a cold compress. If the bone is displaced, the physician reduces the fracture by firmly pressing over the convex side of the nose with one or both thumbs. This forces the displaced bone and septum to return to their correct position. If the fracture cannot be reduced in this manner, the client may be taken to surgery and the reduction made with the client under general anesthesia.

Deviated septum

A deviated nasal septum is a deformity in which the nasal septum has deviated from the midline to one side or the other. Developmental or traumatic factors are most often responsible for producing septal deformities. A developmental defect is generally less serious than one resulting from trauma.

The nasal cartilage is more pliable in the child than in the adult. Thus it is not unusual for small children to injure the anterior portion of the nose from frequent falls and thereby dislocate the septum.

 Assessment. When the trauma occurs later in life, the nose is already formed and the bones have hardened; therefore greater irregularity in the deformity is likely to be noted. The deviation may be so great as to obstruct the airway. Parents therefore should be encouraged to seek medical help at the time any accident occurs, even though the injury seems trivial.

> **Data analysis**
> *Data analysis may reveal nursing diagnoses of ineffective breathing pattern and sensory perception alterations.*

 Planning and implementation. As a form of therapy, a surgical procedure such as a submucous resection (SMR) is performed to straighten a deviated septum and relieve the obstruction. Except in children, this procedure is usually performed with the client under local anesthesia.

After the operative procedure, some type of splint or intranasal pack may be applied for support and to prevent a hematoma from forming postoperatively. The gauze is usually held in place with a nasal bandage secured with adhesive tape across the nares. The packing is generally removed within 1 or 2 days after surgery, and a vasoconstrictor solution may be applied to prevent nasal congestion. Hospitalization may be necessary for only 24 to 48 hours.

Preoperative care. Regardless of the type of surgery performed on the nose, the principles of preoperative and postoperative care are the same. In the preoperative period the client should be informed about the type of surgery and its purpose and how the surgery will affect him. Explanations should cover what can be expected as well as what is expected of the client in the early postoperative period. He should be informed that he will have a nasal pack and a drip pad underneath the nose after surgery. This will require him to breathe through his mouth. It may be helpful to have the client practice mouth breathing before surgery. Some discoloration and swelling of the nose, a dry mouth, difficulty in breathing and talking, nausea, and swelling are expected. The client should be so informed. He should be told not to blow his nose in the postoperative period. The usual preoperative medications, meperidine (Demerol) hydrochloride and atropine, are administered before surgery.

Postoperative care. Postoperative care is planned to facilitate breathing, promote comfort, prevent pain, and monitor for signs of complications. The client should be placed in a semi-Fowler's position to decrease edema at the operative site and to promote drainage. As edema is lessened and drainage is promoted, the client will breathe more comfortably. Because the client becomes a mouth breather, measures to prevent drying of the oral mucosa should be encouraged, such as frequent sips of water and frequent mouth care. Fluids should be given liberally. A liquid diet may be ordered the first postoperative day.

Edema is common; therefore ice compresses are usually prescribed to be applied to the operative site. Such measures reduce edema and bleeding as well as relieve pain. Pain medication should be given as needed.

Because the client breathes through his mouth, the route of taking temperatures will have to be altered. It now becomes necessary to take rectal or axillary temperatures.

Any form of trauma should be avoided. The client should be cautioned not to blow his nose. The child who tends to pick at his nose should be given mittens to wear.

Usually within 12 to 24 hours after the operation the physician removes the nasal packs. During removal of the pack, care is taken to minimize the chance of hemorrhage within the layers of the septum. Formation of a hematoma is likely to prolong convalescence. After the packs are removed, the client should be encouraged to lie quietly for 30 minutes. Nose blowing should be forbidden because it encourages bruising and edema.

Discoloration in the form of ecchymosis is common. It usually reaches a maximum within 24 to 48 hours and then gradually disappears. By the end of the second week, discoloration usually has faded.

During the convalescence period, decongestants may be ordered to reduce the nasal congestion and thus open the nasal airway.

After a submucous resection, hemorrhage, hematoma, falling of the bridge, and flapping septum are common complications. Repeated swallowing, especially by the unconscious surgical client, indicates hemorrhage. Frequent assessments should be made of the vital signs, skin color, and respiratory status. Symptoms that indicate perforation are usually those of rhinitis, sometimes dryness, and crusting with discomfort in the nose or watery discharge.

As the nurse monitors for signs of complications, the position of the pack should be checked at regularly scheduled intervals. This can be accomplished by observing the back of the client's throat. Normally the packing should not be seen. If the packing can be observed, or if bleeding occurs, the amount and character of drainage should be noted.

Rhinoplasty. Rhinoplasty is a plastic surgery procedure performed to reconstruct the external nose. It may involve reshaping the tip, hump, septum, and narrowing the base. It may also be done for cosmetic reasons. Such a procedure may not be performed until the adolescent period unless the child is embarrassed by his appearance and nasal function is impaired. The operation is usually performed under local anesthesia. A nasal splint is usually applied to protect the nose from any form of trauma. Postoperatively the client is placed in a Fowler's position to minimize oozing. An ice pack is applied to the nose to prevent ecchymosis and edema. Because the nasal orifice is closed by a dressing, measures to prevent drying of the oral mucosa should be implemented. For example, oral hygiene measures should be performed at frequent intervals, or sips of water should be offered. The client should be instructed not to remove or bother the dressing. These are generally changed within 3 to 5 days. The client must be helped to maintain his nutritional intake. Although the swelling and ecchymosis gradually disappear within 1 to 2 weeks, it usually takes several weeks before the results of the surgery can be ascertained.

 Evaluation. Evaluation of the nursing care plan for the client having nasal surgery is an ongoing process. Each plan of care must be individualized.

EXPECTED OUTCOMES

The client and/or family can:
1. Describe the health problem.
2. Describe the expected results of the surgery.
3. State posthospital limitations using the specified time frame.
4. Demonstrate postdischarge self-care strategies such as changing dressings or drip pads.
5. Describe posthospital comfort measures.
6. State potential complications and emergency management.
7. Describe plans for follow-up care.

COMMON HEALTH PROBLEMS OF THE YOUNG ADULT

Nasal polyps

Nasal polyps are masses of tissue resembling a bunch of grapes, which result from an allergic reaction that produces prolonged edema in the mucosa of the nose and sinuses. Common in adults, they are generally multiple, always bilateral, and produce nasal blockage. They are rare in children. The submucosa around the middle meatus is especially lax and easily waterlogged; as a result, the tissues tend to swell easily. Swelling is aggravated by the discharge.

Assessment. The many symptoms are those indicative of obstruction to breathing and anosmia (loss of smell). There is generally some discharge, which may be mucoid or purulent if infection occurs. Pain is nil unless infection is present. Occasionally small polyps regress spontaneously if the cause is removed. However, in the vast majority of cases polyps must be removed surgically.

Data analysis

Data analysis may reveal nursing diagnoses of ineffective breathing patterns, potential for injury, and sensory perceptual alterations.

    Planning and implementation. A nasal snare is placed over the polyp, and the growth removed as the snare is closed. The surgical procedure is a *polypectomy* and may be performed in the physician's office, clinic, or hospital. Bleeding is minimal following surgery. The client should be instructed not to blow his nose for 1 to 2 days. When the polyps recur, as they usually do, an ethmoidectomy may be performed. Electrosurgery may be used to remove the remaining tumor.

    Evaluation. The nursing care plan for the client having nasal polyps removed is based on diagnoses that relate to breathing and injury.

EXPECTED OUTCOMES

The client and/or family can:
1. Describe nasal polyps, including the cause.
2. Verbalize the restrictions.
3. State plans for follow-up maintenance and care.

Rhinitis

    Rhinitis is a term used to designate inflammation of the nasal cavities. The inflammatory condition results from interplay of bacteria, viruses, and allergy. It is almost always initiated by one of the viruses that cause upper respiratory tract infections. Two forms of rhinitis may exist: acute or chronic.

    In *acute rhinitis,* sneezing, obstruction to the flow of air, and nasal discharge are characteristic symptoms. The consistency of the discharge ranges from thin and watery to mucopurulent. The latter is produced by invasion of the passages by bacteria.

    The swelling of the nasal mucosa may obstruct the orifices of the air sinuses and cause sinusitis. The bacterially infected cases may, although not common, be complicated by meningitis, brain abscess, or osteomyelitis.

    Chronic rhinitis results from incomplete resolution of acute rhinitis. It may be related to nasal obstruction, allergy, trauma, and endocrine and dietary factors; it may be secondary to sinusitis; or it may result from prolonged use of drops and sprays. Any environmental factors such as dust, fumes, or unsuitable climatic conditions that prevent normal function of the mucous membrane are also considered possible predisposing factors.

    The symptoms are similar in both adults and children. In addition to the appearance of symptoms of the acute form of rhinitis, mouth breathing and snoring may be present as a result of nasal obstruction. In long-standing cases, the voice may become nasal in quality.

    Another form of chronic rhinitis is *atrophic rhinitis,* which is characterized by atrophy of the nasal mucosa as evidenced by dryness and crusting. The crust results from a lack of moisture and nasal secretions and may produce nasal obstruction. Any condition that causes prolonged dryness of the mucous membrane is thought to give rise to atrophic rhinitis. For this reason the condition may

1313

be occupational. In the absence of such obvious causes the etiology is not easily established. Factors such as endocrine dysfunction and dietary deficiencies have been suggested as possible causes. For example, it is more common in women and usually occurs before puberty. It has been demonstrated to be worse during the menstrual period and has a tendency to improve after the menopause. It may occur in several members of the family and is more common in lower socioeconomic groups.

Pharyngitis

Pharyngitis is an acute inflammation of the pharynx that is usually caused by group A hemolytic streptococci or the influenza bacillus. Those caused by *Streptococcus* organisms are of greater concern. An attack of *acute pharyngitis* is manifested by a raw or tickling sensation in the throat, a dry cough, dysphagia, malaise, and an elevated temperature.

Inflammatory conditions of the throat are treated systemically with antibiotics to control infection and with analgesics to relieve pain. Gargles and hot throat irrigations promote comfort. In spite of the sore, irritated throat, nutrition must be maintained. The diet should be nutritious and appetizing. Liquid and soft foods are generally better tolerated.

Because of the serious nature of some sore throats, parents should be encouraged to seek medical help when a sore throat first becomes evident.

Sinusitis

Acute sinusitis is an inflammatory condition of the lining of one or more of the paranasal sinuses. The organisms most often responsible for producing sinusitis are the viruses of acute rhinitis. Any condition that interferes with the drainage and aeration of the sinus renders it liable to infection. For example, conditions that narrow the air passages (such as allergies, chronic edema, thick mucus, and nasal polyps) may interfere with ventilation and drainage of the sinuses. Excessive nose blowing during an acute infection may cause infected material to be driven into the sinus, thus causing an infection.

 Assessment. The symptoms during the early stage are similar to those of acute rhinitis. Headache in the area of one or more of the sinuses is the most characteristic symptom. Postnasal discharge may also be present. An increase or decrease in the amount of secretions generally coincides with an increase or decrease in the severity of pain. Chills and fever may also be present. Chronic sinusitis may follow acute attacks.

 Planning and implementation. The objectives of therapy are to promote drainage and relieve pain. Therefore vasoconstricting medications to shrink the mucous membrane of the nose are usually prescribed. Decongestive drops are used to promote sinus drainage. Analgesics are prescribed to relieve pain and headache. Antibiotics are prescribed to control the infection and prevent complications. When fever is present, bed rest is prescribed, and fluids are forced.

Chronic sinus infections usually require special surgery to facilitate drainage. The two operations that may be performed are an *intranasal antrostomy* and the *Caldwell-Luc operation*. In the former, the maxillary antrum is opened through the nose. The latter is a more radical procedure; the antrum is opened through the mouth. Only a small opening is made in the intranasal approach. The Caldwell-Luc operation permits a more permanent drainage into the nose. Both of these are done with the client under local anesthesia.

Acute bronchitis

Acute bronchitis, an inflammation of the bronchi, is usually caused by viral agents but may be caused by bacterial or chemical agents. It is not uncommon for an upper respiratory tract infection such as the common cold to accompany acute bronchitis. Inhalation of irritating chemical fumes and dusts also causes bronchial irritation and inflammation.

Assessment. The onset of symptoms occurs rapidly and usually includes symptoms indicative of an upper respiratory tract infection: pyrexia, malaise, body aches, and cough. The cough, from stimulation of afferent vagal receptors, at the time of onset is dry and unproductive, but gradually becomes productive. At first the sputum is scanty and tenacious but later becomes abundant and mucopurulent. Both of these symptoms, cough and sputum, may persist 3 to 5 days after the fever and malaise subside.

> **Data analysis**
> *Data analysis may reveal nursing diagnoses of ineffective breathing patterns and alterations in comfort.*

Planning and implementation. Therapy is planned to ensure comfort. Bed rest is an important form of treatment as long as pyrexia is present. Fluids are encouraged to help abate pyrexia. A croup tent may be used to provide inhalation of medicated steam. Analgesic medication may be prescribed to control pain and back and muscle aches. Expectorants, antipyretics, and demulcents may also be prescribed. A liquid or soft diet is usually ordered. Clients with acute bronchitis may be cared for at home or in the hospital. The nurse has a responsibility to educate the client and his family on how to protect an infected individual.

Legionnaire's disease

The term legionnaire's disease originated in the summer of 1976 when approximately 200 individuals were struck by an unknown illness during an American Legion convention.[81] Legionnaire's disease is a febrile respiratory disease. Several risk factors have been identified to predispose to the disease: cigarette smoking,[57,58] advanced age, and being male.[79] Most cases occur in the summer months; however, epidemics have been reported at other times and sporadic cases have been reported in all seasons.[81] An association has also been made between travel and the acquisition of legionnaire's disease, since several cases have been reported after the affected individual traveled.[79] The stress of travel and exposure to sources of etiological agents have been used to explain this association. *Legionella pneumophilia* has been identified as the causative organism.

Assessment. Legionnaire's disease is characterized by a variety of symptoms including malaise, muscle aches, headaches, and an unproductive cough that occurs on the second or third day. A rapidly rising fever, shaking chills, chest pain, dyspnea, abdominal pain, gastrointestinal symptoms (nausea and vomiting, diarrhea) confusion, and changes in affect have also been reported.[86]

Several serum studies are useful in establishing a diagnosis, namely, blood cultures and blood counts, including white cell count and sedimentation rate. The white cell count and sedimentation rates are increased. Serum sodium is decreased. The latter is thought to be related to inappropriate ADH secretion.

> **Data analysis**
> *Data analysis reveals nursing diagnoses of ineffective breathing patterns, fear, and grieving.*

Planning and implementation. Therapy is planned to maintain oxygenation, maintain hydration, control infection, maintain blood pressure and organ perfusion, and promote comfort. Oxygen is administered, and mechanical ventilation with PEEP may be used. Intravenous fluids are administered to maintain hydration status.

To maintain blood pressure, vasoactive drugs are used. For infection control, erythromycin is considered the drug of choice, and it is generally recommended that it be administered for as long as 3 weeks.[81] Antipyretics are prescribed to control temperature and analgesics to control pain. A high temperature is characteristic; therefore the client may be given tepid sponge baths as needed.

The client behavior, vital signs, hydration, and renal status must be assessed at frequent intervals. Accurate intake and output records must be maintained. Because *L pneumophilia* has been isolated from the sputum and transtracheal aspirates,[20] respiratory precautions must be adhered to. The nurse must also be available to answer questions and provide emotional support for the client and the family.

 Evaluation. The client with legionnaire's disease may have problems associated with breathing, fear, and grieving. The nurse and client evaluate the plan on an ongoing basis.

EXPECTED OUTCOMES

The client and/or family can:
1. Describe legionnaire's disease.
2. Describe plans for maintaining health.
3. State indications of health problems requiring health care.
4. State plans for follow-up health care.

Pulmonary embolism

A pulmonary embolus is an intravascular mass of fat or air, but it usually is a blood clot that becomes detached and migrates into the bloodstream until it becomes lodged in a pulmonary vessel too small to permit passage. As a result, the vessel becomes occluded, and a pulmonary embolism exists.

Predisposition to pulmonary embolization. Three factors have been associated with the formation of thrombi: stasis of blood *(venous stasis),* changes in the vessel wall *(endophlebitis),* and changes in coagulation *(hypercoagulability).* Venous stasis is thought to be the most important predisposing factor. Because blood flow decreases by at least one half during periods of bed rest because of diminished muscle tone and pumping action,[67] it is not uncommon for individuals on bed rest for extended periods to develop thrombi.

Contingent with stasis is vein distension with possible disruption of the *endothelial lining*. Any damage to the intima of a vessel alters the antithrombotic properties and subsequently creates an environment for thrombus formation. Hypercoagulability is influenced by factors such as pregnancy, blood disorders, surgery, or trauma. As a result, risk factors identified as likely to produce pulmonary embolism include immobility, advanced age (particularly those immobilized for long periods), obesity, and surgery (especially gynecological, urinary tract, and orthopedic of the lower extremities). Pregnancy, parturition, cardiac disease, varicosities, cancer (especially cancer of the genitourinary, pulmonary, or gastrointestinal systems), oral contraceptives, or estrogen therapy are considered to be risk factors.[55]

Pathophysiology. The dislodgement of an embolus in a pulmonary artery results in varied pulmonary and hemodynamic changes. The immediate *pulmonary changes* include an increased alveolar dead space and pneumoconstriction; loss of alveolar surfactant occurs later. An increase in the dead space results when a portion of the diseased lung no longer participates in gas exchange.

Pneumoconstriction results from alveolar hypocapnea. The major source of alveolar carbon dioxide is pulmonary arterial blood. When an embolism develops, this primary source is interrupted (that is, the region is not properly ventilated), and the response by the distal airways is constriction. Such constriction permits equal distribution of air to those areas that are not affected, thus compensating for the limited gas exchange to the involved areas.

For surfactant to be produced, nutrients must be continuously delivered to the alveoli. Under normal conditions, only pulmonary arterial blood reaches the alveoli; therefore an embolism results in the nutrient supply being cut off and a cessation of the production of surfactant, thus causing the development of alveolar instability and atelectasis. When alveolar instability and atelectasis occur, the embolized area becomes filled with plasma and blood cells. Restoration of the pulmonary arterial circulation or development of bronchial arterial circulation in the involved area results in a return to a normal state.

The immediate *hemodynamic* effect is a decrease in the area of the pulmonary vascular bed and a resultant increase in pulmonary vascular resistance. If the blood flow remains constant, the pressure in the pulmonary arterial system and the work of the right ventricle will rise. A significant increase in workload will cause right ventricular failure.

Resolution of pulmonary emboli. The majority of pulmonary emboli resolve quickly, usually within the first few days, and are well advanced within 2 weeks. The mechanisms responsible for promoting vascular patency include the *fibrinolytic system* and the process of *organization*.[55] The fibrinolytic system dissolves fibrin thrombi and is responsible for the rapid phase of thromboembolic resolution. Organization, on the other hand, is a slower process that requires several days and results in the transformation of the thrombus into a small scar attached to the vascular wall. Failure of some emboli to resolve is thought to be related to impairment in the fibrinolytic system or the fact that the embolus was well organized before it lodged in the lung.

The major origin of pulmonary embolism is the deep veins of the calf muscles of the legs. A second source is the pelvic veins. The mechanisms responsible for dislogement of thrombi are mechanical forces, such as direct trauma, sudden muscle action, or change in the rate of blood flow. These forces may produce changes in the intravascular pressure and cause clot dissolution, which is a natural mechanism.[67]

Assessment. The effect of pulmonary embolism is directly related to the size of the vessel occluded, the age and state of the client, the location, number of emboli, and the percentage of circulation obstructed. Small emboli that lodge in peripheral branches of the pulmonary artery may have no effect. Clients with medium-sized emboli may experience a brief period of dyspnea, mild tachycardia, and diaphoresis. There may or may not be a slight change in blood pressure.[7] If the embolus is large enough to block the main pulmonary artery, or if it lodges at the bifurcation of the right and left branches, sudden death usually results from severe systemic anoxia or from massive right heart strain and a resultant right heart failure.

Nursing process for common health problems

Authorities contend that young clients are more likely to survive a massive attack; whereas elderly clients, especially those with cardiac or pulmonary instability, are likely to die. A small embolus in clients with heart disease (for example, CHF or chronic lung disease) may produce symptoms; whereas a large embolus in relatively healthy clients may only produce mild symptoms.[34]

Likely symptoms of large emboli include severe dyspnea, crushing substernal chest pain, tachypnea, tachycardia, coughing, apprehension, wheezing, and prominent neck veins.

The onset of massive pulmonary emboli may be dramatic. The client may immediately lose consciousness, become cyanotic, and go into shock. Death may occur immediately if the main pulmonary artery is blocked.

The sudden onset of symptoms is helpful in diagnosis. However, several tests may be performed to confirm the diagnosis of pulmonary embolism: blood studies (white blood count, erythrocyte, sedimentation, serum enzymes), chest x-ray films, an electrocardiogram, pulmonary angiography, and arterial blood gases.

> **Data analysis**
> *Data analysis may reveal nursing diagnoses of ineffective breathing patterns, impaired gas exchange, alterations in tissue perfusion, and alterations in cardiac output.*

Planning and implementation. Therapeutic measures are planned to maintain hemodynamic status (measures to maintain blood pressure). The onset of pulmonary embolism demands emergency measures. When symptoms are felt, the bed should be elevated to a semi-Fowler's position and the client should be made as comfortable as possible. Oxygen should be administered to relieve hypoxemia and promote tissue oxygenation. Someone should remain with the client and make frequent assessment of the vital signs and level of consciousness.

The physician should be consulted and will prescribe intravenous fluids with vasopressors to restore normal arterial blood pressure if hypotension occurs. Intravenous fluids must be administered cautiously because of the state of heart failure. Heparin, or some other form of anticoagulant drug, may be prescribed to prevent further thromboembolic formation. Thrombolytic agents (such as streptokinase-streptodornase or urokinase) may be ordered to lyse the emboli; analgesics (such as morphine or meperidine) to relieve pain; sedatives to relieve apprehension; adrenergic drugs (such as atropine) to reduce bronchospasms and decrease secretions; and antibiotics to prevent infection. Oxygen is usually maintained at high concentrations.

During treatment or during resolution, large quantities of fluids should be encouraged orally if possible. To maintain high fluid intake, strategies must be used that will accomplish this, for example, considerations of client likes, use of a variety of fluids, and offering cold liquids.

Prevention of venous thrombi and subsequent embolization. In addition to directing efforts toward treatment, the nurse should plan for prevention. When preventive measures are used, efforts are directed toward altering predisposing conditions: stasis, damage to the lining of the vessel, and hypercoagulability. Surgery may also be performed.

Altering stasis. The nurse has a major responsibility in preventing pulmonary embolization. Clients who have been identified as being most likely to develop embolism and any other person confined to bed should be instructed and encouraged to perform activities that will improve venous circulation. Active leg exercises should be performed hourly throughout the period of confinement. Such exercises involves raising and lowering the legs as well as relaxing and contracting the muscles of the lower extremities. If the client is not able to perform these exercises, passive exercises should be an integral part of the nursing care plan. Frequent changes in position and early ambulation should be encouraged to promote venous drainage. Elastic support stockings are often used for clients after major surgery as well as for those confined to bed. These are valuable in that pressure exerted by the stockings on the superficial veins facilitates venous return in the deeper vessels. As a result, clot formation is lessened. These stockings should be applied before getting the patient out of bed, and they should be removed once each shift to assess and evaluate the condition of the skin and circulation.

Any position that favors venous pooling should be avoided. Clients should be discouraged from sitting for long periods of time. Crossing the legs must not be permitted. Pillows should not be placed directly under the popliteal area, and knee adjustments should not be used because the veins are superficial in this area. Such a strategy may damage the intima lining and obstruct blood flow.

Although less frequently used, elevation of the leg 15 to 20 degrees above horizontal position or elevation of the foot of the bed is thought to improve venous circulation. Recent reports indicate that the process of venous thrombosis begins during surgery. As a result, methods to stimulate blood flow have been used in surgery as a preventive measure. For example, the calf muscles may be stimulated with electrodes while the client is in surgery.[22]

Preventing intima damage. Antiplatelet agents such as aspirin and dextran have been used as a means of preventing the formation of thrombi. Aspirin inhibits platelet-release action, with subsequent blockage of platelet aggregation, whereas dextran reduces platelet adhesiveness to damaged endothelium and reduces blood viscosity.

Preventing coagulation. Studies have revealed a reduction in the incidence of thrombus formation when anticoagulants are administered as a prophylactic measure postoperatively.[38] Anticoagulant therapy (for example, heparin 5000 U) may be administered postoperatively to high-risk clients. The nurse should be aware of the nursing responsibilities related to anticoagulant therapy (see Chapter 20).

Surgical interventions. Frequent recurrences of emboli,[15,34] massive emboli, blood dyscrasias, overt bleeding, and the occurrence of pulmonary embolism during pregnancy[15] contraindicate anticoagulant therapy. In these instances surgery may be performed. Surgical procedures may include *venous interruption* (for example, IVC, or umbrella filter) or an *embolectomy*. The interruption procedures are performed to prevent the thrombi from migrating to the lungs.

Venous interruptions may be performed either at the femoral or caval level. Transvenous filters (for example, the intracaval umbrella filter) is another procedure used (Fig. 21-31). This is a nonsurgical interruption. This filter is generally inserted through the right internal jugular vein, advanced through the superior

FIG. 21-31
Intracaval umbrella filter.

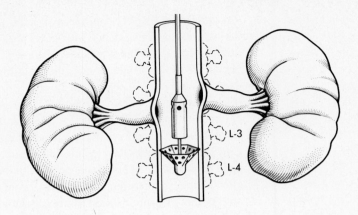

vena cava, into the right atrium, and into the inferior vena cava. The distal end of the capsule is positioned below the level of the more distal renal pelvis.[53] This is accomplished with the aid of fluoroscopy and performed with the client under local anesthesia. It produces a gradual obstruction of the inferior vena cava.[51] The left internal jugular or femoral vein may be used in instances of occlusion or tortosity of the vessel. The procedure generally takes about an hour.

Complications include difficulty with placement, misplacement or detachment of the filter, embolization, and bleeding with hematoma formation.[53]

Preoperative and postoperative care specific to filters. Preoperative strategies should be planned to alleviate stress. Factors such as length of time of the procedure, anesthetic, and postoperative limitations and activities should be explained to the client. The procedure generally takes approximately an hour. Usually the client is allowed nothing by mouth the 6 to 8 hours before surgery. Explanations should also be given as to what to expect during the procedure. The client is attached to a monitor, an intravenous line is inserted, and frequent assessments are made of vital signs. Following the procedure, an x-ray film of the abdomen may be obtained to ascertain the position of the filter.

Bed rest is mandatory the first 24 hours postoperatively to ensure firm placement of the filter in the vena cava. Vital signs should be assessed every 30 minutes until stable. The insertion site should be observed for the presence of hematoma formation. The presence of a hematoma indicates bleeding from the repair of the jugular vein. Daily dressing changes may be prescribed. Exercises, ambulation, and leg exercises (contraction and relaxation) are performed to prevent peripheral venous stasis and edema of the lower extremities. Elastic stockings may be used for the same purpose. Sitting may be discouraged, except during meals and while using the bathroom, because the large leg veins may be compressed from flexion of the hip and subsequently produce stasis.

An *embolectomy* is the removal of an emboli from the heart and, more rarely, from the pulmonary artery, using open heart surgery. Although life saving, most clients with massive emboli die too soon (for example, within 30 min) for surgery to be performed.[13]

Evaluation. The client with pulmonary embolism may exhibit varying degrees of illness. The nurse and client evaluate plans developed to prevent development of further emboli.

EXPECTED OUTCOMES

The client and/or family can:
1. Describe pulmonary embolism.
2. Describe methods for preventing further embolization.
3. Describe plans for health maintenance.
4. State use, dosage, time, route, and side effects of prescribed medications.
5. State plans for follow-up health care.

Pulmonary infarction

Pulmonary infarction (tissue death) is a consolidation of lung tissue from an interrupted blood supply. It may follow embolism. Tissue death occurs because the part of the lung that is normally supplied by the artery no longer receives nourishment. Infarction is thought to be a rare occurrence because usually the involved lung continues to receive adequate oxygenation via the airways and bronchial arterial system.[53] Pleuritic pain, hemoptysis, cough, tachycardia, tachypnea, dyspnea, and low-grade fever are common symptoms of infarction.

Adult respiratory distress syndrome (ARDS)

Adult respiratory distress syndrome (frequently referred to as shock lung, congestive atelectasis, posttraumatic lung, postinfusion lung, and ventilatory lung) is an acute lung condition that produces varied pathophysiological changes in the lung. These changes characteristically resemble those that occur in RDS in the newborn. The difference is that decreased surfactant is the result rather than the cause of the lung damage.

A variety of acute instabilities, both direct and indirect, have been responsible for producing the syndrome. Inhalation of toxic irritants, diffuse alveolar infections, blood-borne toxic substances, aspiration of viral pneumonia, near drowning, and chest trauma are direct conditions that often produce the problem. Conditions indirectly affecting the lung, and often producing ARDS, include traumatic or surgical shock, sepsis with release of endotoxins, disseminated intravascular coagulation, massive blood transfusions, massive fat embolism (possibly secondary to broken ribs), and drug ingestions.

Pathophysiology. Many of the theories explaining the pathogenesis of the syndrome relate that the initial lung damage that occurs is in the alveolar-capillary membrane. Increased capillary permeability occurs and results in fluid leaking into the interstitial spaces, which subsequently affects surfactant activity. As a result, patchy atelectasis occurs. The fluid also fills some of the alveoli and produces pulmonary edema. Plasma and red blood cells escape through the damaged capillaries; hence, hemorrhage is considered a common pathological manifestation.

Assessment. Symptoms occur suddenly within 2 to 3 days after the initial trauma or illness and usually in a young person[84] who has a history of healthy lungs. Signs of marked respiratory distress—dyspnea, tachycardia, cyanosis with or without intercostal retractions, and hypoxemia—are major clinical manifestations. The hypoxemia progressively worsens and responds poorly to oxygen therapy; hence, it is referred to as refractory hypoxemia. A number of other symptoms may occur—hypotension and signs and symptoms of respiratory or metabolic acidosis.[82]

Knowledge of the client's clinical state, difficulty in obtaining adequate ventilation (which is related to decreased compliance), reduced vital capacity, and chest x-ray findings that show patchy alveolar infiltration are significant factors in establishing a diagnosis. Arterial blood gas analysis is also a helpful diagnostic tool.

> **Data analysis**
> *Data analysis may reveal nursing diagnoses of ineffective breathing patterns, alterations in cardiac output, fear, and impaired gas exchange.*

Planning and implementation. Therapy is planned to *maintain adequate tissue oxygenation.*[28,84] This is accomplished by administering high concentrations of oxygen. Mechanical ventilation with PEEP is usually prescribed to deliver high inflation pressures in an effort to overcome lung compliance. PEEP of 5 to 15 cm of water pressure may be used. PEEP maintains the airway pressure above atmospheric pressure throughout the respiratory cycle[84] and subsequently enhances distribution of oxygen throughout the lung by maintaining expansion of the alveoli which would otherwise collapse. As a result, venous admixture (right to-left shunting) and hypoxemia are reduced. The effectiveness of PEEP is monitored by frequent analyses of arterial blood gases. In addition to frequent blood gas determinations, cardiac output is assessed by using a special monitoring device (such as a CVP or Swan-Ganz catheter).

Because PEEP may potentially reduce cardiac output by causing impaired venous return to the heart, the pulse and blood pressure must be monitored frequently. The tendency toward fluid retention during mechanical ventilation and the possibility of pulmonary edema demand frequent assessment of the hydration status (that is, intake and output). Frequent assessments must be made of the flow rate of intravenous fluids, and every possible effort should be directed toward maintaining the flow rate of the prescribed therapy. See Chapter 8 for details about nursing care for intravenous therapy. The client must also be assessed for signs and symptoms indicating circulatory overload. Because of the pathophysiological lung changes, respiratory status (including chest assessments) should be monitored closely.

Another important objective of therapy is to *prevent further pulmonary injury.* In addition to the use of oxygen, corticosteroids are prescribed to decrease the amount of inflammation of the alveolar membrane, thus decreasing pulmonary capillary permeability. Corticosteroids are also thought to improve contractibility of the heart, and improve perfusion of peripheral circulation and of vital organs.[28] Intravenous administration of albumin and high-molecular-weight dextran is also thought to lessen capillary permeability. Diuretics and limitations of fluid are therapeutic measures prescribed to keep the lungs dry. Antibiotics are used to control bacterial infections. Other measures are directed toward correcting the underlying cause of the syndrome.

In addition to frequent assessments, care should be directed toward maintaining airway patency, and promoting psychological and physical comfort.

Secretions should be removed by suctioning as often as necessary. Principles necessary for effective and safe aspiration must be applied during this procedure. The client's position must be changed at frequent intervals, and passive exercises are essential. The environment should be quiet and relaxed. Care should be planned to facilitate adequate rest. See discussion earlier in this chapter for other principles of management for clients with respiratory instabilities.

Tuberculosis

Tuberculosis is an infectious disease caused by the gram-positive aerobic acid-fast bacilli *Mycobacterium tuberculosis*. Tuberculosis is not an inherited disease. Infection with tuberculosis is acquired by inhaling airborne droplet nuclei containing significant numbers of bacilli. The droplets are expelled when a person who is infected with the disease engages in forceful respiration (such as singing, coughing, sneezing, speaking, or laughing). It may also be acquired by direct contact with an infected person for example, from kissing. (Infants and young children may contract tuberculosis from an infected parent, grandparent, friend, or babysitter. Adolescents may also contract tuberculosis from these aforementioned sources as well as from infected persons in the homes of their peers.)

Persons who work in strenuous occupations, are malnourished, or live or work in overcrowded and poorly ventilated environments are more likely to contract the disease. Overwork, excessive play, lack of sleep, chronic fatigue, respiratory tract infections, prolonged stress, and chronic illness may increase susceptibility to the disease. Individuals who are receiving steroid therapy, are pregnant, or have had a gastrectomy are thought to have a higher risk of developing the disease. The disease occurs more in urban areas than in rural areas, and is more common among lower income groups.

Pathophysiology. The bacilli most often affect the lungs, although any part of the body may be affected. It thrives best when there is a Pa_{O_2} of 100 mm Hg or more, and a Pa_{CO_2} of approximately 40 mm Hg. Therefore the organs most commonly affected are those with high oxygen tension. The alveolar surface of the lung parenchyma is the most common site of implantation (Fig. 21-32). In this area the Pa_{O_2} is in the range of 120 to 130 mm Hg in the upright position.[76] The kidneys and growing bones are next in order of being affected; the Pa_{O_2} is approximately 100 mg Hg in those areas.

When the tubercle bacilli on droplet nuclei are inhaled by a susceptible host, infection may occur. The initial reaction produced by the bacilli is an inflammatory reaction. Polymorphonuclear leukocytes phagocytize the bacteria but do not kill the organism. Therefore within a few days macrophages replace the leukocytes. (Macrophages determine whether or not the tuberculous lesion becomes established.[17]) The alveoli that are involved become consolidated and a cellular pneumonia develops, which may resolve the organism, or they may remain and multiply within the cells.

The bacilli are spread through lymphatic channels to the regional lymph nodes. The infiltrating macrophages join together to form the epitheloid cell tubercle. Lymphocytes surround the lymphocytes, a process that takes from 10 to 20 days. The central portion of the lesion becomes necrotic, and forms a cheesy area (named because of its appearance), which is referred to as *caseous necrosis*. Bacilli may grow in the caseous area, but generally the low oxygen tension, low pH, and the accumulation of fatty acids in the area inhibit the growth. Often the bacilli grow intracellularly in the young macrophages of the surrounding tuberculous granulation tissue.[17] This tissue surrounds the caseous center of the tubercle. Whether the lesion will progress or regress depends on the ability of macrophages. Growth of the bacilli results in extension of the caseous necrosis.

Another response that might occur at the site of the necrotic area is *liquefaction,* which occurs when the caseous material softens.[17] This response

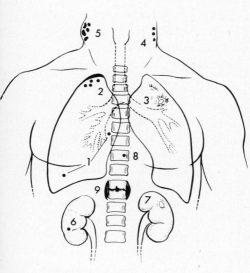

FIG. 21-32
Sites most commonly affected by tuberculosis. (From Stead, William W.: Fundamentals of tuberculosis today, for students in the health professions, ed. 4, 1980, Central Press, Box 251, Milwaukee, Wis. 53201.

may take months, and is believed that proteinases, nucleases, and lipases of live and dead macrophages assist in the liquefying response. Once hydrolyzed, the osmotically active components of caseous material absorb water from the surrounding tissue and become an excellent culture medium for the tubercle bacillus. If the bronchial walls are eroded, air enters and its high oxygen content provides an excellent environment for extracellular growth of the bacilli in the liquid caseous material.

Classification of tuberculosis. The classification of tuberculosis as classed by the American Lung Association is based on quantifiable measures of tubercle bacilli in sputum and the adequacy of chemotherapy. It also covers the total population and is applicable to both children and adults. The classification is as follows:

0. *No tuberculosis exposure, not infected.* No history of exposure, negative tuberculin skin test.
I. *Tuberculosis exposure, no evidence of infection.* History of exposure, negative tuberculin skin test.
II. *Tuberculosis infection, without disease.* Positive tuberculin skin test, negative bacteriological studies (if done), no x-ray findings compatible with tuberculosis, and no symptoms caused by tuberculosis.
III. *Tuberculosis infection, with disease.* The current status of the patient's tuberculosis is described by three characteristics: location of the disease, bacteriological status, and chemotherapy status.

Assessment. The onset of signs and symptoms of pulmonary tuberculosis in many clients may be insidious. In early stages, there may be no symptoms. If symptoms are present, they may be characterized as being *generalized* and *chronic:* low-grade fever, fatigue, malaise, anorexia, weight loss, and irregular menses. It is not unusual for the client to attribute such symptoms to overwork or emotional distress. Generalized symptoms may also occur as manifestations of an acute febrile illness, with the presenting symptoms of chills and fever.

As the disease progresses and as more lung tissue become involved, a cough, which may be dry and progressively become frequent and productive, is characteristic. Chest pain, often described as being aching, dull, or a tightness in the chest, may occur. Although unusual, hemoptysis may be the initial symptom that prompts the client to consult a physician. Pleuritic pain and dyspnea usually result from extensive pulmonary involvement. Both of the types of symptoms described may occur separately or in combination. The diagnosis of tuberculosis is made by tuberculin testing, chest x-ray studies, and bacteriological studies of the sputum.

Data analysis
Data analysis may reveal nursing diagnoses of ineffective breathing patterns, grieving, fear, impaired gas exchange, and ineffective coping.

Planning and implementation. Therapeutic intervention for tuberculosis consists mainly of administration of antimicrobial drugs. These drugs can be used to prevent tuberculosis in individuals who are infected, as well as

DRUGS FOR TREATING TUBERCULOSIS AND THEIR ABBREVIATIONS

First-line drugs

Isonicotinic acid hydrazide (isoniazid)	INH
Ethambutol hydrochloride	EMB
Rifampin	RFN
Streptomycin	SM

Second-line drugs

Ethionamide	ETA
Cycloserine	CS
Pyrazinamide	
Paraaminosalicylic acid	PAS
Capreomycin Sulfate	CAP
Viomycin sulfate	VM
Kanamycin	

RESPIRATORY ISOLATION AND PRECAUTIONS

Respiratory isolation is used for infectious agents that are spread via droplets or by airborne droplet nuclei that get into the environment by breathing, sneezing, or coughing. Pulmonary tuberculosis is a common respiratory problem that requires respiratory isolation. (However, such isolation may also be used for meningococcal meningitis and communicable diseases such as measles and rubella).

1. A private room must be used (the door of which must be kept closed).
2. Masks, gowns, and caps are not needed.
3. Hands must be washed on entering and leaving the room.
4. Vigorous movement of linens should be avoided.
5. Objects contaminated with respiratory tract secretions must be sterilized, disinfected, or discarded.

to treat those with active disease. Preventive therapy includes the use of isonicotinic acid hydrazide (isoniazid, INH) in a single daily dose of 300 mg/day for adults and 10 mg/kg of body weight per day for children. Preventive therapy is usually prescribed for a period of 1 year for both children and adults.

Clients with active disease are treated with first-line drugs. Two-drug combinations are usually used; however, three-drug combinations may also be used. Combination drugs decrease resistance of the organism to the drug. The choice of combination regimens varies and is influenced by factors such as the combination that will most rapidly kill the organisms (as measured by cultures and smears of sputum) and the combination that will prevent drug resistance and prevent relapse. Method of administration, potential side effects, and cost are also considered.

Second-line drugs may be used when the organisms develop resistance to first-line drugs or when there is toxicity or allergy to the first-line drugs. Second-line drugs are also used in retreatment programs.

With the use of antimicrobial therapy, the majority of the clients with tuberculosis may be hospitalized in an acute care facility for as short a period of time as 1 week. It is during this time that adequate instructions should be given to them, their families, and significant friends about the use of antimicrobial agents.

The client should be instructed about the therapeutic and adverse effects of the drugs, as well as the value of uninterrupted therapy. Subsequently the importance of compliance to therapy should be stressed because interruptions encourage the development of resistant bacilli. To facilitate compliance, information should be given about the disease, how it is transmitted, and how to protect oneself and others.

Misconceptions must be cleared and fears allayed. Instructions can be given about the need for adequate ventilation in the environment, and principles of medical asepsis, proper handwashing, covering the mouth and nose on coughing and sneezing or while raising sputum, and proper handling of secretions. Because the disease is transmitted by droplet nuclei, gowns and caps are not necessary. The size of the droplet nuclei is between $1\ \mu$ to $5\ \mu$ and can readily pass through masks. Masks therefore are not needed. The importance of follow-up care should also be stressed.

The nurse should provide nutrition information to the client and family. The client must be instructed to eat a well-balanced diet (high in proteins) to guard against the wasting effects of the disease. Calcium and vitamins B, C, and D must be encouraged. Servings of citrus fruits will increase vitamin C intake. Meats, egg, and milk should be provided generously to increase the protein level of the diet.

The question of bed rest varies with the type of disease. Many individuals can be treated with little disruption in their daily lives. Hospitalization may be necessary only when the client is sick enough to require supportive care, or when special tests are needed. Even when activity is restricted, it is usually for a short time.

 Evaluation. Evaluation of the nursing care plan for the client with tuberculosis is ongoing. Problems may center around breathing, fear, grieving, and ineffective coping.

Nursing process for common health problems

EXPECTED OUTCOMES

The client and/or family can:
1. Describe tuberculosis, including methods of spread.
2. Describe methods for preventing transmission of tuberculosis.
3. Describe plans for maintenance or restoration of respiratory status, including rest, nutrition, and medications.
4. State use, dosage, time, route, and side effects of prescribed medications.
5. State need for compliance with therapy.
6. State plans for compliance with therapeutic plan.
7. State plans for follow-up health care and use of community resources.

Chest trauma

Fractured ribs. Fractured ribs are a common chest injury that usually results from falls, automobile accidents, blows in the chest, or blast injuries. Fractures that result from violent accidents generally result in damage to the internal structures.

Assessment. Severe pain, which is knifelike in character and accentuated by motion of the rib cage and deep inspiration, generally occurs with fractures of the ribs. In fear of evoking pain, the client is reluctant to breathe deeply. As a result breathing is shallow, and rapid. Apprehension is also common. A chest x-ray film is usually obtained to determine the extent of the injury. Complications of rib fractures include atelectasis, pneumothorax and hemothorax.

> *Data analysis*
> *Data analysis may reveal nursing diagnoses of ineffective breathing patterns, impaired gas exchange, and alterations in comfort.*

Planning and implementation. Unless damage is sustained to the internal chest, therapy is directed to controlling pain and preventing pulmonary complications. Medications, such as narcotics, are prescribed to relieve pain. Some form of support may be applied to the chest to minimize pain on breathing. If neither of these measures relieves the pain, an intercostal nerve block may be performed. Such a measure involves infiltrating the spaces above and below the fractured rib with an anesthetic. The nurse should instruct the client on coughing and deep breathing exercises to prevent pulmonary complications. The client's position should be changed frequently, to promote comfort and to enhance adequate ventilation. Frequent assessments must be made to detect any signs that might be indicative of complications.

Flail chest. A flail chest occurs as a result of fractures of multiple (or as few as two) adjacent ribs or fractures of the ribs and sternum. Because of the multiple fractures, the structural integrity of the chest wall is disrupted to the extent that the ribs no longer provide a rigid support. The most serious problems arise from fractures of the first and second ribs because of their association with tears of the thoracic aorta.[60]

Assessment. Visualization of a flail chest is apparent during the process of breathing. During breathing the ribs that are fractured move in the opposite direction of the intact chest wall. For example, during inspiration the affected chest wall moves in and out on expiration *(paradoxical breathing)*. As a result, ventilation is seriously impaired, as is reflected by hypoxia, hypercapnia, and an increased work of breathing. Severe dyspnea and cyanosis are present. Death can occur if measures are not taken to stabilize the chest.

> *Data analysis*
> *Data analysis reveals nursing diagnoses of ineffective breathing pattern, impaired gas exchange, alterations in comfort, alterations in tissue perfusion, and fear.*

Planning and implementation. Therapy is directed toward prompt stabilization of the chest wall. This can be done by either external or internal fixation.

With internal stabilization, continuous ventilatory support is provided. The client is intubated and connected to a volume-controlled ventilator. This setup facilitates lung expansion and adequate ventilation. It may be necessary for the client to remain on the ventilator for a period of 1 to 2 weeks until the chest wall has stabilized. Sedation, if not contraindicated, may be necessary if the client tends to resist the ventilator. See earlier in this chapter for information about the care of a client during ventilatory therapy.

Internal fixation is preferred; however, external stabilization may be accomplished with the use of a pressure dressing and usually the use of traction. A local anesthetic is used for pain to permit the wire to be attached to the rib, thus permitting the chest wall to be pulled outward. A rope is attached to the wire, and a specified number of weights is applied. Traction remains in place until the chest wall becomes rigid, usually 2 to 3 weeks. Towel clips may also be applied to the fractured ribs as a means of external stabilization.

Pneumothorax. Pneumothorax, the presence of air in the pleural space, occurs when there is communication between the atmosphere and pleural space. It can occur spontaneously or as a result of trauma.

A *spontaneous pneumothorax* occurs without any prior trauma to the chest. Spontaneous pneumothoraxes may be classified as primary or secondary. A *primary spontaneous pneumothorax* occurs without known cause. It is most frequently encountered in young adult men between 20 and 40 years of age and predominantly, the tall, asthenic person.[36]

Spontaneous pneumothorax occurs when air enters the pleural space by rupture of the alveolar walls. The upper lobes of the lungs are primarily affected because transpulmonary pressures are greater in these areas than at the bases.[36] The gas then passes along lobular septa either centrally or peripherally. When the air travels centrally, a pneumothorax or subcutaneous emphysema may result. Peripherally, it collects as blebs beneath the pleura. These blebs may later rupture and produce a pneumothorax.[36]

Secondary spontaneous pneumothorax, common in persons over 40 years of age, is associated with an underlying disease process within the lungs or thorax. It usually occurs as a complication of cavitary, fibrotic, or obstructive pulmonary disease. (If it occurs shortly after birth, it is related to the high pressure required to expand the lungs, whereas in infancy it is associated with complicated pneumonia.)

Traumatic pneumothorax occurs as a result of trauma usually from a penetrating or blunt injury, or from surgical procedures. Automobile accidents, stab

1327

or bullet wounds, and crushing injuries are common causes. Surgical causes include procedures (diagnostic or therapeutic) in or near the chest or upper abdomen; for example, thoracentesis and pleural biopsy. Acupuncture has also been reported as a cause.

 Assessment. The symptoms that are experienced depend on the volume size and the degree of collapse of the affected lung. A small pneumothorax may cause no difficulty and may go undetected. However in others, the onset of symptoms is sudden with dyspnea and chest pain, which are experienced in 80% to 90% of clients.[36] Pain may be sharp and severe or mild and dull, and limited to the involved side. A nonproductive cough, hemoptysis and weakness may also be experienced. Breath sounds are decreased or absent on the affected side. A chest x-ray film is helpful in establishing a diagnosis.

> ### Data analysis
> *Data analysis may reveal nursing diagnoses of ineffective breathing pattern, alterations in cardiac output, fear, and impaired gas exchange.*

 Planning and implementation. Therapy is directed toward lung reexpansion. This is achieved either by inserting a needle or pneumothorax catheter in the pleural space, and permitting air to escape (simple aspiration); or with the use of a chest tube and application of negative pressure. Once the lungs reexpand, therapy may be maintained for 24 to 48 hours. By this time it is hoped that the leak seals and pleural adhesions that form will prevent recurrences. Surgical therapy may be considered when the third spontaneous pneumothorax develops. An opened thoracotomy may be performed to resect blebs that may be responsible for the pneumothorax. Other surgical procedures may be performed to produce an adherence to the parietal pleura to visceral pleura, to prevent recurrence. Such procedures include a *pleurectomy,* or *poudrage* (application of irritants to the pleural surfaces).

Complications of pneumothorax

Tension pneumothorax. A tension pneumothorax develops when air enters the pleural space but cannot escape, for example, when pleural pressure exceeds atmospheric pressure.

 ASSESSMENT. It is commonly reported to occur with sucking wounds of the chest. (Air enters during inspiration but cannot escape on expiration because the tissue flap seals the wound and acts as a one-way valve.) However, a tension pneumothorax can also result from a bleb that ruptures spontaneously, particularly if there is a communication between the bleb and an open bronchus. Again, the positive pressure builds up on inspiration, and the air cannot escape because of the one-way valve effect. As the intrapleural pressure continues to build, the lungs continue to collapse, and the heart and great vessels may shift toward the side of decreased pressure and press against the lungs. This is referred to as *mediastinal shift.* Symptoms similar to those of pneumothorax (severe dyspnea, tachypnea) will be experienced. In addition, shock symptoms may be manifested because venous return to the right atrium is impeded. A chest x-ray film is taken to confirm the shift.

> **Data analysis**
> *Data analysis may reveal nursing diagnoses of ineffective breathing patterns, alterations in cardiac output, fear, and impaired gas exchange.*

PLANNING AND IMPLEMENTATION. Therapeutic intervention for tension pneumothorax consists of promptly providing an outlet for the air. Air may be aspirated by a needle or small catheter, or an intercostal drainage tube is inserted in the pleural cavity and is attached to a closed drainage system. Healing usually takes place within a few days.

Hemopneumothorax. Hemorrhage may occur into the pleural space and accompany a pneumothorax. When this occurs, a hemopneumothorax is the result. In a spontaneous pneumothorax, the bleeding is related to tearing of adhesions between the parietal and visceral pleurae. In traumatic pneumothorax, bleeding may be from the chest wall or from the lung. The diagnosis is established at the time the chest tube is inserted. When bleeding is severe and continuous, transfusions are administered and an open thoracotomy is performed to ligate bleeding vessels. The nurse must make frequent assessments of the client's vital signs and respiratory status. Emotional support must be provided.

Evaluation. The client with chest trauma has problems of ineffective breathing, alteration in comfort, ineffective gas exchange, and fear. The nursing care plan focuses on objectives to deal with these problems.

EXPECTED OUTCOMES

The client and/or family can:
1. Describe the specific health problem.
2. Describe plans for health maintenance.
3. State plans for follow-up health care and use of community resources.

COMMON PROBLEMS OF THE MIDDLE-AGED AND OLDER ADULT
Chronic obstructive pulmonary disease

Chronic obstructive pulmonary disease (COPD) is a name given to a group of progressive respiratory tract diseases that cause considerable disability. All diseases result in a similar pathological respiratory pattern, that is, all diseases produce obstruction to air outflow and result in trapping of "stale air" (high in carbon dioxide, low in oxygen) in the alveoli. Included are chronic bronchitis, emphysema, and asthma. Increased resistance to air flow is the most common entity in COPD. Synonyms for the clinical state include chronic obstructive lung disease (COLD) and chronic airway obstruction (CAO).

Chronic bronchitis

Chronic bronchitis is an inflammation of the tracheobronchial tree characterized by excessive mucus production (more than 100 ml per day), cough, airway obstruction, and infection.[37]

Tracheobronchial irritation from smoke, fumes, and dust (air pollutants) has been related to the development of chronic bronchitis. Individuals who smoke and live in an urban environment are at greater risk than individuals who live in rural areas. The incidence is also higher in individuals exposed to dust (for example, those who work in industrial environments such as a coal mine or steel mill). Exacerbations of chronic bronchitis are associated with periods of high pollution. Cigarette smoke inhibits movement of cilia and macrophage activity in the lung and produces hypertrophy of the mucous glands.[2]

Pathophysiology. Hypersecretion of mucus is an early sign. The mucus-

1329

producing bronchial glands and goblet cells within the bronchial wall hypertrophy and increase in number: consequently the increased mucus secretions affect the flow of air and exchange of gas and may predispose the client to plugging and infection.[33] Longstanding infection results in destruction of lung tissue.[37]

Assessment. The onset is usually slow. In the early stages of chronic bronchitis, the client has a cough that is thought to be related to smoking. Colds are also frequent. As the condition progresses, the symptoms of coughing and spitting become more frequent and more severe in the morning, at night, and in cold, damp weather. As the symptoms increase in severity, the quantity of sputum increases. Chronic bronchitis frequently occurs in conjunction with emphysema.

Emphysema

Emphysema is an abnormal and permanent dilatation of the terminal air spaces of the lungs and destruction of their walls.

Although the exact cause of emphysema is obscure, several etiological factors have been identified: smoking, air pollution, and heredity. Cigarette smoking has consistently been related to the development of emphysema. Individuals who smoke cigarettes have about 10 times the risk of nonsmokers of dying of the disease. The mortality rate increases with increased cigarette consumption to over 20 times that of nonsmokers. The role of air pollution has not been as clearly identified. Heredity as an etiological factor relates to a genetic deficiency of alpha antitrypsin, a serum protein of the a_1-globulin fraction. It is associated with a familiar type of emphysema and occurs mainly in women. Emphysema occurs more frequently among persons in the older age group and particularly white men between 50 and 70 years of age.

The mechanisms considered to be responsible for producing the dilation include *hypoplasia, atrophy, overinflation,* and *obstruction.*[56] Hypoplasia is related to growth failure or underdevelopment of the lung. Atrophy is characterized by loss of alveolar surface area and the number of alveoli; whereas with overinflation the alveoli increase in size beyond normal expansion during maximum inspiration. In destruction, alveolar walls are destroyed either partially or completely. Ulceration may also occur.

Types of emphysema, based on the differences in the predominating anatomical site, have been identified: panacinar, centriacinar, periacinar, and irregular. The unit of reference is the acinar, hence the name. In *panacinar (panlobular) emphysema,* there is uniform enlargement and destruction of the entire long lobules and subsequent destruction of alveolar walls and capillary bed. As a result, the air sacs are distended and the normal lung tissue becomes separated by thickened and fibrous septum. The major abnormality therefore is reduction in alveolar capillary bed. Characteristically, the involvement is scattered throughout the lung, but tends to be more severe in the lower zones.[26,33] It is the type common in a_1-antitrypsin deficiency and in compensatory overinflation.

In *centriacinar emphysema* (centrilobular), the most common type, distension is basically limited to the respiratory bronchioles and alveolar ducts. The involvement is more central, and characteristically the air spaces are enlarged and are interposed between small bronchi and alveoli.[26] Impairment of gaseous diffusions within the primary lobule is the major abnormality.[37] It commonly affects the upper zones of the lung and is usually accompanied by inflammation of the bronchioles. It is common among individuals who have no respiratory disability and is especially common in men.

Periacinar (periseptal) *emphysema* involves the periphery of the acinus. The involved air spaces occur under the pleura or along connective tissue septa. *Irregular emphysema* is the type characterized by lack of uniformity, or particular anatomical distribution.

Respiratory tract infections and emphysema. Clients with emphysema are likely to develop respiratory tract infections. This is probably related to a reduction in the cilia and a resultant decrease in their function. The nurse must constantly be alert for signs of increased dyspnea, cough, secretions, and temperature. The appearance of these symptoms should be brought to the attention of the physician because a respiratory tract infection will decrease ventilatory efficiency and further impair gas exchange.

Assessment. Dyspnea is characteristic of emphysema. In the early stages, dyspnea occurs on exertion, but as the disease progresses, it is experienced even at rest. The dyspnea is related to increased difficulty in expelling air from the lungs and to poor distribution of air through them. Often the client leans slightly forward with arms and elbows propped on a table or on the arms of a chair. This position compresses the abdomen and pushes the diaphragm upward, thus increasing intrathoracic pressure and facilitating more efficient expulsion of air. The client may have difficulty eating full meals because of dyspnea.

Coughing, which at first occurs mainly during the morning, later becomes worse and occurs during the day. The cough becomes productive, and thick mucoid secretions are expectorated. Wheezing is also experienced. The abdomen often protrudes because of loss of muscle tone. The chest becomes barrel-shaped because of elevation of the rib cage. Fatigability, anorexia, and weight loss occur.

During an acute episode of emphysema the client appears anxious and tends to speak in short, jerky sentences. The muscles of the neck contract on inspiration, and the neck veins may be noted to stand out during expiration.

Data analysis

Data analysis may reveal nursing diagnoses of ineffective breathing patterns, impaired gas exchange, alterations in tissue perfusion, fear, ineffective coping, alterations in cardiac output, and noncompliance.

Planning and implementation. Therapy for emphysema is directed toward (1) improving ventilation by relieving airway obstruction, maintaining oxygenation, and clearing the air passages of secretions; and (2) controlling infection.

Improving ventilation

Relieving airway obstruction. This may be accomplished with the use of bronchodilators (if asthmatic component is present), steroids, antihistamines, and indirectly by antibiotics. Direct bronchodilators facilitate relaxation of the bronchial mucosa and reduce mucosal edema, thereby permitting the air passages to open. These drugs may be administered orally (oxytriphylline [Choledyl], terbutaline sulfate [Bricanyl], and Tedral), intravenously, rectally (aminophylline), or by nebulization.

Corticosteroid therapy is prescribed to reduce bronchospasms and bronchial inflammation. Prednisolone is a commonly used drug and is usually prescribed on a daily basis. Cartridge-type nebulizers containing dexamethasone are sometimes used.

Nursing process for common health problems

Antihistamines reduce the postnasal drip that often increases both the cough and other symptoms the client may have.

Maintaining oxygenation. Oxygen is administered to maintain normal oxygen levels. The safe administration of oxygen requires it to be given at a rate of 1 to 2 L/min and in concentrations of 24% to 28%—slightly above atmospheric air (21%) but not exceeding 40%. The importance of maintaining a low oxygen concentration cannot be overemphasized.

The respiratory center normally responds to low carbon dioxide concentrations. However in conditions with chronic hypoxia and carbon dioxide retention,

TABLE 21-11

Some drugs used in chronic obstructive pulmonary disease

Drugs	Effects, assessments, and implications

Antibiotics
  Ampicillin
  Cephalexin monohydrate (Keflex)
  Tetracycline
	Suppress growth of or kill bacteria directly, thus useful in preventing and treating infections.
	  Administer drugs on time to maintain blood levels.
	Often prescribed for home use (such as at first sign of infection).
	  Instruct client on signs indicative of infection (such as changes in color of sputum).
	  Encourage client to follow instructions given by physician.
	Hypersensitive reactions can develop.
	  Observe for signs of hypersensitivity.
	  Instruct client about same.

Bronchodilators	Increase size of airways by relaxing spasms of smooth muscles.
	  Observe response to therapy; improvement of symptoms (such as easier breathing or absence of wheezing).
	  Assess respiratory status.
	Increase cardiac action.
	  Monitor pulse and blood pressure before and after administration whether by inhalation or other means.
	  Assess for signs indicative of increased cardiac activity: precordial pain, palpitation, nausea, and dizziness.
	  Be alert to signs of adverse reactions.

Sympathominetramines (adrenergic agonists)
  Terbutaline sulfate (Bricanyl, Brethine)
	May be prescribed for home use.
	  Instruct client and family on proper administration, side effects, and danger of overadministration.
	Refer to effects, assessments, and implications as stated in no. 1 and no. 2 of bronchodilators.

Isoetharine hydrochloride (Bronkosol)	May cause fall in blood pressure.
	  Monitor blood pressure closely.
	  Make same assessments as in no. 2 of bronchodilators.

Ephedrine sulfate	In addition to bronchodilating and cardiac effects as stated above:
	Stimulates central nervous system and may therefore produce mental excitation or insomnia.
	  Refrain from administering medications close to bedtime.
	  Discourage excessive use.
	May produce difficulty in urination in older men and may increase nervousness and palpitations.
	  Make same assessments as in no. 2 of bronchodilators.

Epinephrine (Adrenalin)	Inhibits secretions of bronchial glands and subsequently may increase viscosity of mucus.
	  Maintain adequate fluid intake.
	Produces oropharyngeal dryness when administered by nebulization.
	  Encourage client to rinse mouth following therapy.
	Produces side effects: tachycardia, palpitations, hypertension, anxiety, tremor, nausea, and vomiting.
	  Monitor and evaluate pulse, heart rate, and blood pressure carefully.
	Rapid onset of action. Expect full effect in approximately 20 min.
	  Assess for effects within 10 min.

Isoproterenol hydrochloride (Isuprel)	May be absorbed from the mucosa when administered by nebulization therapy.
	  Instruct client to rinse mouth following therapy to reduce likelihood of sympathomimetic effects: tachycardia, nervousness, cyanosis, or changes in blood pressure (hypotension or hypertension).
	Produces side effects: nausea, excitement, tremors, rapid heart rate, dysrhythmias, and hypotension.
	  Monitor and evaluate heart rate, rhythm, and blood pressure closely.

TABLE 21-11, cont'd

Some drugs used in chronic obstructive pulmonary disease

Drugs	Effects, assessments, and implications
Xanthine-type Aminophylline (theophylline ethylenediamine)	Causes hypotension, dysrhythmias, headache, dizziness, and nausea when administered by rapid infusion. Monitor and evaluate blood pressure and infusion rate carefully during infusion. Produces diuresis in addition to bronchodilating effects. Monitor intake and output. Causes anorectal irritation when suppositories are used repeatedly. Be alert for complaints of pain or discomfort. Periodically assess for signs of rectal irritation.
Oxytriphylline (Choledyl); theophylline (Elixophyllin)	May cause gastrointestinal irritation (such as nausea, vomiting, or epigastric distress), but causes less irritation than other theophylline derivatives. Be alert for side effects. Assess for signs indicative of improvement or worsening of symptoms.
Anticholinergic (parasympatholytic) Atropine	Blocks the muscarinic action of acetylcholine. May cause dryness of mucous membrane.
Corticosteroids Hydrocortisone succinate (Solu-Cortef) Dexamethasone (Decadron) Methylprednisolone sodium succinate (Solu-Medrol)	Possibly effective because of anti-inflammatory activity, thus relieving bronchial obstruction. May produce side effects: hypokalemia, sodium retention, cushingoid signs and symptoms, decreased resistance to infection, and mental changes. Check electrolyte reports; consult physician when indicated. Monitor weights, intake, and output. Provide emotional support as necessary. Protect client from infection. Assess health history and monitor blood pressure; be alert for symptoms associated with ulcers, since those with history of peptic ulcers or hypertension may have flare-ups.
Mucokinetic drugs (oral, commonly referred to as expectorants) Novahistine Dimetane Phenergan	Increase output of respiratory tract secretions. Liquefy thick secretions, thus enhancing removal (such as by coughing). Enhanced by use of adequate fluid intake, since sufficient amount of extracellular fluid facilitates action of drug: certain positions also enhance effects. Fluids lessen viscosity of bronchial secretions and may stimulate respiratory tract fluid. Encourage fluids except immediately after administration. Refrain from giving medications close to mealtime, since increased secretions may precipitate cough and vomiting, hence interfering with nutrition. Position changes facilitate mobilization of secretions to cough-sensitive areas, where they can be coughed up. Encourage frequent position changes, especially sitting position, since it facilitates maximum ventilation. Provide receptacle to facilitate prompt removal. Assess amount and character of secretions.
Ammonium chloride	Enhances mucokinesis.
Saturated solution of potassium iodide (SSKI)	Increases secretory activity of bronchial glands. May produce gastric irritation. Dilute with milk or juice to reduce gastric irritation and to increase hydration.
Mucokinetics (by nebulization or by direct pulmonary instillation, by catheter) N-Acetylcysteine (Acetylcysteine, Mucomyst)	Produces maximum effect approximately 10 min after administration. Encourage coughing approximately 10 min after drug is administered. Aspirate secretions as often as necessary, particularly several minutes after nebulization therapy. May produce side effects such as nausea, vomiting, stomatitis, and bronchospasms (common in asthmatic clients). Assess via stethoscope for development of wheezes. Assess breathing pattern. Consult physician regarding use of bronchodilators if bronchospasms develop and medication has not been prescribed for same.
Hydration Water	Very effective in decreasing viscosity of mucus secretions. May produce circulatory overload. Assess for signs indicative of overload at regular intervals.
Saline	Same effect as water.

such as chronic obstructive lung disease, the opposite effect is observed. Stimulation of the carotid and aortic chemoreceptors by a low Pa_{O_2} activates the medullary respiratory and circulatory centers. Inhalation of high concentrations of oxygen removes the stimulus. Second, the ventilatory exchange of carbon dioxide and oxygen is deficient in clients with chronic emphysema. As a result, the respiratory center becomes insensitive to CO_2 and the high hydrogen ion concentration that is associated with it. Again inhalation of high concentrations of oxygen removes the reflex drive to respiration, and tidal exchange decreases. Subsequently the Pa_{CO_2} approaches narcotic levels and the client may become confused, progressively go into a coma, and die.

ASSESSMENT DURING OXYGEN ADMINISTRATION. During oxygen administration the nurse must therefore observe the client closely for slow, shallow respirations and signs of carbon dioxide narcosis, which may occur if the hypoxic drive is removed. Signs of carbon dioxide narcosis include flushed skin, flaccid or twitching extremities, shallow breathing, mental confusion, depressed sensorium, and falling blood pressure. Thus to determine adequacy of therapy, frequent analyses of blood gases are made.

Clearing air passages of secretions. Adequate *hydration* is essential. Clients, except those with cardiac or renal involvement, are usually encouraged to drink at least 3 liters of fluids per day. Increased fluid intake facilitates liquefication of secretions and loosening of mucus plugs, thereby making them easier to expectorate. Expectorants such as a saturated solution of potassium iodide (SSKI) and ammonium chloride are instrumental in liquefying secretions.

Mucolytic agents and enzymes may also be prescribed to reduce surface tension, thus thinning secretions and facilitating easier expectoration of secretions.

Controlling infection. Antibiotics, also useful forms of therapy, are prescribed prophylactically to control infection. The type of antibiotic prescribed is determined on the basis of the flora of the sputum. Tetracycline and ampicillin are frequently used (Table 21-11).

Chest physiotherapy. Chest physiotherapy, designed to improve distribution of ventilation and efficiency of breathing, and to remove secretions, includes bronchial drainage, percussion, vibration, and breathing and coughing exercises.

Bronchial drainage. Segmental bronchial drainage, commonly referred to as *postural drainage,* is a procedure that facilitates removal of excessive mucus from the bronchial tree by gravity. The secretions drain from the respiratory passages into the pharynx and can easily be expectorated. Its effectiveness is tremendously enhanced after nebulization.

Various positions may be used for bronchial drainage. However, if it is to be effective, it must be done in the position most suitable for drainage of the pulmonary segment involved (Fig. 21-33).

Modifications may be made in position on the basis of the age of the client. The young child may have to be held in the nurse's lap in a head-low position, or a pillow may be used to permit the head to be in a lower position.

PLANNING FOR BRONCHIAL DRAINAGE. Regardless of the position used, the client must be comfortable and relaxed. Measures to *promote safety and comfort* must be provided. The client must be protected from falling.

Periodically during bronchial drainage, the client should be instructed to take deep breaths and cough voluntarily to facilitate removal of secretions. A

FIG. 21-33
Postural drainage.

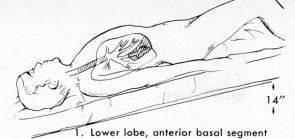

1. Lower lobe, anterior basal segment

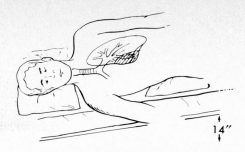

2. Lower lobe, lateral basal segment

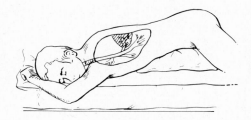

3. Lower lobe, right or left basal

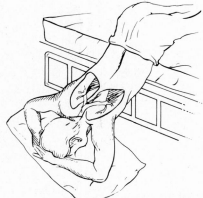

4. Lower lobe, posterior basal segment

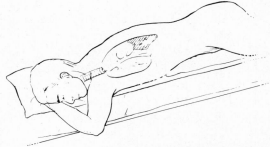

5. Lower lobe, posterior basal segments

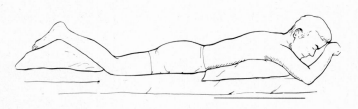

6. Lower lobes, apical segments

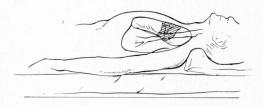

7. Upper lobes, anterior segments

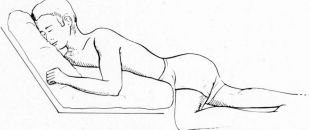

8. Left upper lobe, posterior segment

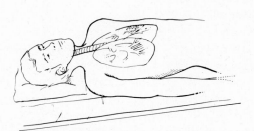

9. Left lingula lobe, posterior segment

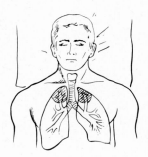

10. Upper lobe, apical segments

sputum receptacle should be provided. The procedure is usually repeated at least four times daily for periods ranging from 10 to 20 min. The time interval is gradually increased to the client's tolerance, up to 20 minutes. The nurse should plan for the drainage procedure to be carried out well in advance of meals so that it does not interfere with food intake. It may also be helpful to perform these at bedtime to facilitate a restful night.

Generally these procedures are performed by a respiratory therapist. However, the nurse should be familiar with the principles of the therapy and specific observations that should be made. The nurse should observe the character and amount of sputum. A change in the color of sputum from the usual white to yellowish often indicates infection, and increased amounts indicate irritation or infection. Observations should also be made regarding the client's tolerance to postural drainage. Any persistent complaint of dizziness should be brought to the physician's attention. On completion of the procedure, the client should be placed in a comfortable position, given oral hygiene measures, and permitted to rest.

Chest percussion and vibrations. In conjunction with bronchial drainage, chest percussion (clapping or tapping) and vibrations may be performed to facilitate removal of secretions. *Percussion* is performed by cupping the hands and giving the section to be drained a succession of short, brisk claps (Fig. 21-34). This breaks up mucus plugs and allows air within the lungs to penetrate behind the secretions, thus facilitating their movement toward the upper respiratory

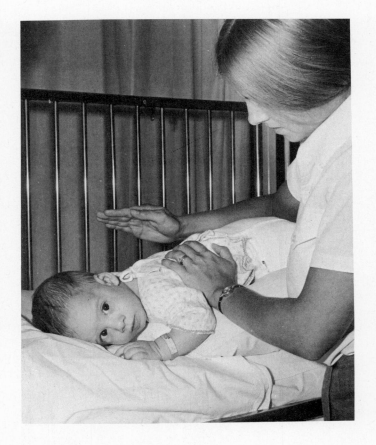

FIG. 21-34
Physical therapist performs cupping and vibration exercises on young client. (Courtesy Children's Health Center, San Diego, Calif.)

tract. For effective percussion, cupping of the hand is important because it forms a cushion of air between the palm and the chest wall, thus changing the pressure within the airway and loosening secretions each time the hands come in contact with the chest wall. A flat, stiff hand should be avoided. Percussion over the breasts, calvicles, spine, scapulae, and vertebrae should also be avoided because of pain. Any form of hemorrhage or pain contraindicates this part of therapy.

Vibrations, which follow percussion, are instrumental in mobilizing secretions to the large airways. Vibrations are performed during the expiratory phase to facilitate movement of secretions from the periphery of the lung with the outflow of ventilation and the narrowing, squeezing action of the airway. The client is instructed to exhale slowly and completely. During expirations, five or six vibrations with the hand are applied over the area. The client is then instructed to cough, and the mucus is expectorated. An electric hand vibrator may be substituted for hand vibrations. These devices are considered more relaxing and provide more uniform vibrations.

MODIFICATIONS FOR INFANTS. Performing percussion and vibration exercises as described above is difficult, if not impossible, to do for the neonate. Special devices have been developed for this age group. One such device developed to assist with percussion is a small plastic cup with a padded rim to prevent skin irritation. Because of the rapid respiratory rate of the infant, vibration by the conventional method is extremely difficult. For this technique, an electric toothbrush whose bristles have been padded can be used. Although the degree of congestion determines how long the exercises are performed, 1 to 2 minutes is considered adequate.

Breathing exercises. Breathing exercises are an important aspect of rehabilitation for chronic obstructive pulmonary emphysema. Instructions about the exercises are usually started in the hospital and continued on an outclient basis. The goals of the breathing exercises are (1) to facilitate maximum ventilation in an effort to produce more effective breathing with less consumption of oxygen; and (2) to improve the strength, coordination, and efficiency of muscles of respiration. As a result, more new air can be taken in, and the client can breathe more efficiently. Included among these exercises are expiratory exercises (including pursed-lip expiration and candle-blowing and bottle-blowing exercises) and diaphragmatic breathing.

All exercises should be carried out within the limits of the client's physical condition and not to the point of exhaustion. As soon as possible, exercises should be incorporated in routine activities such as walking, reaching, bending, and climbing stairs.

PURSED-LIP EXPIRATION. Pursed-lip expiration (Fig. 21-35) functions to slow and coordinate respiration. To accomplish this, the client is instructed to purse the lips as if whistling during expiration and to control the velocity of the exhaled air to the slowest to be consistent with ventilation. When this exercise is performed, resistance to outflow of the lips is produced, intrabronchial pressure is maintained; consequently, airways stay open *longer* on expiration and therefore produce less trapping of air in the alveoli.

ABDOMINAL BREATHING EXERCISES. Abdominal breathing exercises are used to retain and coordinate the breathing pattern. Varied positions may be used to accomplish these exercises; however, the supine position is most commonly used (Fig. 21-36). The principle governing these exercises is based on the fact

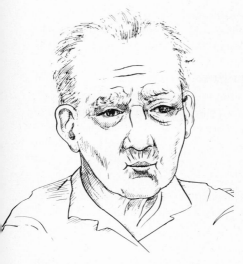

FIG. 21-35
Pursed lip breathing is one means of positive pressure breathing.

FIG. 21-36
Forced exhalation breathing exercises
as client assumes supine position. **A,**
Resting. **B,** Exhalation. **C,** Inhalation.

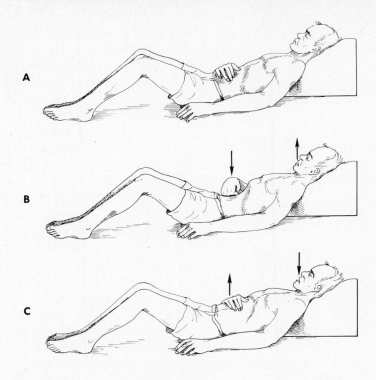

FIG. 21-36
Forced exhalation breathing exercises
as client assumes supine position. **A,**
Resting. **B,** Exhalation. **C,** Inhalation.

that contraction of the abdominal muscles increases the pressure in the abdominal
cavity, which pushes the viscera upward and subsequently displaces and pushes
the diaphragm upward and, as a result, increases its excursion.[33]

GRADED EXERCISES. Walking is also an effective exercise for these clients,
since it helps to improve muscle tone and breathing power. When walking exercises are used, they are planned so that the distance is increased daily. To facilitate relaxation of the shoulder girdle, the client is instructed to swing his arms
loosely in pendulum fashion while he exhales slowly. Playing golf is one way of
accomplishing this exercise. Bicycling exercises and rowing devices can be used
indoors in the exercise program during the winter months. An inclusive and
detailed presentation of all breathing exercises is beyond the scope of this discussion.[27]

Coughing techniques. Effective coughing techniques are described earlier in
this chapter. The same guidelines are essential for the client with a chronic lung
disease (for example, sitting position, relaxed shoulders, feet supported). Some
type of support for the lap is useful. Following this, the client should drop his
head, lean forward, exhale three to four times, and then inhale slowly.[41] If facial
plethora or venous distension of the head or neck is observed, instructions should
be given to breathe more slowly.

Discharge instructions. Teaching for home management should start long
before the client is discharged from the hospital. The nurse should play a major
role in instructing the client about the nature of chronic lung disease. The physician's explanation should be reinforced and the client's questions answered.
They should be instructed to stay as healthy as possible in an effort to keep up
resistance and improve breathing. Persons with upper respiratory tract infections
and crowds should be avoided. They should be aware of signs of upper respira-

tory tract infections, and instructions should be given to seek medical help at the first sign of infection. The U.S. Department of Health and Human Services lists the following danger signals of upper respiratory tract infection: (1) increase in the amount of phlegm, and changes in consistency and color (for example, from clear to gray, brown, yellow, or green [changes in color denote breakdown of polymorphonuclear leukocytes]); (2) increased shortness of breath over a period of days or weeks; (3) coughing, wheezing, or a change in cough; (4) chest pain; (5) excessive drowsiness; and (6) fever. Foul-smelling secretions are also indicative of anaerobic infection.

Instructions should also be given regarding the importance of avoiding inhalation of irritants. Smoking and the use of tobacco are discouraged. Stressful situations should be avoided. All these tend to aggravate the client's condition.

Before the client is discharged from the hospital, instructions should be given on the procedures he will need to carry out at home. As much as possible, the client should be encouraged to perform the activities himself, and family assistance encouraged on those activities that are impossible for him to carry out, for example, clapping and vibrations. The family member who performs these activities must be adequately instructed long before the client is discharged. Portable oxygen units are available and are usually used at night. However, they also permit the client to maintain normal arterial oxygen while he engages in activities in and about the home.

Instructions should be given on how to properly care for sputum. Frequent mouth care is essential, because the sputum is often foul-smelling. Many body proteins are lost through excessive expectoration of sputum; therefore he should be instructed on the value of maintaining adequate nutrition and hydration. Instructions to maintain a diet high in protein and vitamins are essential. Adequate fluids must also be encouraged.

Clients with emphysema should be encouraged to remain as independent as possible. If the client is able to return to his previous employment, this should be encouraged because it undoubtedly helps maintain self-esteem. If modifications or alterations have to be made in the type of work the client is permitted to do or if he has to change jobs completely, a vocational counselor might be consulted to help the client prepare for his return to employment. If he is unable to return to work, the nurse could consult an occupational therapist to assist him in developing outside interests.

Because of the chronic nature of emphysema, full support and cooperation from the family are essential. Family members must be informed of the nature of the disease and the extent of the client's disability. In this way they can better cope with problems as they develop. For example, the family must be made to understand why the client may look well but may not be able to walk through the house without becoming terribly exhausted.

Every opportunity should be provided to allow family members to express their feelings about the condition—whether it be the nuisance of the cough or the physical inactivity of the client.

A burden is often placed on the family's financial resources. The family may not have enough money to meet basic needs. To help the family cope with finances, the nurse must be familiar with community agencies that can assist them.

The community health nurse, visiting nurse, social worker, occupational therapist, or respiratory therapist may be consulted to follow the client in the home, so that progress being made in the home can be assessed.

 Evaluation. The client with chronic obstructive lung disease (for example, emphysema) may demonstrate varying degrees of illness and problems.

EXPECTED OUTCOMES
The client and/or family can:
1. Describe the specific chronic obstructive lung disease.
2. Describe methods for health maintenance and restoration.
3. State use, dosage, time, route, and side effects of prescribed medications.
4. State indications for health care, including infection and weight gain.
5. State the necessity for compliance with therapeutic plan.
6. State plans for compliance with therapeutic plan.
7. State plans for follow-up health care and use of community resources.

Cor pulmonale

Cor pulmonale is an enlargement of the right ventricle secondary to pulmonary diseases, abnormal chest bellows, or a depressed respiratory drive from the respiratory center.[26] Chronic lung disease predisposes cor pulmonale. The incidence tends to be higher in individuals who smoke, in areas where air pollution is a severe problem, and affects men more than women.

Two types of cor pulmonale have been identified: acute and chronic. Acute cor pulmonale is generally associated with dilation of the right side of the heart following acute pulmonary emboli; whereas chronic cor pulmonale is associated with the duration of the pulmonary disease that was responsible for the cardiac enlargement.

Pathophysiology. Pulmonary hypertension, which precedes cor pulmonale, is attributed to an increased cardiac output, tachycardia, an expanded blood volume, increased viscosity (for example, erythrocytosis occurs as a compensatory factor), or myocardial damage from hypoxia and acidosis. However, the most important factor is an increase in pulmonary vascular resistance to blood flow through small arteries and arterioles.[26]

Normally the vascular bed in the pulmonary system is under a lower pressure than that in the systemic circulation. The difference in structure of specific vessels accounts for this. For example, the right ventricular wall is thinner than the left, and the walls of the pulmonary artery are thinner than those of the aorta. Also, in pulmonary disease such as emphysema, some of the alveoli lose elasticity and rupture, and the result is a reduction of the pulmonary vascular bed. However, the same blood volume (5 L/min at rest) must pass through the small vascular bed. Thus pressure in the pulmonary artery rises to accelerate blood flow through the lung and maintain circulation. As a result, the right ventricle hypertrophies. However, according to Fishman, cor pulmonale need not be associated with or terminate in failure of the right side of the heart.[26]

 Assessment. Dyspnea, hypoxia, hypercapnia, and a rise in hematocrit are characteristic. A diagnosis may be made with the use of serial x-ray films to determine heart size, and with electrocardiograms to give evidence to right ventricular enlargement. Rarely, cardiac catheterization may be used.

> **Data analysis**
> *Data analysis may reveal nursing diagnoses of ineffective breathing patterns, impaired gas exchange, and alteration in cardiac output.*

Planning and implementation. The type of therapy planned will depend on the severity of the problem and will be directed toward improving alveolar ventilation. Measures such as hydration, antibiotics, and bronchodilators may be used. Mechanical ventilation may be needed if respiratory failure occurs. Measures for heart failure such as a low-sodium diet, digitalis, and diuretics may be used. Of great importance are measures to decrease circulatory blood volume and hematocrit. To accomplish this, several phlebotomies may be needed to bring hematocrit and volume back to normal. Phlebotomies may be repeated at monthly or bimonthly intervals.

Bronchiectasis   Bronchiectasis is a condition in which the bronchi and terminal bronchioles become irreversibly dilated. The dilation tends to occur in the proximal segmented subdivision.[18] One lobe, a lobe of each lung, or several lobes may be involved. Most dilations occur as a result of infection or an obstruction. The obstruction interferes with the clearance mechanism and enhances the development of infection.

The mechanisms involved in bronchiectasis include (1) damage to the bronchial walls, which may commonly result from infection, occasionally by inhaled noxious particles or gases, or by vascular disease that interferes with bronchial nutrition; or (2) abnormal mechanical forces resulting from atelectasis, loss of lung tissue, and retention of large amounts of heavy secretions in the bronchi.[18] The bronchioles may be slightly or markedly dilated and may assume various shapes: cylindrical (fusiform) or saccular (cystic). A commonly used classification is based on these shapes. *Saccular bronchiectasis* usually occurs in the proximal large bronchi and resembles large sacs, whereas *cylindrical bronchiectasis* generally occurs in the branches.

   Assessment. A dry or slightly productive cough may be the first symptom. As the condition progresses, the cough is precipitated by position change, laughing or talking, and expectoration of a large amount of mucopurulent or blood-tinged sputum. The latter is most likely when an infection is present. Easy fatigability, anorexia, weight loss, and dyspnea on exertion are also common. Diagnosis is established on the basis of the presenting symptoms, chest x-ray study, and bronchography. Sputum cultures are useful in identifying specific organisms.

Data analysis *Data analysis may reveal nursing diagnoses of ineffective breathing patterns and impaired gas exchange.*

   Planning and implementation. Therapy is planned to prevent and control infection and to promote bronchial drainage. Antibiotics are usually prescribed until the sputum production becomes minimal and purulence disappears. Postural drainage and chest physiotherapy facilitate removal of secretions. Adequate hydration and humidification are other measures useful in facilitating bronchial drainage. If sputum is difficult to dislodge because of its viscosity, expectorant drugs such as potassium iodide may be prescribed to enhance the effectiveness of postural drainage.

Resectional surgery is presently limited to those situations where the symptoms significantly interfere with the client's daily lives, or in those who do not respond to medical therapy.

Preventive measures. The nurse should inform clients about the importance of avoiding irritants such as cigarette smoke and industrial or atmospheric pollutions. Clients should be encouraged to seek prompt health care for bacterial infections of the lower respiratory tract to prevent the chronic condition. Prompt removal of foreign bodies or other causes of bronchial obstructions should also be encouraged.

Pneumoconioses

Pneumoconioses refer to a group of occupational pulmonary diseases that are caused by prolonged inhalation of high concentrations of mineral or organic dusts such as silica (silicosis), asbestos (asbestosis), and coal (coal worker's pneumoconiosis). These are the most common, although there seems to be a steady increase in the number of diseases in this category. Persons who work in foundries; pottery and china industries; coal, copper, zinc, and iron mines; sandblasting, sandstone grinding, and granite-cutting industries; and those who work on farms and in fields are commonly affected. Variables such as smoking and air pollution are significant in the development of pneumoconioses.

Normally, by the lungs' defense mechanism, large, inhaled particles are removed by ciliary action of the upper respiratory tract, provided the concentration is 10 or less particles per cubic centimeter. Although the mucus within the alveoli and the lymphocytic cells help remove particles, smaller particles are not as easily expelled. This is especially true if the concentration is increased. Prolonged inhalation of these substances results in the accumulation of particle-laden macrophages in the interstitial tissue where the process of pneumoconioses begins.

Although the pathological reactions in the lung tissue vary, the continued presence of these foreign materials produces changes in the lung tissue and subsequent pulmonary fibrosis.

Characteristic symptoms are dyspnea (partially resulting from increased work of the respiratory muscles as they try to ventilate the fibrotic lung), a chronic cough and excessive sputum production (from irritation), wheezing (from bronchospasms), and cyanosis (from decreased arterial oxygen saturation). Cor pulmonale and spontaneous pneumothorax are common complications of pneumoconioses. Bronchogenic carcinoma often complicates asbestosis, especially in smokers, whereas tuberculosis is the most common complication of silicosis.

Silicosis. Silicosis may occur in acute or chronic forms. Acute forms (acute silicosis) are rare.[8] It occurs in individuals who are exposed to an intense exposure of silica dust over a short period of time. For example, it is common among sandblasters and rock drillers and in individuals who produce finely ground silica.[2]

Chronic silicosis occurs in workers who are exposed to low concentrations of the dust for 10 years or more. Various forms of chronic silicosis may be evident. An early form is characterized by scattered small nodules throughout the lungs. Dyspnea is the leading symptom, whereas a more serious form is characterized by progressive enlargement and increase in the number of nodules. Dyspnea, cough, and sputum production becomes worse. Silicosis may be complicated by progressive massive fibrosis (PMF) that spreads throughout the lungs, restricts lung function, and results in the client developing cor pulmonale. At this point, disability is inevitable.

Prevention of silicosis. Several measures of dust control are used in an effort to eliminate silicosis: wetting down of mines, improved ventilation, special suits, and breathing apparatuses.

Asbestosis. Asbestosis, caused by the mineral dust, is common among shipyard and insulation workers, and among individuals who live near asbestos mines. It slowly develops into pulmonary fibrosis after 10 to 20 years of exposure, but the process continues even after cessation of exposure. The disease primarily affects the lower lobes' bronchioles because the fibers are too large to enter the alveoli.[78] Dyspnea is a major system. Other diseases that may occur as a result of asbestos exposure include bronchogenic carcinoma, mesothelioma, and pleural effusion.[78] Therapy is directed toward prevention. Preventive measures include limiting the concentration of asbestos in the environment, the use of protective devices, and, when possible, limiting the length of employment in industries with high concentration of asbestos.

Coal worker's pneumoconiosis. Coal worker's pneumoconiosis (CWP), commonly referred to as *black lung,* occurs in two forms. Simple CWP results from continued inhalation of coal dust. The dust accumulates in the lungs, most predominantly around terminal respiratory bronchioles, and consequently develops into bronchiolar dilatation as a result of loss of wall structure (for example, centrilobular emphysema). At this point, symptoms may be absent because ventilatory function is normal.

The dust deposits can be seen on chest x-ray film as a nodular opacity. Nodules may be noted on x-ray film after as few as 10 years of exposure. The nodules increase in size with continued exposure.[78]

Complicated CWP occurs in a small percentage (2% to 3%) of individuals. In these individuals fibrosis occurs, most often in the upper lobes.[78] The fibrotic masses continue to spread until most of the lung tissue is involved. Death may occur from respiratory failure, cor pulmonale, or severe infection.[2]

> **Data analysis**
> *Data analysis may reveal nursing diagnoses of ineffective breathing patterns, impaired gas exchange, ineffective coping, knowledge deficit, and grieving.*

Planning and implementation

Therapy. Therapeutic measures are generally symptomatic. Bronchodilators may be prescribed for bronchospasms. Iodides and warm, moist air are essential in reducing the viscosity of the thick, tenacious sputum. Segmental bronchial drainage may be used to remove secretions. Infections are treated with antibiotics.

Prevention. Prevention is an important aspect in the curtailment of pneumoconioses. Some industrial settings have directed efforts toward maintaining healthful working conditions by the use of certified masks and/or ventilation systems. Mining procedures that will result in less dust contamination and lessened worker exposure are being investigated. Engineers have used their skills in creating ways of decreasing dust exposure. Experimental studies have shown the value of certain drugs in eliminating specific dusts from the lungs. In addition to these preventive measures, persons who work in environments where they are exposed to dusts should be encouraged to obtain periodic physical examinations, including chest x-ray films and pulmonary function tests.

 Evaluation. Evaluation of the nursing care plan for the client with pneumoconioses is ongoing as the client's health status changes.

EXPECTED OUTCOMES

The client and/or family can:
1. Describe pneumoconioses.
2. Describe plans for health maintenance.
3. State plans for follow-up health care and use of community resources.

Respiratory failure

Respiratory failure occurs whenever the respiratory apparatus fails to provide adequate tissue oxygenation and to remove carbon dioxide.[71] Numerically, an individual is said to be in respiratory failure when the Pa_{O_2} drops below 50 mm Hg and the Pa_{CO_2} rises above 50 mm Hg. Any conditions that interfere with pulmonary gas exchange between the blood and alveoli may be responsible for producing respiratory failure.

Two basic causes of respiratory failure and two general types have been identified: (1) *alveolar hypoventilation,* which may be experienced in clients with chronic lung or neuromuscular diseases or result from the use of depressant drugs or high-flow oxygen therapy, especially in the presence of chronic lung disorders; (2) *ventilation perfusion* imbalance, which either increases physiological dead space or physiological shunt.[85]

The two types of respiratory failure include (1) the *hypercapneic type,* in which the Pa_{CO_2} is increased and the Pa_{O_2} is lowered; and (2) the *hypoxemic type* in which the Pa_{CO_2} is normal or decreased.[54] These two forms will be discussed.

Hypercapneic respiratory failure. Clients who experience hypercapneic respiratory failure are categorized as either having normal lungs or diseased lungs. In clients with normal lungs, the retention of carbon dioxide is the result of a reduction in alveolar ventilation because of some abnormality in respiratory control, abnormalities in neuromuscular events required to maintain ventilation, or abnormalities of the chest wall.

The second type of hypercapneic respiratory failure occurs in clients with lung disease, especially chronic lung diseases (for example, emphysema, chronic bronchitis, asthma). In these clients, alterations in gas exchange result in inadequate elimination of carbon dioxide. Mixed forms have also been reported to occur in clients with chronic lung diseases who have received respiratory center depressants (sedatives or narcotics). The end result is depressed ventilation, which may lead to respiratory failure, and hypercapneic coma.

Pathophysiology. Some of the consequences of hypercapnia include hypoxemia, respiratory acidosis (especially if the hypercapnia develops rapidly), increased pulmonary resistance, and dilation of the cerebral vessels. The latter is associated with the increased CSF pressure that often accompanies respiratory failure. Hypercapnia results in cerebral vasodilation and increased cerebral blood flow.[71] Consequently, headache and changes in sensorium (such as confusion, irritability, somnolence, and coma) may be evident. Changes in rate or depth of breathing (such as tachycardia, hypertension, retinal vein engorgement, and papilledema) may be noted.

Hypoxemic respiratory failure. Hypoxemic respiratory failure results when an insufficient amount of oxygen is delivered to the pulmonary capillary blood and subsequently results in arterial hypoxemia. The hypoxemia is caused by a ventilation-perfusion imbalance. Carbon dioxide elimination is normal or increased. Any condition responsible for producing adult respiratory distress syndrome may produce hypoxemic respiratory failure.

Assessment. Signs and symptoms of hypoxia include restlessness, confusion, and dizziness, which are indicative of inadequate cerebral oxygenation. Compensatory signs such as tachypnea, tachycardia, and an increase in blood pressure may also occur. These occur as a result of stimulation of the sympathetic nervous system in response to hypoxemia, mediated by the chemoreceptors acting on the vasomotor centers. Peripheral vasoconstriction is also evident. Cyanosis, which is usually a late sign, may also occur. Analysis of blood gases reveals a decreased Pa_{O_2} and a normal Pa_{CO_2}. The presenting symptoms and blood gas values are useful in establishing a diagnosis of respiratory failure. Blood and electrolyte studies may also be obtained.

> *Data analysis*
> *Data analysis may reveal nursing diagnoses of impaired gas exchange, ineffective breathing patterns, and fear.*

Planning and implementation. Because hypoxia can result in brain death within minutes, therapy is planned to *maintain adequate oxygenation.* Oxygen is cautiously administered by varied systems (oxyhood for infants up to 6 to 8 months, plastic hoods for older infants,[16] face tents, cannula, or masks). The Venturi mask is frequently used because it delivers precise concentrations of oxygen. While oxygen is being administered, it must be remembered that complications can occur. The client therefore should be observed closely for signs of carbon dioxide narcosis, which may occur in the first few hours of therapy. The appearance of signs of carbon dioxide narcosis warrants reducing or removing oxygen immediately and consulting the physician. It is not uncommon for oxygen to be titrated by starting at very low flow rates (0.5 to 1.0 L/min), monitoring the response of blood gases, and gradually increasing the flow rate until the desired rate has been achieved.[54]

Apnea and a continual rise in Pa_{CO_2} indicate the need for mechanical ventilation. A cuffed tracheostomy or cuffed endotracheal tube may be inserted, and a ventilator that does the work of breathing is attached to it. With the aid of the ventilator, air is forced into the lungs, and the excess carbon dioxide is blown off. An adequate tidal volume is maintained. When the client is connected to a ventilator, he must be constantly observed, beause the Pa_{CO_2} may drop rapidly and produce respiratory alkalosis. The nurse should be aware of the symptoms of alkalosis (paresthesia, sweating, and tetany) so that they can be promptly reported and proper intervention used.

Other therapeutic measures involve controlling infections and bronchospasms and removing secretions by suctioning. If respiratory failure is accompanied by heart failure, digitalis drugs may be prescribed. Adequate hydration and humidification must be provided.

Nursing process for common health problems

The nurse must continually observe the client for respiratory and circulatory changes and the status of the central nervous system. Emotional support must be provided (allaying apprehension and fear, for example, by answering questions, spending time with the client). If the client is anxious and demanding, the nurse should understand the source of his reactions. He must be encouraged to relax. Nursing measures that facilitate relaxation should be used, because sedatives are contraindicated. The client's position must be changed every 1 to 2 hours. Deep breathing and coughing should be encouraged. The nurse should auscultate the client's chest. The pulse and blood pressure must be monitored frequently. An arterial catheter may be inserted to facilitate monitoring the mean arterial pressure, systolic and diastolic parameters, and sampling of arterial oxygen tension.[16] Frequent temperature assessments are essential. Accurate records must be kept of intake and output.

Respiratory acidosis

Respiratory acidosis, an elevation of Pa_{CO_2}, occurs as a result of *alveolar hypoventilation*. In such instances, ventilation is not adequate to eliminate carbon dioxide from the pulmonary capillary blood as rapidly as it is produced by cellular metabolism. As a result, the level of carbon dioxide and carbonic acid in the blood plasma increases and oxygen concentration decreases. This results in an increase in the hydrogen ion concentration and a reduction in arterial pH.

Pathophysiology. Any condition that interferes with the exchange of gases, subsequently producing retention of carbon dioxide, may cause respiratory acidosis. Common examples include conditions that limit expansion of the thoracic cavity (such as pain following abdominal and thoracic surgery or thoracic deformities), depress the respiratory center (such as narcotics, sedatives, and general anesthetics), limit lung expansion (such as chronic lung diseases or air or fluid in the pleural cavity), produce perfusion failure (such as cardiac arrest or ventricular fibrillation), or obstruct the upper airway (such as croup or foreign body aspiration). It may also occur as a result of neuromuscular instabilities such as poliomyelitis and myasthenia gravis.

Compensation for respiratory acidosis, which may take from a few hours to several days, is the primary function of the kidneys. The kidneys attempt to maintain the 20:1 ratio by increasing (or retaining) the amount of bicarbonates and excreting hydrogen ions. (This is enhanced by the *chloride shift*, whereby with an increase of carbon dioxide in the blood, the chloride moves out of the plasma into the erythrocyte in exchange for bicarbonate.) The specific mechanism by which the kidney maintains a balanced ratio is selective rejection of bicarbonate excretion in the urine (keeping it to be used as a blood buffer) and decrease of sodium excretion (holding on to it so that it can combine with the large amount of bicarbonates). Hence this mechanism is often referred to as the *alkaline reserve*. A second mechanism is removal of increasing amount of hydrogen ions, which in turn reduces the high acid content of the blood. In acute states the kidneys have greater difficulty maintaining the balance, and thus compensation may not be evident for 3 to 4 days. However, in chronic conditions the body's ability to adjust to the changes is increased; therefore the pH is maintained within normal limits.

Assessment. Increased carbon dioxide levels cause dilation of the cerebral vessels and an increase in cerebral blood flow, which results in an increase in cerebrospinal fluid pressure and cerebral edema. Subsequently, symptoms are indicative of alteration in cerebral function and inadequate pulmonary ventilation. Dizziness, headache, and sensorium changes (such as somnolence and confusion) may be associated with the former, whereas dyspnea, tachycardia, and sometimes cyanosis are indicative of the latter.

As the extracellular hydrogen ion concentration increases, hydrogen ions begin to enter the cell. Potassium ions leave the cell to maintain the normal electrical gradient. An increase in the serum potassium level is evident at first, but will later decrease. Therefore symptoms indicative of potassium alteration, including cardiac dysrhythmias such as conduction blocks and ventricular fibrillation, may develop. The nurse should monitor these clients closely. Laboratory assessments include a pH below 7.35, indicating an increase in the carbonic acid, an increase in Pa_{CO_2}.

> **Data analysis**
> *Data analysis may reveal nursing diagnoses of impaired gas exchange, ineffective breathing, and impaired tissue perfusion.*

Planning and implementation. Therapy is directed toward improving alveolar ventilation sufficient to return blood gas levels to normal. To accomplish this the physician will prescribe measures directed toward the cause. For example, mechanical ventilation may be used. Measures may be taken to relieve airway obstruction. A buffer base such as $NaHCO_3$ may be administered until the pH returns to normal.

A number of nursing measures can be implemented to curtail the development of acidosis. For example, before and after administering respiratory depressants the nurse should assess the rate and depth of respiration. A low rate (such as 12 per minute) warrants withholding the medication. Knowledge about the pharmacodynamics of these drugs is essential and must be evaluated in relation to the prescribed dosage and frequency. Clients, especially those who have abdominal or thoracic surgery, should be instructed to cough and breathe deeply to facilitate adequate ventilation and mobilization of secretions. Retained secretions must be removed by suctioning or by means of hydration. Clients receiving ventilatory assistance should be monitored closely (blood gases, vital signs, level of consciousness, and breath sounds).

Respiratory alkalosis

Respiratory alkalosis, low Pa_{CO_2}, occurs as a result of *alveolar hyperventilation*. Hyperventilation usually results when there is an abnormal stimulation of the central nervous system. States such as extremely high fevers, salicylate poisoning, hysteria, hypoxia, and overuse of mechanical ventilation are often responsible.

The renal system attempts to compensate by increasing excretion of bicarbonate, retaining more chloride, forming less ammonia, and excreting less acid salts. As a result, the level of bicarbonate in the blood is lowered, the pH is lowered, and the acid-base ratio approaches 1:20.

Assessment. Calcium ionization is decreased when alkalosis occurs. Subsequently muscular irritability results, and the client may have symptoms such as paresthesias (a feeling often described as pins and needles) of the fingers, toes, and lips; tetany; and seizures. Contraction of the cerebral vessels occurs when there is a rapid reduction in Pa_{CO_2}, which consequently produces an impairment in cerebral circulation. Symptoms that sometimes occur as a result of this effect are slurred speech and muscular paralysis.

The combined factors of vasoconstriction, low carbon dioxide concentration, and reduced cardiac output result in a decreased blood flow to vital organs. Increased respiratory effort causes an increase in the intrathoracic pressure, which in turn impedes cardiac return. Dysrhythmias and palpitations are not uncommon. Tissue hypoxia is usually evident and occurs (1) because the alkalotic condition of the plasma inhibits the release of oxygen from oxyhemoglobin, (2) from vasoconstriction, and (3) from reduced cardiac output.[32] Therefore the client may experience shortness of breath. The brain is highly sensitive to hypoxia; therefore dizziness, feeling of faintness, inability to concentrate, blurred vision, and disorientation may develop. Cerebral ischemia may also be responsible for the seizure activity that is sometimes evident. Laboratory assessments reveal a reduction in the Pa_{CO_2} levels and an increase in arterial pH.

 Planning and implementation. Therapy is planned to increase the level of carbon dioxide in the blood. If overventilation is caused by hysteria, rebreathing into a paper bag or sedation may be prescribed. In salicylate intoxication, therapy is likely to be directed toward administering fluids and electrolytes to facilitate excretion of the drug. Carbon dioxide inhalation of 2% to 4% may also be used. Regardless of the form of therapy, the acid-base must be monitored frequently.

Because clients with respiratory instabilities have alterations in the normal breathing pattern (frequently because of apprehension), their breathing patterns should be observed closely. When abnormal patterns (such as rapid, deep breathing) are noted, instructions should be given to breathe normally. In emotional states, pointing out the relationship between the breathing pattern and the development of symptoms may also prove beneficial.

COMMON HEALTH PROBLEMS OF THE MIDDLE-AGED AND OLDER ADULT
Pleurisy (pleuritis)

Pleurisy is the inflammation of the lining of the pleural cavity. Infectious diseases of the lung, such as pneumonia, viral infections, pulmonary embolism, and tuberculosis, are the most frequent causes of pleurisy. However, tumors and trauma to the chest wall may also be responsible for producing the inflammation. The inflammation usually resolves when the primary disease subsides.[65] Organisms may reach the pleura by way of the bloodstream to cause pleurisy.

Two main types of pleurisy have been identified: *dry* (fibrinous) *pleurisy* and *wet* (serofibrinous) *pleurisy.* The dry type is more common. The accumulation of fluid is called *pleureffusion,* which can occur as a result of exudate or transudate.

The exudate may occur as a result of a number of infectious or inflammatory diseases involving the lung tissue. These may alter membrane permeability and cause excessive fluid to accumulate in the pleural space. Among these diseases are metastatic malignancy and infradiaphragmatic disease (for example, pancreatitis, cirrhosis, pulmonary infarction, trauma, and pneumothorax).[6]

On the other hand, a transudate occurs as a result of a disharmony between the capillary hydrostatic pressure and colloidal osmotic pressure (for example, the fluid formation exceeds fluid reabsorptive capacity). The primary condition is not lung tissue. Disorders such as capillary hypertension, hypoalbuminemia, nephrotic syndrome, immune diseases, congestive heart failure, and ascites may cause transudative trauma.

 Assessment. The pleural lining is richly endowed with pain fibers; as a result, sharp chest pain characterizes dry pleurisy. The pain is aggravated by deep inspiration, coughing, and sneezing and is caused by friction or contact of the inflamed pleural surfaces, hence the name *pleural friction rub.* In an effort to diminish the pain associated with motion, clients usually lie on the affected side and take quick, short, shallow breaths. The friction rub can readily be heard on auscultation of the chest.

When fluid accumulates, the pain subsides because the surfaces no longer rub together. However, because of compression of the lung and displacement of the heart from accumulated fluid, dyspnea becomes a major symptom. The degree of dyspnea depends on the amount of accumulated fluid. In small effusions and slow accumulations, no dyspnea may occur. Pyrexia may be manifested, particularly if the pleurisy results from an infection.

The diagnosis of pleural effusion may be made on the basis of the client's history, findings from physical examination, chest x-ray film, and analysis of pleural fluid.

Data analysis
Data analysis may reveal nursing diagnoses of alterations in comfort, ineffective breathing patterns, and impaired gas exchange.

 Planning and implementation. Therapy for dry pleurisy is directed toward relieving pain and promoting comfort. This may be accomplished by immobilizing the chest with adhesive strapping, analgesics, or mild sedatives. If pyrexia is present, the client is placed on bed rest until the temperature returns to normal. It may be necessary to restrict activity for 1 week. In pleurisy with effusion, the excessive fluid is removed by thoracentesis.

Coughing should be encouraged to prevent further pulmonary complications. Assistance should be given and the client instructed in immobilizing the affected side while coughing exercises are being performed.

 Evaluation. The client with pleurisy may have problems with alterations in comfort, ineffective breathing, and impaired gas exchange.

EXPECTED OUTCOMES

The client and/or family can:
1. Describe pleurisy.
2. State plans for health maintenance.
3. State plans for follow-up health care.

Bronchogenic carcinoma

Bronchogenic carcinoma (carcinoma of the lung) occurs primarily in men between the ages of 40 and 70. Inhalation of smoke, especially cigarette smoke, is most commonly responsible for the development of lung cancer. Other inhaled irritants (for example, environmental pollutants) are thought to act synergistically to enhance the effect of smoking. Acting alone, these substances are rarely thought to produce bronchogenic carcinoma.

Epidemiological studies have demonstrated a higher incidence of lung cancer in men who smoke. Cessation of smoking causes a progressive decrease in the number of cells with atypical nuclei. The extent of the reversal depends on the number of years of nonsmoking. Those who stop smoking reduce the risk of acquiring lung cancer.[4] Reports also indicate that death rates from lung cancer are lower among ex–cigarette smokers.

Bronchogenic carcinoma arises in the bronchial epithelium and may produce extensive metastasis throughout the lung. The tracheal and bronchial lymph nodes are the sites of earliest metastasis. Metastasis to distant lymph nodes and organs, such as the brain, bones, and kidneys, is frequent. Conversely, the breast, gastrointestinal tract, kidneys, testicles, and prostate are also frequent sites of pulmonary carcinoma metastasis.

Pathophysiology. The normal lung, the bronchial epithelium, consists of 2 to 3 layers of cells.[4] Columnar cells that compose the surface layer are mostly ciliated, but may also contain some mucus-containing goblet cells. *Basal cells,* another layer, contain centrally located nuclei. These cells abut the basement membrane. Beneath the basement membrane lies the supporting *stroma,* which contains glands, blood vessels, and lymphatic channels.[49]

The first response to the inhalation of carcinogenic agent (usually contained in cigarette smoke) occurs among the basal cells of the tracheobronchial epithelium. Initially there is an increase in the number of cells. In response, the basal cells enlarge.[4] With continued application of the carcinoma agent, additional layers form. In numerous cells the nuclei are atypical, showing variations in size and shape and in arrangement of chromatin cortex. Continued multiplication results in disorganization of the layering patterns with an increase of atypical cells.

Pleural effusion, which occurs in many clients, is a result of (1) direct involvement of the pleura by the tumor cells; (2) obstruction of mediastinal lymphatics and thoracic duct obstruction; (3) obstruction of pulmonary lymphatics with poor resorption of pleural fluid; and (4) obstructive atelectasis with pneumonitis and pulmonary embolus with pleural effusion.[63]

Assessment. Symptoms of bronchogenic carcinoma are variable and may be those of any pulmonary disease.[59] A cough, which occurs in 90% of clients, often is the first symptom to occur. At that time, however, many clients, particularly heavy smokers, attribute the symptom to cigarette smoking. At first the cough is nonproductive, but later becomes productive. Cessation of smoking usually results in temporary improvement, but the cough later worsens. The cough may be frequent enough to interfere with eating and sleeping. Subsequent weight loss often follows. Chest discomfort, or chest pain, pleuritic in type, is not uncommon. Pain is the result of impingement of the tumor on the nerves or invasion of the chest wall.

Other symptoms that occur relate to extension of the tumor: *infection* (fever and purulent sputum) and *obstruction* (wheezing, dyspnea, dysphagia, hoarseness, and cyanosis). Hoarseness is usually caused by invasion of the tumor on the left laryngeal nerve. The left laryngeal nerve is higher than the right and is therefore infrequently involved. Hemoptysis (for example, from *ulceration*) is usually the symptom responsible for causing the client to consult a physician.

Common tumors of the lung. Five common types of lung cancers have been identified: epidermoid, small cell, adenocarcinoma, large cell, and bronchioloalveolar. Each of these will be discussed.

Epidermoid carcinoma, also referred to as squamous cell epithelioma (SCE) or squamous cell carcinoma, is the most common type of bronchogenic carcinoma.[63] It accounts for 50% to 60% of all cancers of the lung.[59] It generally originates in the first bronchus of the main stem, tends to grow slowly, and forms a nodular mass about the bronchi.[59] As the mass grows, it causes an obstruction, and the subsequent development of atelectasis is not uncommon.

Exfoliative sputum cytology of sputum and secretions from the tracheobronchial tree is useful in establishing a diagnosis. Chemotherapy is one form of therapy commonly used.

Small cell carcinoma, also called oat cell carcinoma and anaplastic small cell cancer, accounts for 20% to 25% of all lung cancers.[31] It originates mainly in the main bronchus, although some arise from near the orifice of a secondary bronchi.[59] It grows rapidly, forms irregular-shaped masses, and has a tendency to spread in all directions at an early stage. It also is highly invasive and usually extends along the bronchus. It is considered to be almost always inoperable,[63] even though the lesion can be surgically resected without apparent involvement of the hilar or mediastinal nodes. However, because of its rapid growth, distal metastasis has usually already occurred.[63] Therefore combination chemotherapy has been used as a form of treatment. For example, cyclophosphamide is often given with either doxorubicin and vincristine, methotrexate and vincristine, or methotrexate and CCNU.[31] Radiotherapy has also been used in combination; however, its value over combination chemotherapy is being studied.[31]

Adenocarcinoma develops peripherally, and because of its peripheral location, is not likely to obstruct a bronchus. Because of the excellent vascular bed in which it originates, hematogenous spread is common. It accounts for 20% to 25% of all lung cancers. Surgery for local disease and radiotherapy for regional disease are common forms of interventions.[59]

Large cell carcinoma, also called undifferentiated or anaplastic carcinoma, also tends to originate in the periphery. It accounts for approximately 15% of all cancer of the lungs.

APPROACHES TO SURGICAL INTERVENTION

Surgical procedures that may be performed include thoracotomy, wedge resection, segmental resection, lobectomy, pneumonectomy, thoracoplasty, and decortication. Usually endotracheal anesthesia is used so that the nonoperated lung will be kept expanded while surgery is being performed.

An *exploratory thoracotomy* may be performed to establish a diagnosis. The chest is opened, a biopsy taken, or an examination made to determine the source of bleeding.

A *wedge resection* is performed to remove a small portion of a lung diseased from a small tumor or certain inflammatory lesions. It is named because of its shape.

A *segmental resection* is the removal of a segment of a diseased lung. The diseased area usually lies close to the surface of the lung. It may be performed to remove an abscess, an emphysematous bleb, or tuberculous cavity.

A *lobectomy* is the removal of a lobe. This surgical procedure is likely to be performed for bronchiectasis, an emphysematous bleb, tumors, and cysts.

A *pneumonectomy,* removal of an entire lung, is most likely to be done for malignant neoplasms of the lung. It may also be a form of treatment for tuberculosis or multiple lung abscesses.

A lung or part of a lung may be made to collapse by removing several ribs. Such procedure is referred to as a *thoracoplasty*. It is performed for tuberculosis or to eliminate an unfilled pleural space created by a lobectomy.

A *decortication* is the removal of a fibrous-restricting membrane from the visceral pleura. It may be performed for hemothorax or empyema. After removal of the membrane, the lungs reexpand.

Bronchioloalveolar cell carcinoma, also known as alveolar cell carcinoma and terminal bronchiolar carcinoma, is thought to originate from type II alveolar cells (surfactant-producing cells). Its occurrence is infrequent and is characterized by slow metastasis. The majority of tumors are thought to rarely metastasize beyond the regional lymph nodes or thorax.[59]

Diagnosis is often made on chest x-ray examination and confirmed with the use of cytological examination of sputum and bronchial secretions, biopsy (for example, lymph node or scalene node), and exploratory thoracotomy. A tomogram and angiogram may also be useful.

 Planning and implementation. *Staging* has become an important part of clinical evaluation of bronchogenic cancer. Its purpose has been documented to estimate the volume of carcinoma in various sites for determining prognosis, planning therapy, and in interpreting results of therapy.[31] Therapeutic intervention, therefore, varies, depending on the cell type, the extent (or stage), and multiple host factors, such as age, general condition, and presence of an active disease such as COPD.

Current therapies include various combinations: surgical resection, radiation therapy, chemotherapy, and immunotherapy.

Surgical removal (see material on p. 1351) of the tumor is a successful way of treating localized carcinoma, provided it is found before it spreads to other parts of the body. Depending on the degree of involvement, a lobectomy (removal of an involved lobe) or pneumonectomy (removal of the involved lung) may offer substantial hope.

Radiation therapy (radiotherapy), a form of high-energy x-rays, is beneficial and may be used after surgery or in cases where surgery has to be delayed or in inoperable cancer. The cumulative effect of the therapy may kill the cancer cells after 10 to 30 treatments.

Chemotherapy involves the use of strong drugs. It may be used in combination with immunotherapy. Drugs used for chemotherapy can damage the cancer cells. Because these drugs are strong, side effects such as nausea, vomiting, hair loss, and damage to the blood are not uncommon.

The nursing care planned for clients with cancer of the lung should be individualized and should be planned to promote physical comfort and psychological support.

Evaluation. The client with bronchogenic carcinoma may exhibit varying degrees of illness and nursing problems.

EXPECTED OUTCOMES

The client and/or family can:
1. Describe bronchogenic carcinoma.
2. Describe plans for health maintenance.
3. State plans for follow-up health care and use of community resources.
4. State importance of follow-up care.
5. State indications for health care.

COMMON HEALTH PROBLEMS THAT OCCUR ACROSS THE LIFE SPAN
Foreign bodies

In the nose. Children around 3 years of age are prone to insert foreign bodies into the nose. Although any object that is small enough may be inserted, beans, peas, nuts, buttons, fluffs from blankets, wads of paper, and pencil erasers are the usual ones. Occasionally, insects are deposited into the nostril, and these usually become impacted in the lower part of the nose. (Foreign bodies can also enter the nasal cavities by the posterior choanae. For example, bullets or gun pellets may penetrate the roof, floor, or wall of the nasal cavity. Foreign bodies of this nature are more likely to be found in adolescents and adults and are usually the result of accidents.)

 Assessment. Smooth objects and objects that are not liable to swell may remain in the nose for weeks or months before they are noted. In infants the presence of a unilateral nasal discharge suggests the possibility of a foreign body. The quantity of discharge may vary, and evidence of increasing irritation may develop as the mucous membrane swells. Edema may cause increasing obstruction, which may be evident by mouth-breathing and snoring.

Planning and implementation. If the object has been present for only a short time, forcibly blowing the nose, with an unaffected nostril compressed, may dislodge it. If the object does not become dislodged, the physician should be consulted. The physician sprays a local anesthetic such as lidocaine (Xylocaine) hydrochloride into the affected nares. Infrequently, a general anesthetic is used, especially if the client is uncooperative. A vasoconstrictor (such as epinephrine or phenylephrine [Neo-Synephrine] hydrochloride) is instilled into the affected side of the nose to shrink the intranasal membranes, thereby making easier the removal of the foreign body. When the foreign body is more securely lodged, the object is removed with the aid of forceps or by irrigation. Suctioning may be needed to keep air passages clear of secretions. The nurse should assist the physician and keep the client as calm as possible.

In the pharynx. Sharp objects and bones often become lodged in the tonsil. A soft-tissue x-ray film may be taken to visualize the foreign body. Once it is visualized, the physician removes it by means of forceps.

In the larynx, trachea, and bronchi. Foreign objects (beans, pins, and food) may also be aspirated into the trachea and bronchi.

Assessment. If the object becomes lodged in the larynx, symptoms similar to croup may be experienced. Aphonia and signs of respiratory distress may also be evident. Symptoms such as hoarseness, cough, dyspnea, and cyanosis may occur if it enters the trachea. Signs of airway obstruction and atelectasis (such as coughing, wheezing, and dyspnea) characterize a foreign body in the bronchus. Laryngospasms and anoxia may develop, thus presenting an emergency.

Data analysis
Data analysis may reveal nursing diagnoses of ineffective airway clearance, ineffective breathing patterns, and potential for injury.

Planning and implementation. The objective of therapy is to dislodge the object and remove it from the air passage (Fig. 21-37).

To attempt to dislodge the obstruction in the conscious choking victim, a series of back blows followed by abdominal thrusts can be administered. For the adult victim the rescuer stands slightly behind the victim and, supporting the torso with one hand, delivers four back blows with the heel of the hand. If the obstruction is not dislodged, the rescuer stands behind the victim and places both arms around the victim's waist, slightly above the waistline. The victim's head, arms, and upper torso are permitted to hang forward. Second, the rescuer grasps

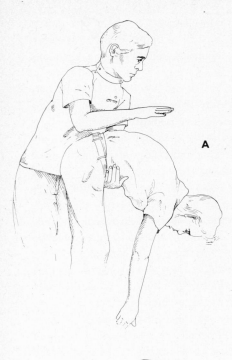

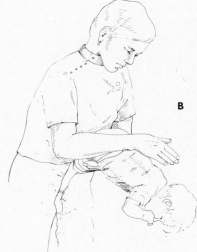

FIG. 21-37
A, Removing a foreign object from the air passages of an adult. The victim assumes a head-down position. The rescuer strikes him on the back between the shoulder blades or compresses the abdomen. This forces air out of the lungs, which facilitates dislodging the obstruction. **B,** Removing a foreign object from the air passage of a child. The same technique is used, but less force is needed.

his wrist, makes a fist, and places the thumb side of his fist against the victim's abdomen. Finally, he rapidly and strongly presses his fist into the victim's abdomen with an upward motion, forcing the diaphragm upward. This may be repeated several times until the object is expelled.

For infants and small children, the victim can be supported in a head-down position on the rescuer's arm with the head and neck supported by the rescuer's hand (Fig. 21-37, *B*). Back blows are given with the heel of one hand, but with less force than required for the adult. If the object is not dislodged after four back blows, the infant or small child can be turned, taking care to support the head and neck, still supported on the rescuer's arm and hand, and given four chest thrusts with two or three fingers placed on the midsternum at the nipple line. If the object causing obstruction can be seen in the mouth, the rescuer can extract it or otherwise continue the sequence of back blows and abdominal thrusts.

If the adult victim becomes or is unconscious, the obstructed airway maneuvers are applied with the victim on a flat surface. The rescuer kneels near the victim, and the back blows are given by logrolling the victim toward the rescuer's knee. Abdominal thrusts are given with the victim supine, and the rescuer places the heels of his hands midway between the umbilicus and xiphoid process and delivers four upward thrusts. Obstructed airway maneuvers for the unconscious infant or child are performed as for the conscious victim.

Another maneuver developed to dislodge an obstructing object from the pharynx is the Heimlich maneuver. It has been endorsed by the American Medical Commission of Emergency Medical Services. First, the rescuer stands behind the victim and places both arms around the victim's waist, slightly above the waistline. The victim's head, arms, and upper torso are permitted to hang forward. Second, the rescuer grasps his wrist, makes a fist, and places the thumb side of his fist against the victim's abdomen. Finally, he rapidly and strongly presses his fist into the victim's abdomen with an upward motion, forcing the diaphragm upward. This may be repeated several times until the object is expelled.

For an infant or small child less force is needed. Another modification is to place the child across the knee so that the leg presses the abdomen below the diaphragm as pressure is applied upward along the lower part of the child's back.

If the object is not removed, the client should be seen by a physician immediately. If breathing stops, a cricothyroidotomy (incision into the cricoid and thyroid cartilages, Fig. 21-38) or tracheotomy may be performed. Inspiratory and expiratory chest roentgenograms may be taken to diagnose the location of the object, and a bronchoscopic examination may be performed to remove the foreign body. Objects that remain lodged in the tracheobronchial tree may cause inflammation and infections, edema, obstructions, and emphysema.

Instructions for prevention. A great deal of the nurse's time should be spent instructing parents and children about safety measures. Parents should be encouraged not to give small children objects to play with that are small enough to be inserted into body orifices. As a precautionary measure, it may be helpful to encourage mothers to sew blankets between sheets to prevent the children form pulling fluff off blankets. Small objects should be kept out of the reach of small children. Children should be instructed not to place objects into their mouths, other than foods and nonplastic eating utensils. Small food particles such as

FIG. 21-38
Site for inserting needle for cricothyroidotomy.

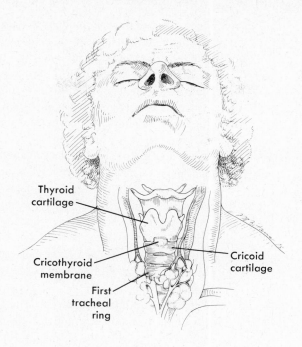

Thyroid
cartilage

Cricothyroid
membrane

First
tracheal
ring

Cricoid
cartilage

nuts, candy, or gum should not be given to the young child. As much as possible, adolescents and adults should be encouraged to maintain care while handling firearms.

Another important teaching point is to instruct parents and other personnel *never* to give a choking individual water, bread, crackers, mashed potatoes, or any form of food, because ingestion of food may complicate matters and delay treatment if anesthetics are required. Second, the client should *never* be pounded vigorously on the back, nor should fingers be rammed down the throat in an attempt to dislodge the article, because of the danger of causing damage to trachea and larynx. Inhaled peanuts have been reported to produce a "vegetable" pneumonia, which results from irritation of the bronchial mucosa by vegetable oils. Therefore the child or adult who has inhaled a peanut should be seen by a physician immediately because any delay will result in increased edema around the object and thereby make removal more difficult.

Epistaxis

Commonly referred to as *nosebleed,* epistaxis usually results from local or systemic conditions. Trauma, the most important local cause of epistaxis, may result from nose picking, a blow on the nose, irritation from foreign bodies and polyps, or operative injury. Capillary or venous congestion such as might result from acute or chronic infections, violent sneezing, and inhalation of irritating chemicals may also cause epistaxis. Hypertension, blood dyscrasias (such as leukemia, hemophilia, purpura, and some anemias), and cardiac abnormalities are among the systemic causes of epistaxis.

Epistaxis occurs in all age groups. However, it occurs about twice as frequently in children as in adults. It rarely occurs before the age of 3 and is infrequent between early childhood and puberty. After puberty, its occurrence tends to decrease. In children and middle-aged clients the course of bleeding is almost always the anterior portion of the septum referred to as Kiesselbach's area. On this portion of the septum is a plexus of arteries that makes it especially liable

1355

to trauma, especially from the fingernails. In the elderly, epistaxis usually arises from an inaccessible site, high and posterior. In these instances the source of bleeding is the ethmoidal artery. Bleeding from the latter area is likely to be severe. It has been reported that as much as a quart of blood may be lost from this area within an hour. Epistaxis in the septum is unassociated with systemic diseases and is likely to be considered more annoying than serious. Whereas, in the ethmoidal artery it is frequently associated with systemic disease and may be profuse and serious.

 Assessment. To completely evaluate the state of the client, a complete assessment must be made concurrently with the initial therapy. The nurse can be instrumental in making these assessments. Answers to the questions found in the assessment guide, opposite, will be valuable as care is planned. The physician will examine the nose to determine the source of the bleeding. Blood (complete blood count) and coagulation (platelet count and partial thromboplastin time) studies may be ordered. If the assessment reveals that trauma has been sustained, x-ray film of the nose and paranasal sinuses will be taken. See assessment guide below.

 Planning and implementation. The aim of therapy is to control the bleeding. Measures to control bleeding may be simple—for example, compressing the nares or slightly packing the nostrils. Most attacks of epistaxis can be controlled by applying pressure to the nares continuously for 10 minutes or until the bleeding stops. This should be done with the client in a sitting or semirecumbent position, with the head tilted slightly forward. This facilitates the formation of a clot by back pressure against the bleeding vessel and prevents blood from running down the pharynx. Generally, pressure is the only form of treatment necessary unless bleeding is severe. If pressure fails, application of an ice collar may be used. A wet compress may be applied to the nose or forehead. Local vasoconstrictors (such as cocaine) may be instilled into the nose to stop the bleeding. If these measures fail, the nostrils may be packed with gauze soaked in epinephrine, or Adrenalin (1:1000), or other hemostatic agents such as Gelfoam or Oxygel may be used as packs. The cellulose pack is usually left in place until it dissolves.

The use of an electric cautery has also proved useful in sealing the bleeding point. Chemical cauterization, as with the use of silver nitrate, has proved effective in sealing the vessel after bleeding has been temporarily controlled.

When bleeding is persistent and the source of bleeding cannot be determined, a postnasal (posterior) packing as well as an anterior packing may be used (Fig. 21-39). General anesthesia is often required, but the packs can be introduced with the use of topical anesthetic agents and sedation. These packs are generally left in place for 48 to 72 hours until the bleeding point is sealed either from edema or a clot. Antibiotics are usually prescribed to prevent infection of the inner or middle ear or sinuses.

Several other devices with inflatable balloons have been used for posterior bleeding. These include a Foley catheter with a 30-ml bag, a postnasal latex balloon, and a double-balloon catheter. The double-balloon catheter has an airway in the center to allow the client to breathe.

Only when local measures fail are systemic measures, vitamins K and C, administered. Fluid replacement using intravenous solutions (whole blood, Ringer's lactate) are indicated after severe blood loss occurs. Ligation of the

---

ASSESSMENT GUIDE FOR THE CLIENT WITH EPISTAXIS

Information should be obtained about the following:
1. Age of the client.
2. The side of the nares from which the blood appears to be coming. One? Both?
3. Whether this is a first episode.
4. Previous episodes? Frequency? Duration?
5. Precipitating factors. Whether any trauma was sustained before the episode.
6. Measures that were used to try to stop the bleeding.
7. Signs of upper respiratory tract infection. Congestion? Sinusitis?
8. Allergic conditions that might have produced nasal inflammation.
9. Medications that the client may be receiving that might influence the clotting mechanism. Anticoagulants? Aspirin?
10. Health history. Is he hypertensive? Does he have a blood dyscrasia? Heart disease? Any recent oral or nasal surgery?

FIG. 21-39
A, Steps used in passing a postnasal pack. **B,** Pack in place. (From De-Weese, David D., and Saunders, William H.: Textbook of otolaryngology, ed. 6, St. Louis, 1982, The C.V. Mosby Co.)

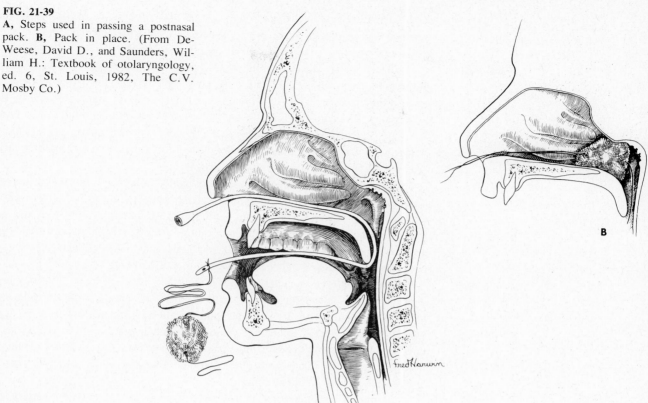

offending artery may also be indicated in severe cases. Such procedure, however, is rarely required.

The nurse should also develop a plan that has as its objective the control of bleeding. If the client is fully clothed, clothing around the neck should be loosened in an effort to lessen pressure on the carotids. In addition to helping control bleeding by the above means, the nurse should also direct efforts toward keeping the client as quiet as possible. Any activity that increases the tendency to bleed should be discouraged. Walking, moving about, laughing, and talking all increase the bleeding tendency. If the client is apprehensive, the nurse should stay with him and provide emotional support. If a client is restless, sedatives may often be prescribed to promote relaxation. He should be cautioned not to blow his nose. A receptacle should be provided so that the client can expectorate any blood, since ingestion of blood may cause nausea and vomiting.

The nurse must also see that the client maintains the position (sitting with head inclined forward) that will facilitate clot formation. In addition, the client should be encouraged to keep his mouth open and cautioned against swallowing. Both of these help keep the nasopharynx closed off, and as a result facilitate the formation of a firm clot. However, if the client is hypovolemic, he should be positioned to facilitate blood flow to the vital organs, while at the same time blood should be prevented from draining into the airway.

During the bleeding episode, a record should be made of the amount of blood lost. Frequent assessments should be made of vital signs and skin color,

1357

especially during periods of prolonged bleeding. Throughout, the nurse should evaluate the effectiveness or ineffectiveness of the treatment and the client's reactions and inform the physician of observations made.

Influenza

Influenza is an acute respiratory tract infection caused by viruses of three immunological types: A, B, and C. Type A virus occurs most frequently and causes epidemics every 2 to 3 years and pandemics approximately every 10 years. Type B occurs every 2 to 4 years and is less severe than influenza by type A. Type C virus rarely causes disease.[2] The incidence of influenza is highest among school-age children and young adults. Individuals with cardiopulmonary diseases are also prone to develop influenza.

Pathophysiology. Influenza is transmitted from human to human by inhalation of droplet nuclei. Although other sites may be involved, the ciliated respiratory epithelium appears to be the principle site of the infection. Following deposit of the inhaled virus on the mucous lining of the tracheobronchial tree, the area becomes inflamed, edematous, and hyperemic. The ciliated epithelium becomes damaged as evidenced by swelling and shrinking of its nuclei.[2]

Assessment. The incubation period is usually 18 to 36 hours, but may last 3 days. A high fever (for example, 101° to 102° F), chills, frontal headache, myalgia (particularly in the legs and lumbosacral area), weakness, and malaise characterize influenza. Sneezing, rhinorrhea, and a productive cough are not uncommon. Severe gastrointestinal symptoms (vomiting, diarrhea) are common in type B influenza.[2] Pneumonia and bacterial infections of the paranasal sinuses and middle ear are frequent complications.

Laboratory examinations of the blood for increasing levels of antibodies and throat cultures are helpful in establishing a diagnosis.

> **Data analysis**
> *Data analysis may reveal nursing diagnoses of alterations in comfort and ineffective breathing.*

Planning and implementation. Measures are planned to promote comfort. Rest and decreasing contacts during the first 3 days are recommended. Analgesics such as aspirin or codeine are sometimes prescribed for pain. In addition, codeine is useful in relieving the cough. Oral fluids are encouraged. Antibiotics are generally not prescribed unless complications develop.

The U.S. Public Health Service recommends annual immunizations with polyvalent influenza vaccine for high-risk groups such as those individuals with chronic rheumatic heart disease, diabetes, cardiovascular disease, and persons 65 years old and older. Such vaccine induces temporary immunity.

Common cold

The common cold (acute coryza) is an acute inflammation of the upper respiratory tract. (In infants it is referred to as acute nasopharyngitis.) It is caused by a filtrable virus, highly contagious, and transmitted from one person to another by droplet infection. Colds are common to all age groups, but children are more frequently affected. Climatic conditions are influential in the causation of colds. This is evidenced by the fact that colds are more common during the winter months. The onset of symptoms is precipitated by lack of immunity, lowered resistance, fatigue, poor nutritional status, and emotional disturbances.

Assessment. Symptoms of the common cold are first experienced in the nasopharynx. The client first experiences a hot, dry, tickling sensation in the pharynx. Shortly after the initial symptoms develop, the nasal passages become congested, and sneezing, coughing, and a nasal discharge become manifest. For the first few days the nasal secretions are copious. The child, particularly, may be irritable and restless. The nasal cavities may become somewhat obstructed, causing conjunctivitis, headache, and mouth-breathing. After the stage of profuse secretion, the nose becomes more obstructed, and the discharge may become thicker and more purulent. Other symptoms are general malaise, chilliness, and aching pains in the shoulders, back, and limbs.

In children under 3 years of age, the symptoms may be more severe. The temperature may increase to as much as 102° to 104° F (38.8° to 40° C). School-age children and adults may have little, if any, fever. Malaise is more common, and anorexia is a problem.

Planning and implementation. The common cold is generally self-limiting. The symptoms may subside within a period of a week, followed by reopening of the nasal passages and normal breathing. Therapeutic measures for the common cold are symptomatic and are aimed at promoting comfort and preventing and controlling infection.

Promoting comfort. A medication such as acetylsalicylic acid (aspirin) or acetaminophen (Tylenol) is prescribed to alleviate the pyrexia, the discomforting headache, and aches of the extremities. Care must be maintained in the use of aspirin in infants because of the immature renal function and subsequent potential for salicylate toxicity. Codeine or medications containing codeine are often prescribed for adults to relieve the cough. Although contraindicated in infants and young children, expectorants may be prescribed to help liquefy secretions. Steam inhalation may be instrumental in soothing the mucous membranes and opening the nasal passages. When the secretions are thick, nasal drops or a nasal inhaler may be useful in shrinking the nasal membranes, thereby facilitating breathing (Fig. 21-40).

Preventing and controlling infection. Adequate rest is essential. If a fever is present, the client may be confined to bed until it subsides. Bed rest is an important measure in that it prevents the spread of infection as well as helps the body defenses control the infection. As much as possible, contacts with others are avoided so that the virus is not spread. Therefore the child should be kept home from school, and the adult should be discouraged from working, since activity is likely to prolong the period of disability. When a client works or a child goes to school, he may pick up bacteria from others and increase his chances of developing complications. Antibiotics are not routinely prescribed. However, they may be prescribed when bacterial extension or such complications as otitis media, sinusitis, pneumonia, or bronchitis are suspected.

Because clients with colds are most often treated at home, nurses have the responsibility of instructing the client and his family regarding how to protect others and prevent infection. The client should be instructed to practice principles of medical asepsis. He is encouraged to cover his mouth and nose when sneezing, coughing, talking, and laughing. Articles that are contaminated with discharge from the nasopharyngeal passages and mouth should be properly disposed of. A bag should be provided for this purpose. The use of disposable tissues and the proper disposal of these also help prevent the spread of microorganisms.

1359

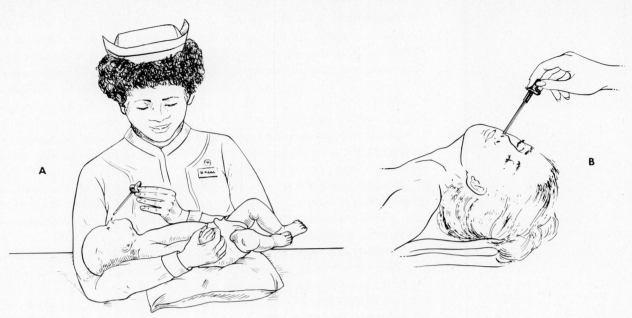

FIG. 21-40
Nasal instillation for the child, **A,** and adult, **B.** Note how the child is restrained for the procedure.

Clothing should be warm and absorbent, but not heavy, and clients should be encouraged to sleep in a well-ventilated room. Each of these is an essential preventive measure.

Maintaining adequate nutrition and hydration. Fluids should be encouraged. Offering the client a different variety of fluids is necessary if the fluid need is to be met. A well-balanced diet consisting of the normal amount of vitamins should be encouraged. An adequate vitamin supply helps raise immunity against respiratory tract infections.

 Evaluation. The client with a common cold may have problems of ineffective airway clearance, ineffective breathing, and alterations in comfort. The nurse and client evaluate plans developed to enhance breathing.

EXPECTED OUTCOMES

The client and/or family can:
1. Describe the common cold.
2. Describe plans for health promotion and maintenance.

Pneumonia

Pneumonia, an acute infection of the parenchyma of the lungs, is most commonly caused by bacteria and less commonly by viruses and fungi. A large percentage of all pneumonias are caused by bacteria, the majority of which are specifically caused by the *Streptococcus* or *Pneumococcus* organisms. *Staphylococcus* and *Klebsiella* organisms may also be responsible. Defense mechanisms of the lungs are essential in maintaining a sterile tracheobronchial tree. Alterations in these mechanisms may be responsible for individuals becoming infected.

Although pneumonia affects all age groups, the two extremes of life, the very young (for example, less than 1 year of age) and the very old are more often affected. The immune system of these individuals is either immature or worn out. It generally develops in chronically debilitated individuals (for example, those with diabetes) and in persons who are immunosuppressed (for example, those receiving steroid or radiation therapy). Immunosuppressive therapy decreases the lymphocytes and an individual's ability to produce antibodies. Persons with pathological involvement of the heart (for example, coronary artery disease) and lungs (for example, cystic fibrosis, COPD) and those exposed to rapidly changing environmental temperatures are thought to be more susceptible to pneumonia than healthy persons in a stable temperature environment.

Other predisposing factors include habitual cigarette smoking because of impaired phagocytic function and impairment of pulmonary defense as might be experienced in persons who are malnourished or consume excessive amounts of alcohol.

The classification of pneumonia may be based on the causative agent (bacterial, virus, *Rickettsia, Mycoplasma*) or anatomical involvement (lobar, bronchopneumonia). Lobar pneumonia involves one or more lobes, whereas bronchopneumonia is manifested as patchy peribronchiolar involvement. Knowledge of the specific organism that causes the infection is basic for the therapy and is therefore commonly used.

Bacterial pneumonias

Pneumococcal pneumonia. Pneumococcal pneumonia is a form of bacterial pneumonia caused by *Streptococcus pneumoniae*. The normal human host is resistant to the induction of pneumonia by the organism. Factors such as mucus secretion and ciliary activity of the mucus membrane, productive cough reflex, and phagocytosis facilitate resistance. Infection with the organism occurs when situations develop that lower defense mechanisms. Clients with pneumococcal pneumonia therefore usually give a history of upper respiratory tract infection. An impairment of the epiglottal reflex, cough reflex, or mucociliary movement may be evident and predispose one to pneumonia.

Seasonal variations are evidenced by the appearance of the pneumonia during the winter and spring. Decreased host resistance and increased crowding of individuals in closed environments during the winter months are also considered to be responsible for the increased incidence.

Pathophysiology. Once the organism enters the alveoli of the lower respiratory tract, there is an outpouring of fluid and neutrophils accumulate and migrate into the alveoli. The infection spreads, and the organisms multiply within the fluid and involve a lobe or lobes. The pleura may also become involved if therapy is not instituted. Infants and young children under 5 years, and older individuals (for example, those over age 50) tend to be more susceptible to developing pneumococcal pneumonia than young adults. The increased susceptibility in the two extremes is possibly related to an ineffective immune response.

Assessment. Pneumococcal pneumonia usually begins suddenly with an abrupt increase in temperature and shaking chills. A corresponding tachycardia (10 beats per minute per degree Fahrenheit), an upper respiratory tract infection, and conjunctival discharge usually precede the pneumonia by several days. Tachypnea, dyspnea, pleuritic chest pain, and a cough are experienced. The cough becomes productive within a few hours and is characterized by pinkish to rusty sputum. Abdominal pain is also common. Atelectasis, with an increasing dyspnea, may develop during any stage of the illness. Hematology studies, blood cultures, chest x-ray films, and analysis of blood gases are useful diagnostic tools.

1361

Streptococcal pneumonia. Streptococcal pneumonia, the most common bacterial pneumonia, is caused by group A or B of beta-hemolytic streptococci. Pneumonias caused by group A streptococci often occur as a complication of viral infections (for example, following childhood diseases) or following streptococcal illnesses such as pharyngitis. When pneumonia occurs as a result of intrapartum infection (factors such as prolonged rupture of the membranes, maternal infection), group B is often responsible.

 Assessment. The onset of pneumonia is sudden and is usually accompanied by cough, which is often productive, chills, usually multiple, and pleuritic pain.

Its incidence is high in infants (particularly group B) less than 5 days of age or in neonates up to 6 weeks of age.[39] In an effort to establish a diagnosis, nose or throat cultures (antistreptolysin [ASO] titer) are taken to identify the specific organism.

Staphylococcal pneumonia. Staphylococcal pneumonia, caused by the *Staphylococcus aureus* organism, usually follows influenza in adults, whereas in children it follows measles or influenza. It generally occurs sporadically, except during epidemics of influenza, and is spread by direct contact with individuals harboring the organism. *Staphylococcus aureus* is carried in the nasal vestibule of many adults and is transiently present in others.

 Assessment. The client may have several symptoms, usually occurring within 5 days following influenza. Chills, high fever, nausea and vomiting, dyspnea, cough, tachycardia, tachypnea, diarrhea, and abdominal distension are common. Cyanosis may also occur.

> ***Data analysis***
> *Data analysis of bacterial pneumonia may reveal nursing diagnoses of impaired gas exchange and ineffective breathing patterns.*

Planning and implementation. Therapy is to (1) relieve respiratory distress; (2) control infection; (3) maintain fluid balance; (4) maintain nutrition; (5) promote rest, activity, and comfort; and (6) prevent pneumonia.

Relieving respiratory distress. The development of hypoxemia demands the administration of oxygen. A high-humidity environment helps loosen a nonproductive cough, thus facilitating cleansing the tracheobronchial tree. This may be administered in the form of steam inhalation. Another adjunct to the removal of secretions is the "stir-up routine"—turning, coughing, and deep breathing (TCDB) exercises. The client is instructed to turn, cough, and breathe deeply every 2 hours. To alleviate the pain that often accompanies the procedure, the nurse should splint the client's chest or instruct him to do so. IPPB therapy may be prescribed if atelectasis is present.

If gastric distension is a problem, neostigmine (Prostigmin) bromide may be prescribed to relieve it. As a result, the client breathes easier because motion of the diaphragm is not impaired.

Controlling infection. Antibiotics are usually administered to prevent pleural extension. The pneumococci organisms are sensitive to penicillin; therefore this is often the drug of choice. Antibiotics such as erythromycin, clindamycin, and the cephalosporins are frequently used for streptococcal pneumonias.

Methicillin sodium (Staphcillin) or erythromycin may be administered if the *Staphylococcus* organism is responsible for the infection.

The nurse also plans with the client to prevent infection in noninfected individuals. If the pneumonia is caused by bacterial agents, the client should be isolated and made aware of principles of medical asepsis.

Maintaining fluid intake. Fluid intake is essential to replace the fluid lost from increased respiration and evaporation during fever and diaphoresis. Fluids are administered according to the client's needs. The nurse should offer frequent sips of a variety of fluids. If the oral intake is inadequate, fluids may be administered intravenously.

Maintaining nutrition. During the acute stage the client with pneumonia usually has a loss of appetite. He should not be forced to eat, nor should large meals be offered. The nurse should provide small, frequent feedings of liquid and soft foods. One measure that will help to improve appetite is frequent oral hygiene. Such a measure relieves dryness and bad taste and, as a result, improves appetite.

After the client's condition and appetite improve, a high-caloric, high-protien diet should be offered in an effort to replace the proteins lost during the acute phase of the illness.

Promoting rest, activity, and comfort. Physical and mental rest are essential for healing of diseased tissue. Rest should be provided in a room with a constant temperature to avoid extra work for heat regulation. The demands for entertainment and worry should be minimal. Visitors should be kept to a minimum. Provisions for a clean, cheerful environment are also important.

Clients with pneumonia are likely to maintain a position that is most comfortable for them. Some may breathe better in a semi-Fowler's position. Others may prefer to lie on the affected side to lessen pain. The nurse must allow the client to assume the position that is most comfortable to him.

A narcotic analgesic such as codeine may be needed to control the pain without depressing respiratory and cough reflex mechanisms. More potent narcotics (for example, morphine and Demerol) are contraindicated. Pain relief is not only important for comfort of the client, but it also facilitates more effective breathing and coughing. When narcotics are ordered, they should be administered with caution because they have a depressant effect on the respiratory center. If chest pain is a problem, chest strapping with adhesive tape may be necessary. Antipyretics are prescribed to control temperature.

Diaphoresis is frequently a problem; therefore the client should be bathed at least daily to maintain the integrity of the skin and prevent skin breakdown. Bed linen and clothing should be changed as often as necessary, and the client should be protected from drafts. Frequent mouth care should be given to alleviate dryness experienced from mouth breathing.

Activity should be encouraged as soon as the condition warrants. Whenever activity is increased, the nurse should observe the client's tolerance to increased activity. Data that may be useful in determining a client's tolerance to activity include pulse rate.

Preventing pneumonia. A vaccine, pneumococcal vaccine polyvalent, is available for pneumococcal pneumonia. The vaccine has been found to induce formation of antibodies in recipients 2 years old and older with healthy immune tissue. To date, it is recommended that the vaccine be administered to individuals over 2 years of age with chronic, systemic disease (for example, diabetes and cardiorespiratory, hepatic, or renal disease), those over age 50, and especially those living in chronic care institutions, those in boarding schools, those with splenic dysfunctions, including those induced by sickle cell anemia or those who have had their spleens removed.

Indirect methods such as prevention of influenza through immunization are considered helpful for streptococcal pneumonia. In addition to immunization for influenza, helpful preventive measures for staphylococcal pneumonia include controlling staphylococcal infections.

Viral pneumonia. Viral pneumonia is commonly caused by a number of viruses, including *respiratory syncytial virus* (RSV); *parainfluenza viruses 1, 2, and 3; adenoviruses;* and *influenzas A* and *B.* The incidence of viral pneumonia varies with age; however, it tends to be highest in children 5 years old and under. Respiratory syncytial virus is the most common cause of pneumonia in infancy, occurring usually in the first 3 years of life, and most commonly in boys. Its occurrence during winter and spring months is frequent.

Parainfluenza 3 is second to *RSV* as a cause of viral pneumonia in infants and children. *Adenoviruses* occur less frequently, but are responsible for many episodes of pneumonia.

Assessment. Several days before developing the pneumonia the client experiences upper respiratory symptoms such as fever, coryza, hoarseness, and cough. Headaches, malaise, and myalgia may also occur.

Planning and implementation. Therapeutic intervention includes bed rest, analgesics, antipyretics, maintenance of fluid intake, and increased humidification.

Aspiration pneumonia. Aspiration pneumonia is a pneumonia that results when a foreign substance is aspirated into the lung. Aspiration occurs in a wide variety of situations. It may occur during the birth process, or it may occur later in life. When it occurs at birth, amniotic fluid is aspirated by the neonate. In later life, gastric content (for example, vomitus and various food particles) may be aspirated into the lung. It is not uncommon in the client with a drug overdose, alcoholism, neurological deficits, and surgical clients. It is also common in clients with a depressed cough or gag reflex and in unconscious clients (for example, during the induction of anesthesia, especially following surgical emergencies where preoperative preparation is less than ideal). Postoperative clients with a depressed sensorium from narcotic sedation as well as those with a Levine tube in place are also at risk of aspirating. The reason for the latter being at risk is the fact that the presence of a tube in the esophagus renders the upper and lower esophageal sphincters incompetent.[9]

Pathophysiology. The pneumonia that occurs following the aspiration is caused by chemical bacteria. The degree of lung injury is related to the size of the material that may either partially or completely obstruct the airway. A complete obstruction causes hypoxia and death within minutes, whereas a partial obstruction retards ventilation and causes the arterial oxygen saturation to fall and CO_2 to be retained. Materials that pass into the mainstem bronchi produce atelectasis. An immediate injury to the pulmonary capillary occurs when acid comes in contact with the respiratory epithelium. As a result, a large volume of protein-rich extracellular fluid becomes exudated, and symptoms indicative of pulmonary edema develop. The pulmonary edema symptoms result from a

1364

chemical burn or injury to the lung. Such injury increases capillary permeability and fluid exudation. The hematocrit also increases following a large aspiration because of depletion of intravascular volume, which occurs because the fluid escapes in the injured lung.[10] Pneumonia or atelectasis may develop within 12 to 24 hours, and is usually distributed in the lower lobes.[9]

Assessment. Symptoms depend on whether the aspirate is solid or liquid. Signs of acute respiratory distress (for example, stridor, cyanosis) are likely in individuals who aspirate solids. The basis for the distress is obstruction of the upper airway. Clients more likely to experience such trauma are victims in whom an unexpected accident occurred in the presence of a full stomach.

Symptoms occurring from the aspiration of liquid gastric contents, although more frequent, are not as dramatic. The symptoms depend on the quantity and pH of the fluid.[9] Symptoms may range from being barely unrecognizable to those of acute pulmonary edema. The former is likely to be the case if a small amount of fluid with a low pH is aspirated. If the amount of gastric fluid that is aspirated is large and if the pH is low, signs of acute pulmonary edema (blood-tinged frothy secretions, tachypnea, dyspnea, cyanosis) may develop within minutes. Hypotension and a decrease in cardiac output may also occur.[9] A fever also develops. The mortality rate is high in those who sustain a massive aspiration.

> *Data analysis*
> *Data analysis may reveal nursing diagnosis of ineffective breathing, impaired gas exchange, ineffective airway clearance, alteration in tissue perfusion, and fear.*

Planning and implementation. Therapy is planned to facilitate airway patency. The material should be removed immediately. The measure used will be based on whether the aspirate is liquid or solid. If the client does not spontaneously evacuate the aspirate, liquid gastric content should be suctioned. Although the amount obtained from suctioning might be minimal, because of the absorptive capacity of the respiratory tree,[9] stimulation of coughing reflexes by the catheter may facilitate expulsion of small fragments of particulate matter. A bronchoscopy or laryngoscopy and possibly a tracheostomy may be performed.

Oxygen is administered, often in conjunction with mechanical ventilation. Intravenous fluid may also be prescribed. Parameters such as central venous pressure readings, urinary output, and vital signs are used to determine the amount of fluid needed. Antibiotics are prescribed from the outset, especially if the aspirate is intestinal content, because of the high content of bacterial and endotoxin in such aspirated material.[9]

Prevention. The nurse has a major role in preventing aspiration pneumonia. Clients who are at risk should be observed at frequently scheduled intervals. On observing, attention should be given to factors that predispose one to aspirate. The unconscious client or one with a depressed cough or gag reflex should be positioned properly (for example, side-lying position). These clients should not be positioned in a supine position. When a Levine tube is in place, the adequacy of functioning should be assessed. Improper functioning may be the result of the holes in the tube being plugged with mucus and gastric secretions. Measures must therefore be used to maintain patency. Tube feedings must be administered slowly to permit satisfactory gastric emptying.

 Evaluation. Evaluation of the nursing care plan for the client with pneumonia is ongoing as the client's health status changes. Nursing problems may include impaired gas exchange and ineffective breathing.

EXPECTED OUTCOMES

The client and/or family can:
1. Describe the specific pneumonia.
2. Describe strategies for prevention.
3. Describe plans for health maintenance or restoration.
4. State the necessity for compliance with therapy.
5. State use, dosage, time, route, and side effects of prescribed medications.
6. State plans for follow-up health care and use of community resources.

Asthma

Asthma is an intermittent airway obstruction caused by constriction of the bronchial smooth muscle, excess mucus secretions, and mucosal edema. The subsequent end result is increased resistance to air flow.

Pathophysiology. The increased resistance to air flow in the tracheobronchial tree, evident in asthma, occurs as a result of constriction of smooth muscle. The excessive mucus, which is difficult for the client to expel because of the ineffective cough, further hinders the flow of air. The mucus usually becomes thick and tenacious. The altered resistance is not evenly distributed throughout the lungs, which results in an unequal distribution of inspired air.[80] As a result, the ventilation-perfusion ratio becomes altered and causes a reduction in the Pa_{O_2} and oxygen saturation.

Asthma may appear at any age, but usually begins in childhood (the majority before age 8). It may persist through adulthood. Until puberty, boys are affected twice as frequently as girls; however, the trend may be reversed after this period.

HEALTH ASSESSMENT GUIDE FOR THE ASTHMATIC CLIENT

The nurse may find the following information useful in developing a plan of care. Such data can be obtained from interview or observation.
1. Length of illness (in other words, how long client has had asthma).
2. Usual reaction to crisis.
3. Current life situation.
4. Previous episodes: frequency, severity, and duration of treatment.
5. Duration and course of current state.
6. Events leading to present attack, such as geographic location, infection, exposure to known allergens, air pollution, unusual exertion, and stress.
7. Changes in characteristics of cough.
8. Mucus production: change in character, such as changes from thin to thick (increased airway obstruction) or changes from clear to purulent (infection).
9. Medications: type, amount, frequency, increase in use, and use of any type of spray.
10. Ability to talk: short, jerky sentences or long sentences without interruptions.
11. Color: pale or cyanotic.
12. Skin: moist or dry.
13. Sounds: any wheezing.
14. Level of awareness, such as aware of surroundings or lethargic.
15. Respiratory status: dyspnea, retractions, or engorgement of neck veins.

The incidence of asthma has been estimated as occurring in 1% of the population.

The bronchial constriction that occurs in asthma may occur when the client is exposed to parasympathetic drugs, allergens (especially IgE substances), or irritants (for example, chemicals, odors, smoke); from sudden irritation of cold air; or the pressure of a respiratory tract infection (viral or bacterial). Strenuous exercise, especially if associated with breathlessness and emotional factors, may also have an influence on the development of an asthma attack.

 Assessment. Asthma attacks may occur gradually or abruptly. They are characterized by increasing dyspnea with prolonged expirations, coughing, and wheezing. Wheezing, which occurs in the large airways, is caused by air rushing past a narrowed area in enough force to generate air vibrations that are perceived as sound. Its movement through the small airways does not produce sound because the air moves too slowly. Symptoms commonly evident are increases in respiratory and heart rates. Restlessness, fatigue, and diaphoresis are not uncommon. The sputum is tenacious. Chest tightness is experienced, with a feeling of inability to take in air. The client maintains a sitting position and focuses attention on each breath. (See health assessment guide, p. 1366.)

Data analysis
Data analysis may reveal nursing diagnoses of ineffective breathing, impaired gas exchange, fear, and ineffective coping.

Planning and implementation. Therapy is based on avoidance of factors that are commonly responsible for attacks and includes principles of care related to avoid known inciting agents, including cats, dogs, feathers, dust, smoke, cold, infection, exercise, and emotional disturbances; hyposensitization, which provides added protection when the specific antigen has been identified; and counteracting histamine effects, which are accomplished with the administration of bronchodilators—epinephrine, 1:1000, in a single dose of 0.1 to 0.5 ml, may be administered subcutaneously; isoproterenol in a 1:100 aqueous solution by inhalation; and aminophylline, 250 to 500 mg, diluted for intravenous administration. Oral theophylline drugs and sometimes aminophylline suppositories may be prescribed.

Cromolyn sodium (disodium cromoglycate) is a drug used prophylactically to *prevent* attacks of asthma. It is not to be taken during an attack. The medication, administered by inhalation, is in the form of a dry, white, crystalline powder. A spinhaler is used to deliver the medication. The nurse should stress the usefulness of this drug as preventive therapy. Some clients experience bronchospasm after cromolyn use. To counteract this effect, they often take a puff on a bronchodilator after using the spinhaler.

Measures are also taken to prevent disability and minimize physical and psychological morbidity. Attention is directed to the social adjustment of the child and his family and the adjustment of the child to school and the community, including normal participation in recreational activities.

Status asthmaticus. Status asthmaticus is a prolonged asthmatic episode that does not respond to treatment and is of such severity as to threaten life.[70]

Nursing process for common health problems

Episodes of status asthmaticus often emerge gradually from a less severe potentially responsive asthmatic attack.

The development of status asthmaticus is related to changes in bronchial secretion rather than bronchial constriction alone.[70] Large amounts of mucus are produced. Additionally, plasma protein, which can contribute to increased viscosity of secretions transudates into bronchial secretions. Subsequently the increased viscosity and increased amount of secretions in conjunction with an impaired mucociliary apparatus make movement of secretions difficult.

Status asthmaticus occurs in 10% of adults hospitalized for asthma and has a mortality rate of approximately 1 in 100,000 persons. It usually develops in those whom asthma is poorly controlled and is preceded by days or weeks of progressive worsening symptoms.

Assessment. Wheezing, which is audible without a stethoscope, dyspnea, and marked respiratory effort characterize the attack. The development of these symptoms is thought to occur because of a marked increase in airway resistance and a heightened respiratory drive that stimulates hyperventilation.[70]

Using the accessory muscle, the client works hard to move air through the obstructed air passages. The chest appears to be in a fixed distended position. To facilitate breathing, a sitting position is maintained. The client typically appears anxious, is restless and diaphoretic, and finds it difficult to complete sentences without pausing. Dehydration and fatigue are common. Fatigue is caused by the increased work of breathing and sleep interference. Breath sounds may become almost inaudible because of poor air movement. Respiratory acidosis ensues, and death, from respiratory arrest, may occur if treatment is delayed.

Arterial blood gas levels are obtained to determine the level of alveolar ventilation. Chest x-ray films may be taken to detect any complication (for example, mucoid impaction, pneumothorax). Sputum specimens may be obtained to detect eosinophils and bacteria. Blood studies (for example, of hematocrit, hemoglobin, and electrolytes) are helpful for determining fluid and electrolyte status. Electrocardiograms are also taken.

> **Data analysis**
> *Data analysis may reveal nursing diagnoses of ineffective breathing patterns, fear, and impaired gas exchange.*

Planning and implementation. During an acute attack of asthma, the client's distress is likely to be so great that the immediate goal will be to *decrease airway resistance by relieving bronchial spasms, reducing edema of the bronchial mucosa, and liquefying the thick secretions.* Initially, epinephrine, which has both beta-1 and beta-2 adrenergic activity, is administered subcutaneously. It produces relaxation of the smooth muscles and vasoconstriction in the bronchial mucosa, subsequently causing bronchodilation and reduced congestion and edema.

Generally, intravenous fluid is started with bronchodilating agents such as aminophylline. Bronchodilators are given to relax the bronchial mucosa, thereby decreasing airway resistance.

In addition to providing a vehicle for medication, intravenous fluid serves to correct dehydration and electrolyte disturbance, because these clients have a

Lerner, A. Martin: Systemic effects of pulmonary infections. In Fishman, Alfred P., editor: Pulmonary diseases and disorders, vol. 2, New York, 1980, McGraw-Hill Book Co.

Mandel, S.R.: Surgical methods of preventing recurrent pulmonary emboli. In Rutherford, R.B., editor: Philadelphia, 1977, W.B. Saunders Co.

McCabe, William R., and Kibrick, Sidney: Infections of the respiratory tract. In Keefer, Chester S., and Wilkins, Robert W.: Medicine: essentials of practice, Boston, 1970, Little Brown and Co.

McFadden, E. Regis Jr., and Ingram, Roland H. Jr.: Asthma perspectives, definitions and classification. In Fishman, Alfred P., editor: Pulmonary diseases and disorders, vol. 2, New York, 1980, McGraw-Hill Book Co.

Mountain, Clifton F.: Surgical therapy. In Fishman, Alfred P., editor: Pulmonary diseases and disorders, New York, 1980, McGraw-Hill Book Co.

Mulder, G. Arnold: Diagnostic procedures in lung cancer, Chest **71:**629-634, May 1977.

Murphy, Raymond L.H., and Holford, Stephen K.: Lungs, Basics Respir. Dis. **8:**41-46, March 1980.

Murray, Henry W., and others: Fever and pulmonary thromboembolism, Am. J. Med. **67:**232-235, August 1979.

Murray, John F.: Bronchiectasis, lung abscess and bronchiolithiasis. In Harrison's principles of internal medicine, ed. 9, Philadelphia, 1980, McGraw-Hill Book Co.

Neff, Thomas A.: Biopsy procedures. In Fishman, Alfred P., editor: Pulmonary diseases and disorders, vol. 1, New York, 1980, McGraw-Hill Book Co.

Newth, Christopher J.L.: Recognition and management of respiratory failure, Pediatr. Clin. North Am. **26:**617-643, August 1979.

Norman, Philip S.: Asthma, hay fever and other manifestations of allergy. In Harrison's principles of internal medicine, ed. 9, New York, 1980, McGraw-Hill Book Co.

Organ, Alan E.: Lower respiratory tract infection in childhood, Issues Comprehens. Pediatr. Nurs. **3:**13-23, August 1978.

Peter, Richard M.: Staging of lung cancer, Chest **71:**633-634, May 1977.

Pierce, Alan K.: Recent advances in the therapy of asthma, Hosp. Formulary **14:**1,32-37, January 1979.

Pinney, Margo: Foreign body aspiration, Am. J. Nurs. **81:**521-522, March 1981.

Proctor, Donald F., and Stitik, Frederick P.: Bronchography. In Fishman, Alfred P., editors: Pulmonary diseases and disorders, vol. 1, New York, 1980, McGraw-Hill Book Co.

Rendle-Short, John: The child, ed. 2, London, 1977, Billing and Sons Ltd.

Riley, Richard: The changing scene in tuberculosis. In Fishman, Alfred P., editor: Pulmonary diseases and disorders, vol. 2, New York, 1980, McGraw-Hill Book Co.

Rohatgi, Prashant, and Massaro, Donald: The chemotherapy of pulmonary tuberculosis, Hosp. Formulary **13:**665-669, September 1978.

Sanford, Jay P.: Pneumonias caused by gram-positive bacteria. In Fishman, Alfred P., editor: Pulmonary diseases and disorders, vol. 2, New York, 1980, McGraw-Hill Book Co., pp. 1130-1137.

Sheldon, George: Fractured ribs and flail chest, Emerg. Med. **12:**49-50, January 15, 1980.

Simkins, Rosemary: Reactive airways disease, Am. J. Nurs. **81:**522-526, March 1981.

Stead, William W., and Bates, Joseph H.: Epidemiology and prevention of tuberculosis. In Fishman, Alfred P., editor: Pulmonary diseases and disorders, vol. 2, New York, 1980, McGraw-Hill Book Co., pp. 1234-1253.

Sturgess, Jennifer M.: Mucous secretion in the respiratory tract, Pediatr. Clin. North Am. **26:**481-501, August 1979.

Van DeWater, Joseph: Preoperative and postoperative techniques in the prevention of pulmonary complications, Surg. Clin. North Am. **60:**1339-1348, December 1980.

Wayman, Tom: Factors affecting capillary blood-gas values, Respir. Ther. **10:**21-23, January/February 1980.

Weill, Hans, and Ziskind, Morton M.: Occupational pulmonary diseases. In Fishman, Alfred P., editor: Pulmonary diseases and disorders, vol. 2, New York, 1980, McGraw-Hill Book Co.

Weinberger, Miles: Theophylline for treatment of asthma, J. Pediatr. **92:**1-7, January 1978.

Wilson, William L.: Cancer of the lung. In Nealon, Thomas F.: Management of the patient with cancer, Philadelphia, 1976, W.B. Saunders Co.

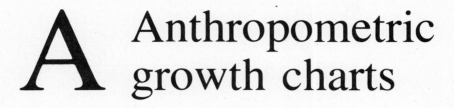

A Anthropometric growth charts

TABLE A-1

Height and weight tables for adults: desirable weights for persons age 25 and over*
(weight in pounds according to frame [in indoor clothing])

Men						Women†		
Height (with shoes on) 1-inch heels		Small frame (lb)	Medium frame (lb)	Large frame (lb)	**Height (with shoes on) 2-inch heels**		Small frame (lb)	Medium frame (lb)	Large frame (lb)
ft	in				ft	in			
5	2	112-120	118-129	126-141	4	10	92-98	96-107	104-119
5	3	115-123	121-133	129-144	4	11	94-101	98-110	106-122
5	4	118-126	124-136	132-148	5	0	96-104	101-113	109-125
5	5	121-129	127-139	135-152	5	1	99-107	104-116	112-128
5	6	124-133	130-143	138-156	5	2	102-110	107-119	115-131
5	7	128-137	134-147	142-161	5	3	105-113	110-122	118-134
5	8	132-141	138-152	147-166	5	4	108-116	113-126	121-138
5	9	136-145	142-156	151-170	5	5	111-119	116-130	125-142
5	10	140-150	146-160	155-174	5	6	114-123	120-135	129-146
5	11	144-154	150-165	159-179	5	7	118-127	124-139	133-150
6	0	148-158	154-170	164-184	5	8	122-131	128-143	137-154
6	1	152-162	158-175	168-189	5	9	126-135	132-147	141-158
6	2	156-167	162-180	173-194	5	10	130-140	136-151	145-163
6	3	160-171	167-185	178-199	5	11	134-144	140-155	149-168
6	4	164-175	172-190	182-204	6	0	138-148	144-159	153-173

*Metropolitan Life Insurance Company, New York.
†For girls between 18 and 25, subtract 1 pound for each year under 25.

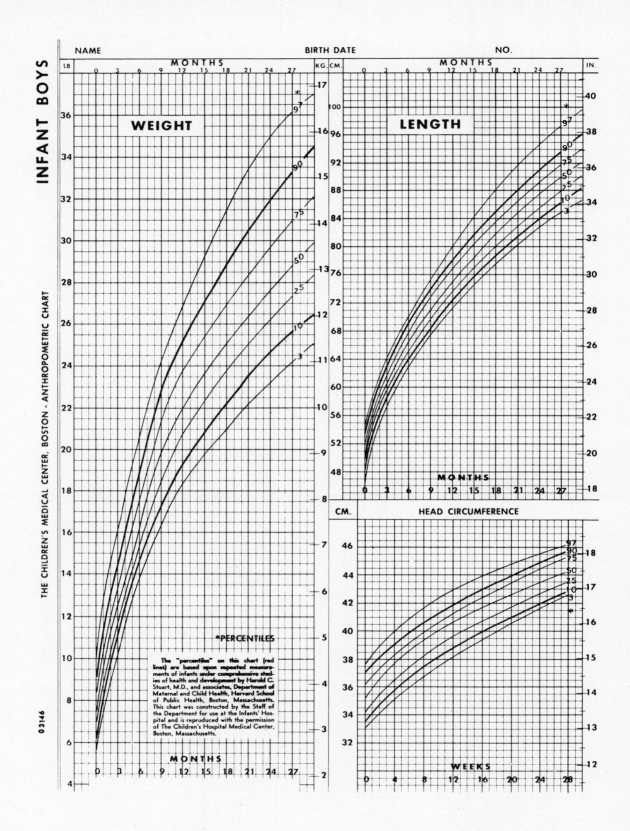

INFANT BOYS

THE CHILDREN'S MEDICAL CENTER, BOSTON - ANTHROPOMETRIC CHART

NAME   BIRTH DATE   NO.

WEIGHT

LENGTH

HEAD CIRCUMFERENCE

*PERCENTILES

The "percentiles" on this chart (red lines) are based upon repeated measurements of infants under comprehensive studies of health and development by Harold C. Stuart, M.D., and associates, Department of Maternal and Child Health, Harvard School of Public Health, Boston, Massachusetts. This chart was constructed by the Staff of the Department for use at the Infants' Hospital and is reproduced with the permission of The Children's Hospital Medical Center, Boston, Massachusetts.

03146

MONTHS

WEEKS

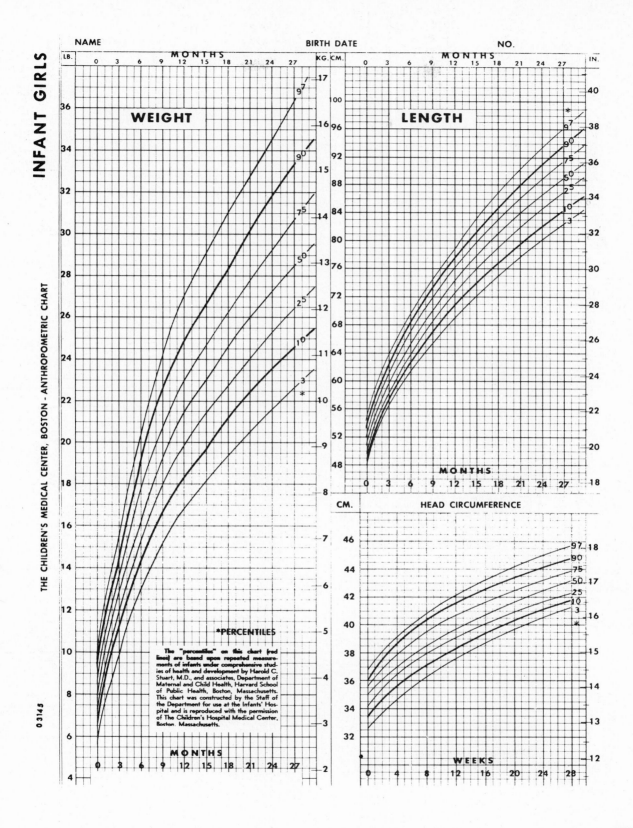

INFANT GIRLS

THE CHILDREN'S MEDICAL CENTER, BOSTON - ANTHROPOMETRIC CHART

WEIGHT

LENGTH

HEAD CIRCUMFERENCE

*PERCENTILES

The "percentiles" on this chart (red lines) are based upon repeated measurements of infants under comprehensive studies of health and development by Harold C. Stuart, M.D., and associates, Department of Maternal and Child Health, Harvard School of Public Health, Boston, Massachusetts. This chart was constructed by the Staff of the Department for use at the Infants' Hospital and is reproduced with the permission of The Children's Hospital Medical Center, Boston, Massachusetts.

03145

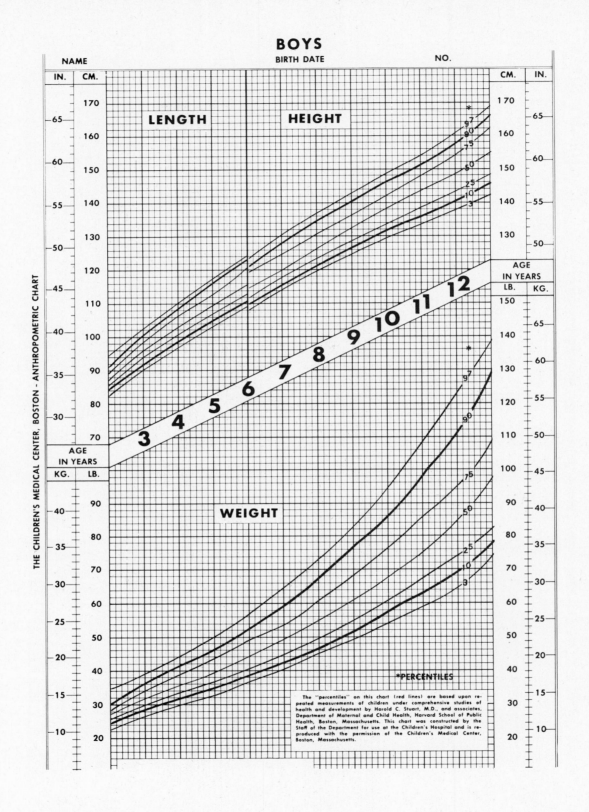

BOYS

NAME   BIRTH DATE   NO.

LENGTH   HEIGHT

AGE IN YEARS

WEIGHT

*PERCENTILES

THE CHILDREN'S MEDICAL CENTER, BOSTON - ANTHROPOMETRIC CHART

The "percentiles" on this chart (red lines) are based upon repeated measurements of children under comprehensive studies of health and development by Harold C. Stuart, M.D., and associates, Department of Maternal and Child Health, Harvard School of Public Health, Boston, Massachusetts. This chart was constructed by the Staff of the Department for use at the Children's Hospital and is reproduced with the permission of the Children's Medical Center, Boston, Massachusetts.

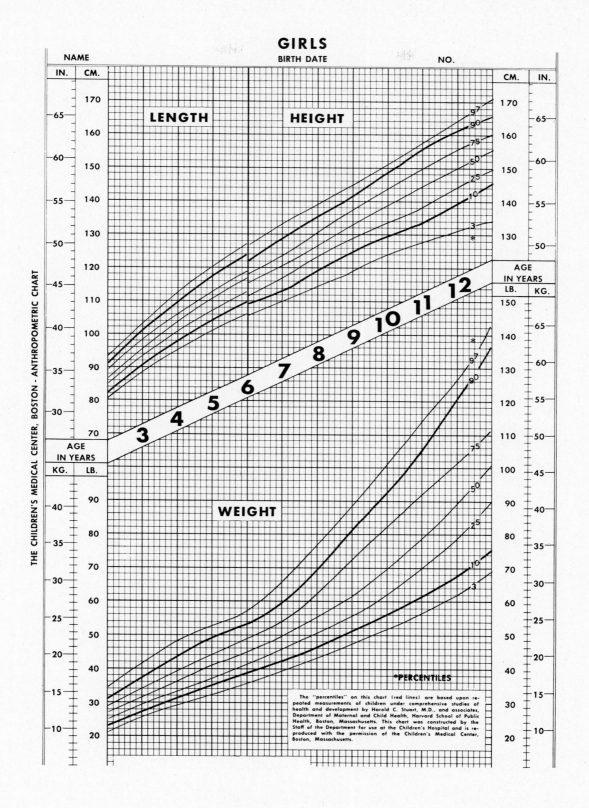

B Denver Developmental Screening Test

1. Try to get child to smile by smiling, talking or waving to him. Do not touch him.
2. When child is playing with toy, pull it away from him. Pass if he resists.
3. Child does not have to be able to tie shoes or button in the back.
4. Move yarn slowly in an arc from one side to the other, about 6" above child's face. Pass if eyes follow 90° to midline. (Past midline; 180°)
5. Pass if child grasps rattle when it is touched to the backs or tips of fingers.
6. Pass if child continues to look where yarn disappeared or tries to see where it went. Yarn should be dropped quickly from sight from tester's hand without arm movement.
7. Pass if child picks up raisin with any part of thumb and a finger.
8. Pass if child picks up raisin with the ends of thumb and index finger using an over hand approach.

         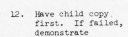

9. Pass any enclosed form. Fail continuous round motions.
10. Which line is longer? (Not bigger.) Turn paper upside down and repeat. (3/3 or 5/6)
11. Pass any crossing lines.
12. Have child copy first. If failed, demonstrate

When giving items 9, 11 and 12, do not name the forms. Do not demonstrate 9 and 11.

13. When scoring, each pair (2 arms, 2 legs, etc.) counts as one part.
14. Point to picture and have child name it. (No credit is given for sounds only.)

 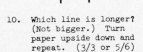 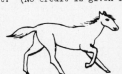

15. Tell child to: Give block to Mommie; put block on table; put block on floor. Pass 2 of 3. (Do not help child by pointing, moving head or eyes.)
16. Ask child: What do you do when you are cold? ..hungry? ..tired? Pass 2 of 3.
17. Tell child to: Put block on table; under table; in front of chair, behind chair. Pass 3 of 4. (Do not help child by pointing, moving head or eyes.)
18. Ask child: If fire is hot, ice is ?; Mother is a woman, Dad is a ?; a horse is big, a mouse is ?. Pass 2 of 3.
19. Ask child: What is a ball? ..lake? ..desk? ..house? ..banana? ..curtain? ..ceiling? ..hedge? ..pavement? Pass if defined in terms of use, shape, what it is made of or general category (such as banana is fruit, not just yellow). Pass 6 of 9.
20. Ask child: What is a spoon made of? ..a shoe made of? ..a door made of? (No other objects may be substituted.) Pass 3 of 3.
21. When placed on stomach, child lifts chest off table with support of forearms and/or hands.
22. When child is on back, grasp his hands and pull him to sitting. Pass if head does not hang back.
23. Child may use wall or rail only, not person. May not crawl.
24. Child must throw ball overhand 3 feet to within arm's reach of tester.
25. Child must perform standing broad jump over width of test sheet. (8-1/2 inches)
26. Tell child to walk forward, ⬤⬤⬤⬤➡ heel within 1 inch of toe. Tester may demonstrate. Child must walk 4 consecutive steps, 2 out of 3 trials.
27. Bounce ball to child who should stand 3 feet away from tester. Child must catch ball with hands, not arms, 2 out of 3 trials.
28. Tell child to walk backward, ⬅⬤⬤⬤⬤ toe within 1 inch of heel. Tester may demonstrate. Child must walk 4 consecutive steps, 2 out of 3 trials.

DATE AND BEHAVIORAL OBSERVATIONS (how child feels at time of test, relation to tester, attention span, verbal behavior, self-confidence, etc,):

Appendix

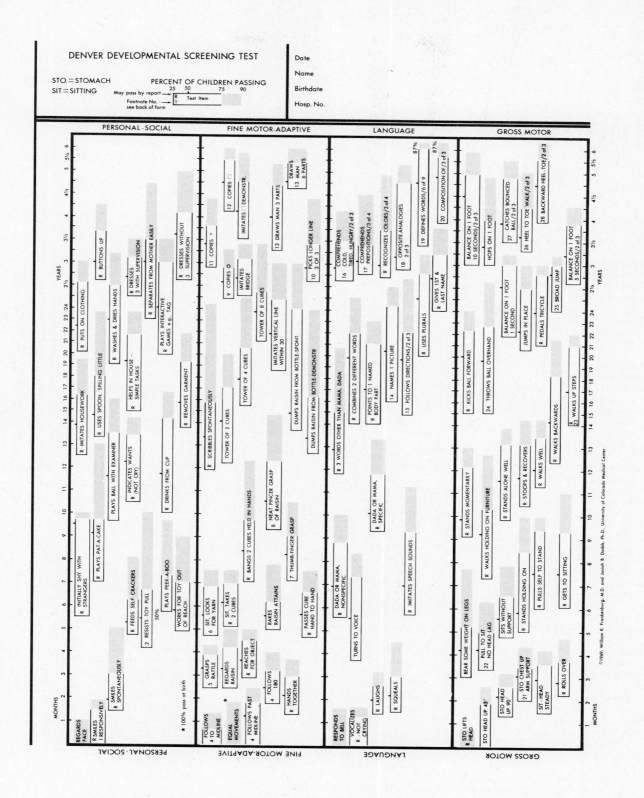

Index

A

ABCs and burns, 835
Abdomen, quadrants of, 900, 901
Abdominal breathing, 1240
Abdominal hysterectomy, 641
Abdominal injury masking, 476
Abdominal tap and cirrhosis, 962
Abdominal thrusts, 1353-1354
Abducens nerve, 669
  testing of, 365, 367-368
    for comatose client, 370
Abduction, 396
ABE, 1150-1151
Abortion, 649-652
  complete, 649
  criminal, 649
  drug-induced, 651
  habitual, 649
  imminent, 650
  incomplete, 649
  induced, 649, 650-652
  inevitable, 650
  mini, 651
  missed, 649
  saline, 651
  spontaneous, 649-650
  therapeutic, 649
  threatened, 649-650
Abrasions, 172, 776
  of eye, 713
Abscess, 168
  as cause of unconsciousness, 391
  of central nervous system, 505-506
  rectal, 1016
Absorption, prevention of, in poisoning, 111
Abuse, drug, 118
Abused woman, 575-577
Academic failure in adolescence, 42
Acceptance, 58
Accident liability, 104
Accident prevention, 107
Accident prone, 104
Accident repetitiveness, 103
Accident risks and precautions, 106
Accidental amputation, 577
Accidents, 103-105

Accidents—cont'd
  and age, 104-105
Accommodation-convergence reflex, 368
Acestix, 345
Acetaminophen
  and arthritis, 560
  and common cold, 1359
  and headache, 500
  and peptic ulcer disease, 944
  and teething, 890
  and vaccines, 786
Acetazolamide
  for electrolyte imbalance, 109
  and glaucoma
    closed-angle, 702
    open-angle, 700
  and poison victims, 114
Acetest, 345
Acetohexamide, 338
Acetone, urine tests for, 345
Acetylcholine, 1086
  and sleep, 235-236
Acetylcysteine, 1269
Achilles tendon reflex, 374
Acholic stools, 984
Acid(s)
  in eye, 714-715
  hydrochloric, 884
Acid-base regulation, 184-185
Acid burns, 850-851
Acid poisoning, 109-110
Acidosis
  and idiopathoc respiratory distress syndrome,
    1298-1299
  hyperchloremic metabolic, and total paren-
    teral nutrition, 919
  lactic, 350
  respiratory, 1346-1347
Acini, 586
Acne vulgaris, 806-810
  surgery for, 809
Acoustic nerve testing, 365, 369
  for comatose client, 370
Acromegaly, 303-304
ACTH, 288, 291, 296
  for chemotherapy, 161
Actinic keratosis, 820
Activated charcoal, 113
Active acquired immunity, 171
Active assistance exercises, 397

Activities of daily living, 442-443
  rating scale for, 223
    instrumental, 224
Activity
  after chest surgery, 1289
  and diabetes mellitus, 331
  and metabolism, 331
  after myocardial infarction, 1165-1166
  and pneumonia, 1363
  and rest
    after cardiac surgery, 1138-1139
    and dyspnea, 1258-1259
    and hypertension, 1197
  and sleep and nephrosis, 1055
  and water loss, 862
Activity theory, 14
Actual problem, 196-197
Acuity, visual; see Visual acuity
Acupuncture, 246
Acute pain, 242
Adaptation
  and coping, 138-142
  to stress, 6
Adaptation syndrome
  general, 139-140
  local, 139-140
Adaptive behavior, 21
  of adolescent, 82
  of adult, older, 84
  of child
    preschool, 74-77
    school-age, 78-80
  of neonate, 64-71
  of preadolescent, 81
  of toddler, 72-74
Addict personality, 118-119
Addiction, drug, 118
Addisonian crisis, 320-321
Addison's disease, 319-320
Adduction, 396
Adenocarcinoma, 151, 153
  of lung, 1351
Adenohypophysis, 289
Adenoidectomy, 1305-1307
Adenoiditis, 1305-1307
Adenoma, 151, 152
Adenomastectomy, 627
Adenoviruses, 1300
  and pneumonia, 1364
ADH, 289, 859

Aurothioglucose, 559
Auscultation
　of blood vessels, 1098
　of gastrointestinal system, upper, 900-901
　of heart, 1093-1095
　of respiratory system, 1241-1244
Autism, 33-34
Autograft, 846
Autoimmune theory, 15
Automaticity, 1086
Automatism, reflex, 476
Autonomic hyperreflexia, 474-475
Autonomy versus shame and doubt, 6, 11, 27-28
Autoregulation, 1026
Autosomes, 146
Aveeno, 791
Azathioprine
　and arthritis, 560
　and colitis, 997
　and lupus erythematosus, 813
　and renal transplant, 1079
Azoospermia, 619
Azotemia, 1069
　and head injuries, 454
　prerenal, 919
Azulfidine; see Sulfasalazine
Azuresin test, 905

B
Babinski's reflex, 372
　and spinal shock, 469
Babybird, 1271
Bacille Calmette-Guerin, 166
Bacilli, Doderlein, 586
Bacillus proteus, 1059
Bacitracin
　and conjunctivitis of newborn, 692
　and impetigo, 797
Back blows, 1353-1354
Bacterial conjunctivitis, 716
Bacteriological studies and respiratory system,
　1250-1252
BAL; see Dimercaprol
Balanced traction, 527, 531
Balanitis, 600
Baldness, 771
Ball squeezing, 631
Balloon pump, intraaortic, 1176-1177
Balloon septostomy, 1131-1132
"Band-Aid surgery," 608
Barbiturate coma, 492
Barbiturates
　as cause of unconsciousness, 391
　diuresis for overdose of, 122
　effects of, 120
　and epilepsy, 421
　and toxic hepatitis, 957
Bargaining, 58
Barium, 902
Barium enema, 987
Barometric pressure, effects of, 127
Barrel chest, 1237
Bartholinitis, 623
Bartholin's gland, 586
Basal cell carcinoma, 151, 153, 818-819
Basal metabolic rate, 885
Base, data, 198
Basedow's disease, 308-312
Baseline, wandering, 1100
Basic metabolic rate, 294

Basic need theory, 5-6
Basophils, 1088
Bathing, 781
　self-maintenance scale of, 223
Bathroom activities, 446
Baths, 790-791
Battered child syndrome, 575-577
Battered wife syndrome, 575
Battering, 575-577
Battery acid, antidote for, 109
Battle's sign, 451
BCG, 166
Bed board, 394
Bed-wetting, 31-32
Beef tapeworm infection, 995, 996
Behavior
　adaptive, 21
　fine motor, 21
　gross motor, 21
　health, 137-138
　illness, 138
　language, 21
　personal-social, 21
Behavior modification and obesity, 972
Behavioral changes and dehydration, 868
Behavioral risks, 134
Belladonna
　and colitis, 997
　and Parkinson's disease, 427
Benadryl; see Diphenhydramine
Bence-Jones protein, 568
Benemid; see Probenecid
Benign neoplasms, 152
Benign prostatic hypertrophy, 655-659
Bennett ventilators, 1271
Benzathine penicillin
　and rheumatic fever, 1147
　and syphilis, 617
Benzoyl peroxide, 809
Berkow's method, 836-837
Beta rays, 156
Beta adrenergic blockers, 700
Betamethasone, 301
Betazole, 905
Bicillin; see Benzathine penicillin, 617
BiCNU; see Carmustine
Biceps tendon reflex, 374
Bile, 884
　lithogenic, 950
Bile ducts, radiographs of, 902-903
Biliary atresia, 935
Biliary drainage, 905-906
　and gallbladder surgery, 952-953
Bilirubin, 906
Bilirubin assay, 906-907
Bill of rights for nonsmoker, 123-124
Biochemical parameters of nutrition, 899, 900
Biofeedback
　and migraine, 499
　and pain, 244
Biographical data, 194
Biological death, 1187
Biological theories of aging, 15
Bio-med MVP-10, 1271
Biopsy(ies)
　endometrial, and infertility, 620
　of gastrointestinal system, upper, 904-905
　liver, 904
　lung, 1250
　percutaneous renal, 1037

Biopsy(ies)—cont'd
　pleural, 1250
　punch, 779
　of reproductive system, 599-600
　　breast, 600
　　cervical, 599
　　dilation and curettage as, 599
　　testicular, 600
Biotin, 911
Biot's respirations, 455, 1239
　spirogram of, 1240
Bird ventilator, 1271
Birnberg bow, 609
Birth control pills, 608-609
Birth control planning, 607-611
Birth weight, low, 926-929
Black eye, 681, 713
Black food customs, 893, 894-897
Black lung, 1343
Blackheads, 807
Bladder, 1025
　effects of epinephrine and norepinephrine on,
　　290
　exstrophy of, 1050
　neurogenic, 1064-1065
　　electronic stimulation of, 1068
Bladder atony and spinal cord injury, 476
Bladder function
　and spinal shock, 469-471
　of unconscious client, 402
Bladder spasms and prostate surgery, 657-658
Bladder tap, percutaneous, 1030
Bladder tumors, 1058-1059
Blalock-Hanlen procedure, 1132
Blalock-Taussig procedure, 1131
Bland diet, 944
Blanching and decubiti, 393
Bleach, household, antidote, for, 109
Bleb, 776
Bleeding; see also Hemorrhage
　after amputation, 580
　after surgery, 280
　and Curling's ulcer, 848-849
　from eye, 681
　gastrointestinal, and chemotherapy, 165
　managing, and leukemia, 1221
　and multiple trauma, 576
　and open-heart surgery, 1139
Blenoxane; see Bleomycin
Bleomycin, 160
　and cancer of testis, 661
Blepharitis, 696
Blepharoplasty, 706
Blindness, 685, 686-691
　of child, 687
　eclipse, 716
　education for, 687-688
　of hospitalized client, 689-691
　night, 670
　reactions to, 686
　rehabilitation of, 688-689
Blinking, excessive, 672
Blinking reflex of unconscious client, 401
Blister, 168, 776
Blistering and radiation, 158
Blood, 1088-1089
　administration of, 264-267
　　complications following, 265-267
　　　air embolism as, 266, 267
　　　allergic reaction as, 266, 267

1400

Epinephrine—cont'd
and open-angle glaucoma, 700
and peptic ulcer disease, 946
and pheochromocytoma, 325
physiological effects of, 290
and plasma glucose level, 343
and rhinoscopy, 1247
and shock, 183
and status asthmaticus, 1368
and urticaria, 827
Epiphora, 672
Epiphysis, 512
slipped femoral capital, 554
Epiphysitis of tibial tubercle, 554
Episodic care, 202
Epispadias, 612
Epistaxis, 1355-1358
Epithelial sloughing and radiation, 158
Epithelium, neoplasms arising from, 151
Epstein-Barr virus, 1149-1150
Epstein's pearls, 900
Equalizer ground bus, 233
Equilibrium, 5
Equine encephalitis, 502-503
Equanil; see Meprobamate
Equinus, 546
Ergocalciferol, 317
Ergotamine tartrate, 498
plus caffeine, 498
Erikson, Erik, 6, 11
Ernst applicator, 639
Erosion, 776
ERS, 650
ERV, 1254
Erythema
palmar, and cirrhosis, 961
and radiation, 158
Erythema marginatum, 1146
Erythroblastosis fetalis, 1216
and hearing loss, 744
Erythrocyte sedimentation rate, 1109
Erythrocytes, 1088
Erythromycin
and acne, 807, 809
and impetigo, 797
and legionnaire's disease, 1316
and meningitis, 501
and pneumonia, 1362, 1363
Erythropenia, 164
Eschar, 844
formation of, 848
Escharotomy, 844
Escherichia coli, 501
and cholecystitis, 954
and cystic fibrosis, 1307
and diarrhea, 1016
and urinary tract infections, 1059
and vaginitis, 621, 622
Esophageal defects, 933-934
Esophageal speech, 763
Esophageal varices, 964-966
Esophagitis, 939
and radiation, 159
Esophagogastric tube, 964
Esophagoscopy, 903-904
Esophagostomy feedings, 925
Esophagus, 884
cancer of, 939-940
radiographs of, 902
Esophoria, 693

Esotropia, 693
ESR, 1109
Establishment phase of family, 95-96
Estrogen(s), 292, 586
and advanced breast cancer, 634
and cancer of prostate, 660
for chemotherapy, 161
and menopause, 606
and osteoporosis, 568
and rape, 663
and sodium retention, 291
Ethambutol, 1325
Ethanol, effects of, 120
Ethchlorvynol, effects of, 120
Ether, 277
topical, 616
Ethinamate, effects of, 120
Ethionamide, 1325
Ethmoidectomy, 1313
Ethnic influences on food, 894-897, 898
Ethylene, 277
Ethyl chloride, 277
Eustress, 6
Euthroid; *see* Liotrix
Eutonyl; *see* Parglyline
Evacuation
during fire, 231
of retained secundines, 650
Evaluation
of acne, 809-810
of adrenocortical insufficiency, 320
of anaphylaxis, 829
of anemia, 1217-1218
of aneurysm, 1204
of assisted locomotion, 537
of asthma, 1370
of atelectasis, 1372
of auditory system and speech, 765
of breast cancer, 636
of bronchogenic carcinoma, 1352
of carbuncle, 811
of carcinoma of larynx, 764-765
of cardiogenic shock, 1177
of cardiovascular system, 1223-1224
of casts, 524
of cataracts, 706
of cerebrovascular disease, 447
of chest trauma, 1329
of cholelithiasis and cholecystitis, 955
of chronic obstructive pulmonary disease,
1340
of cirrhosis, 966
of cleft lip and palate, 933
of colorectal cancer, 1013
of common cold, 1360
of congenital heart disease, 1140-1141
of congenital hip dysplasia, 545
of conjunctivitis of newborn, 693
of cradle cap, 795-796
of croup, 1303
of cystic fibrosis, 1309
of dehydration, 869-870
of dermatitis
atopic, 805
contact, 806
of diabetes, 354
of diaper rash, 794
of dysmenorrhea, 649
of dysrhythmias, 1193
of ecthyma, 798

Evaluation—cont'd
of edema, 873
of encephalitis, 503
of endocrine imbalance, 880-881
of endocrine system, 355
of fluid and electrolyte balance, 881
of foreign bodies in ear, 736-737
of fracture, 573
of gastrointestinal system
lower, 1022-1023
upper, 978
of glaucoma, 703
of glomerulonephritis, 1052-1053
of head injury, 464-465
of heart failure, 1174-1175
of hemangiomas, 793
of hemophilia, 1145
of hepatitis, 959-960
of Hodgkin's disease, 1149
of hypertension, 1199
of hyperthyroidism, 312
of hypothermia, 817
of hysterectomy, 644
of idiopathic respiratory distress syndrome,
1299
of impetigo, 798
of integumentary system, 852-853
of intertrigo, 796
of legionnaire's disease, 1316
of leukemia, 1222-1223
of lupus erythematosus, 815
of malignant melanoma, 822
of Meniere's disease, 741
of miliaria, 794-795
of multiple sclerosis, 424
of musculoskeletal system, 582
of myasthenia gravis, 426
of myocardial infarction, 1167
of myxedema, 307-308
of nasal polyps, 1313
of nasal surgery, 1312
of nephrosis, 1055-1056
of neurological system, 506-507
of obesity, 973
of otitis externa, chronic, 742
of otitits media, 735
chronic, 735
of otosclerosis, 740
of Parkinson's disease, 427-428
of pediculosis, 802
of peptic ulcer disease, 949-950
of pheochromocytoma, 327
of pleurisy, 1349
of pneumoconiosis, 1344
of pneumonia, 1366
of presenile dementia, 449-450
of prostate surgery, 659
of psoriasis, 812
of pulmonary embolism, 1320-1321
of renal calculi, 1058
of renal failure, 1080-1081
of reproductive system, 664
of respiratory system, 1372
of retinal detachment, 698
of retinoblastoma, 696
of retrolental fibroplasia, 692
of rheumatic fever, 1146-1147
of rheumatoid arthritis, 566
of scoliosis, 552
of seizures, 497

Griseofulvin, 800
Grooming, self-maintenance scale of, 223
Gross motor behavior, 21
Ground equalization, 232-233
Grounding, 232
Growth(s), 17
   in adolescence, 40-41
   assessment of, 19-20
   on conjunctiva, 673
   and development, 10-86
      assessment of, 19-21
      and cerebral edema, 487
      principles of, 17-19
      and seizures, 494
      table of, 64-84
   on eyelid, 672
Growth charts, anthropometric, 1379-1383
Growth hormone and dwarfism, 303
Growth hormone releasing factor, 289
Guaiac examination, 987
Guanethidine, 1197
Guide dog, 688
Guidelines for bowel training, 989
Guillain-Barré syndrome, 503
Guillotine amputation, 578
Guilt, 29
Gummas, 617
Gynecogram, nitrous oxide, 600
Gynecomastia, 587
Gynergen; see Ergotamine tartrate

H

HA$_s$Hg, 958
Habitual abortion, 649
Haemophilus influenzae, 501
   and croup, 1302
   and cystic fibrosis, 1307
   and osteomyelitis, 547
   and otitis media, 734
Haemophilus ducreyi, 614, 618
Hageman factor, 1109
Hair, 774, 775
   in neonates, 19
Half-cord lesion, 466
Half-life, 156
Half-ring splint, 572
Hall-Stone ring, 609
Halo traction, 478
Halo-femoral traction, 551
Halo-pelvic traction, 551-553
Halothane, 277
Halter, head, 477
Hammock sling, 531
Hand care after mastectomy, 634
Hand rolls, 394
Hands, arthroplasty of, 565
Haptens, 170
Harrington rod, 552, 553
Hartmann's solution, 253
Harvey-Rand-Rittler plates, 676
Hashimoto's thyroiditis, 316
Havighurst, Robert, 7-8
Hay fever, 716-717
Hazards, developmental, 21-23
   of adolescent, 42-43
   of adult, 51-52
   of child
      preschool, 29-32
      school-age, 33-37
HB$_e$Ag antigens, 956

HB$_s$Ag antigens, 956
HBIG, 956
HBV, 956
HDL, 1114
Head circumference, chart for, 18, 1380
Head cold, 168
Head halter, 477
Head injury(ies), 450-465
   cardiovascular factors in, 455-456
   as cause of unconsciousness, 391
Head injuries
   closed, 452
   emergency care of, 457-459
   and eye movements and oculovestibular re-
      sponse, 462
   gastrointestinal factors in, 456
   and level of consciousness, 461
   metabolic factors in, 453-454
   and motor functioning, 463
   and pupil size and reaction, 462
   respiratory factors in, 454-455
   and respiratory pattern, 461-462
Head measurements of child, 366
Heat tilt/chin lift maneuver, 1121
   for infant, 1122
Head tilt/neck lift maneuver, 1121
   for infant, 1122
Headache, 497-500
   and cerebral edema, 488
   cluster, 499-500
   inflammatory, 499
   and meningitis, 500
   migraine, 497-499
   muscle contraction, 499
   nasomotor reaction, 499
   sinus, 499
   traction, 499
   vascular, 497-499
Headstart, 92
Healing of wounds; see Wounds, healing of
Health/behavior, 137-138
Health
   and health problems, 133-143
   and high-level wellness, 133-134
   and illness
      determinants of, 136-137
      perceptions of, 137
Health Belief Model, 138
Health care delivery systems, 202-210
   and government, 209-210
   organization and location of, 203-209
      disaster, 204-209
      emergency, 204
      regionalization of, 204
Health hazard appraisal, 135
Health history, 194
   of auditory system, 722-723
   of cardiovascular system, 1089-1090
   of endocrine system, 291-292
   of gastrointestinal system
      lower, 983-984
      upper, 885-886
   of integumentary system, 769
      focus questions for, 770
   of musculoskeletal system, 512-513
   of neurological system, 363
   of reproductive system, 590-591
   of respiratory system, 1231-1234
   of urinary system, 1026
   of visual system, 669-670

Health-illness continuum, 133-136
Health maintenance organizations, 202-
   203
Hearing of unconscious client, 401
Hearing aids, 746-748
   body, 746
   caring for, 747-748
   eyeglass, 746
   in-the-ear, 746-747
   postauricular, 746
   selection of, 747
Hearing impairment, 744-751; *see also* Hearing
      loss
   caring for client with, 732-733
   conductive, 744
   coping with, 745-746
   education for client with, 750-751
   mixed, 744
   noise-induced, 131
   reactions to, 744-745
   rehabilitation for, 746-751
   sensorineural, 744
   suggestions for clients with, 745
Hearing problems, detection of, 730-731
Heart, 1085-1087
   auscultation of, 1093-1095
   blood supply of, 1085
   conduction system of, 1085-1086
   increased workload of, and immobility,
      539
   inspection of, 1092
   nervous system control of, 1086
   output of, 1086-1087
   palpation of, 1092
   percussion of, 1093
   rate and rhythm of, 1093
Heart blocks, 1179, 1182-1183
   first-degree, 1182
   second-degree, 1182-1183
   third-degree, 1183
   Wenchebach, 1182-1183
Heart defects
   acyanotic, 1127-1130
   cyanotic, 1130-1132
Heart disease; *see also* Cardiovascular system,
      problems of
   atherosclerotic, 1152
   congenital, 1127-1141
      acyanotic, 1127-1130
      cyanotic, 1130-1132
   ischemic, 1152-1153
   valvular, 1211-1212
Heart failure, 1167-1175
   acute, 1168
   causes of, 1168
   chronic, 1168
   left-sided, 1167
   right-sided, 1167-1168, 1169
Heart rate, 1090
Heart sounds, 1093-1094
   anatomical areas used to locate, 1094
Heat
   and degeneration, 186
   and humidity, effects of, 126
Heat rush, 794-795
Heat therapy and arthritis, 560
Hedulin; *see* Phenindione
Heel walking, 377
Heel-to-knee-to-toe test, 376
Heimlich chest drainage valve, 1292

Hydrocephalus—cont'd
  surgery for, 405-406
Hydrochloric acid, 884
  antidote for, 109
Hydrocortisone
  and adrenocortical insufficiency, 319
  and chronic obstructive pulmonary disease, 1333
  and otitis externa, 740
    chronic, 741
  and pruritus, 791
  side effects of, 301
Hydrocortisone ointment and allergic conjunctivitis, 717
Hydrocortisone sodium succinate
  and adrenal crisis, 321
  and anaphylaxis, 829
Hydrophilic lenses, 683
Hydrostatic forces, 859
Hydrotherapy, 845
Hydrothorax, 872
Hydroxychloroquine
  and arthritis, 559
  and discoid lupus erythematosus, 814
17-Hydroxycorticosteroid tests, 295-296
Hydroxyzine, 827
Hygiene, personal, and reproductive system, 601-605
  female, 601-604
  male, 604-605
Hykinone; see Menadione sodium bisulfite
Hymen, 586
Hyperadrenocorticism, 321
Hyperalimentation
  enteral, 916
  and head injuries, 454
  parenteral, 916-918
Hyperammonemia, 919
Hyperbaric oxygen, 1268
Hypercalcemia, 879-880
Hypercapnia, 1255
Hypercholesterolemia, 1114-1115
  prevention of, 1114-1115
  risk management of, 1115
Hypercoagulability and pulmonary embolism, 1316
Hyperemia and decubiti, 393
Hyperextension, 396
Hyperglycemia, 919
Hyperglycemic, hyperosmolar, nonketotic coma, 350
Hyperhemolytic crisis, 1142
Hyperkalemia, 874, 877
Hyperkalemic reaction to blood transfusion, 266
Hyperkinesias, 376
Hypermagnesemia, 880
Hypernasality, 759
Hypernatremia, 875, 878-879
Hyperopia, 671, 711
Hyperosmolar coma, 350
Hyperosmolar nonketotic dehydration, 919
Hyperparathyroidism, 317-319
  primary, 317-318
  secondary, 319
Hyperphoria, 693
Hyperpigmentation, 774
Hyperpituitarism, 303-304
Hyperplasia, 146, 187
Hyperpnea, 1239

Hyperreflexia, autonomic, 474-475
Hypersensitivity reactions, 823-826
Hyperstat; see Diazoxide
Hypertension, 1193-1199
  benign, 1193, 1194
  complications of, 1199
  drugs for, 1197-1198
  essential, 1193, 1194
  and hemodialysis, 1077
  intracranial, 486-492
  malignant, 1193, 1194
  portal, 963-964
  preventing, 1041, 1114
  primary, 1193, 1194
    diagnostic standards for, 1196
    phases of, 1194
    risk factors of, 1195
  pulmonary, and cor pulmonale, 1340
  as risk factor in cardiovascular disease, 1113-1114
  risk management of, 1114
  secondary, 1193, 1194
  and sodium regulation, 1194, 1197
  after surgery, 275
Hypertet; see Hyperimmune globulin
Hyperthermia and cranial surgery, 486
Hyperthermia blanket, 122
Hyperthyroidism, 308-312
Hypertonic solutions, 503
Hypertonicity, 375
  solute-loading, 870
Hypertrophy, 146, 187, 375
Hypertropia, 693
Hyperuricemia, 165
Hyperventilation, 1237
  alveolar, 1347
  and head injury, 454-455
  spirogram of, 1239
Hypnosis and pain, 244-245
Hypnotics and alcohol, 252
Hypoaldosteronism, 324
Hypocalcemia, 874, 879
  and hypoparathyroidism, 316
Hypocalcemic reaction to blood transfusion, 266
Hypocapnia, 1255
Hypodermoclysis, 864
Hypoglossal nerve testing, 365, 369-370
  for comatose client, 370
Hypoglycemia, 338, 345-348
  as cause of unconsciousness, 391
  exercise-induced, 348
  and low birth weight, 927-928
  and total parenteral nutrition, 919
Hypoglycemic drugs and diabetes mellitus, 337-338
Hypoglycemic reactions
  and diabetic coma, 347
  warning symptoms of, 346
Hypogonadism, 303
Hypokalemia, 874, 875-877
  drug-induced, 252
  and total parenteral nutrition, 919
Hypomagnesemia, 874, 880
  and total parenteral nutrition, 919
Hyponasality, 759
Hyponatremia, 875, 877-878
  and total parenteral nutrition, 919
Hypoparathyroidism, 316-317
Hypophosphatemia, 919

Hypophysectomy
  and breast cancer, 636
  and cancer of prostate, 660
  transphenoid, 304
Hypophysis gland, 288
Hypopigmentation, 774
Hypopituitarism, 302-303
Hypoplasia, 187
Hyposensitization, 824
Hyposmia, 366
Hypospadias, 611-612
Hypotension
  and hemodialysis, 1077
  orthostatic, and syncope, 493
  postural, and immobility, 539, 540
  and spinal shock, 471
  after surgery, 275
Hypothalamus, 359, 885
Hypothermia, 817-818
  accidental, 823
  and cerebral edema, 490-491
  after surgery, 276
  open-heart, 1133
Hypothermic reaction from blood transfusion, 264, 266
Hypothyroidism, 305
  juvenile, 306
Hypotonicity, 375
Hypotropia, 693
Hypoventilation, 1239
  alveolar
    and respiratory acidosis, 1346
    and respiratory failure, 1344
  and multiple trauma, 576
  spirogram of, 1239
  after surgery, 275
Hypovolemic shock, 178
Hypoxemia, 1255
  and head injury, 454, 455
Hypoxia, 1263
  hypoxic, 1263
Hypoxic test, 1298
Hysterectomy, 641-644
  and sterility, 608
Hysterogram, 600
Hysterosalpingogram, 600
Hysterotomy, 652

I

^{131}I, 294
Iatrogenic disease, 251-252
Ibuprofen
  and arthritis, 559
  and dysmenorrhea, 648
  and osteoarthritis, 569
IC, 1254
ICSH, 288
Icterus, 1091
Icterus index, 906
Ictus, 495
Id, 25
Id level, 11
Identity
  versus diffusion, 41, 43
  versus role confusion, 6, 11
Idioventricular rhythm, low, 1186
IDL, 1114
IF, 289
IgA, 170, 171
IgD, 170

IgE, 170, 171
IgG, 170, 171
IgM, 170, 171
Ileal conduit, 1047-1049
Ileocecal valve, 983
Ileostomy, 991, 998-1003
    collecting drainage from, 1000-1001, 1002-
        1003
    complications of, 1001
    continent, 998, 999
    Koch, 998
    and nutrition, 1001-1002
    and partial colectomy, 998
    pouch, 998, 999
Ileum, 983
Ileus
    meconium, 993-994
    paralytic, 1022
        and spinal shock, 471
Illiterate E test, 675
Illness, 136
    and health
        determinants of, 136-137
            environment as, 136-137
            heredity and life-style as, 136
        perceptions of, 137
    and nutrition, 898
    pathophysiological processes of, 144-188
    precursors of, 133, 134-136
        risk as, 134-135
        vulnerability as, 136
    psychosomatic, 140
Illness behavior, 138
Illumination, 681-682
Imferon; see Iron-dextran
Immersion scald burns, 830
Imminent abortion, 650
Immobility, 537-542
    and decubitus ulcer, 538
    developmental considerations of, 541-542
    and foot drop, 537
    hazards of, 537-541
    after hip arthroplasty, 563-564
    and sensory alterations, 537, 538
    and skin breakdown, 537-540
    after surgery, 281
Immobilization and fracture, 571-572
Immune competence, 899, 900
Immune system, 170-172
Immunity, 171-172
    active acquired, 171
    natural, 171
    passive acquired, 171-172
    species, 171
Immunization, 782-788
    assessment guide for, 787
    schedules for, 782-783
Immunization card, 788
Immunoglobulins, 170
Immunosuppressive agents and arthritis, 560
Immunosuppressive responses to renal trans-
    plant, 1079-1080
Immunotherapeutic agents, 166
Immunotherapy for cancer, 163-166
Impact stage of disaster, 205
Impacted fracture, 569
Impaction, 989
    and immobility, 539, 540
    removal of, 989-990
Impetigo, 796-798

Implant
    breast, 634
    corneal, 708
    radioactive, and pituitary tumor, 304
Implementation; see also Planning and imple-
        mentation
    for allergy, 825
    for auditory system, 733-751
    for cardiovascular system, 1127-1224
    for endocrine system, 302-354
    for endotracheal intubation, 1276
    for fluid and electrolyte balance, 865-881
    for gastrointestinal system
        lower, 992-1022
        upper, 926-978
    for integumentary system, 791-852
    for musculoskeletal system, 542-582
    for neurological system, 403-506
    for reproductive system, 611-664
    for respiratory system, 1295-1372
    for speech, 757-765
    as stage of nursing process, 199-200
    for urinary system, 1049-1081
    for visual system, 691-712
Impotence and diabetes, 352
Imuran; see Azathioprine
Incentive spirometry, 1270
Incised wound, 172
Incisional hernia, 978
Incontinence, 1040, 1064
    overflow, 1064
    stress, 1059, 1064
    and unconscious client, 402
    urgency, 1064
Incubator, 1264, 1265
Indentation tonometer, 677, 678
Independence, promoting after cardiovascular
        disease, 442-444
Inderal; see Propranolol
Index, icterus, 906
Indian, American, food customs of, 894-897
Indocin; see Indomethacin
Indomethacin
    and arthritis, 559
    and dysmenorrhea, 648
    and gout, 567
    and patent ductus arteriosus, 1127-1128
Induced abortion, 649, 650-652
Induction, menstrual, 651
Industry versus inferiority, 6, 11, 32
Inevitable abortion, 650
Infant, 24-27
    accident risks of, 106
    adaptive behavior of, 64-71
    auditory system of, 723
        problems of, 734-737
    and immersion scald burns, 830
    cardiac surgery for, 1135
    cardiovascular system of, 1091
        problems of, 1127-1145
    chest percussion and vibrations for, 1337
    congenital heart disease of, 1134
    dentition of, 66-68, 890
    developmental tasks of, 28
    feeding patterns of, 889-890
    gastrointestinal system of
        lower, 984
            problems of, 992-994
        upper, 889-890
            problems of, 926-938

Infant—cont'd
    hearing ability of, 725
    hospitalized, 214-219
        admission of, 216-217
        planning for, 215
        psychological impact on, 218-219
        visiting and rooming-in with, 217-218
    and immobility, 541
    integumentary system of, 770
        problems of, 793-806
    musculoskeletal system of, 513
        problems of, 542-547
    neurological system of, 364
        problems of, 403-410
    personal-social development of, 64-71
    physical development of, 64-71
    reproductive system of, 591
        problems of, 611-613
    respiratory system of, 1235-1236
        problems of, 1300-1310
    sensorimotor development of, 64-71
    and sleep, 235
    speech of, 754
        development of, 64-71
    urinary system of, 1026-1027
        problems of, 1049-1050
    urinary tract infections of, 1061
    visual system of, 670-671
        problems of, 693-696
    weight gain of, 890
Infantile reflexes, disappearance of, 373
Infantile seizures, 494
Infarct, 185
Infarction
    cerebral, 433-434
    myocardial; see Myocardial infarction
    pulmonary, 1321
Infection
    beef tapeworm, 995, 996
    and bronchogenic carcinoma, 1350
    and burns, 842
    under cast, 524
    and common cold, 1359-1360
    and diabetes, 351
    and dyspnea, 1262
    and emphysema, 1334
    of eye, 716-717
    and glomerulonephritis, 1052
    after hip arthroplasty, 564
    hookworm, 995
    and hydrocephalus, 406
    kidney, 1062-1063
    prevention of
        and cardiovascular disease, 1119
        and leukemia, 1221
    and nephrosis, 1055
    of neurological system, 500-506
    and open-heart surgery, 1139
    parasitic, 994-996
    pinworm, 994, 995
    and pneumonia, 1362-1363
    puerperal, 624
    of reproductive system, 621-624
    and status asthmaticus, 1369
    urinary tract, 1059-1062
        preventing, 1040-1041
    vaginal, 621-622
Infertility, 619-621
Infiltration of intravenous infusion, 260
Inferiority, 32

1414

Mesh graft, 846
Metabolic demands, reducing, and dyspnea, 1258-1262
Metabolic equivalents, 1165, 1166
Metabolic factors in head injuries, 453-454
Metabolic rate, decreased, and immobility, 538
Metabolic studies of pituitary function, 294-295
Metabolism and burns, 833
Metamorphopsia, 670
Metaplasia, 146, 187
Metaraminol
  and anaphylaxis, 829
  and shock, 183
Metastasis, 152
  of breast cancer, 625
    advanced, 635
Methadone and drug addiction, 119
Methanol-extracted residue of BCG, 166
Methdilazine, 789
Methicillin, 1363
Methimazole, 310
Method, Credé, 1067
Methotrexate, 160, 162
  and breast cancer, 636
  and leukemia, 1219
  and lung cancer, 1351
  and osteogenic sarcoma, 554
  and psoriasis, 812
Methoxamine, 183
Methoxyflurane, 277
Methyldopa
  and enzyme indicators, 345
  and hypertension, 1197
Methylphenidate, 417
Methylprednisolone, 301
  and COPD, 1333
  and shock, 183
Methysergide, 499
Metoprolol, 1197
Metronidazole, 617
Metrorrhagia, 638
METS, 1165, 1166
Mexican food customs, 893, 894-897
MH, 288
Microcirculation, 1087
Micrococcus and vaginitis, 621
Micronazole
  and moniliasis, 618
  and herpes genitalis II, 616
Microphthalmos, 673
Microsporum canis, 800
Microtia, 733
Microwaves, effects of, 126
Midbrain, 359
Middle childhood, 32-37
Middle years stage of family, 99
Midlife crisis, 52
Midstream specimen, 1029
MIFR, 1254
Migraine headache, 497-499
Miliaria, 794-795
Milibis; *see* Glycobiarsol
Military antishock trousers, 178
Milk
  for gastric lavage, 113
  of magnesia, 942
Milk-alkali syndrome, 943
Miller-Abbott tube, 990
Milliequivalent, 860
Milliosmol, 860

Milwaukee brace, 532, 550-551
Mineralocorticoid hormone, 291
Mineralocorticord suppression tests, 296
Mineralocorticoids, 301
  and fluid balance, 859-860
Minimal brain dysfunction, 415-417
Minipress; *see* Prazosin
Minute volume, 1254
Mirror biopsy, 600
Miscarriage, 649
Missed abortion, 649
Mist tent
  and croup, 1300, 1301-1302
  and cystic fibrosis, 1308
Mistogen test, 1265
Mithracin; *see* Mithramycin
Mithramycin, 160
  and hypercalcemia, 880
Mixed tumor, 151
MMR, 783
Mobile intensive care unit, 204
Mobile spasm, 376
Mobility and arthritis, 561-562
Mobility, impaired physical
  and arterial aneurysm, 436
  and arthritis, 557
  and cerebral embolism, 433
  and cerebral infarction, 433
  and cerebral thrombosis, 431
  and congenital hip dysplasia, 544
  and fracture, 571
  and hypothermia, 817
    accidental, 823
  and integumentary system, 781, 852
  and lupus erythematosus, 813
  and musculoskeletal system, 517, 582
  and immobility, 538, 540
  and intracerebral hemorrhage, 434
  and neurological system, 389, 506
  and scoliosis, 550
Modeling, 572
Models, nursing, 200-202
  adaptation, 201-202
  life process, 202
  self-care, 201
Modification, behavior, and obesity, 972
Mold, 825
Molestation, sexual, 661
Molybdenum, 911
Mongolian spots, 792
Mongolism, 147
Moniliasis, 614, 618
Monistat; *see* Myconazole
Monitoring of intracranial pressure, 488-489
Monoamine oxidase inhibitors; *see* MAO inhibitors
Monocytes, 1088
Mononucleosis, infectious, 1149-1150
Monoplegia, 375
Montgomery's glands, 586
Mons pubis, 586
MOPP, 1148
Moral development, theory of, 15-17
Morbidity and smoking, 123
"Morning-after" pill, 611
Morning glory seeds, effects of, 121
Moro's reflex, 371
Morphine
  and burns, 838
  and closed-angle glaucoma, 702

Morphine—cont'd
  and heart failure, 1171
  and meningitis, 502
  and myocardial infarction, 1161
  and pulmonary embolism, 1318
  and toxic hepatitis, 957
Mortality and smoking, 123
Motivators, needs as, 5
Motor ability, assessment guide for, 377
Motor aphasia, 438
Motor functioning
  assessment of, 374-379
    and spinal cord abnormality, 409
  changes in, 378-379
  loss of, and cerebral edema, 488
Motor strength and power, 375
Motrin; *see* Ibuprofen
Mourning, 57-58
Mouth, 884
  cancer of, 938-939
  inflammations of, 969-970
  radiographs of, 902
Mouth care and radiation, 160
Movements, clonic, 495
Moving, crises of, 140-141
MUAC, 899
Mucomyst; *see* Acetylcysteine
Mucosa, protecting, and peptic ulcer disease, 943
Mucous membranes
  as defense, 167
  and dehydration, 868
  and oxygen, 1264
Mucous patches and syphilis, 616
Multiple births, 24
Multiple myeloma, 151, 568
Multiple sclerosis, 422-424
Multiple sclerosis personality, 423
Multiple trauma, 575
Mummy restraint, 268
Mumps, 784-785
  vaccine for, 782, 783
Mumps toxoid, 166
Murmurs, 901, 1094-1095
  intensity of, 1095
  location of, 1095
  pitch of, 1095
  quality, 1095
  timing of, 1095
Muscle(s), 512
  effects of epinephrine and norepinephrine on, 290
  electrical impulses of, 378-379
  neoplasms arising from, 151
Muscle contraction headache, 499
Muscle contractures and immobility, 538
Muscle cramp, 376-377
Muscle-setting exercises, gluteal, 518
Muscle relaxants and hip arthroplasty, 564
Muscle spasm and fracture, 571
Muscle tone, assessment of, 375
Muscle volume and contour, assessment of, 375
Muscular dystrophy, 147, 419
Musculoskeletal assessment for poisoning, 111
Musculoskeletal system, 511-584
  assessment of, 512-517
  data analysis of, 517
  evaluation of, 582
  overview of, 512

Trichomoniasis, 614, 617-618
Trichophyton tonsurans, 800
Tricuspid atresia, 1127, 1132
Triethylene-thiophosphoramide, 161
Trigeminal nerve testing, 365, 368-369
  for comatose client, 370
Trigeminal neuralgia, 428
Triglycerides, 1114
  serum, 1109
Triiodothyronine, 289
Triiodothyronine concentration test, 294
Triiodothyronine suppression test, 294
Trimeprazine
  and atopic dermatitis, 805
  and pruritus, 789
Trisomy 21, 419
TRH, 289
Trochanter rolls, 394
Trochlear nerve, 669
Trochlear nerve testing, 365, 367-368
  for comatose client, 370
Trophectoderm, neoplasm of, 151
Tropia, 676
Tropic hormones of pituitary, 288
Trousseau's sign, 311-312
TRP, 295
Truncus arteriosus, 1127, 1132
Truss, 977
Trust
  versus mistrust, 6, 11, 26
  promoting in infant, 89
Tryptamines, effects of, 121
L-Tryptophan and sleep, 235
TSF, 899
TSH, 288, 289, 294
TSH-RF, 289
Tubal insufflation, 620
Tubal ligation, 608
Tube(s)
  Cantor, 990
  cuffed tracheostomy, 1277-1278
  Dennis, 990
  double-lumen, 990, 991
  endotracheal, 1277
  esophagogastric, 964
  Ewald, 964
  gastrointestinal, 990, 991
  Kaslow, 990
  Keofeed, 924
  Miller-Abbott, 990
  nephrostomy, 1042-1043
  Sengstaken-Blakemore, 964, 965
  ureterostomy, 1042
Tubercle, 776
Tuberculin, old, 1252
Tuberculosis, 1323-1326
  classification of, 1324
  drugs for, 1325
  miliary, 1309-1310
  pneumonectomy and, 1351
  respiratory isolation and precautions for, 1325
  sites affected by, 1323
  skin tests for, 1252-1253
  and thoracoplasty, 1351
Tuberculous meningitis, 501
Tubular function tests, 1036-1037
Tubular reabsorption of phosphate, 295
Tubules, 1026
Tumor(s), 150-166, 775, 776
  adrenal, 321

Tumor(s) — cont'd
  of adrenal medulla, 325-327
  benign, 150
  bladder, 1058-1059
  brain, 482-486
  as cause of unconsciousness, 391
  classification of, 151
  Ewing's, 151
  intracranial, complications of, 482
  and ischemia, 185
  of larynx, 760-765
  malignant, 150
  mixed, 151
  pituitary, 304-305
  primary, 152
  renal, 1058-1059
  spinal cord, 492-493
  of thyroid, 314-315
  Wilms', 1056
Tuning fork tests, 729-730
TUR, 656
Turgor, skin, 778
  and dehydration, 866
Turnbuckle cast, 551, 552
Turning client in cast, 521, 522
TV, 1254
Twins, 24
Two-person carry
  with chair, 230
  with rolled bedding, 230
Two-point gait, 536
Tylenol; *see* Acetaminophen
Tympanic membrane, rupture of, 742-743
Tympanitic sound, 1240
Tympanoplasty, 743
Typhoid bacillus and cholecystitis, 954
Typhoid fever, 1018
Tyramine, 498

U

U wave, 1097
Ulceration and radiation, 158
Ulcerative colitis; *see* Colitis, ulcerative
Ulcer(s), 776
  Curling's, 848-849, 941
  Cushing's, 941
  and decubiti, 393
  decubitus; *see* Decubitus ulcer
  duodenal, 940
  gastric, 940
  peptic, 940-950
  stress, 848-849, 941
    and spinal shock, 471
  varicose, 1211
Ulnar deviation, 556
Ultrasonics, effects of, 127
Ultrasonography of eye, 679
Ultrasound
  and gastrointestinal system, upper, 903
  of heart, 1110
Ultraviolet burns of eye, 716
Ultraviolet light and acne, 809
Ultraviolet radiation, effects of, 126
Umbilical hernia, 976
Uncinariasis, 995
Unconscious client, 390-403
  bladder and bowel function of, 402
  fluid status of, 401-402
  and incontinence, 402
  maintaining airway of, 391

Unconscious client — cont'd
  maintaining joint mobility of, 393-401
  nasogastric tube and, 401
  nutritional status of, 401-402
  sensory function of, 401
  skin care of, 392-393
  vital signs and, 391-392
Unconsciousness, 390
  caused by drug overdose, 122
  causes of, 390-391
Underweight, 973-975
Union of fracture, 573
Universal antidote, 113
Unmarried couples, 87-88
Unresponsiveness, 1120
Urea
  and cerebral edema, 490
  and skin destruction, 393
Urea clearance, 1035-1036
Uremia, 1068-1069
  as cause of unconsciousness, 391
Uremic syndrome, 1068-1069
Ureteral catheter, 1042-1043
Ureterostomy tubes, 1042
Ureterotomy, 1046
Ureters, 1025
Urethra, 587, 1025
Urethral catheters, 1041
Urethritis, 624
Urethrovaginal fistula, 652
Urethrovesical reflux, 1060
Urgency incontinence, 1064
Uricosuric drugs and gout, 566
Urinalysis, 1028-1031
Urinary assessment for poisoning, 111
Urinary calcium, 295
Urinary diversion, 1047-1049
Urinary elimination
  in adults, 1039-1041
  in children, 1038-1039
  after surgery, 281
Urinary elimination, alterations in patterns of
  and benign prostatic hypertrophy, 655
  and dehydration, 868
  and edema, 872
  and electrolyte imbalances, 873
  and endocrine system, 298, 355
  and fluid and electrolyte balance, 862, 881
  and glomerulonephritis, 1051
  and hyperparathyroidism, 318
  and immobility, 539, 540
  and nephrosis, 1054
  and renal calculi, 1057
  and renal failure, 1071
  and reproductive system, 601, 664
  and urinary system, 1038, 1081
  and urinary tract infection, 1061
Urinary output and shock, 182
Urinary retention and immobility, 539, 540
Urinary stasis
  and immobility, 539
  and spinal cord injury, 476
Urinary studies
  of adrenal cortex function, 295-296
  of parathyroid function, 295
Urinary system, 1025-1083
  assessment of, 1026-1037
  data analysis of, 1037-1038
  evaluation of, 1081

Visceral protein status, 899, 900
Visceromegaly, 303
Visit Vision, 542
Vision
    color, assessment of, 676
    peripheral, 679
Visual acuity, 670
    assessing, 675-676
    after cataract surgery, 705
    and cataracts, 704
    development of, 671
    and strabismus, 694
Visual disturbance, 670
Visual disorders, danger signals of, 681
Visual impairment, 685-691; *see also* Blind-
    ness
Visual system, 668-719
    assessment of, 666-679
    data analysis of, 679
    evaluation of, 718
    implementation for, 691-712
    overview of, 668-669
    planning for, 679-691
    problems of
        blepharitis as, 696
        burns as, 714-716
        cataracts as, 703-706
            congenital, 693-695
        conjunctivitis of newborn as, 692-693
        errors of refraction as, 711-712
        eye injuries as, 713-714
        eye surgery as, 706-710
        foreign bodies in eye as, 712-713
        glaucoma as, 699-703
        infections and inflammation as, 716-717
        retinal detachment as, 696-698
        retinoblastoma as, 695-696
        retrolental fibroplasia as, 691-692
Visualization of auditory canal, 724, 725
Vital capacity, 1254
    of lungs and cardiovascular disease, 1118
Vital signs
    age-related, 1090
    monitoring in unconscious client, 391-392
    and multiple trauma, 576
Vitamin(s)
    A
        and cystic fibrosis, 1307, 1308
        daily intake of, 912
        and infertility, 620
    B and tuberculosis, 1325
    B_6
        daily intake of, 913
        and nervous system, 390
    B_{12}
        daily intake of, 913
        and gastric surgery, 949
        and gastritis, 975
        and nervous system, 390
        and pernicious anemia, 1214
        and red blood cell production, 1088
        and Schilling's tests, 1111
    and burns, 841
    C
        and Clinitest, 344
        daily intake of, 912
        and epistaxis, 1356
        and resistance to inflammation, 169
        and tuberculosis, 1325
        and wound healing, 175

Vitamin(s) — cont'd
    D, 512
        and cystic fibrosis, 1307, 1308
        daily intake of, 912
        and hypoparathyroidism, 317
        and osteomalacia, 567
        and renal failure, 1072
        and rickets, 549
        and tuberculosis, 1325
    D_2 and hypoparathyroidism, 317
    E
        and cystic fibrosis, 1307, 1308
        daily intake of, 912
        and infertility, 620
    fat-soluble, daily intake of, 912
    K, 911
        and cystic fibrosis, 1307, 1308
        and epistaxis, 1356
        and gallbladder surgery, 952
        and prothrombin production, 1091
        and thrombophlebitis, 1208
        and tonsillectomy, 1306
    and minerals, daily intake of, 911, 912-913
    water-soluble, daily intake of, 912-913
Vitreous humor, 669
Vitreous transplant, 708
VLDL, 1114
VMA, 1111
VMA test, 296
Vocal fremitus, 1240
Vocalization, 756
Vocational preparation after cerebrovascular ac-
    cident, 447
Voice production after laryngectomy, 763-764
Voice quality, 1233
    deviations in, 759
Voice sounds, assessment of, 1241-1242
Voice test, 726-728
Voided specimens, 1029
Voiding cinecystourethrography, 1034-1035
Volume, pulse, 1239-1240
Volume-cycled ventilator, 1271
Volunteers, 46
Volvulus, 1022
Vomiting
    and cerebral edema, 488
    and chemotherapy, 164
    and migraine headache, 498
    and radiation therapy, 159
    after surgery, 276, 280
VSD, 1129
Vulnerability, 136
Vulva, 586
    examination of, 604
    cancer of, 646-647
Vulvectomy, 647-648

W

Waldeyer's ring, 1304
Walker, 533, 534
Walking, tandem, 377
Wall climbing, 631, 632
Wandering baseline, 1100
Warfarin
    and myocardial infarction, 1163
    and stroke in evolution, 431
    and thrombophlebitis, 1207, 1208
Warmth after cardiac surgery, 1137
Warmup, 1116
Warning stage of disaster, 205

Wart(s), 798-800
    plantar, 798
Wasserman test, 617
Waste theory, 15
Water compartments, maintenance of, 859-860
Water intoxication, 870
    after prostate surgery, 658
Water loss and activity and environmental in-
    fluences, 862
Water pollution, 128
Waterson procedure, 1131
Wear and tear theory, 15
Weber test, 729
Wedge resection and lung cancer, 1351
Weed, Lawrence, 197-198
Weight bearing after hip arthroplasty, 564
Weight gain
    of infant, 889-890
    of neonate, 888-889
Weight loss and dehydration, 866
Weight Watchers, 972
Wellness centers, 202-203
Wet dressings; *see* Dressings, wet
Wet lung syndrome, 1203-1204
Wet soaks and burns, 845
Wheal, 775, 776
Wheelchairs, 536-537
Wheezes, 1243
Whiplash injury, 478-480
Whipple procedure, 968
Whistle-tip catheter, 1280
White matter of brain, 359
Whiteheads, 807
Whooping cough, 784-785
Wife abuse, 575-577
Wilms' tumor, 1056
Withdrawal, from alcohol, 125
Wood's light, 780
    and ringworm, 800
Work ethic, 47
Workout, 1116
Wound evisceration and dehiscence, 280
Wound precautions for burns, 842
Wounds, 172-175
    healing of, 173-175
        by first intention, 173
        by second intention, 173-175
        by third intention, 175
        variables affecting, 175
Wrist, exercises for, 398
Wryneck, 547

X

Xenografts and burns, 846
Xeromammograms, 601
Xiphisternal junction, 1123
X-ray films, sinus, 1247
Xylocaine; *see* Lidocaine

Y

Y board, 268
Young adult; *see* Adult, young
Y-tubing hookups, 261-262
Y valve, 1281

Z

Zinc, daily intake of, 913
Zonulolysis, enzymatic, 704
Z-track technique for iron-dextran, 1214-1215
Zyloprim; *see* Allopurinol